TEXTBOOK OF
ARTHROSCOPY

TEXTBOOK OF
ARTHROSCOPY

Editors

Mark D. Miller, MD
Associate Professor of Orthopaedic Surgery
Co-Director of Sports Medicine
University of Virginia Health System
Charlottesville, Virginia

Brian J. Cole, MD, MBA
Associate Professor of Orthopedics and Anatomy
Director, Rush Cartilage Restoration Center
Rush University Medical Center
Chicago, Illinois

Associate Editors

Steven B. Cohen, MD
Resident Physician
Department of Orthopaedic Surgery
University of Virginia Health System
Charlottesville, Virginia

Junaid A. Makda, BS
Research Assistant
Department of Orthopedic Surgery
Rush University Medical Center
Chicago, Illinois

SAUNDERS
An Imprint of Elsevier

SAUNDERS
An Imprint of Elsevier

The Curtis Center
Independence Square West
Philadelphia, Pennsylvania 19106

TEXTBOOK OF ARTHROSCOPY   ISBN 0-7216-0013-1
© 2004 Elsevier. All rights reserved.

Notice

Orthopedics is an ever-changing field. Standard safety precautions must be followed but as new research and clinical experience broaden our knowledge, changes in treatment and drug therapy may become necessary or appropriate. Readers are advised to check the most current product information provided by the manufacturer of each drug to be administered to verify the recommended dose, the method and duration of administration, and contraindications. It is the responsibility of the treating physician, relying on experience and knowledge of the patient, to determine dosages and the best treatment for each individual patient. Neither the Publisher nor the author assumes any liability for any injury and/or damage to persons or property arising from this publication.

The Publisher

Library of Congress Cataloging-in-Publication Data
Textbook of arthroscopy / [edited by] Mark D. Miller, Brian J. Cole; associate editors,
   Steven B. Cohen, Junaid A. Makda.—1st ed.
        p. ; cm.
   ISBN 0-7216-0013-1
   1. Arthroscopy. 2. Joints—Endoscopic surgery. I. Miller, Mark D. II. Cole, Brian J.
[DNLM: 1. Arthroscopy—methods. WE 304 T355 2004]
RD686.T43 2004
617.4′720597—dc22   2004041767

Acquisitions Editor: Richard Lampert
Developmental Editor: Heather Krehling
Project Manager: Amy Norwitz

Printed in China

Last digit is the print number: 9   8   7   6   5   4   3   2   1

To our patients—athletes of all levels and abilities—for it is the people that we treat, not the joints that we scope, that make this profession an honor to be a part of.

CONTRIBUTORS

Frank G. Alberta
Sports Medicine Fellow
Kerlan-Jobe Orthopaedic Clinic
Los Angeles, California
Ch 4: Arthroscopic Knot Tying
Ch 9: Shoulder: Diagnostic Arthroscopy

Answorth A. Allen, MD
Assistant Professor of Orthopedic Surgery
Weill Medical College of Cornell University
Assistant Attending Orthopedic Surgeon
Hospital for Special Surgery
New York, New York
Ch 11: Single-Point Fixation for Shoulder Instability

Christina R. Allen, MD
Assistant Clinical Professor of Orthopaedic Surgery
University of California, San Francisco, School of
    Medicine
San Francisco, California
*Ch 67: Posterior Cruciate Ligament: Diagnosis and Decision
    Making*

D. Greg Anderson, MD
Assistant Professor of Orthopaedic Surgery
University of Virginia School of Medicine
Charlottesville, Virginia
Ch 79: Posterior Endoscopic Lumbar Surgery
Ch 80: Thoracoscopic Surgery of the Spine
Ch 81: Laparoscopic Surgery of the Spine

Özgür Ahmet Atay, MD
Associate Professor
Hacettepe University Medical Center
Orthopedics and Traumatology
Ankara
Turkey
Ch 5: Grafts

Michail N. Avramov, MD
Department of Anesthesiology
Rush University Medical Center
Chicago, Illinois
Ch 7: Anesthesia and Postoperative Pain

Bernard R. Bach, Jr., MD
Professor of Orthopedic Surgery
Rush Medical College
Director, Sports Medicine Section
Department of Orthopedic Surgery
Rush University Medical Center
Chicago, Illinois
*Ch 62: Anterior Cruciate Ligament: Diagnosis and Decision
    Making*
Ch 63: Patellar Tendon Autograft for ACL Reconstruction
*Ch 66: Revision ACL Reconstruction: Indications and
    Technique*

Shyamala Badrinath, MD
Associate Professor of Anesthesiology
Rush Medical College
Senior Attending Anesthesiologist
Rush University Medical Center
Medical Director
Rush Surgical Center
Chicago, Illinois
Ch 7: Anesthesia and Postoperative Pain

Craig M. Ball, FRACS
Shoulder and Elbow Specialist
Department of Orthopaedic Surgery
Waitemata Health, North Shore Hospital
Shoulder and Elbow Specialist
Auckland Bone and Joint Surgery
Ascot Integrated Hospital
Auckland
New Zealand
Ch 34: Arthroscopic Management of Elbow Stiffness

F. Alan Barber, MD
Plano Orthopedic and Sports Medicine Center
Plano, Texas
Ch 3: Implants

Mark J. Berkowitz
Resident in Orthopaedic Surgery Service
Tripler Army Medical Center
Honolulu, Hawaii
*Ch 74: Arthroscopically Assisted Fracture Repair for Intra-
    articular Knee Fractures*

Kevin F. Bonner, MD
Assistant Professor of Surgery
Uniformed Services University of the Health Sciences
F. Edward Hébert School of Medicine
Bethesda, Maryland
Jordan-Young Institute
Virginia Beach, Virginia
Ch 60: Osteochondral Allografting in the Knee

Craig R. Bottoni, MD
Assistant Professor of Surgery
F. Edward Hébert School of Medicine
Uniformed Services University of the Health Sciences
Bethesda, Maryland
Chief, Sports Medicine
Orthopaedic Surgery Service
Tripler Army Medical Center
Honolulu, Hawaii
Ch 74: Arthroscopically Assisted Fracture Repair for Intra-articular Knee Fractures

William D. Bugbee, MD
Assistant Professor of Orthopaedic Surgery
University of California, San Diego
Chief, Joint Reconstruction
Director, Cartilage Transplantation Program
University of California, San Diego, Medical Center
University of California, San Diego, Thornton Hospital
San Diego, California
Ch 60: Osteochondral Allografting in the Knee

Stephen S. Burkhart, MD
Clinical Associate Professor of Orthopaedic Surgery
University of Texas Health Science Center
Director of Orthopaedic Education
The Orthopaedic Institute
San Antonio, Texas
Ch 22: Rotator Cuff: Diagnosis and Decision Making
Ch 23: Arthroscopic Repair of Crescent-Shaped, U-Shaped, and L-Shaped Rotator Cuff Tears

Charles A. Bush-Joseph, MD
Associate Professor of Orthopaedic Surgery
Associate Director, Rush Orthopaedic Sports Medicine
  Fellowship Program
Rush University Medical Center
Chicago, Illinois
Ch 48: Arthroscopic Synovectomy in the Knee

J. W. Thomas Byrd, MD
Assistant Clinical Professor of Orthopaedics and
  Rehabilitation
Vanderbilt University School of Medicine
Orthopaedic Surgeon
Nashville Sports Medicine and Orthopaedic Center
Nashville, Tennessee
Ch 43: Hip: Patient Positioning, Portal Placement, Normal Arthroscopic Anatomy, and Diagnostic Arthroscopy
Ch 44: General Techniques for Hip Arthroscopy: Labral Tears, Synovial Disease, Loose Bodies, and Lesions of the Ligamentum Teres

David N. M. Caborn
Professor of Orthopaedic Surgery
University of Louisville
Orthopedic Surgeon
Jewish Hospital
Louisville, Kentucky
Ch 51: Arthroscopic Meniscus Repair

Raymond M. Carroll, MD
Clinical Instructor of Orthopaedic Surgery
Georgetown University Medical Center
Washington, DC
Ch 25: Arthroscopic Management of Glenoid Arthritis

A. Bobby Chhabra, MD
Assistant Professor of Orthopaedic Surgery
University of Virginia Health System
Charlottesville, Virginia
Ch 29: Arthroscopic Management of Osteochondritis Dissecans of the Elbow

James Chow, MD
Clinical Assistant Professor of Surgery
Southern Illinois University School of Medicine
Springfield, Illinois
Director of Orthopaedics
Department of Surgery
St. Mary's Good Samaritan, Inc.
President and Founder
Orthopaedic Center of Southern Illinois
Orthopaedic Research of Southern Illinois
Mt. Vernon, Illinois
Ch 42: Arthroscopic Management of Triangular Fibrocartilage Complex Tears

Steven B. Cohen, MD
Resident Physician
Department of Orthopaedic Surgery
University of Virginia Health Sciences Center
Charlottesville, Virginia
Ch 70: PCL Tibial Inlay and Posterolateral Corner Reconstruction

Brian J. Cole, MD, MBA
Associate Professor of Orthopaedics and Anatomy
Director, Rush Cartilage Restoration Center
Rush University Medical Center
Chicago, Illinois
Ch 4: Arthroscopic Knot Tying
Ch 8: Shoulder: Patient Positioning, Portal Placement, and Normal Arthroscopic Anatomy
Ch 9: Shoulder: Diagnostic Arthroscopy
Ch 18: Arthroscopic Repair of SLAP Lesions
Ch 53: Arthroscopic Meniscus Transplantation: Bridge in Slot Technique
Ch 54: Knee Cartilage: Diagnosis and Decision Making
Ch 56: Microfracture Technique in the Knee
Ch 61: Autologous Chondrocyte Implantation in the Knee

David R. Diduch, MD
Associate Professor of Orthopaedic Surgery
Co-Director of Division of Sports Medicine, Associate
 Team Physician, and Fellowship Director for Sports
 Medicine
Department of Orthopaedic Surgery
University of Virginia
Charlottesville, Virginia
Ch 46: Knee: Patient Positioning, Portal Placement, and
 Normal Arthroscopic Anatomy
Ch 47: Knee: Diagnostic Arthroscopy
Ch 58: Avascular Necrosis Drilling in the Knee

Bassem T. Elhassan, MD
Orthopedic Resident
University of Illinois at Chicago
University of Illinois Hospital
Chicago, Illinois
Ch 41: Arthroscopy of the First Carpometacarpal Joint

Andrew J. Elliott, MD
Assistant Professor of Orthopaedic Surgery
Weill Medical College of Cornell University
Assistant Attending in Orthopaedic Surgery
Hospital for Special Surgery
New York-Presbyterian Hospital
New York, New York
Ch 78: Arthroscopy of the First Metatarsophalangeal Joint

Gregory C. Fanelli, MD
Full-time faculty
Geisinger Health System Orthopaedic Surgery
 Residency Program
Chief, Arthroscopic Surgery and Sports Medicine
Department of Orthopaedic Surgery
Geisinger Health System Medical Center
Danville, Pennsylvania
Ch 68: Transtibial Tunnel PCL Reconstruction
Ch 71: Multiligament Injuries: Diagnosis and Decision
 Making
Ch 72: Multiligament Injuries: Surgical Technique

Gary S. Fanton, MD
Clinical Assistant Professor of Orthopedics
Stanford University School of Medicine
Team Physician
Stanford University
Stanford, California
Partner, Sports Orthopedic and Rehabilitation
 Medicine Associates
Redwood City, California
Team Orthopedist
San Francisco Giants
San Francisco, California
Ch 15: Radiofrequency Technique for Shoulder Instability

Jack Farr, MD
Clinical Associate Professor of Orthopedic Surgery
Indiana University School of Medicine
Director, Cartilage Restoration Center of Indiana
OrthoIndy
Indianapolis, Indiana
Ch 53: Arthroscopic Meniscus Transplantation: Bridge in
 Slot Technique
Ch 73: Lateral Release and Medial Repair for Patellofemoral
 Instability

Michael D. Feldman, MD
Clinical Professor of Orthopaedic Surgery
Brown University School of Medicine
Providence, Rhode Island
Team Physician
Bryant College
Smithfield, Rhode Island
Orthopedic Group, Inc.
Pawtucket, Rhode Island
Ch 35: Arthroscopic Fracture Management in the Elbow

John J. Fernandez, MD
Assistant Professor of Orthopaedic Surgery
Rush Medical College
Rush University Medical Center
Chicago, Illinois
Ch 38: Wrist and Hand: Patient Positioning, Portal
 Placement, Normal Arthroscopic Anatomy, and Diagnostic
 Arthroscopy
Ch 39: Arthroscopic Management of Scapholunate Injury

Larry D. Field, MD
Clinical Associate Professor of Orthopaedic Surgery
University of Mississippi School of Medicine
Co-Director, Upper Extremity Service
Mississippi Sports Medicine and Orthopaedic Center
Jackson, Mississippi
Ch 14: Arthroscopic Rotator Interval Closure
Ch 31: Arthroscopic Management of Soft Tissue Impingement
 in the Elbow
Ch 32: Arthroscopic Management of Valgus Extension
 Overload of the Elbow

David C. Flanigan, MD
Resident, Department of Orthopedic Surgery
McGraw Medical School at Northwestern University
Northwestern Memorial Hospital
Chicago, Illinois
Ch 20: Acromioclavicular Joint Pathology

Evan L. Flatow, MD
Bernard J. Lasker Professor of Orthopaedic Surgery
Mount Sinai School of Medicine
Chief of Shoulder Surgery and Attending
Department of Orthopaedics
Mount Sinai Medical Center
New York, New York
Ch 21: Biceps Tendinitis

Kyle R. Flik, MD
Resident in Sports Medicine
Hospital for Special Surgery
New York, New York
Ch 11: Single-Point Fixation for Shoulder Instability

Jeff A. Fox, MD
Clinical Faculty
Department of Orthopedics
University of Oklahoma School of Medicine
Tulsa, Oklahoma
Ch 24: Arthroscopic Subscapularis Repair
Ch 54: Knee Cartilage: Diagnosis and Decision Making

Kevin B. Freedman, MD, MSCE
Assistant Professor of Orthopaedic Surgery
Stritch School of Medicine
Loyola University of Chicago
Co-Director, Section of Sports Medicine
Department of Orthopaedic Surgery and
    Rehabilitation
Loyola University Medical Center
Maywood, Illinois
*Ch 53: Arthroscopic Meniscus Transplantation: Bridge in
    Slot Technique*
Ch 54: Knee Cartilage: Diagnosis and Decision Making
Ch 56: Microfracture Technique in the Knee
Ch 61: Autologous Chondrocyte Implantation in the Knee

Freddie Fu, MD
David Silver Professor and Chairman
Department of Orthopaedic Surgery
University of Pittsburgh
Chief of Orthopaedics
Department of Orthopaedic Surgery
University of Pittsburgh Medical Center–Presbyterian
Hospitals
Pittsburgh, Pennsylvania
*Ch 46: Knee: Patient Positioning, Portal Placement, and
    Normal Arthroscopic Anatomy*
Ch 47: Knee: Diagnostic Arthroscopy

John P. Fulkerson, MD
Clinical Professor of Orthopedic Surgery
Sports Medicine Fellowship Director
University of Connecticut
Head Team Physician
AHL Hartford Wolfpack Hockey Club
Orthopedic Associates of Hartford, PC
Farmington, Connecticut
*Ch 65: Central Quadriceps Free Tendon for ACL
    Reconstruction*

Leesa M. Galatz, MD
Assistant Professor of Orthopaedic Surgery
Washington University School of Medicine at Barnes-
Jewish Hospital
St. Louis, Missouri
Ch 34: Arthroscopic Management of Elbow Stiffness

Gary M. Gartsman, MD
Clinical Professor of Orthopaedics
University of Texas Health Science Center
Fondren Orthopedic Group
Texas Orthopedic Hospital
Houston, Texas
Ch 26: Arthroscopic Management of Shoulder Stiffness

Jonathan A. Gastel, MD
Miriam Hospital
Providence, Rhode Island
Orthopedic Surgeon
Orthopedic Group, Inc.
Pawtucket, Rhode Island
Ch 35: Arthroscopic Fracture Management in the Elbow

Sanjitpal S. Gill, MD
The Emory Spine Center
Department of Orthopaedic Surgery
Emory University School of Medicine
Atlanta, Georgia
*Ch 70: PCL Tibial Inlay and Posterolateral Corner
    Reconstruction*

James N. Gladstone, MD
Assistant Professor Orthopaedic Surgery
Mount Sinai School of Medicine
Chief of Sports Medicine
Department of Orthopaedic Surgery
Mount Sinai Medical Center
New York, New York
Ch 21: Biceps Tendinitis

E. Marlowe Goble, MD
Adjunct Professor of Orthopedics
University of Utah
Salt Lake City, Utah
Staff, Department of Orthopedics
Cache Valley Specialty Hospital
Logan Regional Hospital
Logan, Utah
*Ch 52: Arthroscopic Meniscus Transplantation: Plug and
    Slot Technique*

Mark H. Gonzalez, MD
Professor and Chief, Section of Joint Arthroplasty
Department of Orthopedic Surgery
University of Illinois
Chairman of Orthopedic Surgery and Chief of Hand
Surgery, Department of Orthopedic Surgery
Cook County Hospital
Chicago, Illinois
Ch 41: Arthroscopy of the First Carpometacarpal Joint

Daniel J. Gurly, MD
Surgeon
Kansas City Bone and Joint Clinic
Kansas City, Missouri
*Ch 31: Arthroscopic Management of Soft Tissue Impingement
in the Elbow*
*Ch 32: Arthroscopic Management of Valgus Extension
Overload of the Elbow*

Brett J. Hampton, MD
Fellow, Arthritis and Reconstructive Surgery
Massachusetts General Hospital
Wang Ambulatory Care Center
Boston, Massachusetts
Ch 58: Avascular Necrosis Drilling in the Knee

Michael H. Handy, MD
Chief Resident, Department of Orthopaedic Surgery
University of Virginia Health System
Charlottesville, Virginia
Ch 37: Arthroscopic Management of Olecranon Bursitis

Christopher D. Harner, MD
Professor of Orthopedic Surgery
University of Pittsburgh School of Medicine
Chief, Division of Sports Medicine
University of Pittsburgh Medical Center
Center for Sports Medicine
Pittsburgh, Pennsylvania
*Ch 57: Primary Repair of Osteochondritis Dissecans in the
Knee*
*Ch 67: Posterior Cruciate Ligament: Diagnosis and Decision
Making*
Ch 69: Transtibial Double-Bundle PCL Reconstruction

Michael G. Hehman, BA
Research Assistant
Sports, Orthopedic and Rehabilitation Medicine
Associates
Redwood City, California
Ch 15: Radiofrequency Technique for Shoulder Instability

Peter W. Hester
Orthopaedic Surgeon
St. Joseph Hospital
Lexington, Kentucky
Ch 51: Arthroscopic Meniscus Repair

Stephen M. Howell, MD
Associate Professor of Mechanical and Aeronautical
Engineering
University of California, Davis
Davis, California
Orthopedic Surgeon
Methodist Hospital
Sacramento, California
Ch 64: Hamstring Tendons for ACL Reconstruction

Jim C. Hsu, MD
Resident Physician
Department of Orthopaedic Surgery
Washington University School of Medicine
Barnes-Jewish Hospital
St. Louis, Missouri
*Ch 28: Elbow: Anesthesia, Patient Positioning, Portal
Placement, Normal Arthroscopic Anatomy, and Diagnostic
Arthroscopy*

William M. Isbell, MD
Fellow, Hospital for Special Surgery
New York, New York
Ch 5: Grafts

Yasuyuki Ishibashi, MD
Assistant Professor of Orthopaedic Surgery
Hirosaki University School of Medicine
Hirosaki, Aomori
Japan
Ch 1: The History of Arthroscopy

Laith M. Jazrawi, MD
Assistant Professor of Orthopedic Surgery
New York University School of Medicine
Hospital for Joint Diseases
New York, New York
Ch 19: Arthroscopic Subacromial Decompression

Darren L. Johnson, MD
Professor and Chair
Department of Orthopaedic Surgery
Director of Sports Medicine
University of Kentucky
Lexington, Kentucky
Ch 5: Grafts

Don Johnson, MD
Director of Sports Medicine
Carleton University
Attending Surgeon
Department of Orthopedic Surgery
Ottawa Hospital
Ottawa, Ontario
Canada
Ch 6: Digital Imaging

David M. Kahler, MD
Associate Professor and Director of Orthopaedic
Trauma
University of Virginia Health System
Associate Team Physician
Department of Orthopaedic Surgery
University of Virginia
Charlottesville, Virginia
*Ch 45: Arthroscopic Removal of Post-traumatic Loose Bodies
and Penetrating Foreign Bodies from the Hip*

Leonid I. Katolik, MD
University of Washington School of Medicine
Fellow in Hand and Microvascular Surgery
Harborview Medical Center
Seattle, Washington
*Ch 38: Wrist and Hand: Patient Positioning, Portal
    Placement, Normal Arthroscopic Anatomy, and Diagnostic
    Arthroscopy*
Ch 39: Arthroscopic Management of Scapholunate Injury
*Ch 42: Arthroscopic Management of Triangular
    Fibrocartilage Complex Tears*

John G. Kennedy, MD
Assistant Professor of Orthopaedic Surgery
Weill Medical College of Cornell University
Assistant Attending Foot and Ankle Surgeon
Hospital for Special Surgery
New York, New York
*Ch 75: Ankle: Patient Positioning, Portal Placement, and
    Diagnostic Arthroscopy*
Ch 76: Ankle Arthrodesis and Anterior Impingement

Warren Kuo, MD
Visiting Shoulder Fellow
Mount Sinai Medical Center
New York, New York
Ch 21: Biceps Tendinitis

Mark A. Kwartowitz, DO
Department of Orthopedics
North Suburban Medical Center
Thornton, Colorado
Department of Orthopedics
Platte Valley Medical Center
Brighton, Colorado
Ch 55: Debridement of Articular Cartilage in the Knee

Keith W. Lawhorn, MD
Assistant Professor of Surgery
F. Edward Hébert School of Medicine
Uniformed Services University of the Health Sciences
Bethesda, Maryland
Staff Orthopedic Surgeon
Malcolm Grow Medical Center
Andrews Air Force Base, Maryland
Ch 64: Hamstring Tendons for ACL Reconstruction

Ronald A. Lehman, Jr., MD
Teaching Fellow in Surgery
F. Edward Hébert School of Medicine
Uniformed Services University of the Health Sciences
Bethesda, Maryland
PGY-5, Senior Resident
Walter Reed Army Medical Center
Washington, DC
Ch 36: Arthroscopic Management of Lateral Epicondylitis

William N. Levine, MD
Assistant Professor of Orthopaedic Surgery
Columbia University College of Physicians and
    Surgeons
Assistant Attending in Orthopaedic Surgery
New York-Presbyterian Hospital
Director of Sports Medicine
Assistant Director, Center for Shoulder, Elbow and
    Sports Medicine
Columbia-Presbyterian Medical Center
New York, New York
Ch 25: Arthroscopic Management of Glenoid Arthritis

Ian K. Y. Lo, MD
Assistant Professor of Surgery
Division of Orthopaedics
University of Calgary
Arthroscopic and Reconstructive Shoulder Surgery
Calgary, Alberta
Canada
Ch 22: Rotator Cuff: Diagnosis and Decision Making
*Ch 23: Arthroscopic Repair of Crescent-Shaped, U-Shaped,
    and L-Shaped Rotator Cuff Tears*

Victor Lopez Jr., DO
Research Intern
Sports Medicine and Shoulder Service
Hospital for Special Surgery
New York, New York
Medical Intern
Department of Medicine
Peninsula Hospital Center
Far Rockaway, New York
Ch 11: Single-Point Fixation for Shoulder Instability

Augustus D. Mazzocca, MD
Assistant Professor of Orthopaedic Surgery
University of Connecticut School of Medicine
Farmington, Connecticut
Ch 4: Arthroscopic Knot Tying
*Ch 8: Shoulder: Patient Positioning, Portal Placement, and
    Normal Arthroscopic Anatomy*
Ch 9: Shoulder: Diagnostic Arthroscopy

Mark D. Miller, MD
Associate Professor of Orthopaedic Surgery
Co-Director of Sports Medicine
University of Virginia Health System
Charlottesville, Virginia
Ch 30: Arthroscopic Synovectomy of the Elbow
Ch 59: Osteochondral Autologous Plug Transfer in the Knee
*Ch 70: PCL Tibial Inlay and Posterolateral Corner
    Reconstruction*

Peter J. Millett, MD, MSc
Clinical Instructor of Orthopaedic Surgery
Harvard Medical School
Harvard Shoulder Service/Sports Medicine
Brigham and Women's Hospital
Massachusetts General Hospital
Boston, Massachusetts
*Ch 27: Arthroscopic Management of Scapulothoracic
    Disorders*

Michael J. Moskal, MD
Clinical Instructor of Orthopedic Surgery and Sports
    Medicine
University of Washington
Seattle, Washington
Shoulder and Elbow Surgeon
Shoulder and Elbow Center
New Albany, Indiana
Ch 10: Shoulder: Diagnosis and Decision Making
Ch 12: Suture Anchor Fixation for Shoulder Instability

Kevin P. Murphy, MD
Assistant Professor of Surgery
F. Edward Hébert School of Medicine
Uniformed Services University of the Health Sciences
Director, Sports Medicine
Chief, Orthopaedic Surgery Service
Walter Reed Army Medical Center
Washington, DC
Ch 36: Arthroscopic Management of Lateral Epicondylitis

Volker Musahl, MD
Resident Physician
Department of Orthopaedic Surgery
University of Pittsburgh School of Medicine
Pittsburgh, Pennsylvania
*Ch 46: Knee: Patient Positioning, Portal Placement, and
    Normal Arthroscopic Anatomy*
Ch 47: Knee: Diagnostic Arthroscopy

Akbar Nawab, MD
Clinical Faculty
Department of Orthopaedic Surgery
University of Louisville
Orthopaedic Surgeon
Jewish Hospital
Louisville, Kentucky
Ch 51: Arthroscopic Meniscus Repair

Eric S. Neff, MD
Orthopaedic Surgeon
Orthopaedic Associates of Virginia, LTD
Norfolk, Virginia
Ch 59: Osteochondral Autologous Plug Transfer in the Knee

Shane J. Nho, BA
Medical Student
Rush Medical College
Rush University Medical Center
Chicago, Illinois
*Ch 62: Anterior Cruciate Ligament: Diagnosis and Decision
    Making*

Mayo A. Noerdlinger, MD
Adjunct Associate Professor
Team Physician
University of New Hampshire
Durham, New Hampshire
Portsmouth Regional Hospital
Portsmouth, New Hampshire
Ch 24: Arthroscopic Subscapularis Repair

Gordon W. Nuber, MD
Professor of Clinical Orthopaedic Surgery
Northwestern University Medical School
Chicago Illinois
Ch 20: Acromioclavicular Joint Pathology

James D. O'Holleran, MD
Fellow, Harvard Shoulder Service
Brigham and Women's Hospital
Massachusetts General Hospital
Boston, Massachusetts
*Ch 27: Arthroscopic Management of Scapulothoracic
Disorders*

Martin J. O'Malley, MD
Associate Professor of Orthopaedic Surgery
Weill Medical College of Cornell University
Associate Attending in Orthopaedic Surgery
Hospital for Special Surgery
New York Presbyterian Hospital
New York, New York
*Ch 75: Ankle: Patient Positioning, Portal Placement, and
    Diagnostic Arthroscopy*
Ch 76: Ankle Arthrodesis and Anterior Impingement
Ch 78: Arthroscopy of the First Metatarsophalangeal Joint

Bernard C. Ong, MD
Sports Medicine and Shoulder Fellow
Center for Sports Medicine
University of Pittsburgh Medical Center
Pittsburgh, Pennsylvania
*Ch 46: Knee: Patient Positioning, Portal Placement, and
    Normal Arthroscopic Anatomy*
Ch 47: Knee: Diagnostic Arthroscopy
*Ch 57: Primary Repair of Osteochondritis Dissecans in the
    Knee*

Michael L. Pearl, MD
Clinical Instructor of Orthopaedics
University of Southern California
Shoulder and Elbow Surgeon
Kaiser-Permanente Medical Center
Los Angeles, California
Ch 10: Shoulder: Diagnosis and Decision Making
Ch 12: Suture Anchor Fixation for Shoulder Instability

Gary G. Poehling, MD
Professor and Chairman
Department of Orthopaedic Surgery
Wake Forest University Health Sciences
North Carolina Baptist Hospital
Winston-Salem, North Carolina
*Ch 33: Arthroscopic Management of Degenerative Joint
    Disease in the Elbow*

Kornelis A. Poelstra, MD, PhD
Resident Physician
Department of Orthopaedic Surgery
University of Virginia
Charlottesville, Virginia
Ch 59: Osteochondral Autologous Plug Transfer in the Knee

Bruce Reider, MD
Professor of Surgery
Director of Sports Medicine
University of Chicago
University of Chicago Hospitals
Chicago, Illinois
Ch 55: Debridement of Articular Cartilage in the Knee

David P. Richards, MD
Arthroscopic Surgery and Sports Medicine
Institute for Bone and Joint Disorders
Phoenix, Arizona
Ch 3: Implants

Jeffrey A. Rihn, MD
Resident Physician
Department of Orthopaedic Surgery
University of Pittsburgh School of Medicine
Pittsburgh, Pennsylvania
*Ch 67: Posterior Cruciate Ligament: Diagnosis and Decision
Making*

Andrew S. Rokito, MD
Associate Professor of Orthopaedic Surgery
New York University School of Medicine
Chief, Shoulder Service
Associate Director, Sports Medicine Service
Hospital for Joint Diseases
New York, New York
Ch 19: Arthroscopic Subacromial Decompression

Anthony A. Romeo, MD
Associate Professor of Orthopaedic Surgery
Rush Medical College
Attending Staff
Orthopaedic Surgery
Rush University Medical Center
Chicago, Illinois
Ch 4: Arthroscopic Knot Tying
*Ch 8: Shoulder: Patient Positioning, Portal Placement, and
Normal Arthroscopic Anatomy*
Ch 9: Shoulder: Diagnostic Arthroscopy
Ch 16: Arthroscopic Repair of Posterior Shoulder Instability
Ch 18: Arthroscopic Repair of SLAP Lesions
Ch 24: Arthroscopic Subscapularis Repair

Marc R. Safran, MD
Associate Professor of Orthopaedic Surgery
Director, Sports Medicine
University of California, San Francisco
San Francisco, California
Ch 49: Meniscus: Diagnosis and Decision Making
Ch 50: Arthroscopic Meniscectomy

Lisa M. Sasso, BS
Research Assistant
Rush University Medical Center
Chicago, Illinois
Ch 24: Arthroscopic Subscapularis Repair

Felix H. Savoie III, MD
Clinical Associate Professor of Orthopaedic Surgery
University of Mississippi School of Medicine
Co-Director, Upper Extremity Services
Mississippi Sports Medicine and Orthopaedic Center
Jackson, Mississippi
Ch 14: Arthroscopic Rotator Interval Closure
*Ch 31: Arthroscopic Management of Soft Tissue Impingement
in the Elbow*
*Ch 32: Arthroscopic Management of Valgus Extension
Overload of the Elbow*

Jon K. Sekiya, MD
Assistant Professor of Surgery
Department of Surgery
F. Edward Hébert School of Medicine
Bethesda, Maryland
Staff Orthopaedic Surgeon
Team Physician and Surgeon
Naval Special Warfare Development Group
Bone and Joint/Sports Medicine Institute
Naval Medical Center Portsmouth
Portsmouth, Virginia
*Ch 57: Primary Repair of Osteochondritis Dissecans in the
Knee*
Ch 69: Transtibial Double-Bundle PCL Reconstruction

Robert Sellards, MD
Assistant Professor of Orthopaedic Surgery
Louisiana State University Health Sciences Center
New Orleans, Louisiana
Ch 16: Arthroscopic Repair of Posterior Shoulder Instability
Ch 48: Arthroscopic Synovectomy in the Knee

Francis H. Shen, MD
Assistant Professor of Orthopaedic Surgery
Division of Spine Surgery
University of Virginia School of Medicine
Charlottesville, Virginia
*Ch 46: Knee: Patient Positioning, Portal Placement, and
Normal Arthroscopic Anatomy*
Ch 47: Knee: Diagnostic Arthroscopy
Ch 79: Posterior Endoscopic Lumbar Surgery
Ch 80: Thoracoscopic Surgery of the Spine
Ch 81: Laparoscopic Surgery of the Spine

Charlotte Shum, MD
Post-Doctoral Fellow, Hand and Upper Extremity
Surgery
Department of Orthopaedic Surgery
Hospital for Special Surgery
New York, New York
Attending Physician and Clinical Instructor
San Francisco Orthopaedic Residency Program
St. Mary's Hospital
San Francisco, California
Ch 40: Endoscopic Carpal Tunnel Release

Gordon Slater, FRACS (Ortho)
Albury Wodongo Private Hospital
Albury Base Hospital
Head, Foot and Ankle Surgery
Alpine Orthosport
New South Wales
Australia
*Ch 75: Ankle: Patient Positioning, Portal Placement, and
Diagnostic Arthroscopy*
Ch 76: Ankle Arthrodesis and Anterior Impingement

Gabriel Soto, MD
Chief Resident, Department of Orthopaedic Surgery
University of California, San Francisco
San Francisco, California
Ch 49: Meniscus: Diagnosis and Decision Making
Ch 50: Arthroscopic Meniscectomy

Patrick St. Pierre, MD
Assistant Professor of Surgery
F. Edward Hébert School of Medicine
Uniformed Services University of the Health Sciences
Bethesda, Maryland
Associate Director, Nirschl Orthopedic and Sports
Medicine Fellowship
Virginia Hospital Medical Center
Arlington, Virginia
Ch 2: Instrumentation and Equipment

Kathryne J. Stabile, MS
Research Engineer
Department of Orthopaedic Surgery
Center for Sports Medicine
University of Pittsburgh Medical Center
Pittsburgh, Pennsylvania
Medical Student
Drexel University College of Medicine
Philadelphia, Pennsylvania
Ch 69: Transtibial Double-Bundle PCL Reconstruction

Rodney Stanley, MD
Orthopaedic Surgery Resident
Louisiana State University Health Sciences Center
New Orleans, Louisiana
Ch 16: Arthroscopic Repair of Posterior Shoulder Instability
Ch 48: Arthroscopic Synovectomy in the Knee

Scott P. Steinmann, MD
Assistant Professor of Orthopedics
Mayo Medical School
Consultant
Department of Orthopedic Surgery
Mayo Clinic
Rochester, Minnesota
Ch 25: Arthroscopic Management of Glenoid Arthritis

James P. Tasto, MD
Clinical Professor of Orthopaedics
University of California, San Diego
Orthopaedic Surgeon
San Diego Sports Medicine and Orthopaedic Center
San Diego, California
Ch 77: Arthroscopic Subtalar Arthrodesis

Joseph C. Tauro, MD
Clinical Assistant Professor of Orthopaedic Surgery
New Jersey Medical School
Newark, New Jersey
Attending Orthopedic Surgeon
Community Medical Center
Toms River, New Jersey
*Ch 17: Arthroscopic Repair of Multidirectional Shoulder
Instability*

Raymond Thal, MD
Assistant Clinical Professor of Orthopaedic Surgery
George Washington University School of Medicine
Washington, DC
Orthopedic Surgeon
Town Center Orthopaedic Associates
Reston, Virginia
*Ch 13: Knotless Suture Anchor Fixation for Shoulder
Instability*

Richard J. Thomas, MD
Resident Physician
Department of Orthopaedic Surgery
University of Virginia Health System
Charlottesville, Virginia
*Ch 29: Arthroscopic Management of Osteochondritis
Dissecans of the Elbow*

Jonathan B. Ticker, MD
Assistant Clinical Professor of Orthopaedic Surgery
College of Physicians and Surgeons of Columbia
University
New York, New York
Active Attending Staff
New Island Hospital
Bethpage, New York
North Shore University Hospital–Plainview
Plainview, New York
*Ch 17: Arthroscopic Repair of Multidirectional Shoulder
Instability*

James A. Tom, MD
Department of Orthopedic Surgery
Drexel University College of Medicine
Philadelphia, PA
Ch 30: Arthroscopic Synovectomy of the Elbow

Scott W. Trenhaile, MD
Orthopaedic Surgeon
Orthopaedic Associates of North Illinois
Rockford, Illinois
Ch 14: Arthroscopic Rotator Interval Closure

Nikhil N. Verma, MD
Sports Medicine Fellow
Hospital for Special Surgery
New York, New York
Ch 18: Arthroscopic Repair of SLAP Lesions

Jon J. P. Warner, MD
Associate Professor
Harvard Medical School
Chief, Harvard Shoulder Service
Massachusetts General Hospital
Brigham and Women's and Children's Hospital
Boston, Massachusetts
Ch 27: Arthroscopic Management of Scapulothoracic Disorders

Andrew J. Weiland, MD
Professor of Orthopaedic Surgery and Professor of
  Surgery (Plastic)
Weill Medical College of Cornell University
Attending Orthopaedic Surgeon
Hospital for Special Surgery
New York, New York
Ch 40: Endoscopic Carpal Tunnel Release

Ethan R. Wiesler, MD
Assistant Professor of Orthopaedic Surgery
Wake Forest University School of Medicine
Winston-Salem, North Carolina
*Ch 33: Arthroscopic Management of Degenerative Joint
  Disease in the Elbow*

Stephan V. Yacoubian, MD
Orthopaedic Surgeon/Sports Medicine Specialist
Providence St. Joseph Medical Center
Burbank, California
*Ch 65: Central Quadriceps Free Tendon for ACL
  Reconstruction*

Ken Yamaguchi, MD
Associate Professor and Chief, Shoulder and Elbow
  Service
Department of Orthopaedic Surgery
Washington University School of Medicine at Barnes-
  Jewish Hospital
St. Louis, Missouri
*Ch 28: Elbow: Anesthesia, Patient Positioning, Portal Place-
  ment, Normal Arthroscopic Anatomy, and Diagnostic
  Arthroscopy*
Ch 34: Arthroscopic Management of Elbow Stiffness

Yuji Yamamoto, MD
Department of Orthopaedic Surgery
Hirosaki University School of Medicine
Hirosaki, Aomori
Japan
Ch 1: The History of Arthroscopy

Brad A. Zwahlen, MD
Sports Medicine Fellow
Sports, Orthopedic and Rehabilitation Medicine Associ-
  ates
Redwood City, California
Ch 15: Radiofrequency Technique for Shoulder Instability

FOREWORD

Textbook of Arthroscopy offers a state-of-the-art and comprehensive approach to arthroscopic surgical procedures. Drs. Mark Miller and Brian Cole have enlisted many of the world's leading sports medicine experts as well as talented younger practitioners. They have written brief, tightly focused chapters that will interest both novice and experienced arthroscopists.

It is a privilege to write this Foreword, because both Mark Miller and Brian Cole trained with us at the Sports Medicine fellowship at University of Pittsburgh. I enjoyed working with both of them during their time here, and I have also enjoyed following their flourishing careers.

This work reflects their energy and talents as surgeons, communicators, and individuals committed to the education of other orthopedic surgeons. This text provides a fresh perspective on this ever-changing field.

FREDDIE H. FU, MD, DSc (Hon), DPs (Hon)

PREFACE

But optics sharp it needs, I ween, to see what is not to be seen.

JOHN TRUMBUL (1750–1831)
MCFINGAL. CANTO I. LINE 67

The arthroscope is possibly the most widely used tool in all of orthopedic surgery. Initially utilized only as a means to *visualize* intra-articular structures, it has become the most important *facilitator* for the majority of surgical techniques in virtually every joint in the body. New techniques continue to be developed, humbling even the most technically adept arthroscopist who finds himself suddenly thrust to the bottom of the learning curve. It has become increasingly difficult to keep up on all of these developments. Thus, now more than ever, a definitive resource is desperately needed.

Textbook of Arthroscopy was specifically written to fill this void. The book, written by some of the most respected arthroscopic surgeons and educators, is up-to-date, comprehensive, and thorough. The authors have selflessly shared their masterful knowledge through real case presentations, representative arthroscopic images, and one-of-a-kind illustrations.

Textbook of Arthroscopy uses a standardized format in each anatomic area; this format is concise, is easy to follow, and offers the greatest opportunity to take newly acquired skills directly into the arthroscopy suite. The book is divided into eight parts. The introductory part, *Equipment and Materials*, is composed of several chapters that provide the most complete foundation for arthroscopic surgery ever written. A quick perusal will make the arthroscopic an expert in everything from knot tying to digital imaging. The subsequent parts are head-to-toe joint-specific chapters on shoulder, elbow, wrist and hand, hip, knee, ankle, and spine. Each chapter follows an identical format, most beginning with a *Nutshell*, a summary of the chapter and techniques. Because there is more than one way to "scope a cat," each chapter includes a variety of procedures and techniques. Many chapters are authored by the original developers of specific arthroscopic techniques or by well-respected educators who provide the most accurate depiction of "how to" perform virtually any arthroscopic procedure.

If a picture is worth a thousand words, then perhaps a video clip is worth ten thousand. We are proud to include some clips of several arthroscopic procedures with this text. These clips have been extensively edited and are a valuable addition to the text.

Textbook of Arthroscopy is a natural product of our education. Both of us were fortunate to have learned from some of the greatest contemporary arthroscopists, including our mentors, Drs. Freddie Fu, Chris Harner, J P Warner, Russell Warren, and David Altchek, to name only a few. These and others have inspired us to become teachers ourselves, and we hope to share some of the same knowledge that we have taught our residents, fellows, and colleagues through this book. We are deeply indebted to the contributors to this textbook. They have made a Herculean effort to create what we envision to be a landmark textbook in this field. We also sincerely thank our editor and the Vice President of Global Surgery at Elsevier, Richard Lampert, for his constant prodding that kept the project on time and completed with the excellence that this publisher is known for. Finally, we would like to thank you for your efforts in the pursuit of improving your arthroscopic skills—we know your patients approve!

MARK D. MILLER, MD

BRIAN J. COLE, MD, MBA

CONTENTS

Equipment and Materials

The History of Arthroscopy

Yasuyuki Ishibashi and Yuji Yamamoto

Endoscopy

According to Jackson's chapter on arthroscopy,[5] the earliest references to the exploration of body cavities are found in the ancient Hebrew literature. Later, proctoscopes were discovered in the ruins of Pompeii. The desire to explore the bladder spurred the development of endoscopic devices. Botzini presented a "Lichtleiter" endoscope to the Joseph Academy of Medical Surgery in Vienna in 1806, but it was not well accepted. The Lichtleiter used a candle to reflect light into the bladder through a tube while the surgeon looked through another tube. The gazogene endocystoscope produced by Désormaux in 1853 used turpentine and alcohol to fuel a fire in a small combustion chamber to light the bladder through a tube, which was also used for visualization. The first modern cystoscope, consisting of a platinum loop heated by electricity and surrounded by a water–cooled goose quill, was developed by Nitze in 1876. Edison's invention of the carbon filament light bulb in 1880 facilitated illumination and proved to be a turning point in the science of endoscopy. Great progress followed, with applications in various areas of medicine, including the laparoscope designed by Jacobaeus in 1910. Endoscopy of joint cavities, however, lagged behind.

Development of Arthroscopy

In Japan

In 1918, in the first instance of endoscopy of a joint, Dr. Kenji Takagi (Fig. 1–1) of Tokyo University viewed the interior of a cadaver knee joint using a Charrier number 22 (7.3mm) cystoscope.[11] In 1920, he modified a cystoscope and thereby developed the first joint scope. With this device, he observed the interior of a tubercular knee

joint filled with saline. However, the diameter at 7.3mm was too large for the knee joint, which is narrow and has a complicated structure as well as solid cartilaginous walls, unlike the bladder or stomach. Takagi then developed a more practical arthroscope with a smaller diameter. In 1931, the Takagi number 1 scope (3.5mm in diameter) was produced (Fig. 1–2).[9] In 1932, Takagi presented this scope at the meeting of the Japanese Orthopaedic Association and later applied it clinically in a knee joint filled with saline.

Subsequently, Takagi designed other instruments, including 11 arthroscopes (numbers 2 through 12) and several types of trocar sheaths for specialized purposes. The adjustable focus of the number 4 arthroscope enabled a close-up view of up to 3mm, and in 1937, it was exhibited at the International Exhibition in Paris. The numbers 7, 10, and 11 arthroscopes were smaller, with a diameter of 2.7mm. The number 12 arthroscope consisted of two telescopes, a flexible biopsy punch, and cautery, making it possible to perform a biopsy under arthroscopic visualization. Takagi continually improved his arthroscope and progressively reduced the diameter, but the instruments were fragile.

In 1932, Takagi was successful in obtaining a black-and-white photograph through the arthroscope. In 1936, he and Dr. Saburo Iino obtained color photographs and a 16-mm black-and-white movie film. Basic research for the clinical application of arthroscopy was carried out by Iino, Masashi Miki, Fumihide Koike, and others under the direction of Takagi. Iino documented reliable methods of knee joint puncture and visualization of the knee joint and associated pathology. He was also the first to describe and name the various plicae, or folds, of the synovium.

Takagi also used the arthroscope as a panendoscope in other body cavities. For instance, he used it as a myeloscope in the case of spina bifida, to observe the interior of a tubercular abscess in the iliac fossa, and to evaluate the effects of phonation training after surgery for cleft

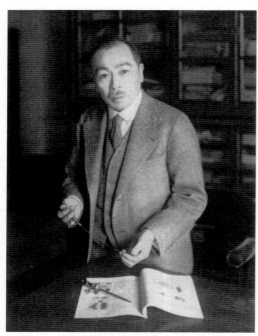

Figure 1–1   **Dr. Kenji Takagi (1888-1963).** (From Watanabe M, Takeda S, Ikeuchi H: Atlas of Arthroscopy. Tokyo, Igaku-Shoin, 1957.)

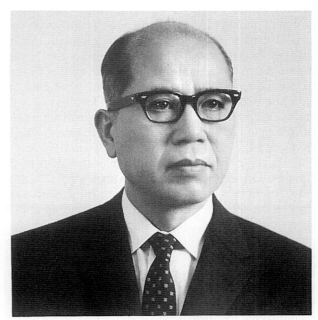

Figure 1–3   **Dr. Masaki Watanabe (1921-1994).** (From McGinty JB, Jackson RW [eds]: Operative Arthroscopy, 2nd ed. Philadelphia, Lippincott-Raven, 1996.)

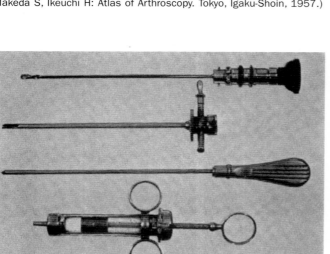

Figure 1–2   **The Takagi number 1 arthroscope, with a diameter of 3.5 mm.** (From Watanabe M, Takeda S, Ikeuchi H: Atlas of Arthroscopy. Tokyo, Igaku-Shoin, 1957.)

palate. In addition to the knee joint, he applied the technique of arthroscopy to the shoulder, elbow, and ankle joints. Further study of arthroscopy was interrupted by World War II, and during the immediate postwar period, the scale of study was reduced.

Following World War II, Dr. Masaki Watanabe (Fig. 1–3) took over for Takagi and continued to develop more useful arthroscopes. In 1951, he developed the number 13 arthroscope (4 mm in diameter) by modifying a pediatric cystoscope. With this arthroscope, side and oblique views were possible; it had sufficient strength, but it was difficult to observe the meniscus and to take color photographs. As the result of 300 arthroscopic observations using this arthroscope, the first edition of the *Atlas of Arthroscopy* was published in 1957.[11] Because the photographs and observations by the number 13 arthroscope were unclear, however, the atlas was illustrated with intra-articular views painted by Shinichiro Fujihashi, who specialized in making endoscopic paintings under direct observation.

In 1954, the number 14 arthroscope (5 mm in diameter) was designed, and Watanabe and Takeda succeeded in taking color photographs and 16-mm color movies with it. Subsequently, for knee arthroscopy in children, the number 15 arthroscope (2.9 mm in diameter) was designed.

In 1958, after making several more trial arthroscopes, Watanabe developed the first truly successful arthroscope, the Watanabe number 21. The diameter was 4.9 mm, and the depth of focus ranged from 1 mm to infinity. The visual angle was 100 degrees in air, which was wide enough to see the in situ structural relationships. The incandescent light bulb at the end of the scope provided good illumination and also functioned as a retractor. Excellent photographs and clear views of the meniscus could be obtained consistently using the number 21 arthroscope. The *Atlas of Arthroscopy* was completely revised, and a second edition with actual color photographs was published in 1969.[12] That same year, a movie made with the number 21 arthroscope was shown at a meeting of the International Society of Orthopedic Surgery and Traumatology in Mexico City. After that, arthroscopic procedures in the knee gained worldwide attention.

Arthroscopic surgery also began in Japan. Watanabe removed a xanthomatous giant cell tumor under arthroscopic control on March 9, 1955. He and Ikeuchi performed the first arthroscopic meniscectomy on May 4, 1962, in a 17-year-old basketball player with a medial meniscal tear of the right knee. It was partially resected under arthroscopy, and the boy was playing basketball again 6 weeks after surgery.

In the West

On the other side of the world, another pioneer was independently exploring the knee joint using endoscopy at almost the same time as Takagi. In 1921, Dr. Eugen Bircher (Fig. 1–4), a Swiss surgeon, published the first report on clinical arthroscopy.[1] He introduced the Jacobaeus laparoscope into a knee filled with gas and called the procedure "arthroendoscopy." In 1922, he reported the successful diagnosis of eight of nine meniscal injuries in 20 cases of post-traumatic arthritis examined arthroscopically.

In 1925, Dr. Phillip H. Kreuscher of Chicago published the first U.S. report on arthroscopy in the *Illinois Medical Journal*.[7] This article was a plea for the early recognition of meniscal lesions by the use of arthroscopy and their early treatment. Although his paper provided a picture of the arthroscope, it did not describe in detail the arthroscope that he developed and used.

In 1930, Dr. Michael Burman (Fig. 1–5) at the Hospital for Joint Disease in New York began studying arthroscopy. In 1931, he reported his experimental cadaver study in every joint of the body using a 4-mm-diameter arthroscope constructed by Wappler.[2] A constant irrigation system with Ringer's solution was used.

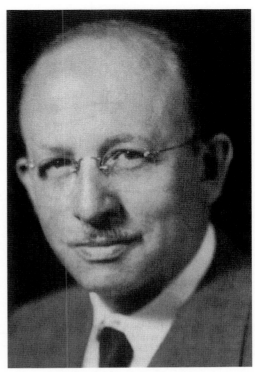

Figure 1–5 Dr. Michael Burman (1901-1975). (From McGinty JB, Jackson RW [eds]: Operative Arthroscopy, 2nd ed. Philadelphia, Lippincott-Raven, 1996.)

In the German literature, Sommer[8] and Vaubel[10] published articles in 1937 and 1938, respectively. Possibly because of the turmoil surrounding World War II, there were no significant advances in arthroscopy from 1939 to 1945.

In 1955, Hurter,[3] writing in French, reported a new method of examining joints with an arthroscope, and Imbert[4] also published articles in the French literature in the mid-1950s.

The First Arthroscopist

Until recently, it had generally been accepted that Takagi was the first to perform arthroscopy in 1918 and that Bircher published the first paper about arthroscopy in 1921. However, a record of arthroscopic activity before World War I has been discovered.[6] In 1912, the Proceedings of the 41st Congress of the German Society of Surgeons at Berlin contained a presentation entitled "Endoscopy of Closed Cavities by the Means of My Trokart-Endoscope." The author was a Danish surgeon from Aarhus named Severin Nordentoft (Fig. 1–6). He had constructed an endoscope similar to the Jacobaeus thoracoscope, consisting of a trocar 5 mm in diameter, a fluid valve, and an optic tube. In addition to cystoscopy and laparoscopy, he reported that it could be used for endoscopy of the knee joint, especially for the early detection of meniscal lesions. Nordentoft used the term *arthroscopy* (Latin, *arthroscopia genu;* German, *Arthroscopia*) and described the handling of the instrument and

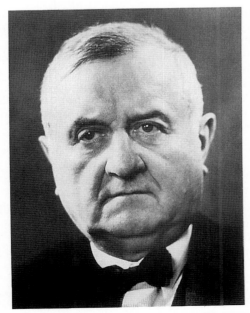

Figure 1–4 Dr. Eugen Bircher (1882-1956). (From McGinty JB, Jackson RW [eds]: Operative Arthroscopy, 2nd ed. Philadelphia, Lippincott-Raven, 1996.)

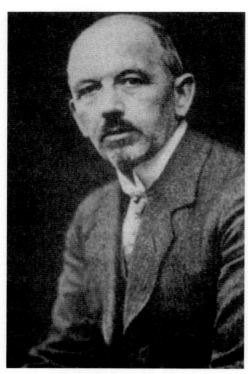

Figure 1–6 **Severin Nordentoft (1866-1922).** (From Kieser CW, Jackson RW: Severin Nordentoft: The first arthroscopist. Arthroscopy 17:532-535, 2001.)

the view of the anterior region of the knee, including the articular cartilage, synovial membrane, villi, and plicae. He used sterile saline as the optical medium during arthroscopy. However, it is unclear whether he performed arthroscopy on patients or on cadaver knees. In subsequent years, his interest changed to radiotherapy, and today he is well known as a pioneer in radiation treatment of mammary carcinoma and brain tumors.

Nordentoft not only performed endoscopy of a knee joint 6 years earlier than Takagi but also published a description of an endoscopic view of a knee joint 9 years earlier than Bircher. In addition, he created the term *arthroscopy*. Thus, he must be considered the first arthroscopist.

Internationalization

Many Europeans and Americans visited Tokyo Teishin Hospital to learn arthroscopic procedures from Watanabe. In 1964, Robert W. Jackson arrived in Japan and learned the technique of arthroscopy.[5] He then returned to Canada and began to practice arthroscopy using the Watanabe number 21 arthroscope in cooperation with Dr. Isao Abe, who had just relocated from Tokyo. Jackson gave an instructional lecture on arthroscopy at a meeting of the American Academy of Orthopaedic Surgeons in 1968, as well as many other lectures at various places in the West, and he greatly contributed to the spread of arthroscopy.

In England, rheumatologists such as Jason and Dixon introduced the Watanabe number 21 arthroscope for the treatment of rheumatic knees. In 1969, Dr. Richard O'Connor visited Watanabe in Tokyo to be trained in arthroscopy and then developed a clinic specializing in arthroscopy in Los Angeles, thus laying the foundations of arthroscopic surgery.

The International Arthroscopy Association (IAA) was founded in Philadelphia by Jackson, O'Connor, Casscells, and Joyce in 1974, and Watanabe was elected its first chairman and was given the name "father of arthroscopy." After that, arthroscopy courses were given in various places in the United States. In 1975, the second meeting of the IAA was held in Copenhagen, and in 1978, the third meeting was in Kyoto.

In 1995, the IAA was dissolved for various reasons and started afresh as the International Society of Arthroscopy, Knee Surgery, and Orthopaedic Sports Medicine (ISAKOS).

Modifications and Improvements

The Watanabe number 21 arthroscope was a bulky instrument with a large diameter and a light bulb attached to the end; this created the risk of injury from heat or breakage of the light bulb. After the Hopkins rod-lens with a high resolution was developed in 1966, a new telescope using this system was introduced into the Watanabe number 21 arthroscope.

In 1970, the Watanabe number 24 arthroscope (Selfoc arthroscope), 1.7 mm in diameter, was developed for smaller joints in collaboration with the Nippon Sheet Glass Company. With former optical systems, it had been impossible to create an arthroscope less than 2 mm in diameter. The Selfoc (for "self-focus") was a glass rod 1 mm in diameter and was used as a lens in the number 24 arthroscope. Smaller-diameter arthroscopes have now been developed, and we can observe almost all joints in the body.

In 1975, McGinty introduced a television system into the arthroscope. Thanks to the development of a small television camera using a charge-coupled device (CCD), several operators can visualize the joint cavity through the TV monitor simultaneously, contributing to advances in arthroscopic surgery.

Conclusion

Arthroscopic surgery is acknowledged as minimally invasive surgery, and new techniques for its use are constantly being developed. We must be grateful to the above-mentioned pioneers of arthroscopy for all their efforts.

References

1. Bircher E: Die Arthroendoskopie. Zentralbl Chir 40:1460-1461, 1921.

2. Burman MS: Arthroscopy or direct visualization of joints: An experimental cadaver study. J Bone Joint Surg 13:669-695, 1931.

3. Hurter E: L'arthroscopie, nouvelle méthode d'exploration du genou. Rev Chir Orthop 41:763-766, 1955.

4. Imbert R: Arthroscopy of the knee: Its technique. Mars Chir 8:368, 1956.

5. Jackson RW: History of arthroscopy. In McGinty JB, Jackson RW (eds): Operative Arthroscopy, 2nd ed. Philadelphia, Lippincott-Raven, 1996.

6. Kieser CW, Jackson RW: Severin Nordentoft: The first arthroscopist. Arthroscopy 17:532-535, 2001.

7. Kreusher P: Semilunar cartilage disease, a plea for early recognition by means of the arthroscope and early treatment of this condition. Ill Med J 47:290-292, 1925.

8. Sommer R: Die Endoskopie des Kniegelenkes. Zentralbl Chir 64:1692, 1937.

9. Takagi K: Practical experience using Takagi's arthroscope. J Jpn Orthop Assoc 8:132, 1933.

10. Vaubel E: Die Arthroskopie (Endoskopie des Kneigelenkes) eibeitrag zur Diagnostiek der Gelenkkrankheiten. Z Rheumaforsch 1:210-213, 1938.

11. Watanabe M, Takeda S, Ikeuchi H: Atlas of Arthroscopy. Tokyo, Igaku-Shoin, 1957.

12. Watanabe M, Takeda S, Ikeuchi H: Atlas of Arthroscopy, 2nd ed. Tokyo, Igaku-Shoin, 1969.

2

Instrumentation and Equipment

PATRICK ST. PIERRE

Arthroscopic Surgery

In 1918, Takagi of Japan used a 7.3-mm cystoscope to examine a cadaveric knee.[6] It was more than 40 years before Watanabe reported on the efficient use of an arthroscope to diagnose conditions in the knee.[8] Today, arthroscopy is the technique of choice for many procedures in the knee, shoulder, elbow, wrist, ankle, and hip. Once on the cutting edge of orthopedic surgery, arthroscopic surgery is now a mainstay and a focus of training programs for orthopedic surgeons. The Arthroscopy Association of North America has led the way in education and the development of new techniques to perform arthroscopic surgery more safely, faster, and with less morbidity than in the past. Arthroscopy should not be thought of as a procedure in itself; rather, it is a better method of performing the same operations that were traditionally performed open. Arthroscopic procedures should be of equal quality and effectiveness as those done open, and the goal of every arthroscopic surgeon should be to perform the procedure better than he or she could have with an arthrotomy.

Surgical Environment

There are several different places where a surgeon can perform arthroscopic surgery. Which one to use is determined primarily by the availability of the different

No benefits in any form have been received or will be received from a commercial party related directly or indirectly to the subject of this article. The views expressed are the views of the author and do not necessarily represent the views of the United States Army or Department of Defense.

options and by the surgeon's desire to expand beyond the hospital setting. The quality of the arthroscopic procedure must not be compromised by the location. Each surgeon should be able to do the same operation in a hospital, surgical center, or office setting. It is the surgeon's responsibility to ensure that the surgical environment is safe and meets all regulations and safety requirements.

Hospital Surgical Suite

The traditional site for arthroscopic surgery has been the hospital surgical suite. Standard-sized rooms are usually adequate, but extra space may be needed for the equipment. The primary additional requirement is the arthroscopy tower (Fig. 2–1). Orthopedic surgeons are not the sole users of this type of equipment. Because of the increased use of endoscopy in general surgery and obstetrics and gynecology, most hospitals have developed storage areas and procedures to facilitate the easy transfer of towers in and out of rooms. Periodic in-service training programs may be necessary to facilitate the team effort required between the nursing team and surgeons to manage the arthroscopic environment. Utilization committees may be mandated to streamline the use of equipment and to cut costs and inventory.

Outpatient Ambulatory Surgical Center

Outpatient surgical centers are being developed all over the country. Many have been created by individual or shared practices to provide increased access to surgery. Because such centers are owned by surgeons with similar practices, scheduling, standardization of equipment, and day-to-day management may be easier. For patients,

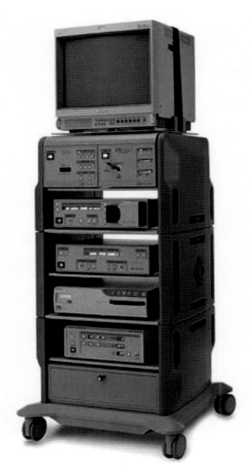

Figure 2–1 Arthroscopy tower.

ambulatory settings offer several advantages over a traditional hospital setting. These centers are newer, so the design is more conducive to the easy flow of patients from the waiting area to the preoperative holding area, the operating room, and finally the recovery room. There is a more relaxed atmosphere, allowing patients to have surgery without the stress of a hospital admission and stay. Because these centers are used primarily for arthroscopic, endoscopic, and minor procedures, patients expect to have surgery and go home with little discomfort and few complications. This atmosphere encourages patients' rapid recovery and independence from the health care system.

The outpatient center must provide all the features of a standard hospital room, including anesthesia support, power, lighting, and suction. OSHA guidelines must still be met, and the same level of care and safety must be provided.[7]

Office

The use of office arthroscopy is growing among surgeons who have primarily arthroscopic surgery practices and want the convenience of performing their procedures in the same setting. Generally, office arthroscopy takes the idea of the outpatient surgical center one step further.

However, the office setting must meet the same guidelines for safety and space that apply to larger facilities. For the surgeon, the office setting obviously offers more access and control, but also more responsibility. In an office setting, the surgeon may also be the anesthesia provider and must be capable of handling any emergency. The setup and management of these arthroscopy suites must meet state regulations.

Sterilization of Equipment

Adequate sterilization of arthroscopy equipment is crucial. Ethylene oxide gas sterilization has been the gold standard for years.[3] However, gas sterilization requires 6 hours for exposure and then aeration to prevent toxicity. This method is usually reserved for overnight sterilization of equipment that will be used the next day. Because of the toxicity of ethylene oxide,[3] other methods of gas sterilization are being developed. Currently, sterilization with 58% hydrogen peroxide is rapidly replacing ethylene oxide; it is safer and just as efficient. Steam autoclaving is the standard method of rapid sterilization, and equipment companies have come a long way in making the equipment durable enough to withstand the high temperature and water exposure required with such techniques. In the past, this was not true, and other methods, such as cold soaking of instruments, were necessary. Glutaraldehyde was the first chemical used extensively, but it is very toxic to health care workers and patients inadvertently exposed to it.[5] Newer techniques using peracetic acid are now available. Peracetic acid is less toxic than glutaraldehyde, more effective, and noncorrosive.[2] It does not require high heat, so it can be applied to heat-sensitive instruments. This is the most common method of sterilizing arthroscopy cameras.

Instruments

Arthroscopic technology is changing rapidly, with new instruments and equipment being developed yearly. Thus, the information in this chapter may be obsolete a few years after publication. The illustrations are representative of the type of instruments available and are not intended to promote a specific company. It is in the best interest of all arthroscopic surgeons to stay abreast of new developments by reading the literature provided by the various manufacturers and to visit their booths when attending conferences. However, it must be remembered that the goal of these companies is to sell products, not necessarily to provide the most cost-effective intervention for patients. It is the surgeon's responsibility to keep up-to-date on outcomes reported for the different devices and equipment in peer-reviewed literature.

Arthroscopes and Cameras

The development of newer and better arthroscopes and cameras has enhanced our ability to see within the joints and bursae. The triple-chip camera head has quickly

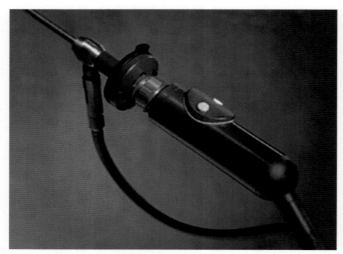

Figure 2–2 Triple-chip camera system.

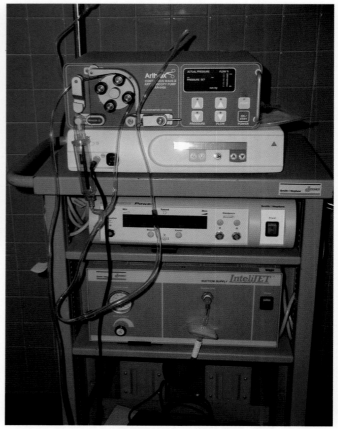

Figure 2–3 Arthroscopy pump.

become the standard in the operating room and provides excellent resolution (Fig. 2–2). Some camera heads can be autoclaved, thus reducing sterilization costs and turn-around time. Most companies now offer this feature.

New arthroscopes are being developed and marketed that offer an increasing field of view with smaller scope diameters, better depth of field with improved optics, and better flow through the sheaths. There are now steer-able arthroscopes for getting into hard-to-see spaces.

Irrigation Systems

Water flow is now managed with computerized consoles that are more adept at detecting pressure and flow within a joint. Certain systems can adjust for the pressure changes associated with the use of suction devices and shavers. Although some surgeons continue to hang bags of saline and use gravity, most have changed to pumps and computerized systems (Fig. 2–3). The utility of these devices has been enhanced by the development of car-tridges to connect the tubing to the monitors. This has also been effective at increasing the consistency of pres-sure. Being able to adjust the pressure with a pump is advantageous when trying to obtain hemostasis. Adding epinephrine to the fluid can be effective but may be counterproductive if the anesthesiologist is trying to lower the blood pressure.

Motorized Shaving Systems

Motorized shavers (Fig. 2–4) have been instrumental in increasing the surgeon's ability to remove large amounts of tissue in a short amount of time. Shavers are dispos-able and come in many different sizes and shapes. Based on trial and error, surgeons can determine which ones are most useful for common surgeries. Different angles and blades are available from all the manufacturers (Fig. 2–5). Some shavers are more aggressive and can remove bone as efficiently as a bur. Some have protective sheaths to prevent too much tissue from being removed,

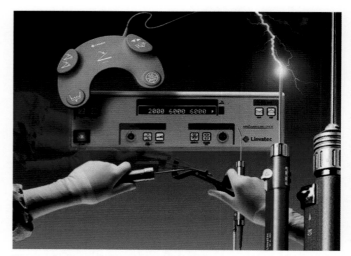

Figure 2–4 Motorized shaver system.

such as whisker blades. These are helpful to prepare the capsule for plication. Some companies now market blades that are combined with electrocautery to decrease the need to change instruments back and forth.

Hand Instruments

A set of hand instruments, including basket forceps, graspers, and scissors, is necessary to perform

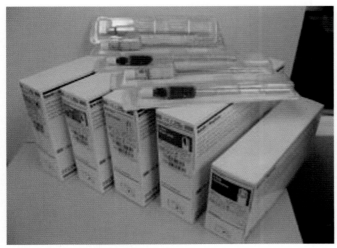

Figure 2–5   Shaver blades.

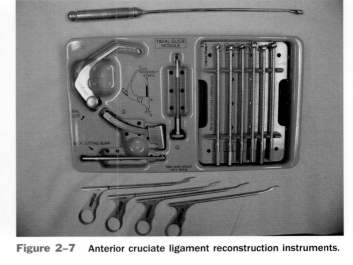

Figure 2–7   Anterior cruciate ligament reconstruction instruments.

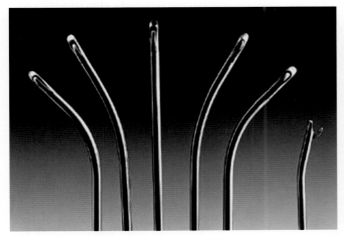

Figure 2–6   Hand instruments.

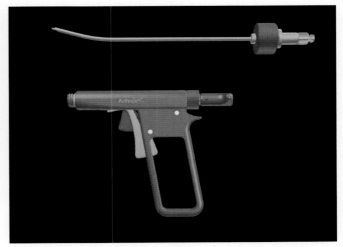

Figure 2–8   Meniscal dart.

arthroscopic surgery (Fig. 2–6). Manufacturers have developed instruments with different angles, sharper blades, and smaller diameters to get to difficult areas. Most hospitals have these sets available. It is important to investigate the variety of instruments offered, as well as the ability to get them serviced, before selecting a product for a specific practice.

Specialized Procedure Instruments

Manufacturers have developed instrument sets that can speed the performance of many common procedures, including anterior or posterior cruciate ligament reconstruction (Fig. 2–7), meniscal repair (Figs. 2–8 and 2–9), osteochondral transplantation (Fig. 2–10), hip arthroscopy (Fig. 2–11), and others. Many of these sets are technique specific and promote the manufacturer's own implant. These sets are extremely helpful in performing the procedures, but sound surgical principles are required for success. Again, it is the surgeon's responsibility to ensure that the technique meets the demand of the injury.

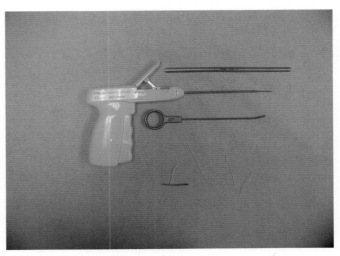

Figure 2–9   Meniscal RapidLoc system.

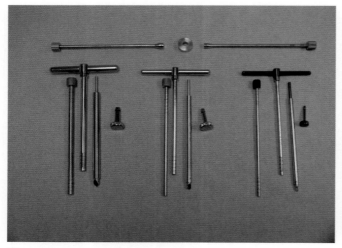

Figure 2–10   Osteochondral system.

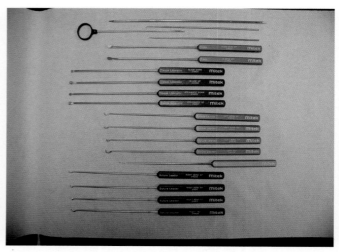

Figure 2–12   Shoulder arthroscopy instruments.

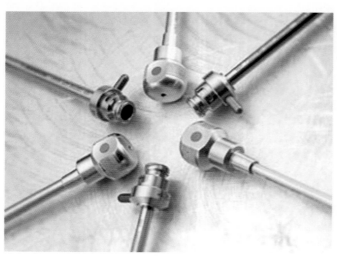

Figure 2–11   Hip arthroscopy instruments.

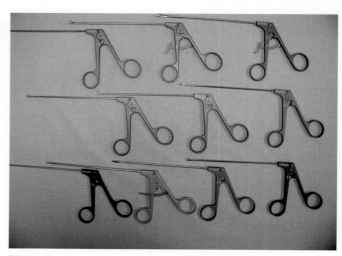

Figure 2–13   Shoulder arthroscopy instruments.

Specialized Suture Instruments

With the increased use of suture anchors, especially in the shoulder, there is an increased need for tools to manage sutures in the joint and to tie arthroscopic knots (specific techniques are discussed in other chapters). New products are available that assist with the passage of suture through tissue (Figs. 2–12 and 2–13). These instruments carry the suture through tissue, use a wheel device to pass suture relay systems, or puncture through tissue to grasp the suture on the other side. This is a rapidly changing market, and the ideal device has not been developed. For surgeons who do frequent arthroscopic repairs, several different types of suture management devices will be needed.

Laser and Radiofrequency Systems

The use of laser and radiofrequency systems with arthroscopy has increased dramatically over the past 10 years.[4] Laser was first used as an ablation device and has the advantage of being smaller and causing less mechanical injury to articular cartilage than radiofrequency systems. However, there have been reports of subchondral bone injury and necrosis associated with laser use. Lasers have also been used for capsular shrinkage in the shoulder.[1] The biggest downside of laser use is its costs. The surgeon or the institution must decide whether its benefits are cost effective.

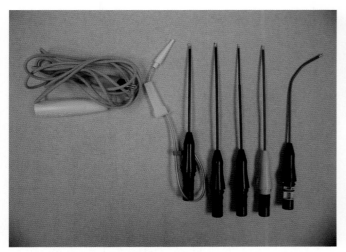

Figure 2–14 Bipolar radiofrequency unit.

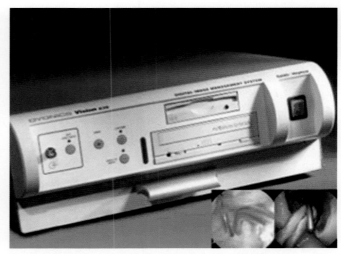

Figure 2–16 Digital imaging management system.

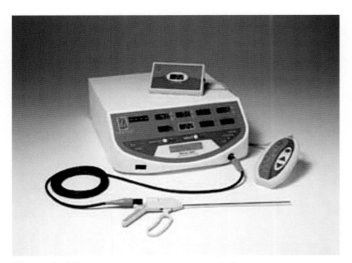

Figure 2–15 Monopolar radiofrequency device.

Radiofrequency systems have been marketed as a way to produce similar heat energy at a fraction of the cost of a laser. They are also used for tissue ablation, electrocautery, and capsular shrinkage. The two types available are bipolar (Fig. 2–14) and monopolar (Fig. 2–15) devices. The advantage of the bipolar design is that the energy is transferred between electrodes at the site of treatment. Monopolar devices must use a grounding pad and draw energy through the body. Current controversies include the depth of tissue penetration, the amount of cell death, and the ability of each device to monitor and control temperature.

Documentation Systems

Another major advantage of arthroscopic surgery is the ability to document with pictures both the pathology and the treatment. Having actual pictures of the injury and the final treatment outcome can help patients understand their injuries and their prognosis for recovery. This is also an indispensable tool for referral surgeons providing subsequent care, allowing them to see what has been done before. Although printing photographs directly has been the standard method of documentation, many surgeons record a videotape of the full or partial procedure. Companies now produce CD-writable systems that enable digital recording of the pictures as well as small amounts of video (Fig. 2–16). I have found that pictures and videos are very helpful during preoperative counseling and when obtaining informed consent. Patients have a better understanding of their injuries and the treatment when they are able to compare their pictures with pictures of normal anatomy.

Surgical Positioning and Preparation

How the patient is positioned and the ease of access to the joint can often determine the success of surgery. Many devices are available to assist with optimal patient positioning. Leg holders and lateral posts have been available for years, and new lower-profile devices that are easier to use have been designed. Traction units are available for wrist, hip, and ankle arthroscopy, and single-use sterile attachments are now available for the wrist and ankle. These are especially useful if the surgeon does not have an assistant available. Traction devices are designed to be attached to standard operating tables.

Shoulder arthroscopy can be performed equally well in either the lateral decubitus or the beach chair position. With the lateral decubitus position, a traction unit is used to keep the arm abducted and flexed forward slightly. Traction injuries have been reported, but this is generally a safe position and provides excellent exposure, especially in the glenohumeral joint. Shoulder arthroscopy in the beach chair position is safe and much easier with new table attachments that allow better access to the posterior shoulder (Fig. 2–17). In the beach chair

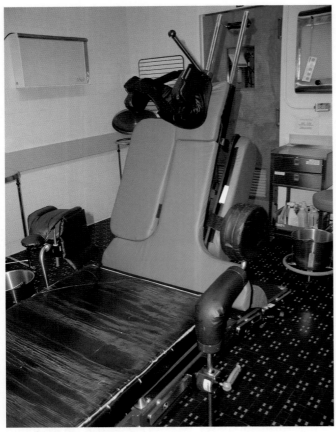

Figure 2–17 Beach chair.

position, it is easier to rotate the shoulder, but an assistant is needed to position the shoulder to allow adequate inspection and treatment within the joint. Sterile armholder attachments are available to adjust and hold the shoulder in place during arthroscopy. This device is indispensable if an assistant or extra scrub technician is not available.

References

1. Arnoczky SP, Aksan A: Thermal modification of connective tissues: Basic science considerations and clinical implications. J Am Acad Orthop Surg 8:305-313, 2000.
2. Crow S: Peracetic acid sterilization: A timely development for a busy healthcare industry. Infect Control Hosp Epidemiol 13:111-113, 1992.
3. Ethylene Oxide Fact Sheet. OSHA Fact Sheet No. 95-17 (January 1, 1995).
4. Hayashi K, Markel D: Thermal modification of joint capsule and ligamentous tissues: The use of thermal energy in sports medicine. Op Tech Sports Med 6:120-125, 1998.
5. Johnson LL, Shneider DA, Austin MD: Two percent glutaraldehyde; a disinfectant in arthroscopy and arthroscopic surgery. J Bone Joint Surg Am 64:237-239, 1982.
6. Sisk TD: Arthroscopy of knee and ankle. In Crenshaw AH (ed): Campbell's Operative Orthopedics, 7th ed. St. Louis, CV Mosby, 1987, pp 2547-2608.
7. U.S. Department of Labor, Occupational Safety and Health Administration. www.osha.gov. 2002.
8. Wantanabe M, Takeda S: The number 21 arthroscope. J Jpn Orthop Assoc 34:1041, 1960.

3

Implants

F. Alan Barber and David P. Richards

The advent of arthroscopic surgery led to the need for more appropriate surgical implants that could take advantage of these minimally invasive techniques. Initially content to observe pathology and later to remove torn cartilage, arthroscopic surgeons soon began to develop techniques that called for both repair and fixation of tissue. This effort to expand the proven surgical options has led to an increasing demand for new technology, which has driven the development of these devices.

Numerous implants, both metal and biodegradable, are used in arthroscopic surgery today. These include suture anchors, meniscal repair devices, and soft tissue (tendon and ligament) fixation devices, as well as techniques for articular cartilage repair. These devices are not specific to any single joint. Although suture anchors are most often used in the shoulder, they can also be applied elsewhere in the body (knee, wrist, foot, and ankle). Nor are these devices restricted to use in arthroscopic techniques. Suture anchors are widely used in both open and arthroscopic orthopedic surgery, as well as by other surgical specialists.

The need for more stable and less invasive devices to restore normal joint biomechanics has generated numerous implants, some of which are made from biodegradable materials. Many different types of polymers are used; newer ones continue to be introduced, and older forms are replaced. A surgeon selecting a biodegradable implant should be aware of the characteristics of the material and its strength loss and degradation profile. This chapter describes the characteristics, benefits, and uses of current arthroscopic implants.

Suture Anchors

In the past, attaching soft tissue (ligaments and tendons) to bone was accomplished by passing sutures through tunnels in the bone. These tunnels were created by awls,

drills, or needles that passed the suture. Although this technique worked well for open procedures, it was impractical as an arthroscopic technique, so an alternative method was sought. Mitek provided the first-generation suture anchor, which was called the G1 anchor. This anchor, which resembled a fishhook, allowed the arthroscopic surgeon to attach a suture to the bone without the use of a tunnel.

Many other anchoring devices have followed this first anchor. At about the same time the Mitek G1 was developed, Marlowe Goble developed a screw suture anchor known as the Statak anchor. Today, there are many screw and nonscrew suture anchors. Although the designs differ and the insertion techniques vary, they are all designed to accomplish the same task: attaching a suture to the bone.

The initial site of suture anchor use was the shoulder. Anchors are currently used for glenohumeral instability procedures, biceps tendon procedures (superior labral anterior to posterior [SLAP] repairs and tenodesis), and rotator cuff repairs. Over time, anchor applications have expanded to include other joints and other disciplines. Anchors are used for the reattachment of tendons and ligaments in the hand and elbow,[21,34,40,47,85,109] foot,[32,38,60,80] and knee.[46] Anchors are also being used in other disciplines such as gynecology,[100] urology,[54,65] craniofacial surgery,[39] and plastic surgery.[87]

Shoulder

When evaluating a suture anchor, several components must be considered. The fundamental characteristics of a good anchor are that it must fix the suture to the bone, not pull out of the bone, permit an easy surgical technique (i.e., the ability to tie an arthroscopic slipknot), and not cause long-term problems. Other desirable features include biocompatibility, adequate strength, easy insertion, and the ability to allow early rehabilitation. Although suture anchors have many advantages over a conventional bone tunnel, they require special instrumentation that is specific for each anchor and may present storage problems. Other disadvantages of anchors include cost, learning curves, and retained foreign material. For convenience, lists of anchoring devices are provided, including both traditional suture anchors and tissue fixation tacks; these are divided into nonbiodegradable (Table 3–1) and biodegradable (Table 3–2) devices.

Anchor Selection

An evaluation of a suture anchor must consider the anchor size, the number of sutures and the suture size it can accommodate, the anchor material, the anchor type, and the insertion technique (the procedure and anatomic location).

ANCHOR SIZE

Suture anchors come in a wide assortment of sizes (Fig. 3–1), ranging from very small for the sutures used in hand surgery to very large anchors that can accommodate multiple strands of number 5 suture. Size should be considered in terms of both the outside anchor measurement (major diameter) and the size of the bone hole made (minor diameter for a screw or drill hole). Anchor size also depends on the surgical application. For example, for Bankart, SLAP, and biceps tendon repairs, number 2 is usually the largest suture chosen; therefore, the anchor does not need to take several number 5 sutures. In contrast, a large anchor that offers excellent fixation in osteoporotic bone and can take many sutures is advantageous in rotator cuff repairs. Additionally, the anchor should fit securely in the glenoid without either

Table 3–1
Nonbiodegradable Suture Anchors

Company	Anchor	Size (mm)	Material	Sutures
Arthrex	Corkscrew	3.5, 5.0, 6.5	Titanium	2 (#2)
Arthrex	FASTak	2.8	Titanium	1 (#2)
Arthrex	Parachute	5.0 screw, 6.5 PLLA button	Titanium and PLLA	N/A (#4 suture attaches button to screw)
Arthrotek	Harpoon	3.4	Stainless steel	#5
Arthrotek	MiniHarpoon	2.0	Stainless steel	#1
Arthrotek	Ti Screw	3.0, 5.0	Titanium	2 (#2)
Arthrotek	LactoScrew	3.5, 5.5	PLLA (82%), PGA (18%)	N/A
Mitek	G2	2.4	Nickel titanium	#2
Mitek	Superanchor	2.9	Nickel titanium	#5
Mitek	Rotator cuff	2.9	Nickel titanium	#2
Mitek	MiniMitek	2.1 drill	Nickel titanium	#0
Mitek	MicroMitek	1.3	Nickel titanium	#3-0
Mitek	Fastin 3, 4, 5.2	3.0, 4.0, 5.2	Titanium	1 (#2)
Mitek	Fastin RC		Titanium	2 (#2)
Mitek	ROC EZ	2.3, 2.8, 3.5	Polyethylene	1 (#2)
Mitek	Tacit 2.0	1.7 drill	Titanium	#2-0
Mitek	Knotless anchor	2.9	Titanium	#1
Linvatec	Revo	4.0	Titanium	1 (#2)
Linvatec	MiniRevo	2.7	Titanium	1 (#2)
Linvatec	SuperRevo	5.0	Titanium	2 (#2)
Linvatec	UltraFix RC	3.2 hole	Stainless steel	2 (#2)
Linvatec	UltraFix MiniMite	2.4 hole	Stainless steel	1 (#2)
Linvatec	UltraFix MicroMite	1.8 hole	Stainless steel	1 (#2-0)
Multitak	Titanium anchor	3.0 × 6.0, 1.8 × 3.7	Titanium	1 (#2), 1(#2-0)
Smith & Nephew	MiniTac	2.0	Titanium	2 (#3-0)
Smith & Nephew	Twinfix Ti	2.0, 2.8, 3.5, 5.0	Titanium	2.8 has #1; 3.5 has 2 (#2); 5.0 has 2 (#2)
Smith & Nephew	Twinfix Ti 4.0, 6.5	4.0, 6.5	Titanium	Large eyelet allows for multiple sutures
Stryker Endoscopy	Mainstay (Zip)	2.7, 3.5, 4.5	Titanium	2.7 has #0; 3.5 has #2; 4.5 has 2 (#2) or 1 (#5)
Stryker Endoscopy	Cuff anchor	5.0	Titanium	2 (#2)
Stryker Endoscopy	Glenoid anchor	3.0	Titanium	#2
Surgical Dynamics	Ogden	2.5, 3.5, 4.5, 5.5, 7.4	Titanium	#0, #1, #2, 2 (#2)
Zimmer	Statak	2.5, 3.5, 5.0, 5.2	Stainless steel	1 (#2)

N/A, not applicable; PGA, polyglycolic acid; PLLA, poly-L-lactic acid.

Table 3–2
Biodegradable Suture Anchors

Company	Anchor	Size (mm)	Material	Sutures
Arthrex	BioCorkscrew	5.0, 6.5	PDLLA	2 (#2)
Arthrex	Bio-Fastak	3.0	PDLLA	1 (#2)
Arthrex	Bio-SutureTak	3.0	PDLLA	1 (#2)
Arthrex	TissueTak	3.0	PDLLA	N/A
Arthrotek	Lactosorb anchor	5.5	PGA, PLLA	2 (#2)
Arthrotek	Bio-Phase	2.0, 3.0	PGA, PLLA	2 mm, #1; 3 mm, #2
Bionx	Duet anchor	6.0 OD, 3.3 CD	PDLA (4%), PLLA (96%); or PLLA	2 (#2)
Bionx	Bankart Tack	3.5	PDLA (4%), PLLA (96%); or PLLA	N/A
Bionx	BioCuff C	5.7 × 18, 28, 36	PDLA (4%), PLLA (96%); or PLLA	N/A
Bionx	Contour labral nail	3.5 × 20	PDLA (4%), PLLA (96%); or PLLA	N/A
Linvatec	BioAnchor	3.5 OD, 2.1 CD	PLLA	1 (#2)
Linvatec	BioTwist	2.9	PLLA	N/A
Linvatec	Ultrasorb	3.5	PLLA	2 (#2)
Mitek	BioKnotless	2.9	PLLA	#2-0
Mitek	BioROC EZ	2.8, 3.5	PLLA	1 (#2)
Mitek	CuffTack	4.5 body, 8.9 wings	PLLA	N/A
Mitek	ConTack	3.5	PLLA body, PDLLA washer	N/A
Mitek	PanaLok	3.5	PLLA	1 (#2)
Mitek	PanaLok RC	3.5	PLLA	1 (#2)
Multitak	Bone Button	3.0 × 6.0, 1.8 × 3.7	Allograft bone	1 (#2), 1 (#2-0)
Orthopedic Biosystems	Phoenix Allograft	5.0 OD, 3.0 CD	Allograft bone	2 (#2)
Regeneration Technologies	AlloAnchor RC	5.0	Allograft cortical bone	2 (#2)
Smith & Nephew	Phoenix 5.0	4.85 OD, 3.1 CD	Allograft	2 (#2)
Smith & Nephew	Twinfix PMR	5.0 OD, 3.2 CD	Polyacetyl	2 (#2)
Smith & Nephew	Twinfix AB	5.0 OD, 3.2 CD	PLLA	2 (#2)
Smith & Nephew	RotorloC	4.5 drill	PLLA	2 (#2)
Smith & Nephew	Suretac 6.0, 8.0	3.4 , 3.7	PGA-TMC	N/A
Smith & Nephew	Suretac II/spikes	3.4	PGA-TMC	N/A
Smith & Nephew	TAG Wedge 3.7	3.7	PGA-TMC	1 (#2)
Smith & Nephew	TAG Rod II	3.7	PGA-TMC	1 (#2)
Surgical Dynamics	SDsorb 2, 3	2.2, 3.2	PGA, PLLA	1 (#2)
Surgical Dynamics	SDsorb EZ Tac	3.5	PGA, PLLA	N/A
Zimmer	BioStatak	5.0 OD, 2.5 CD	PLLA	1 (#2)

CD, core diameter; N/A, not applicable; OD, outside diameter; PDLA, poly-D-lactic acid; PDLLA, polydextrolevolactic acid; PGA, polyglycolic acid; PLLA, poly-L-lactic acid, TMC, trimethylcarbonate.

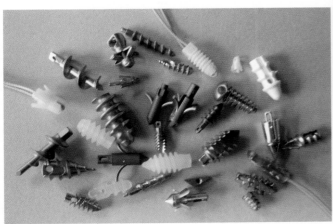

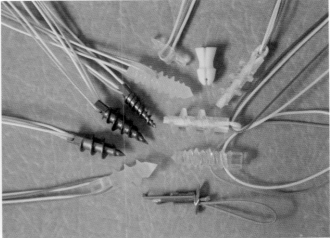

A B

Figure 3–1 Suture anchors have eyelets for the suture and hold the suture in the bone. They come in various sizes, shapes, designs, and materials.

breaking out during insertion or being so small that it cannot gain adequate purchase.

SUTURE SIZE, NUMBER, AND MATERIAL

The size of the suture is related to the repair strength, and the number of sutures an anchor can accommodate has an impact as well. Anchors that allow the use of two or more sutures have clear advantages in rotator cuff surgery, whereas this is less of an advantage in Bankart repairs. The desired suture size and number influence the anchor selected. Using more fixation points provides statistically better strength in anterior shoulder stabilization procedures. At least two anchors are needed to exceed the strength of the anterior shoulder capsule and ligaments.[69]

Additionally, anterior-inferior translation with the shoulder in 90 degrees abduction is statistically reduced by the use of three fixation points compared with two fixation points.[19] Using smaller anchors allows the insertion of more fixation points.

Suture material is another issue to consider. Both absorbable and nonabsorbable sutures are used for these repairs. In the shoulder, a commonly used nonabsorbable suture is Ethibond. It is a braided polyester suture (like Mersiline) but is coated with polybutylate, which allows for superior arthroscopic knot tying, better suture handling, greater loop security, and thus a better knot. Monofilament polydioxanone (PDS) suture is absorbable, and although it is easily placed by suture hooks and punches, it retains only 40% of its original strength at 6 weeks and is gone 9 weeks after implantation.[9] Other absorbable materials are available, including Panacryl.

ANCHOR MATERIAL

Most current anchors are metal, which provides both strength and ease of insertion. The anchors can be easily seen radiographically, and because most are titanium, they do not interfere with postoperative imaging studies. Although the biodegradable anchors demonstrate lower failure loads and are not as easy to insert, they are stronger than the sutures for which they are designed. The softer eyelet of the biodegradable anchor is less likely to fray a suture, and biodegradable anchors offer several other advantages over nonbiodegradable materials: easier revision, better imaging, eventual anchor resorption, and pediatric applications.

ANCHOR TYPE

The many different anchor designs can all be categorized as either screw or nonscrew types.[11,12] In addition, tack-like devices eliminate the need to tie sutures. Screw anchors (see Tables 3–1 and 3–2) are very efficient, with excellent failure load characteristics. All screw anchors have eyelets that accommodate a variety of suture sizes, allow for the substitution of suture, and permit the tying of slipknots. The nonscrew anchors have many different designs, including expanding anchors, toggle anchors, and wedges. They also allow sliding knots, although some nonscrew anchors do not permit suture substitution.

Some screw anchors have equipment that allows the surgeon to "unscrew" and remove the anchor. Nonscrew anchors do not allow for removal after insertion unless it is done by drilling out a biodegradable or plastic anchor. The nonscrew anchors require a hole to be drilled or punched to allow anchor insertion. These holes are sometimes large, and if the anchor pulls out of osteoporotic bone, it can create a large defect. The screw anchors usually create their own holes that are no larger than the minor diameter of the screw.

Insertion Technique

No evaluation of a suture anchor is complete without considering the insertion technique. Several technical points must be contemplated, including the steps and equipment needed to place the anchor in the bone (does a hole need to be drilled or punched? how is the anchor deployed? how are the sutures managed?). For devices that are used with a suture, the surgeon must also anticipate the technique used to pass the suture through the tissue and for tying the knot.

There are three techniques available for passing the suture through the tissue (tendon or ligament), and these have implications for anchor selection. The three techniques are anchor first (in which the anchor is placed in the bone and then the suture is passed through the tissue), suture first (in which the suture is passed through the tissue and threaded onto the anchor, and then the anchor is inserted), and the transtissue technique (in which the anchor threaded with a suture is passed through the tissue). The suture-first technique cannot be used with any screw suture anchor. The transtissue technique requires an anchor sharp enough to pass through the tissue as it carries the suture into place, which usually means that it must be a screw anchor. The anchor-first technique is applicable to both screw and nonscrew anchors.

A new variety of suture anchor (the "knotless" anchor) is a hybrid that attempts to solve the knot-tying issue by having a loop suture attached to the anchor, which is deployed in a novel fashion. This is a version of the suture-first technique.

Suture anchors should be thought of as a system with many parts. Clinical failure of this suture anchoring system can occur at the ligament, bone, suture anchor, or suture. Either the suture or the anchor can fail, but the weakest point is the suture-tendon interface. The key steps in arthroscopic anchor use include site exposure, drill hole placement, anchor insertion, suture placement, and knot tying. With an appropriately selected suture and anchor, the most likely failure situations are either knot failure due to poor knot security or the suture cutting through the tendon.

Elbow

Elbow reconstructions have not traditionally used implantable devices. Instead, reconstructions use suturing techniques and bone tunnels. The recent literature describes the use of suture anchors in the repair of chronic or acute biceps tendon ruptures,[4,62,103] repair of ruptured triceps tendons,[83] and avulsion fractures associated with ulnar collateral ligament injuries.[91]

Lynch et al.[62] demonstrated that using suture anchors to repair the biceps tendon to the radial tuberosity led to an excellent functional outcome based on biomechanical parameters. Vardakas et al.[103] also demonstrated that patients in their series had an acceptable functional outcome after repairing the biceps tendon with suture anchors. Salvo et al.[91] described the use of suture anchor fixation for ulnar collateral ligament instability secondary to an avulsion fracture of the sublime tubercle. Their data suggested that individuals treated with suture anchor fixation returned to their preinjury levels of sports activity and had no elbow pain or instability. Because of the limited access to the elbow, arthroscopic fixation applications are infrequent. The anchors selected tend to be the smaller metallic anchors.

Wrist and Hand

The arthroscopic indications for suture anchor use in the wrist and hand are also limited. However, with the development of smaller (micro) implants, their use may become more common. Although most of the current literature deals with the biomechanical assessment of suture anchor fixation in cadaveric models,[1,34,41] two small studies demonstrated the usefulness of suture anchor repairs in the wrist and hand region.[71,102] Both Mitsionis et al.[71] and Tuncay and Ege[102] demonstrated very good outcomes with the use of suture anchors to repair collateral ligament injuries. Mitsionis's group showed minimal loss of stability, range of motion, or pinch strength in patients who had gamekeeper's thumb surgically repaired with suture anchors.

Foot and Ankle

Suture anchors are being applied in ligamentous reconstructions around the ankle. Reconstruction of the peroneal retinaculum can be facilitated with the use of Mitek suture anchors. Safran et al.[90] described this technique in acute, symptomatic, and subacute injuries involving the peroneal tendons. Lateral ankle instability can be managed using suture anchors as well. Messer et al.[70] assessed the results of a modified Brostrom procedure using suture anchors and found that 91% of their patients had good or excellent outcomes.

Knee

The use of suture anchors in the knee is very limited. There are few arthroscopic applications, although there is some application in the treatment of anterior tibial spine avulsions. Given the various injuries that can occur about the knee, a significant number of implants have been designed. The most common type of arthroscopic implant used in the knee is associated with either ligament reconstruction or meniscal repair, but other devices can be used for specific knee lesions.

Meniscal Repair Devices

Meniscal tears are a common knee injury, with an incidence of approximately 70 in 100,000.[50,77] The desirability of repairing rather than removing the meniscus is well established because of its influence on articular compressive forces, load transmission, shock absorption, joint congruity in both flexion and extension, cartilage nutrition, and joint lubrication, as well as its contribution to joint stability, especially in anterior cruciate ligament (ACL)–deficient knees. Meniscal repair avoids the degenerative changes that follow removal of the meniscus. Arthroscopically, inside-out, outside-in, and all-inside techniques are available.

Both absorbable and nonabsorbable sutures play a key role in these repairs, as do different suturing techniques.[84,86] The gold standard for meniscal repair is a vertically oriented suture repair, and most techniques require the passage of a suture through a skin incision and through the underlying structures posterolaterally or posteromedially. Because of the problems associated with suture passage, there has been an effort to come up with alternative techniques. Bioabsorbable meniscal repair devices are the result (Table 3–3). These devices, with varying designs and failure characteristics, permit an all-inside meniscal repair without the need for accessory portals or incisions (Fig. 3–2). In this section, all-inside meniscal repairs are discussed as "generations," roughly reflecting their development over time but also the general categories of techniques or devices.

First Generation

The first generation of all-inside meniscal repair techniques used either spinal needles or the spectrum suture hook. Morgan[74] described an all-inside technique that

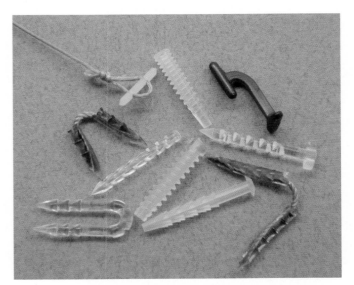

Figure 3–2   Meniscal repair devices vary in design and permit an all-inside meniscal repair without the need for accessory portals or incisions.

Table 3–3

Meniscal Repair Devices

Device	Material	Length	Strength (N)
Arthrotek staple	PGA (18%), PLLA (82%)	10 mm	27
Arthrotek screw	PGA (18%), PLLA (82%)	11 mm	28
Mitek system	Prolene/PDS	6–8 mm	30
Clearfix screw	PLLA	10 mm	32
T-Fix	Plastic bar	3-mm bar #2-0 suture	50
SDsorb staple	PGA (18%), PLLA (82%)	7 mm (10 mm)	31
Arrow (Bionx)	PDLA (20%), PLLA (80%)	10, 13, 16 mm	33
BioStinger	PLLA	10, 13, 16 mm	57
Dart	PDLA (30%), PLLA (70%)	12 mm	62 (2)
FasT-Fix	2 plastic bars	5-mm bars #0 suture	72
RapidLoc	PLLA TopHat and bar	#2-0 suture	43
Horizontal suture	Braided polyester	#2-0	56
Vertical suture	Braided polyester	#2-0	81
Double vertical suture	Braided polyester	#2-0	113

PDLA, poly-D-lactic acid; PDS, polydioxanone suture; PGA, polyglycolic acid; PLLA, poly-L-lactic acid.

was developed to allow the safe repair of the posterior horn by alleviating the risk of neurovascular injury. PDS was best suited for this repair technique.

Second Generation

The second generation of meniscal repair devices was a modification of the suture technique. A toggle suture anchor was passed through the peripheral capsule by a spinal needle, leaving a single suture through the meniscus and out in the joint. Placing two of these T-Fix devices side by side allowed the surgeon to tie them arthroscopically, creating a repair. This T-Fix meniscal repair device (Smith and Nephew Endoscopy, Andover, MA) allowed the repair of torn menisci without the need for a secondary incision. The T-Fix anchor consists of a 3-mm polyacetal bar with a 2-0 braided polyester suture attached to its midpoint. After deployment of the device, arthroscopic knot tying is used to secure the fixator in place. Barrett et al.,[14] in their series of 62 patients, found that the T-Fix was an effective way to repair torn menisci. The subjects in the prospective study by Escalas et al.[42] also had favorable outcomes when the T-Fix was used. A cadaveric study by Coen et al.[35] demonstrated that other soft tissue, besides the meniscus, could be plicated by the T-Fix. Barber and Herbert[10] found that T-Fix had a load to failure of 50N, which was similar to the 48N that Bellemans et al.[16] demonstrated in their study.

Third Generation

A large number of meniscal repair devices fall into this classification. These devices are tacklike or screw fixators that eliminate the need to tie an arthroscopic knot because they fix the inner rim of the meniscal tear to the outer rim. These devices are either pushed or screwed into place and hold the inner rim in position against the

outer rim. After the appearance of the first of these devices (the Bionx Arrow), the use of meniscal repair devices became widespread.[2] This popularity was due to the elimination of the need for arthroscopic knot tying, incisions, or accessory portals.

Meniscal Arrow

The meniscal arrow has a barbed shaft and a crossbar, or "T," and is made of self-reinforced poly-L-lactic acid (PLLA). The shaft is machined from a solid bar of polymer; it is rigid and sharpened to a point. The barbs are cuts placed in two sides of the shaft. These devices come in 10-, 13-, and 16-mm lengths and are placed at 5-mm intervals in the meniscal tear. The arrow insertion instrumentation has been refined and now includes both hand insertion and gun options. Many studies have examined the arrow load-to-failure strength, and the reported results vary somewhat.

Song and Lee[94] demonstrated a pullout strength of 38N for a single arrow and 53N for a double arrow. Bellemans et al.[16] demonstrated that the longer arrow (16 mm) has a slightly greater load-to-failure strength (39N) than the 13-mm arrow (33N) and a significantly greater load-to-failure strength than the 10-mm arrow (19N). Other studies showed a failure load of 30 to 44N.[3,5,8,20,25,44] Barber and Herbert[10] demonstrated that the meniscal arrow failed by pulling through the meniscal fragment. Petsche et al.[82] recently looked at the meniscal arrow and assessed their patients retrospectively. Their subjects' Lysholm[63] and Tegner[101] scores improved significantly after meniscal repair. They noted no surgical complications, such as infection or neurovascular injury. They did, however, state that five patients had mild subcutaneous irritation caused by the arrow tips, which resolved in approximately 5 months. The complications of arrow migration to a subcutaneous position, synovitis, and chondral excoriation have been documented.[49,78,88,95]

Meniscal Screws

Two meniscal screws are on the market. The Clearfix screw has a graduated pitch to compress the meniscal fragments together as the screw is advanced; the Arthrotek screw has a constant pitch. The Clearfix is made of PLLA, and the Arthrotek screw is made of the "Lactosorb" material (a copolymer with 18% polyglycolic acid [PGA] and 82% PLLA). Both screws are 10 mm long. Becker et al.[15] tested the Clearfix screw and found it to have a load failure of approximately 15 N. In the study by Arnoczky and Lavagnino,[5] the Clearfix screw failed at 35 N. Barber et al.[10,13] studied both the Clearfix and the Arthrotek screws, which failed at 32 and 28 N, respectively. The most common means of failure for both screws is the head pulling through the inner rim while remaining in the outer rim. Like the meniscal arrow, the meniscal screw (Clearfix) has been implicated in chondral damage.[58]

BioStinger

The BioStinger (Linvatec, Largo, FL) is another tacklike device. It is composed of molded rather than machined PLLA (more amorphous than the self-reinforced material) and is inserted into the meniscal tissue over a needle. This cannulated design results in a flexible device with a blunted tip and four rows of molded fins. The crossbar has a rounded low profile. It comes in 10-, 13-, and 16-mm lengths and is deployed by either a gun or a plunger insertion device.

Becker et al.[15] found that the failure load of this device was 25 N. Barber and Herbert[10] also studied this meniscal fixator, and their load-to-failure result was 56 N. Arnoczky and Lavagnino[5] found that the BioStinger failed at 35 N. At present, there are no reports of complications associated with BioStinger fixation.

Dart

The meniscal Dart (Arthrex Corporation, Naples, FL) is a headless device available in 10-, 12-, and 14-mm lengths. Arthrex Darts are inserted by a gun that places these devices below the meniscal surface. The Dart possesses a double-reverse barb design without a head and is used as a pair. It is made of a copolymer (30% poly-D-lactic acid and 70% PLLA) that is gamma irradiated.

Other Devices

Other third-generation devices do not easily fit into a specific category. These include staple devices (Biomet staple, SDsorb meniscal staple) and the Mitek meniscal repair system. These devices are inserted using a gun. Barber and Herbert[10] found that the Biomet staple failed at 27 N, SDsorb failed at 31 N, and the Mitek meniscal repair system failed at 30 N. Arnoczky and Lavagnino[5] found that the SDsorb staple failed at 9 N and the Mitek meniscal repair system failed at 27 N. They also found that the SDsorb staple demonstrated a significant decrease in failure strength at 12 and 24 weeks. Walsh et al.[104] reported that the failure load of the SDsorb staple was 18 N, and Bellemans et al.[16] reported a 4-N failure load.

Fourth Generation

FasT-Fix and RapidLoc

The fourth-generation devices combine a biodegradable implant that is locked with a sliding knot and allows for "adjustable" fixation. The meniscal repair device comes preloaded with the sliding knot, thus eliminating the need to tie an arthroscopic knot. The FasT-Fix (Smith and Nephew Endoscopy, Andover, MA) is an updated version of the T-Fix and incorporates twin 3-mm polyacetal bars and double number 0 braided polyester suture. It is completely nonabsorbable. It can be deployed in both horizontal and vertical configurations. The strength of the double suture of the FasT-Fix is reflected in the load-to-failure strength for both vertical and horizontal deployments (71 and 72 N, respectively).[13]

The RapidLoc device (Mitek Products, Westwood, MA) consists of a PLLA or PDS "TopHat" and bar that are connected by either 2-0 Ethibond or Panacryl suture. The bar serves as an anchor, which is passed through the meniscal substance into the peripheral capsule. The TopHat is backed up by a sliding knot; when this knot is advanced by pulling the suture and pushing the TopHat using a single-lumen knot pusher, it slides down to dimple the meniscal surface. Its load-to-failure strength was 43 N.[13]

Both these devices allow adjustment of the tension of the inner meniscal rim against the outer meniscal rim. The nonabsorbable FasT-Fix leaves no polyacetyl bars in the joint, whereas the RapidLoc leaves the PLLA TopHat in the joint. Whether this will cause articular cartilage abrasion or synovitis remains to be seen.

Future Generations

It is difficult to predict how meniscal injuries will be dealt with in the future. A recent study[43] evaluated the use of chemically unaltered porcine small intestine submucosa as a scaffold for meniscal tissue regeneration. This study demonstrated that the submucosal graft allowed cellular repopulation, which led to the healing of meniscal deficits in the rabbit model by 24 weeks. Tissue engineering may also hold some answers with regard to meniscal repair.[52]

Anterior Cruciate Ligament Fixation

ACL injuries occur in 1 of 3000 Americans, commonly as a result of sports that require pivoting, cutting, and acceleration and deceleration.[72] Torn ACLs frequently occur from skiing and football injuries. Paletta and Warren[79] documented 0.6 ACL injuries per 1000 skier days, and Speer et al.[96] noted 0.7 ACL injuries per 1000 college football player days. Bach et al.[6] stated that 100,000 ACL reconstructions are performed each year. Because of the high number of ACL injuries and the morbidity associated with an unstable knee, there has been a significant amount of research in ACL fixation.

The goal is to fix the graft in place securely while allowing early knee function. As a frame of reference, it is helpful to list the various functional activities and the respective forces applied to the ACL[27,75,76]:

Level walking = 169 N
Ascending stairs = 67 N
Descending stairs = 445 N
Descending ramp = 93 N
Ascending ramp = 27 N
Normal walking = 400 N
Sharp cutting = 1700 N

The method of ACL fixation is determined in part by the graft selection. Bone-to-bone fixation is different from soft tissue (tendon)–to–bone tunnel fixation. Additionally, there are both biodegradable (Table 3–4) and nonbiodegradable materials (Table 3–5) available for fixation. This section discusses the various fixation options for each of the commonly used grafts.

Bone–Patellar Tendon–Bone Autograft

The bone–patellar tendon–bone (B-PT-B) autograft is the historical gold standard for ACL reconstruction. The natural ACL has an ultimate strength to failure of 2160 N and a stiffness of 242 N/mm,[108] whereas the B-PT-B graft has an ultimate strength of 2977 N and a stiffness of 455 N/mm.[36] To ensure that the biomechanics of the graft are similar to those of the normal ACL, appropriate fixation must occur during the healing process.

Tibial Fixation

Numerous types of tibial fixation for B-PT-B autografts have been documented in the literature. Kurosaka et al.[59] assessed the biomechanical properties of distal fixation using a number 5 suture tied to a button. They found that grafts fixed in this manner had a load-to-failure strength of 248 N and a stiffness of 12.8 N/mm. The same study assessed the strength of the patellar tendon stapled to the proximal tibia; the failure load of this graft fixed with staples was 129 N, with a stiffness of 10.8 N/mm. These authors also studied interference fixation using 6.5- and 9-mm AO screws. The 6.5-mm AO screw pro-

Table 3–4

Biodegradable Ligament Fixation

Company	Type of Fixation	Material	Diameter (mm)	Length (mm)
Alaron Surgical	Bilok screw	PLLA (75%), βTCP (25%)	7–10	20, 22, 25, 30, 35
Arthrex	Full thread screw	PLLA	7–12	28
Arthrex	Sheathed Bio interference screw	PLLA	7–10	23
Arthrex	Bio-Transfix	PLLA	9–12	35
Arthrex	BioTenodesis	PLLA	4, 5.5, 7, 8, 9	
Bionx	SmartScrew ACL	PDLA (4%), PLLA (96%); or PLLA	7, 8, 9, 10, 11	20, 25, 30
Bionx	The Wedge	PDLA (4%), PLLA (96%); or PLLA	5, 7, 9	20, 25
Biomet (Arthrotek)	Gentle threads interference screw	PLLA (82%), PGA (18%)	7–12	20, 25, 30 (for 7–10) 25 (for 11 and 12)
Mitek	PHANTOM screw	PLLA	7, 8, 9	20, 25, 30
Mitek	PHANTOM SOFTHREAD	PLLA	7, 8, 9, 10	25
Mitek	Biocryl	TCP, PLLA	7, 8, 9, 10, 11	23, 30
Mitek	RIGIDfix cross pin	PLLA	2.7, 3.3	42
Linvatec	BioScrew, Guardsman BioScrew	PLLA	7, 8, 9, 10, 11	20, 25, 30
Linvatec	BioScrew XtraLok	PLLA	9, 10, 11	35, 40
Linvatec	Absolute	PLLA	7, 8, 9, 10, 11	23, 30
Regeneration Technologies	CorIS HT	Allograft cortical bone	7, 8, 9	15, 20, 25
Regeneration Technologies	CorIS ST	Allograft cortical bone	7, 8, 9	15, 20, 25
Smith & Nephew	Endo-fix Screw	PGA, TMC	7, 9	20, 25, 30
Smith & Nephew	BioRCI	PLLA	7, 8, 9, 10	25, 30, 35
Smith & Nephew	BioRCI-HA	PLLA-HA	7, 8, 9, 10, 11, 12	20, 25, 30, 35
Stryker Endoscopy	Bioabsorbable ACL interference screw	PLLA	7, 8, 9, 10	23, 28
Stryker Endoscopy	Biosteon HA/PLLA ACL screw	PLLA (75%), HA (25%)	7, 8, 9, 10	23, 28

HA, hydroxyapatite; PDLA, poly-D-lactic acid; PGA, polyglycolic acid; PLLA, poly-L-lactic acid; TCP, tricalcium phosphate; TMC, trimethylcarbonate.

Table 3–5

Nonbiodegradable Ligament Fixation

Company	Type of Fixation	Material	Diameter (mm)	Length (mm)
Arthrex	Sheathed screw	Titanium	6, 7, 8, 9	15, 20, 25, 30
Arthrex	Nonsheathed screw	Titanium	10	20, 25, 30
Arthrex	Tibial screw	Titanium	5 × 20, 7, 8, 9, 10	20, 25, 30
Arthrex	Soft screw (blunt thread)	Titanium	7, 8, 9, 10	25, 30, 35
Arthrotek	Bone Mulch screw	Titanium	10.5	20, 25, 30, 35
Arthrotek	WasherLoc screw	Titanium	4.5 cortical or 6.0 cancellous	24-60 (2-mm increments)
Arthrotek	Tunneloc	Titanium	5, 6, 7, 8, 9, 10, 11	20, 25, 30
Arthrotek	Blunt-nose setscrew	Titanium	9	20, 25, 30, 35, 40
Linvatec	Cannulated IS	Titanium	7, 8, 9	20, 25, 30, 35, 40
Linvatec	Propel Cannulated IS (original or taper tip)	Titanium	7, 8, 9	20, 25, 30
Linvatec	Guardsman femoral IS (original or taper tip)	Titanium	7, 8, 9	20, 25, 30
Mitek	Advantage	Titanium	7, 9	15, 20, 25, 30, 35, 40
Mitek	Profile	Titanium	7, 8, 9	20, 25, 30
Mitek	Big Advantage	Titanium	11, 13	20, 25, 30
Smith & Nephew	Endobutton	Titanium	Attached with continuous loop	
Stryker Endoscopy	Cross-Screw System	Titanium	8	40, 50, 60
Stryker Endoscopy	Universal ACL Wedge	Titanium	7, 8, 9, 10	20, 25, 30

vided a pullout strength of 215 N and a stiffness of 23.5 N/mm; the 9-mm AO screw resulted in 476 N of strength and 57.9 N/mm of stiffness.

Sutures around a post have also been used to stabilize the B-PT-B graft distally. Steiner et al.[99] found that this technique provided a load-to-failure strength of 396 N and a stiffness of 27 N/mm. They found that graft stability was increased when interference fixation was added to post fixation (674 N strength and 50 N/mm stiffness). Other studies have assessed B-PT-B fixation using interference screw fixation. With greater screw diameter, there was an overall increase in pullout strength and stiffness. Kohn and Siebert[55] assessed tibial fixation with interference screw fixation. They found that with the 7-mm interference screw, the strength of the graft was 461 N and its stiffness was 47 N/mm. With the 9-mm interference screw, the strength of the graft was increased to 678 N, with greater stiffness as well. Gerich et al.[44] found similar biomechanical data when they assessed a 9- by 30-mm interference screw (758 N). Brand et al.[22,23] found that with a 9- by 25-mm biodegradable interference screw, the overall strength of the graft was 293 N, with a stiffness of 42 N/mm.

Femoral Fixation

A number of methods of fixing the femoral side of the B-PT-B graft have been described. Brown et al.[25,26] reported femoral fixation using an Endobutton and a Mitek anchor. The Endobutton had a failure load of 554 N and a stiffness of 27 N/mm, and the Mitek anchor had similar fixation characteristics (511 N and 27 N/mm). They also described the strength of a press-fit graft within the femoral tunnel. These results (350 N and 37 N/mm) were slightly less than those achieved with other modes of fixation.

Several studies have looked at interference screw fixation. Steiner et al.[99] and Brown et al.[25,26] examined interference screw fixation from an outside-in position. Their results were somewhat different, in that Steiner's group found that the fixation strength using an outside-in screw was greater than that demonstrated by Brown's group (423 N vs. 235 N). Insertion of the interference screw endoscopically, from inside out, has also been evaluated. These studies reported a failure load of 256 to 640 N and a stiffness of 33 to 77 N/mm.[25,26,29,53,81,99] Studies have also attempted to compare the differences between metal and biodegradable interference screw fixation. The fixation strength with bioabsorbable implants appears to be similar to the load to failure of metal screws (Fig. 3–3), with failure loads ranging from 418 to 565 N.[29,53,81]

Recent Literature

Mariani et al.[67] assessed the difference between interference screw fixation and transcondylar screw fixation. The functional outcomes (IKDC, Lysholm, Tegner) of the two groups were not significantly different. The initial strength of bioabsorbable interference screw fixation (837 and 605 N) was similar to that of titanium interference screw fixation (863 and 585 N) during single-cycle load to failure and cyclic loading to failure, respectively.[56] In another study that compared conventional interference screw fixation and a bioabsorbable plug (a shortened screw), the cyclic loading to failure of the bioabsorbable plug was 994 N, compared with 1001 N for the interference screw.[57] Interference screw length appears to have no effect on tibial tunnel fixation, and there was no biomechanical difference among interference screws measuring 9 mm by 12.5, 15, and 20 mm.[18]

Bioabsorbable screws appear to be well tolerated and incorporate well with bone, with no evidence of tunnel

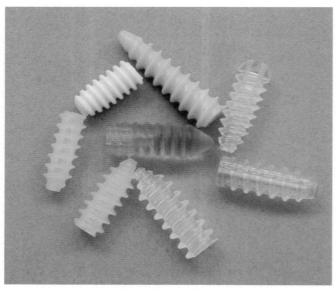

Figure 3–3 Bioabsorbable interference screws provide fixation strengths that are similar to those of metal interference screws.

widening. A 5-year follow-up on bone tunnel remodeling by Lajtai et al.[61] demonstrated minimal reaction to bioabsorbable interference screw fixation, with complete replacement of the bone tunnel with bone. Barber et al.[8] found that BioScrew fixation of patellar tendon autografts had a similar functional outcome, with similar KT 1000/2000 differences and no evidence of bony changes associated with the bioabsorbable screw.

Graft mechanics have been assessed based on B-PT-B graft modifications. The mechanical properties of tubularization of the B-PT-B graft demonstrated that tubularized grafts stretched more on loading than did flat grafts, but there was no significant difference in stiffness.[73] Barber[7] assessed a flipped patellar tendon autograft and found that these patients had good functional outcomes, with a maximum KT 1000/2000 difference of 0.7 mm and no radiographic changes in the bone tunnels. Hoffmann et al.[51] studied the biomechanics of flipped B-PT-B autografts fixed with interference screws and found that the highest load-to-failure strength was achieved with interference screw fixation at the lateral aspect of the bone plug for both RCI screw fixation (479 N) and biodegradable screw fixation (610 N).

Hamstring (Semitendinosus-Gracilis) Autograft

ACL reconstruction using autogenous hamstring tendons is gaining popularity, and the graft material has favorable mechanical properties. A quadrupled semitendinosus-gracilis graft has a load-to-failure strength of 4140 N and a stiffness of 807 N/m.[48] The limiting factor with hamstring autografts is the fixation, which must be secure enough to allow the formation of Sharpey's fibers as the tendon heals to bone.

Tibial Fixation

The hamstring graft can be fixed with a staple securing it to the proximal tibia. Kurosaka et al.[59] found that the strength of this fixation was 137 N, with a stiffness of 8.8 N/mm. Steiner et al.[99] found that a hamstring graft fixed with a screw and soft tissue washer had superior fixation than a graft using a suture and post technique. The screw and soft tissue washer failed at 821 N, and the suture and post technique failed at 573 N. Another study[66] assessed the security of a washer plate and compared it with a graft fixed with an RCI titanium screw. The washer plate failed at 905 N and had a stiffness of 273 N/mm; the RCI titanium screw lost fixation at 350 N and was significantly less stiff. Weiler et al.[106] also assessed hamstring grafts fixed with an RCI titanium screw and reported similar results, with a failure load of 201 N. Brand et al.[24] assessed whether graft security was affected by tunnel size mismatch and demonstrated superior fixation when the biodegradable screw and graft were inserted into a hole that was mismatched by only 0.5 mm, as opposed to 1 mm.

Femoral Fixation

Femoral fixation has also been thoroughly assessed. Proximal fixation of the hamstring graft may occur either within the bone tunnel or external to it. Brown et al.[25] studied proximal fixation of hamstring grafts, assessing the transfixion pin, Endobutton with Mersiline tape, Endobutton with Endotape, Endobutton with sutures, and Endobutton with a double loop of Endotape. They found that the load-to-failure strength of these various fixation techniques ranged from 520 to 699 N. Rowden et al.[89] also studied the security of Endobutton fixation and found that this construct, when used with a tibial post, provided a load-to-failure strength of 612 N and had a stiffness of 47 N/mm. Clark et al.[33] found that the functional outcome of the transfixion pin was excellent, and the pullout strength of this type of fixation was 725 to 1600 N. Using a Mitek anchor to fix the graft proximally has also been described.[25] Fixing the graft in this manner provides adequate fixation strength (412 N), but it is slightly less strong than other modes of fixation. Interference fixation has also been assessed. The failure load of an RCI titanium screw (242 N) was not as high as that achieved with a bioabsorbable screw (341 and 530 N).[24,28]

Recent Literature

Selby et al.[92] showed a significant difference in the load to failure of hamstring grafts based on interference screw length. The failure load of the 28-mm screw was 594 N; it was 825 N for the 35-mm screw. The EndoPearl device increased the fixation strength of hamstring grafts that used interference screw fixation.[107] The interference screw alone failed at 386 N, while the EndoPearl–interference screw construct failed at 659 N. The EndoPearl group also had greater stiffness (42 vs. 26 N/mm) and sustained a greater number of cycles (389 vs. 153).

Biodegradable screw fixation is commonly used to supplement hamstring graft fixation. A recent study demonstrated that tunnel expansion decreases with the use of a biodegradable interference screw.[93] Screw geometry has a significant effect on interference fixation of hamstring grafts. Weiler et al.[105] demonstrated that when the screw diameter was equal to the graft diameter, the pullout strength was 367 N. When the screw diameter was 1 mm greater than the graft diameter, the load-to-failure strength was 479 N. They also found that increasing the screw length was more important than oversizing the screw diameter in improving fixation. However, Stadelmaier et al.[97] found no relationship between pullout strength and screw length in a study assessing 7- by 25-mm and 7- by 40-mm screws.

Quadriceps Tendon Autograft

The quadriceps tendon is a strong graft with an ultimate load to failure of 2353 N and a corresponding stiffness of 313 N/mm.[98] The quadriceps graft can be used with one bone block or as a complete soft tissue graft. Fixation of this type of graft can be done using any of the previously described techniques for bone block fixation and soft tissue fixation.

Recent Literature

The quadriceps autograft is unique in that the tendon itself has excellent biomechanical characteristics and can be fixed in a variety of ways, depending on whether there is a bone block. Brand et al.[22] assessed the quality of fixation of the soft tissue end of the quadriceps tendon fixed with either an Endobutton or an interference screw and compared it with a B-PT-B graft fixed with a biodegradable interference screw. They found that failure load was superior with interference screw fixation compared with the Endobutton and that the overall stiffness of the interference screw construct was similar to that of the same construct using B-PT-B.

Allografts

Allograft fixation depends on the type of graft selected. Allografts come in the form of bone-tendon-bone, bone-tendon, or tendon. Fixation needs to be secure, because the healing of allograft bone to host bone is slightly slower than that of autogenous bone.

Posterior Cruciate Ligament Reconstruction

The arthroscopic reconstruction of the posterior cruciate ligament has evolved considerably over time. Graft attachment locations and techniques, as well as the number of bundles of graft to use, continue to be challenges in posterior cruciate ligament reconstruction. The techniques of arthroscopic fixation, however, are essentially the same as for ACL reconstruction. Whether it is soft tissue–to–bone tunnel fixation or bone block in a tunnel fixation, the devices and their properties are the same.

Articular Cartilage Repair

Although a majority of implants used around the knee were specifically designed for meniscal repair and cruciate ligament reconstruction, the arthroscopic repair of osteochondral lesions is another increasingly common implant technology.

Osteochondral lesions can be fixed in many ways. Traditionally, cortical bone pegs were used to fix unstable osteochondral lesions.[45] Internal fixation of these lesions with K-wires,[30] Herbert screws,[64] cortical screws,[31] and cannulated screws[37] has also been described. Biodegradable pin fixation can be an effective means of managing unstable osteochondral lesions. Matsusue et al.,[68] in a small series, found that the use of a biodegradable PLLA pin was safe and helpful in the repair of osteochondral lesions.

One challenge when reattaching osteochondral fragments is that the bone of the fragment is often devitalized and will not heal back into place. Placing a dead graft into a defect on the femoral condyle serves little purpose. To address this situation, osteochondral autografting was developed. Three techniques have been advanced to solve this problem, and they have different commercial names: mosaicplasty (Smith and Nephew Endoscopy), OATS (Arthrex), and the COR technique (Mitek).[17] Berlet et al.[17] used a mosaicplasty technique to graft an osteochondral lesion with one or multiple autologous osteochondral plugs. They found that this provides excellent results, with evidence of healing on magnetic resonance imaging scans at 6 to 9 months.

Acknowledgment

The authors thank Morley A. Herbert, PhD, Advanced Surgical Institutes, Medical City Dallas Hospital, Dallas, Texas.

References

1. Abboud JA, Bozentka DJ, Soslowsky LJ, Beredijiklian PK: Effect of implant design on the cyclic loading properties of mini suture anchors in carpal bone. J Hand Surg [Am] 27:43-48, 2002.

2. Albrecht-Olsen P, Kristensen G, Törmälä P: Meniscus bucket-handle fixation with an absorbable Biofix tack: Development of a new technique. Knee Surg Sports Traumatol Arthrosc 1:104-106, 1993.

3. Albrecht-Olsen P, Lind T, Kristensen G, Falkenberg B: Failure strength of a new meniscus Arrow repair technique: Biomechanical comparison with horizontal suture. Arthroscopy 13:183-187, 1997.

4. Aldridge JW, Bruno RJ, Strauch RJ, Rosenwasser MP: Management of acute and chronic biceps tendon rupture. Hand Clin 16:497-503, 2000.

5. Arnoczky SP, Lavagnino M: Tensile fixation of absorbable meniscal repair devices as a function of hydrolysis time: An in-vitro experimental study. Am J Sports Med 29:118-123, 2001.

6. Bach BR Jr, Tradonsky S, Bojchuk J, et al: Arthroscopically assisted anterior cruciate ligament reconstruction using

patellar tendon autograft: Five- to nine-year follow-up evaluation. Am J Sports Med 26:20-29, 1998.

7. Barber FA: Flipped patellar tendon autograft anterior cruciate ligament reconstruction. Arthroscopy 16:483-490, 2000.

8. Barber FA, Elrod BF, McGuire DA, Paulos LE: BioScrew fixation of patellar tendon autografts. Biomaterials 21:2623-2629, 2000.

9. Barber FA, Herbert M: Suture anchors—update 1999. Arthroscopy 15:719-725, 1999.

10. Barber FA, Herbert MA: Meniscal repair devices. Arthroscopy 16:613-618, 2000.

11. Barber FA, Herbert MA, Click JN: Suture anchor strength revisited. Arthroscopy 12:32-38, 1996.

12. Barber FA, Herbert M, Click JN: Internal fixation strength of suture anchors—update 1997. Arthroscopy 13:355-362, 1997.

13. Barber FA, Herbert MA, Richards DP: Failure strengths of new meniscal repair techniques [abstract]. Proceedings of 21st annual meeting of the Arthroscopy Association of North America, April 2002.

14. Barrett GR, Treacy SH, Ruff CG: The T-Fix technique for endoscopic meniscus repair: Technique, complications, and preliminary results. Am J Knee Surg 9:151-156, 1996.

15. Becker R, Schroder M, Starke C, et al: Biomechanical investigations of different meniscal repair implants in comparison with horizontal sutures on human meniscus. Arthroscopy 17:439-444, 2001.

16. Bellemans J, Vandenneucker H, Labey L, Van Audkercke R: Fixation strength of meniscal repair devices. Knee 9:11-14, 2002.

17. Berlet GC, Mascia A, Miniaci A: Treatment of unstable osteochondritis dissecans lesions of the knee using autogenous osteochondral grafts (mosaicplasty). Arthroscopy 15:312-316, 1999.

18. Black KP, Saunders MM, Stube KC, et al: Effects of interference fit screw length on tibial tunnel fixation for anterior cruciate ligament reconstruction. Am J Sports Med 28:846-849, 2000.

19. Black KP, Schneider DJ, Yu JR, Jacobs CR: Biomechanics of the Bankart repair: The relationship between glenohumeral translation and labral fixation site. Am J Sports Med 27:339-344, 1999.

20. Boenisch UW, Faber KJ, Ciarelli M, et al: Pull-out strength and stiffness of meniscal repair using absorbable arrows of Ti-Cron vertical and horizontal loop sutures. Am J Sports Med 27:626-631, 1999.

21. Bovard RS, Derkash RS, Freeman JR: Grade III avulsion fracture repair on the UCL of the proximal joint of the thumb. Orthop Rev 23:167-169, 1994.

22. Brand J, Hamilton D, Selby J, et al: Biomechanical comparison of quadriceps tendon fixation with patellar tendon bone plug interference fixation in cruciate ligament reconstruction. Arthroscopy 16:805-812, 2000.

23. Brand J, Weiler A, Caborn DNM, et al: Graft fixation in cruciate ligament reconstruction. Am J Sports Med 28:761-774, 2000.

24. Brand JC Jr, Pienkowski D, Steenlage E, et al: Interference screw fixation strength of a quadrupled hamstring tendon graft is directly related to bone mineral density and insertion torque. Am J Sports Med 28:705-710, 2000.

25. Brown CH, Sklar JH, Hecker AT, et al: Endoscopic anterior cruciate ligament graft fixation [abstract]. Presented at the 10th Combined Orthopaedic Association meeting, 1998, New Zealand.

26. Brown GA, Pena F, Grontvedt T, et al: Fixation strength of interference screw fixation in bovine, young human, and elderly human cadaver knees: Influence of insertion torque, tunnel-bone block gap, and interference. Knee Surg Sports Traumatol Arthrosc 3:238-244, 1996.

27. Butler DL, Grood ES, Noyes FR, Sodd AN: On the interpretation of our anterior cruciate ligament data. Clin Orthop 196:26-34, 1985.

28. Caborn DNM, Coen M, Neef R, et al: Quadrupled semitendinosus-gracilis autograft fixation in the femoral tunnel: A comparison between a metal and a bioabsorbable interference screw. Arthroscopy 14:241-245, 1998.

29. Caborn DN, Urban WP Jr, Johnson DL, et al: Biomechanical comparison between BioScrew and titanium alloy interference screws for bone–patellar tendon–bone graft fixation in anterior cruciate ligament reconstruction. Arthroscopy 13:229-232, 1997.

30. Cahill B: Treatment of juvenile osteochondritis and osteochondritis of the knee. Clin Sports Med 4:367-384, 1985.

31. Cetik O, Bilen FE, Sozen YV, Hepgur G: A 2-staged method for treatment of deep osteochondral lesions of the knee joint. Arthroscopy 17:E35, 2001.

32. Chen DS, Wertheimer SJ: Centrally located osteochondral fracture of the talus. J Foot Surg 31:134-140, 1992.

33. Clark R, Olsen RE, Larson BJ, Goble EM: Cross-pin femoral fixation: A new technique for hamstring anterior cruciate ligament reconstruction of the knee. Arthroscopy 14:258-267, 1998.

34. Cluett J, Milne AD, Yang D, Morris SF: Repair of central slip avulsions using Mitek Micro Arc bone anchors: An in vitro biomechanical assessment. J Hand Surg [Br] 24:679-682, 1999.

35. Coen MJ, Caborn DN, Urban W, et al: An anatomic evaluation of T-Fix suture device placement for arthroscopic all-inside meniscal repair. Arthroscopy 15:275-280, 1999.

36. Cooper DE, Deng XH, Burstein AL, Warren RF: The strength of the central third patellar tendon graft: A biomechanical study. Am J Sports Med 21:818-824, 1993.

37. Cugat R, Garcia M, Cusco X, et al: Osteochondritis dissecans: A historical review and its treatment with cannulated screws. Arthroscopy 9:675-684, 1993.

38. Dawson DM, Julsrud ME, Erdmann BB, et al: Modified Kidner procedure utilizing a Mitek bone anchor. J Foot Ankle Surg 37:115-121, 1998.

39. DeRowe A, Gunther E, Fibbi A, et al: Tongue-base suspension with a soft tissue–to–bone anchor for obstructive sleep apnea: Preliminary clinical results of a new minimally invasive technique. Otolaryngol Head Neck Surg 122:100-103, 2000.

40. Dervin GF, McBride D, Keene GCR, Downing K: Failure strengths of suture versus biodegradable arrow for meniscal repair. Arthroscopy 13:296-300, 1997.

41. Dunn MJ, Johnson C: Static scapholunate dissociation: A new reconstruction technique using a volar and dorsal approach in a cadaver model. J Hand Surg [Am] 26:749-754, 2001.

42. Escalas F, Quadras J, Caceres E, Benaddi J: T-Fix anchor sutures for arthroscopic meniscal repair. Knee Surg Sports Traumatol Arthrosc 5:72-76, 1997.

43. Gastel JA, Muirhead WR, Lifrak JT, et al: Meniscal tissue regeneration using a collagenous biomaterial derived from porcine small intestine submucosa. Arthroscopy 17:151-159, 2001.

44. Gerich TG, Cassim A, Lattermann C, Lobenhoffer HP: Pullout strength of tibial graft fixation in anterior cruciate ligament replacement with a patellar tendon graft:

Interference screw versus staple fixation in human knees. Knee Surg Sports Traumatol Arthrosc 5:84-89, 1997.

45. Gillespie HS, Day B: Bone peg fixation in the treatment of osteochondritis dissecans of the knee joint. Clin Orthop 143:125-130, 1979.

46. Gillquist J: Reconstruction of the anterior cruciate ligament: Indications, operative technique, and rehabilitation. Op Tech Orthop 2:104-111, 1992.

47. Hallock GG: The Mitek mini GII anchor introduced for tendon reinsertion in the hand. Ann Plast Surg 33:211-213, 1994.

48. Hamner DL, Brown CH Jr, Steiner ME, et al: Hamstring tendon grafts for reconstruction of the anterior cruciate ligament: Biomechanical evaluation of the use of multiple stands and tensioning techniques. J Bone Joint Surg Am 81:549-557, 1999.

49. Hartley RC, Leung YL: Meniscal arrow migration into the popliteal fossa following attempted meniscal repair: A report of two cases. Knee 9:69-71, 2002.

50. Hede A, Jensen DB, Blyme P, Sonne-Holm S: Epidemiology of meniscal lesions in the knee: 1215 open operations in Copenhagen 1982-84. Acta Orthop Scand 61:435-437, 1990.

51. Hoffmann RF, Peine R, Bail HJ, et al: Initial fixation strength of modified patellar tendon grafts for anatomic fixation in anterior cruciate ligament reconstruction. Arthroscopy 15:392-393, 1999.

52. Ibarra C, Koski JA, Warren RF: Tissue engineering meniscus: Cells and matrix. Orthop Clin North Am 31:411-418, 2000.

53. Johnson LL, vanDyk GE: Metal and biodegradable interference screws: Comparison of failure strength. Arthroscopy 12:452-456, 1996.

54. Klutke JJ, Bullock A, Klutke CG: Comparison of anchors used in anti-incontinence surgery. Urology 52:979-981, 1998.

55. Kohn D, Siebert W: Meniscus suture techniques: A comparative biomechanical cadaver study. Arthroscopy 5:324-327, 1989.

56. Kousa P, Jarvinen TL, Kannus P, Jarvinen M: Initial fixation strength of bioabsorbable and titanium interference screws in anterior cruciate ligament reconstruction: Biomechanical evaluation by single cycle and cyclic loading. Am J Sports Med 29:420-425, 2001.

57. Kousa P, Jarvinen TL, Kannus P, et al: A bioabsorbable plug in bone-tendon-bone reconstruction of the anterior cruciate ligament: Introduction of a novel fixation technique. Arthroscopy 17:144-150, 2001.

58. Kumar A, Malhan K, Roberts SN: Chondral injury from bioabsorbable screws after meniscal repair. Arthroscopy 17:34, 2001.

59. Kurosaka M, Yoshiya S, Andrish JT: A biomechanical comparison of different surgical techniques of graft fixation anterior cruciate ligament. Am J Sports Med 15:225-229, 1987.

60. Kuwada GT: Use of the ROC anchor in foot and ankle surgery: A retrospective study. J Am Podiatr Med Assoc 89:247-250, 1999.

61. Lajtai G, Schmiedhuber G, Unger F, et al: Bone tunnel remodeling at the site of biodegradable interference screws used for anterior cruciate ligament reconstruction: 5 year follow-up. Arthroscopy 17:597-602, 2001.

62. Lynch SA, Beard DM, Renstrom PA: Repair of distal biceps tendon ruptures with suture anchors. Knee Surg Sports Traumatol Arthrosc 7:125-131, 1999.

63. Lysholm J, Gilquist J: Evaluation of knee ligament surgery results with special emphasis on use of a scoring scale. Am J Sports Med 10:150-154, 1992.

64. Mackie IG, Pemberton DJ, Maheson M: Arthroscopic use of the Herbert screw in osteochondritis dissecans. J Bone Joint Surg Br 72:1076, 1990.

65. Madjar S, Wald M, Halachmi S, et al: Minimally invasive per vaginam procedures for the treatment of female stress incontinence using a new pubic bone anchoring system. Artif Organs 22:879-885, 1998.

66. Magen HE, Howell SM, Hull ML: Structural properties of six tibial fixation methods for anterior cruciate ligament soft tissue grafts. Am J Sports Med 27:35-43, 1999.

67. Mariani PP, Camillieri G, Margheritini F: Transcondylar screw fixation in anterior cruciate ligament reconstruction. Arthroscopy 17:717-723, 2001.

68. Matsusue Y, Nakamura T, Suzuki S, Iwasaki R: Biodegradable pin fixation of osteochondral fragments of the knee. Clin Orthop 322:166-173, 1996.

69. McEleney ET, Donovan MJ, Shea KP, Nowak MD: Initial failure strength of open and arthroscopic Bankart repairs. Arthroscopy 11:426-431, 1995.

70. Messer TM, Cummins CA, Ahn J, Kelikian AS: Outcome of the modified Brostrom procedure for chronic lateral ankle instability using suture anchors. Foot Ankle Int 21:996-1003, 2000.

71. Mitsionis GI, Varitimidis SE, Sotereanos GG: Treatment of chronic injuries of the ulnar collateral ligament of the thumb using a free tendon graft and bone suture anchors. J Hand Surg [Br] 25:208-211, 2000.

72. Miyasaka KC, Daniel DM, Stone ML, Hirshman P: The incidence of knee ligament injuries in the general population. Am J Knee Surg 4:3-8, 1991.

73. Moore DC, Belanger MJ, Crisco JJ, et al: The effect of tubularization on the mechanical properties of patellar tendon grafts. Am J Knee Surg 13:211-217, 2000.

74. Morgan CD: The all inside meniscus repair. Arthroscopy 7:120-125, 1991.

75. Morrison JB: Function of the knee joint in various activities. Biomed Eng 4:573-580, 1969.

76. Morrison JB: The mechanics of the knee joint in relation to normal walking. J Biomech 3:51-61, 1970.

77. Nielsen AB, Yde J: Epidemiology of acute knee injuries: A prospective hospital investigation. J Trauma 31:1644-1648, 1991.

78. Oliverson TJ, Litner DM: Biofix Arrow appearing as a subcutaneous foreign body. Arthroscopy 16:652-655, 2000.

79. Paletta GA, Warren RF: Knee injuries and alpine skiing. Sports Med 17:411-423, 1994.

80. Pederson B, Wertheimer SJ, Tesoro D, Coraci M: Mitek anchor system: A new technique for tenodesis and ligamentous repair of the foot and ankle. J Foot Surg 30:48-51, 1991.

81. Pena F, Grontvedt T, Brown GA, et al: Comparison of failure strength between metallic and absorbable interference screws: Influence of insertion torque, tunnel-bone block gap, bone mineral density, and interference. Am J Sports Med 24:329-334, 1996.

82. Petsche TS, Selesnick H, Rochman A: Arthroscopic meniscus repair with bioabsorbable arrows. Arthroscopy 18:246-253, 2002.

83. Pina A, Garcia I, Sabater M: Traumatic avulsion of the triceps brachii. J Orthop Trauma 16:273-276, 2002.

84. Post WR, Akers SR, Kish V: Load to failure of common meniscal repair techniques: Effects of suture technique and suture material. Arthroscopy 13:731-736, 1997.

85. Rehak DC, Sotereanos DG, Bowman MW, Herndon JH: The Mitek bone anchor: Application to the hand, wrist and elbow. J Hand Surg [Am] 19:853-860, 1994.

86. Rimmer MG, Nawana NS, Keene GCR, Pearcy MJ: Failure strengths of different meniscal suturing techniques. Arthroscopy 11:146-150, 1995.

87. Rinehart GC: Mandibulomaxillary fixation with bone anchors and quick-release ligatures. J Craniofac Surg 9:215-221, 1998.

88. Ross G, Grabill J, McDevitt E: Chondral injury after meniscal repair with bioabsorbable arrows. Arthroscopy 16:754-756, 2000.

89. Rowden NJ, Sher D, Rogers GJ, Schindhelm K: Anterior cruciate ligament graft fixation: Initial comparison of patellar tendon and semitendinosus autografts in young fresh cadavers. Am J Sports Med 25:472-478, 1997.

90. Safran MR, O'Malley D Jr, Fu FH: Peroneal tendon subluxation in athletes: New exam technique, case reports, and review. Med Sci Sports Exerc 31(7 Suppl):S487-S492, 1999.

91. Salvo JP, Rizio L, Zvijac JE, et al: Avulsion fractures of the ulnar sublime tubercle in overhead throwing athletes. Am J Sports Med 30:426-431, 2002.

92. Selby JB, Johnson DL, Hester P, Caborn DN: Effect of screw length on bioabsorbable interference screw fixation in a tibial bone tunnel. Am J Sports Med 29:614-619, 2001.

93. Simonian PT, Monson JT, Larson RV: Biodegradable interference screw augmentation reduces tunnel expansion after ACL reconstruction. Am J Knee Surg 14:104-108, 2001.

94. Song EK, Lee KB: Biomechanical test comparing the load to failure of the biodegradable meniscus arrow versus meniscal suture. Arthroscopy 15:726-732, 1999.

95. Song EK, Lee KB, Yoon TR: Aseptic synovitis after meniscal repair using the biodegradable meniscus arrow. Arthroscopy 17:77-80, 2001.

96. Speer KP, Warren RF, Wickiewicz TL, et al: Observations on the injury mechanism of anterior cruciate ligament tears in skiers. Am J Sports Med 23:77-81, 1995.

97. Stadeimaier DM, Lowe WR, Ilahi OA, et al: Cyclic pullout strength of hamstring tendon graft fixation with soft tissue interference screws: Influence of screw length. Am J Sports Med 27:778-783, 1999.

98. Staubli HU, Schatzmann L, Brunner P, et al: Quadriceps tendon and patellar ligament: Cryosectional anatomy and structural properties in young adults. Knee Surg Sports Traumatol Arthrosc 4:100-110, 1996.

99. Steiner ME, Hecker AT, Brown CH Jr, Hayes WC: Anterior cruciate ligament graft fixation: Comparison of hamstring and patellar tendon grafts. Am J Sports Med 22:240-247, 1994.

100. Takeda M, Hatano A, Kurumada S, et al: Bladder neck suspension using percutaneous bladder neck stabilization to the pubic bone with a bone-anchor suture fixation system: A new extraperitoneal laparoscopic approach. Urol Int 62:57-60, 1999.

101. Tegner Y, Lysholm J: Rating systems in the evaluation of knee ligament injuries. Clin Orthop 198:43-49, 1985.

102. Tuncay I, Ege A: Reconstruction of chronic collateral ligament injuries to fingers by use of suture anchors. Croat Med J 42:539-542, 2001.

103. Vardakas DG, Musgrave DS, Varitimidis SE, et al: Partial rupture of the distal biceps tendon. J Shoulder Elbow Surg 10:377-379, 2001.

104. Walsh SP, Evans SL, O'Doherty DM, Barlow IW: Failure strength of suture vs biodegradable arrow and staple for meniscal repair: An in vitro study. Knee 8:151-156, 2001.

105. Weiler A, Hoffmann RF, Siepe CJ, et al: The influence of screw geometry on hamstring tendon interference fit fixation. Am J Sports Med 28:356-359, 2000.

106. Weiler A, Hoffmann RF, Stähelin AC, et al: Hamstring tendon fixation using interference screws: A biomechanical study in calf tibial bone. Arthroscopy 14:29-37, 1998.

107. Weiler A, Richter M, Schmidmaier G, et al: The EndoPearl device increases fixation strength and eliminates construct slippage of hamstring tendon grafts with interference screw fixation. Arthroscopy 17:353-359, 2001.

108. Woo SL, Hollis JM, Adams DJ, et al: Tensile properties of the human femur–anterior cruciate ligament–tibia complex: The effects of specimen age and orientation. Am J Sports Med 19:217-225, 1991.

109. Woods DA, Hoy G, Shimmin A: A safe technique for distal biceps repair using a suture anchor and a limited anterior approach. Injury 30:233-237, 1999.

Arthroscopic Knot Tying

Frank G. Alberta, Augustus D. Mazzocca,
Brian J. Cole, and Anthony A. Romeo

Knot tying is a basic surgical skill that has been practiced for centuries. The knots used today have their roots in fishing and sailing. These basic knots have been tailored and customized into thousands of variations with both specific and general uses. The advent of endoscopic surgery placed new demands on surgeons and their ability to tie effective knots. Endoscopic and arthroscopic knots must be delivered over a distance to tissue with limited manual access. This presents new technical challenges, requiring surgeons to learn new techniques while still adhering to sound principles.

Despite the large number of knot options, all effective knots must meet two criteria: (1) the knot must be properly formed so the suture does not slip or cut into itself, and (2) it must be easily tightened to ensure maximum strength. The arthroscopic knot is simply a knot that must be formed at a distance and then tightened at the level of the target tissue. This is generally where the difficulty arises. Maintaining tension is more important than the knot configuration chosen.

The purpose of this chapter is to define the nomenclature associated with arthroscopic knots, provide a framework for successful and reproducible suture management and knot tying, review various techniques, and provide examples of currently used knots and sutures.

Definitions

When a suture has been passed through tissue (or the eyelet of a suture anchor), it creates two limbs. The *post* is the limb of suture that the other limb will be looped or passed around. This limb is generally held under tension during the tying and delivery of knots. The post defines the side of the tissue where the knot will ultimately sit. The *loop* is the limb that is passed around the post to create the knot. It is also known as the *nonpost* or *wrapping* suture. Although these limbs can be assigned

arbitrarily by the surgeon, some thought should be given to where the knot stack will sit. For labral fixation in the glenohumeral joint, for instance, it is beneficial to choose the limb away from the glenoid articular surface as the post limb, so that the knot stack does not articulate with the humeral head. Similarly, during arthroscopic rotator cuff repair, the post limb should be the limb passing through the tendon so that the knot stack will approximate the tissue to the greater tuberosity.

When knots are constructed from consecutive loops tied around a post, certain concepts become important. *Post switching* or *reversing* is a technique by which the post and loop are alternated for each successive loop. Similarly, *reversing throws* refers to the direction around the post in which the loop is formed. Loops are generally referred to as underhand or overhand (overhand being on top of the post). These techniques have benefits that are discussed in detail later.

Basic Knot Types

Arthroscopic surgeons must learn to tie two basic types of knots: nonsliding and sliding knots. Nonsliding knots are constructed in single loops outside the joint and are pulled or led down sequentially into the joint. The ultimate construction and tensioning of nonsliding knots are performed *at the tissue site* in a stepwise manner. Examples of nonsliding knots are the square knot and the Revo knot.[18] The square knot is the most difficult to tie arthroscopically because, if tension is applied asymmetrically, it can convert to a sliding knot (stacked half hitches). This can result in loss of tension at the tissue site.

Sliding knots are constructed *completely outside the cannula* or joint around the post limb. They are delivered to the tissue site through tension on the post limb that allows the knot to slide into place. The Duncan loop (hangman's knot),[14] Roeder knot,[17] Tennessee slider, Weston knot,[22] and SMC knot[8] are just a few examples of sliding knots. A prerequisite for tying a sliding knot is the suture's ability to pass freely through the tissue (or eyelet of the suture anchor). If, after passage of the suture through the tissue, both limbs of the suture flow smoothly and freely back and forth, a sliding knot can be tied. If the limbs do not pass freely (because of tension or capture in the tissue or routing of the suture), a nonsliding knot must be tied. Sliding knots are a better option for securing tissue under tension. However, they may impart a higher degree of suture trauma, leading to failure during or after knot tying.

Sliding knots are further subdivided into locking and nonlocking knots. Locking knots are constructed in such a way that when they arrive at the tissue, a different tensioning sequence takes place and the knot can be "locked" as the loop strand captures the post. These knots maintain their tension and position at the tissue. Most sliding knots have some ability to lock. Examples of these knots are the taut line hitch,[12] Tennessee slider, Weston, and SMC knot. It is important to understand that the locking mechanism may result in loss of initial tension at the tissue as the knot folds back on itself.

Nonlocking knots require further throws for security after they have been delivered and tensioned at the tissue. Examples of nonlocking knots are the Duncan loop, overhand loop, and multiple half hitches. Tension must be maintained on the post limb to keep these knots in place. Additional throws can be passed around the post and advanced down into place.

A final category of sliding knots is the ratchet knot. These knots allow movement in only one direction. Examples of these knots are Nicky's knot,[5] the Lafosse knot, the giant knot,[6] and certain modifications of the taut line hitch.[12]

Loop and Knot Security

All knots rely on two principles for their effectiveness and their ability to securely hold and approximate tissue. The first concept is *loop security*, which is defined as the ability of the length of suture passed through the tissue (loop) to maintain the initial tension and length as the knot is

delivered and tightened. Loop security can never be greater than when the knot is originally tensioned. It is therefore essential to maintain loop security while completing the knot (Fig. 4–1).[1] If, for example, a knot needed to be tied around a piece of tissue that measured 1 cm in circumference, a completely secure loop would have a circumference of 1 cm or, preferably, less. *Knot security* is the ability of the completed knot to resist slippage and, therefore, loosening. These two concepts are interrelated and partially dependent on each other. For example, a completely secure knot can be tied behind a loop that is 3 mm too long. Although the knot may not slip, it will not approximate the tissue effectively, because loop security was never achieved. Conversely, if an insecure knot is tied behind a completely secure loop, the knot will eventually slip under load, and tissue approximation will be lost. Biomechanical studies have assumed that 3 mm of knot slippage causes loss of soft tissue fixation.[11] So it is safe to assume that an initial loop that slips 3 mm while it is being tied will lose soft tissue apposition as well.[1]

Suture Management and Optimal Knot Tying

A distinct set of principles and techniques needs to be adhered to for successful knot tying, especially early in the learning process.[4,15] If a step is missed, problems can multiply quickly. Further, successful arthroscopic knot tying begins long before a knot is delivered to the target tissue. If the arthroscopist adheres to these fundamental principles, suture management and delivery of sound arthroscopic knots will be less intimidating.

Cannulas

It is important to note that effective and efficient cannula usage begins with portal placement. Arthroscopic knots must be tied through a cannula, which should be placed directly over, or as close as possible to, the area to be tied to avoid soft tissue interposition. Maintenance of the cannula over the proposed knot area and in line with the sutures minimizes suture chafing on the edge of the

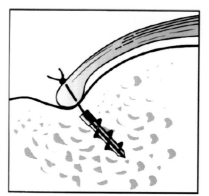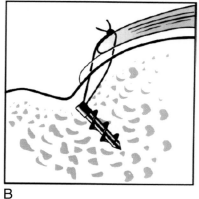

A   B

Figure 4–1 *A,* Secure initial loop holds the soft tissue tightly apposed. *B,* Lack of initial loop security leads to loss of apposition, regardless of knot security. (From Burkhart SS, Wirth MA, Simonick M, et al: Loop security as a determinant of tissue fixation security. Arthroscopy 14:773–776, 1998.)

cannula. Clear cannulas improve visualization of sutures and knots along their entire course. It is easier to avoid and correct tangles if the suture can be seen through the cannula with both the arthroscope and the naked eye outside the joint. Threaded cannulas prevent inadvertent dislodgment due to fluid pressure or instrument passage. Cannula size is determined by the largest instrument required to pass through it.

Anchor Orientation and Suture Passage

Thought should be given to the orientation of the suture limbs as they pass through the tissue alone or through the eyelet of an anchor and the tissue. If anchors are used, the eyelet of the anchor should be oriented with its open face perpendicular to the path of the suture through the tissue (i.e., parallel to the tissue to be sutured) (Fig. 4–2). If the anchor is rotated 90 degrees, the suture can be frayed as it passes acutely around the eyelet into the tissue. These problems occur primarily with anchors that have metal eyelets and less commonly with bioabsorbable or suture eyelets.

The surgeon must be familiar with whatever anchor device he or she is using to ensure that the correct limb arrangement is maintained in the cannulas during passage. Specifically, the limb exiting the eyelet of the anchor closest to the tissue to be sutured should be passed. This ensures easy and smooth sliding and avoids twists (see Fig. 4–2). If a double-loaded anchor is used, care should be taken not to overlap the sutures as they exit the eyelet. Passing and tying the distal suture first minimizes friction on the second, more proximal suture during passage.

Single Suture Sets Inside a Cannula

Only one set of suture limbs should be inside an operative cannula during knot tying and delivery. If multiple sutures are being used, a second portal can "store" the sutures, or they can be placed adjacent to the cannula in the subcutaneous tissue. This principle holds true even for double-loaded suture anchors.

Avoidance of Twists

The suture limbs must not be crossed inside the cannula. If the knot is twisted during delivery, it can lead to loss of loop or knot security and premature knot failure. First, the knot pusher should be advanced down either limb of suture into the joint under arthroscopic vision; this can avoid or correct any crossed or twisted sutures and help identify the post limb. After confirming that there are no twists in the suture limbs, the separated limbs can be placed off to respective sides of the cannula to keep them from twisting later. At this point, a clamp can be placed behind the knot pusher on the post strand to remind the surgeon which side of the cannula the post is on and to avoid confusion between the strands. To avoid suture twisting while actually tying the knots, have an assistant place a finger in the junction of the post and loop while the loops are formed to keep them separated (Fig. 4–3). Double-loaded anchors with same-color sutures should be differentiated by marking one suture with a sterile marking pen at the level of the anchor and at both tips

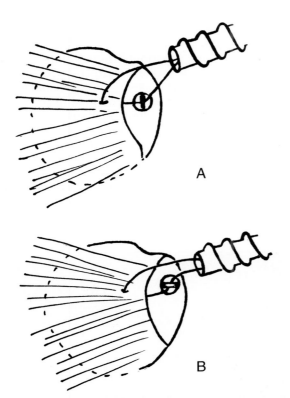

A

B

Figure 4–2 *A,* Correctly rotated suture anchor allows suture to pass perpendicularly into tissue edge without twisting. Note appropriate passage of limb closest to tissue to optimize sliding characteristics and minimize potential fraying of suture through eyelet. *B,* Anchor rotated 90 degrees produces twist as suture passes through eyelet; when tensioned, this can lead to decreased loop security and poor suture sliding.

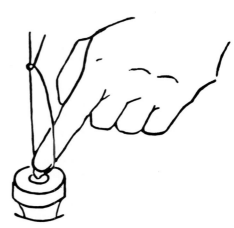

Figure 4–3 Placing a finger in the axilla formed by the suture limbs close to the cannula keeps the limbs separated and makes complex wrapping easier.

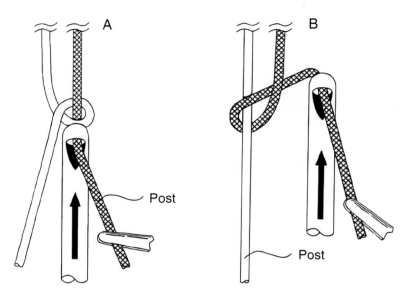

Figure 4–4 *A,* Pushing an overhand loop down the post with the knot pusher results in jerky tensioning, which can lead to tangles and passage of the knot pusher through the loop. *B,* Without switching the knot pusher, the post strand can be converted to the nonpost by pushing the knot pusher past the loop along the post. The result is an underhand loop around the original nonpost limb that can now be pulled smoothly into the joint. (From Chan KC, Burkhart SS: How to switch posts without rethreading when tying half-hitches. Arthroscopy 15:444–450, 1999.)

of the same suture to identify them as they lie outside the cannula.

Appropriate Use of Knot Pusher

Knots should be advanced to the target with a knot pusher and by appropriate tension on the limbs. For sliding knots, the knot pusher should be on the post limb and the knot *pushed* down to the target. Tension should be maintained on the post strand alone while these knots are delivered. This technique ensures initial loop security and allows the knot to be progressively tightened through simultaneous tension on the post and pressure with the knot pusher. Care is used to avoid a mismatch of tension and pressure and to deliver the knot without residual slack between the anchor and knot.

When the knot pusher is used to push half-hitch loops down a cannula (i.e., placing the knot pusher on the post limb to push the loop into the joint), several problems can arise. The knot pusher can easily slip through the loop and not advance it at all. Tension has to be applied alternately on and off both strands to advance the knot. This can lead to fraying of braided suture. These problems in combination can result in a greater chance of tangles within the cannula. Finally, with the knot pusher on the post strand, effective past-pointing cannot be achieved. When passing half hitches, therefore, the knot pusher is most effectively used to *pull* or lead the loops down to the target, much like an index finger is used during open single-handed knot tying in a deep wound. This method ensures smooth delivery of the individual knot loop down the post and allows for effective past-pointing. As the knot pusher is advanced, tension is applied to the post and nonpost in an alternating fashion. It is important to realize that by pulling a loop into the joint, the surgeon can "switch" the post limb and nonpost limb simply by pushing the knot pusher past the loop without moving the knot pusher to the nonpost limb (Fig. 4–4).[2] This achieves two goals: it allows the surgeon to pull a loop into the joint without switching

the knot pusher from limb to limb, and it can provide a convenient way to tie alternating post half hitches. The technique of pulling or leading half-hitch loops down a post is used in a number of nonsliding knots (e.g., Revo knot). Effective past-pointing of the loop limb at 180 degrees to the post limb between sequential loops maximizes the tension and security of the final knot.

There are many commercially available knot pushers. Simple, single-holed knot pushers are most commonly used and are sufficient for all types of knots. Other types of knot pushers include double-holed and cannulated double-diameter knot pushers (Surgeon's Sixth Finger, Arthrex, Naples, FL) (Fig. 4–5). Double-diameter knot pushers allow the initial loop to be held in place by the inner pusher while another loop is advanced by the outer one. A comparison of hand-tied knots and knots tied with either a standard single-holed knot pusher or a cannulated double-diameter knot pusher showed that knots tied with the double-diameter pusher achieved similar loop security to hand-tied knots and significantly better

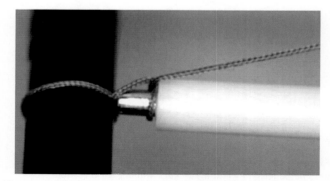

Figure 4–5 Double-diameter knot pusher holds the initial loop secure while subsequent loops are advanced down with the outer pusher. (From Burkhart SS, Wirth MA, Simonick M, et al: Loop security as a determinant of tissue fixation security. Arthroscopy 14:773-776, 1998.)

loop security than those tied with the standard knot pusher.[1] The double-diameter pusher is an excellent tool to help maintain a secure initial loop while additional half hitches are thrown, but it is somewhat difficult to use initially.

Suture Materials

A variety of suture materials has been used in arthroscopic surgery. Choice of suture material should be based on the inherent suture characteristics and the surgeon's familiarity with the material. Suture material is classified by its absorbability and whether it is monofilament or braided.

The absorbable sutures used in arthroscopic knot tying can be braided (Panacryl, Ethicon, Somerville, NJ) or monofilament (PDS [polydioxanone suture]). Absorbable sutures, by design, lose strength as they are degraded but usually start out at a lower tensile strength than nonabsorbable sutures of the same caliber. The most commonly used nonabsorbable suture material in arthroscopy is braided polyester. Recently, braided polyester suture reinforced with Kevlar (Fiberwire, Arthrex, Naples, FL) has become popular. The principal limitation of nonabsorbable suture is its permanency inside the joint and its possible mechanical or abrasive effects.

Tying characteristics are dependent more on the suture construction than on the material properties. Braided suture is more pliable, less ductile, stiffer,[10] and generally easier to tighten. It tends to fray with handling, however, and its rough surface may decrease its ability to slide but improve internal frictional ability and decrease the likelihood of loop loosening. Monofilament suture is smooth and therefore tends to slide better. It is stiffer to work with, however, and knot security is difficult to maintain. Monofilament suture (PDS in particular) has memory and recoil, making it more ductile. In one biomechanical study, the most important factor affecting knot security was suture material.[14] A high percentage of knots tied with monofilament suture failed due to knot slippage, even when tied with alternating post and throw half hitches. In contrast, knots tied with braided material failed more often by suture breakage. In a specific comparison of the same stacked half-hitch knots tied with either number 2 PDS II or number 1 Ethibond (Ethicon, Somerville, NJ), the Ethibond knots had a 50% higher knot-holding capacity.[3]

Specific Knot-Tying Techniques

At a minimum, the arthroscopist must be able to tie a nonsliding knot, because there are times when the limbs will not slide. Because loop security can be improved with sliding knots (which may or may not lock), the surgeon should also learn to tie a sliding knot. The specific knot used is immaterial; it is only important to be able to achieve loop and knot security in a reproducible fashion. Therefore, it is recommended that the arthroscopist practice knot-tying techniques outside the operating room to master this skill (see also reference 13).

Nonsliding Knots

Nonsliding knots can be used any time during arthroscopy; there are no absolute prerequisites for their use. Nonsliding knots may not be the ideal choice when tissue is under tension, however. They are also more difficult to secure when using monofilament suture, owing to the low coefficient of friction and its stiffness. All nonsliding knots are combinations of half-hitch loops. Therefore, the surgeon must learn how to throw and secure half-hitch loops effectively. The knots described here are stacked half hitches and the Revo knot.

Stacked Half Hitches

Half hitches are the surgeon's workhorse. They are familiar to most surgeons owing to their routine use in open surgery. Stacked half hitches can be tied with alternating posts or throws or any combination of the two. Biomechanical studies have evaluated the importance of reversing posts or throws for knot security.[3,11,12] The most secure half-hitch knots are those in which the post and direction of throw are alternated. When using half hitches to back up sliding knots, the surgeon should reverse either the throws or the post to maximize knot security.[11] As described earlier, single loops can be pushed into the joint (down the post) or pulled (led) into place with the knot pusher on the nonpost limb. Pulling the loops into place results in smoother passage and minimizes suture fraying and tangles.[15] Remember also that the post limb can be switched by alternate tensioning while the knot is being advanced.

To tie stacked half hitches:

1. Maintain the limbs of the suture at equal lengths. Determine which limb is the post by sliding the knot pusher down into the joint and removing all twists. Tag the post with a clamp to identify the suture limbs and separate them.
2. Throw an overhand loop around the post, and pull the knot down to the target with the knot pusher on the nonpost. As the knot pusher is advanced, keep continuous tension on the post, and alternately apply tension and release it on the nonpost. Past-point the post and loop limbs at 180 degrees to each other with the knot pusher.
3. Switch the knot pusher to the other strand (the original post) and throw an underhand loop around the new post. Pull this loop into the joint and apply tension by past-pointing while maintaining tension on the post strand.
4. Continue in this fashion with reversing posts and alternating throws for a total of five loops.

This method of tying half hitches is the most effective at maintaining knot security.[3,11] However, different strategies are frequently and effectively employed. To help improve loop security, a surgeon's knot can be tied initially. Two identical loops around the same post create the surgeon's knot and allow the tissue loop to be further tensioned after the first throw. Internal friction between the two same-direction throws is usually sufficient to maintain the loops in place. Subsequent loops can then be thrown with reversing posts and throws to increase knot security.

Revo Knot

As stated earlier, all nonsliding knots are a combination of various half-hitch loops. The Revo knot (Fig. 4–6) is no exception.[18] To tie a Revo knot:

1. Throw an overhand loop around the post with the knot pusher on the post and advance it down into the joint.
2. Maintain continuous tension on the post, throw a second identical half hitch (i.e., overhand) around the same post, and advance it down on top of the initial loop (effectively throwing a surgeon's knot).
3. Tension both loops by applying continuous tension on the post and pushing on the knot stack while tensioning the nonpost.
4. Wrap a third half-hitch loop in the opposite direction (i.e., underhand) around the post limb, advance it to the knot stack, and tension as above.
5. Switch posts, throw an overhand loop, advance to the knot stack, and tension it as above with past-pointing. This throw effectively locks the initial three loops thrown around the original post. Therefore, it is paramount that all slack in the knot stack be removed before this throw.
6. To complete the knot, reverse the post again, tie an underhand loop around the new post, and tension as above.

Sliding Knots

The basic requirement for tying a sliding knot (locking or nonlocking) is that the suture must slide through the tissue and anchor freely. If the suture does not slide, the surgeon must use a nonsliding knot. Sliding knots have a number of advantages over serial half-hitch throws. These knots can be constructed completely outside the cannula and joint and then slid down into place. They have better loop security and require fewer steps to tie once the wrapping sequence is learned. Problems with sliding knots are usually encountered when the suture

does not slide as planned. Locking sliding knots can lock prematurely and bind in the cannula; this problem may not be recoverable.

Sliding knots are generally more complicated to tie than are half hitches and other nonsliding knots. Successful use of sliding knots depends on smooth sliding of the knot, easy passage through the cannula, and maintenance of loop tension while the knot is secured in place. There is a significant learning curve associated with these knots. In addition, their sliding and holding characteristics vary from surgeon to surgeon, underscoring their technique-dependent nature.[7]

Nonlocking Sliding Knots

Nonlocking sliding knots cannot prematurely lock and bind the post before they are tensioned at the tissue. These knots require backup half hitches to secure the knot once it is in place. If no backup loops are thrown, these knots will lose loop security by sliding back up the post limb. Here we describe the Duncan loop (hangman's knot) and the Roeder knot.

Duncan Loop

To tie the Duncan loop (Fig. 4–7)[14]:

1. As always, identify the post and ensure that there are no twists or tangles along the sutures in the cannula. Slide the suture so that the nonpost is about twice as long as the post strand. Place a knot pusher and clamp on the post limb, and hold both limbs between the thumb and long finger.
2. Wrap the loop strand over the thumb, creating a loop, and then wrap it over and around both limbs four times.
3. Pass the free end of the loop strand back through the loop formed around the thumb.
4. Remove excess slack (i.e., dress or set) in the knot by pulling on the free end of the loop strand and then tensioning the loop strand from the knot to the cannula. This is facilitated by placing an index finger just distal to the loop stack in the axilla at the junction of the post and loop limb.
5. The knot can now be slid into place by simply pulling on the post limb. As it is advanced, push it into

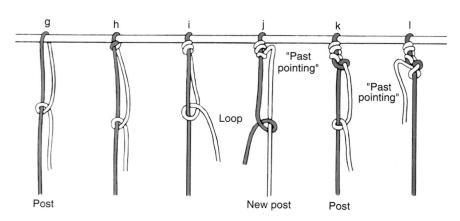

Figure 4–6 Revo knot. (From Nottage WM, Lieurance RK: Arthroscopic knot tying techniques. Arthroscopy 15:515-521, 1999.)

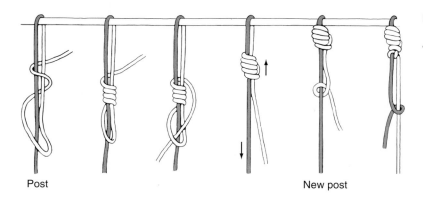

Figure 4–7 Duncan loop. (From Nottage WM, Lieurance RK: Arthroscopic knot tying techniques. Arthroscopy 15:515-521, 1999.)

Post   New post

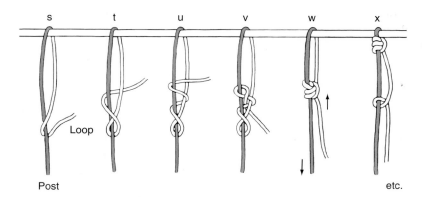

Figure 4–8 Roeder knot. (From Nottage WM, Lieurance RK: Arthroscopic knot tying techniques. Arthroscopy 15:515-521, 1999.)

s   t   u   v   w   x

Loop

Post   etc.

place with the knot pusher to minimize suture trauma.

6. Continue pushing on the knot as the post is tensioned. While keeping continuous tension on the post, throw a half hitch around the post and advance it into place behind the Duncan loop.

7. Continue throwing a minimum of three reversing half hitches on alternate posts to secure the knot.

ROEDER KNOT

The Roeder knot (Fig. 4–8) is a modification of the Duncan loop.[17] It consists of the same number of loops and has the same characteristics as the Duncan loop. To tie the Roeder knot:

1. As always, identify the post and ensure that there are no twists or tangles along the sutures in the cannula. Slide the suture so that the nonpost is about twice as long as the post strand. Place a knot pusher and clamp on the post limb, and hold both limbs between the thumb and long finger.

2. Throw a loop over and around the post strand.

3. Throw a second loop over both strands.

4. Throw the third loop over only the post strand.

5. Pass the free end of the loop strand down between the second and third loops from above the knot.

6. Dress the knot and slide it into place by pulling on the post strand and pushing the knot down with the knot pusher. Secure the knot with a series of three alternating post and throw half hitches.

Locking Sliding Knots

The advantages of locking sliding knots are that they can be constructed completely outside the joint and, once delivered to the tissue, provide loop and knot security without further steps. Most surgeons throw additional locking loops behind these knots to ensure knot security, however. Potential problems are related to the knots' complexity. They rely on multiple loops around one or both limbs and proper sequencing of the loops. Additionally, these knots can lock prematurely if tension is applied on the nonpost limb before the knot is seated. Unfortunately, this problem usually cannot be fixed and may require starting with a new anchor. Despite the potential shortcomings, these knots are excellent choices for tissues under tension. They can be used effectively any time the suture slides freely through the anchor.

TENNESSEE SLIDER

The Tennessee slider (Fig. 4–9) has all the advantages of locking sliding knots,[15] plus the added advantages of being low profile and low volume. Unfortunately, it is difficult to tie and can bind prematurely. To tie the Tennessee slider:

1. As always, identify the post and any twists with a knot pusher and mark the post with a clamp.

2. Slide the suture until the nonpost limb is twice as long as the post, and grasp both limbs of the suture between the thumb and index finger.

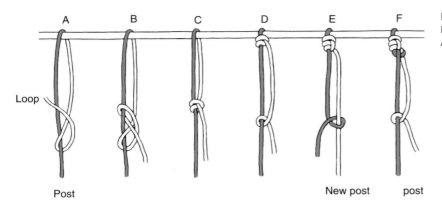

Figure 4–9 **Tennessee slider.** (From Nottage WM, Lieurance RK: Arthroscopic knot tying techniques. Arthroscopy 15:515-521, 1999.)

3. Pass the wrapping strand over the post, and continue wrapping outside and proximal (closer to the surgeon) to the loop just created.

4. Pass the wrapping strand back over the post.

5. Reach between the wrapping strand and the post and pull the free end of the suture up through the loop created by the second overthrow.

6. Dress the knot and remove slack, but *do not tension the loop strand.*

7. Place the knot pusher on the post strand and advance the knot into the joint by pulling on the post and pushing with the knot pusher.

8. Maintain tension on the post, and tension the wrapping strand to capture the post and lock it into place.

It is critical to maintain tension on the post, because this knot has a tendency to lose some of its initial tension as it is locked.

9. Throw a minimum of three additional half hitches on alternating posts to ensure security.

SMC KNOT

The SMC knot (Fig. 4–10) was recently described as a new type of locking sliding knot.[8] It provides excellent initial loop and knot security and has a low profile. It can be backed up with half hitches to improve on its already excellent inherent security. It also relies on an internal locking mechanism to capture the post once it is deliv-

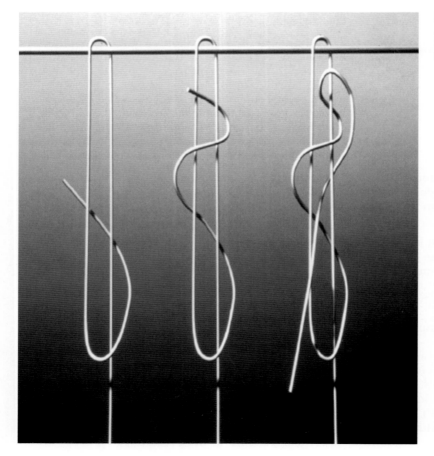

Figure 4–10 **SMC knot.** (From Kim SH, Ha KI, Kim JS: Significance of the internal locking mechanism for loop security enhancement in the arthroscopic knot. Arthroscopy 17:850-855, 2001.)

ered to the tissue. Unlike the Tennessee slider, it does not tend to "back off" the tissue as it is being locked and therefore maintains its loop security. In biomechanical studies, this knot fails through suture breakage rather than knot slippage.[9]

To tie the SMC knot:

1. As always, identify the post and any twists with a knot pusher and mark the post with a clamp.
2. Slide the suture until the nonpost limb is twice as long as the post, and grasp both limbs of the suture between the thumb and index finger. Have an assistant place a finger between the strands to keep them separated as the knot is tied.
3. Begin the knot by passing the loop strand over the post strand and then over both strands again (see Fig. 4–10A and B).
4. Reach between the post and loop strands, grab the free end of the loop strand, and pass it over only the post strand (see Fig. 4–10B).
5. Pass the free end of the suture under the post between the first two throws, and leave a loop of suture. Lightly dress the knot, but *do not pull on the loop strand* (see Fig. 4–10C).
6. Advance the knot to the tissue by pulling on the post and pushing the knot into place with the knot pusher. The knot can then be locked by pulling on the loop strand to incorporate the locking loop into the knot and capturing the post. The loop strand now becomes the new post.
7. Additional half hitches can be thrown to further secure the knot.

Knot-Tying Alternatives

Many devices have been developed to avoid knot tying in arthroscopic surgery. Staples and tacks have been used with mixed results in the fixation of labral and rotator cuff repairs. Recently, knotless suture anchors have been developed that combine the benefits of suture through tissue and a bone anchor.[19–21] These knotless anchors compare favorably with standard suture anchors in pull-through strength because when they are implanted, there are effectively two strands of suture through the tissue (Fig. 4–11).[20] Although this is an attractive option, there are limitations. Only a fixed and maximal amount of tissue volume can be captured, leading to a theoretically limited ability to address capsular redundancy. The somewhat larger insertion cannulas required may also limit inferior placement in some conditions. These anchors, however, can provide secure fixation and avoid the need for arthroscopic knot tying.

Ultrasonic suture welding seeks to retain the benefits of suture passage through tissue without the need to tie knots. This technique employs an ultrasonic wand that imparts heat to a loop of polypropylene (monofilament, nonabsorbable) suture to "weld" it together (Fig. 4–12). It can be passed down a cannula and used arthroscopically. Biomechanical studies have shown that a number 2 suture welded together has better strength, less elongation at failure, and a higher load to failure under cyclic loading conditions than the same suture tied with traditional knots.[16] This technique is operator dependent, however, and involves additional equipment and

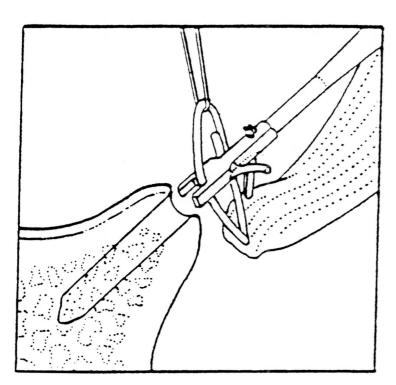

Figure 4–11 Knotless suture anchor. The anchor has a utility suture fed through the loop attached to the anchor. A shuttle is passed through the tissue, and the loop is pulled through via the utility suture. The pronged end of the anchor is then used to grab the loop and advanced into the tunnel. (From Thal R: A knotless suture anchor: Technique for use in arthroscopic Bankart repair. Arthroscopy 17:213-218, 2001. With permission from The Arthroscopy Association of North America.)

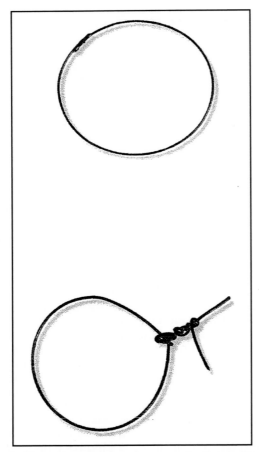

Figure 4–12 **Welded suture (top) compared with a traditionally tied suture.** (From Richmond JC: A comparison of ultrasonic suture welding and traditional knot tying. Am J Sports Med 29:297-299, 2001.)

cost. It also cannot be used with braided nonabsorbable sutures.

Conclusion

We have presented a framework for successful arthroscopic knot tying. This chapter is intended to be a guide for surgeons to organize their thoughts and plan accordingly for surgery. Proficiency with these techniques, like any other surgical skill, requires practice and meticulous attention to detail. The steps involved in effectively and efficiently tying arthroscopic knots start with portal placement and do not end until the suture is cut.

References

1. Burkhart SS, Wirth MA, Simonick M, et al: Loop security as a determinant of tissue fixation security. Arthroscopy 14:773-776, 1998.

2. Chan KC, Burkhart SS: How to switch posts without rethreading when tying half-hitches. Arthroscopy 15:444-450, 1999.

3. Chan KC, Burkhart SS, Thiagerajen P, et al: Optimization of stacked half-hitch knots for arthroscopic surgery. Arthroscopy 17: 752-759, 2001.

4. De Beer JF: Arthroscopic Bankart repair: Some aspects of suture and knot management. Arthroscopy 15:660-662, 1999.

5. De Beer JF, van Rooyen K, Boezaart AP: Nicky's knot—a new slip knot for arthroscopic surgery. Arthroscopy 14:109-110, 1998.

6. Fleega BA, Sokkar SH: The giant knot: A new one-way self-locking secured arthroscopic slip knot. Arthroscopy 15:451-452, 1999.

7. Hughes PJ, Hagan RP, Fisher AC, et al: The kinematics and kinetics of slipknots for arthroscopic Bankart repair. Am J Sports Med 29:738-745, 2001.

8. Kim SH, Ha KI: The SMC knot—a new slip knot with locking mechanism. Arthroscopy 16:563-565, 2000.

9. Kim SH, Ha KI, Kim JS: Significance of the internal locking mechanism for loop security enhancement in the arthroscopic knot. Arthroscopy 17:850-855, 2001.

10. Lee TQ, Matsuura PA, Fogolin RP, et al: Arthroscopic suture tying: A comparison of knot types and suture materials. Arthroscopy 17:348-352, 2001.

11. Loutzenheiser TD, Harryman DT 2nd, Yung SW, et al: Optimizing arthroscopic knots. Arthroscopy 11:199-206, 1995.

12. Loutzenheiser TD, Harryman DT 2nd, Ziegler DW, et al: Optimizing arthroscopic knots using braided or monofilament suture. Arthroscopy 14:57-65, 1998.

13. McMillan E: Arthroscopic Knot Tying Manual. Arthroscopy Association of North America, 1999.

14. Mishra DK, Cannon WD Jr, Lucas DJ, et al: Elongation of arthroscopically tied knots. Am J Sports Med 25:113-117, 1997.

15. Nottage WM, Lieurance RK: Arthroscopic knot tying techniques. Arthroscopy 15:515-521, 1999.

16. Richmond JC: A comparison of ultrasonic suture welding and traditional knot tying. Am J Sports Med 29:297-299, 2001.

17. Sharp HT, Dorsey JH, Choven JD, et al: A simple modification to add strength to the Roeder knot. J Am Assoc Gynecol Laparosc 3:305-307, 1996.

18. Snyder SJ: Technique of arthroscopic rotator cuff repair using implantable 4-mm Revo suture anchors, suture shuttle relays, and no. 2 nonabsorbable mattress sutures. Orthop Clin North Am 28:267-275, 1997.

19. Thal R: Knotless suture anchor: Arthroscopic Bankart repair without tying knots. Clin Orthop 390:42-51, 2001.

20. Thal R: A knotless suture anchor: Design, function, and biomechanical testing. Am J Sports Med 29:646-649, 2001.

21. Thal R: A knotless suture anchor: Technique for use in arthroscopic Bankart repair. Arthroscopy 17:213-218, 2001.

22. Weston PV: A new clinch knot. Obstet Gynecol 78:144-147, 1991.

Grafts

Darren L. Johnson, William M. Isbell, and Özgür Ahmet Atay

The ideal graft material for ligament reconstruction of the knee would be strong, be readily available, cause no morbidity to the patient, and allow for early, aggressive rehabilitation. There is no single "ideal" graft material for every patient. All the currently available choices have distinct advantages and disadvantages that are often patient specific. The decision of which graft to use must take into account the patient's age, activity level, and associated injuries; the availability of graft materials; and the surgeon's comfort level. After considering all these factors, the surgeon may be able to choose the ideal graft for a particular patient.

In 1998, the members of the ACL Study Group reported that 73% of them used patellar tendons, 23% used hamstring tendons, and 4% used "others," including allografts, for ligament reconstruction.[4] Of the 14 members of the ACL Reconstruction Panel at the Eighth Panther Symposium, 8 (57%) reported using hamstring tendons, 5 (36%) preferred patellar tendon, and 1 (7%) used quadriceps tendon exclusively. Allograft is used in only 2% of primary anterior cruciate ligament (ACL) reconstructions. Eleven of the 14 panelists reported using more than one type of graft, depending on the context of the injury; the majority, however, had a preferred graft that they used in more than 90% of their cases.[9]

When attempting to choose the ideal graft for a particular patient, it is important to review the properties of each graft type and compare them in terms of biomechanical properties, healing, fixation, graft site morbidity, and associated complications. An intimate knowledge of the profile of each graft material allows the surgeon to match graft and patient for the best possible outcome.

Autografts

An autograft is tissue taken from the patient's own body. Autogenous tissue is used in the majority of ligament reconstructions. In general, autografts are inexpensive

and readily available and have no risk of an immune response. The disadvantages are increased operative time for harvest of the graft, potential complications associated with the harvest, and graft site morbidity. Common autogenous tissue used for ligament reconstruction includes bone–patellar tendon–bone, quadrupled hamstring tendons, and quadriceps tendon–bone. Each of these graft ligament substitutes has different biomechanical properties, incorporation issues, and graft site morbidities that need to be considered.

Four stages of ligamentization of autografts have been described. Repopulation with fibroblasts occurs over the first 2 months, with the graft being viable as early as 3 weeks after implantation. Over the next 10 months, rapid remodeling occurs, with more fibroblasts, neovascularity, and a reduction in mature collagen. Over the next 2 years, there is a maturation of the collagen. By 3 years, the graft appears to be ligamentous histologically.[17] In an animal model, examination of hamstring ACL grafts showed that the initial random collagen fiber orientation at 4 weeks progressed to a longitudinal orientation from the peripheral to the central areas of the graft at 12 weeks after surgery. At 24 weeks, a uniform sinusoidal crimp pattern similar to that seen in the normal ACL was identified under polarized light in only half the grafts examined. Histologic examination of the grafts at 52 weeks revealed this uniform sinusoidal crimp pattern in 75% of grafts, with the remaining tissue having a disorganized pattern similar to immature collagen.[7] It is important to consider this evolving process of ligamentization when determining the appropriate intensity of postoperative rehabilitation. The rehabilitation must be sensitive to the biology of the graft during its incorporation to avoid early catastrophic failure of the graft.

The strength of a graft declines shortly after its insertion. Therefore, it is important that the graft initially be as strong as or stronger than the native ligament it is replacing. The relative strengths of each of the graft types most commonly used in ACL reconstruction are listed in Table 5–1. A working knowledge of these values aids in

Table 5–1

Accepted Values for Ultimate Tensile Load

Graft Type	Ultimate Tensile Load (N)
Native anterior cruciate ligament	2160
Bone–patellar tendon–bone (10 mm)	2977
Quadrupled semitendinosus and gracilis	3880
Quadriceps tendon (10 mm)	2352
Bone–patellar tendon–bone allograft	2552

graft selection. It should be remembered, however, that these values represent maximum values achieved in the laboratory under ideal testing conditions, which may be higher than those achieved in vivo.

Patellar Tendon

The central third of the patellar tendon has been referred to as the gold standard for ACL reconstruction. More clinical studies with long-term follow-up have been reported using this graft than any other. It has been touted for its ultimate strength and stability. Routinely, a 10-mm central portion of the patellar tendon is harvested with bone blocks from both the patella and the tibial tubercle of the ipsilateral knee. This provides a large, stable graft that is often thought to be the ideal choice for ACL reconstruction. In spite of its obvious strengths, however, this graft may not be ideal for every patient. A thorough knowledge of its mechanical properties and potential morbidities is essential to determine the appropriateness of a patellar tendon autograft for a particular patient.

The patellar tendon autograft has its own set of distinct advantages. Cooper et al. showed that a 10-mm patellar tendon graft has both a high ultimate tensile load (2977 N) and greater stiffness (455 N/mm) when compared with the ultimate tensile load (2160 N) and stiffness (242 N/mm) of a native ACL.[6] The ultimate load to failure of patellar tendon autograft has been shown to be 53% of the original insertion strength at 3 months following implantation, 52% at 6 months, 81% at 9 months, and 81% at 12 months.

The presence of bone blocks on each end of the tendon allows for rapid bone-to-bone healing of the graft as early as 6 weeks.[23] These bone blocks also act as a mechanical block initially; in combination with the interference screws, they provide rigid fixation of the graft in the bone tunnels. Both of these factors lead to early stability of the graft, which allows for aggressive rehabilitation.

Some surgeons are reluctant to use the patellar tendon for ligament reconstruction because of the potential for anterior knee pain after graft harvest. The cause of this pain may be multifactorial, including the initial injury that resulted in the ACL tear, the surgery itself, and factors associated with harvesting of the graft. Some reports indicate that the incidence of anterior knee pain may be greater after patellar tendon ACL reconstruction than after hamstring tendon ACL reconstruction.[18] This increased incidence is an early postoperative phenomenon, however, and there is no significant difference in anterior knee pain at 2 years after reconstruction. Also, the increased incidence of anterior knee pain in this population is likely a function of the much less aggressive rehabilitation program these patients participate in postoperatively. With early, aggressive rehabilitation following bone–patellar tendon–bone ACL reconstruction, the incidence of anterior knee pain is not increased compared with quadrupled hamstring tendon ACL reconstruction.

Other concerns include the potential loss of quadriceps strength following allograft patellar tendon ACL reconstruction. It has been shown that any initial postoperative reduction in quadriceps strength appears to return over time. At 6 months following surgery, Indelicato et al. showed that only 12% of patients with patellar tendon autograft had 80% of their contralateral quadriceps strength, compared with 77% of the patients who had allograft reconstruction.[11] At 1 year, there was no difference in quadriceps strength in these two groups of patients.

Rare complications of patellar tendon graft harvest include patellar fracture, both with harvesting and postoperatively, and patellar tendon rupture. In addition, the incision required for harvesting the patellar tendon graft may expose the infrapatellar branch of the saphenous nerve to injury. Despite these risks, the patellar tendon remains a stable and reliable graft source for ligament reconstruction.

Quadrupled Hamstring Tendon

The semitendinosus and gracilis tendons are the most commonly used hamstring tendons for ligament reconstruction. These tendons have been used as single strands, doubled, and quadrupled, with a quadrupled semitendinosus and gracilis graft having the highest ultimate load to failure. Hamner et al.[8] reported that combined strands of hamstring tendons have the additive tensile properties of each of the individual strands. In the laboratory under ideal testing conditions, four combined strands of two gracilis and two semitendinosus strands equally tensioned (3880 N) were shown to be stronger than a 10-mm patellar tendon graft (2977 N).[8] This value may be difficult to reproduce clinically, with current technology.

The shape of a quadrupled hamstring graft (Fig. 5–1) is cylindric, in contrast to the rectangular shape of a patellar tendon. As a result of this physical characteristic, hamstring tendon grafts have a 26% greater cross-sectional area than patellar tendon grafts of the same size. To compare, a 15.9- by 4-mm patellar tendon graft must be harvested to equal the surface area of a 9-mm hamstring tendon graft. The ability to bundle multiple strands of hamstring tendons further increases the cross-sectional area of the graft, thereby increasing its ultimate strength. The cylindric shape of hamstring tendons matches that of the bone tunnels, allowing for increased

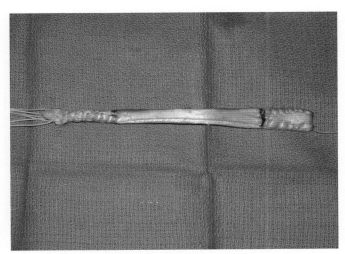

Figure 5–1 Quadrupled hamstring autograft used for anterior cruciate ligament reconstruction.

"fill" of the tibial and femoral tunnels, which minimizes the dead space and maximizes graft incorporation.

As mentioned previously, there may be less anterior knee pain associated with hamstring autografts compared with patellar tendon autografts, because the anterior knee and its extensor mechanism are not violated when harvesting the graft. Any local pain in the area of the hamstring tendon harvest usually resolves early in the postoperative course. The all–soft tissue nature of this graft makes passage of the graft technically easier, which may be of increased importance in posterior cruciate ligament reconstruction, where the graft may have to "turn the corner." The soft tissue nature of this graft also makes it ideal for ACL reconstruction in skeletally immature patients. Autogenous hamstring ACL reconstruction in this population has been shown to have a low risk of growth disturbance, making it an ideal graft choice.[14]

One of the primary disadvantages of a hamstring autograft is that the initial fixation relies on a soft tissue–bone interface, versus the bone-to-bone interface of the patellar tendon graft. This implies that the initial strength of a hamstring ACL reconstruction relies primarily on the strength of the fixation device. Another disadvantage is that the incorporation process of a hamstring autograft is slower compared with bone-to-bone healing. Animal studies have shown that hamstring grafts fail by pulling out of the bone tunnel at up to 12 weeks after implantation, indicating a lack of early graft-to-tunnel healing.[16] As a result, some surgeons are cautious when considering an aggressive rehabilitation program of early motion and weight bearing following hamstring ACL reconstruction.

The potential for loss of hamstring strength following harvest for ACL reconstruction is a concern. This may be important early in the postoperative course; an approximately 10% difference in hamstring strength may be present up to 1 year after surgery. However, with long-term follow-up, there appears to be little or no loss of hamstring power.[13] For athletes who participate in more hamstring-dependent activities, the use of quadrupled

hamstring tendons for ACL reconstruction may be less desirable than other graft options. For example, female basketball players are thought to have an increased risk of ACL tears, partly because of the relative weakness of their hamstrings in comparison with their quadriceps musculature. Weakening the hamstrings further by taking them for ACL reconstruction may result in an increased risk of reinjury to the ACL-reconstructed knee, leading to higher failure rates in these quadriceps-dependent female athletes.

Bone tunnel enlargement, or tunnel lysis, may be increased with hamstring autografts. This tunnel lysis has been attributed to both mechanical and biologic factors. Proposed causes are related to the soft tissue nature of the graft, including motion of the graft in the tunnel and bathing of the graft by synovial fluid. Regardless of the mechanism, this tunnel enlargement does not appear to affect the clinical outcome of quadrupled hamstring autograft ACL reconstruction.[22] A quadrupled hamstring tendon autograft remains a viable alternative for ligament reconstruction owing to its high strength and low morbidity.

Quadriceps Tendon

The central third of the quadriceps tendon can be used for ligament reconstruction. It is harvested with a section of the superior pole of the patella (Fig. 5–2). This provides a bulky graft requiring soft tissue fixation on one end and bony fixation on the other. The quadriceps tendon has almost twice the strength and has twice the cross-sectional area of a patellar tendon autograft of the same width. The mean cross-sectional area of a 10-mm quadriceps tendon averages $65\,mm^2$, compared with $37\,mm^2$ for a 10-mm patellar tendon graft. Staubli et al.[21] reported the ultimate tensile load of a 10-mm quadriceps tendon graft to be 2352 N, making it as strong as or stronger than a native ACL.

The advantages of the quadriceps tendon include its strength, the ability to achieve bony fixation on one end, and its availability after other graft sources have been

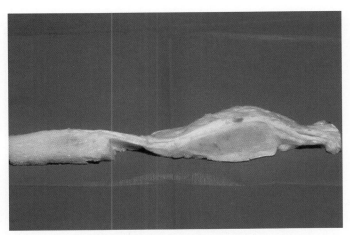

Figure 5–2 Quadriceps tendon–patella–patellar tendon–bone allograft.

used. This graft may be technically more difficult to harvest than other graft types, and many surgeons are unfamiliar with the technique. Harvesting bone from the patella is associated with the same risks reported for harvesting patellar tendon autografts, including the potential for fracture and anterior knee pain. The biggest disadvantage of this graft may be quadriceps weakness. The strength of the quadriceps in the donor knee has been reported to be as low as 80% of normal 1 year after surgery.[5]

Allografts

An allograft is any tissue harvested from a cadaver. Orthopedic surgeons have used bony and soft tissue allografts successfully in various applications. Shino et al.[19] described 22 different grafts that can be harvested from a human donor that are acceptable for ligament reconstruction. The five most common allograft tissue types used in ligament reconstruction are bone–patellar tendon–bone (Fig. 5–3), Achilles tendon (Fig. 5–4), anterior tibialis tendon (Fig. 5–5), fascia lata, and quadrupled hamstring tendon (semitendinosus and gracilis).

Allograft tissue functions as a scaffold, providing a structure that is rapidly incorporated and remodeled by the host. At the time of insertion, allografts are similar to autografts both histologically and biomechanically; however, the ligamentization process may be less uniform and more prolonged with allografts. The initial stages progress very rapidly. Jackson et al.[12] demonstrated the complete replacement of donor cells by host cells in the goat ACL by 4 weeks after transplantation. The remodeling phase of an allograft is lengthy; it may take up to one and a half times as long as an autograft to complete remodeling and regain comparable strength. Once the remodeling phase is complete, implanted allograft ligament tissue appears similar to the native ACL. In animal studies, by 52 weeks after implantation, bone–patellar tendon–bone allografts had regained a

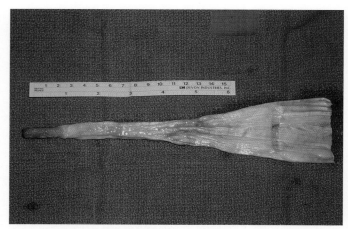

Figure 5–4 Achilles tendon–bone allograft.

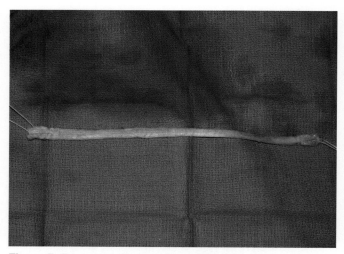

Figure 5–5 Anterior tibialis tendon allograft used for anterior or posterior cruciate ligament reconstruction.

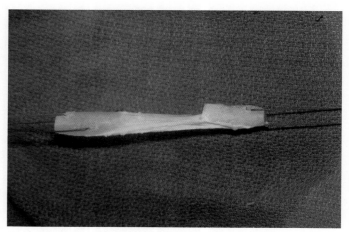

Figure 5–3 Bone–patellar tendon–bone allograft.

fibrous framework that was histologically similar to that seen in normal ligament.

The clinical outcome after allograft ACL reconstruction has been compared with that after autograft reconstruction, with conflicting results. Some studies found no significant differences between graft types, and others reported significant differences in anterior stability. Overall, the results of primary reconstruction with allografts are similar to those obtained with autografts. Some concern has been expressed that allografts may begin to show increased laxity or rerupture rates 5 years or more after surgery, but no series with data showing this has been published. Noyes and Barber-Westin[15] found no significant change in knee laxity or in the overall knee score when assessing their patients 3 and 7 years after allograft ACL reconstruction.

Some advantages are common to all allograft tissue types. In most instances, the tissue is readily available, and there is obviously no donor site morbidity. The operative time is shorter, and the need for large incisions is eliminated. The use of allograft tissue allows the placement of a large, strong graft without removing other supporting structures or risking injury to harvest sites.

The use of autogenous tissue may be constrained by its limited size, shape, and availability, making allograft tissue ideal for revision surgery. In revision ACL reconstruction, larger bone plugs may be needed and are usually available with bone–patellar tendon–bone or Achilles tendon allografts (Figs. 5–6 and 5–7). This may eliminate the need for another source of bone graft to fill a large defect and avoid a staged procedure.

Allograft tissue also has its disadvantages. A potential disastrous complication of allogeneic tissue use is the transmission of disease, including infection, hepatitis, and human immunodeficiency virus (HIV).[20] All allografts should come with the highest possible assurance that they are free of pathogens. Buck et al.[3] calculated that the risk of HIV transmission in properly screened and tested donors was 1 in 1.6 million and stated that adequate serologic testing and histopathologic examinations are most important in securing safe, sterile grafts.

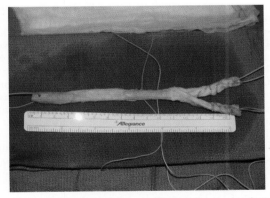

Figure 5–6 Quadriceps tendon–patella–patellar tendon–bone allograft used for revision anterior cruciate ligament surgery with tibial tunnel lysis and compromised tibial tunnel fixation.

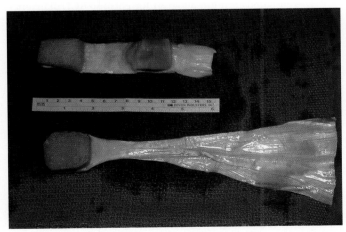

Figure 5–7 Bone–patellar tendon–bone and Achilles tendon–bone allograft before preparation.

Recently, the Centers for Disease Control and Prevention (CDC) reported two cases of *Clostridium* infections in patients who had undergone knee reconstruction using musculoskeletal allografts. In one case, the patient died from septic shock, with postmortem blood cultures growing *Clostridium sordellii*. As of March 2002, the CDC had received 26 reports of bacterial infections associated with musculoskeletal tissue allografts. Of these 26 patients, 13 were infected with *Clostridium* species, and 11 patients were infected with gram-negative bacilli. The majority of the musculoskeletal allografts (18) were used for ACL reconstruction. The CDC continues to investigate these cases.[1]

Unfortunately, most of the methods used to sterilize operative materials are unsuitable for human tissue. Viruses that transmit diseases are not eradicated by the freezing of tissue. Heat and high doses of gamma radiation (3 Mrad) are effective but weaken the collagen structure. The current irradiation dose recommended by the American Association of Tissue Banks is between 1.5 and 2.5 Mrad, although it acknowledges that some resistant spore-forming organisms and viruses may survive 2.5 Mrad. Chemical agents such as ethylene oxide, though effective in removing unwanted microorganisms, leave behind a chemical residue that may cause chronic synovitis and graft failure.

The remodeling and mechanical properties of allograft tissue may be affected by both immune reactions and graft preparation. In the canine model, Arnoczky et al.[2] showed that fresh patellar tendon allografts incite a marked inflammatory and rejection response in the knee. Frozen patellar tendon allografts appeared to be benign and were comparable with autogenous tendon grafts in this study. Harner et al.[10] analyzed the synovial fluid of patients following allograft and autograft ACL reconstruction. At 6 months postoperatively, 60% of the patients who received allograft tissue had evidence of an intra-articular humoral response; none of the autograft patients had a humoral immune response. Both groups showed a mild intra-articular cellular response without evidence of a systemic response. None of these patients had a frank rejection of the allograft. The clinical significance of this immune response is not fully known; however, there are reports of allografts being removed following a marked inflammatory response.

With regard to graft preparation, freeze-drying seems to be superior to deep-freezing for reducing the immunogenicity of allograft tissue. However, freeze-drying has been shown to dramatically alter the mechanical properties of the graft. Some patients have developed delayed toxic and inflammatory intra-articular reactions from the use of freeze-dried allograft sterilized with ethylene oxide; therefore, ethylene oxide sterilization of allografts should be avoided. Freezing the tissue to −80°C degrees has been shown to decrease the immune response. In light of this, fresh-frozen allograft tissue seems to be the best at preserving both the biologic and the biomechanical properties of the graft.

Despite the attractions of no morbidity from graft harvest and satisfactory mechanical properties, many factors enter into the decision to use an allograft. These include the preference of the patient and the surgeon, the risk of disease transmission, the availability of tissue, the method of tissue preparation, and the potential for increased laxity.

Synthetic Grafts

The use of synthetic ligament substitutes has fallen out of favor, but a discussion of them shows the progress we have made in ligament reconstruction. Artificial ligaments have several theoretic advantages. They are readily available and eliminate any graft harvest morbidity. Their strength can exceed that of any biologic tissue, and they have no risk of disease transmission. The return to activities following ligament reconstruction is not limited by the need to wait for the graft to mature.

Three main types of synthetic grafts were used in the past: permanent prostheses, ligament scaffolds, and ligament augmentation devices (LADs). Permanent prostheses made of Gore-Tex (Gore and Co., Flagstaff, AZ) and Stryker Dacron (Stryker Endoscopy Co., Sunnyvale, CA) generally exhibit high ultimate tensile strength at implantation and have limited potential for ingrowth. Ligament scaffolds (Leeds-Keio and carbon fiber ligament) theoretically allow ingrowth of tissue over time. LADs (Kennedy LAD, 3M, St. Paul, MN) are intended to serve as load-sharing devices, shielding the biologic graft substitute from potentially deleterious loads during the revascularization and remodeling phase, when the graft is at its weakest.

The experience with fully prosthetic grafts has been disappointing. They have not proved to be durable, and the materials have exhibited marked short- and long-term fatigue or failure, leading to recurrent instability. They also have an increased rate of infection, as well as frequent effusions, synovitis, and tunnel osteolysis due to the generation of intra-articular particulate debris.

Several studies have evaluated the efficacy of LADs used with either hamstring or patellar tendon grafts. None of these studies has shown clinical results superior to those achieved with an isolated autograft or allograft. It has been shown that fixation of the LAD at both ends of the graft can lead to failure as a result of stress shielding. The use of LADs cannot be advocated at this time.

Conclusion

No longer is there one best graft for all patients needing ACL reconstruction. The gold-standard graft must be patient specific. Patellar tendon autograft is not the ideal graft choice for every patient, and there are several viable alternatives for ligament reconstruction of ACL-deficient knees. A thorough knowledge of the mechanical and clinical properties of each of these graft types, as well as an understanding of the techniques used for their harvest and implantation, is essential to select the best graft for a particular patient. A thorough knowledge of the biologic properties of each graft type also allows the

tailoring of a graft-specific rehabilitation program. All these factors are used in concert to obtain the best possible clinical outcomes for patients undergoing ACL reconstruction.

References

1. Archibald LK, Jernigan DB, Kainer MA: Update: Allograft-associated bacterial infections—United States, 2002. MMWR Morb Mortal Wkly Rep 51:207-210, 2002.
2. Arnoczky SP, Warren RF, Ashlock MA: Replacement of the anterior cruciate ligament using a patellar tendon allograft: An experimental study. J Bone Joint Surg 68:376-385, 1986.
3. Buck BE, Malinin TI, Brown MD: Bone transplantation and human immunodeficiency virus: An estimate of risk of acquired immunodeficiency syndrome (AIDS). Clin Orthop 240:129-136, 1989.
4. Campbell JD: The evolution and current treatment trends with anterior cruciate, posterior cruciate, and medial collateral ligament injuries. Am J Knee Surg 11:128-135, 1998.
5. Chen CH, Chen WJ, Shih CH: Arthroscopic anterior cruciate ligament reconstruction with quadriceps tendon–patella bone autograft. J Trauma 7:111-117, 1999.
6. Cooper D, Deng X, Burstein A, Warren R: The strength of the central third patellar tendon graft. A biomechanical study. Am J Sports Med 21:818-824, 1993.
7. Gordia VK, Rochat MC, Kida M, Grana WA: Natural history of a hamstring tendon autograft used for anterior cruciate ligament reconstruction in a sheep model. Am J Sports Med 28:40-46, 2000.
8. Hamner DL, Brown CH, Steiner ME, et al: Hamstring tendon grafts for reconstruction of the anterior cruciate ligament: Biomechanical evaluation of the use of multiple strands and tensioning techniques. J Bone Joint Surg 81:549-557, 1999.
9. Harner CD, Fu FH, Irrang JJ, Vogrin TM: Anterior and posterior cruciate ligament reconstruction in the new millennium: A global perspective. Knee Sports Traumatol Arthrosc 9:330-336, 2001.
10. Harner CD, Thompson W, Jamison J, et al: The immunologic response to fresh frozen patellar tendon allograft ACL reconstruction. Paper presented at the American Academy of Orthopaedic Surgeons, Feb 24–Mar 1, 1995, New Orleans, LA.
11. Indelicato PA, Linton RC, Hoegel M: The results of fresh frozen patella tendon allograft for chronic ACL deficiency of the knee. Am J Sports Med 20:118-121, 1992.
12. Jackson DW, Simon TM, Kurzweil PR, et al: Survival of cells after intra-articular transplantation of fresh allografts of the patellar and anterior cruciate ligaments: DNA-probe analysis in a goat model. J Bone Joint Surg 74:112-118, 1992.
13. Libscomb AB, Johnson RK, Snyder RB, et al: Evaluation of hamstring strength following the use of semitendinosus and gracilis tendons to reconstruct the anterior cruciate ligament. Am J Sports Med 10:340-342, 1983.
14. Marder RA, Raskind JR, Carroll M: Prospective evaluation of arthroscopically assisted anterior cruciate ligament reconstruction: Patellar tendon versus semitendinosus and gracilis tendons. Am J Sports Med 19:478-484, 1991.
15. Noyes FR, Barber-Westin SD: Reconstruction of the anterior cruciate ligament with human allograft: Comparison of early and late results. J Bone Joint Surg 78:524-537, 1996.
16. Rodeo SA, Arnoczky SP, Tozilli PA: Tendon healing in a bone tunnel: A biomechanical and histological study in the dog. J Bone Joint Surg 75:1795-1803, 1993.

17. Rougraff B, Shelbourne KD, Gerth PK, Warner J: Arthroscopic and histologic analysis of human patellar tendon autografts used for anterior cruciate ligament reconstruction. Am J Knee Surg 21:277-284, 1993.

18. Shaieb MD, Kan DM, Chang SK, et al: A prospective randomized comparison of patellar tendon versus semitendinosus and gracilis tendon autografts for anterior cruciate ligament reconstruction. Am J Sports Med 30:214-220, 2002.

19. Shino K, Kimura T, Hirose H, et al: Reconstruction of the anterior cruciate ligament by allogenic tendon graft: An operation for chronic ligamentous insufficiency. J Bone Joint Surg 68:739-746, 1986.

20. Simonds RJ, Holmberg SD, Hurwitz RL, et al: Transmission of human immunodeficiency virus type 1 from a seronegative organ and tissue donor. N Engl J Med 326:726-732, 1992.

21. Staubli HU, Schatzmann L, Brunner P, et al: Mechanical tensile properties of the quadriceps tendon and patella ligament in young adults. Am J Sports Med 27:27-34, 1999.

22. Webster KE, Feller JA, Hameister KA: Bone tunnel enlargement following anterior cruciate ligament reconstruction: A randomized comparison of hamstring and patellar tendon grafts with 2-year follow up. Knee Surg Traumatol Arthrosc 9:86-91, 2001.

23. Yoshiya S, Nagano M, Korosaka M, et al: Graft healing in the bone tunnel in anterior cruciate ligament reconstruction. Clin Orthop 372:278-286, 2000.

6

Digital Imaging

DON JOHNSON

It has been said that a picture is worth a thousand words, and this is especially true in a visual field such as arthroscopy. It makes sense to capture digitally the images we view daily on the monitor. This improves the documentation of the pathology and its subsequent treatment. It makes it much easier to communicate to the patient what the problem was and what was done to correct it. It also makes a review of the patient in 6 months more relevant. Viewing an image of the chondral surface is better than reading a textual description of the chondromalacia. This information is easily transferred to a referring physician or to another consultant for ongoing treatment. The images can also be used to communicate to others about the patient's pathology in a PowerPoint presentation for rounds or in an instructional course. Now that the importance of the digital image has been established, the method of image acquisition must be examined.

Digital Still Image and Video Acquisition

The digital image can be acquired by scanning in the photographs taken with the Sony printer present on most arthroscopy carts. This is somewhat time-consuming and results in the loss of some image quality. An improvement is to use an image capture unit available from one of the three main suppliers of arthroscopy equipment: Linvatec, Smith and Nephew Dionics, and Stryker (Figs. 6–1 to 6–3). These units are all similar in hardware and software operation. The unit plugs into the back of the arthroscopy camera and is activated by a button on the camera head. When this button is pushed, the image on the screen is captured to a hard disk (Fig. 6–4) and stored in a patient file on the hard drive of a computer. The patient's demographic information has been entered beforehand, and the images are stored in a file folder under the patient's name. At the end of the case or end of the day, the data are written to a compact disk (CD). Short video segments can also be captured, stored, and written to a disk in a similar fashion.

The least inexpensive method to capture digital video is directly from the arthroscopy camera with a video camcorder. This requires a mini-DV camcorder with an SVHS video cable input. The SVHS cable is plugged into the back of the arthroscopy camera and to the digital camcorder. The images and video are recorded by using the camcorder remote to the mini-DV tape or to the memory stick of the Sony camera. The images and video are then titled and archived in the patient's file.

Digital Imaging in the Operating Room

Images of pathology can be acquired by a digital camera. Any digital camera with three megapixels of resolution and a macro function (e.g., those made by Nikon, Olympus, or Sony) is suitable. The most common uses are to photograph patients in the clinic (Fig. 6–5); to take intraoperative photographs, such as of the patellar tendon–bone graft (Fig. 6–6); to photograph magnetic resonance imaging scans (Fig. 6–7) or plain radiographs (Fig. 6–8); and to document the setup for a surgical procedure (Fig. 6–9). If these images are photographed at a high resolution (300 dpi), they can be printed or archived in the patient's file. Use of high resolution requires a high-capacity storage card and plenty of hard disk space, but both are inexpensive. It is recommended that the images be saved at a high resolution initially, because it is difficult to get enough pixels from a low-resolution photograph to print it later (e.g., for publication).

Editing Digital Images

Digital still images can be edited in several inexpensive programs, such as PhotoImpact (www.ulead.com) and PhotoDeluxe (www.adobe.com), or in an expensive professional program, such as PhotoShop (www.adobe.com). The image is imported into the

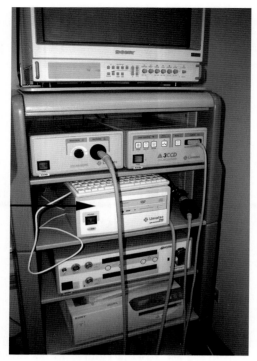

Figure 6–1 Linvatec digital image capture unit.

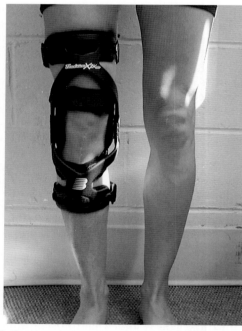

Figure 6–4 Captured digital arthroscopy image of a chronic anterior cruciate ligament tear.

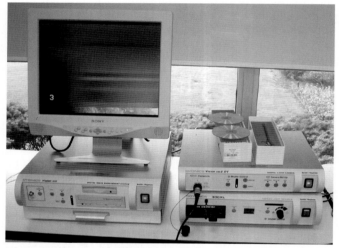

Figure 6–2 Smith and Nephew Dionics digital image capture unit.

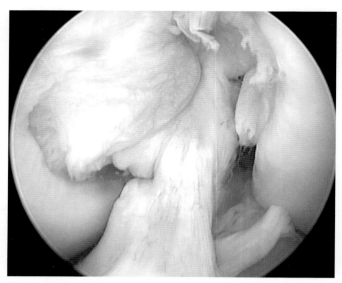

Figure 6–5 Use of a brace to unweight the medial compartment of the knee.

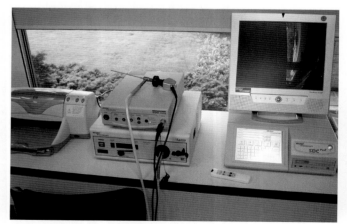

Figure 6–3 Stryker digital image capture unit.

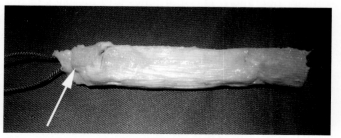

Figure 6–6 Patellar tendon graft.

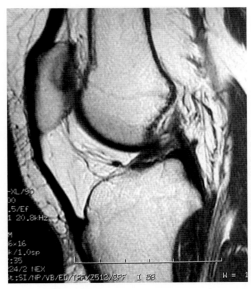

Figure 6–7   Magnetic resonance imaging scan demonstrating an anterior cruciate ligament tear.

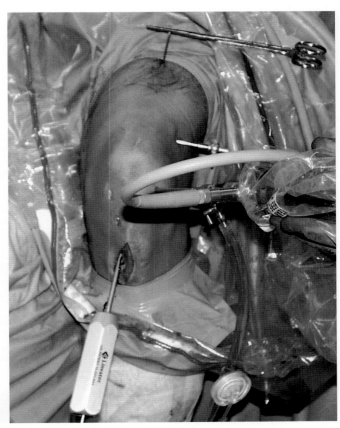

Figure 6–9   Setup for the femoral tunnel guide.

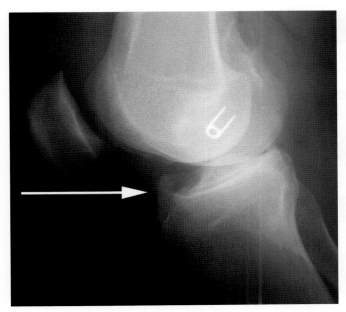

Figure 6–8   Plain lateral radiograph of a knee with an anterior osteophyte.

Archiving the Digital Images

In the long term, it is worthwhile to have a system for archiving the images. There is nothing more frustrating than trying to find that beautiful picture of an anterior cruciate ligament (ACL) tear that you wanted to present at rounds tomorrow morning.

There are a variety of ways to keep track of photographs. The first step is to make folders on the hard drive to store the photos temporarily (Fig. 6–11). The arthroscopy folder is divided into ankle, knee, and shoulder. The knee folder is subdivided into ACL, chondral, meniscus, other, posterior cruciate ligament (PCL), and patellofemoral (PF) joint. The figure shows the knee-ACL folder open. In Win ME, Win 2000, and Win XP, thumbnails of all the images in the folder are displayed. The images from the captured patient file should be copied into these folders. Once you have built up an extensive file of representative images, you can copy only the more interesting or unusual examples. The main file of patient images on the CD or ZIP disk should be printed or inserted into an operative report and stored in a safe place. The file can be stored on a large server for later access, if necessary.

If you have only a few hundred images in each folder,

program, and the common functions such as crop, lighten, darken, and adjust color are performed (Fig. 6–10). The image is then given a name and saved to the hard drive. The low-end programs, costing $50 to $100, perform these common functions just fine, making the $600 PhotoShop program unnecessary.

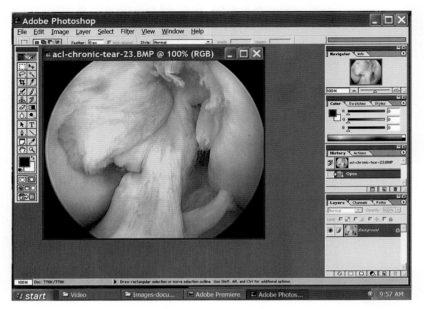

Figure 6–10 PhotoShop editing of the image of a chronic anterior cruciate ligament tear.

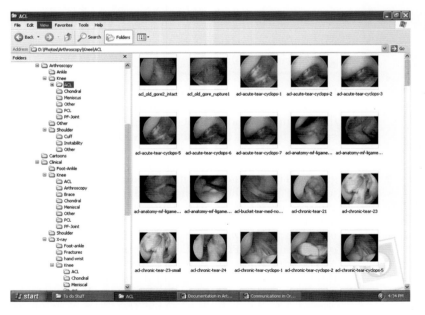

Figure 6–11 Organization of file folders on the hard drive.

using the thumbnail display function is a reasonable way to scan the folder to find the image you want. If you have thousands of images in a folder, however, a program such as ThumbsPlus can be used to search by keywords, for example, "ACL chronic tear" (Fig. 6–12). By assigning each image a keyword or -words, a large database of, say, 25,000 images containing multiple folders can be quickly searched.

Editing and Archiving Digital Video

Similar to the editing programs for still images, digital imaging programs for video range from the inexpensive

VideoStudio (www.ulead.com), Pinnacle studio (www.pinaclesys.com), and Premiere (www.adobe.com) to the expensive professional software such as Final Cut Pro (www.apple.com). These programs are not intuitive, and it takes a considerable investment of time to learn how to use them properly. The best advice is to buy a relatively inexpensive program to cut the captured video into small segments for use in PowerPoint (Fig. 6–13).

When capturing the video file in the operating room, it should be rough edited by filming only the important segments. This initial editing makes the files smaller and much easier to handle later. The file is imported into the timeline in Premier (see Fig. 6–13) and cut into small

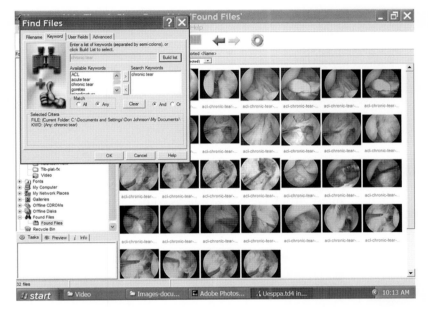

Figure 6–12 Results of a search in ThumbsPlus for chronic anterior cruciate ligament tear.

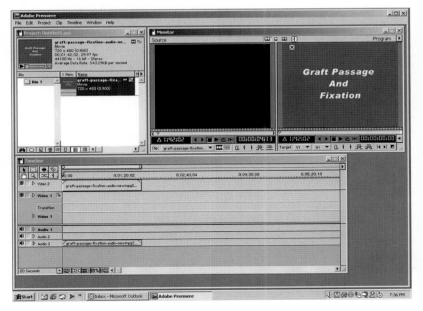

Figure 6–13 Working window of Premiere.

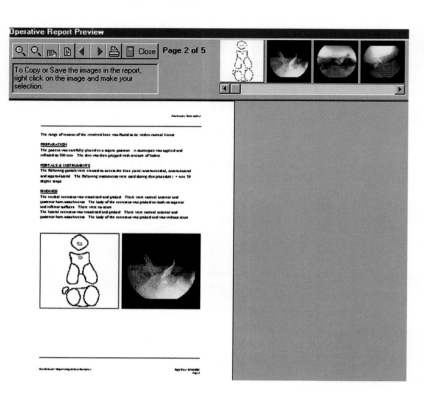

Figure 6–14 Notematic, with the digital images inserted next to the text in a templated operative report.

segments by using the razor tool. The clip is then exported and compressed using a variety of codes. The easiest method is to purchase an Mpeg plug-in for Pre-miere from Ligos (www.ligos.com); Mpeg1 is the standard for PowerPoint presentations.

Importing Digital Images and Video into an Operative Note

One method to keep the images and video organized is to import the appropriate images into an operative report such as Notematic (www.puremed.com) (Fig. 6–14). After the images are imported and printed for the patient's chart, the CD with the original images is stored according to date or patient name. Notematic is a text-based operative report that can be templated for common surgical procedures. The images are imported into the appropriate position in the text; for example, the image of the torn meniscus is placed next to the text description of the meniscal tear. The completed form is stored electronically and printed for insertion into the patient's chart. The video is stored as a compressed file in the electronic record. The original file from the CD must be accessed to edit video for PowerPoint presentations.

Operative Documentation on a Personal Digital Assistant

Data from the operating room can also be documented on a personal digital assistant (PDA) (Fig. 6–15). The PDA touch screen is ideal for entering data with

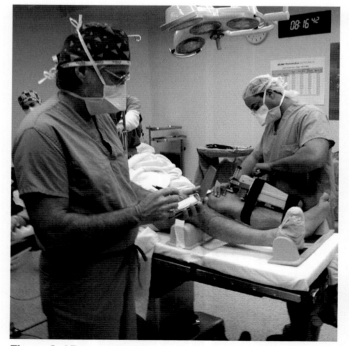

Figure 6–15 Documentation of operative data on a personal digital assistant.

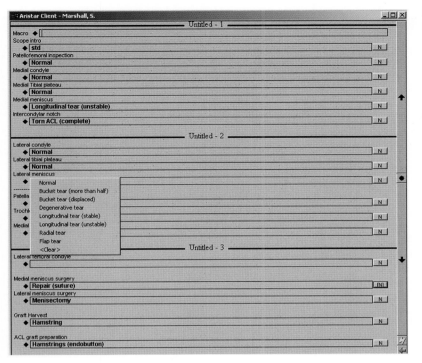

Figure 6-16   Personal digital assistant touch screen with drop-down menus to document operative findings.

pull-down menus (Fig. 6–16). This software, Orthostar (www.aristar.com), can be integrated into the office record or printed out for the traditional patient chart. Which method is better depends on whether you want a stand-alone operative report with images integrated into the printed report or you prefer to have a report that can be part of the office electronic medical record.

Anesthesia and Postoperative Pain

Michail N. Avramov and Shyamala Badrinath

Advances in technology and innovations in surgical technique have led to a steady increase in the number of arthroscopic orthopedic procedures over the last decade. The less invasive nature of arthroscopic surgery allows most of these procedures to be performed on an outpatient or short-admission (<24 hours) basis. Although arthroscopic surgery patients are generally young, active, and healthy, issues related to the outpatient nature of this surgery are major considerations in the choice of anesthetic and perioperative management. Prompt recovery from anesthesia with minimal side effects is essential for early discharge home; however, moderate to severe postoperative pain may be experienced for several days by the majority of patients, especially those undergoing more extensive reconstructive surgery. Thus, an aggressive pain management strategy must be incorporated in the treatment plan. Our modern understanding of the pathophysiology of pain has influenced clinical practice, and concepts such as "preemptive" and "multimodal" analgesia are best implemented as an integrated perioperative and postoperative pain management plan involving both the anesthesiologist and the surgeon. Our goal in this chapter is to provide an overview of the anesthetic aspects of arthroscopic surgery, with an emphasis on outpatient management.

Preoperative Evaluation

Patients presenting for arthroscopic surgery are generally young and otherwise healthy. However, with the growing popularity of arthroscopic procedures, an increasing number of patients have significant comorbidities that could have a significant impact on their perioperative management and outcome. The ultimate goal of the preoperative evaluation is to determine the patient's risk for undergoing surgery and anesthesia and to help optimize his or her preoperative condition.

Although the preoperative evaluation is done by the surgeon and other primary care providers, it is ultimately the anesthesiologist's responsibility to determine the patient's fitness for the administration of anesthesia and to decide on the appropriate anesthetic technique. Taking a history, conducting a physical examination, and performing preoperative testing do not constitute "clearance" for surgery; they do, however, provide information that the anesthesiologist can use to make his or her decision. For patients with chronic medical conditions, the input from primary care providers is especially useful; they have likely been managing such patients for long periods and are familiar with the natural history of their patients' conditions.

The risk to the patient is a function of his or her preoperative physical status (Table 7–1), the nature of the surgical procedure (low, medium, or high risk), and the nature of the planned anesthetic technique (e.g., monitored anesthesia care, regional anesthesia, general anesthesia, or a combination). Patients with no or few well-controlled medical conditions (American Society of Anesthesiologists [ASA] classes I and II) are classified as low risk, and patients with major and potentially life-threatening medical problems (ASA classes III and IV) are classified as high risk. With regard to operative procedure, low-risk procedures are those imposing minimal physiologic stress and risk (independent of medical condition); medium-risk procedures are associated with moderate physiologic stress and risk, with minimal blood loss, fluid shifts, or postoperative changes in normal physiology; and high-risk procedures are associated with significant perioperative and postoperative physiologic stress. Arthroscopic procedures generally fall into the low- to moderate-risk groups, and low-risk patients can usually have their preanesthetic assessment on the day of surgery. Prior consultation with the anesthesiologist may be required for major ambulatory procedures (e.g., extensive shoulder and knee reconstruction), as well as for all high-risk patients, especially those being

Table 7–1 American Society of Anesthesiologists' Physical Status Classification

Class I	A healthy patient
Class II	A patient with mild systemic disease
Class III	A patient with severe systemic disease that limits activity but is not incapacitating
Class IV	A patient with incapacitating systemic disease that is a constant threat to life
Class V	A moribund patient not expected to survive 24 hours with or without operation

"E" is added for procedures performed on an emergency basis.

considered for outpatient procedures. Ultimately, the determination of whether a patient is fit to undergo arthroscopic surgery on an outpatient basis is based on his or her physical status and functional capacity in the context of the expected invasiveness of the procedure; the type of anesthesia; and, not least, the type of outpatient surgery facility (e.g., freestanding versus hospital based).

If the history and physical examination detect a condition that may adversely affect the safe performance of the proposed procedure or its outcome, further preoperative testing is indicated. Testing without a specific indication, however, is of low utility and may only contribute to morbidity and excessive costs. The usual approach to preoperative testing in patients undergoing outpatient procedures includes the following:

- Electrocardiogram—for patients with hypertension, other current or past significant cardiovascular disease, or diabetes mellitus.
- Chest radiograph—for patients with asthma or chronic obstructive pulmonary disease with a change in symptoms or an acute episode within the past 6 months.
- Serum chemistry—for patients with kidney disease or adrenal or thyroid disorders and those undergoing therapy with diuretics.
- Complete blood count—for patients with hematologic disorders or undergoing chemotherapy.
- Coagulation studies—for patients undergoing anticoagulation therapy.
- Pregnancy testing—for patients of uncertain pregnancy status by history and examination.

Patients with comorbidities that significantly increase their operative risk for major surgery may be able to safely undergo a minor procedure (e.g., diagnostic arthroscopy) on an outpatient basis and be discharged home 2 to 3 hours after its completion. The most common comorbidities that influence patient selection for outpatient procedures are respiratory disease (reactive airway disease), heart disease (ischemic or valvular), and obesity. The most important question is whether the coexisting condition is well controlled. Patients with reactive airway disease need to be evaluated with regard to the severity of symptoms, recent or current upper respiratory tract infection, and history of previous responses to anesthesia. For such patients, the need for general anesthesia versus regional or local anesthesia with sedation may be the decisive factor in whether the procedure can be safely performed on an outpatient basis. Patients with heart disease who have poor exercise tolerance, signs of unstable angina, decompensated congestive heart failure, or arrhythmia require further assessment even for minor procedures, including stress testing and echocardiogram to evaluate ventricular function. Because of the prevalence of obesity, outpatient surgery facilities often impose eligibility limits based on body mass index; however, additional considerations, such as the presence and severity of sleep apnea, preoperative use of analgesics, and expected need for postoperative opioid analgesics, are no less important than weight itself.

Anesthetic Techniques

Arthroscopic procedures can be categorized as upper extremity procedures and lower extremity procedures. Upper extremity procedures include arthroscopy of the shoulder, elbow, and wrist. The most common lower extremity procedures are arthroscopy of the knee and ankle. Such an anatomic classification is useful, because it relates to the distinct regional anesthetic techniques used—brachial plexus blocks for the upper extremity versus central neuraxial (spinal, epidural) or peripheral nerve blocks for the lower extremity. Because virtually all regions involved in arthroscopic procedures of the upper and the lower extremities are amenable to some kind of regional anesthetic technique, the choice of anesthesia for these procedures has traditionally included both general and regional techniques.

The advent of newer, shorter-acting intravenous (propofol) and inhaled (sevoflurane, desflurane) anesthetics that allow rapid recovery and have a low incidence of postoperative nausea and vomiting has had a significant impact on outpatient anesthetic management. Not surprisingly, in contrast to previous studies that used older inhaled agents and found regional (e.g., epidural) techniques to be advantageous,[14] it is now generally accepted that rapid turnover and prompt recovery with a low incidence of adverse effects can be easily achieved with general anesthesia. However, the main factors that prolong recovery and delay discharge after ambulatory surgery are pain, nausea and vomiting, urinary retention, and unresolved neuraxial blocks. Orthopedic procedures are associated with a high incidence of pain (16%) during the immediate postoperative recovery period in ambulatory patients,[5] and pain accounted for half the unanticipated hospital admissions in a series of 1996 patients undergoing outpatient orthopedic surgery.[10] Therefore, postoperative pain remains a major concern, especially after extensive reconstructive surgery. Although regional techniques can provide superior pain relief, they must be chosen carefully so that they do not cause a significant delay in discharge. Ultimately, the choice of anesthetic technique is based on the intraoperative and postoperative demands of the surgical procedure and the preferences of the patient, surgeon, and anesthesiologist. In our practice, the combined use of regional and general anesthesia is most popular.

Arthroscopic shoulder surgery comprises a variety of diagnostic and reconstructive procedures notable for causing significant, persistent postoperative pain. When such procedures are performed on an outpatient basis, inadequate pain control is a primary reason for unanticipated hospital admissions,[12] and regional (e.g., interscalene block) techniques are commonly used. The interscalene approach to brachial plexus block (ISB) was introduced by Winnie.[18] It provides adequate sensory and motor block for procedures over the shoulder and proximal upper extremity. There are several excellent descriptions of the anatomic landmarks and technique of ISB (Fig. 7–1).[3,4] The efficacy and safety of this technique have been demonstrated in numerous studies. However, potential serious complications include central nervous system toxicity (e.g., seizures); cardiac toxicity (e.g., cardiac arrest); pneumothorax; high spinal or epidural block due to accidental injection; hematoma formation; and phrenic, laryngeal, or vagal nerve injury. ISB produces ipsilateral diaphragmatic paresis, decreasing forced vital capacity by up to 30%.[16] It is contraindicated in patients who would be unable to tolerate respiratory compromise, such as those with severe chronic obstructive pulmonary disease, contralateral phrenic nerve palsy, or pneumonectomy.

Although ISB is a commonly used technique, few large-scale studies have carefully evaluated the incidence of complications associated with its use. In a survey of major complications of regional anesthesia in France,[1] ISB appeared to be quite safe: there was only one case of peripheral neuropathy in 3459 blocks performed (for an incidence of 2.9 per 10,000). Borgeat et al.[2] conducted one of the most extensive outcome studies of complications associated with ISB. It included 521 patients who were observed for 10 days postoperatively and followed up for 9 months. The overall incidence of acute and severe chronic complications was 0.4%. Acute complications included pneumothorax in one patient (0.2%); central nervous system intoxication, expressed as incoherent speech shortly after administration of the drug, in one patient (0.2%); and aspiration of blood on injection in three patients (0.6%), which did not preclude successful performance of the block after redirecting the needle. At 10 days postoperatively, there was a relatively high incidence (up to 14%) of transient problems consisting of paresthesia, dysesthesia, and pain. Other nonacute complications included sulcus ulnaris syndrome (1.5%), complex regional pain syndrome (1%), carpal tunnel syndrome (0.8%), and plexus neuropathy (0.2%). In addition, one patient (0.2%) suffered severe plexus

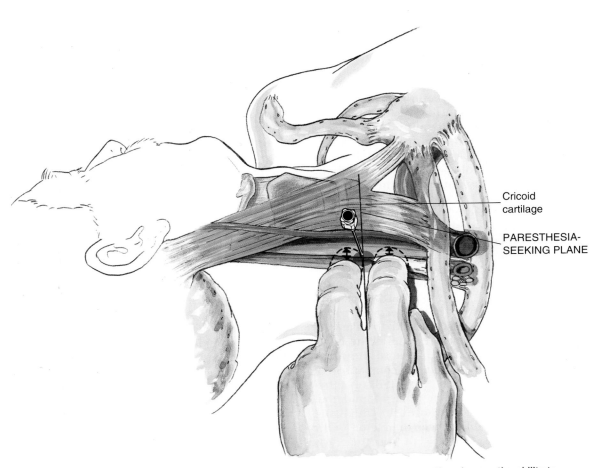

Cricoid
cartilage

PARESTHESIA-
SEEKING PLANE

Figure 7–1   Interscalene block: paresthesia-seeking plane. The use of a stimulator greatly enhances the ability to position the tip of the needle close to the nerve. (From Brown DL: Atlas of Regional Anesthesia, 2nd ed. Philadelphia, WB Saunders, 1999.)

damage after an apparently uneventful ISB without paresthesia or pain on injection; this was the only patient who remained symptomatic at 9 months. All other patients with longer-term complications had spontaneous resolution during the sixth to ninth postoperative months.

The potential for serious complications with ISB was recently reinforced by Weber and Jain[17] in a retrospective study of a series of 218 patients. Two patients developed temporary neurologic injuries that persisted at 6 weeks; one patient had a full recovery by 12 weeks, but the other had persistent weakness and numbness 2 years after the procedure. In addition, one patient suffered a grand mal seizure. There was one episode of cardiovascular collapse and four episodes of severe respiratory distress. The same authors surveyed members of the American Shoulder and Elbow Society and found 57 temporary and 25 permanent nerve injuries related to ISB.[17] However, it may be difficult to confirm a causal relationship between neurologic injury of the brachial plexus and ISB during shoulder surgery. Factors other than those related to the block itself (e.g., direct needle trauma, intraneural injection of local anesthetic, local anesthetic toxicity) may be involved, including stretching and compression of the plexus due to positioning and surgical technique. Unpublished outcome data from our outpatient surgical center indicate that the incidence of new-onset neurologic symptoms (e.g., numbness, tingling, muscle twitching) at 7 days after surgery is essentially the same for patients having general anesthesia combined with ISB (14%) and those having general anesthesia without block (18%). This underscores the importance of accounting for non-ISB-related factors when estimating the impact of anesthesia on neurologic complications after shoulder surgery. However, given the lack of extensive outcome data in the literature and medicolegal considerations that may lead to underreporting of complications, the potential for serious complications with ISB, including neurologic injury, should be included in the risk-benefit assessment and in discussions with the patient.

As pointed out earlier, our current practice is to combine ISB with general anesthesia. This provides for reliable intraoperative conditions without a delay for a complete evaluation of the block's efficacy preoperatively. The reported failure rate of ISB (requiring supplemental opioids, conversion to general anesthesia) is on the order of 9% to 13%.[3,17] Up to a third of patients may require intravenous opioids in the recovery room, and virtually all patients are encouraged to take oral opioids to avoid experiencing severe pain as the block starts to wear off. This is essential, because the mean duration of ISB is usually 6 to 15 hours. A comparison of patients managed postoperatively with ISB or intravenous patient-controlled analgesia (PCA) found that ISB provided superior pain relief only during the first 4 to 6 hours; there were no differences thereafter.[20] Our own experience indicates that except for the early postanesthesia care unit (PACU) recovery period, pain scores and oral analgesic requirements are similar in patients with and without ISB. Thus it is not surprising that some practitioners, especially at smaller community hospitals, are reevaluating the utility of ISB. Lewis and Buss[12] reported excellent outcomes and a high level of patient satisfaction with the use of general anesthesia alone and concluded that, given its costs and risks, the marginal benefit of adding ISB may not be justified for routine use. However, their readmission rate of 5% (for pain or intractable nausea) is considerably higher than the overall readmission rate for ambulatory surgery facilities (<1%). So, in the setting of a busy outpatient surgery center, the use of ISB during the first few postoperative hours may actually be quite beneficial. It would minimize the need for intraoperative and postoperative intravenous opioids, thereby reducing the risk of postoperative nausea and vomiting and provide for a smooth, pain-free recovery and prompt discharge home. Future outcome data may help resolve the question of the ideal approach to anesthetic management for arthroscopic shoulder surgery.

For procedures below the shoulder, axillary block is commonly used. It involves the injection of a large volume of local anesthetic (40 to 50 mL) into the perivascular sheath of the axillary artery using either the transarterial approach or paresthesia. A nerve stimulator can be used to identify the different nerves (median, radial, ulnar, and musculocutaneous) and decide where to inject the local anesthetic or place a catheter (Fig. 7–2). Complications associated with axillary block in a series of 11,024 blocks included seizures in one patient (for an incidence of 0.9 per 10,000) and peripheral neuropathy in two patients (1.8 per 10,000).[16] Axillary block is popular because it is efficacious and simple to perform. Arthroscopy of the elbow and wrist can be done using this anesthetic method, with intravenous sedation added as required. This ensures prompt recovery, excellent postoperative pain control, and early discharge home.

Knee arthroscopy is one of the most commonly performed outpatient orthopedic procedures. The nature of the procedure may differ significantly—from "one-look" diagnostic arthroscopy to various degrees of repair or arthroscopically assisted reconstruction (e.g., allograft, anterior cruciate ligament reconstruction). Accordingly, virtually all kinds of anesthetic techniques, including local anesthesia alone or in combination with intravenous sedation, regional anesthesia, central neuraxial (epidural, spinal) or general anesthesia, and combinations thereof, have been used and recommended. It is important to realize that there is considerable bias in patients' and surgeons' preferences regarding the optimal anesthetic technique.

Some consider intra-articular administration of local anesthetic the technique of first choice for knee arthroscopy.[6] It is simple to perform, is inexpensive, and provides good postoperative pain control for less extensive procedures. However, it does not provide adequate muscle relaxation, and patient acceptance is generally low. For these reasons, we routinely use general anesthesia (propofol–nitrous oxide), with intra-articular instillation of local anesthetic for postoperative pain control. The addition of clonidine and morphine to the intra-articular local anesthetic solution has been shown to improve postoperative analgesia.[8]

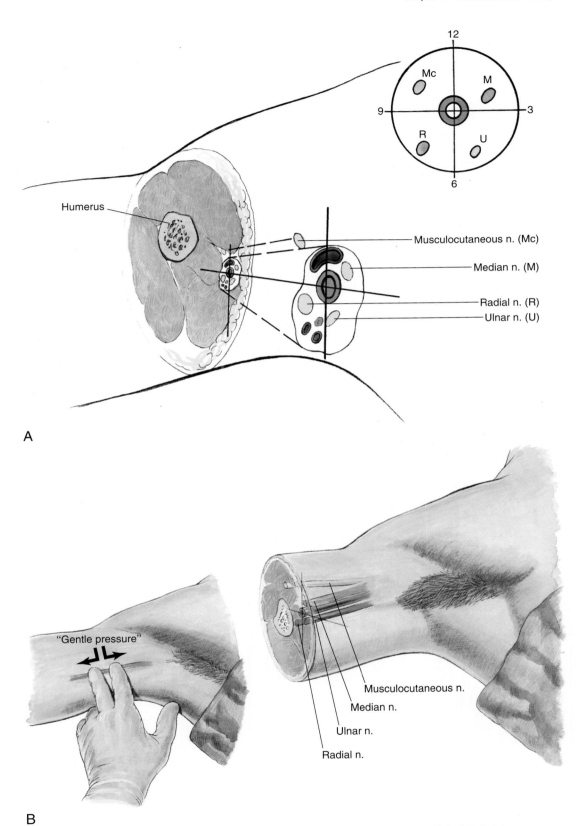

A

B

Figure 7–2   **Axillary block. *A*, Functional anatomy at the level of the distal axilla. *B*, Clinical technique— positioning of the arm and palpation of the artery (lower panel).** (From Brown DL: Atlas of Regional Anesthesia, 2nd ed. Philadelphia, WB Saunders, 1999.)

Peripheral blocks of the lumbar plexus nerves, combined with sciatic nerve block, can provide excellent conditions for performing almost any lower extremity procedure. The advantages of peripheral nerve blocks include adequate muscle relaxation, intense and prolonged analgesia, low incidence of urinary retention, and preservation of contralateral leg strength, which allows almost immediate ambulation with crutches and early discharge. The most commonly used techniques are femoral nerve block (Fig. 7–3), "three-in-one" block, lateral femoral cutaneous nerve block, and fascia iliaca compartment block. Peripheral nerve blocks take longer to perform than other anesthetic techniques, and experience is required to improve their success rate. The availability of catheters and single-use pumps has produced a resurgence in their use, especially for postoperative pain control. Conversely, modern protocols for postoperative physical therapy often require active participation early after surgery, and the persistence of

motor block may be a limiting factor to the use of nerve blocks.

Neuraxial blocks are relatively easy to perform and widely used. Spinal anesthesia is simple and reliable but is limited by the injection of a single dose. Administering larger doses results in delayed discharge (requiring longer stays than with general anesthesia); reducing the dose shortens the recovery time but increases the failure rate. The occurrence of transient neurologic symptoms after the use of spinal lidocaine and the increased incidence of such complications when procedures are performed in positions that stretch the spinal nerve roots (e.g., arthroscopy) have limited its use. Numerous studies have attempted to find the optimal dose and drug for subarachnoid block.[7,15] This search has continued with the introduction of selective spinal anesthesia—a technique of using minimal doses of hyperbaric local anesthetics to provide only segmental block for the roots supplying the relevant area. This requires longer

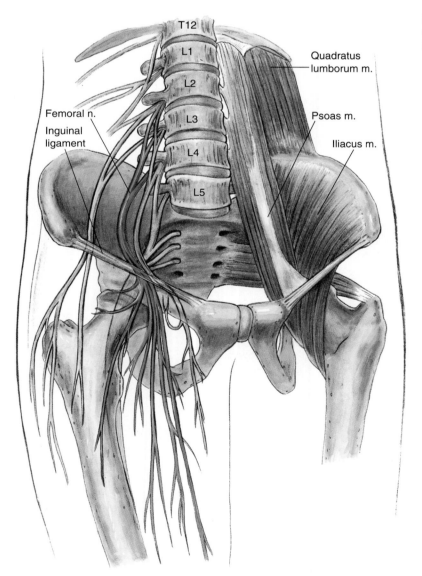

Figure 7–3 **Femoral nerve block: anatomic landmarks.** (From Brown DL: Atlas of Regional Anesthesia, 2nd ed. Philadelphia, WB Saunders, 1999.)

preparation (maintenance of the lateral decubitus position for 10 minutes), and the success rate is not 100%. Epidural block with a shorter-duration local anesthetic (e.g., chloroprocaine) is another alternative. Mulroy et al.[13] concluded that epidural block provides recovery and discharge times comparable to those obtained with general anesthesia. However, in common with spinal anesthesia, epidural block takes longer to perform than to start general anesthesia, and the risk of postdural puncture headache is always present.

The anesthetic of choice for general anesthesia is intravenous propofol–nitrous oxide, supplemented with an opioid such as sufentanil. We try to avoid inhalation agents to minimize the risk of postoperative nausea and vomiting. Also, with inhalation techniques, patients are less alert and oriented shortly after the procedure than they are with intravenous techniques.

The choice of anesthesia for lower extremity arthroscopy depends largely on the nature of the procedure, as well as patient, surgeon, and anesthesiologist preferences. There is a variety of choices, and satisfactory anesthesia can be provided for both the patient who would like to be awake and alert during surgery and the patient who would prefer to be unaware.

Postoperative Pain Management

Pain management is a critical part of the perioperative care of arthroscopy patients, because the majority of patients experience moderate to severe pain for at least 2 to 3 days postoperatively. Adequate postoperative pain control before discharge, with successful conversion to oral analgesics, is essential in the outpatient setting. Advances in the understanding of postoperative pain pathophysiology have led to a more rational approach to pain management in these patients.

Although not completely elucidated, the changes in pain processing induced by surgery and the perioperative use of analgesics have a significant impact on patients' postoperative opiate requirements and pain experience. The trauma of arthroscopic surgery stimulates free nerve endings and afferent nociceptors. This barrage of activity is augmented by the effects of tissue inflammation factors such as bradykinin, histamine, and serotonin, which are released from the damaged cells. In addition to direct stimulation, these neuroactive peptides act in concert with prostaglandins (specifically the arachidonic acid derivative prostaglandin E_2) to sensitize the peripheral primary nociceptive afferents, by decreasing their activation threshold and shortening their response latency, and alter the central processing of sensory stimuli by facilitating nociceptive transmission in the spinal cord dorsal horn. This sensitization is considered the neurophysiologic basis for the state of exaggerated pain sensation characterized clinically by the phenomena of hyperalgesia—a state of increased sensitivity to stimuli that are painful under normal conditions—and allodynia—painful sensation caused by normally innocuous stimuli such as light touch. Although the effect of sustained nociceptive activity is

essential for the establishment of primary hyperalgesia, the action of the tissue mediators of pain and inflammation is diffuse—not limited to the projection area of the initial pain—and "spreads" the pain by secondary hyperalgesia involving areas farther away from the skin incision. This sequential mechanism is important not only for understanding the pathophysiology of hyperalgesia but also for making rational choices among the techniques and drugs available for postoperative pain management.

The concept of preemptive analgesia is based on the initiation of treatment *before* the onset of surgical pain to prevent peripheral and central sensitization in the first place.[19] Numerous studies have explored this concept, especially with the use of epidural analgesia; however, not all outcomes are consistent, and the concept remains debatable.[11] The realization that postoperative pain involves multiple pathophysiologic mechanisms and mediators and that achieving optimal pain relief using a single drug can be associated with significant side effects has led to the principle of "multimodal" or "balanced" analgesia.[9] It involves combination therapy with different analgesic drugs and different treatment techniques. In the setting of arthroscopic surgery, this involves nonsteroidal anti-inflammatory drugs, nerve blocks (peripheral and central neural), opioids, N-methyl-D-aspartate agonists (ketamine), local anesthetics, infiltration with local anesthetic at incision sites (before and after surgery), intra-articular local anesthetics or opioids, and postoperative opioids and nonsteroidal anti-inflammatory drugs (around the clock for the first 24 to 48 hours, then on an as-needed basis).

References

1. Auroy Y, Benlamon D, Bargues L, et al: Major complications of regional anesthesia in France. Anesthesiology 97:1274-1280, 2002.
2. Borgeat A, Ekatodramis G, Kalberer F, Benz C: Acute and nonacute complications associated with interscalene block and shoulder surgery. Anesthesiology 95:875-889, 2001.
3. Brown AR, Weiss R, Greenberg C, et al: Interscalene block for shoulder arthroscopy: Comparison with general anesthesia. Arthroscopy 9:295-300, 1993.
4. Brown DL: Interscalene block. In Atlas of Regional Anesthesia, 2nd ed. Philadelphia, WB Saunders, 1999, pp 23-29.
5. Chung F, Ritchie W, Su J: Postoperative pain in ambulatory surgery. Anesth Analg 85:808-816, 1997.
6. Goranson BD, Lang S, Cassidy JD, et al: A comparison of three regional anesthetic techniques for outpatient knee arthroscopy. Can J Anaesth 44:371-376, 1997.
7. Iskander H, Benard A, Ruel-Raymond J, et al: Femoral block provides superior analgesia compared with intra-articular ropivacaine after anterior cruciate ligament reconstruction. Reg Anesth Pain Med 28:29-32, 2003.
8. Joshi W, Reuben SS, Kilaru PR, et al: Postoperative analgesia for outpatient arthroscopic knee surgery with intraarticular clonidine and/or morphine. Anesth Analg 90:1102-1106, 2000.
9. Kehlet H, Dahl JB: The value of "multimodal" or "balanced analgesia" in postoperative pain treatment. Anesth Analg 77:1048-1056, 1993.

10. Kinnard P, Lirette R: Outpatient orthopedic surgery: A retrospective study of 1996 patients. Can J Surg 34:363-366, 1991.

11. Kissin I: Preemptive analgesia. Anesthesiology 93:1138-1143, 2000.

12. Lewis RA, Buss DD: Outpatient shoulder surgery: A prospective analysis of a perioperative protocol. Clin Orthop 390:138-141, 2001.

13. Mulroy ME, Larkin KL, Hodgson PS, et al: A comparison of spinal, epidural, and general anesthesia for outpatient knee arthroscopy. Anesth Analg 91:860-864, 2000.

14. Parnass SM, McCarthy RJ, Bach BR, et al: Beneficial impact of epidural anesthesia on recovery after outpatient arthroscopy. Arthroscopy 9:91-95, 1993.

15. Pawlowski J, Sukhani R, Pappas AL, et al: The anesthetic and recovery profile of two doses (60 and 80 mg) of plain mepivacaine for ambulatory spinal anesthesia. Anesth Analg 91:580-584, 2000.

16. Urmey WF, McDonald M: Hemidiaphragmatic paresis during interscalene brachial plexus block: Effects on pulmonary function and chest wall mechanics. Anesth Analg 74:352-357, 1992.

17. Weber SC, Jain R: Scalene regional anesthesia for shoulder surgery in a community setting; an assessment of risk. J Bone Joint Surg 84:775-779, 2002.

18. Winnie AP: Interscalene brachial plexus block. Anesth Analg 49:455-466, 1970.

19. Woolf CJ, Chong M: Preemptive analgesia: Treating postoperative pain by preventing the establishment of central sensitization. Anesth Analg 77:362-379, 1993.

20. Wu CL, Rouse LM, Chen JM, Miller RJ: Comparison of postoperative pain in patients receiving interscalene block or general anesthesia for shoulder surgery. Orthopedics 25:45-48, 2002.

ARTHROSCOPY OF THE SHOULDER

Shoulder: Patient Positioning, Portal Placement, and Normal Arthroscopic Anatomy

Augustus D. Mazzocca, Brian J. Cole, and Anthony A. Romeo

The concept of shoulder arthroscopy was introduced in 1931 by Burman[4] when he reported on the direct visualization of cadaver joints. Our understanding of and experience with this valuable tool have increased significantly since that time. The anatomy of the shoulder can be examined in detail, allowing analysis of its structure and form. This ability can confirm diagnoses, provide information about particular shoulder pathologies, and improve patient care. In addition, because less soft tissue dissection is required, arthroscopic procedures can result in decreased postoperative pain and generally better early rehabilitation. Patient positioning, portal placement, and fluid management are critical elements in performing effective, reproducible shoulder arthroscopy. This chapter reviews these elements to provide a basic understanding of the performance of other procedures presented in this book.

Preoperative Considerations

A combination of interscalene block and general anesthesia is preferred, leading to a reduced need for inhalation agents and the achievement of postoperative pain relief. Maintenance of a mean arterial pressure of 70 to 90 mm Hg or a systolic blood pressure of 100 mm Hg maximizes visualization.[18]

Obesity is a factor that should be considered before shoulder arthroscopy. A patient with a large abdomen who is placed in a beach chair position runs the risk of superior vena cava compression, causing decreased venous return and resulting in uncontrollable hypotension. The physician must be willing to lower the back of the table to facilitate the proper return of blood flow to the heart and restore adequate cardiac output if this problem arises. Another consideration for obese patients is that most operating room beds are rated for 400 pounds. Patients weighing more than 400 pounds require two operating room beds placed together, with the patient in the lateral position with a distraction device.

Examination under Anesthesia

An examination under anesthesia (EUA) is performed with the patient in a supine position. Particular attention is paid to the range of motion (ROM) and stability of the affected shoulder. Comparison between the affected and unaffected limbs should be carried out before the patient is positioned. The EUA is used to support the diagnosis based on the preoperative history, physical examination, and radiographic studies.

Range of Motion

Internal and external rotation with the arm abducted to 90 degrees and at the side should be recorded. An increase in external rotation with the arm at the side may indicate a subscapularis tear, and an increase of internal rotation of the arm abducted to 90 degrees may indicate a posterior rotator cuff tear (infraspinatus or teres minor). Limited external rotation with the arm at the side is seen in osteoarthritis or adhesive capsulitis. Limited internal rotation with the arm abducted is evidence of a tight posterior capsule.

Stability

Labral pathology can be detected during the EUA. A click or grind with loading of the glenohumeral joint can often be elicited in an anesthetized patient who may have been too apprehensive to allow this physical finding to occur while conscious. Increased pathologic translation can also be detected with the EUA. Posterior instability testing can be carried out with the shoulder flexed to 140 degrees (allowing the greater tuberosity to clear the acromion) and adducted to 15 degrees as a posterior-directed axial force is applied. The scapula must be stabilized with the opposite hand when performing this test (Fig. 8–1). Anterior instability can be demonstrated by abducting the arm to 90 degrees and applying an axial and anterior force while stabilizing the scapula. Some other forms of instability may not be apparent with these

maneuvers because such extremes of motion tend to tighten the shoulder capsule. In this case, the arm should be held in neutral with the capsule relaxed, and the humeral head should be grabbed by the examiner's fingers and translated anteriorly and posteriorly. Translation to the glenoid rim is classified as grade I instability, translation over the glenoid rim with spontaneous reduction is grade II, and translation over the rim that is locked and irreducible is classified as grade III.[1] Once the EUA is completed, the patient is positioned.

Patient Positioning

Beach Chair

In the beach chair position (Fig. 8–2), the patient is aligned on the edge of the table so that the affected shoulder is not supported by it (i.e., the medial scapula is parallel and adjacent to the table's edge). Some operating room tables are equipped with headrests with removable backs so that the entire posterosuperior quadrant of the patient is easily accessible. The operating room table is flexed approximately 45 to 60 degrees, and the patient's legs are lowered so that they are parallel to the floor. Lowering the legs beyond the horizontal would allow operative equipment placed on the patient's thighs to slide down to the floor. This is easily remedied by having a Mayo stand positioned over the patient's thighs to hold any operative equipment. The back of the table is completely elevated, which positions the acromion at an approximately 90-degree angle to the floor and places the glenohumeral joint in an anatomic position. The table back is lowered to 30 degrees if conversion to an open procedure is required.

Lateral Decubitus

In the lateral position, the patient must be placed on a beanbag or other stabilizing device, with all bony prominences padded. The patient's torso is rolled posterior 25 to 30 degrees to position the glenoid parallel to the floor (Fig. 8–3). This also opens up the joint and facilitates access into the shoulder joint with the arthroscope. An axillary roll is placed under the thorax distal to the axilla to protect the brachial plexus, and the patient's torso is secured. Once positioned, the arm is suspended so that it can be prepared and draped in a sterile surgical fashion. With the lateral decubitus position, the arm is placed in a foam traction sleeve and connected to the traction device (Fig. 8-4). It is positioned in 45 degrees of abduction and 15 degrees of forward flexion. This arm position is adequate for visualization of both the glenohumeral joint and the subacromial space, obviating the need for repositioning during the procedure. Some surgeons prefer to increase the angle of the arm to 70 degrees, allowing the greater tuberosity to be in a more abducted position and taking tension off the deltoid muscle. Traction is then applied with the arm in neutral. If the arm is rotated, traction should not be placed. Ten pounds is placed for arm distraction, and 10 pounds is

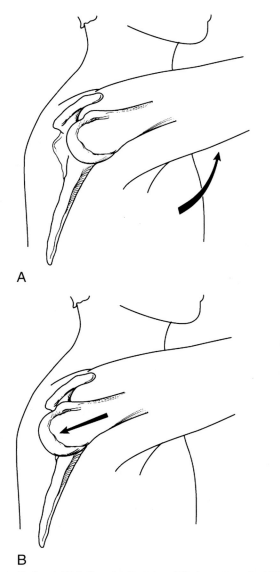

A

B

Figure 8–1 *A*, With the arm flexed to 140 degrees and adducted 15 degrees, the greater tuberosity clears the acromion. *B*, Posterior-directed axial force with stabilization of the scapula allows the testing of posterior restraints.

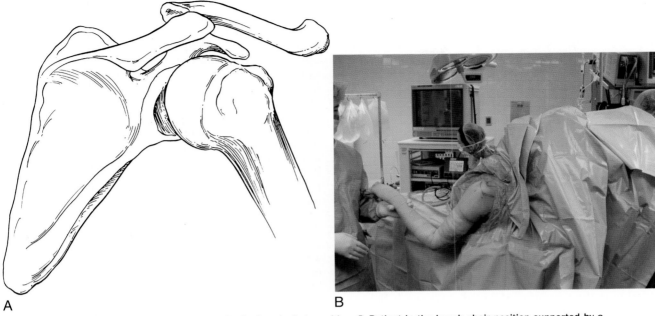

Figure 8–2   *A,* Scapular-humeral articulation in the beach chair position. *B,* Patient in the beach chair position supported by a McConnell headrest and side plate.

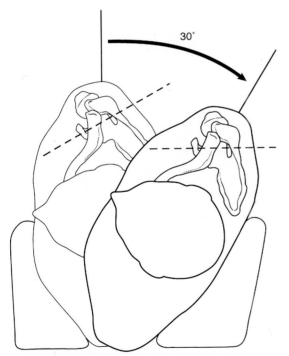

Figure 8–3   Lateral decubitus position with the patient angled 30 degrees posteriorly to place the glenoid parallel to the floor.

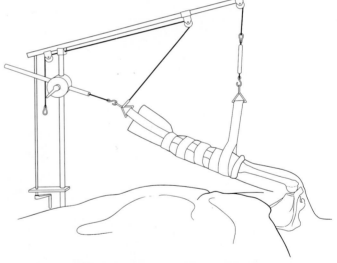

Figure 8–4   Lateral decubitus position with the arm in a foam sleeve. For glenohumeral surgery, the arm is abducted to 45 degrees. For subacromial surgery, the arm is abducted only 20 to 30 degrees. (Courtesy of Arthrex, Naples, FL.)

Skin Preparation and Draping

There are numerous commercially available bacteriostatic solutions for use in operating rooms and surgery centers. There is no consensus about the necessity of shaving the axilla at the time of surgery. Having the least amount of skin accessible to the surgical wound is desirable.

Draping for shoulder arthroscopy follows the same principles as for other operative procedures. The basic

placed for abduction traction. The humerus is allowed to float away from the glenoid. Optimal traction is achieved when the arm is in a neutral position so that the shoulder capsule ligaments are relaxed. More than 20 pounds of weight is not recommended because a neurapraxia may develop as traction weight increases.[8,14]

difference is the potential for a tremendous amount of fluid to be distributed about the surgical field. Plastic U drapes with water bags or receptacles placed proximally and distally to the axilla may limit this phenomenon. Inadvertently draping out the surgical field during preparation must be avoided.

Equipment Setup

After the completion of patient positioning, equipment setup is considered. A tower containing a video monitor, control box, light source, shaver power source, videotape recorder, and irrigation pump is placed opposite the surgeon at the level of the shoulder on the opposite side of the patient (Fig. 8–5A). This positioning provides for visualization of the video monitor and allows the equipment to be serviced without interfering with the arthroscopist. A Mayo stand is placed distal to the first assistant and should contain the basic or more frequently used equipment necessary to complete the case (Fig. 8–5B). A back table is then positioned within easy reach behind

the first assistant; this should contain procedure-specific equipment (Fig. 8–5C).

With the patient in the beach chair position, the surgeon stands slightly behind the shoulder, and the operating table is moved slightly away from the anesthesiologist to give the surgeon more room. The arthroscopy monitor is positioned on the opposite side of the patient at the level of the shoulders for easy viewing by the surgeon. The arthroscopy pump and electrocautery unit are positioned just distal (toward the patient's feet) from the arthroscopy tower. The assistant surgeon stands next to the operating surgeon in front of the patient's shoulder. The assistant's role is to position the arm as required by the specific surgical procedure. Surgical scrub technicians stand behind the surgeon and the assistant.

With the patient in the lateral position, the head of the table is turned away from the anesthesiologist. The surgeon stands above the patient's shoulder, and the assistant is below the surgeon. The surgical scrub technician is positioned behind the surgeon. The table can be rotated 180 degrees so that the anesthesiologist is situated at the patient's feet, but the anesthesiologist has

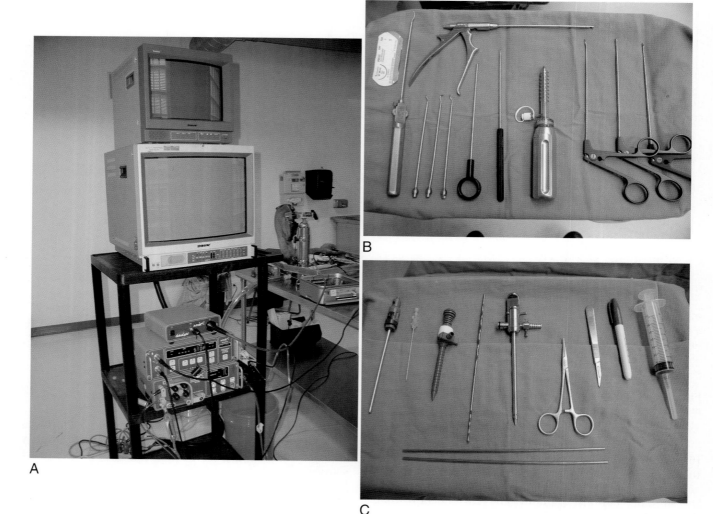

Figure 8–5 *A,* Arthroscopy tower. *B* and *C,* Basic arthroscopic instrumentation.

to be comfortable with this technique. The benefit of this position is that it allows the surgeon complete access to the anterior and posterior aspect of the shoulder by walking around the head of the table.

For diagnostic arthroscopy, a 30-degree arthroscope, cannula, tubing, and probe are the only items needed. For any debridement work, a motorized shaver, bur, and electrocautery or ablation device are used. For reconstructive procedures, the necessary cannulas and fixation devices must be available.

Pumps and Fluid System

Fluid management is critical to shoulder arthroscopy, and understanding fluid dynamics is vital for the performance of advanced arthroscopic procedures. Despite the success of laparoscopy, the fear of pneumomediastinum made isotonic fluid the preferred choice over carbon dioxide.[3,6,7,11–13] Glycine is another fluid that allows excellent visualization, but it is more expensive than sterile saline. In general, the fluid pressure within the glenohumeral joint is kept close to 30 mm Hg; it increases to between 40 and 70 mm Hg in the subacromial space, allowing adequate visualization of the anatomy. Maintenance of a mean arterial pressure around 70 to 90 mm Hg or a systolic blood pressure of 100 mm Hg improves visualization of the shoulder, especially in the subacromial space.[18] Increasing the pressure or flow may cause extravasation of fluid into the soft tissues, distortion of the anatomy, and a gradually decreasing field due to the swollen tissues. Therefore, achieving a balance between fluid pressure or flow and the patient's vital signs is valuable during shoulder arthroscopy.

Fluid management during shoulder arthroscopy is critical for visualization and to minimize postoperative morbidity. There are four basic parameters in fluid management: flow, flow rate, resistance, and pressure. Flow is determined by Poiseuille's law (flow = pressure/resistance), leading to fluid inflow during arthroscopy.[16] Flow rate is the amount of fluid that moves past a specific point over a specified period; it is measured in liters per minute and is dependent on inflow (flow of fluid into the joint space) and outflow (flow of fluid out of the joint space). Resistance is based on the diameter of the tube and the diameter of the cannula. Pressure is a measure of force over a certain area; it is measured in millimeters of mercury, and when the inflow equals the outflow, the pressure is stable or in equilibrium. Flow in shoulder arthroscopy is important for keeping the field of view clear, because it flushes blood and debris from the field. It also increases blade-cutting efficiency. Pressure in shoulder arthroscopy distends the joint and helps control bleeding. The two main goals of fluid management systems are to maintain the desired pressure to provide for adequate distention and to control bleeding by means of flow rates to keep the surgical field clear.

Outflow is another critical element in the shoulder arthroscopy system, and it aids in preventing extravasation of fluid into the tissues. Fluid in any system takes the path of least resistance. The subacromial region is a potential space, and a higher pressure forces fluid out through the point of least resistance. Outflow to gravity allows fluid to exit in this path, decreasing the amount exiting into the tissue. Over time, extravasation into the tissue also has to do with tissue compliance. Younger, more compliant tissues have a tendency to hold more fluid than do older, less compliant tissues.

Two main fluid management systems can be used: a mechanical (motor-driven) pump system in which fluid is "driven" into the joint, and a gravity (passive) system. Peristaltic and centrifugal are the two basic types of mechanical pump systems.

The gravity system works on hydrostatic pressure (1 foot = 22 mm Hg). Increasing the height of the bags or decreasing the height of the joint being worked on increases the pressure in the system. The advantages of a gravity system are that it is simple and relatively inexpensive. A potential disadvantage is that when there is a large flow demand, gravity cannot keep up, and the system can "drain the joint."

The peristaltic pump system works by "pinching" inflow tubing as the pump head turns, allowing the introduction of a discrete fluid quantity (individual packets of fluid). This allows for positive fluid displacement by controlling the revolutions per minute of the pump head, thus controlling the amount of pressure and flow. The motor drives rollers that compress the inflow tubing against a race (a metal guard that allows the tubing to be compressed in a uniform fashion). The pump then forces fluid (flow) into the joint, creating a pressure. The inflow tube is a closed system, so the pressure in the tube is the pressure in the joint. However, owing to the momentum of the rollers, there are short peaks and valleys of pressure in a dynamic situation. Flow rate determines how fast the desired pressure is achieved and is measured as a percentage of maximum flow rate. One of the problems with this type of system is that it leads to a pulsing type of action, potentially causing a pressure spike at high flow rates.

The centrifugal pump works on the basis of a rotating impeller in which a continuous volume of fluid is sent. This continuous flow of fluid allows for smoother control of pressure, without any spiking. The problem, however, is that there is a constant fluid flow, so that an uncontrolled or potential space (the subacromial space) may lead to distention of the surrounding soft tissue.

The control of fluid into and out of the joint is critical for shoulder arthroscopy. In basic glenohumeral shoulder arthroscopy, inflow is connected to the camera, and outflow is generally established through the anterior portal. The relationship between inflow and outflow is especially important in the subacromial space, because the area is less confined than the glenohumeral joint, and fluid dynamics greatly affect the surgical field.

Portal Placement and Anatomy

The importance of accurate portal placement cannot be overstated. Because the operative field is limited to the view of a 30- or 70-degree lens, the angle at which this lens is inserted is critical. This is true for all portals but is especially true for the posterior portal, which is usually the main visualization portal for most procedures.

Accurate tracing of the patient's bony anatomic landmarks is necessary. The anterior and posterior borders of the acromion can be palpated. Marks are then placed at each of these landmarks, and, with the use of an index finger, a line is drawn between them to delineate the lateral border of the acromion. Next, an index finger is placed in the soft spot between the posterior aspect of the distal clavicle and the anterior aspect of the scapular spine. The outline of the clavicle can be drawn from this point, as well as the scapular spine. The acromioclavicular joint is also palpated and drawn, along with the coracoid process, which generally lies 2 to 3 cm inferior to the acromioclavicular joint; these two points mark the level of the glenohumeral articulation. A line marking the path of the coracoacromial ligament is then placed. After all these anatomic areas are palpated and drawn, portal placement can commence.

Posterior Portal

Shoulder arthroscopy begins with the creation of the posterior portal, through which the arthroscope is inserted into the shoulder joint and subacromial space. Depending on the findings observed through this portal, certain accessory portals may be added during the case.

In the beach chair position, the posterior portal is typically placed approximately 2 cm inferior and 1 cm medial to the posterolateral acromion.[12] Although relatively specific coordinates have been reported in the literature, it is important to use all anatomic landmarks as well as various coordinate systems to maintain the ideal position of this portal. The posterior portal is extremely important, as it is the initial viewing portal. This portal "sets the tone" for the rest of the procedure. It is also important to realize that coordinate systems are given for the "normal" shoulder. In extremely small or large shoulders, these coordinates must be modified.

Coordinate systems, bony landmarks, and palpation should all be used to obtain appropriate placement. One method of ensuring correct placement of this portal involves palpation of the bony landmarks with the same hand as the shoulder being operated on. The middle finger is placed on the coracoid process, the index finger is placed into the notch directly posterior to the acromioclavicular joint and anterior to the scapular spine, and the thumb feels for the "soft spot," which is the muscular interval between the infraspinatus and teres minor muscle groups (Fig. 8–6). Another useful method is to grasp the proximal humerus with one hand while stabilizing the scapula with the other and to feel the motion interface at the glenohumeral joint. Once the correct placement has been determined, a mark is made where the posterior portal should go.

The skin is injected with a local anesthetic, and a 1-cm incision is made through the dermis with a number 11 or 15 blade. Depending on the surgeon's preference, a sharp or dull trocar within the cannula for the arthroscope is used next. If a sharp trocar is used, it is advanced

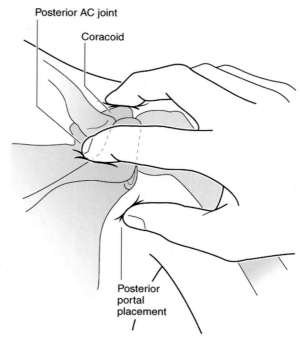

Posterior AC joint

Coracoid

Posterior portal placement

Figure 8–6 **Romeo three-finger shuck.** This is one method of ensuring the correct placement of the posterior portal. It involves palpation of the bony landmarks with the same hand as the shoulder being operated on. The middle finger is placed on the coracoid process, the index finger is placed into the notch directly posterior to the acromioclavicular (AC) joint and anterior to the scapular spine, and the thumb feels for the "soft spot," which is the muscular interval between the infraspinatus and teres minor muscle groups.

only past the deltoid musculature before being exchanged for a dull trocar. A constant, steady pressure is used to advance the trocar from the posterior skin puncture in line with the tip of the coracoid process, which is being palpated. The amount of resistance encountered at this point varies from shoulder to shoulder. There may be quite a bit of resistance in patients who have adhesive capsulitis or thick posterior capsules, whereas little resistance may be encountered in those with multidirectional instability or thin posterior capsules. If the trocar does not "pop in," it should not be forced, as this may cause injury. To help with insertion, an assistant rotates the arm to localize the joint space by means of the surgeon's palpation of the moving humeral head contrasted with the stationary glenoid. Another method involves having the assistant grab the arm just distal to the axilla, creating an abduction distraction force. This, in essence, creates slightly more glenohumeral space, allowing the trocar to be easily slipped into the joint. Ideally, the cannula is introduced into the shoulder joint at the midequator of the glenoid to provide ideal visualization of the intra-articular structures at the top and bottom of the joint. An upward motion should be used at this time to avoid iatrogenic injury to the articular cartilage of the posterior humeral head. Any bony resistance encountered during insertion should be considered either the posterior aspect of the humeral head or the posterior glenoid. If bony resistance is experienced, it is safer to take a moment to reassess the anatomic landmarks and then reapply steady pressure at a slightly different angle rather than to attempt forceful insertion and risk possible iatrogenic cartilage injury.

Creation of the posterior portal in the lateral decubitus position is slightly different. There is a natural tendency to enter the joint medially, but this would force the arthroscopist to come over and around the glenoid to view the joint, which could be problematic with some procedures. In general, the portal should be placed slightly more lateral and proximal than the beach chair posterior portal. It is recommended that the portal be placed 3 cm inferior and in line with the posterolateral corner of the acromion (Fig. 8–7).

Distention of the glenohumeral joint with fluid before entering it may have some advantages. The humeral head and glenoid are separated by the fluid, leaving a wider glenohumeral space and allowing the medial trocar to be inserted with less risk of iatrogenic injury. Filling the joint with fluid also puts the posterior capsule in tension and makes entering the joint easier. A theoretic limitation of this technique is the potential for injury to the humeral head during spinal needle placement.

For diagnostic glenohumeral arthroscopy, the entrance for the posterior portal is the same skin incision that can be used for posterior entry into the subacromial space. There are many ways to enter the subacromial space; however, the primary factor is visualization. The technique described here is based on establishing a "room with a view."

After complete glenohumeral arthroscopy, the posterior portal cannula and trocar are withdrawn through the interval between the infraspinatus and teres minor muscles. The trocar is withdrawn in such a way that no rotator cuff musculature is brought in when entering the subacromial space. The trocar and cannula are angled more superiorly than with glenohumeral arthroscopy, and the posterior border of the acromion is palpated with the trocar. The trocar is then placed underneath the acromion and inserted in an anterior direction. Palpation of the anterior joint with the opposite hand aids in understanding how large the acromion is in relation to the length of the cannula. Both these factors give the surgeon feedback about how far the trocar has been advanced into the space. The subacromial bursa is an anterior structure (Fig. 8–8). After initially aiming anteromedially, the trocar is placed as lateral as possible (Fig. 8–9A). The trocar is removed, and the arthroscope is inserted. When fluid is allowed to distend this potential space, a "room with a view" should be seen (Fig. 8–9B). If soft tissue obscures the view, the surgeon must withdraw and reposition the arthroscope. There is a tendency to be either too medial or too anterior. If this is the case, the anatomic references should be reassessed, and the procedure should be repeated. The posterior portal must be low enough to allow a smooth transition into and out of the subacromial space. If the posterior portal is too close to the scapular spine, a shaver placed through this portal will have to be aimed inferiorly to get under the acromion before it can be aimed superiorly to perform the anterior acromioplasty. Also, if an arthroscopic distal clavicle excision is part of the planned procedure, the posterior portal can be made slightly medial so that the angle of attack is more in line with the acromioclavicular joint.

Alternatively, the anterior portal can be used by passing the arthroscope and trocar through the posterior portal and out the anterior aspect of the shoulder. A plastic outflow cannula is placed over and withdrawn to the center of the subacromial space. Following reinsertion of the camera into its sheath, a spinal needle can be used for triangulation to establish the standard lateral working portal (described later).

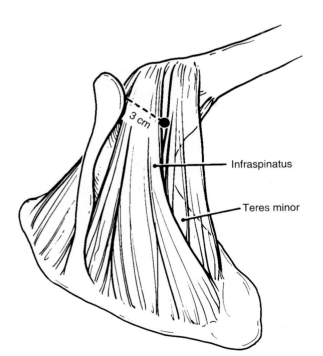

Figure 8–7   Posterior portal placement through the infraspinatus and teres minor interval in the lateral decubitus position.

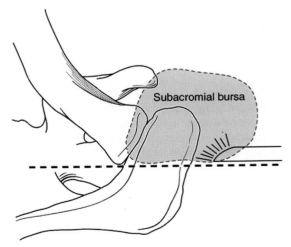

Figure 8–8   Subacromial bursa.

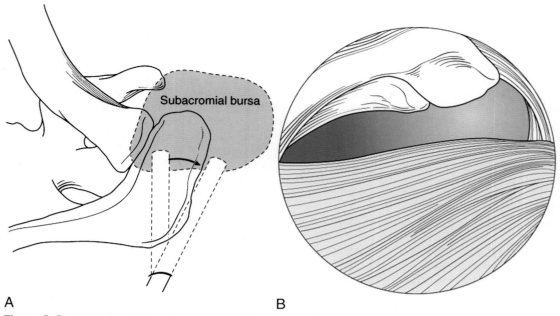

A

B

Figure 8–9 *A,* Initial angulation of the trocar medially to enter the subacromial bursa, followed by manipulation of the trocar laterally. *B,* "Room with a view"—the arthroscopic view inside the subacromial bursa.

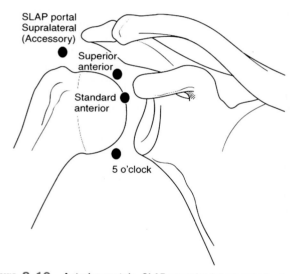

Figure 8–10 Anterior portals. SLAP, superior labral anterior to posterior.

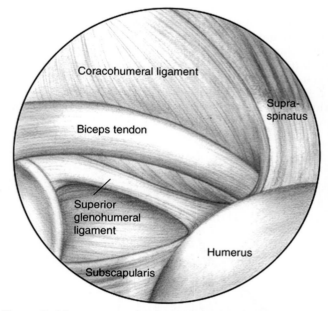

Figure 8–11 Arthroscopic view of the biceps sling anatomy of a right shoulder with the arthroscope in the posterior portal.

Anterior Portal

The standard anterior portal (Fig. 8–10) is generally placed in the rotator interval or triangle created by the subscapularis tendon, the humeral head, and the biceps tendon superiorly. It is important to assess the competence of the superior glenohumeral and coracohumeral ligaments and the stability of the long head of the biceps tendon before creating this portal. The coracohumeral ligament, along with the superior glenohumeral ligament, forms the medial sling of the biceps, thereby creating medial stability for the long head of the biceps tendon. The supraspinatus creates a bumper, or sling, for the biceps on its lateral side (Fig. 8–11). Creation of the anterior portal can be done with an inside-out or outside-in technique. The inside-out technique involves "driving" the arthroscope into the anterior triangle and placing it with some force into that area so that it does not move. The arthroscope is then removed, and a stout Wissinger rod is placed through the cannula. The rod is then forcefully pushed through the interval tissue, tensing the skin anteriorly. This tented skin should be directly lateral to the tip of the coracoid process. If it is medial, the rod should immediately be withdrawn and the anatomic structures reassessed. The musculocutaneous nerve exits 1 cm medial and 3 cm distal to the coracoid process. A scalpel (number 11 blade) is used to create a 1-cm incision, and the Wissinger rod is pushed through this incision. A plastic cannula can then be placed over the rod. The arthroscope is advanced into the space, and the position is checked visually (Fig. 8–12).

The outside-in technique uses direct visualization. A spinal needle is placed from the lateral aspect of the coracoid process through the rotator interval (Fig. 8–13). The spinal needle is then removed, and a number 11 blade is used to make the 1-cm skin incision. Under direct visualization, the plastic cannula and plastic trocar

are advanced through this tissue bounded by the long head of the biceps tendon superiorly, humeral head laterally, and subscapularis inferiorly. Care should be taken not to place the portal through the subscapularis tendon. Depending on the pump system being used and the fluid dynamics, the outflow can be changed from the posterior portal to this anterior portal to improve visualization of the shoulder joint.

When creating the anterior portal with the patient in the lateral decubitus position, the tendency is to make the anterior portal too medial, so an effort must be made to ensure that the portal is lateral enough. When establishing the portal, if it is difficult to determine the correct site for needle insertion, the anterior aspect of the shoulder can be palpated while viewing through the arthroscope to observe capsular indentation due to the palpating finger.

In a diagnostic arthroscopic procedure, the anterior portal can be placed anywhere in the rotator cuff interval. If, according to the preoperative plan, various procedures are going to be performed, special attention should be paid to where the initial anterior portal goes. For arthroscopic distal clavicle excision, placing the anterior portal slightly medial is useful to gain access to the acromioclavicular joint. For arthroscopic labral stabilization, the anterior portal may be put slightly higher than usual because a second anterior portal will be needed. It is important to realize that with two anterior portals, crowding can occur. Increasing the distance between these portals helps with triangulation and decreases congestion.

If the selected procedure requires two anterior portals, both can be placed into the rotator interval. The anterosuperior portal is close to the acromion, even with the acromioclavicular joint, and the standard antero-inferior portal is adjacent to the coracoid (Fig. 8–14).

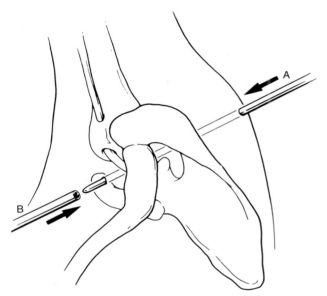

Figure 8–12   Rod being directed anteriorly through the skin (A). Retrograde placement of an arthroscopic cannula into the joint over a Wissinger rod (B).

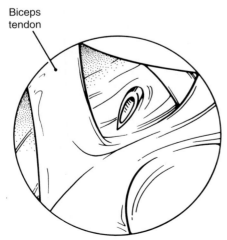

Figure 8–13   Intra-articular view of a spinal needle entering the anterior capsule at the proper site for the anterior portal.

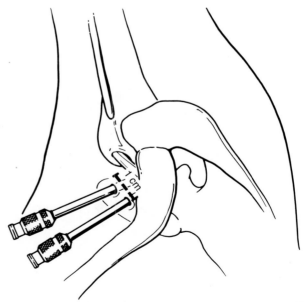

Figure 8–14   Placement of two anterior portals with a 1-cm skin bridge between them.

Standard Lateral Portal

The standard lateral portal (Fig. 8–15) is strictly a sub-acromial space portal. This exclusive role is due to the fact that the supraspinatus and infraspinatus tendons, depending on internal and external rotation, protect the glenohumeral joint from access by this portal. The axillary nerve anatomy is an important consideration when establishing the direct lateral portal. Many descriptions of the axillary nerve in relation to the lateral edge of the acromion have been provided. Hollinsehead[9] determined that the position of the axillary nerve was 1.5 to 2 inches (3.8 to 5.1 cm) below the acromion. Hoppenfeld and deBoer[10] reported that the axillary nerve was 7 cm from the acromion. Beals et al.[2] found that the mean distances from all points of the acromion to the axillary nerve averaged approximately 5 cm.

To localize this portal, an index finger is placed in the notch between the posterior aspect of the clavicle and the spine of the scapula, and a line is drawn from this notch laterally past the lateral edge of the acromion for approximately 2 cm. This places the line in the midportion of the acromion. A spinal needle is used to localize this portal under direct visualization. The needle is placed in position, and once it is manipulated so that all areas of the subacromial space can be accessed with it, a 1-cm incision is made either vertically or horizontally, depending on the surgeon's preference. A dull trocar is used to enter the subacromial space first, and the position is checked again. If this portal is placed too close to the acromion, as the shoulder swells, introducing instruments will become more difficult as they are forced in a caudad direction. This misplacement also raises the relative position of the portal, making contact with the medial acromion difficult. These factors should always be considered when making this portal.

Accessory Anterior Portals

To aid in performing the multitude of arthroscopic shoulder procedures, various portals have been described (see Fig. 8–10). As already stated, correct placement of portals is critical to the success of the procedure. A spinal needle can be used in the glenohumeral joint to localize and ascertain the correct angle and position of the proposed portal site. One can then create a portal site that is specific to both the patient's anatomy and the proposed procedure. When creating accessory portals, knowledge of the neurovascular anatomy is important. The musculocutaneous nerve exits 2 cm inferior and 1 cm medial to the coracoid process (Fig. 8–16). The cephalic vein is found in the deltopectoral interval, and the anterior humeral circumflex vessel travels along the inferior border of the subscapularis tendon to send branches into the biceps sheath and humeral head. Beals et al.[2] reported that the axillary nerve is, on average, 5 cm from the acromion. This can be thought of as a "safe zone" for the application of accessory portals.

Superolateral Portal

The superolateral portal (see Fig. 8–10) has been defined by Laurencin et al.[15] It is placed at a position just lateral to the acromion on a line drawn from the acromion to the coracoid. A spinal needle is placed to enter the subacromial space or joint obliquely. This portal is useful for anterior shoulder procedures, but it is especially important in arthroscopic rotator cuff repair for anchor placement and suture shuttling (Fig. 8–17).

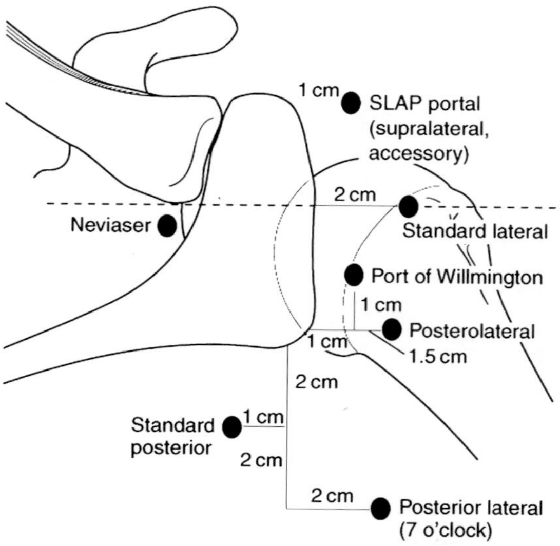

Figure 8–15 Posterior and lateral portals.

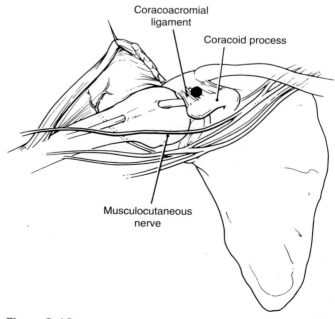

Figure 8–16 Anterior portal placement in relation to the coracoid process and musculocutaneous nerve.

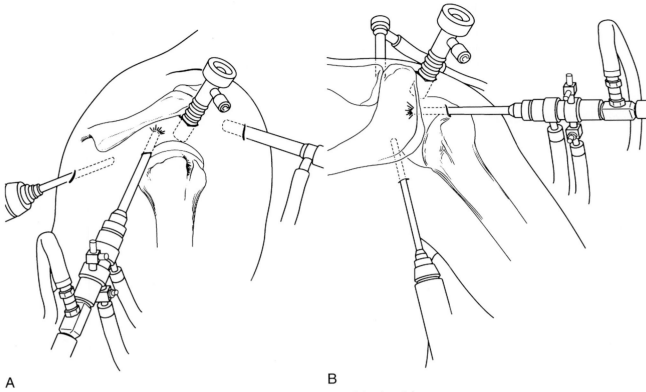

A   B

Figure 8–17   Lateral *(A)* and posterior *(B)* views of an accessory superolateral portal.

Neviaser Portal

This portal (see Fig. 8–15) is placed in the notch between the posterior acromioclavicular joint and the spine of the scapula. It is useful for the repair of anterior supraspinatus rotator cuff injuries, as well as for arthroscopic distal clavicle resection (Fig. 8–18). The suprascapular nerve and artery traverse the floor of the supraspinatus fossa, approximately 3 cm medial to the portal.

Anteroinferior, or 5 O'clock, Portal

This portal is especially useful for glenohumeral reconstructive procedures such as arthroscopic labral stabilization. Davidson and Tibone[5] described the anteroinferior 5 o'clock portal for shoulder arthroscopy (see Fig. 8–10). This provides direct linear access to the glenoid rim at the critical anteroinferior site of Bankart capsulolabral detachment. This portal passes lateral to the musculocutaneous nerve and superolateral to the axillary nerve. The mean portal-to-nerve distance for the musculocutaneous nerve is 22.9 mm, and for the axillary nerve it is 24.4 mm.[9] This portal passes within 10 mm of the deltopectoral groove, slightly lateral to the conjoined tendon in the lower third of the subscapularis muscle. The portal can be placed from the inside out or outside in. With an inside-out technique, the humerus is maximally adducted, the upper third of the subscapularis is pierced, and a Wissinger rod is passed through the capsule with the exiting tip directed as far laterally as possible. A plastic cannula is then placed over the rod anteriorly to provide access to the 5 o'clock position.

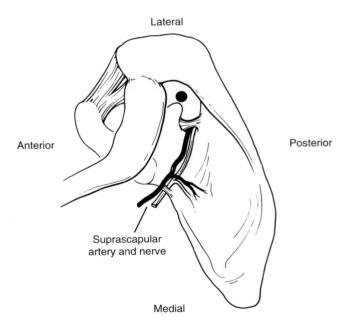

Lateral

Anterior

Posterior

Suprascapular
artery and nerve

Medial

Figure 8–18   Neviaser portal in relation to the suprascapular nerve and artery, acromion, clavicle, and spine of the scapula.

Anterolateral Portal

This is a useful portal for placing anchors to repair anteriorly located superior labral tears. It is placed 1 cm lateral to the anterior acromion. Accessing the glenohumeral joint from this position violates the supraspinatus tendon. Recent advances in anchor placement have allowed smaller incisions to be made. Anchor cannulas are smaller than the standard arthroscopic cannulas. Small incisions in the supraspinatus tendon have not been reported to cause difficulties; however, damage to the rotator cuff tendon should be minimized (see Fig. 8–15).

Accessory Posterior Portals

The anterior portals do not provide a satisfactory angle of approach for the placement of suture anchors in the posterior aspect of the superior or inferior labrum.

Portal of Wilmington

This portal is used for labral repair in the posterosuperior quadrant of the glenoid.[17] The skin incision is made 1 cm lateral and 1 cm anterior to the posterolateral corner of the acromion, and the portal is made with a 45-degree angle of attack. No cannula is placed in this portal site, to avoid iatrogenic injury to the infraspinatus tendon. For this reason, once the spinal needle is localized to the correct trajectory, the labral fixation device is placed percutaneously under direct visualization (see Fig. 8–15).

Posterolateral, or 7 O'clock, Portal

Placement of plication sutures or anchors into the posteroinferior glenoid is difficult through standard portals. This necessitates the use of an accessory posterior portal. Morrison et al.[18] described a portal that is placed 2 cm inferior to the standard posterior portal at approximately the 7 o'clock position (Fig. 8–19). This facilitates easy access to the axillary pouch by entering the joint below the equator of the glenoid. The average distance

between the accessory posterior portal and the axillary nerve is 3.7 cm. The distance to the suprascapular nerve is 2.88 cm. Another accessory posterolateral portal has been described. The incision for this posterolateral portal is placed 1.5 cm lateral to the acromion at its posterior third. The reported average distance between the posterolateral portal and the axillary nerve is 14.4 to 24.1 mm. Although these coordinates are helpful, a spinal needle for localization of the portal is essential (see Fig. 8–15).

Once multiple portals have been established, care must be taken not to widen the portal openings excessively. Cannulas can help keep portals a standard size. If portal distention occurs, this can lead to extravasation of fluid into the soft tissues. Switching sticks or rods can be used to move the arthroscope from one portal to another while maintaining the same portal configuration (Figs. 8–20 and 8–21).

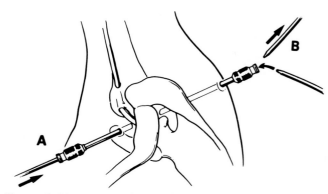

Figure 8–20 Use of switching sticks (A and B) to interchange working portals.

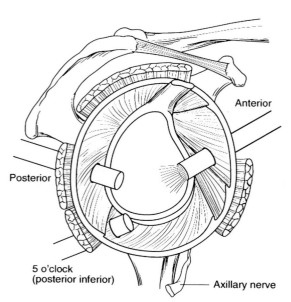

Figure 8–19 Posterolateral (7 o'clock) portal.

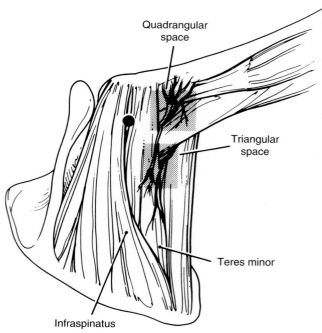

Figure 8–21 View of the posterior portal in relation to the infraspinatus, teres minor, quadrangular space, and triangular space.

Conclusion

Shoulder arthroscopy is an excellent method for treating various pathologies. Attention to detail during patient positioning, portal placement, and fluid management will enhance the success of all arthroscopic procedures of the shoulder.

References

1. Altchek DW, Warren RF, Skyhar MJ, Ortiz G: T-plasty modification of the Bankart procedure for multi-directional instability anterior and inferior types. J Bone Joint Surg Am 73:105-112, 1991.
2. Beals TC, Harryman DT, Lazarus MD: Useful boundary of the subacromial bursa. Arthroscopy 14:465-470, 1998.
3. Bert JM, Posalaky Z, Snyder S, et al: Effect of various irrigating fluids on the ultrastructure of articular cartilage. Arthroscopy 6:104-111, 1990.
4. Burman MS: Arthroscopy or direct visualization of joints: Experimental cadaver study. J Bone Joint Surg 13:669-695, 1931.
5. Davidson PA, Tibone JE: Anterior inferior (5 o'clock) portal for shoulder arthroscopy. Arthroscopy 11:519-525, 1995.
6. Gradinger R, Träger J, Klauser RJ: Influence of various irrigation fluids on articular cartilage. Arthroscopy 11:263-269, 1995.
7. Hamada S, Hamada M, Nishiue S, Doi T: Osteochondritis dissecans of the humeral head [case report]. Arthroscopy 8:132-137, 1992.
8. Hennrikus WL, Mapes RC, Bratton MW, et al: Lateral traction during shoulder arthroscopy: Its effect on tissue perfusion measured by pulse oximetry. Am J Sports Med 23:444-446, 1995.
9. Hollinsehead WH: Anatomy for Surgeons, vol 3, 2nd ed. Philadelphia, Harper & Row, 1969, p 316.
10. Hoppenfeld S, deBoer P: Surgical exposures. In Orthopaedics, 2nd ed. Philadelphia, JB Lippincott, 1994, pp 25-29.
11. Jobe FW, Giangarra CE, Kvitne RS, Glousman RE: Anterior capsulolabral reconstruction of the shoulder in athletes in overhand sports. Am J Sports Med 19:428-434, 1991.
12. Johnson LL: Arthroscopic Surgery: Principles and Practice, 3rd ed. St Louis, CV Mosby, 1986.
13. Johnson LL, Schneider DA, Austin MD, et al: Two-percent glutaraldehyde: A disinfectant in arthroscopy and arthroscopic surgery. J Bone Joint Surg Am 64:237-239, 1982.
14. Klein AH, France JC, Mutschler TA, et al: Measurement of brachial plexus strain in arthroscopy of the shoulder. Arthroscopy 3:45-52, 1987.
15. Laurencin CT, Detsh A, O'Brien SJ, Altchek DW: The superior lateral portal for arthroscopy of the shoulder. Arthroscopy 10:255-258, 1994.
16. Morgan C: Fluid delivery systems for arthroscopy. Arthroscopy 3:288-291, 1987.
17. Morgan CD, Burkhart SS, Palmeri M, Gillespie M: Type II SLAP lesions: Three subtypes and their relationships to superior instability and rotator cuff tear. Arthroscopy 14:553-555, 1998.
18. Morrison DS, Schaefer RK, Friedman RL: The relationship between subacromial space pressure, blood pressure, and visual clarity during arthroscopic subacromial decompression. Arthroscopy 11:557-560, 1995.

9

Shoulder: Diagnostic Arthroscopy

Augustus D. Mazzocca, Frank G. Alberta,
Brian J. Cole, and Anthony A. Romeo

The diagnostic examination is a key component of all shoulder arthroscopy. The arthroscope gives the surgeon the ability to visually inspect and palpate the intra-articular and subacromial anatomy. The arthroscopic shoulder examination should proceed in a stepwise fashion, and it is important that all structures be evaluated consistently. To ensure that this is done in a reproducible manner, the glenohumeral joint can be divided into sectors.

The *anterosuperior sector* includes the rotator interval, consisting of the coracohumeral ligament (CHL), superior glenohumeral ligament (SGHL), and biceps tendon; the *superior sector* includes the superior labrum and superior glenoid articular surface; the *posterior sector* includes the posterior labrum, posterior band of the inferior glenohumeral ligament (IGHL), and posterior glenoid articular surface; the *inferior sector* includes the axillary pouch; the *anterior sector* includes the subscapularis tendon and its insertion on the humerus, middle glenohumeral ligament (MGHL), anterior labrum, anterior glenoid articular surface, and anterior band of the IGHL; and the *humerus* includes the rotator cuff insertion, bare area, and entire humeral articular surface.

Surgical Technique

Diagnostic arthroscopy of the shoulder starts with insertion of the arthroscope into the glenohumeral joint through the posterior portal. The arthroscope passes through the skin, the posterior deltoid, and the infraspinatus–teres minor interval. The position of the posterior portal is variable but is generally established 2 cm inferior and 1 cm medial to the posterolateral edge of the acromion, avoiding the neurovascular structures located in the quadrangular space, triangular space, and triangular interval (Fig. 9–1). These spaces are located 7 to 8 cm inferior to the posterolateral corner of the acromion. The quadrangular space is formed by the teres minor superiorly, the teres major inferiorly, the long head of the triceps medially, and the humeral shaft laterally. The posterior humeral circumflex vessels and the axillary nerve pass through the quadrangular space. The triangular space contains the circumflex scapular vessels, and the triangular interval contains the radial nerve and the deep brachial artery. The triangular space is bounded by the long head of the triceps laterally and the two teres muscles medially.

The anterior portal is created through the rotator interval, and a cannula is inserted to be used for outflow (Fig. 9–2). This portal is generally in line with the acromioclavicular joint, approximately 2 or 3 cm inferior to the anterolateral edge of the acromion. The musculocutaneous nerve can generally be found 3 to 5 cm distal and just medial to the coracoid process.

Superior Sector

Upon entering the joint, the surgeon should see the triangle formed by the biceps tendon superiorly, the humeral head laterally, and the subscapularis inferiorly. The biceps tendon and the glenoid labrum surrounding the entire glenoid have the appearance of an inverted comma or Q.[5] The biceps tendon attaches to the supraglenoid tubercle at the posterosuperior aspect of the glenoid rim. The biceps origin either is attached to the superior labrum or sends fibers to the anterosuperior and posterosuperior labrum (Fig. 9–3). The first portion of this examination can be done before distention of the capsule with fluid. This allows visualization and quantification of the amount of erythema on the biceps tendon. Once the fluid has been introduced, the pressure

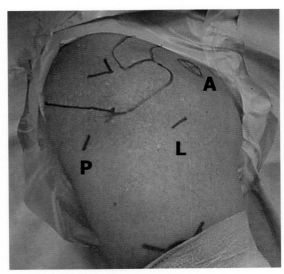

Figure 9–1   Intraoperative photograph of standard shoulder portals drawn before the incision. A, anterior portal; L, lateral subacromial working portal; P, posterior portal.

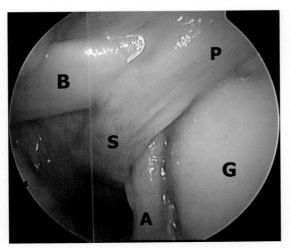

Figure 9–3   Arthroscopic image from a posterior viewing portal. The biceps tendon (B), superior glenohumeral ligament (S), and the labrum, both anterior and posterior, are intimately related. A, anterior labrum; G, glenoid surface; P, posterior labrum.

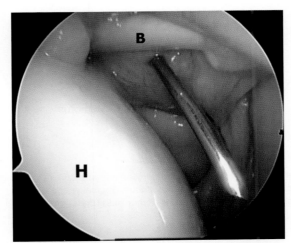

Figure 9–2   Arthroscopic image from a posterior viewing portal. The spinal needle marks the position of the anterior rotator interval portal. B, biceps tendon; H, humeral head.

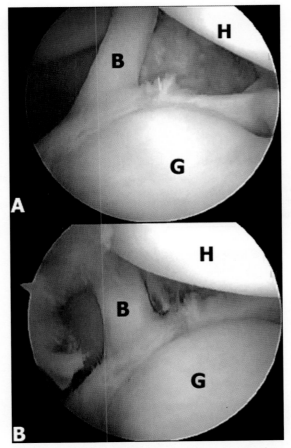

Figure 9–4   In abduction and external rotation, the superior labrum can rotate posterior and medially from the superior glenoid (peel-back phenomenon). *A,* Superior labrum with the arm in neutral position. *B,* Superior labrum with the arm in abduction and external rotation, demonstrating peel back. Note the change in the orientation of the biceps tendon (B). G, glenoid; H, humeral head.

tamponades the microinflammation and "washes" it out. This can be a helpful adjunct to the diagnosis of biceps tendinosis.[15]

The superior labrum should be evaluated for tears, detachment, or other abnormalities that could represent the clinical entity known as the superior labral anterior to posterior (SLAP) lesion.[13] A probe can be used from the anterior portal to look under the labrum to evaluate whether it is detached. Burkhart and Morgan[3] described the peel-back phenomenon in evaluating overhead athletes. When the arm is abducted and externally rotated, the superior labrum may rotate off the superior glenoid posteriorly and superiorly (Fig. 9–4).

Anterosuperior Sector

The CHL should be evaluated as it encircles the biceps tendon. This ligament originates at the base of the cora-coid and then spans out, sending fibers that circle the biceps tendon, intertwine with the supraspinatus tendon, and insert in front of the subscapularis tendon insertion. The SGHL also attaches to the superior portion of the glenoid but is in a different plane from the CHL. The SGHL runs from the anterosuperior aspect of the glenoid to the upper part of the lesser tuberosity and is considered by some to be the floor of the bicipital groove (Fig. 9–5). The SGHL works with the CHL in preventing anterior translation of the humeral head with the arm adducted and externally rotated. The SGHL also pre-vents inferior subluxation of the humeral head (sulcus sign) with the arm at the side. The biceps can be followed distally into the bicipital groove. Forward elevation with the elbow flexed, combined with internal rotation of the arm, may assist in viewing the biceps as it passes under-neath the transverse humeral ligament. To visualize the biceps tendon, which is located in the intertubercular groove, the probe can be placed superior to the tendon and used to "pull" the tendon down into the joint (Fig. 9–6).

The bicipital groove is further bordered by the sub-scapularis tendon medially and the supraspinatus tendon laterally (Fig. 9–7). The supraspinatus tendon can be seen adjacent to the biceps with abduction and external rotation (Fig. 9–8). The SGHL and CHL form the medial

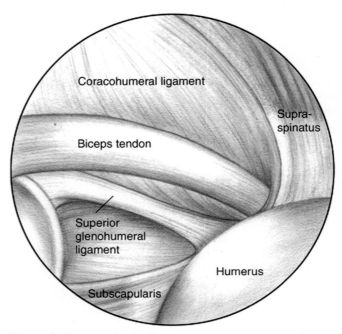

Figure 9–7 Relationship of anterosuperior structures to the biceps tendon and its groove. The subscapularis (medially) and the supraspinatus (laterally) tendons border the bicipital groove.

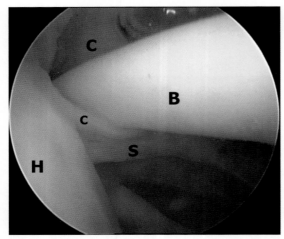

Figure 9–5 Arthroscopic image from a posterior viewing portal demonstrating the biceps tendon sling. B, biceps tendon; C, coracohumeral ligament; H, humeral head; S, superior glenohumeral ligament.

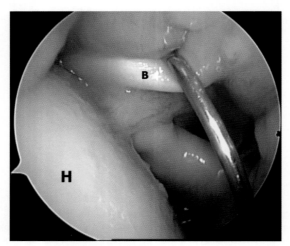

Figure 9–6 The biceps tendon (B) can be examined by pulling it into the joint with a hook probe. This allows full evaluation of the tendon distal to its intra-articular portion. H, humeral head.

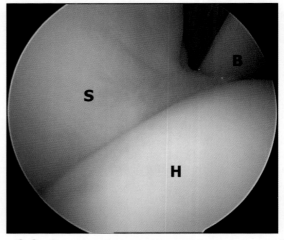

Figure 9–8 The supraspinatus tendon contributes to the stability of the biceps tendon (B) in its groove, a relationship that is especially appreciated in abduction and external rotation. H, humeral head; S, superior glenohumeral ligament.

sling of the biceps. Damage to these structures can result in biceps instability or pain.

Finally, the anterosuperior labrum can be evaluated. The labrum has been described as being triangular in cross section, with its free edge directed at the glenoid center. It is made up of dense, fibrous connective tissue and anchored to the osseous rim of the glenoid. The hyaline cartilage of the glenoid articular surface frequently extends under and beyond this free edge. Significant normal variability exists in the appearance of the anterosuperior labrum; this can include physiologic detachment and confluence with the MGHL (Buford complex), simple detachment (sublabral hole), or complete absence. A probe can be inserted through the anterior portal as previously described and used to examine all labral and ligamentous structures. Notation of labral atrophy, fraying, and amount of movement should always be made, as this information may aid in diagnosis.

Anterior Sector

With the arthroscope in the posterior portal and the 30-degree objective facing laterally, the rolled upper edge of the subscapularis is examined. The MGHL is variable in thickness and intersects the subscapularis at a 60-degree angle (Fig. 9–9).[6] It can be a veil of tissue or a cordlike structure, as in the Buford complex. This normal anatomic variant consists of a cordlike MGHL with a high origin off the glenoid at the base of the biceps tendon. Frequently, the anterosuperior labrum is absent in these cases.[14] The MGHL arises from the anterior humeral neck just medial to the lesser tuberosity and inserts on the medial and superior glenoid rim and scapular neck. Its function is to resist anterior translation of the humeral head at 45 degrees of abduction.[8] In diagnostic glenohumeral arthroscopy, it is also important to examine the subscapularis recess. Loose bodies can be lodged here and will not be discovered unless this area is actually visualized. Inferiorly, the anterior and anteroinferior labrum can be inspected. Sublabral defects of the anterosuperior labrum can be seen in 60% of patients. In 10%, the defect is a complete hole and communicates with the subscapularis recess. These are normal variants and should not be mistaken for labral pathology. Any detachment of the labrum below the glenoid equator (at the level of the rolled edge insertion of the subscapularis), however, is generally considered pathologic.

The articular surface of the glenoid and humerus must be examined in detail. The articular cartilage of the glenoid thins at the center. The surrounding cartilage should be examined for full-thickness lesions, fibrillation, and softening. The treatment of such lesions is still controversial, but they must be noted. Large articular lesions can manifest as a feeling of instability as the humeral head articulates with the lesion and the sensation of "clunks" in various positions of rotation and abduction (Fig. 9–10).

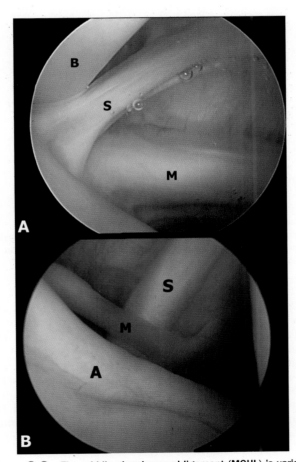

Figure 9–9 The middle glenohumeral ligament (MGHL) is variable in its appearance and consistency. It crosses the superior rolled edge of the subscapularis tendon at a 60-degree angle. *A*, Cordlike MGHL with a high takeoff from the superior glenoid. *B*, Thin MGHL with its typical relationship to the subscapularis tendon. A, anterior labrum; B, biceps; M, middle glenohumeral ligament; S, superior glenohumeral ligament.

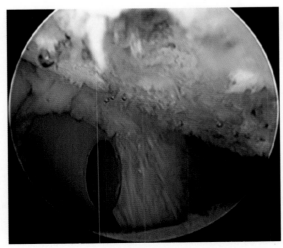

Figure 9–10 Large humeral head articular cartilage defect that can cause mechanical symptoms.

Inferior Sector

The inferior sector is examined for evidence of synovitis and the presence of loose bodies. As the assistant holds traction in 20 to 30 degrees of abduction with the arm in a beach chair position, the anterior band of the IGHL can be inspected. The IGHL runs from the glenoid to the anatomic neck of the humerus (Fig. 9–11). The anterior band of the IGHL prevents anterior translation of the humeral head when the arm is abducted 90 degrees and externally rotated. It also restricts inferior translation when the arm is abducted and internally rotated. The humeral attachment of the anterior band is best visualized from the anterior portal. It is from this view that a humeral avulsion of the glenohumeral ligament (HAGL) can be seen (Fig. 9–12). The axillary pouch is then inspected. The capsule of the axillary pouch is thin, and beneath it lies the axillary nerve. This relationship should always be considered when performing suture capsular plication or thermal capsulorrhaphy (Fig. 9–13).

Posterior Sector

The posteroinferior labrum and the posterior band of the IGHL can be inspected sequentially. The posterior band of the IGHL prevents inferior translation of the

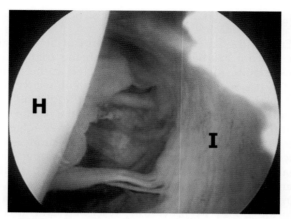

Figure 9–12   Humeral avulsion of the glenohumeral ligament (HAGL). Typically, the anterior structures of the shoulder are damaged at their glenoid insertions during dislocation. An HAGL lesion develops when they fail at their humeral insertion instead. H, humeral head; I, inferior glenohumeral ligament.

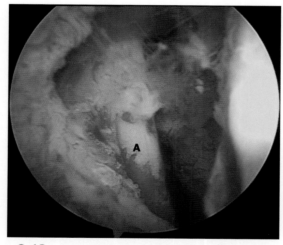

Figure 9–13   Arthroscopic view of the axillary nerve (A) just outside the inferior capsule. The nerve lies just inferior to the inferior pouch and can be injured during capsular release, suture plication, and other anterior or inferior procedures.

humeral head when the arm is abducted 90 degrees and externally rotated. It also prevents posterior translation when the arm is abducted and internally rotated (Fig. 9–14).[9] From this position, the posterior insertion of the rotator cuff can be evaluated for fraying associated with internal impingement. The arm should be abducted to 90 to 110 degrees and maximally externally rotated. Fraying and contact of the posterior labrum and the rotator cuff tendon in a patient with pain can be indicative of internal impingement.

Humerus and Rotator Cuff Insertion

Evaluating the supraspinatus tendon insertion beginning just posterior to the biceps tendon is performed with slight forward elevation and external rotation of the humerus (see Fig. 9–8). Placing an 18-gauge spinal

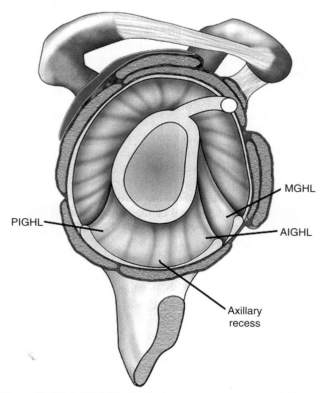

Figure 9–11   The inferior glenohumeral ligament (IGHL) forms a sling that cradles the inferior portion of the shoulder joint, with thickenings at its anterior and posterior edges. Its function is dependent on the position of the arm. AIGHL, anteroinferior glenohumeral ligament; MGHL, middle glenohumeral ligament; PIGHL, posteroinferior glenohumeral ligament.

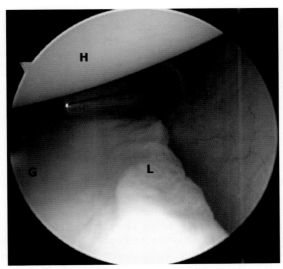

Figure 9–14   Anterior arthroscopic view showing the posterior labrum and capsule. The cannula is in the posterior portal. G, glenoid; H, humeral head; L, labrum.

needle percutaneously and passing a monofilament suture into the joint assists in identifying partial-thickness tears by viewing the suture from within the subacromial space following intra-articular arthroscopy (Fig. 9–15).

By observing the posterior and inferior humerus, the bare area can be visualized. This is an area of bare bone with remnants of old vascular channels. This bare area also correlates with the attachment of the infraspinatus tendon. It can be used as a landmark in rotator cuff surgery to align the infraspinatus to its footprint (Fig. 9–16).

Subacromial Evaluation

After complete glenohumeral arthroscopy, the posterior portal cannula and trocar are withdrawn through the interval between the infraspinatus and teres minor muscles. The trocar is withdrawn so as not to bring in any of the rotator cuff musculature when entering the subacromial space. The trocar and cannula are angled more superiorly than with glenohumeral arthroscopy, and the posterior border of the acromion is palpated with the trocar. The trocar is then placed underneath the acromion and inserted in an anterior direction. Palpation of the anterior joint with the opposite hand aids in determining how large the acromion is in relation to the length of the cannula. Both these factors give the surgeon feedback about how far the trocar has been advanced into the space. The subacromial bursa is an anterior structure (Fig. 9–17*A*). After initially aiming anteromedially, the trocar is placed as lateral as possible (Fig. 9–17*B*). The trocar is removed, and the arthroscope is inserted. When fluid is allowed to distend this potential space, a "room with a view" should be seen (Fig. 9–17*C*). If soft tissue obscures the view, the surgeon must withdraw and reposition the arthroscope. There is a tendency to be either too medial or too anterior. The anatomic references are reassessed, and the procedure is

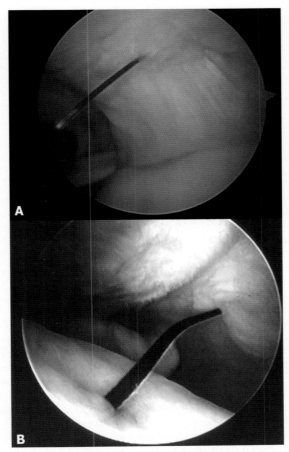

Figure 9–15   A suture can be used to mark the intra-articular location of a partial-thickness rotator cuff tear (A), which can be located in the subacromial space (B), to evaluate the extent of the tear.

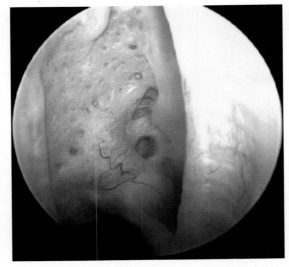

Figure 9–16   Bare area of the humeral head. This landmark corresponds to the insertion of the infraspinatus tendon and can serve as a guide in rotator cuff surgery.

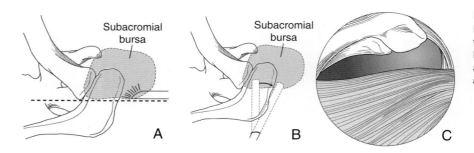

Figure 9–17   *A and B,* The subacromial bursa is an anterior structure that is easily viewed from either the posterior or lateral portal. *C,* Posterior view of the subacromial space provides a "room with a view" once the scope is inserted and distention is achieved.

repeated. The posterior portal must be low enough to allow a smooth transition into and out of the subacromial space. If the posterior portal is too close to the scapular spine, a shaver placed through this portal must be aimed inferiorly to get under the acromion, therefore limiting access to the anterior acromion. If an arthroscopic distal clavicle excision is part of the planned procedure, the posterior portal can be made slightly medial so that the angle of attack is more in line with the acromioclavicular joint.

Alternatively, the anterior portal can be used by passing the arthroscope and trocar through the posterior portal and out the anterior aspect of the shoulder. A plastic outflow cannula is placed over the scope sheath and withdrawn to the center of the subacromial space. Following reinsertion of the camera into its sheath, a spinal needle can be used for triangulation to establish the lateral working portal (described next).

The lateral subacromial working portal is essential for subacromial decompression and other work in the bursal space. It should be made at the junction of the anterior one third and posterior two thirds of the acromion (corresponding to the posterior border of the clavicle) and approximately 2 to 3 cm lateral to the lateral edge of the acromion (see Fig. 9–1). This position provides excellent access and angle of attack for instrument use during subacromial decompression. If the cutting block technique for decompression is used, the arthroscope can easily be switched to this lateral portal. Viewing from the lateral portal gives excellent perspective and helps the surgeon judge the extent and plane of resection.

Considerations and Complications

Shoulder arthroscopy is a minimally invasive procedure with significantly less postoperative pain compared with many similar open procedures. The decreased pain with shoulder arthroscopy is due to the lack of layer-by-layer dissection, minimizing the morbidity of soft tissue damage. One disadvantage of arthroscopy is the visual distortion caused by the parallax of the 30- or 70-degree arthroscope. This distortion makes it difficult to determine the smoothness of certain surfaces, especially when dealing with the anterior acromion.

Bleeding in the subacromial space is a problem that has been studied extensively. Morrison et. al.[11] reported that maintaining a pressure difference (systolic blood pressure minus subacromial space pressure) equal to or less than 49 mm Hg can prevent bleeding. The acromial branch of the coracoacromial artery is usually transected just lateral to the acromioclavicular joint as the coracoacromial ligament is being resected. Thermal ablation electrocautery devices can facilitate the coagulation of these vessels and help control generalized subacromial bleeding. If bleeding obscures the field of view, the arthroscope should be advanced against the suspected area of bleeding so that the fluid coming from the inflow sheath dilutes the blood enough to allow visualization of the bleeding vessel and the use of electrocautery to control the hemorrhage.

Articular damage can be caused by the sharp corners of the arthroscope or by thermal ablation devices. Such damage can be caused on entrance to the joint and is more likely in the case of inaccurate portal placement.

Other difficulties with shoulder arthroscopy include the extravasation of fluid into the soft tissues.[10] Older patients with poor tissue quality have a greater risk of extravasation because their fascia and capsule are not strong enough to contain the fluid in the glenohumeral or subacromial space. This is rarely a clinical problem, but it can make working with portals and cannulas difficult.

True complications are rare, especially if the surgeon pays strict attention to detail. Proper portal placement avoids the majority of neurovascular complications of shoulder arthroscopy. With the patient in the lateral decubitus position, traction in the operative limb may cause neurapraxia.[7] The position that seems to result in the greatest traction on the brachial plexus is 30 degrees of forward elevation and 70 degrees of abduction.[7] The risk of infection is rare in shoulder arthroscopy and has been reported to occur in less than 1% of cases.[1]

Other general areas of concern include the effect of epinephrine in the arthroscopic irrigation solution. This could cause an arrhythmia or generalized vasoconstriction, increasing the systemic vascular resistance and pulmonary pressure and causing pulmonary edema.

If large individuals with thick necks are extubated too quickly, they can experience laryngospasm. The force generated by the accessory muscles of inspiration can cause a negative-pressure pulmonary edema.

Other complications can be caused by anesthesia. Interscalene blocks have proved to be a successful method of pain control. Reported complications include hematoma formation, phrenic and recurrent laryngeal nerve block, vasovagal attack, pneumothorax, total spinal anesthesia, high epidural block, Horner syndrome, and cardiac arrest.[12] Dietzel and Ciullo[4] reported four cases of spontaneous pneumothorax after shoulder arthroscopy. All these patients had a history of smoking or asthma, and all had been operated on in the lateral decubitus position.

A patient with deep venous thromboembolism was reported by Burkhart.[2] This patient had pain and swelling 3 days after surgery, and venography showed thrombosis of the basilic vein. Because deep vein thrombosis is so rare, its occurrence should prompt investigation for a hypercoagulable state.

Conclusion

Diagnostic arthroscopy is a critical and necessary component of any arthroscopic shoulder procedure. An understanding of normal anatomy helps determine appropriate treatment for pathoanatomy found to be present in specific clinical scenarios. Although arthroscopy provides a sensitive mechanism for evaluating intra-articular anatomy, the risk of overdiagnosing an anatomic finding as a pathologic entity is a real concern. Clearly, attention to the history, mechanism of injury, physical findings, and examination under anesthesia is necessary to associate the arthroscopic findings with clinically relevant pathology.

References

1. Armstrong RW, Bolding F, Joseph R: Septic arthritis following arthroscopy: Clinical syndromes and analysis of risk factors. Arthroscopy 8:213-223, 1992.
2. Burkhart SS: Deep venous thrombosis after shoulder arthroscopy. Arthroscopy 6:61-63, 1990.
3. Burkhart SS, Morgan CD: The peel back mechanism: Its role in producing and extending posterior type II SLAP lesions and its effect on SLAP repair rehabilitation. Arthroscopy 14:637-640, 1998.
4. Dietzel DP, Ciullo JV: Spontaneous pneumothorax after shoulder arthroscopy: A report of four cases. Arthroscopy 12:99-102, 1996.
5. Ellman H, Gartsman GM: Arthroscopic Shoulder Surgery and Related Procedures. Philadelphia, Lea & Febiger, 1993, p 67.
6. Gohlke F, Essigkrug B, Schmitz F: The pattern of the collagen fiber bundles of the capsule of the glenohumeral joint. J Shoulder Elbow Surg 3:111-128, 1994.
7. Hamada S, Hamada M, Nishiue S, Doi T: Osteochondritis dissecans of the humeral head [case report]. Arthroscopy 8:132-137, 1992.
8. Jobe CM: Posterior superior glenoid impingement: Expanded spectrum. Arthroscopy 11:530-536, 1995.
9. Jobe FW, Giangarra CE, Kvitne RS, Glousman RE: Anterior capsulolabral reconstruction of the shoulder in athletes in overhand sports. Am J Sports Med 19:428-434, 1991.
10. Jurvelin JS, Jurvelin JA, Kiviranta I, Klauser RJ: Effects of different irrigation liquids and times on articular cartilage: An experimental, biomechanical study. Arthroscopy 10:667-672, 1994.
11. Morrison DS, Schaefer RK, Friedman RL: The relationship between subacromial pressure, blood pressure, and visual clarity during arthroscopic subacromial decompression. Arthroscopy 11:557-560, 1995.
12. Schaffer BS, Tibone JE: Arthroscopic shoulder instability surgery complications. Clin Sports Med 4:737-767, 1999.
13. Snyder SJ, Karzel RP, del Pizzo W, et al: SLAP lesions of the shoulder. Arthroscopy 6:274-279, 1990.
14. Williams MM, Snyder SJ, Buford D: The Buford complex—the "cord-like" middle glenohumeral ligament and absent anterosuperior labrum complex: A normal anatomic capsulolabral variant. Arthroscopy 10:241-247, 1994.
15. Yamaguchi K. Personal communication, AAOS Advanced Shoulder Course, July 2002.

CHAPTER

10

Shoulder: Diagnosis and Decision Making

MICHAEL J. MOSKAL AND MICHAEL L. PEARL

Instability is defined as an inability to hold the humeral head centered on the glenoid, resulting in *unwanted* excessive translation. The patient's history and physical examination can determine the degree, direction, and frequency of unwanted excessive humeral head translation on the glenoid.

Classification schemes of shoulder instability have been based on the energy of the injury, whether it is atraumatic or traumatic, the compromised stability mechanism, and the direction of the resultant instability. Concomitantly, instability may be organized by the arm positions associated with excessive translation and therefore the direction of humeral translation on the glenoid, as well as whether the instability occurs with the arm at the extremes of motion or in the midrange.

In this chapter, the basic mechanisms of shoulder stability are detailed first. In the unstable shoulder, one or more of these mechanisms have failed. An understanding of the failed mechanism or mechanisms allows treatment to be directed, regardless of the specific surgical technique employed. Next, an instability-directed clinical evaluation is detailed. The final section summarizes the compromised stability mechanisms, physical examination and radiographic findings, and reconstruction techniques to restore stability.

Anatomy and Biomechanics

Glenohumeral stability combines both dynamic and static anatomic stabilizing factors that exist in combination and may be additive in failure, leading to instability or unwanted excessive translation of the humeral head on the glenoid.[11]

Balance

The glenoid can be positioned such that net humeral joint reaction forces pass through the glenoid fossa.[3] The alignment of joint reaction forces is determined by the position of the glenoid (scapula) relative to the humerus; greater stability is present if net forces pass closely through the glenoid centerline as opposed to near the edge. The greater the angle between the humeral shaft and the glenoid, the greater the tendency for instability, because the net joint reaction forces summate near the periphery of the glenoid.[10,12] Decreased glenoid length or depth decreases the "allowable" motion that is stable, because the joint reaction forces align beyond the glenoid support.

Balance requires neuromuscular control of the scapula and the humerus relative to the scapula.[13,17] The range of directions of force supported by the glenoid is directly related to the arc length of the glenoid.

A glenoid fracture can shorten the glenoid arc length, limiting the range of forces supported by the glenoid and therefore the arm positions that allow the humeral head to remain located (Fig. 10–1). Poor scapular control can result in inferior tilting of the scapula, leading to subluxation of the humerus (Fig. 10–2). Finally, muscle imbalance, such as that seen in Erb's palsy, in which internal rotation forces (subscapularis) are more powerful than external rotation forces (supraspinatus and infraspinatus), causes the humeral head to subluxate posteriorly. Similarly, diminished superior stability can exist in the context of rotator cuff disease due to muscle imbalance, as the superiorly directed forces of the deltoid overcome the compression of the diseased rotator cuff.

Concavity Compression

Compression of the convex humeral head into the concave glenoid resists translation forces. The rotator cuff compresses the humeral head into the glenoid throughout the range of motion. Stability is increased by increasing the depth of the concavity, which is accomplished by both the "hard tissue" anatomy (bone and

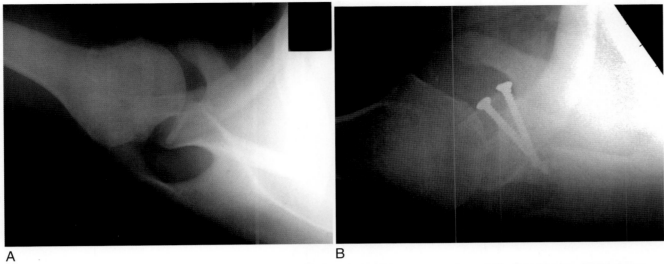

Figure 10–1   *A,* Glenoid fracture limits the range of motion in which the humeral head remains stabilized against the glenoid due to the foreshortened arc length. *B,* Glenoid arc length has been restored by anterior extracapsular bone grafting, restoring stability without altering the capsular length.

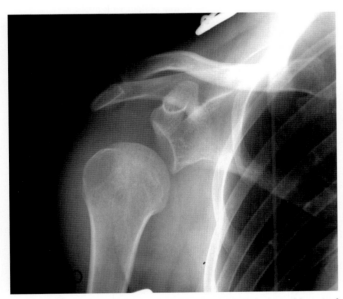

Figure 10–2   This patient's scapula is tilted inferiorly and is out of balance, resulting in inferior subluxation of the humeral head despite normal neurologic function. Interestingly, this patient failed six previous soft tissue operations designed to limit capsular length.

articular cartilage) and the soft tissue labrum. Theoretically, excessive unwanted translation of the humeral head on the glenoid can occur in any direction. Other anatomic factors such as the coracoacromial arch limit the magnitude of humeral displacement; therefore, certain directions of instability may be more subtle in their manifestations due to the minimal humeral translation.[16]

The bony anatomy of the glenoid is such that there is greater concavity in the superoinferior direction than in the anteroposterior direction. Further, the depth of articular cartilage increases toward the periphery, thus increasing the depth of the concavity. The capsulolabral complex, which attaches to the glenoid such that the labrum is on the surface of the glenoid fossa, increases the depth significantly at the periphery. The magnitude of compressive forces created by the rotator cuff increases glenohumeral stability.[18,20] However, the edge of the glenoid (cartilage and labrum) is deformable, and repeated excessive translation can decrease the height and minimize the concavity when the humeral head has excessively translated over the glenoid fossa edge[7,8,14,15] (Fig. 10–3).

After a patient suffers an anteroinferior dislocation of the shoulder, the capsulolabral complex typically avulses from the glenoid. If the anteroinferior labrum and capsule do not heal in their anatomic positions, the depth of concavity will be lost in that isolated area. When a patient's arm is placed in the abducted and externally rotated position, the summary forces across the glenoid align near the periphery. With a loss of concavity, excessive unwanted translation of the humeral head occurs, despite compression by the rotator cuff. The patient feels unwanted translation of the humeral head and reports "apprehension." Similarly, placing the arm in an adducted, internally rotated position places joint reaction forces at the posteroinferior portion of the glenoid. The adducted, internally rotated position may also result in apprehension due to unwanted, excessive posterior translation. Further, if there is a concomitant fracture of the glenoid bone, the arm position of abduction and external rotation tolerated by the patient would necessarily be less owing to the lack of support, because the joint reaction forces summate outside of the bone (see the earlier discussion of balance).

Another clinical example is the "load and shift" test. The patient relaxes to minimize the compressive effect of the rotator cuff. The examiner manually compresses the humeral head into the glenoid and then attempts to translate the humeral head (a tangential force).

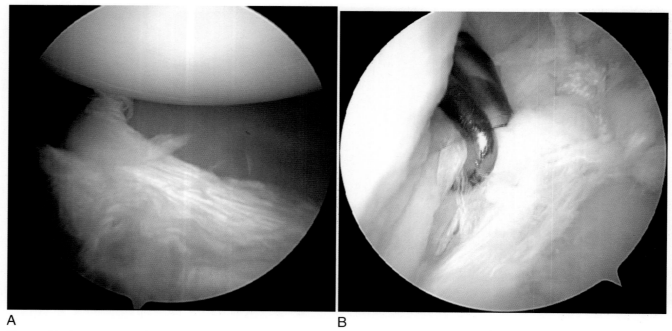

A   B

Figure 10–3   *A,* As seen from the posterior portal, the posterior labrum is flattened and attenuated in this patient with posterior instability. Also note the relative posteroinferior subluxation of the humeral head. *B,* In addition to rotator interval shortening, this patient underwent a capsulolabral augmentation by capsular plication. The first inferior suture (in this case, anchors were used) incorporates the patulous capsule and the split labrum. The probe demonstrates the split in the labrum.

Normally, to translate, the humeral head must move laterally over the glenoid edge and labrum. If the labrum has been avulsed or flattened, translation is easier due to the lost concavity. The deformable nature of the glenoid periphery serves to enhance stability when the humeral head is centered by a suction cup–like effect.

Suction Cup Effect

The labrum and capsule form a seal around the humeral head. Like a rubber suction cup, the glenoid is noncompliant in the center and increasingly compliant toward the periphery. The cartilage thickens toward the periphery, and the labrum and capsule at the periphery are more compliant. With compression, the interposed fluid is expressed to the periphery. Graduated flexibility allows the glenoid (cartilage, labrum, and capsule) to seal around the humeral head.

The suction cup effect helps center the humeral head independently of muscular forces and is significant in the midrange, where capsule and ligaments are not under tension. If the glenoid labrum is torn or the articular cartilage is eroded, the ability of the capsulolabral complex to "seal" around the humeral head is limited. Just as wetting a rubber suction cup often improves the compressive effect, in the shoulder, the synovial fluid in the glenohumeral joint facilitates stability by the "adhesion-cohesion" phenomenon.[12]

Adhesion-Cohesion

An adhesive fluid is one in which the molecules are attracted to like molecules. A cohesive surface is one to which fluid adheres. So when two cohesive surfaces (articular cartilage) come into contact with adhesive (synovial) fluid, the adhesion of the fluid and the cohesion of the surfaces tend to keep the surfaces together. This phenomenon is similar to the forces seen when two wet glass microscope slides are stuck together. Adhesion-cohesion functions in any joint position. The magnitude of the stabilizing force is predicated on the synovial fluid present, as well as the conformity of the contacting surfaces.

The loss of articular cartilage and labral tears limit both adhesion-cohesion and the suction cup effect. Articular cartilage irregularity diminishes the integrity of the contact surfaces, and labral tears do not allow a conforming seal to form around the humeral head (Fig. 10–4). Inflammatory changes in the synovial fluid alter the cohesive properties. Further, the volume of fluid and the volume of the glenohumeral joint (determined by capsular length) affect glenohumeral stability.[12]

Limited Joint Volume

The synovia removes free fluid and maintains the negative intra-articular pressure. The joint capsule is sealed, and the length is fixed. The humeral head is held with increasing force to the glenoid by the relative vacuum created as it is distracted away, increasing the negative pressure and adding to the resistance to displacement. Stability is enhanced by the close apposition of the joint surfaces, independent of muscular action.

Simply venting the glenohumeral capsule increases translation ease.[4] Glenohumeral venting is common in shoulder biomechanical studies to minimize the limited

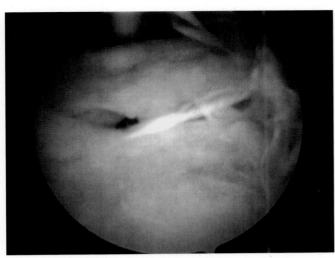

Figure 10–4   Loss of cartilage on the anterior glenoid. This patient, a competitive baseball player, never dislocated his shoulder but rather had straight anterior instability. The detached labrum and middle glenohumeral ligament are present.

joint space effect. Stability is compromised by factors that increase the amount of fluid, such as the presence of a hemarthrosis after fractures of the proximal humerus. Not uncommonly, the humeral head is subluxated inferiorly after a fracture, and with fracture healing and hemarthrosis resolution, the humeral head centers on the glenoid. Furthermore, the amount of "drive-through" present during arthroscopy should be interpreted with caution because of the necessary venting and the instillation of arthroscopy fluid. The degree of separation is predicated on capsular length and the amount of traction present.

Patients vary in the degree of ligamentous laxity. A very compliant capsule may stretch and be pulled into the joint. This greater compliance minimizes the increase in the negative pressure with distraction. The capsule and ligaments may actually infold into the joint between the humerus and glenoid and diminish the stability mechanisms that rely on conformity, thus contributing to the lack of centering in the midrange. The capsular length also contributes to glenohumeral stability at the extremes of motion and has been referred to as the capsuloligamentous constraint mechanism.

Capsuloligamentous Constraint

The capsule and ligaments are checkreins to rotation and translation. The magnitude of rotation, elevation, and translation is predicated on capsular length and compliance.[16] The capsule and ligaments are in continuity with the glenoid articular surface and, under tension, provide a smooth continuation of the glenoid concavity.

The greater the angle between the humeral shaft and the glenoid, the greater the tendency for instability, owing to the fact that summating forces align near the periphery of the glenoid fossa as opposed to the center. Coincidentally, the positions that result in the joint reaction forces falling *outside* the glenoid concavity are those positions in which the capsuloligamentous structures become tight. This mechanism is not activated in the midrange of motion because no tension is present in the capsulolabral complex. At the extremes of motion, tension is rapidly generated to impart a stabilizing force to both limit rotation and exert a force on the humeral head to normalize joint reaction forces. The ligaments are well placed to tolerate the large torques encountered at the extremes of common motions such as overhead throwing.

After a dislocation, the capsule is detached (typically along with the labrum) and functionally lengthened, and it does not exert a centering force to minimize the restraint to translation (in addition to the loss of concavity due to the labral avulsion). With repeated trauma, the capsule may become lengthened[1,2,9,19] while attached to the labrum and glenoid. Independent of humeral version, excessive rotation of the humerus may occur and increase normal contact forces between the undersurface of the rotator cuff and the posterosuperior labrum. Shortening of the anterior capsule can limit rotation and minimize such contact.

One of the primary goals of the clinical evaluation is to differentiate between *mechanical laxity* and *clinical instability*. Laxity refers to the amount (distance) of translation of the humeral head on the glenoid away from the center and therefore reflects the length and compliance of the capsule. Translation requires lateral displacement of the humeral head over the intact labrum. A "normal" amount of laxity does not exist, and there is tremendous individual variation. Translation is limited at the extremes of motion by tension and shortening of the capsule as it wraps around the humeral head. Increased or decreased laxity does not *necessarily* imply instability or stability, respectively. Stable shoulders can be extremely lax, whereas unstable shoulders can be minimally lax. Typical laxity tests require the patient to relax (and therefore minimize concavity compression) and position the humerus in the midrange of motion (to maximize capsular length).[5]

In certain circumstances, increased laxity may allow the humeral head to be positioned in extremes before the stretched capsule tightens, limiting translation.

Rotator Interval Capsule

The rotator interval is a triangular structure whose base is the coracoid process; the coracohumeral ligament originates from the base, and the transverse humeral ligament is the apex. The structural contents of the rotator interval are the capsule, coracohumeral ligament, and superior glenohumeral ligament. The rotator interval capsule plays a major role in the range of certain motions, in obligate translation, and in allowed translation of the glenohumeral joint.[6,21]

Shortening of the rotator interval decreases posterior and inferior translation. The length of the rotator interval does *not* have a significant effect on anterior translation in the midrange and, interestingly, *augments* obligate anterior and superior translation at extremes of flexion. When repairing the rotator cuff, cutting the rotator interval can diminish the anterosuperior translation with elevation and minimize tension on the cuff repair.

Clinical Evaluation

History

The basic functions of the history are to determine the circumstances in which the problem began and that presently cause symptoms and to correlate the arm position or positions that produce symptoms. Other components of the history can refine the diagnosis and add to the understanding of the deficient stabilizing mechanism. Associated numbness or tingling of the arm should be ascertained.

Patient Age

Unwanted excessive humeral translation can occur at any age. For instance, the sequelae of a stroke may paralyze the shoulder girdle muscles and allow the humeral head to subluxate inferiorly on the glenoid. The most common age of presentation, however, is between 15 and 40 years. Patients with "atraumatic" or repetitive low-level injuries tend to be younger and are typically 10 to 30 years old, whereas patients with "traumatic" unidirectional instability tend to be 16 to 40 years old.

Injury

The type of trauma has been used to classify these injuries and to help understand patient characteristics and the underlying faulty stabilizing mechanisms. If the initial traumatic event was a fairly violent mechanism with large applied forces, the instability pattern can be classified as a "traumatic" type. The humeral head translates significantly, but the humerus does not necessarily dislocate. Some form of reduction maneuver is common. These traumatic types of injuries result in an instability in which the humerus translates excessively in a single direction and are associated with labral detachments; the instability pattern is duplicated by unique, typically singular arm positions. This common form of antero-inferior instability is referred to as the "TUBS" type (*t*raumatic *u*nidirectional instability *B*ankart lesion, often improving with *s*urgery). Should a posterior dislocation occur, the "B" of the acronym would refer to the labral detachment corresponding to the posteroinferior quadrant of the glenoid.

In other forms of instability, a clear-cut high-energy injury is not present in the history. Rather, the patient recounts a series of events that individually do not cause clinical instability but rather cause a number of stability mechanisms to eventually decompensate. The patient may recall a specific low-energy event, such as an awkward lift, as the decompensating injury and may report that "popping" the shoulder provides comfort. The clinical instability is such that the humeral head translates excessively in multiple directions. A reduction maneuver is almost never needed. Instability with multiple directions of excessive translation is referred to as the

"AMBRII" type (*a*traumatic *m*ultidirectional instability with *b*ilateral findings, often improving with *r*ehabilitation, and should surgery be needed, a *r*otator interval capsule–coracohumeral ligament plication with tightening of the *i*nferior capsule is needed).

Importantly, one should try to understand the instability in terms of the mechanisms of stability that have failed, so that treatment can be directed toward correcting each one. The broad classifications remain useful and highlight the fact that in certain instability patterns, rehabilitation is critical because associated muscular weakness and imbalance are typically present.

Arm Position

Arm position at the time of injury and the arm positions that reproduce the symptoms are critical to understanding the type of instability and the underlying failed mechanisms of stability.

In traumatic instability, a common mechanism of injury is an indirect loading to the capsulolabral complex, glenoid, and rotator cuff through the arm, which acts as a lever arm to transmit and augment energy to the structures. Commonly, the arm is at the extremes of elevation and rotation. Placing the humerus in abduction and external rotation tightens the anteroinferior glenohumeral ligament. The arm is forcefully extended and externally rotated, avulsing the anteroinferior labrum via the anteroinferior glenohumeral ligament.

In traumatic instability, the subsequent arm positions that provoke symptoms (instability) are typically similar to the position of the arm at the time of injury. The ease of translation and therefore symptoms of instability may increase with time, progressing to subluxation during sleep.

Patients with atraumatic or repetitive low-level instability often give a history of repetitive arm positions at extremes of motion in multiple positions. Common sport histories are swimming and volleyball. A patient may complain of mild symptoms that increase significantly after a seemingly trivial event.

In atraumatic or multidirectional instability, patients often (but not always) complain of symptoms with the arm in the midrange of motion, and sometimes in combination. The predominant arm positions that increase symptoms are in front of the body.

Physical Examination

The physical examination for shoulder instability is confirmatory or elaborative in nature based on the patient's history. A comprehensive musculoskeletal examination is also important. The following description is weighted primarily toward an instability examination.

Observation and Palpation

Observe the overall posture, with the patient both seated and standing, from posterior and anterior viewpoints. Look for shoulder girdle ptosis and scapular position asymmetry. In the chronic state, tenderness is unusual in patients with isolated instability.

Range of Motion

The range of motion of both shoulders should be measured, and it is typically symmetrical. Significantly greater range of motion than population norms may suggest the possibility of multidirectional instability, as capsular length is proportionate to elevation and rotation.

Provocative Positions

Observe as the patient demonstrates the arm positions that feel unstable, with special reference to associated faulty scapular mechanics. Following the demonstration, combine arm positions with force applications (rotation and translation) to produce or "threaten" instability (excessive unwanted translation).

The apprehension test places the arm in abduction and external rotation. A patient response of impending subluxation is positive and suggestive of anterior instability. In contrast, the jerk test, which places the arm in forward elevation, internal rotation, and adduction, can cause the humeral head to subluxate with reduction as the arm is abducted and externally rotated.

Translation

With the patient relaxed, the arm is positioned in the midrange of motion. The humerus is translated (tangential force to the glenoid) in the anterior, posterior, and inferior (sulcus test) directions to observe the magnitude of distance traveled. The mechanical laxity demonstrated by these translations is not specific for instability. One should observe the patient's response with each direction. A catch or a pop may be indicative of a torn labrum. Finally, the "feel" of the glenoid concavity can be appreciated, as can the accompanying lateral displacement of the humeral head, with translation in the anterior, posterior, and inferior directions.

Noting the ease of translation is also important. With the patient relaxed, the examiner compresses the humeral head medially to mimic the cuff and then translates the humeral head. With a competent labrum, translation is typically minimal. Without a labrum present to increase the concavity, the humeral head can be felt to move tangentially on the glenoid (translate) without appreciable lateral displacement.

Neuromuscular Examination

As described earlier, scapulothoracic motion and static scapular posture should be observed. A lateral "droop" or retraction with anterior elevation predisposing to excessive translation is typical in multidirectional instability. The periscapular muscles, including the protractors, elevators, and lower trapezius, should be tested.

Manual muscle testing of the rotator cuff can be done in external rotation at the side, in internal rotation at the side, and with the arm elevated 90 degrees in the scapular plane. Associated tears of the rotator cuff are unusual but become more common after a dislocation as patient age increases. Greater or lesser tuberosity fractures may occur and result in weakness.

Brachial plexus injuries are not uncommon but are typically minor and transient. Older age is associated with clinically observable sequelae of neural injury. In addition to examining peripheral pulses, signs of atrophy should be documented. Weakness without fracture or rotator cuff tendon tear raises the suspicion of neural injury.

Imaging

An anteroposterior view in the scapular plane and an axillary lateral view are the basic radiographs obtained. Specialized views, such as the apical oblique view, may be added based on the clinical situation.

Ancillary studies such as magnetic resonance imaging or computed tomography may be helpful but are not needed on a routine basis. Computed tomography is useful to evaluate the glenoid arc length after fracture. Magnetic resonance imaging with or without a gadolinium arthrogram is useful to determine subtle labral or capsular tearing, as well as the integrity of the rotator cuff tendons.

Summary

Traumatic Anterior Instability

History

1. Typically, the humerus is elevated beyond 90 degrees and externally rotated. The force is applied at a distance, such as when the forearm is trying to block a shot in basketball. The arm is forcefully externally rotated.
2. If the humerus dislocates, a reduction maneuver is often required.
3. The arm is stable at the side. Abduction and external rotation increase symptoms.

Physical Examination

1. Normal appearance in the chronic state.
2. Absence of rotator cuff weakness.
3. Apprehension with the arm in 90 degrees of abduction and 90 degrees of external rotation.
4. Load and shift test is positive (ease of translation).

Radiographs

1. Anteroposterior: observe for periosteal changes inferiorly, and ensure that the joint space is visible.
2. Axillary: observe for glenoid fracture and humeral fracture.
3. Apical oblique: observe for humeral impaction fracture and inferior glenoid avulsion fracture.

Primary Failed Stability Mechanisms

1. Concavity compression:
   a. Loss of concavity (labrum or cartilage).
   b. Compression by rotator cuff is typically normal.
2. Capsuloligamentous constraint.
3. Adhesion-cohesion and suction cup.
4. Balance if a fracture significantly shortens the arc length of the glenoid.

Treatment: Nonoperative

1. Sling for comfort.
2. Strengthening.
3. Avoid abducted, externally rotated arm position.

Treatment: Operative

1. Examination under anesthesia.
2. Labral repair to the peripheral margin of the glenoid fossa.
3. Capsulorrhaphy:
   a. If the capsule is significantly lengthened.
   b. If there is no labral avulsion, the capsule can be shifted and repaired to the labrum, which increases the depth of the glenoid and shortens the capsule.
4. Glenoid fracture:
   a. Acute: open reduction and internal fixation.
   b. Chronic glenoid deficiency: bone graft (Bristow-Laterjet or iliac crest) to lengthen glenoid arc.

Traumatic Posterior Instability

History

1. Humerus elevated to about 90 degrees and internally rotated (as in blocking in football).
2. If the humerus dislocates, a reduction may be needed.
3. Arm stable at the side; elevation, internal rotation, and adduction increase symptoms.

Physical Examination

1. Normal in chronic state.
2. Absence of rotator cuff problems.
3. Apprehension with arm elevated 90 degrees, internally rotated, and adducted across the chest.
4. Jerk test positive:
   a. The arm is subluxated in the position described for apprehension
   b. The arm is reduced with abduction and external rotation.

Radiographs

1. Anteroposterior: ensure joint space is present; overlap suggests chronic dislocation.
2. Axillary: observe for glenoid and humeral fracture.

Primary Failed Stability Mechanisms

1. Concavity compression:
   a. Concavity loss due to labral avulsion; more commonly, repeated humeral subluxations flatten the labrum.
   b. Compression by the rotator cuff is typically normal.
2. Capsuloligamentous constraint.
3. Adhesion-cohesion and suction cup.
4. Balance:
   a. Fracture significantly shortens the arc length of the glenoid.
   b. Abnormal scapular movement (tilting) with glenohumeral motion.

Treatment: Nonoperative

1. Sling for comfort.
2. Strengthening.
3. Avoid adducted, elevated, and internally rotated arm position.

Treatment: Operative

1. Labral repair similar to that for anterior instability.
2. Capsulorrhaphy—posterior instability typically has an attenuated labrum rather than avulsion of the capsule and labrum, as in traumatic anterior instability:
   a. Shortening of lengthened capsule.
   b. Capsule plicated to the labrum to shorten the capsule and increase the depth of the glenoid concavity.
3. Rotator interval plication:
   a. Reduces flexion, adduction, and external rotation.
   b. Minimizes posterior and inferior humeral translation.

Multidirectional "Atraumatic" Instability

History

1. Repetitive activities requiring excellent coordination, strength, endurance, and often extremes of motion, such as swimming or volleyball.
2. Pain, occasional paresthesias (commonly ulnar nerve distribution); if the humerus dislocates, a reduction may be needed.
3. Arm stable at the side.
4. Symptoms typically in the midrange of motion as well as at extremes.

Physical Examination

1. Poor shoulder posture and associated shoulder girdle ptosis.
2. Rotator cuff weakness.
3. Apprehension with arm elevated 90 degrees, internally rotated, and adducted across the chest.
4. Jerk test positive:
   a. The arm is subluxated in the position described for apprehension.
   b. The arm is reduced with abduction and external rotation.

Radiographs

1. Anteroposterior and axillary views are typically normal.

Primary Failed Stability Mechanisms

1. Concavity compression:
   a. Concavity loss due to repeated humeral subluxations that flatten the labrum.
   b. Compression by the rotator cuff is typically diminished.
2. Capsuloligamentous constraint: loose, stretchy capsular tissue is common and may predispose to lengthening.

3. Adhesion-cohesion and suction cup:
   a. Possible capsular inflolding between humeral head and glenoid due to increased capsular length and compliance.
   b. When infolded, the redundant capsule may act as a skid to facilitate humeral subluxation.
4. Limited joint volume: loose, stretchy capsule minimizes negative intra-articular pressure with distraction.
5. Balance: abnormal scapular movement (tilting) with glenohumeral motion.

Treatment: Nonoperative

1. Avoid provocative positions and inciting activities.
2. Strengthening:
   a. Scapular strengthening and positioning exercises.
   b. Postural exercises.
   c. Avoid rotator cuff strengthening until manual muscle testing is pain free.

Treatment: Operative

1. Labrum is typically attenuated but attached; if torn, repair to surface of glenoid periphery.
2. Capsulorrhaphy:
   a. Concentric shortening with repair to labrum.
   b. Symmetrically tighten anteriorly and posteriorly.
   c. Capsule plicated to labrum to shorten capsule and increase depth of glenoid concavity.
3. Rotator interval plication:
   a. Reduces flexion, adduction, and external rotation.
   b. Minimizes posterior and inferior humeral translation.

References

1. Bigliani LU, Flatow EL, Kelkar R, et al: The effect of anterior capsular tightening on shoulder kinematics and contact. J Shoulder Elbow Surg 3:S65, 1994.
2. Bigliani LU, Kelkar R, Flatow EL, et al: Glenohumeral stability: Biomechanical properties of passive and active stabilizers. Clin Orthop 330:13-30, 1996.
3. Gerber A, Ghalambor N, Warner JJ: Instability of shoulder arthroplasty: Balancing mobility and stability. Orthop Clin North Am 32:661-670, 2001.
4. Gibb TD, Sidles JA, Harryman DT 2nd, et al: The effect of capsular venting on glenohumeral laxity. Clin Orthop 268:120-127, 1991.
5. Harryman DT, Sidles JA, Clark JM, et al: Translation of the humeral head on the glenoid with passive glenohumeral motion. J Bone Joint Surg Am 72:1334-1343, 1990.
6. Harryman DT 2nd, Sidles JA, Harris SL, Matsen FA 3rd: The role of the rotator interval capsule in passive motion and stability of the shoulder. J Bone Joint Surg Am 74:53-66, 1992.
7. Kelkar R, Wang VM, Flatow EL, et al: Glenohumeral mechanics: A study of articular geometry, contact, and kinematics. J Shoulder Elbow Surg 10:73-84, 2001.
8. Lazarus MD, Sidles JA, Harryman DT 2nd, Matsen FA 3rd: Effect of a chondral-labral defect on glenoid concavity and glenohumeral stability: A cadaveric model. J Bone Joint Surg Am 78:94-102, 1996.
9. Levine WN, Flatow EL: The pathophysiology of shoulder instability. Am J Sports Med 28:910-917, 2000.
10. Lippitt S, Matsen F: Mechanisms of glenohumeral joint stability. Clin Orthop 291:20-28, 1993.
11. Matsen FA 3rd: The biomechanics of glenohumeral stability. J Bone Joint Surg Am 84:495-496, 2002.
12. Matsen FA, Lippit SB, Sidles JA, Harryman DT: Practical Evaluation and Management of the Shoulder. Philadelphia, WB Saunders, 1994, pp 213-214.
13. McClure PW, Michener LA, Sennett BJ, Karduna AR: Direct 3-dimensional measurement of scapular kinematics during dynamic movements in vivo. J Shoulder Elbow Surg 10:269-277, 2001.
14. Metcalf MH, Duckworth DG, Lee SB, et al: Posteroinferior glenoplasty can change glenoid shape and increase the mechanical stability of the shoulder. J Shoulder Elbow Surg 8:205-213, 1999.
15. Metcalf MH, Pon JD, Harryman DT 2nd, et al: Capsulolabral augmentation increases glenohumeral stability in the cadaver shoulder. J Shoulder Elbow Surg 10:532-538, 2001.
16. Moskal MJ, Harryman DT 2nd, Romeo AA, et al: Glenohumeral motion after complete capsular release. Arthroscopy 15:408-416, 1999.
17. Pearl ML: Dynamic electromyographic analysis of the throwing shoulder with glenohumeral instability. J Bone Joint Surg Am 70:1428-1429, 1988.
18. Schiffern SC, Rozencwaig R, Antoniou J, et al: Anteroposterior centering of the humeral head on the glenoid in vivo. Am J Sports Med 30:382-387, 2002.
19. Ticker JB, Bigliani LU, Soslowsky LJ, et al: Inferior glenohumeral ligament: Geometric and strain-rate dependent properties. J Shoulder Elbow Surg 5:269-279, 1996.
20. Warner JJ, Bowen MK, Deng X, et al: Effect of joint compression on inferior stability of the glenohumeral joint. J Shoulder Elbow Surg 8:31-36, 1999.
21. Warner JJ, Deng XH, Warren RF, Torzilli PA: Static capsuloligamentous restraints to superior-inferior translation of the glenohumeral joint. Am J Sports Med 20:675-685, 1992.

Single-Point Fixation for Shoulder Instability

KYLE R. FLIK, VICTOR LOPEZ JR.,

AND ANSWORTH A. ALLEN

SINGLE-POINT FIXATION FOR SHOULDER INSTABILITY IN A NUTSHELL

Background:
The Suretac device is a bioabsorbable cannulated tack that has been used successfully in the shoulder for single-point fixation of Bankart lesions in patients with anterior instability.

History:
Most patients have had a traumatic anteroinferior shoulder dislocation with an associated Bankart lesion but without other shoulder pathology or significant laxity.

Physical Examination:
Anterior instability is demonstrated on anterior drawer testing. Apprehension and relocation tests are positive. There is no significant sulcus sign, which would be evidence of multidirectional instability.

Imaging:
Radiographs include true anteroposterior, scapular Y view, Stryker notch (for Hill-Sachs), and West Point axillary (for bony Bankart). Magnetic resonance imaging can be used to document labral detachment and to rule out other pathology.

Indications:
Suretac is used for patients with (1) pure anteroinferior instability, (2) a discrete labral tear, (3) a healthy anteroinferior glenohumeral ligament complex without significant stretch or fraying, (4) no evidence of multidirectional instability, and (5) the ability to comply with rehabilitation restrictions.

Technique:
Important technical points include (1) examination under anesthesia and diagnostic arthroscopy, (2) careful selection of portal position, (3) adequate preparation of the glenoid neck, (4) appropriate tissue tensioning, (5) avoidance of medialization of the implant, and (6) elimination of the drive-through sign.

Postoperative Management:
Weeks 0-4: sling; weeks 4-8: active assisted range of motion; weeks 8-12: rotator cuff strengthening; weeks 12-16: passive stretch, especially external rotation; weeks 16-24: nonoverhead sports; after 24 weeks: unrestricted.

Results:
Reported rates of recurrence range from 0% to 38%. Lower rates occur when stricter indications are applied. Compared with open stabilization, there is a higher recurrence rate, improved range of motion, improved cosmesis, and shorter hospital stay.

Complications:
Reactive synovitis can occur, which may require arthroscopic synovectomy. Technical errors leading to failure include medialization of implant, resulting in loss of external rotation; inadequate compression of capsular tissue by the implant; and articular damage from poorly placed implants or misdirected drilling.

Many innovative techniques have been developed for the arthroscopic repair of the Bankart "essential lesion" in patients with anterior shoulder instability. Currently, the most commonly used methods for repair of a detached anterior labrum and anteroinferior glenohumeral ligament (AIGHL) complex are metal or biodegradable knotless suture anchors (Mitek Products, Westwood, MA) and FASTak suture anchors (Arthrex, Naples, FL), which require arthroscopic knot tying and bioabsorbable tack systems such as the Suretac (Smith and Nephew, Andover, MA). Two-pronged metal staple fixation has lost its role in the armamentarium because of its increased risk of loosening, injury to the joint surface, and recurrent instability.[13,18,24,28] Transglenoid sutures are rarely used because of the increased risk of suprascapular nerve injury.[16,17,37,44]

Before deciding which technique to use, one must determine that the injured capsulolabral complex can be adequately and anatomically repaired arthroscopically. This requires an accurate history, thorough physical examination, and proper imaging studies. Ultimately, the decision to employ an arthroscopic technique for repair is made in the operating room after an examination under anesthesia (EUA) and diagnostic arthroscopy are performed.

Regardless of which method is used, the goal is to provide adequate stability, function, and early rehabilitation without loss of motion. Although a variety of arthroscopic techniques have proved effective in achieving these objectives, this chapter focuses on single-point fixation with the Suretac device.

History

Traumatic anterior glenohumeral dislocation has an incidence of approximately 1.7% in the general population.[21] It is one of the most common shoulder injuries in athletes. The reported incidence of a Bankart lesion after acute dislocation ranges from 85% to 100%.[6,27,30,41] Risk of recurrence is directly related to activity level and inversely related to age.

A patient with anterior shoulder instability may present in a variety of ways, ranging from frank dislocation with pain and deformity to subtle complaints of pain or a vague sense of instability. The latter is more common in patients with multidirectional instability. When obtaining a patient history, it is important to try to ascertain the arm position and direction of force at the time of injury and the method used for reduction to help confirm the direction of instability. It is also important to determine whether there is a prior history of subluxation, dislocation, surgery, or other injury and the chronicity of the complaint. A history of multiple dislocations or subluxations implies a higher likelihood of capsular deformation and stretch, which, if significant enough, may require an open capsular shift procedure for proper tensioning of the tissue.

Another important factor in an athlete's history is the type of sport in which he or she participates. Patients who return to collision or contact sports may be at greater risk

for recurrent instability episodes. In addition, the age of the patient is a critical factor. If treated nonoperatively, the risk for recurrent instability in patients younger than 20 years is greater than 90%, compared with 10% in patients older than 40.[36]

Physical Examination

Typically, a patient who has suffered an acute traumatic anterior shoulder dislocation presents in severe pain, with the arm usually in slight abduction and internal rotation. Axillary nerve injury is possible, and motor and sensory examination of the nerve should be documented. More commonly, the patient presents with minimal pain days after being treated acutely with a reduction maneuver and placed in a sling.

After taking a thorough history, the clinician should have a definite sense of the direction and type of instability pattern that may be present. The shoulder examination is then performed systematically. This includes inspection, palpation, range of motion, strength testing, and provocative maneuvers. A thorough neurovascular examination to evaluate for possible concomitant brachial plexus or vascular injury is also executed, as well as an examination of the cervical spine. Finally, specific tests for instability should be performed, including the apprehension test, relocation test, anterior and posterior drawer maneuvers, and sulcus sign.

The apprehension test is performed by placing the arm in a position of abduction with external rotation. This causes a feeling of uneasiness and an uncomfortable sense of imminent dislocation. The relocation maneuver, which simply places a posterior-directed force on the proximal humerus, is positive if it relieves the apprehension.[31] According to Romeo,[35] a history of a traumatic event with a documented anterior dislocation and a positive apprehension sign is associated with a greater than 95% incidence of a Bankart lesion. These patients also have increased anterior translation with drawer testing.[3] The amount of translation is graded based on the final position of the humerus in relation to the glenoid.

The sulcus sign is demonstrated by a depression visualized between the inferior border of the lateral acromion and the superior aspect of the humeral head while pulling longitudinal traction on the arm. The presence of a sulcus sign greater than 2 cm suggests inferior laxity to the degree commonly found in patients with multidirectional instability.[29]

Imaging

The plain radiographs used in the routine evaluation of shoulder instability include a true anteroposterior view of the shoulder in internal and external rotation, a lateral view of the scapula (scapula Y view), a West Point axillary view, and a Stryker notch view. The West Point axillary view clearly shows the condition of the anteroinferior glenoid rim, where a bony Bankart may be found. The Stryker notch view is the best radiograph to demonstrate a Hill-Sachs lesion (impaction of the posterolateral aspect of the humeral head).

Magnetic resonance imaging is excellent for the detection of labral injuries, chondral defects, capsular detachments, rotator cuff tears, or biceps anchor injuries. Stabilization with the Suretac device is best suited for pure, isolated Bankart lesions, so detection of concomitant pathology is important. (An example of a Bankart lesion is shown in Figures 11–1 and 11–2.)

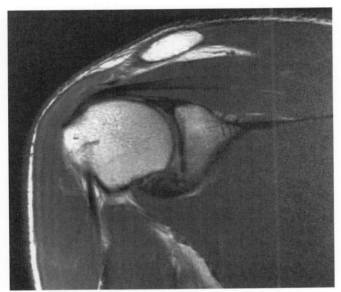

Figure 11–1   Coronal oblique magnetic resonance imaging scan of a glenohumeral joint with a Bankart lesion.

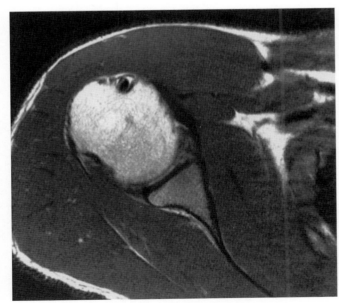

Figure 11–2   Axial magnetic resonance imaging scan of a glenohumeral joint with a Bankart lesion.

Decision-Making Principles

The most crucial step in arthroscopic stabilization with the Suretac device is patient selection. The ideal patient has a discrete Bankart lesion, a robust and well-developed AIGHL complex, no significant capsular laxity or intraligamentous injury, and no other intra-articular pathology.[39,40] Single-point fixation with a biodegradable implant such as Suretac was devised to provide an efficient method of reestablishing the integrity of the soft tissue–glenoid interface by reattaching the detached labrum while simultaneously retensioning the AIGHL complex. However, the preoperative decision-making process is crucial to determining which patients will have good results with this technique.

An EUA that reveals pure 2+ or 3+ anterior translation is an indication of a good candidate for arthroscopic stabilization. Diagnostic arthroscopy that shows an isolated Bankart lesion without significant degeneration or fraying and no significant capsular laxity probably indicates a good candidate for Suretac fixation. In contrast, a history of long-standing subluxations coupled with physical findings of generalized ligamentous laxity or a large sulcus sign suggests multidirectional instability, which requires open stabilization. Additional reasons to choose an alternative to the Suretac system include the presence of poor-quality labral tissue or the lack of a well-defined anterior band of the inferior glenohumeral ligament (IGHL). Some authors consider participation in contact sports to be a relative contraindication to arthroscopic stabilization with the Suretac device.[1]

Surgical Technique

Suretac is the first generation of bioabsorbable transfixing devices with a bioabsorption profile similar to that of native healing tissue. The device is a cannulated tack made of polyglyconate. There are two sizes: the 8-mm tack has a core diameter of 4.3 mm and a head diameter of 7.5 mm, and the 6-mm tack has a core diameter of 3.5 mm and a head diameter of 6 mm; both sizes are 16 mm long. Each has undersurface spikes that help hold the soft tissue while minimizing tissue necrosis. It contains concentric ribs along its shaft, which help provide initial pullout strength of approximately 100 N. The device loses one quarter of its strength each week, until it no longer plays a mechanical role at 4 weeks.[15]

Positioning

We prefer to use the beach chair position with regional or interscalene block anesthesia for most arthroscopic shoulder surgeries. This position is especially useful in instability cases when conversion to an open procedure may be necessary. There is no need for traction devices, so the arm can rest freely and the shoulder can be easily examined in the anatomic position.

2 Shoulder

Examination under Anesthesia

To confirm the instability pattern, we always perform drawer testing during the EUA. If significant inferior laxity exists, as evidenced by grade 3+ inferior translation or sulcus sign, the patient should be evaluated further for significant capsular laxity and considered for a formal capsular shift procedure. Excellent correlation has been reported between the findings on EUA and the findings at surgery.[8,9,32]

Diagnostic Arthroscopy

We use an arthroscopic pump to circulate saline with epinephrine within the joint to provide constant distention, minimize bleeding, and improve visualization during the procedure. A diagnostic arthroscopy is the first step in the procedure. The arthroscope is placed through a standard posterior portal located 2 cm distal and medial to the posterolateral border of the acromion. A superolateral portal is created by placing a spinal needle under direct visualization from outside in at the superolateral aspect of the acromion to the intra-articular edge of the supraspinatus tendon, as described by Laurencin et al.[25] This portal is used for inflow and anterior visualization of the joint. A second anterior portal, the anteroinferior portal, is created just lateral to the coracoid and immediately adjacent to the superior edge of the subscapularis. This portal will receive the large 7-mm cannula for the fixation system. Proper placement of this portal is important for access to the anteroinferior rim of the glenoid. To help improve accuracy, we insert the cannulas by first placing the blunt end of a Steinmann pin into the joint and then advancing the cannula over the pin.

A full diagnostic arthroscopy is performed, specifically looking for anatomic lesions such as a suspected detached anteroinferior glenoid labrum, chondral lesion, rotator cuff injury, or Hill-Sachs lesion. The ideal lesion for fixation with Suretac is a discrete detachment of a healthy labrum with little capsular stretch. Therefore, the condition of the labrum should be evaluated, and the capsule should be assessed for redundancy. A grasper can be used through the anteroinferior portal to pull the labrum to its planned position on the glenoid rim. After the labrum is positioned appropriately, the arthroscope is driven from posterior into the anteroinferior pouch. This "drive-through" test, described by Pagnani and Warren,[33] can be used to assess whether the proposed fixation will accomplish the goal of re-creating enough stability. The ease of passage of the arthroscope is used to assess capsular tension. The drive-through sign is obliterated if appropriate tension is restored. Transferring the arthroscope to the superolateral portal is helpful to assess the anterior ligaments. The decision to proceed with Suretac fixation is made after this initial arthroscopic evaluation, which should reveal a robust capsulolabral complex that can be adequately tensioned. The arm is positioned in adduction and slight internal rotation for the procedure.

Specific Surgical Steps

Glenoid Preparation

The first step in the procedure is preparation of the glenoid neck. The labrum is dissected from the glenoid neck with a sharp-tipped rasp to mobilize the tissue to the 6 o'clock position (Fig. 11–3). An arthroscopic bur is used to create a bleeding bone bed for reattachment of the labrum approximately 10 to 15 mm from the edge of the glenoid (Figs. 11–4 and 11–5).

Tissue Tensioning and Glenoid Drilling

The drill and guidewire are assembled with approximately 5 to 10 mm of the guidewire protruding and inserted through the large cannula in the anteroinferior portal. The capsulolabral complex is captured with the tip of the guidewire and advanced superiorly along the scapular neck. It may be helpful to use a grasper through the superolateral portal to tension the tissue before fixation (Fig. 11–6). Place the first Suretac as low as possible (usually around the 4 o'clock position in a right shoulder) on the anteromedial aspect of the prepared glenoid neck. Avoid placing the labrum medially on the glenoid neck, which can lead to failure and recurrence of instability. Advance the drill and guidewire into the glenoid at an oblique angle, and avoid the articular surface (Fig. 11–7). The drill should be advanced in the

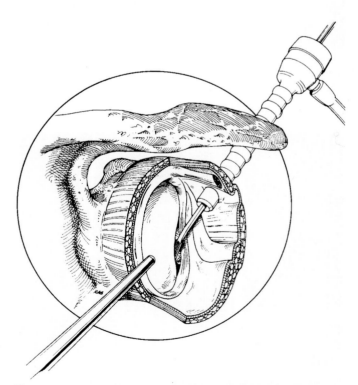

Figure 11–3 Glenoid attachment site preparation. The labrum and capsule may require further detachment initially to allow proximal positioning of the tissue. Dissecting the capsule and labrum off the neck of the glenoid may be required.

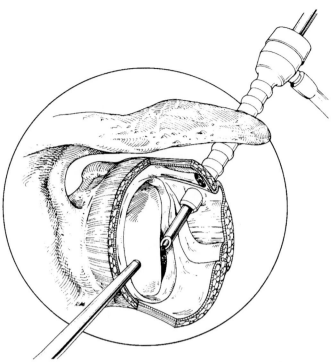

Figure 11–4 The bone is prepared using an Acufex knife rasp that has a cutting edge to facilitate capsular detachment. A shaver and bur complete the preparation of the bone to a depth of 10 to 15 mm from the edge of the glenoid, to promote soft tissue healing.

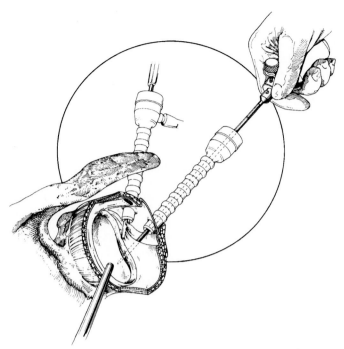

Figure 11–6 The tissue tensioner is inserted into a superior portal to grasp the edge of the labrum and inferior ligament, advancing it proximally. The cannula (7 mm) is placed into the joint space proximal to the edge of the subscapularis tendon. The Suretac drill, guidewire, and drill handle are assembled and placed through the cannula and against the capsule or labrum at a point that puts maximal tension on the soft tissue.

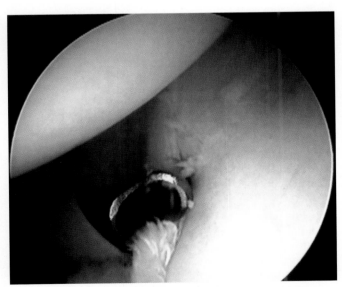

Figure 11–5 Intraoperative view of glenoid preparation using an arthroscopic bur.

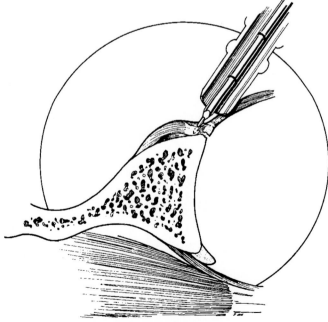

Figure 11–7 The drill and guidewire are then advanced (either manually with the drill handle or power assisted) into the glenoid at an oblique angle, avoiding the articular surface.

bone to a depth equal to one length of the Suretac implant (16 mm) or one marking on the drill (Fig. 11–8). Carefully withdraw the drill bit over the wire after releasing the locking screw. Tap the guidewire with a mallet to secure it within the bone while the drill is removed.

Implant Placement

Insert a Suretac over the guidewire, and impact it through the cannula using the cannulated driver (Figs. 11–9 and 11–10). This transfixes the labrum to the glenoid neck. When tapping the Suretac into the glenoid, avoid overpenetrating the ligament (Fig. 11–11). Remove the guidewire through the driver. Figure 11–12 shows a well-seated device. The entire process is then repeated, typically in the 3 o'clock and 2 o'clock positions, to restore tension adequately in the IGHL complex (Fig. 11–13). From the superolateral portal, the anterior aspect of the shoulder can be viewed to ensure adequate soft tissue purchase. From the posterior portal, the drive-through sign can now be eliminated.

Pearls and Pitfalls

Most of the potential problems with the use of the Suretac device are related to errors in patient selection, inadequate technical execution of the procedure, and less than optimal postoperative rehabilitation.

Patients who have the best outcomes after surgery are those with traumatic unidirectional anterior instability,

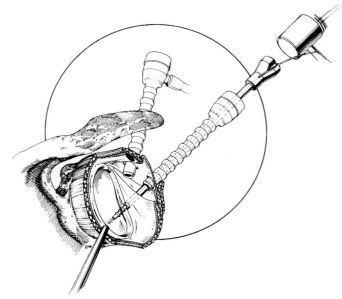

Figure 11–9 After the drill is removed, the Suretac is placed over the guidewire, and the Suretac driver is used to seat the Suretac.

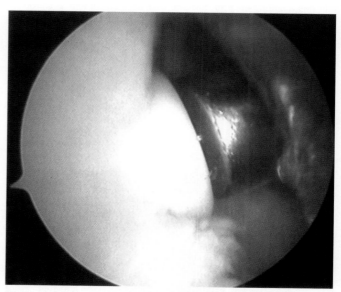

Figure 11–10 Intraoperative arthroscopic image showing placement of a Suretac anchor, with the Suretac driver seating the device.

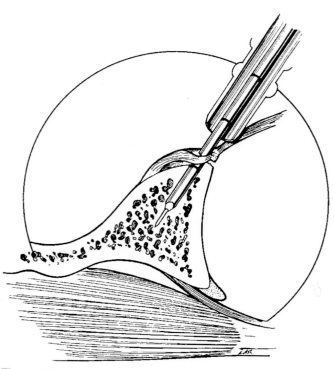

Figure 11–8 The drill is placed in the bone to a depth equal to one length of the Suretac implant (16 mm) or one marking on the Suretac drill. (It is imperative to use the specially designed Suretac drill to create a bone hole of the appropriate depth.)

a Bankart lesion, and a well-developed IGHL. With a first-time dislocation, surgery should not be performed between 10 and 30 days after injury. During this period, there is a biologic response as the tissue attempts to heal. It becomes soft and friable and will not hold the anchor.

In patients with chronic recurrent anterior instability, Suretac fixation is advisable only if there is a well-developed capsulolabral complex and no excessive capsular laxity. For these patients, we generally recommend

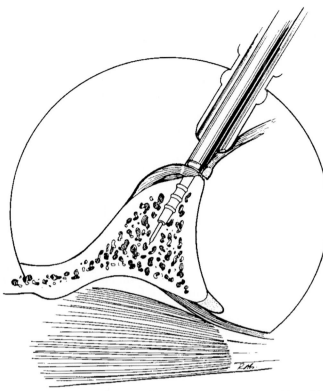

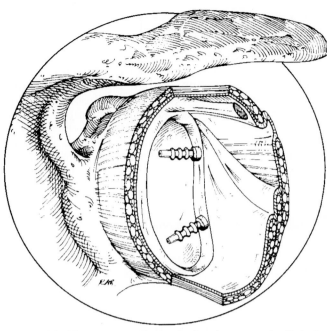

Figure 11–11 When tapping the Suretac into the glenoid, avoid overpenetrating the ligament. The guidewire is then removed through the driver to ensure its easy removal.

Figure 11–13 A second Suretac is placed more proximally in a similar manner. After inserting the Suretacs, they should be viewed anteriorly to ensure that they are holding the tissue properly. Sometimes, a third Suretac is needed. A probe is used to assess the tension on the ligament, and the position of the humeral head is noted. The tension on the ligament is set with the arm adducted and at neutral to slight external rotation.

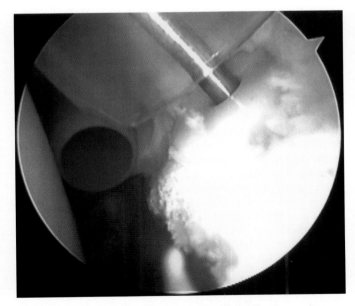

Figure 11–12 Arthroscopic image of a placed Suretac anchor, with the guidewire visible, to the anatomically correct anterior lip of the glenoid.

another procedure that can decrease capsular laxity more reliably.

Although the technique of Suretac fixation is relatively simple, some caveats can lead to better results.

Proper portal placement is essential for optimal execution of the procedure. The anteroinferior portal is most important. This portal is made with the arm in adduction and internal rotation. This permits the subscapularis muscle to relax, allowing more inferior placement of the portal. Trans-subscapularis tendon portals have been described, but we would hesitate to place a large cannula through the tendon.

Preparation of the glenoid neck and mobilization of the labrum-IGHL complex are also crucial to the success of the procedure. The capsulolabral complex should be mobilized from the glenoid until the subscapularis muscle belly is visible. The capsulolabral complex can then be grasped and pulled superiorly and laterally on the glenoid neck from the anterosuperior portal before tack placement.

The guidewire and drill should be assembled so that approximately 1 cm of the guidewire is available to spear the tissue. We recommend spearing the tissue and visualizing the tip of the guidewire before placement on the glenoid. The drill should be angled with the retroversion of the glenoid in mind and should be placed at the bone–articular surface junction to avoid articular surface injury.

When the drill is removed from the guidewire, the wire should be tapped slightly farther into the glenoid to prevent inadvertent dislodgment from the bone. When the tack is finally placed, we recommend advancing the cannula along the wire to avoid capturing the soft tissue during impaction of the anchor. In addition, overly aggressive impaction can lead to fracturing of the implant.

To prevent complications, it is essential that patients be given appropriate postoperative instructions. Early unprotected motion can lead to recurrent instability. Extensive immobilization can lead to adhesive capsulitis.

Suretac synovitis has been documented in case reports. If this is suspected, it can be documented with imaging studies and should be treated with anti-inflammatory medications and aggressive rehabilitation. Arthroscopic debridement may be required in selected cases.

Postoperative Management

Postoperatively, we place patients in a sling and swath for 4 weeks. During this period, the patient is instructed to remove the sling and support the arm with the other hand while flexing and extending at the elbow. We also encourage grip and pendulum exercises. The sling is removed at 4 weeks, and active assisted range of motion is initiated. Therabands are then introduced for external and internal range of motion. At 6 weeks, external rotation at 90 degrees is allowed. At 8 to 10 weeks, patients begin resistive strengthening of the rotator cuff and scapular stabilizers. At 12 weeks, we allow passive stretching, especially external rotation, and permit swimming and gentle throwing. Nonoverhead athletics can be resumed after 16 weeks. If motion and strength are fully restored, contact and overhead sports can begin at 24 weeks (Table 11–1).

Results

Initial results from the authors' institution revealed a recurrence rate of 21% (either dislocations or subluxations) in an initial group of 52 patients treated with the Suretac device.[40] When the indications for Suretac were refined to include only patients with (1) traumatic anterior instability, (2) a Bankart lesion, (3) a robust IGHL complex, and (4) minimal to mild bony erosion at the glenoid, Laurencin et al.[26] reported a 10% recurrence rate. Other reported recurrence rates range from 0% to 38%.* Resch et al.[34] found a 9% recurrence rate in 98 shoulders using an inferior trans-subscapularis portal to better reach the anteroinferior glenoid. In 1998, Karlsson et al.[22] reviewed 82 patients and reported a 10% recurrence rate. Three years later, they compared arthroscopic to open repair and found a 15% recurrence rate in the arthroscopic group, compared with 10% in the open group. However, the range of motion was better in the group repaired arthroscopically.[23] They concluded that the Suretac produces reliable results if it is used in patients with appropriate pathology and anatomy. In true anteroinferior dislocations, Segmuller et al.[38] reported

---

*See references 2, 4, 5, 10-12, 14, 15, 20, 22, 23, 34, 38, 43.

Table 11–1

Rehabilitation Schedule

Postoperative Week	Rehabilitation Focus
0-4	Sling removed for pendulum, forward flexion, elbow and hand range of motion, grip strengthening
4-8	Discontinue sling; active assisted external rotation, Theraband
8-12	Rotator cuff strengthening program
12-16	Swimming; passive stretching, especially external rotation
16-24	Nonoverhead athletics
>24	Contact sports and overhead sports

only a 3.2% rate of recurrent dislocation or subluxation in 31 shoulders after a 12-month follow-up. Arciero et al.[4] reported on the acute repair of Bankart lesions with a cannulated bioabsorbable tack in cadet athletes. There were no recurrent dislocations in their group of 19 patients with a 19-month follow-up. Several authors suggest that acute stabilization of initial anterior shoulder dislocations is an effective treatment option in the young athletic population, which is known to have high recurrence rates.[4,14]

Cole et al.[12] compared arthroscopic to open repair and concluded that the results are equivalent if the decision is made intraoperatively, based on arthroscopic evaluation of the pathology. Among the 37 (of 59) patients chosen for arthroscopy, there was a 16% rate of recurrent dislocation or subluxation; all recurrences were secondary to contact sports or falls less than 2 years postoperatively. Table 11–2 summarizes some of the results gathered from the literature.

Complications

Complications associated specifically with the Suretac device include synovitis, which has a reported incidence of 5%.[11] Fealy et al.[15] also reported several cases of synovitis in which the patient presented with a diffuse loss of motion and shoulder pain after the procedure. If early treatment (with nonsteroidal anti-inflammatory medications) is ineffective, treatment with arthroscopic debridement and synovectomy is recommended.[15] Burkart et al.[7] concluded that the Suretac device might be prone to early failure, particularly in superior labral anterior to posterior (SLAP) lesions, because of its biodegradability profile.

Technical errors may also be a cause of complications. Warner et al.[42] studied the use of Suretac in a cadaver model; by dissection, they evaluated the placement of the device relative to the articular margin and scapular neck. The errors detected included inadequate abrasion of the anterior and inferior glenoid neck, inadequate shift of the AIGHL superomedially before placement of the lowest Suretac, medial placement relative to the articular surface, and inadequate compression of the capsular tissue after being caught by the Suretac. When the

Table 11-2

Results of Arthroscopic Bankart Repair with Suretac Device

Author (Date)	No. of Patients	Mean Follow-up (mo.)	Results/ Rate of Redislocation or Resubluxation
Karlsson et al. (2001)[23]	66	28	15% recurrence in this prospective comparison of open vs arthroscopic repair
Cole et al. (2000)[10]	37	54	16% recurrence—all following a fall or contact sports
Karlsson et al. (1998)[22]	82	27	10% recurrence; compared favorably with open repair group
Resch et al. (1997)[34]	98	35	9% recurrence using an inferior trans-subscapularis portal to reach the anteroinferior glenoid
Segmuller et al. (1997)[38]	31	12	3.2% recurrence in those patients selected as having true anteroinferior dislocation
Laurencin et al. (1996)[26]	19	24	10% recurrence when patients limited to those with traumatic anterior instability, Bankart lesion, robust inferior glenohumeral ligament, and minimal glenoid erosions
Speer et al. (1996)[40]	52	42	21% recurrence; of 11 failures, 2 were traumatic, 7 were atraumatic; this study led to refinements in indications for Suretac use
Arciero et al. (1995)[4]	19	19	0% recurrence in this preliminary report when repair performed within 10 days of acute dislocation

Suretac is placed too medially, the Bankart lesion is repaired in a nonanatomic site, and only partial healing takes place. The result is loss of external rotation and early clinical failure, with return of glenohumeral instability.

Other technical complications can result from placing too few Suretacs, inadequately mobilizing the labrum and AIGHL, damaging the articular cartilage, or failing to abide by appropriately conservative rehabilitation protocols.[19]

Future Considerations

The next generation of Suretac devices has not been released as of this writing; however, the new Suretac (QuickT) will combine two new appealing features. The head of the device will be self-aligning, so that once the anchoring portion is set, the head will sit flush with the glenoid. It will also contain the pretied knot technology of the FasT-Fix device used currently for meniscal repairs.

References

1. Allen AA, Warner JJ: Shoulder instability in the athlete. Orthop Clin North Am 26:487-504, 1995.
2. Altchek DW: Arthroscopic shoulder stabilization using a bioabsorbable fixation device. Instr Course Lect 45:91-96, 1996.
3. Altchek DW, Warren RF, Skyhar MJ, Ortiz G: T-plasty modification of the Bankart procedure for multidirectional instability of the anterior and inferior types. J Bone Joint Surg Am 73:105-112, 1991.
4. Arciero RA, Taylor DC, Snyder RJ, Uhorchak JM: Arthroscopic bioabsorbable tack stabilization of initial anterior shoulder dislocations: A preliminary report. Arthroscopy 11:410-417, 1995.
5. Arciero RA, Wheeler JH, Ryan JB, McBride JT: Arthroscopic Bankart repair versus nonoperative treatment for acute, initial anterior shoulder dislocations. Am J Sports Med 22:589-594, 1994.
6. Baker CL Jr: Arthroscopic evaluation of acute initial shoulder dislocations. Instr Course Lect 45:83-89, 1996.
7. Burkart A, Imhoff AB, Roscher E: Foreign-body reaction to the bioabsorbable Suretac device. Arthroscopy 16:91-95, 2000.
8. Cofield RH, Irving JF: Evaluation and classification of shoulder instability: With special reference to examination under anesthesia. Clin Orthop 223:32-43, 1987.
9. Cofield RH, Nessler JP, Weinstabl R: Diagnosis of shoulder instability by examination under anesthesia. Clin Orthop 291:45-53, 1993.
10. Cole BJ, L'Insalata J, Irrgang J, Warner JJ: Comparison of arthroscopic and open anterior shoulder stabilization: A two to six-year follow-up study. J Bone Joint Surg Am 82:1108-1114, 2000.
11. Cole BJ, Romeo AA, Warner JJ: Arthroscopic Bankart repair with the Suretac device for traumatic anterior shoulder instability in athletes. Orthop Clin North Am 32:411-421, 2001.
12. Cole BJ, Warner JJ: Arthroscopic versus open Bankart repair for traumatic anterior shoulder instability. Clin Sports Med 19:19-48, 2000.
13. Coughlin L, Rubinovich M, Johansson J, et al: Arthroscopic staple capsulorrhaphy for anterior shoulder instability. Am J Sports Med 20:253-256, 1992.
14. DeBerardino TM, Arciero RA, Taylor DC: Arthroscopic stabilization of acute initial anterior shoulder dislocation: The West Point experience. J South Orthop Assoc 5:263-271, 1996.
15. Fealy S, Drakos MC, Allen AA, Warren RF: Arthroscopic Bankart repair: Experience with an absorbable, transfixing implant. Clin Orthop 390:31-41, 2001.
16. Geiger DF, Hurley JA, Tovey JA, Rao JP: Results of arthroscopic versus open Bankart suture repair. Clin Orthop 337:111-117, 1997.
17. Goldberg BJ, Nirschl RP, McConnell JP, Pettrone FA: Arthroscopic transglenoid suture capsulolabral repairs: Preliminary results. Am J Sports Med 21:656-664, discussion 664-665, 1993.
18. Hawkins RB: Arthroscopic stapling repair for shoulder instability: A retrospective study of 50 cases. Arthroscopy 5:122-128, 1989.

19. Higgins LD, Warner JJ: Arthroscopic Bankart repair: Operative technique and surgical pitfalls. Clin Sports Med 19:49-62, 2000.
20. Horns HJ, Laprell HG: Developments in Bankart repair for treatment of anterior instability of the shoulder. Knee Surg Sports Traumatol Arthrosc 4:228-231, 1996.
21. Hovelius L, Eriksson K, Fredin H, et al: Recurrences after initial dislocation of the shoulder: Results of a prospective study of treatment. J Bone Joint Surg Am 65:343-349, 1983.
22. Karlsson J, Kartus J, Ejerhed L, et al: Bioabsorbable tacks for arthroscopic treatment of recurrent anterior shoulder dislocation. Scand J Med Sci Sports 8:411-415, 1998.
23. Karlsson J, Magnusson L, Ejerhed L, et al: Comparison of open and arthroscopic stabilization for recurrent shoulder dislocation in patients with a Bankart lesion. Am J Sports Med 29:538-542, 2001.
24. Lane JG, Sachs RA, Riehl B: Arthroscopic staple capsulorrhaphy: A long-term follow-up. Arthroscopy 9:190-194, 1993.
25. Laurencin CT, Deutsch A, O'Brien SJ, Altchek DW: The superolateral portal for arthroscopy of the shoulder. Arthroscopy 10:255-258, 1994.
26. Laurencin CT, Stephens S, Warren RF, Altchek DW: Arthroscopic Bankart repair using a degradable tack: A followup study using optimized indications. Clin Orthop 332:132-137, 1996.
27. Lintner SA, Speer KP: Traumatic anterior glenohumeral instability: The role of arthroscopy. J Am Acad Orthop Surg 5:233-239, 1997.
28. Matthews LS, Vetter WL, Oweida SJ, et al: Arthroscopic staple capsulorrhaphy for recurrent anterior shoulder instability. Arthroscopy 4:106-111, 1988.
29. Neer CS 2nd, Foster CR: Inferior capsular shift for involuntary inferior and multidirectional instability of the shoulder: A preliminary report. J Bone Joint Surg Am 62:897-908, 1980.
30. Norlin R: Intraarticular pathology in acute, first-time anterior shoulder dislocation: An arthroscopic study. Arthroscopy 9:546-549, 1993.
31. Norris TR: Diagnostic techniques for shoulder instability. Instr Course Lect 34:239-257, 1985.
32. Oliashirazi A, Mansat P, Cofield RH, Rowland CM: Examination under anesthesia for evaluation of anterior shoulder instability. Am J Sports Med 27:464-468, 1999.
33. Pagnani MJ, Warren, RF: Arthroscopic shoulder stabilization. Oper Tech Sports Med 1:276-284, 1993.
34. Resch H, Povacz P, Wambacher M, et al: Arthroscopic extra-articular Bankart repair for the treatment of recurrent anterior shoulder dislocation. Arthroscopy 13:188-200, 1997.
35. Romeo A: Traumatic anterior shoulder instability. Orthop Clin North Am 32:399-409, 2001.
36. Rowe CR: Acute and recurrent anterior dislocations of the shoulder. Orthop Clin North Am 11:253-270, 1980.
37. Savoie FH 3rd, Miller CD, Field LD: Arthroscopic reconstruction of traumatic anterior instability of the shoulder: The Caspari technique. Arthroscopy 13:201-209, 1997.
38. Segmuller HE, Hayes MG, Saies AD: Arthroscopic repair of glenolabral injuries with an absorbable fixation device. J Shoulder Elbow Surg 6:383-392, 1997.
39. Speer KP, Warren RF: Arthroscopic shoulder stabilization: A role for biodegradable materials. Clin Orthop 291:67-74, 1993.
40. Speer KP, Warren RF, Pagnani M, Warner JJ: An arthroscopic technique for anterior stabilization of the shoulder with a bioabsorbable tack. J Bone Joint Surg Am 78:1801-1807, 1996.
41. Taylor DC, Arciero RA: Pathologic changes associated with shoulder dislocations: Arthroscopic and physical examination findings in first-time, traumatic anterior dislocations. Am J Sports Med 25:306-311, 1997.
42. Warner JJ, Miller MD, Marks P: Arthroscopic Bankart repair with the Suretac device. Part II. Experimental observations. Arthroscopy 11:14-20, 1995.
43. Warner JJ, Miller MD, Marks P, Fu FH: Arthroscopic Bankart repair with the Suretac device. Part I. Clinical observations. Arthroscopy 11:2-13, 1995.
44. Youssef JA, Carr CF, Walther CE, Murphy JM: Arthroscopic Bankart suture repair for recurrent traumatic unidirectional anterior shoulder dislocations. Arthroscopy 11:561-563, 1995.

Suture Anchor Fixation for Shoulder Instability

MICHAEL J. MOSKAL AND MICHAEL L. PEARL

SUTURE ANCHOR FIXATION FOR SHOULDER INSTABILITY IN A NUTSHELL

History:
Documented dislocation; apprehension with arm positioned at extremes of motion, such as external rotation in abduction for anterior instability

Physical Examination:
Load and shift demonstrate loss of glenoid concavity; apprehension in abduction–external rotation or flexion adduction–internal rotation

Imaging:
Anteroposterior and axillary; apical oblique; magnetic resonance imaging in questionable cases

Indications:
Symptomatic unwanted translations

Contraindications:
Voluntary dislocation; scapular dumping syndrome

Diagnostic Arthroscopy:
Evaluate position of labrum and glenoid arc length, referencing the bare spot; humeral head fractures

Arthroscopic Release:
Release capsulolabral complex from glenoid neck to 6 o'clock position to allow superomedial shift

Anchor Placement:
On glenoid face at the periphery, spaced to allow for suture capture inferior to anchor site

Tissue Capture:
6 o'clock capture site sets tension for remainder of repair

Capture Devices:
Suture shuttle useful for 6 o'clock position; retrograde retrievers better suited in more superior positions

Concavity Restoration:
Labrum should be firmly attached on glenoid periphery

Postoperative Management:
Traumatic: early protected motion without putting tension on repair with isometric strengthening; check for unwanted stiffness; full motion at 6 weeks with concentric strengthening
Atraumatic: 8-12 weeks, neutral rotation brace, scapular isometrics and position/posture biofeedback, isometric strengthening; 12 weeks, concentric strengthening, sequential placement of arm in positions that require greater balance control during rehabilitation

Glenohumeral instability, or excessive unwanted humeral translation on the glenoid, can result from failed stabilizing mechanisms such as the loss of glenoid concavity compression and the capsulolabral constraint arising after a specific traumatic event (dislocation) or repetitive microtraumatic events (subluxation or plastic deformation). Compared with earlier methods (i.e., tacks, staples), the use of suture anchors in arthroscopic surgery allows more precise approximation of the capsular tissues to a specific anchor site, facilitating the secure restoration of the capsulolabral complex.

History

After a single traumatic event such as a dislocation, there is typically a loss of glenoid concavity and capsulolabral tension. The patient often describes shoulder stability as being "threatened" in a position similar to that held at the time of the dislocation (Table 12–1). That position is typically at the extremes of motion, with few or no symptoms occurring in the midranges of motion or with the arm at the side. In contrast, patients with unwanted subluxation who do not recall a high-energy traumatic event often complain of popping and pain after a relatively minor event or after exposure to repetitive high-endurance activities such as swimming, in which compression by the rotator cuff is compromised and scapular positioning is poor due to muscle fatigue. Subsequently, the glenohumeral joint may experience increases in translation without dislocation, leading to instability in the midranges of motion—often characterized as atraumatic instability.[6]

Physical Examination

Often in cases of traumatic anterior and posterior instability, the rotator cuff is strong. The patient typically describes feeling apprehensive when the arm is placed in abduction and external rotation (anterior) or elevated, internally rotated, and adducted (posterior). With anterior instability, this sense of apprehension is reduced with a posteriorly directed force on the abducted and externally rotated arm. With posterior instability, patients may complain of pain and not true apprehension. Diminished rotator cuff strength or endurance and poor scapulohumeral rhythm are common in atraumatic instability. Although not a prerequisite for or synonymous with instability, relatively increased humeral translation, implying excessive capsular redundancy and increased

Table 12–1	Instability Patterns Based on Direction and Arm Position
Direction	**Arm Position**
Anterior	Abduction, external rotation
Posterior	Elevated, internally rotated, adducted
Multidirectional	Midelevation

compliance, is a common characteristic in patients with atraumatic instability.

Imaging

An anteroposterior radiograph in the scapular plane and an axillary lateral view are typically sufficient in the workup of instability. An apical oblique or Stryker notch view may also be useful to evaluate for glenoid or humeral bone loss (e.g., bony Bankart or Hill-Sachs defect). Magnetic resonance imaging with or without contrast can be helpful to evaluate the rotator cuff or labrum; this may be most important in young athletes or in elderly patients following instability episodes.

Indications and Contraindications

The indications and contraindications for arthroscopic reconstruction for glenohumeral instability are essentially the same as for open reconstruction. With current technology and procedures, most pathoanatomy, except for excessive bone loss of the glenoid or humerus, can be addressed entirely arthroscopically.

Indications are as follows:

1. Symptomatic excessive, unwanted humeral translation unresponsive to conservative care.
2. Loss of concavity compression due to decompensation of the capsulolabral complex.
3. Sufficient quality and quantity of capsulolabral tissue.
4. Motivated patient who understands and is willing to comply with the postoperative rehabilitation and precaution protocol.

Contraindications are as follows:

1. Loss of sufficient bony glenoid arc length, such that despite restoration of the soft tissue stabilizers, the joint reaction forces align outside the arc of bony glenoid support (i.e., >25% to 30% anteroinferior glenoid bone loss).[2]
2. Engaging Hill-Sachs lesion, despite efforts at soft tissue stabilization.
3. Static, inferiorly tilted scapula, also known as "scapular dumping" or voluntarily tilted scapula.
4. Poorly motivated patient or one who voluntarily subluxates his or her shoulder for secondary gain (which should not be confused with the ability to demonstrate the position that threatens stability).

Surgical Technique

Positioning

Patients can be positioned in either the lateral decubitus or the beach chair position; the choice is based largely on surgeon preference. However, it is often easier to address the inferior or posterior capsulolabral complex with the patient in the lateral decubitus position. The arm is placed in various positions of external rotation and abduction, depending on the portion of the capsule being addressed, such that excessive tensioning of the capsulolabral complex does not lead to motion loss.

Examination under Anesthesia

Side-to-side comparisons with the normal shoulder are routinely performed. Because of the inherent problems of examining an awake patient, the examination under anesthesia should concentrate on the following:

1. Concavity compression: The humeral head is manually compressed into the glenoid and then translated in the anterior, posterior, and inferior directions to detect ease of translation.[5]
2. Capsulolabral complex: The humerus is rotated, and translation is tested in varying degrees of humeral elevation. Because the capsulolabral complex is a checkrein to motion, translation should diminish with increasing humeral rotation and with increasing elevation.
3. Range of motion: Capsular length corresponds directly to humeral rotation (range of motion). Losses of motion in certain planes can be expected if capsular plication is performed during stabilization surgery.

Diagnostic Arthroscopy

Diagnostic arthroscopy is useful to fine-tune the preoperative diagnosis while noting the status and condition of the following:

1. Labrum—its location, position, and stability
2. Capsule and rotator interval
3. Long head of the biceps tendon
4. Humeral head impaction fractures
5. Rotator cuff
6. Bony glenoid arc length (i.e., bony Bankart lesion)

Specific Surgical Steps

Anterior Surgical Reconstruction

1. Anterior portal position. An outside-to-inside technique ensures the position and trajectory of the portals created.
   a. Low anterior portal (Fig. 12–1): created just superior to the subscapularis tendon, which is critical for capsular release and mobilization, as well as placement of the 5 o'clock anchor.
   b. Superoanterior portal: created just anterior to the biceps tendon, allowing a secondary suture management portal or superior labral anterior to posterior (SLAP) reconstruction.
2. Capsular release and anterior glenoid neck preparation.
   a. Through the low anterior portal, release the capsulolabral complex from the glenoid neck to the 6 o'clock position for a distance of 1 to 2 cm medially along the glenoid neck (Fig. 12–2).

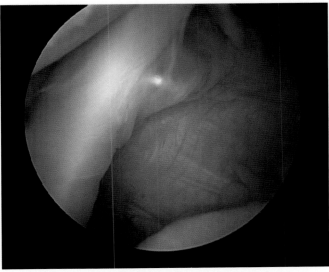

Figure 12–1   The cannula and obturator are piercing the thin tissue superior to the subscapularis tendon. Note that the entry site is in a lateral position in relation to the glenoid to ensure an appropriate trajectory of the suture anchor into the glenoid. The glenoid labrum is seen below and to the right.

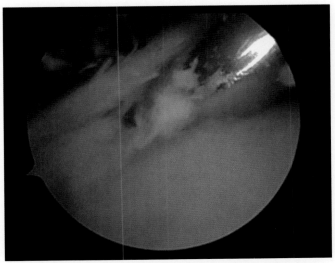

Figure 12–2   The bur is located at the inferior (6 o'clock) position of the glenoid. The capsulolabral complex has been released to approximately the 7 o'clock position to ensure adequate superior shift.

   b. Decorticate the anterior glenoid neck using an arthroscopic bur.
   c. Grasp the labrum to ensure that it can be readily shifted superiorly and onto the glenoid fossa into its normal position. Adequate mobilization is achieved when the underlying subscapularis muscle is seen (Fig. 12–3).
3. Anchor position and suture passing.
   a. Anchors are inserted onto the glenoid face near the periphery at the 3, 4, and 5 o'clock positions when necessary (right shoulder). Anchors are placed one at a time, and the sutures are passed and tied before subsequent anchor placement.

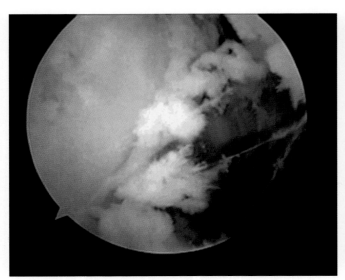

Figure 12–3 As seen from the anterior portal, the anterior glenoid neck has been debrided of soft tissue. The subscapularis muscle can be visualized to the right.

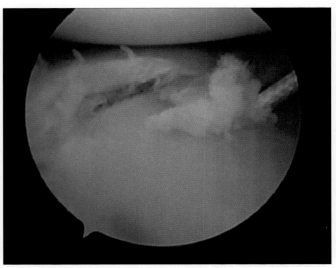

Figure 12–5 The 5 o'clock anchor has been placed. Note its position relative to the capsulolabral release, which has been extended posterior to the most inferior portion of the glenoid. The capsulolabral tissues will be shifted superiorly to this anchor site.

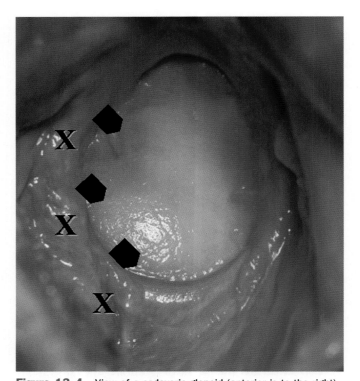

Figure 12–4 View of a cadaveric glenoid (anterior is to the right). The blocks represent suture anchor placement at the 5, 4, and 3 o'clock positions. The X's represent the point where sutures should pass through the capsulolabral complex.

    b. The capsulolabral complex is captured at the 6, 5, and 4 o'clock positions corresponding to the 5, 4, and 3 o'clock anchor positions, respectively. This tissue capture management effectively shifts the capsulolabral tissue superiorly and onto the glenoid fossa (Fig. 12–4).

    c. The 5 o'clock anchor is placed, and its security in the osseous tunnel is confirmed (Fig. 12–5). Placement of the 5 o'clock anchor and its suture passage are the most critical steps; they will determine the amount of subsequent tissue captured by the more proximal anchors. Lateral and posterior translation of the humerus is helpful during 5 o'clock anchor and suture placement.

    d. Use of a commercially available suture shuttle or use of a 48-inch looped Prolene suture allows for capture of the tissue at the 6 o'clock position for the 5 o'clock suture anchor (Fig. 12–6). Suture management is improved by placing the "articular" suture through the superior cannula, so as to shuttle the capsular suture through the low anterior portal. If desired, shifting of the labrum is facilitated by placing a grasper through the superior portal during suture passage. Knot tying is performed based on the surgeon's preference. These simple sutures typically slide easily without fraying or hanging up at the soft tissue–anchor interface.

    e. The 4 and 3 o'clock anchors are placed with sequential tension created in the capsulolabral complex following suture passage and knot tying (Fig. 12–7). At these higher positions, retrograde suture retrievers placed through the anteroinferior portal work well for suture passage (Fig. 12–8).

Posterior Reconstruction

The sequence of soft tissue release, anchor placement, and capsulolabral capture are similar to anterior reconstruction in the case of a posterior Bankart repair. More commonly, two anchor sites at 7 and 9 o'clock are sufficient. Suture passage incorporates the posteroinferior capsule, which is repaired to the labrum or "tucked" to itself. Rotator interval closure is usually performed simultaneously in cases of posterior instability.[1,7]

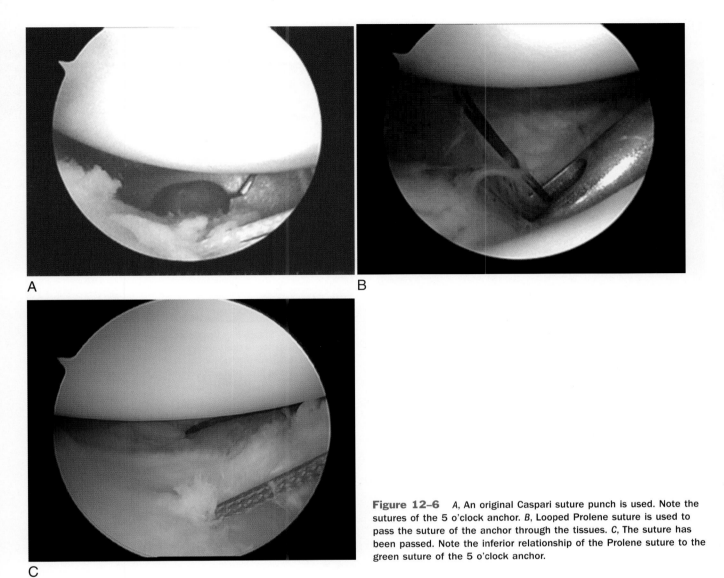

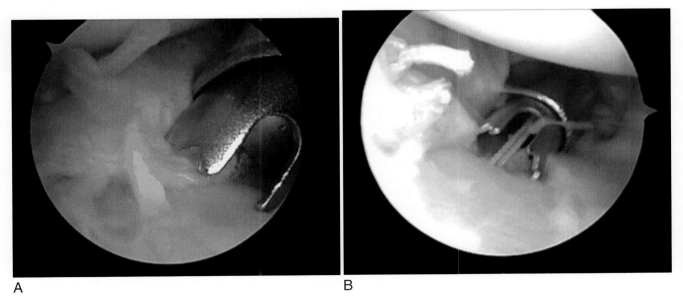

Figure 12–6 *A,* An original Caspari suture punch is used. Note the sutures of the 5 o'clock anchor. *B,* Looped Prolene suture is used to pass the suture of the anchor through the tissues. *C,* The suture has been passed. Note the inferior relationship of the Prolene suture to the green suture of the 5 o'clock anchor.

Figure 12–7 *A,* The drill guide is on the glenoid face at the 3 o'clock position. Note the suture knot positioned at 5 o'clock and the intervening capsulolabral tissue, which would correspond to the 4 o'clock position. *B,* The 3 o'clock anchor has been inserted. Note its relationship to the suture knot and intervening tissue (see Fig. 12–4 as a reference).

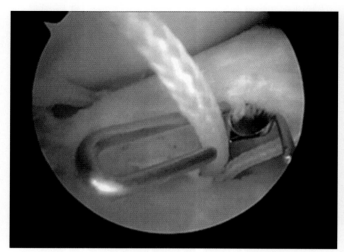

Figure 12– 8   A retrograde wire loop suture retriever captures the suture limb and retrieves it from the anteroinferior cannula.

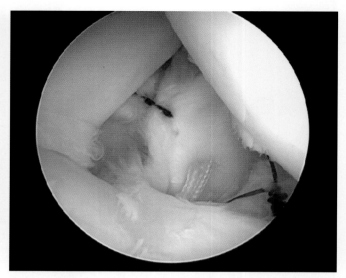

Figure 12–9   Suture has been passed through the rotator interval starting just anterior to the biceps tendon and through the middle glenohumeral ligament. Interval shortening is typically performed during posterior and multidirectional instability reconstruction.

Capsular Tensioning

As already alluded to, capsular reduction is performed, when necessary, with suture shuttle techniques, taking intra-articular "tucks" of capsule following local abrasion using a manual rasp. The capsule is plicated either directly to the labrum or to itself.[3]

Rotator Interval Closure

Rotator interval capsule closure or plication is important to treat residual inferior translation in cases of traumatic anterior instability or to complement posterior labral reconstruction in cases of posterior instability.[4] The interval, which is triangular in shape, is closed by passing one or two sutures from the middle glenohumeral ligament to the capsule just anterior to the biceps tendon. Thus, the triangle's base and tip are in the same position, but the sides of the triangle are approximated (Fig. 12–9). Various techniques have been described; however, the common goal is capsular reduction.

1. The capsule is lightly debrided with a rasp or slotted shaver.
2. A spinal needle is placed just anterior to the biceps tendon, and a suture is passed through the needle.
3. From the anterior portal, a retrograde retriever is passed through the middle glenohumeral ligament, and the suture is retrieved through the portal.
4. The second limb of the suture is retrieved through the anterior portal outside the glenohumeral joint, and the sutures are tied blindly against the capsule.

Multidirectional Instability Repair

Capsular shortening with repair to the labrum (capsulolabral augmentation) reduces capsular volume while increasing glenoid concavity. Use of suture anchors instead of sutures is based on surgeon preference. However, if the labrum is significantly frayed, sutures alone may not be secure. Anchors placed into the

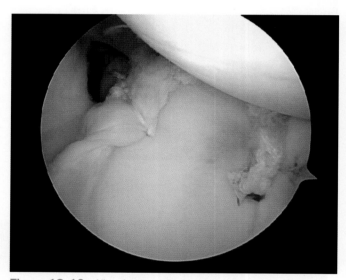

Figure 12–10   View from a superoanterior portal. Five suture anchors were used to perform a capsulolabral augmentation in this patient with multidirectional instability. Note the position of the posteroinferior cannula. The 3 and 9 o'clock anchors are readily seen.

glenoid can provide a secure attachment point for capsulolabral augmentation (Fig. 12–10).

▌ Postoperative Management

Anterior Reconstruction

The patient's arm is placed in a simple sling for 4 to 6 weeks. Range of motion is initially limited to 90 degrees of elevation in neutral rotation and 0 degrees of rotation at the side. Older patients may benefit from earlier

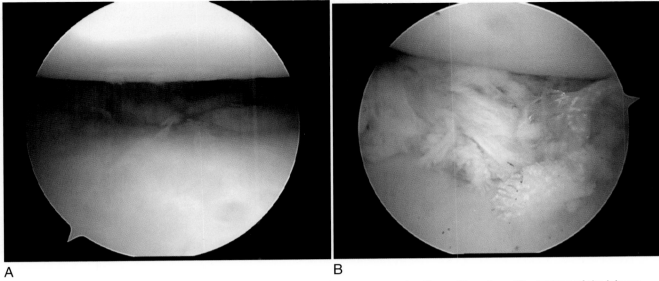

A   B

Figure 12–11 *A,* This patient had recurrent instability after two failed open reconstructions with anchors. The position of the labrum is at the level of the glenoid face because the anchors were placed in a medialized position on the anterior glenoid neck. The failed stabilizing mechanisms are concavity compression and capsular constraint. *B,* An arthroscopic revision capsulolabral Bankart repair was performed. Note the position of the labrum on the glenoid fossa at the periphery. The glenoid concavity is restored. Suture remnants and metal fragments from the previous surgeries can be seen.

mobilization because of the propensity for stiffness. At 3 weeks, if the patient is having difficulty achieving motion beyond 0 degrees of rotation and 90 degrees of elevation, motion beyond the restrictions should be allowed. If motion is easily achieved at 3 weeks, sling immobilization and continued motion limits remain in place until 6 weeks after surgery.

Concentric internal and external rotation strengthening (within motion limits) is begun as soon as tolerated. Isometric strengthening can be instituted as soon as possible after repair.

At 6 weeks after surgery, unrestricted motion is allowed. Rotator cuff and periscapular muscle strengthening and endurance training are continued and maximized. Sports- and activity-related rehabilitation is instituted, with a goal of maximizing function at 3 to 4 months.

Posterior and Multidirectional Reconstruction

Neutral rotation in abduction bracing is critical to postoperative rehabilitation. Brace immobilization is individualized but is typically in place for approximately 8 to 12 weeks after surgery.

Isometric strengthening, scapular retraction, and postural cuing exercises are instituted within a week after surgery. Internal and external rotation strengthening begins at 12 weeks after surgery. At 16 weeks after surgery, humeral elevation with the arm close to the chest ("ceiling punch"), with special attention to maintaining appropriate scapular-humeral rhythm, is instituted. At 4 to 6 months after surgery, sports- or activity-specific rehabilitation ensues, with return to unrestricted activities at 6 months.

Complications

Rarely, the anchor may become dislodged from its osseous tunnel and cause mechanical complications, such as cartilaginous injury or failure of the capsulolabral tissue to heal to the glenoid. Prevention is the best management. The bone tunnel should be within the glenoid, and after suture placement, the sutures are pulled to ensure that they are firmly in bone. Early recognition followed by removal of the anchor helps minimize cartilaginous injury.

The anchor entry site into bone should be on the glenoid face at the periphery. Medial neck placement puts the capsulolabral tissue at or below the glenoid face and predisposes to recurrent instability or external rotation loss (Fig. 12–11).

Finally, care should be taken to avoid excessive decreases in capsular length with capsulolabral repair. An individual's tolerance for capsular length reduction can be estimated by assessing preoperative motion. Capsular length reduction of 1 cm is associated with an approximate 20-degree loss of angular rotation. A patient who can passively externally rotate the arm to 70 degrees (or greater) may tolerate similar angular motion losses better than a patient who can rotate to only 40 degrees at the side.

References

1. Antoniou J, Duckworth DT, Harryman DT: Capsulolabral augmentation for the management of posteroinferior instability of the shoulder. J Bone Joint Surg Am 82:1220-1230, 2000.

2. Churchill RS, Moskal MJ, Lippitt SB, Matsen FA III: Extra-capsular anatomically contoured glenoid bone grafting for complex glenohumeral instability. Tech Shoulder Elbow Surg 2:210-218, 2001.

3. Duncan R, Savoie FH III: Arthroscopic inferior capsular shift for multidirectional instability: A preliminary report. Arthroscopy 9:24-27, 1993.

4. Harryman DT, Sidles JA, Harris SL, Matsen FA III: The role of the rotator interval capsule in passive motion and stability of the shoulder. J Bone Joint Surg Am 74:53-66, 1992.

5. Lippitt SB, Vanserhoost JE, Harris SL, et al: Glenohumeral stability from concavity-compression: A quantitative analysis. J Shoulder Elbow Surg 2:27-35, 1993.

6. Matsen FA III, Lippitt SB, Sidles JA, Harryman DT II: Practical Evaluation and Management of the Shoulder. Philadelphia, WB Saunders, 1994.

7. Metcalf MH, Pond JD, Harryman DT II, et al: Capsulolabral augmentation increases glenohumeral stability in the cadaver shoulder. J Shoulder Elbow Surg 10:532-538, 2001.

Knotless Suture Anchor Fixation for Shoulder Instability

R AYMOND T HAL

KNOTLESS SUTURE ANCHOR FIXATION FOR SHOULDER INSTABILITY IN A NUTSHELL

Portal Placement:
Posterior portal
Anteroinferior portal—"hug" subscapularis tendon
Anterosuperior portal—anterolateral corner of acromion

Pathoanatomy Assessment:
Bankart, anterior labroligamentous periosteal sleeve avulsion, humeral avulsion of glenohumeral ligament, anterior glenoid bone loss

Ligament Preparation and Mobilization:
Completely detach glenohumeral ligament and shift it superiorly to restore appropriate ligament position

Glenoid Preparation:
Abrasion of anterior glenoid

Drill Hole Placement:
Corner drill holes onto articular margin; 1, 3, and 5 o'clock position

Utility Loop Passage:
Pass utility suture through glenohumeral ligament at 2, 4, and 6 o'clock to provide superior shift; pass suture from articular side to nonarticular side of ligament for inferior 2 anchors; pass suture through anteroinferior portal and out anterosuperior portal

Anchor Loop Passage:
Use utility loop to pull anchor loop through glenohumeral ligament

Anchor Loop Capture:
Ensure appropriate anchor and anchor loop orientation

Anchor Insertion into Drill Hole:
Ensure proper anchor alignment

Repair Tension:
Slowly tap anchor to tension repair; assess tension by pulling on utility suture and probing repair site

Completion:
Remove inserter rod and utility suture

Arthroscopic Bankart repair procedures have been developed in an effort to restore stability to the shoulder while avoiding some of the morbidity associated with an open repair.[12,18] An arthroscopic Bankart repair must provide secure ligament fixation, similar to that obtained with an open repair, if it is to achieve comparable recurrence rates. The fixation methods used in early arthroscopic repairs[1,3,6-15,17,19,20,29-31] (tacks, staples, transglenoid sutures) were different from those described for open repairs (suture anchors, osseous tunnels). More recent arthroscopic repair studies describe the use of suture anchors with arthroscopic knot tying.[2,5,18,22,32-34] Although an arthroscopic suture anchor repair has the appeal of using a fixation method identical to that used in an open repair, the quality and consistency of arthroscopic knots and the technical difficulty associated with tying them are concerns.[16] Satisfactory knot tying requires significant practice with special knot-tying devices, and unfamiliar, bulky knot designs are often used. This skill can be difficult to master and time-consuming to perform.

A knotless suture anchor and a technique that does not require arthroscopic knot tying have been described.[24,25,28] Secure, consistent suture anchor fixation is achieved arthroscopically using the knotless suture anchor. Increased superior capsular shift and a low-profile repair can be achieved.[4,26,27] The procedure is simplified by the elimination of arthroscopic knot tying, and knotless suture anchor fixation eliminates the potential weakness associated with arthroscopic knots.

Case History

The patient is a 21-year-old, right-hand-dominant man with a 2-year history of right shoulder instability. He had an initial abduction–external rotation injury during a fall while snowboarding, which resulted in an anterior glenohumeral dislocation requiring physician reduction. The patient did well for 6 months following this injury until a second dislocation occurred during a sudden abduction–external rotation movement while playing basketball, again requiring physician reduction. The patient reports five subluxations over the subsequent year with trivial movements such as gesturing or reaching. A third dislocation, requiring physician reduction, occurred during a fall playing soccer, almost 2 years after the initial injury.

Physical Examination

There is a positive apprehension sign with a 5-degree loss of external rotation at 90 degrees of abduction. Anterior excursion is increased, with full range of motion in all other planes. There are no rotator cuff symptoms or weakness. The following test results were obtained: positive Jobe relocation test, negative O'Brien test, negative liftoff test, negative belly-press test, negative sulcus sign,
negative biceps tension test. There is no posterior or inferior instability.

Imaging

Prereduction radiographs revealed an anteroinferior glenohumeral ligament (AIGHL) dislocation. Postreduction radiographs showed concentric reduction of the glenohumeral joint. A Hill-Sachs lesion was evident. No other associated bony lesions or fractures were noted. Particular attention should be given to evaluating the anterior glenoid rim for evidence of significant bone deficiency.

Indications and Contraindications

The patient was treated with arthroscopic anterior shoulder stabilization owing to the recurrent nature of his symptoms. The bony anterior glenoid rim was well preserved. The presence of a significant anterior glenoid bone defect may require an anterior bone graft to address this structural deficiency.[5] The uncommonly encountered humeral avulsion of the glenohumeral ligament requires repair when present. These lesions are difficult to treat arthroscopically and may require an open repair. Capsular redundancy can be addressed by superior capsular shift, capsular plication, or selective capsular resection, as indicated.

Knotless Suture Anchor Design

The knotless suture anchor (Fig. 13–1) consists of a titanium body with two nitinol arcs. The arcs have a memory property that creates resistance to anchor pullout after insertion into bone through small drill holes. Although the knotless suture anchor looks similar to the GII anchor (Mitek Products, Westwood, MA), it differs structurally in several ways. A channel or slot is located at the tip of the knotless suture anchor. A short loop of green, number 1 Ethibond suture (Ethicon, Somerville, NJ), called the anchor loop, is attached to the tail end of the anchor instead of the long suture strands used in the GII anchor. A second, longer loop of white 2-0 Ethibond suture, called the utility loop, is linked to the anchor loop and serves as a passing suture.

An absorbable version of the knotless suture anchor, the BioKnotless suture anchor (Fig. 13–2), is also available. The BioKnotless suture anchor looks similar to the Mitek Panalok anchor. The BioKnotless suture anchor has a wedge-shaped, poly-L-lactic acid anchor body with a slot located at the tip. The anchor loop is white number 1 Panacryl, and the utility loop is green 2-0 Ethibond.

The sides of both anchor designs are flat to create space for the captured suture loop to pass without suture abrasion.

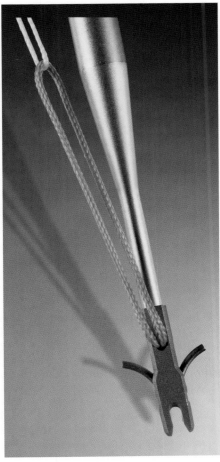

Figure 13–1   Metallic knotless suture anchor design.

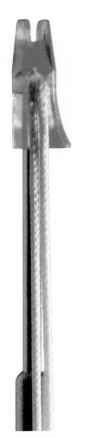

Figure 13–2   BioKnotless suture anchor design.

Surgical Technique

Positioning and Examination under Anesthesia

The procedure is performed with the patient in a modified lateral decubitus position, with a 30-degree posterior tilt. Either general anesthesia or interscalene block is used. Examination under anesthesia demonstrates anterior glenohumeral instability. There is no evidence of posterior or inferior instability. A complete glenohumeral arthroscopic examination is performed with the arthroscope in the posterior portal. Dual anterior portals are established for instrumentation. The anteroinferior portal is placed as close as possible to the superior edge of the subscapularis tendon to allow access to the anterior and inferior aspect of the glenoid rim. The anterosuperior portal is placed in the rotator cuff interval just anterior to the biceps tendon.

Diagnostic Arthroscopy

A thorough arthroscopic evaluation is done, including examination of the articular surfaces, labrum, biceps tendon, rotator cuff, and glenohumeral ligaments. Visualization through both the posterior and anterior portals is performed, with particular attention to the anterior labrum and AIGHL.

Preparation of the AIGHL complex depends on the pathology encountered. Instrumentation via the anteroinferior and anterosuperior portals is useful. The exposed labral edge of a Bankart lesion is debrided with a motorized shaver to promote healing after repair. Care is taken to adequately release and mobilize the AIGHL from the glenoid and underlying subscapularis tendon. When an anterior labroligamentous periosteal sleeve avulsion (ALPSA) lesion[21] (Fig. 13–3) is the cause of instability, the periosteum should be incised to release the AIGHL from the glenoid (Fig. 13–4). This essentially converts an ALPSA lesion to a Bankart lesion. The AIGHL is often scarred to the subscapularis muscle, requiring dissection and mobilization in this area. After mobilization, a grasper is used to pull the ligament superiorly and to the articular margin while capsular tension and mobility are evaluated. The degree of capsular laxity can be assessed at this time as well (Fig. 13–5). This is a critical step in the procedure that greatly affects the final outcome.

A motorized bur is used to decorticate the anterior glenoid neck from the edge of the articular cartilage medially 1 to 2 cm. Abrasion of the articular surface, a few millimeters from the edge, is also performed to promote healing.

The anteroinferior cannula is replaced by a larger 8-mm cannula to accommodate the drill guide, suture

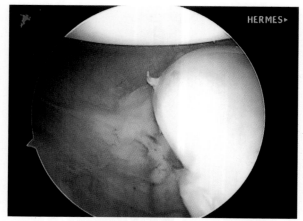

Figure 13–3 Anterior labroligamentous periosteal sleeve avulsion (ALPSA) lesion (anterior view).

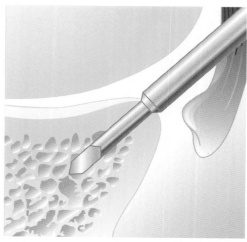

Figure 13–6 Three 2.9-mm drill holes are created in the anterior glenoid rim.

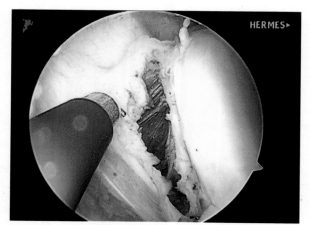

Figure 13–4 Anterior labroligamentous periosteal sleeve avulsion (ALPSA) lesion during mobilization (anterior view).

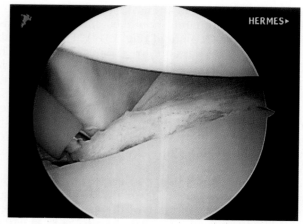

Figure 13–5 A grasper is used to pull the ligament superiorly and to the articular margin while capsular tension and mobility are evaluated. The degree of capsular laxity can also be assessed at this time (posterior view).

passer, and knotless anchors. Three drill holes are created in the anterior glenoid rim using the Mitek drill guide and a Mitek 2.9-mm drill (Fig. 13–6). These drill holes are spaced as far apart as possible (1, 3, and 5 o'clock positions on a right shoulder) and at the edge of the articular cartilage. It is important to direct the drill bit medially, away from the articular surface of the glenoid, by at least a 15-degree angle to avoid damaging the articular surface. The drill holes are marked with a suction punch to make anchor insertion easier.

Specific Surgical Steps

Knotless Suture Anchor Repair Procedure

The knotless suture anchor or BioKnotless suture anchor is used to repair the AIGHL to the glenoid rim. A superior shift of the ligament is done as well.

Suture Passage

The utility loop of the knotless suture anchor assembly is passed through the AIGHL at a selected site via the anteroinferior portal (Fig. 13–7). This can be achieved using various arthroscopic suture-passing techniques.

The utility loop is used to pull the anchor loop through the AIGHL (Fig. 13–8). As the utility loop pulls the anchor loop through the ligament, the attached anchor is passed down the anteroinferior cannula while being controlled on the threaded inserter rod.

Once the anchor loop has passed through the AIGHL, one strand of the anchor loop is captured or snagged in the channel at the tip of the anchor (Fig. 13–9). When the metallic knotless anchor is used, the anchor is rotated so that the arc positioned inside the anchor loop is rotated toward the utility loop. The utility loop is used to pull the anchor loop over one of the anchor arcs. The anchor is then inserted and tapped into the glenoid drill hole to the desired depth to achieve appropriate tissue tension (Fig. 13–10). This process pulls the AIGHL to the

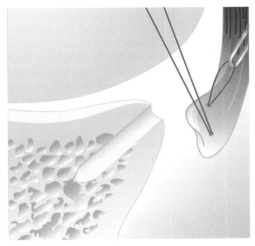

Figure 13–7   The utility loop of the knotless suture anchor assembly is passed through the anteroinferior glenohumeral ligament at a selected site.

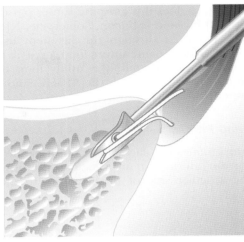

Figure 13–10   The anchor is inserted and tapped into the glenoid drill hole to the desired depth to achieve appropriate tissue tension.

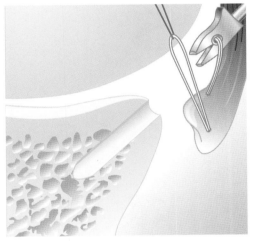

Figure 13–8   The utility loop is used to pull the anchor loop through the anteroinferior glenohumeral ligament.

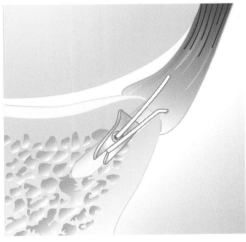

Figure 13–11   The utility loop and inserter rod are removed after a secure, low-profile repair is achieved.

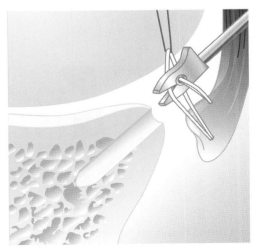

Figure 13–9   One suture strand of the anchor loop is captured or snagged in the channel at the tip of the anchor.

appropriate position. The ligament shifts superiorly and securely approximates to the glenoid rim. The utility loop and inserter rod are removed. A secure, low-profile repair is achieved, with a superior shift of the AIGHL (Fig. 13–11).

Suture Loop Shuttle Technique for Arthroscopic Passage of Utility Loop

Arthroscopic passage of the utility loop can be achieved using a previously described suture loop shuttle technique.[23] The passage of the utility loop through the ligament at a precise location using this technique allows for proper capsule shift. The location of suture loop placement is determined by grasping the ligament with the Shutt suture punch (Linvatec, Largo, FL) and pulling it superiorly to the drill hole site while ligament tension is assessed. A needle-type or penetrating suture passer does not grasp the ligament or allow for assessment of superior shift, as does this grasping suture passer. A 48-inch-long, 2-0 Prolene (Ethicon, Somerville, NJ) suture loop is then passed through the ligament using the suture punch. The Prolene suture loop serves as a suture shuttle and is used to pull the utility loop into the anteroinferior portal, through the AIGHL, and out the anterosuperior portal (Fig. 13–12).

Pearls and Pitfalls

Several techniques can facilitate capture of the anchor loop. For the inferior two anchors, pass the suture loop from the articular side of the ligament to the extra-articular side. For the superior anchor, pass the suture loop from the extra-articular side of the ligament to the articular side. Pull the utility loop through the anterosuperior portal to orient the anchor loop at a better angle with respect to the anchor and thus ease loop capture (Fig. 13–13). Intermittently, pull the utility loop to test the tension of the anchor loop during insertion. Too much tension can cause the anchor loop to tear through the ligament.

Where the utility loop and anchor loop are passed through the AIGHL is very important. This location should be inferior to the glenoid drill hole so that a superior shift of the ligament is achieved when the anchor is

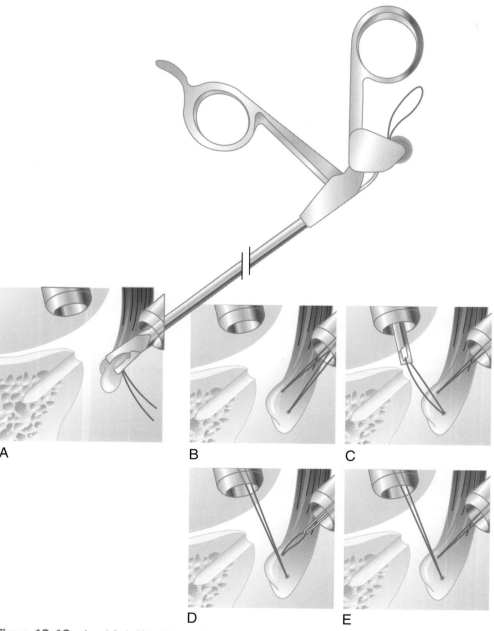

A

B

C

D

E

Figure 13–12 *A* and *B*, A 48-inch-long, 2-0 Prolene suture loop is passed through the ligament using a suture punch. *C*, The free ends of the Prolene suture loop are pulled out the anterosuperior portal while the loop remains out the anteroinferior portal. *D* and *E*, The Prolene suture loop is used as a suture shuttle to pull the utility loop through the ligament.

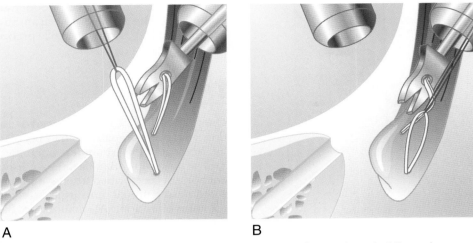

Figure 13–13   *A*, The utility loop is pulled out the anterosuperior portal to orient the anchor loop at a better angle with respect to the anchor and thus facilitate loop capture. *B*, Loop capture is more difficult when the loop is pulled toward the same portal as the anchor.

inserted into the drill hole. The anchors are inserted in the most inferior site first, progressing to more superior sites.

The utility loop can be used to facilitate the passage of one of the anchor arcs through the anchor loop with the metallic knotless suture anchor. Pull the utility loop to hold the anchor loop safely away from the arcs during the first stages of anchor insertion. Tension on the anchor loop is relaxed once the arcs have entered the bone.

Several anchor loop configurations can lead to anchor loop breakage with the metallic anchor and should be avoided. One arc must be passed through the anchor loop before anchor insertion. If this is not done, the anchor loop will be cut on insertion into bone (Fig. 13–14). The anchor loop must pass directly from the base

of the anchor into the ligament. If, instead, the anchor loop is allowed to wrap around the body of the anchor, the anchor loop will be at risk of being cut by the closing anchor arc as the anchor is inserted into bone (Figs. 13–15 and 13–16).

Postoperative Management

The postoperative rehabilitation protocol involves the use of a sling for 4 weeks. During that time, pendulum exercises, range-of-motion exercises of the shoulder and elbow, and isometric exercises of the forearm are performed. External rotation is limited to neutral. At 4 weeks postoperatively, progressive active and passive range-of-motion exercises are begun. External rotation is

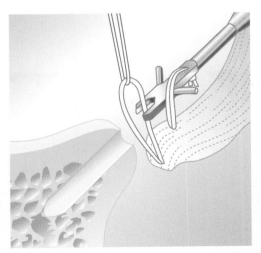

Figure 13–14   One anchor arc has not been passed through the anchor loop and will cut the anchor loop when the anchor is inserted into bone. (From Thal R: Knotless suture anchor: Arthroscopic Bankart repair without tying knots. Clin Orthop 390:46-47, 2001.)

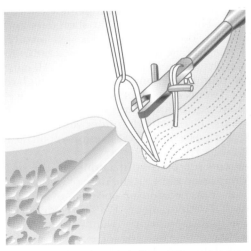

Figure 13–15   The anchor loop is incorrectly wrapped around the anchor. (From Thal R: Knotless suture anchor: Arthroscopic Bankart repair without tying knots. Clin Orthop 390:46-47, 2001.)

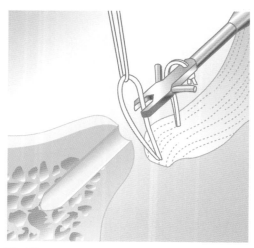

Figure 13–16 The anchor loop is incorrectly wrapped around the anchor. (From Thal R: Knotless suture anchor: Arthroscopic Bankart repair without tying knots. Clin Orthop 390:46-47, 2001.)

limited to 45 degrees. In addition, isometric deltoid exercises and periscapular exercises are begun. At 6 weeks postoperatively, progression to a full, active range of motion is allowed. At 8 weeks, resistive training with the use of isotonic and isokinetic modalities is performed in a progressive manner, but with no limitation on the patient. Participation in contact and overhead sports is not allowed until 5 months postoperatively.

Results

A prospective evaluation of the first 27 consecutive patients with traumatic anterior shoulder instability treated with arthroscopic Bankart repair using the knotless suture anchor was done; results were reported at an average 29 months' follow-up (range, 24 to 39 months).[25,27,28] The study population consisted of 24 males and 3 females, with an average age of 28 years (range, 17 to 59 years); 12 of the patients were 22 years or younger. There were 16 right shoulders and 11 left shoulders; the dominant shoulder was involved in 18 patients. The average duration of preoperative symptoms was 66 months (range, 3 to 192 months). All patients had an initial traumatic event, and they all had recurrent instability. Twenty-one patients had preoperative dislocations (an average of four), and six patients had recurrent subluxations. Five patients underwent superior labral anterior and posterior (SLAP) lesion repair at the time of the Bankart repair.

All patients reported satisfaction with the surgery. All patients remained stable at the time of follow-up, without feelings of apprehension or episodes of subluxation or dislocation. Twenty patients (74%) regained full range of motion postoperatively. Twenty-five patients (93%) had less than 5 degrees' loss of external rotation at 90 degrees of abduction. Two patients had a 10-degree loss of external rotation at 90 degrees of abduction. The average loss of external rotation was 2 degrees. The average Rowe score was 36 preoperatively and 96 postoperatively. The average American Shoulder and Elbow Society (ASES) score was 62 preoperatively and 94 postoperatively.

Complications

One patient (3.7%) experienced a traumatic redislocation 1 year after repair. He had been asymptomatic until he dislocated his shoulder when he fell skiing. Revision arthroscopic Bankart repair using knotless suture anchors was performed when symptoms of instability persisted despite initial nonsurgical treatment with a period of immobilization. A small bony Bankart lesion was encountered at revision surgery. This patient remains stable 25 months after revision surgery. No other patient had signs or symptoms of recurrent dislocation or subluxation. No other complications of treatment occurred in any other patient.

Three anchor loops broke during insertion of the 92 anchors used in this study. Two of the three broken anchor loops occurred in the first three cases performed. Repair was successfully achieved by stacking another knotless anchor into the same drill hole in each case. Review of the videotape of these broken anchor loops revealed that the loop had been allowed to wrap around the base of the anchor and had been cut by the closing anchor arc on insertion into the bone.

Conclusion

The described technique for arthroscopic Bankart repair using the knotless suture anchor is much simpler than other methods of arthroscopic suture anchor repair. Cumbersome knot tying is avoided, excellent capsular shift can be achieved, and a more secure, low-profile repair can be created (Fig. 13–17).

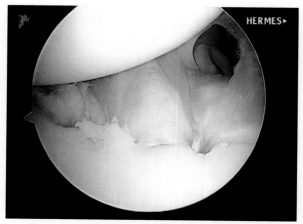

Figure 13–17 Bankart repair with knotless suture anchors.

References

1. Arciero RA, Taylor DC, Snyder RJ, Uhorchak JM: Arthroscopic bioabsorbable tack stabilization of initial anterior shoulder dislocations: A preliminary report. Arthroscopy 11:410-417, 1995.

2. Bacilla P, Field LD, Savoie FH: Arthroscopic Bankart repair in a high demand patient population. Arthroscopy 13:51-60, 1997.

3. Benedetto KP, Glotzer W: Arthroscopic Bankart procedure by suture technique: Indications, technique, and results. Arthroscopy 8:111-115, 1992.

4. Berg JH, Thal R, Tamai J: A comparison of capsular shift in medially based repairs for glenohumeral instability: A cadaveric study. Paper presented at the 19th annual meeting of the Arthroscopy Association of North America, Apr 16, 2000.

5. Burkhart SS, DeBeer JF: Traumatic glenohumeral bone defects and their relationship to failure of arthroscopic Bankart repairs. Arthroscopy 16:677-694, 2000.

6. Caspari RB: Shoulder arthroscopy: A review of the present state of the art. Contemp Orthop 4:523-531, 1982.

7. Caspari RB: Arthroscopic reconstruction for anterior shoulder instability. Tech Orthop 3:59-66, 1988.

8. Coughlin L, Rubinovich M, Johansson J, et al: Arthroscopic staple capsulorrhaphy for anterior shoulder instability. Am J Sports Med 20:253-256, 1992.

9. Detrisac DA, Johnson LL: Arthroscopic shoulder capsulorrhaphy using metal staples. Orthop Clin North Am 24:71-88, 1993.

10. Elrod BF: Arthroscopic reconstruction of traumatic anterior instability. Oper Tech Sports Med 5:215-225, 1997.

11. Grana WA, Buckley PD, Yates CK: Arthroscopic Bankart suture repair. Am J Sports Med 21:348-353, 1993.

12. Green MR, Christensen KP: Arthroscopic versus open Bankart procedures: A comparison of early morbidity and complications. Arthroplasty 9:371-374, 1993.

13. Hawkins RB: Arthroscopic stapling repair for shoulder instability: A retrospective study of 50 cases. Arthroscopy 5:122-128, 1989.

14. Johnson LL: Arthroscopy of the shoulder. Orthop Clin North Am 11:197-204, 1980.

15. Lane JG, Sachs RA, Riehl B: Arthroscopic staple capsulorrhaphy: A long-term follow-up. Arthroscopy 9:190-194, 1993.

16. Loutzenheiser TD, Harryman DT II, Yung SW, et al: Optimizing arthroscopic knots. Arthroscopy 11:199-206, 1995.

17. Matthews LS, Vetter WL, Oweida SJ, et al: Arthroscopic staple capsulorrhaphy for recurrent anterior shoulder instability. Arthroscopy 4:106-111, 1988.

18. Metcalf MH, Savoie FH, Smith KL, Matsen FA: Meta-analysis of surgical reconstruction for anterior shoulder instability: A comparison of arthroscopic and open techniques. Paper presented at the 21st annual meeting of the Arthroscopy Association of North America, Apr 26, 2002.

19. Morgan CD: Arthroscopic transglenoid Bankart suture repair. Oper Tech Orthop 1:171-179, 1991.

20. Morgan CD, Bodenstab AB: Arthroscopic Bankart suture repair: Technique and early results. Arthroscopy 3:111-122, 1987.

21. Neviaser TJ: The anterior labroligamentous periosteal sleeve avulsion lesion: A cause of anterior instability of the shoulder. Arthroscopy 9:17-21, 1993.

22. Tauro JC: Arthroscopic inferior capsular split and advancement for anterior and inferior shoulder instability: Technique and results at 2- to 5- year follow-up. Arthroscopy 16:451-456, 2000.

23. Thal R: A technique for arthroscopic mattress suture placement. Arthroscopy 9:605-607, 1993.

24. Thal R: A knotless suture anchor: Technique for use in arthroscopic Bankart repair. Arthroscopy 17:213-218, 2001.

25. Thal R: Arthroscopic anterior stabilization of the shoulder with a knotless suture anchor: Technique and results. Paper presented at the 27th annual meeting of the American Orthopaedic Society for Sports Medicine, June 30, 2001.

26. Thal R: A knotless suture anchor: Design, function, and biomechanical testing. Am J Sports Med 29:646-649, 2001.

27. Thal R: Knotless suture anchor: Arthroscopic Bankart repair without tying knots. Clin Orthop 390:42-51, 2001.

28. Thal R: Arthroscopic anterior stabilization of the shoulder with a knotless suture anchor: Technique and results. Arthroscopy (in press).

29. Warner JJP, Miller MD, Marks P, Fu FH: Arthroscopic Bankart repair with the Suretac device. Part I. Clinical observations. Arthroscopy 11:2-13, 1995.

30. Warner JJP, Miller MD, Marks P, Fu FH: Arthroscopic Bankart repair with the Suretac device. Part II. Experimental observations. Arthroscopy 11:14-20, 1995.

31. Warner JJP, Pagnani M, Warren FF, et al: Arthroscopic Bankart repair utilizing a cannulated absorbable fixation device. Orthop Trans 15:761-762, 1991.

32. Wolf EM: Arthroscopic anterior shoulder capsulorrhaphy. Tech Orthop 3:67-73, 1988.

33. Wolf EM, Eakin CL: Arthroscopic capsular plication for posterior shoulder instability. Arthroscopy 14:153-163, 1998.

34. Wolf EM, Wilk RM, Richmond JC: Arthroscopic Bankart repair using suture anchors. Oper Tech Orthop 1:184-191, 1991.

Arthroscopic Rotator Interval Closure

Scott W. Trenhaile, Larry D. Field,
and Felix H. Savoie III

ARTHROSCOPIC ROTATOR INTERVAL CLOSURE IN A NUTSHELL

History:
  Patients may present with pain, fatigue, weakness, recurrent instability, and numbness; symptoms may follow an acute traumatic event or have a gradual onset secondary to associated multidirectional instability

Physical Examination:
  Presence of a significant sulcus sign with the arm in adduction and internal rotation that persists with external rotation; anterior or posterior instability may also be present with load and shift testing, depending on associated labral pathology

Imaging:
  Anteroposterior radiograph can demonstrate inferior subluxation of the humeral head with a significant rotator interval lesion; arthrography may demonstrate dye in the rotator interval

Indications:
  Significant functional impairment, pain, and continued instability despite an adequate rehabilitation program

Contraindications:
  Loss of motion secondary to capsular contracture

Surgical Technique:
  Superior and middle glenohumeral ligaments are approximated along with the anterior capsule using #1 Prolene or #2 Ethibond suture; adjacent borders of the subscapularis and supraspinatus tendons may be incorporated into the interval closure if additional stability is required

Postoperative Management:
  Immobilization in a sling with limited pain-free passive exercises for the first 3 weeks postoperatively; active exercises are continued for an additional 3 weeks before range-of-motion and strengthening exercises are started 6 to 8 weeks postoperatively

Results:
  83% to 100% success when performed alone or with other stabilization procedures

Complications:
  Loss of external rotation with overtightening of rotator interval capsule; persistent instability can occur with overly aggressive postoperative rehabilitation

The rotator interval has been described as a space between the superior border of the subscapularis tendon and the anterior border of the supraspinatus tendon.[16] The rotator interval has two capsular layers. The superficial layer is an expansion of the coracohumeral ligament between the subscapularis and supraspinatus tendons, and the deep layer is between the superior glenohumeral ligament (SGHL) and middle glenohumeral ligament (MGHL).[7] Between the rotator interval, these capsular layers can be lax or deficient secondary to traumatic injury, repetitive microtrauma, or congenital ligamentous laxity.[2,5,16,17,20]

A number of reports have examined the rotator interval's role in glenohumeral stability. Ovenson and Nielsen[13] found that in the adducted shoulder, the structures within the rotator interval were the most important in preventing inferior subluxation of the humeral head. Harryman et al.[7] demonstrated that anterior, posterior, and inferior translation of the glenohumeral joint increased after sectioning the interval capsule in a cadaveric model. Warner et al.[21] demonstrated that the SGHL limits inferior translation and external rotation of the humeral head when the arm is adducted. Posterior translation is also limited by the SGHL with the shoulder flexed, adducted, and internally rotated. The MGHL limits anterior glenohumeral translation in abduction and external rotation, as well as inferior translation when the arm is adducted and externally rotated.[12,21] Van der Reis and Wolf[20] demonstrated that suturing the SGHL to the MGHL reduces glenohumeral elevation, external rotation, and extension. Numerous authors have described open and arthroscopic techniques of rotator interval closure alone and in conjunction with other stabilization procedures to decrease the capsular volume and increase shoulder stability.[4-6,10,11,14,18,19-22]

History

Patients often report a traumatic subluxation or dislocation event. Symptoms of pain, popping, and early fatigue are associated with repetitive heavy activity, including weight lifting, swimming, rowing, volleyball, tennis, and baseball. Patients may also report the inability to use the arm in overhead activity secondary to the "dead arm syndrome," characterized as recurrent numbness and tingling.[16] Recurrent subluxation events may occur with active forward elevation, abduction–external rotation, or adduction with a load applied to the glenohumeral joint. The direction of glenohumeral translation that produces the symptoms is related to the pathology within the shoulder joint. Patients may also report weakness in elevated positions if a significant component of scapular winging is present.

Physical Examination

Significant inferior translation of the glenohumeral joint is found when a sulcus sign is present. This test is performed by applying a downward force to the arm while it is in an adducted position (Fig. 14–1). When the coracohumeral ligament is present, the sulcus sign should decrease or disappear with external rotation of the humerus. A rotator interval defect is suspected if the sulcus sign persists. Generalized ligamentous laxity may be present and can be tested according to the criteria of Marshall et al.[8]

The load and shift test can be used to assess ligamentous stability for anterosuperior, straight anterior, anteroinferior, and posterior directions. With the patient

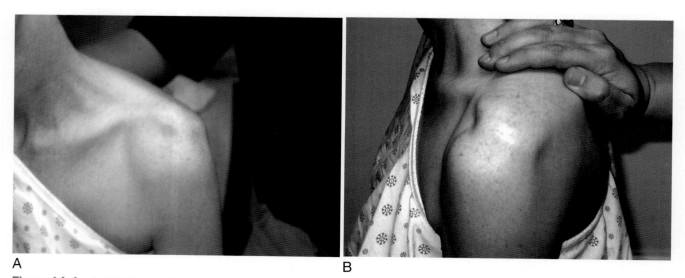

A   B

Figure 14–1 *A,* With downward traction on the upper extremity, an obvious inferior subluxation is present with a rotator interval lesion. *B,* The rounded contour of the shoulder is lost, and the deltoid flattens.

in the supine position, an axial load is applied to the arm to center the humeral head. The other hand is used to translate the humerus in the anterior and posterior directions. Additional provocative maneuvers may be used, including the Jobe apprehension, reduction, and augmentation test. Scapular dyskinesis may also be present with considerable long-standing glenohumeral instability.

Imaging

Standard radiographs of the shoulder should be obtained to identify any evidence of a bony Bankart or Hill-Sachs lesion. An anteroposterior radiograph may demonstrate inferior subluxation of the humeral head that persists despite external rotation in the presence of a rotator interval defect (Fig. 14–2). In addition, an anteroposterior radiograph with active elevation may show posteroinferior subluxation. Nobuhara and Ikeda[10] used shoulder arthrography to demonstrate radiopaque dye filling the rotator interval with active elevation and external rotation. Although magnetic resonance imaging may help define labral pathology, rotator interval defects are not well detected, as reported by Field et al.[5]

Indications and Contraindications

General surgical indications begin with ensuring that the correct diagnosis has been made. History, physical examination, and radiographic examinations are mandatory when making the diagnosis of glenohumeral instability with a rotator interval lesion. Patients must have significant functional impairment, pain, and continued instability despite an adequate rehabilitation program for

surgery to be indicated. Patients with a 2+ sulcus sign with the humerus subluxating over the glenoid rim or frank inferior dislocation are considered possible candidates for interval closure. This is particularly true if the sulcus sign does not diminish with humerus adduction and external rotation. Earlier surgical intervention may be indicated in high-demand athletes, overhead workers, or military personnel who continue to perform activities related to their dislocation or subluxation events. Contraindications may include patients unfit for surgery, active infection, humeral head fracture, or loss of motion secondary to capsular contracture.

Surgical Technique

Positioning and Examination under Anesthesia

Either general anesthesia or interscalene block can be used. Examination under anesthesia is then performed before positioning the patient. Care is taken to assess the range of motion and anterior, posterior, and inferior stability of the operative and nonoperative shoulders. The patient is then positioned in the lateral decubitus position with the arm in 10 to 15 pounds of traction or in the beach chair position.

Diagnostic Arthroscopy

A standard posterior portal is established, and diagnostic arthroscopy is performed. The rotator interval is carefully assessed for laxity either in the interval itself or in the SGHL. Chondromalacia of the superior glenoid may indicate evidence of anterosuperior instability. A wide rotator interval in the presence of inferior capsular laxity or subluxation of the humeral head inferiorly can indicate rotator interval problems. These findings may be correlated with the examination under anesthesia, particularly the presence of a sulcus sign with the arm in adduction and external rotation. Diagnostic arthroscopy should also include careful evaluation of the attachments of the middle and inferior glenohumeral ligaments, including the anterior and posterior bands. Rotator cuff pathology should also be identified at this time.

Specific Surgical Steps

An anterior instrument portal is established under direct visualization. The portal is localized first with a spinal needle just superior to the subscapularis tendon within the rotator interval. The portal is created, and an instrument cannula is inserted. Pathologic conditions within the glenohumeral joint are addressed from an inferior to superior fashion, repairing any anterior or posterior Bankart lesions or inferior capsular laxity. Once the arthroscopic reconstruction is completed, attention is turned to the rotator interval (Fig. 14–3).

The rotator interval is prepared for closure by gently abrading the capsule with a synovial shaver with the

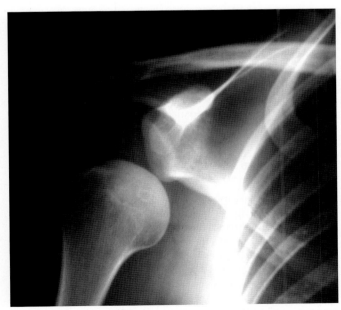

Figure 14–2   Anteroposterior radiograph of the glenohumeral joint shows inferior subluxation in the presence of a rotator interval lesion.

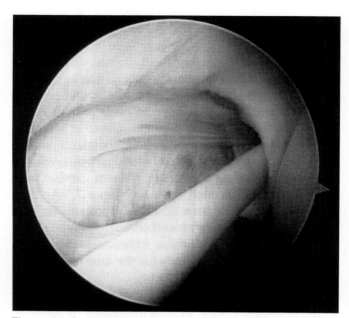

Figure 14–3 The rotator interval is visualized within the glenohumeral joint of the right shoulder between the supraspinatus and subscapularis tendons.

suction in the off position. The goal of this step is to incite a healing response once the interval has been closed. No tissue is removed with the shaver. The rotator interval can then be closed. While viewing the glenohumeral joint through the posterior portal, a suture retrieval device is inserted through the anterior cannula. Depending on the angle of the suture retrieval device, a 5- or 8-mm-diameter cannula is used to accommodate arthroscopic instruments. The cannula is retracted enough to place the suture retrieval device through the anterior capsule adjacent to the subscapularis tendon and through the MGHL. Occasionally the superior portion of the subscapularis may be included in this repair, but it is important to include the capsule anterior to the subscapularis tendon and the MGHL.

A spinal needle is then placed through the skin or the anterosuperior portal (if used) just lateral to the anterolateral edge of the acromion. The needle is directed through the capsule just anterior to the edge of the supraspinatus tendon. Care is taken to direct the needle anterior to the biceps tendon to avoid incorporating it into the interval closure. A number 1 Prolene or number 2 Ethibond suture is then passed through the spinal needle and retrieved out the anterior portal using the suture retrieval device (Fig. 14–4). The suture closes or plicates the more lateral portion of the rotator interval. The suture retriever is placed back down the anterior cannula and through the capsule, medial and superior to the previous stitch, and then through the SGHL. A spinal needle is introduced in a similar fashion to the first stitch, but more medially. The number 1 Prolene or number 2 Ethibond suture is placed through the spinal needle and retrieved through the anterior cannula (Fig. 14–5). A third stitch can be placed more medially, if necessary, in a similar fashion. The order of

suture placement is always from lateral to medial. Once the sutures have been properly positioned, they can be put under tension to ascertain tensioning of the rotator interval and elimination of intra-articular instability. The surgeon may choose to tie the first stitch laterally to determine whether additional, more medial stitches are required (Fig. 14–6).

Two methods of tying the stitches can be used. The first method allows direct visualization of the arthroscopic knot tying. The arthroscope is placed through the posterior portal into the subacromial space. The anterior cannula is placed in the subacromial space as well. The sutures are identified in the subacromial space and retrieved out of the anterior portal using a crochet hook. Care is taken to tie the lateral sutures first (Fig. 14–7). The more medial stitches are then retrieved and tied in a sequential fashion. The arthroscope can then be placed through the posterior portal into the glenohumeral joint to evaluate the rotator interval capsular closure.

The second method of tying the stitches is done with the arthroscope in the glenohumeral joint. This method allows direct visualization of the rotator interval as it is closed during knot tying. However, it requires that the stitches be placed and tied before placing an additional stitch more medially. With the arthroscope through the posterior portal in the glenohumeral joint, a switching stick is placed through the anterior cannula in the joint. The cannula and switching stick are then retracted anteriorly until they both reach just outside the capsule. The switching stick, followed by the cannula, is advanced into the subacromial space and above the rotator cuff. While viewing the rotator cuff from within the glenohumeral joint, the rotator cuff is blotted with the switching stick and cannula until it is directly over the superior Prolene stitch near the anterior edge of the supraspinatus tendon. The switching stick is then removed, and the crochet hook is inserted along the same path used for the switching stick's removal. The suture is snared with the crochet hook and delivered out of the anterior portal. With the inferior limb of suture already out of the anterior portal, the knot can be tied with a locking sliding knot (Fig. 14–8). The rotator interval is evaluated for proper closure and the need to place additional interval closure sutures. Care must be taken to avoid the arthroscopic knots when performing a subacromial bursectomy after interval closure.

Postoperative Management

For the first postoperative week, the shoulder is maintained in a sling with a small abduction pillow. The patient is then started on a home exercise program consisting of shoulder shrugs, passive forward flexion of the shoulder to 90 degrees, and passive external rotation to neutral. All exercises should be done in a pain-free manor. These exercises are continued for 2 weeks. At 3 weeks, active internal and external rotation exercises are commenced at the waist level with a Theraband and continued for an additional 3 weeks. At 6 weeks, physical

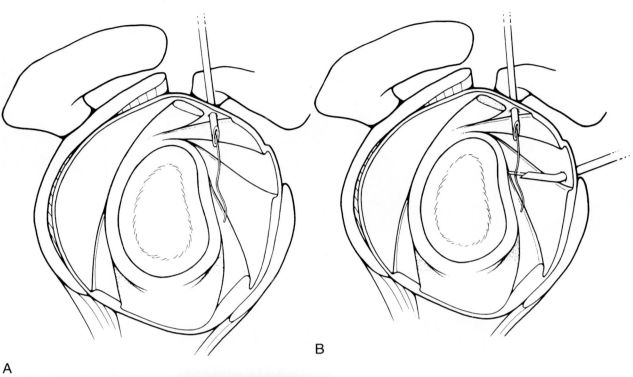

B

A

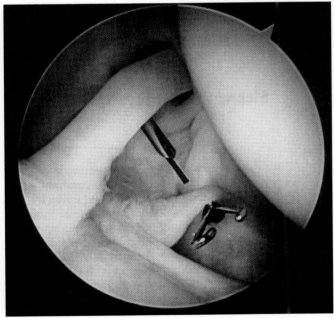

C

Figure 14–4   *A*, Initiation of intra-articular rotator interval closure. A spinal needle is seen beside the anterior margin of the supraspinatus tendon and through the superior portion of the rotator interval capsule. A number 1 Prolene suture is being advanced through the spinal needle. *B*, The retrieval device has already been passed through the inferior portion of the anterior capsule of the rotator interval. *C*, Note that the suture retrieval device is through the subscapularis tendon and the middle glenohumeral ligament in this example.

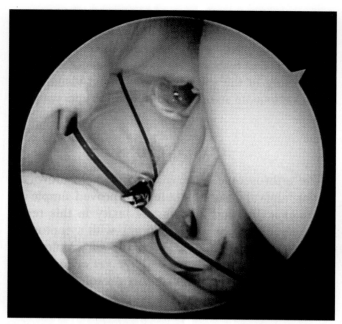

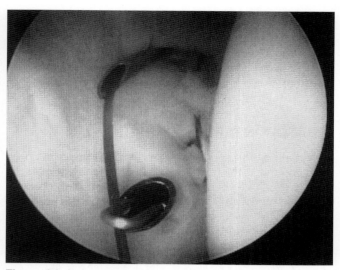

Figure 14–6   A lateral plication stitch has been tied, and a second plication stitch is being placed more medially.

Figure 14–5   A lateral plication stitch is seen in place. A second, more medial stitch is being completed as the transporter device retrieves the suture out of the anterior portal.

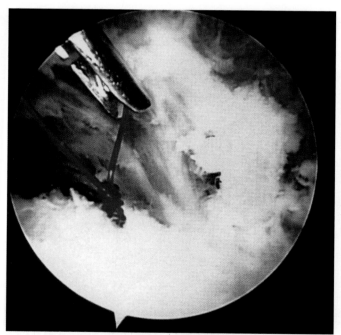

Figure 14–7   An arthroscopic knot tied through the lateral portal completes the lateral plication stitch in the rotator interval.

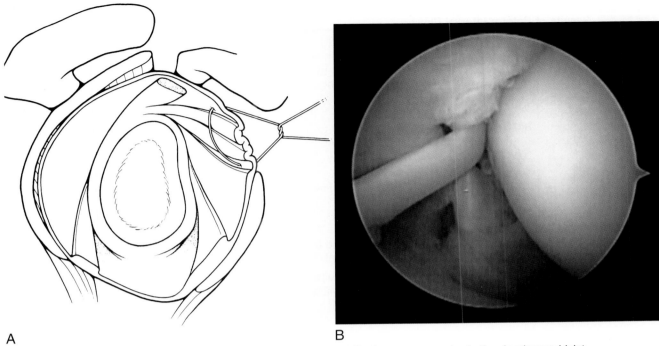

A   B

Figure 14–8   *A* and *B,* Arthroscopic knot tying above the rotator cuff while the camera remains in the glenohumeral joint.

therapy is started, emphasizing active range of motion with rotator cuff strengthening. Plyometric exercises can begin at 2 months, followed by a return to low-velocity throwing at 3 months. Return to contact sports and aggressive sports-specific drilling is determined on an individual basis but is usually delayed until 4 months postoperatively.

Results

Numerous authors have reported their results with rotator interval closure (Table 14–1). In 1981, Rowe and Zarins[16] identified 20 of 37 patients suspected of having a rotator interval lesion. The overall population consisted of 50 patients with either a Bankart lesion or capsular laxity. At a 2-year minimum follow-up, 94% had achieved good to excellent results using the Rowe score.

In 1987, Nobuhara and Ikeda[10] reported the results in 84 patients with looseness and instability secondary to the rotator interval. An open technique was used in which the supraspinatus was closed to the subscapularis tendon and the coracohumeral ligament was advanced over the rotator interval closure. A rate of 96% good to excellent results was reported, but this included a second group of patients who underwent release for a rotator interval contracture.

Warner et al.[22] reported the results of 18 patients requiring open capsulorrhaphy for traumatic anterior instability. All patients had capsular laxity or frank disruption of the capsule. A discrete Bankart lesion was noted in six patients, and seven patients were found to have a rotator interval capsular defect. Those patients with rotator interval defects were repaired using an "inverted L" superolateral capsular shift. At an average of 27 months' follow-up, 83% of the patients were completely satisfied with the procedure. Symmetrical or near-symmetrical external rotation was noted in 78%, and 75% of patients could perform recreational overhead sports without limits.

In 1995, Field et al.[5] treated 15 patients with open repair of the superficial and deep layers of the rotator interval for isolated defects. The rotator interval defect averaged 2.75 cm wide and 2.3 cm high. All patients had good to excellent outcomes using the American Shoulder and Elbow Society (ASES) and Rowe outcome scores at an average of 3.3 years' follow-up.[1,5,15]

In 1997, Treacy et al.[19] reported an arthroscopic technique for closure of superficial and deep layers of the rotator interval performed on 50 patients. Rotator interval closure was performed in conjunction with various procedures for labral pathology, producing "encouraging" results but with limited short-term follow-up.

Noojin et al.[11] reported a similar arthroscopic technique in 2000 for rotator interval closure to supplement the repair of labral pathology. At an average of 2 years' follow-up, patients had a 97% success rate and a Bankart score of 93.[11,15]

Savoie and Field[18] reported their results using a combination of capsular shrinkage and the rotator interval closure technique described by Treacy et al.[19] in a population of patients with multidirectional instability. Only

Table 14–1

Results of Rotator Interval Closure

Author (Date)	No. of Patients	Follow-up	Results	Surgery Type	Interval Plication	Other Factors
Rowe and Zarins (1981)[16]	20	2 yr minimum	94% good to excellent	Open	Deep layer	Mixed population of Bankart and capsular laxity pathology
Nobuhara and Ikeda (1987)[10]	84	—	96% good to excellent	Open	Superficial layer	Included those with contracture and instability of rotator interval
Warner et al. (1995)[22]	18	27 mo average	83% satisfied	Open	Deep layer	Mixed population of Bankart and capsular laxity pathology
Field et al. (1995)[5]	15	3.3 yr average	100% good to excellent	Open	Superficial and deep layers	Isolated interval defects only
Treacy et al. (1997)[19]	50	Short term	"Early results encouraging"	Arthroscopic	Superficial and deep layers	Varied procedures for labral pathology plus rotator interval closure
Noojin et al. (2000)[11]	35	2 yr average	97% success, Bankart score 93	Arthroscopic	Superficial and deep layers	Varied procedures for labral pathology plus rotator interval closure
Savoie and Field (2000)[18]	30	25 mo average	93% satisfactory	Arthroscopic	Superficial and deep layers	Multidirectional instability patients, thermal plus rotator interval closure

three patients experienced instability after a single traumatic event, whereas 91% of patients had evidence of generalized ligamentous laxity as defined by Marshall et al.[8] At an average of 25 months' follow-up, 93% of patients had satisfactory results according to the UCLA, Rowe, and Neer-Foster outcome scales.[3,9,15]

Complications

Patients undergoing rotator interval closure alone or in conjunction with other stabilization procedures may encounter loss of motion postoperatively. If adequate stability is achieved with labral reconstruction procedures alone, overtightening of the glenohumeral joint should be avoided by electing not to perform a rotator interval closure. If an interval closure is needed at the time of surgery, care must be taken to avoid excessive internal rotation or forward elevation to avoid loss of external rotation or extension, respectively. Conversely, instability may persist despite performing a rotator interval closure or other stabilization procedure. Overaggressive rehabilitation should be avoided in the early postoperative period.

References

1. Barett WP, Frankin JL, Jackins SE, et al: Total shoulder arthroplasty. J Bone Joint Surg Am 69:865-872, 1987.
2. Cole BJ, Rodeo SA, O'Brien SJ, et al: The anatomy and histology of the rotator interval capsule of the shoulder. Clin Orthop 390:129-137, 2001.
3. Ellman H: Arthroscopic subacromial decompression: Analysis of 1 to 3 year results. Arthroscopy 3:173-181, 1987.
4. Field LD, Savoie FH: Anterosuperior instability and the rotator interval. Oper Tech Sports Med 5:257-263, 1997.
5. Field LD, Warren RF, O'Brien SJ, et al: Isolated closure of rotator interval defects for shoulder instability. Am J Sports Med 23:557-563, 1995.
6. Gartsman GM, Taverna E, Hammerman SM: Arthroscopic rotator interval repair in glenohumeral instability: Description of an operative technique. Arthroscopy 15:330-332, 1999.
7. Harryman DT II, Sidles JA, Harris SL, et al: The role of the rotator interval capsule in passive motion and stability of the shoulder. J Bone Joint Surg 74:53-66, 1992.
8. Marshall JL, Johanson N, Wickiewicz TL, et al: Joint looseness: A function of the person and the joint. Med Sci Sports Exerc 12:189-195, 1980.
9. Neer CS, Foster CR: Inferior capsular shift for involuntary inferior and multidirectional instability at the shoulder. J Bone Joint Surg Am 62:897-908, 1980.

10. Nobuhara K, Ikeda H: Rotator interval lesion. Clin Orthop 223:44-50, 1987.

11. Noojin FK, Savoie FH, Field LD: Arthroscopic Bankart repair using long-term absorbable anchors and sutures. Orthop Today 20:18-20, 2000.

12. O'Connell PW, Nuber GW, Mileski RA, et al: The contribution of the glenohumeral ligaments to anterior stability of the shoulder joint. Am J Sports Med 18:579-584, 1990.

13. Ovenson J, Nielsen S: Experimental distal subluxation in the glenohumeral joint. Arch Orthop Trauma Surg 104:78-81, 1985.

14. Rook RT, Savoie FH, Field LD: Arthroscopic treatment of instability attributable to capsular injury or laxity. Clin Orthop 390:52-58, 2001.

15. Rowe CR, Patel D, Southmayd WW: The Bankart procedure: A long-term end result study. J Bone Joint Surg Am 60:1-16, 1978.

16. Rowe CR, Zarins B: Recurrent transient subluxation of the shoulder. J Bone Joint Surg Am 63:863-872, 1981.

17. Rowe CR, Zarins B, Ciullo JV: Recurrent anterior dislocation of the shoulder after surgical repair. J Bone Joint Surg Am 66:159-168, 1984.

18. Savoie FH, Field LD: Thermal versus suture treatment of symptomatic capsular laxity. Clin Sports Med 19:63-75, 2000.

19. Treacy SH, Field LD, Savoie FH: Rotator interval capsule closure: An arthroscopic technique. Arthroscopy 13:103-106, 1997.

20. Van der Reis W, Wolf EM: Arthroscopic rotator cuff interval capsular closure. Orthopedics. 24:657-661, 2001.

21. Warner JJ, Deng XH, Warren RF, et al: Static capsuloligamentous restraints to superior-inferior translation of the glenohumeral joint. Am J Sports Med 20:675-685, 1992.

22. Warner JJ, Johnson D, Miller M, et al: Technique for selecting capsular tightness in repair of anterior-inferior shoulder instability. J Shoulder Elbow Surg 4:352-364, 1995.

15

Radiofrequency Technique for Shoulder Instability

GARY S. FANTON, BRAD A. ZWAHLEN, AND MICHAEL G. HEHMAN

RADIOFREQUENCY TECHNIQUE FOR SHOULDER INSTABILITY IN A NUTSHELL

History:
Recurrent subluxations or a sensation of the joint "popping out" of the socket; symptom exacerbation with abduction–external rotation activities

Physical Examination:
Positive apprehension sign and mild to moderate sulcus

Imaging:
Capsulolabral detachment with attenuated capsule on magnetic resonance imaging

Indications:
(1) Mild to moderate recurrent instability, (2) positive apprehension sign and symptomatic subluxation, (3) no major bony defects, (4) sufficient anterior capsular ligamentous structures, (5) anterior capsulolabral detachment repairable with attenuated capsule on magnetic resonance imaging

Surgical Technique:
Examination under anesthesia
Diagnostic arthroscopy: lateral decubitus or beach chair position; assess capsular tissue, labral integrity
Surgical steps: bend radiofrequency probe 25 degrees and place through anterior portal; begin anteroinferiorly in pouch and work superiorly; use striping technique, leaving 3 to 4 mm between treated tissue; continue striping to top of middle glenohumeral ligament; reattach anterior capsulolabral complex; place probe in posterior portal to tighten posteroinferior glenohumeral ligament; keep probe moving while in pouch to avoid injuring axillary nerve

Postoperative Management:
Immobilization for 2 to 4 weeks; limit abduction to 90 degrees and external rotation to 45 degrees until 6 weeks; rotator cuff and scapular stabilization exercises

Results:
85% success at 4 years' follow-up; better results with mild to moderate instability

Complications:
Axillary neuritis (rare, occurring in 1% to 2% of patients treated) usually resolves in 6 to 8 weeks when treated with physical therapy and anti-inflammatory drugs; capsulitis should be treated with appropriate physical therapy and anti-inflammatory drugs and possibly manipulation under anesthesia in severe cases

Shoulder instability is one of the most common causes of shoulder pain in young, active patients presenting to the orthopedic surgeon. Because traditional open stabilization is associated with morbidity, such as loss of range of motion, arthroscopic techniques have been developed to reattach the capsulolabral complex. However, arthroscopic procedures that address only the capsulolabral detachment have resulted in high failure rates, possibly due to the failure to treat the patulous capsule and stretched ligaments. In the past 20 years, the concept of using heat to alter the structure of collagen has generated considerable interest. By thermally changing the structure of collagen, the surgeon can decrease capsular volume without incurring the associated morbidity seen after an open procedure.[2,3,6,8-12]

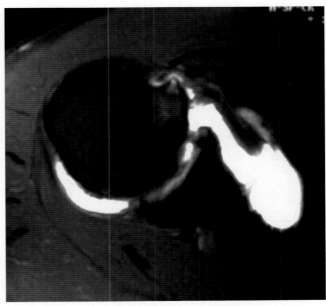

Figure 15–1 Axial magnetic resonance imaging scan demonstrating anteroinferior capsulolabral detachment.

Case History

The patient is a 21-year-old man whose initial shoulder instability and pain began 2 years earlier when his right arm was pulled into extension during a rugby tackle. He felt his shoulder "pop out" and pop back in again spontaneously. He now has recurrent episodes of shoulder subluxation with his arm in extension and abduction.

Physical Examination

The patient has full range of motion of the right shoulder but is apprehensive with an anterior force on the humeral head when his arm is placed in more than 90 degrees of abduction and external rotation. He has a mild sulcus sign and no posterior laxity.

Imaging

Plain radiographs are normal, but magnetic resonance imaging suggests an anteroinferior capsulolabral detachment with capsular attenuation (Fig. 15–1).

Indications and Contraindications

The primary indication for surgical stabilization is recurrent instability that fails to respond to a conservative program of strengthening. Thermal stabilization is considered in patients who have mild to moderate instability and no major bony defects in either the anterior glenoid (bony Bankart lesion) or the posterior humeral head (large Hill-Sachs lesion). Thermal stabilization is often used as an adjunct to arthroscopic anterior capsulolabral repair or in patients with an attenuated capsule, with or without an associated superior labral anterior to posterior (SLAP) lesion. Contraindications to this procedure include major bony defects or a thin or ruptured capsule, especially at the anterior middle and inferior glenoid humeral ligament complex.

Surgical Technique

Examination under Anesthesia

The patient's shoulder is examined in both the supine and the operative position. The shoulder demonstrates a full range of motion with an anterior "shift" with full abduction–external rotation associated with a subtle "clunk." In this case, a frank dislocation was not demonstrated.

Positioning

The patient is transferred to the lateral decubitus position, and the arm is suspended using 7 pounds of longitudinal traction. The arm is positioned in approximately 40 degrees of abduction, and the torso is tilted backward (toward the surgeon) approximately 10 to 15 degrees. The back of the table is also elevated approximately 20 degrees (Fig. 15–2). The beach chair position can also be used, depending on the surgeon's preference.

Diagnostic Arthroscopy

Standard diagnostic arthroscopy is performed. In this case, it revealed an anterior capsulolabral detachment with a capacious anteroinferior capsular pouch (drive-through sign) (Fig. 15–3).

Specific Surgical Steps

1. The radiofrequency (RF) probe is bent approximately 25 degrees near the tip using a probe bender before inserting it through the anterior cannula.

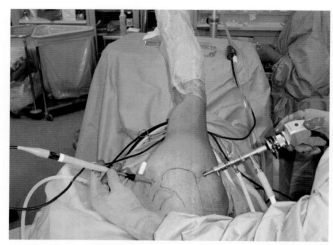

Figure 15–2 Clinical photograph of arthroscopy performed with the patient in the lateral decubitus position.

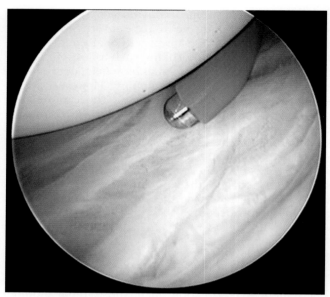

Figure 15–4 The probe is swept in a medial to lateral direction, beginning in the anteroinferior pouch.

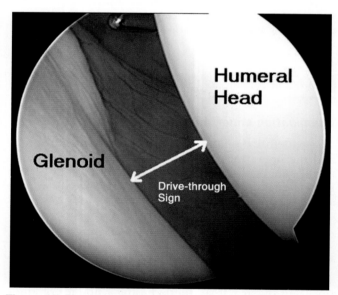

Figure 15–3 Arthroscopic example of the drive-through sign in a patient with a capacious anteroinferior capsular pouch.

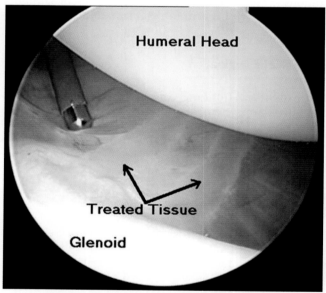

Figure 15–5 A linear striping technique is used, leaving approximately 3 to 4 mm of untreated tissue between the stripes.

2. The probe is directed down to the anteroinferior glenohumeral ligament area. The RF generator is set at 75° C and 40 watts.
3. The RF probe is activated using a foot pedal. The probe is swept in a medial to lateral direction beginning at the anteroinferior capsule and working superiorly (Fig. 15–4).
4. A linear striping technique is used, leaving approximately 3 to 4 mm of untreated tissue between the linear stripes (Fig. 15–5). The striping technique is continued laterally as far as possible, with attention to tightening the lateral capsule recess near the humeral attachment.
5. Striping is continued superiorly to the top of the middle glenohumeral ligament (Fig. 15–6). In this patient, the RF treatment was *not* continued all the way to the glenoid margin of the capsule. The capsule should be preserved and left untreated along the glenoid margin if a capsular reattachment or suturing technique is to be performed. This maintains the integrity of the tissue used for the capsulolabral repair.
6. The anterior capsule is reattached to the glenoid rim using bioabsorbable anchors. Arthroscopic suturing techniques and suture anchors can also be employed, depending on the surgeon's preference. The rotator interval is closed if necessary.
7. The arthroscope is introduced anteriorly and directed toward the posteroinferior capsule (Fig. 15–7).

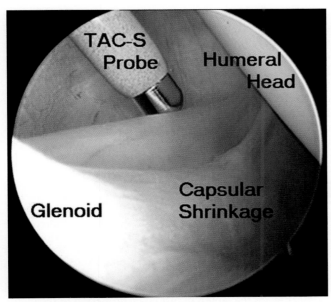

Figure 15–6   Striping continues superiorly to the top of the middle glenohumeral ligament.

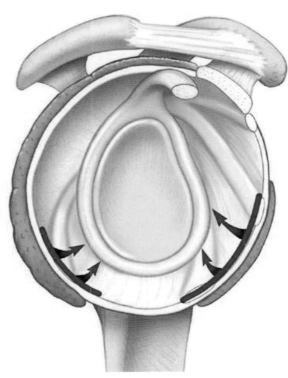

Figure 15–8   Schematic demonstrating avoidance of the inferior capsular recess and treatment with the striping technique antero- and posteroinferiorly.

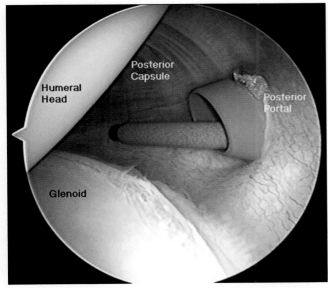

Figure 15–7   The probe is inserted through the posterior portal to treat the posteroinferior glenohumeral ligament.

Through the posterior portal, a striping pattern is used to tighten the posteroinferior glenohumeral ligament.

Pearls and Pitfalls

It is important to keep the RF probe moving during thermal treatment. The axillary nerve can be injured by excessive treatment in the axillary pouch (between the 5 and 7 o'clock positions), especially in patients with a thin capsule. Avoid treatment in this area, or use substantially reduced power settings (Fig. 15–8). Painting the entire capsule surface is infrequently required. Studies have shown that healing is faster and more complete if viable tissue is left between the treatment stripes.

Postoperative Management

Postoperative immobilization is important after thermal capsulorrhaphy. The capsule is weakest at 2 weeks postoperatively and gradually regains strength over the next 3 to 4 months. The capsule should be protected during this early postoperative phase. A shoulder immobilizer is used for 2 to 4 weeks, depending on the amount of preoperative laxity and the use of supplemental fixation. As a general rule, the looser the shoulder was preoperatively, the longer immobilization is maintained postoperatively. Physical therapy is begun after immobilization to restore range of motion. However, abduction is limited to 90 degrees and external rotation to 45 degrees until 6 weeks postoperatively. Range of motion is then progressed as tolerated, but external rotation is limited to −15 degrees compared with the opposite side to avoid restretching the repaired capsule. Scapular stabilization and rotator cuff strengthening are also emphasized.

Results

As with most surgical procedures designed to address shoulder instability, results depend on a variety of factors, including the degree and direction of preoperative instability, the presence of bony defects of the glenoid or humeral head, and whether the patient is returning to collision sports versus "repetitive use" sports such as throwing or swimming. Even the cause of instability, such as traumatic versus congenital laxity, significantly affects the success of any procedure. It is appealing to think that all shoulder instabilities can be treated thermally, but such is not the case. We have seen higher failure rates in patients with large Hill-Sachs lesions that engage on the anterior glenoid rim when the shoulder is fully externally rotated. Likewise, patients with severe instability and large rotator interval defects, a centrally deficient capsule, humeral avulsion lesions, or a large bony avulsion of the capsule at the anterior glenoid rim are probably best treated with other arthroscopic or open procedures.

Thermal stabilization is best suited to patients who have mild to moderate instability and as an adjunct to other arthroscopic stabilization procedures. In this patient population, we have achieved an overall success rate of 85% at 4 years, with a patient satisfaction rate of more than 90%.[5,7] In patients with thin joint capsules and severe multidirectional instability, the long-term success rate is lower, at 70%.[1] Thermal contraction of collagen is limited (maximum 35%).[2] In patients with severe laxity, the amount of ligament reduction may not be enough to overcome greater degrees of instability. In these patients, suture plication techniques or rotator interval closure should be considered as arthroscopic adjuncts or alternatives to thermal capsulorrhaphy. Alternatively, open procedures to perform a capsule shift can be considered.

Complications

Thermal capsulorrhaphy is technically easy, but there are some procedure-specific complications.[4] Axillary neuritis occurs in 1% to 2% of the patients treated.[13,14] This is usually sensory and presents as a numbness or tingling along the axillary nerve distribution on the lateral deltoid. Motor weakness can also occur but is rare. Axillary neuritis should be treated with anti-inflammatory medications and physical therapy. In most cases, full sensory recovery occurs within 6 to 8 weeks, but some patients may take up to 6 months to fully recover.

Capsulitis of the shoulder can occur after any shoulder operation, including thermal stabilization. This usually does not result in a loss of range of motion but can cause capsule and joint line pain lasting up to 6 months after surgery. Again, this is treated with appropriate physical therapy and anti-inflammatory medications. It is rare for patients to undergo manipulation under anesthesia after arthroscopic thermal stabilization, and the necessity of this procedure is no greater than with other shoulder procedures.

Finally, capsule deficiency syndrome has been reported. All surgical procedures, including thermal capsulorrhaphy, can affect the compliance of the shoulder capsule, resulting in increased stiffness. If trauma to the capsule occurs during the early recovery period, the capsule may rupture and require a secondary surgical repair. This can happen with any surgical procedure that causes scarring of the capsule. The term *capsule necrosis* has been applied to these areas of capsule deficiency, but to date, there has been no biopsy evidence that capsule deficiency is a result of a loss of viability of the capsule. It is also seen after other nonthermal shoulder procedures. Further studies are required to evaluate this uncommon finding.

References

1. Bradley JP: Thermal capsulorrhaphy for instability of the shoulders: Multidirectional (MDI) and posterior instabilities. Paper presented at the American Academy of Orthopaedic Surgeons Symposium: Mar 19, 2000, Orlando, FL.
2. Hayashi K, Thabit G, Massa KL, et al: The effect of thermal heating on the length of histologic properties of the glenohumeral joint capsule. Am J Sports Med 25:107-112, 1997.
3. Hecht P, Hayashi K, Cooley AL, et al: The thermal effect of monopolar radiofrequency energy on the properties of joint capsule: An in vivo histologic study using a sheep model. Am J Sports Med 26:808-814, 1998.
4. Jensen K: Management of Complications Associated with Thermal Capsulorrhaphy. Orlando, FL, American Shoulder and Elbow Society, 2000.
5. Khan AM, Fanton GS: Electrothermal assisted shoulder capsulorrhaphy—monopolar. Clin Sports Med 21:599-618, 2002.
6. Lopez MJ, Hayashi K, Fanton GS, et al: The effect of radiofrequency on the ultrastructure of joint capsule collagen. Arthroscopy 14:495-501, 1998.
7. Mishra DK, Fanton GS: Two year outcome of arthroscopic Bankart repair and electrothermal assisted capsulorrhaphy for recurrent traumatic anterior shoulder instability. Arthroscopy 17:844-849, 2001.
8. Naseef GS, Foster TE, Trauner K, et al: The thermal properties of bovine joint capsule: The basic science of laser and radiofrequency induced capsular shrinkage. Am J Sports Med 25:670-674, 1997.
9. Osmond C, Hecht P, Hayashi K, et al: Comparative effects of laser and radiofrequency energy on joint capsule. Clin Orthop 375:286-294, 2000.
10. Tibone JE, McMahon PJ, Shrader TA, et al: Glenohumeral joint translation after arthroscopic, nonablative, thermal capsuloplasty with a laser. Am J Sports Med 26:495-498, 1998.
11. Vangsness CT, Mitchell W, Nimni M, et al: Collagen shortening: An experimental approach with heat. Clin Orthop 337:267-271, 1997.
12. Wall MS, Deng XH, Torzilli PA, et al: Thermal modification of collagen. J Shoulder Elbow Surg 8:339-344, 1999.
13. Weber SC: Surgical management of failed arthroscopic thermal capsulorraphy. Paper presented at the 20th Annual Meeting of the Arthroscopy Association of North America, Apr 22, 2001, Seattle.
14. Williams GR, Wong KL: Complications of thermal capsulorrhaphy of the shoulder. Paper presented at the 68th Annual Meeting of the American Academy of Orthopaedic Surgeons, Feb 28, 2001, San Francisco.

Arthroscopic Repair of Posterior Shoulder Instability

ROBERT SELLARDS, RODNEY STANLEY, AND ANTHONY A. ROMEO

ARTHROSCOPIC REPAIR OF POSTERIOR SHOULDER INSTABILITY IN A NUTSHELL

Physical Examination:
Apprehension with forward flexion, internal rotation adduction
Jerk test: abduct shoulder with arm in forward flexion, internal rotation, adduction

Imaging:
Shoulder radiographs, including an axillary lateral
Computed tomography scan to determine articular head involvement

Decision Making:
Traumatic or atraumatic posterior instability
Dislocation or subluxation
Acute or chronic posterior dislocation

Surgical Technique:
Examine both shoulders under anesthesia
Perform arthroscopic reduction if dislocated
Create standard arthroscopic portals, with 7 o'clock portal in posteroinferior position
Place camera in anterior portal
Use suture shuttle technique with suture hook in 7 o'clock portal
Place anchors posterior to anterior
Place plication stitches anterior and posterior
Plicate rotator interval

Postoperative Management:
Splint in abduction brace
Adhere to traumatic or atraumatic rehabilitation protocol

Case History

A 26-year-old, left-hand-dominant man presented 3 weeks after being attacked in a robbery. During the assault, he suffered an injury to his left shoulder. He was seen in the emergency room, had radiographs taken, and was told that he had no fracture (Fig. 16–1). The diagnosis was a shoulder contusion, and he received follow-up treatment from his primary care physician. The patient was started on a physical therapy program but failed to make any progress in range of motion. The concerned physician referred the patient to an orthopedic surgeon for evaluation (Table 16–1).

Physical Examination

This patient's range of motion was assessed. With his shoulder locked in 20 degrees of internal rotation, the patient could raise the arm to only 80 degrees of forward flexion. He was not able to abduct the shoulder. The

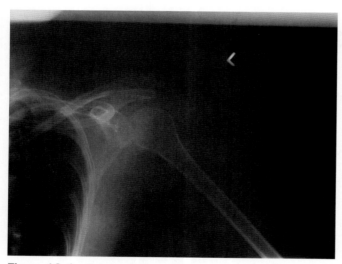

Figure 16–1   Anteroposterior radiograph of left shoulder taken in the emergency department.

Table 16–1	Important Points in History Taking—Posterior Instability

Mechanism of Injury

Direct: force directed at proximal humerus
Indirect: flexion, internal rotation, adduction (most common mechanism)

Associated Causes

Dislocation: 3 Es (ethanol, epilepsy, electricity)
Subluxation: joint laxity

Recurrent Instability

Where is the arm position when these events occur?
How often do these events occur?
Is this voluntary?

Table 16–2	Examination Findings—Locked Posterior Dislocation

Arm fixed in internal rotation, limited abduction
Prominent coracoid process
Inability to fully supinate forearm

Table 16–3	Examination Findings—Posterior Instability

Positive posterior stress test or jerk test
Symptoms reproduced with arm flexed, internally rotated, adducted

coracoid process was noted to be prominent anteriorly, and the patient was unable to supinate his forearm. Neurologic examination of the extremity was normal.

Posterior dislocations of the shoulder often have a subtle presentation (Table 16–2). The shoulder may appear normal, with little loss of symmetry, when viewed anteriorly. Only when viewed laterally or from above is the coracoid prominence evident.[15] With regard to range of motion, there is usually no external rotation. The arm is fixed in 10 to 60 degrees of internal rotation, and forward elevation is limited to less than 100 degrees.[8] A neurologic injury of the brachial plexus can occur with acute dislocations, so a thorough neurologic examination of the extremity is important.

In patients with posterior instability without a locked dislocation, provocative tests can re-create the patient's discomfort. The mechanism of injury for posterior instability is usually forward flexion, adduction, and internal rotation. When this movement is performed with posterior force directed at the patient's elbow, apprehension can be elicited.[3] From this same position, the jerk test can be performed (Fig. 16–2). With the scapula stabilized, posterior force is directed on the elbow to posteriorly displace the humeral head. The humerus is then abducted, eliciting a palpable "jerk" or "clunk" of the humeral head as it passes over the labral rim into the glenoid (Table 16–3).[12]

Imaging

A complete series of shoulder radiographs was obtained in this patient, including true anteroposterior, lateral scapular, and axillary views. The standard axillary radiograph revealed a locked posterior dislocation of the humeral head on the glenoid, with a significant reverse Hill-Sachs lesion (Fig. 16–3). There was no evidence of posterior glenoid erosions or calcifications and no evidence of excessive glenoid retroversion. The following day, a computed tomography scan was performed, revealing approximately 20% involvement of the articulating surface of the humeral head (Fig. 16–4). The scan did not demonstrate glenoid hypoplasia or abnormal humeral head retrotorsion.

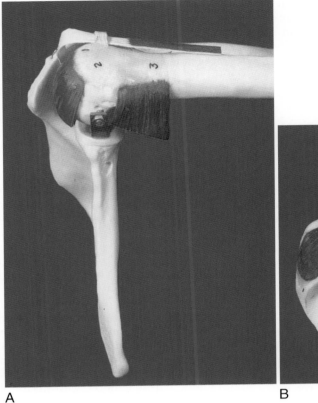
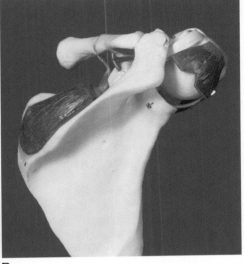

A   B

Figure 16–2   Model illustrating the provocative position of posterior instability. The humerus is forward flexed, internally rotated, and adducted. This position is viewed laterally *(A)* and posteriorly *(B)*.

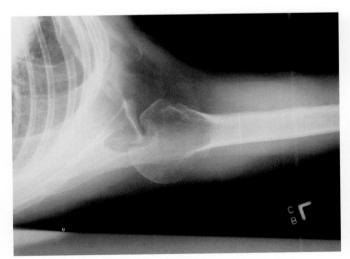

Figure 16–3   Axillary radiograph revealing a locked posterior shoulder dislocation.

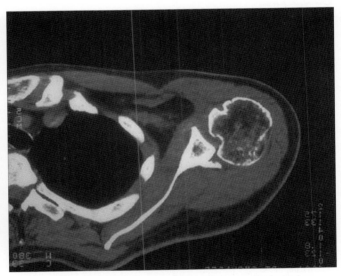

Figure 16–4   Axial computed tomography scan of a locked posterior shoulder dislocation. Approximately 20% of the humeral head articular surface is damaged.

In many emergency rooms, a routine shoulder series may not include an axillary view; thus, the glenohumeral joint may appear reduced to the untrained eye, and a patient may be discharged with a missed dislocation. The diagnosis is eventually made when the patient is seen by an orthopedic consultant and proper radiographs are obtained, sometimes weeks or months after the injury.[5,11]

Decision-Making Principles

It is important to determine the cause of the patient's instability. The first determination is whether the injury is traumatic or atraumatic (Table 16–4). In traumatic dislocations, it is possible that reduction alone will stabilize the shoulder joint. However, there is likely to be a complete disruption of the posterior capsulolabral structures, and instability may persist.[2] There is also a varying amount of humeral head involvement, which can be determined from the computed tomography scan. If more than 40% of the humeral head is damaged, hemiarthroplasty is the procedure of choice to restore an articulating surface with the glenoid (Table 16–5).[9,10]

Arthroscopic management enables the surgeon to address all aspects of the intra-articular soft tissue pathology associated with these traumatic injuries. An open anterior procedure does not allow adequate exposure for treatment of the posterior pathology, so the recommended procedure is to compensate for the posterior capsulolabral injury by transferring the lesser tuberosity

---

Table 16–4

Classification of Posterior Dislocations

Acute posterior dislocation: <6 weeks
Chronic posterior dislocation: >6 weeks
Recurrent subluxation
   Traumatic
   Atraumatic
      Voluntary
      Involuntary

Table 16–5

Management of Posterior Dislocations

<40% Articular Surface

Reduce
Evaluate stability
   Stable
      Splint in 10 degrees of external rotation
   Unstable
      Arthroscopy
      Repair capsule and labral avulsion
      Splint in 10 degrees external rotation

>40% Articular Surface

Reduce
Hemiarthroplasty

---

and limiting internal rotation (McLaughlin procedure).[13] This approach does not adequately address the posterior capsulolabral complex, which contributes to the instability (Fig. 16–5). Analogous to the Bankart lesion of anterior dislocations, this reverse Bankart lesion should be repaired to restore posterior stability and provide the best opportunity for reestablishing normal function.

In the case of recurrent subluxation, it is important to determine whether there is a traumatic or atraumatic cause. If the cause is atraumatic, one must distinguish between voluntary and involuntary subluxation. Careful physical examination is necessary to rule out a multidirectional instability component, which would alter management of the injury. Atraumatic subluxation is often seen in the athletic population, especially those engaging in overhead sports.[4] The pathology varies from that of traumatic dislocations. In acute subluxation, there is an avulsion of the posterior band of the inferior glenohumeral ligament. In chronic subluxation, there is a large capsular redundancy, with stretching of the rotator interval (Fig. 16–6).[3,4] Traditional open methods have been described to address posterior instability in these individuals.[14] These procedures use a posterior open approach with a capsulorrhaphy. These atraumatic patients can also be managed arthroscopically, accomplishing the goal of reducing capsular laxity and restoring stability. This is achieved with suture plication of the posteroinferior capsule in combination with closure of the rotator interval.[1,16,19]

The treatment plan for the patient described earlier was a closed reduction under anesthesia. Then, if the stability was acceptable, he would be treated in a brace. If there was significant instability, the plan was to proceed with posterior stabilization.

Surgical Technique

Positioning

The patient was brought into the operating room, intubated, and placed in the right lateral decubitus position. An axillary roll was secured beneath his right axilla, and the beanbag was deflated, stabilizing the patient on the table. Patient positioning is specifically addressed in Chapter 8.

Examination under Anesthesia

Before the patient is secured in the lateral position, both shoulders should be carefully evaluated. This provides an opportunity to compare the laxity between the injured and uninjured shoulders. It is also important to determine whether there is a component of multidirectional instability.

In this patient, closed reduction was attempted. The shoulder was externally rotated with one hand, and the other hand was placed on the medial aspect of the proximal humerus, providing lateral distraction. This maneuver was not successful in achieving a reduction.

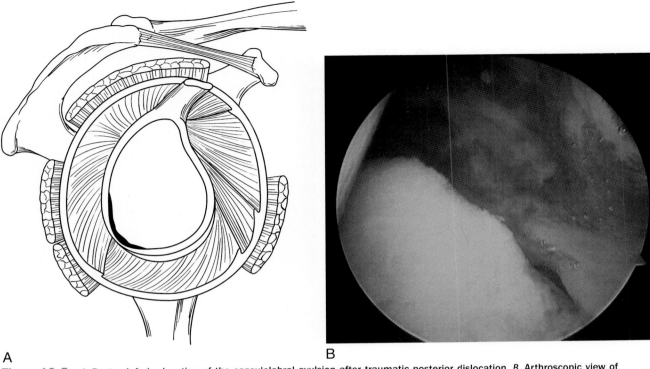

A   B

Figure 16–5   *A*, Posteroinferior location of the capsulolabral avulsion after traumatic posterior dislocation. *B*, Arthroscopic view of the labrum, which is separated from its glenoid insertion. This is visualized from the posteroinferior arthroscopic portal.

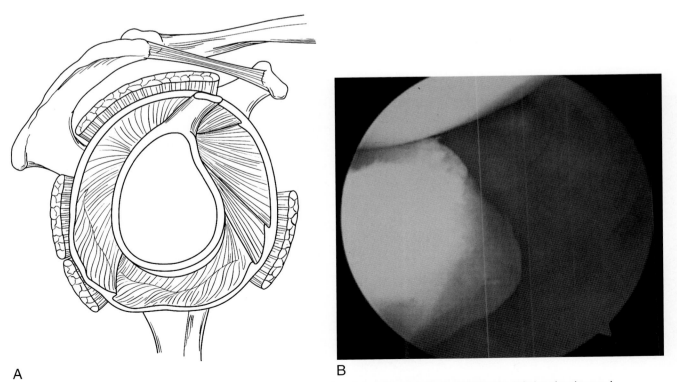

A   B

Figure 16–6   *A*, Inferior capsular redundancy resulting from chronic, atraumatic posterior instability. The inferior glenohumeral ligament has lost its tension after repeated episodes of humeral head subluxation. *B*, Arthroscopic visualization of the posteroinferior glenoid. The inferior capsule is patulous and incompetent.

An arthroscopic reduction was then attempted. Through a small posterior skin incision made at the site of the posterior arthroscopic portal, a 4-mm metal rod, commonly referred to as a switching stick, was introduced into the glenohumeral joint. It was placed medial and superior to the humeral head, resting on the anterior rim of the glenoid. After complete relaxation of the shoulder with paralysis by the anesthesiologist, a reduction maneuver was performed. The assistant provided lateral and slight distal traction of the extremity while the surgeon slowly levered the switching stick anteriorly using the anterior rim of the glenoid as a fulcrum. The switching stick provided a direct lateral force through the rotator cuff tissue, not the humeral articular surface, separating the humeral impaction fracture from the posterior glenoid rim. As the arm was gently externally rotated, the humeral head was felt to reduce within the glenohumeral joint. This was confirmed on clinical examination. The arm was placed on the patient's side and was easily dislocated a second time with the humerus in neutral rotation. Based on this instability, the plan was to proceed with arthroscopic surgical stabilization.

Diagnostic Arthroscopy

One should carefully evaluate the condition of the posteroinferior quadrant. This includes an assessment of the labrum, joint capsule, and glenoid bone stock. In this case, there was a significant amount of blood within the joint, with obvious cartilage fragments. The large reverse Hill-Sachs lesion was identified on the anterior aspect of the humerus, seen best from the anterior portal (Fig. 16–7). The capsulolabral complex had been completely disrupted off the posteroinferior glenoid rim (Fig. 16–8).

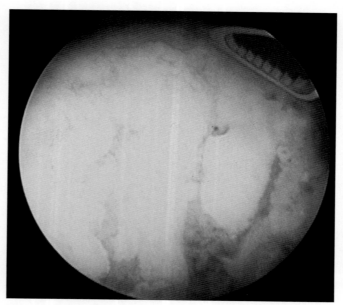

Figure 16–7 Arthroscopic view of a reverse Hill-Sachs lesion of the humeral head.

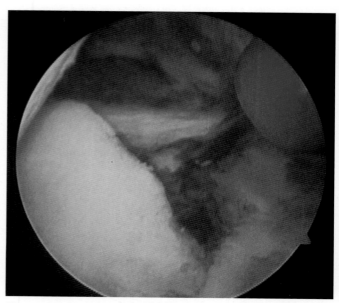

Figure 16–8 Traumatic disruption of the posteroinferior glenoid labrum after a posterior dislocation. The arthroscopic instrument illustrates the extent of the lesion.

Specific Surgical Steps

1. Establish a standard posterior portal.
2. Establish an anterior portal in the rotator interval.
3. Perform glenohumeral diagnostic arthroscopy.
4. Using switching sticks, place the camera in the anterior portal.
5. Carefully examine the posteroinferior quadrant.
6. Establish the 7 o'clock portal[6] with a large-bore screw-in cannula, which will accommodate an angled suture hook (Linvatec, Largo, FL) (Fig. 16–9).
7. Prepare the glenoid for soft tissue reattachment with an arthroscopic rasp and bur. Be sure to debride the entire glenoid neck to provide a large surface for tissue repair.
8. Plicate the capsule beyond the tear, both posteriorly and anteriorly. This is performed by passing the suture hook through the capsule and then exiting at the labral articular cartilage junction (Fig. 16–10). The PDS suture is then advanced into the joint and pulled through the posterosuperior portal. A number 2 nonabsorbable suture is passed through a loop in the PDS. The PDS is then used as a suture shuttle, pulling the nonabsorbable suture through the capsulolabral complex.
9. The suture limb is retrieved from the posterosuperior cannula with a crochet hook. This limb is then pulled out through the posteroinferior cannula, and an arthroscopic knot is tied (Fig. 16–11). The goal of this stitch is twofold. It functions in plicating the capsule and also prevents propagation of the labral tear.
10. The suture anchor is placed at a 45-degree angle to the plane of the glenoid. The anchor should be slightly on the articular surface. This ensures restoration of the labral "bumper" (Fig. 16–12).

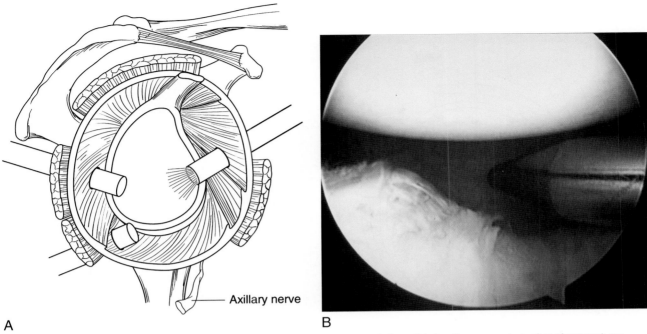

A   B

Figure 16–9   *A,* Schematic representation of the 7 o'clock arthroscopic portal. From this location, accurate anchor placement can be achieved on the glenoid. This portal is also used for suture passage and knot tying. Note that the axillary nerve is a safe distance from the cannula. *B,* Arthroscopic insertion of the 7 o'clock cannula as viewed from the posterosuperior portal.

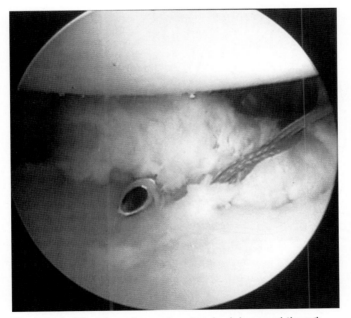

Figure 16–10   The arthroscopic suture hook is passed through the capsulolabral complex, exiting at the edge of the glenoid. The number 1 PDS is then advanced and pulled through the posterosuperior cannula.

2 Shoulder

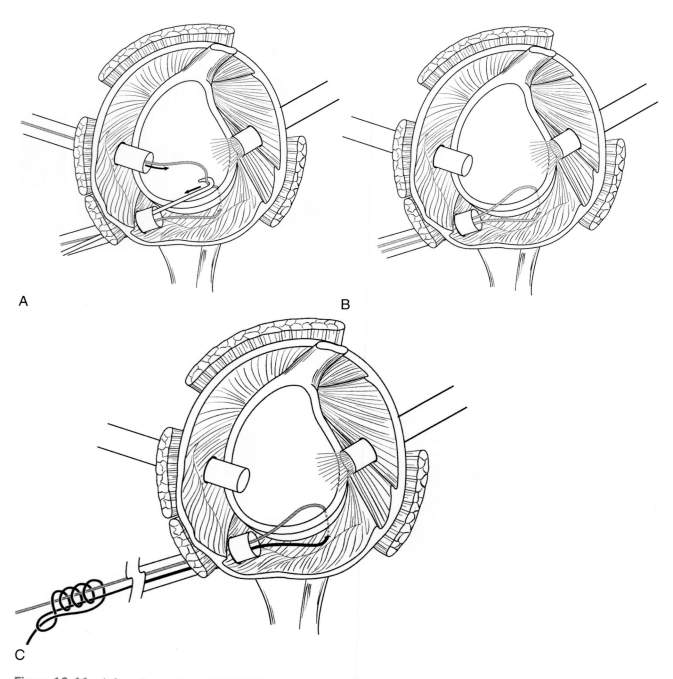

Figure 16–11   *A*, Once the nonabsorbable plication stitch has been shuttled through the labrum with the PDS, the limb exiting the posterosuperior cannula is retrieved with a crochet hook. *B*, The limb is pulled out through the posteroinferior cannula in preparation for knot tying. *C*, If the suture slides freely through the capsulolabral complex, a sliding knot may be used for stabilization. The knot-tying post should be the limb that pierces the soft tissue.

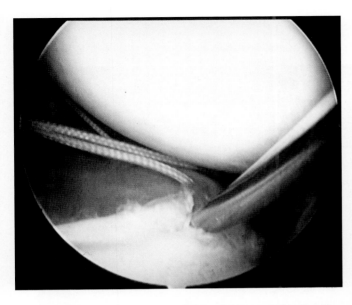

Figure 16–12 The arthroscopic anchor is placed on the glenoid rim, slightly on the articular surface. The anchor is angled 45 degrees to the plane of the glenoid surface. This location ensures restoration of the labral "bumper" when the arthroscopic knot is secured.

11. The number of suture anchors used depends on the size of the lesion. Proceed with anchor placement in a posterior to anterior direction.

12. Place the first anchor at the most posterior extent of the lesion through the 7 o'clock portal. Both suture ends are pulled with a crochet hook through the posterosuperior portal. A suture hook is placed in the 7 o'clock portal and then through the capsulolabral complex. A number 1 PDS suture is advanced with the device into the joint and then pulled out through the superoposterior portal. Using the suture shuttle technique, a simple loop is thrown with the PDS, and this is tied around one of the ends of the anchor suture. Attempt to pull the suture end nearest the capsulolabral complex. This gives the surgeon the option of tying a sliding knot or alternating half hitches.

13. The suture hook is removed from the portal, and the PDS is pulled through the 7 o'clock portal. This brings one end of the anchor suture through the capsulolabral complex. The other end of the anchor suture is also pulled through the 7 o'clock portal with a crochet hook.

14. An arthroscopic knot is tied. If both ends of the anchor suture slide freely, a sliding knot may be used. If not, alternating half hitches should be thrown to secure the knot. In either case, the post will be on the side of the capsulolabral complex.

15. This sequence is repeated for the additional suture anchors. The anchors should be spaced approximately 1 cm apart, and there should be an anchor at the apex of the transition between the labral tear and normal labrum. In most cases, the site of injury extends from the 6 o'clock to 9 o'clock position. This is usually repaired with three suture anchors with

plication stitches at either end. If subluxation persists, the rotator interval can be closed with a number 1 PDS suture to further decrease the glenohumeral joint volume and prevent subluxation of the humeral head (Fig. 16–13).

Pearls and Pitfalls

Our technique of reducing locked posterior dislocations uses traditional methods of reduction along with the assistance of an arthroscopic switching stick to separate the humerus from the glenoid, translate the articular surface laterally, and then gently reduce the humeral articular surface into the glenoid. The leverage is applied through the soft tissues, primarily the rotator cuff and capsule, not the articular surface. The advantage of this technique is that it eliminates the need for an open procedure to reduce the joint. One can proceed immediately with arthroscopy after reduction is achieved to address the capsulolabral complex.

One should work in an expedient manner. The longer the case progresses, the more difficult it becomes. Soft tissue fluid extravasation becomes greater as time progresses, decreasing the joint volume and limiting the amount of work space.

Suture management is also important. In general, one should progress from a posterior to an anterior direction, tying down one anchor at a time. Multiple anchor placement leaves too many sutures in the joint at one time, which may make knot tying unnecessarily difficult and increase case time.

Soft tissue dilators should be used when placing large-bore cannulas. The dilators are cannulated and slide easily over the switching stick at the site of the proposed portal. Care must be taken to keep the cannula pointing toward the posteroinferior glenoid, slightly lateral to the labrum. This allows the suture hook to gain purchase in the capsulolabral complex and also permits accurate anchor placement on the glenoid.

Postoperative Management

Appropriate rehabilitation for traumatic and atraumatic posterior instability is extremely important for a successful surgical outcome (Tables 16–6 and 16–7). For the first 6 weeks after a traumatic posterior dislocation, the patient should be splinted in 10 degrees of external rotation with a brace. During this period, isometric abduction and internal rotation exercises are allowed. After 6 weeks, external rotation and forward flexion in the plane of the scapula, as well as internal rotation without assistance, are begun. At 3 months, the patient may progress to range of motion as tolerated and shoulder strengthening with a Theraband or springs. In 4 to 5 months, motion is continued, and weight strengthening is allowed. Return to noncontact, nonoverhead sports is permitted at 6 months after surgery. If function is greater than 85% that of the opposite shoulder at 9 months, the patient is allowed full range of motion without restrictions.

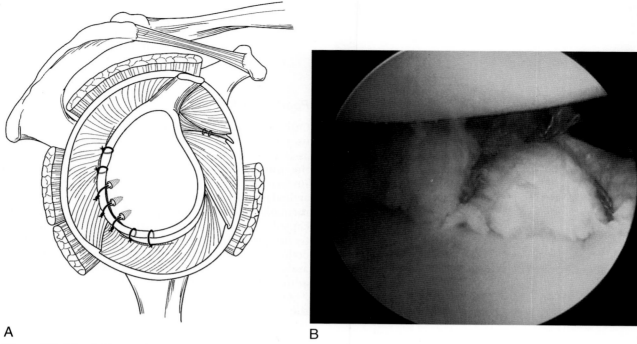

A   B

Figure 16–13   *A,* Diagram illustrating the final repair. Two plication stitches have been placed at either end of the labral repair. Three arthroscopic anchors were used to attach the capsulolabral complex to the glenoid. Note that the rotator interval was also closed with two absorbable sutures. *B,* Arthroscopic view of the completed repair at the posteroinferior glenoid.

Table 16–6	**Rehabilitation Protocol for Traumatic Posterior Instability**

Weeks 1-6

Patient splinted in 10 degrees ER in brace
Active ROM only to regain FF and ER at side as tolerated
IR in ABD permitted if active only
Begin isometrics with arm at side—ER, IR, ABD, ADD; no resisted FF or biceps motion until 12 wk postop
Start strengthening scapular stabilizers (trapezoids, rhomboids, levator scapulae)
No passive motion of posterior capsule
Physical modalities at physical therapist's discretion

Weeks 6-12

Increase posterior capsule ROM gently (active ROM)
Advance strengthening as tolerated: isometrics → bands → weights; 10 repetitions/1 set per rotator cuff, deltoid, and scapular stabilizers
Do strengthening only 3 times/wk to avoid rotator cuff tendinitis

Months 3-12

Advance to full ROM as tolerated
Begin eccentrically resisted motions, plyometrics, proprioception, body blade, and closed chain exercises at 16 wk
Resume sports and throwing at 9 mo postop

ABD, abduction; ADD, adduction; ER, external rotation, FF, forward flexion; IR, internal rotation; ROM, range of motion.

Rehabilitation after atraumatic posterior instability differs slightly. For the first 3 weeks, the patient remains in the abduction brace without any shoulder motion. At week 3, the patient begins active range of motion for forward flexion and external rotation, with limitations to prevent stress on the posterior capsule. More aggressive range of motion in all planes is started at week 8, including some shoulder strengthening. The goal is to return the patient to preinjury athletic participation at 6 months postoperatively.

Results

At 24 months' follow-up, the patient described earlier had full range of motion compared with his contralateral shoulder. There was no evidence of posterior laxity or subluxation, and the patient had returned to his presurgical level of recreational athletic participation.

Arthroscopic stabilization of posterior instability has had favorable results. Most series have included only small groups of patients without long-term follow-up. Further, some series have included patients without any signs of posterior instability, some of whom may be more appropriately classified as having multidirectional instability.

Antoniou et al.[1] reviewed 41 consecutive patients with primary posteroinferior instability for an average of 28 months. Their goal was to describe the pathologic morphology of the posteroinferior aspect of the glenolabral

Table 16–7	Rehabilitation Protocol for Atraumatic Posterior Instability

Weeks 0-3

No motion! Patient in handshake orthosis (gunslinger brace) at all times
Grip strengthening and supination, pronation of forearm

Weeks 3-8

Active ROM only to regain FF and ER at side as tolerated
IR-ADD limited to stomach or active cross-body ADD without pain
IR in ABD permitted if active only
Begin isometrics with arm at side—ER, IR, ABD, ADD; no resisted FF or biceps motion
Start strengthening scapular stabilizers (trapezoids, rhomboids, levator scapulae)
No passive motion of posterior capsule

Weeks 8-12

Increase posterior capsule ROM gently (active ROM)
Advance strengthening as tolerated: isometrics → bands → weights; 10 repetitions/1 set per rotator cuff, deltoid, and scapular stabilizers; no resisted FF or biceps motion yet
Do strengthening only 3 times/wk to avoid rotator cuff tendinitis

Months 3-12

Advance to full ROM as tolerated
Begin eccentrically resisted motions, plyometrics, proprioception, body blade, and closed chain exercises at 16 wk
Resume sports, throwing at 6 mo postop

ABD, abduction; ADD, adduction; ER, external rotation, FF, forward flexion; IR, internal rotation; ROM, range of motion.

fossa and to prospectively examine the efficacy of managing this instability with an arthroscopic capsulolabral augmentation procedure. Thirty-five patents had improved stability, and all patients had significant improvement of physical examination findings. Twenty-eight patients had a perception of residual stiffness.

Similarly, Wolf and Eakins[19] performed a retrospective study of 14 patients who had undergone arthroscopic repair of the posterior capsule and labrum. Posterior capsular laxity was present in all cases and was believed to be the primary pathology. Twelve patients showed some form of labral pathology as well. Twelve patients had excellent results, and two had fair results. There was one recurrence. All 14 were satisfied with the results of their surgery.

Savoie and Field[16] described five arthroscopic techniques to address various lesions associated with posterior instability. The preliminary results among 61 patients with 1- to 7-year follow-up indicated a 90% success rate.

There are limited data to support the use of thermal capsulorrhaphy at this time. Results are limited to a few non–peer-reviewed articles and unpublished reports.[7] These reports had short-term follow-up, and the results

of patients with posterior instability were grouped with those of patients with anterior and multidirectional instability.

Savoie and Field[17] reported on 30 patients with multidirectional instability treated with thermal capsulorrhaphy and arthroscopic suture plication of the rotator interval. At a follow-up of 22 to 28 months, the patients were assessed using the UCLA and Rowe and Neer rating scales. They reported 28 patients (93%) with satisfactory results and 2 (7%) with unsatisfactory results. Both patients with unsatisfactory results had recurrent instability that required open capsular repair.

Thabit[18] reports on 41 shoulders with multidirectional and unidirectional instability treated with laser-assisted capsulorrhaphy. There were 27 patients with anterior instability, 12 with multidirectional instability, and 2 with posterior instability. Follow-up ranged from 2 to 12 months. Results were assessed with the Rowe instability scale, with an average postoperative score of 88.2 out of 100 points.

Complications

Complications are similar to those encountered with any other surgical procedure involving the shoulder. These include infection, neurovascular injury, pain, stiffness, and recurrence of instability. Preoperative antibiotics should be administered to prevent infection. Accurate placement of the 7 o'clock portal avoids damage to the axillary nerve, which is near the inferior glenohumeral capsule. A well-supervised postoperative physical therapy regimen decreases the chance of shoulder stiffness. A premature return to sporting activities may compromise the repair and place the patient at an increased risk of recurrent dislocation.

References

1. Antoniou J, Duckworth DT, Harryman DT: Capsulolabral augmentation for the management of posteroinferior instability of the shoulder. J Bone Joint Surg Am 82:1220-1230, 2000.
2. Antoniou J, Harryman DT: Posterior instability. Orthop Clin North Am 32:463-473, 2001.
3. Bigliani L, Pollock R, McIlveen S, et al: Shift of the posteroinferior aspect of the capsule for recurrent posterior glenohumeral instability. J Bone Joint Surg Am 77:1011-1020, 1995.
4. Fronek J, Warren R, Bowen M: Posterior subluxation of the glenohumeral joint. J Bone Joint Surg Am 71:205-216, 1989.
5. Gerber C: Chronic locked anterior and posterior dislocations. In Warner J, Iannotti JP, Gerber C (eds): Complex and Revision Problems in Shoulder Surgery. Philadelphia, Lippincott-Raven, 1996, pp 99-113.
6. Goubier JN, Iserin A, Augereau B: The posterolateral portal: A new approach for shoulder arthroscopy. Arthroscopy 17:1000-1002, 2001.
7. Griffin JR, Annunziata CC, Bradley JP: Thermal capsulorrhaphy for instability of the shoulder: Multidirectional and posterior instabilities. Instr Course Lect 20:23-28, 2001.

8. Harryman D, Sidles J, Harris S, et al: Laxity of the normal glenohumeral joint: A quantitative in vivo assessment. J Shoulder Elbow Surg 1:66-76, 1992.

9. Hawkins RJ, McCormack RG: Posterior shoulder instability. Orthopedics 11:101-107, 1988.

10. Hawkins RJ, Neer CS 2nd, Pianta RM, Mendoza FX: Locked posterior dislocations of the shoulder. J Bone Joint Surg Am 69:9-18, 1987.

11. Loebenberg MI, Cuomo F: The treatment of chronic anterior and posterior dislocations of the glenohumeral joint and associated articular surface defects. Orthop Clin North Am 31:23-34, 2000.

12. Matsen FA III, Thomas SC, Rockwood CA Jr: Anterior glenohumeral instability. In Rockwood CA Jr, Matsen FA III (eds): The Shoulder. Philadelphia, WB Saunders, 1998, pp 611-754.

13. McLaughlin H: Posterior dislocation of the shoulder. J Bone Joint Surg Am 34:584-590, 1952.

14. Misamore GW, Facibene WA: Posterior capsulorrhaphy for the treatment of traumatic recurrent posterior subluxations of the shoulder in athletes. J Shoulder Elbow Surg 9:403-408, 2000.

15. Petersen SA: Posterior shoulder instability. Orthop Clin North Am 31:263-274, 2000.

16. Savoie FH II, Field LD: Thermal versus suture treatment of symptomatic capsular laxity. Clin Sports Med 19:63-75, 2000.

17. Savoie FH, Field LD: Arthroscopic management of posterior shoulder instability. Oper Tech Sports Med 5:226-232, 1997.

18. Thabit G III: The arthroscopically assisted holmium:YAG laser surgery in the shoulder. Oper Tech Sports Med 6:131-138, 1998.

19. Wolf EM, Eakin CL: Arthroscopic capsular plication for posterior shoulder instability. Arthroscopy 14:153-163, 1998.

Arthroscopic Repair of Multidirectional Shoulder Instability

JOSEPH C. TAURO AND JONATHAN B. TICKER

ARTHROSCOPIC REPAIR OF MULTIDIRECTIONAL SHOULDER INSTABILITY IN A NUTSHELL

History:
Young, active patient with increasing pain, feeling of subluxation or "dead arm"; history may be atraumatic, microtraumatic, or sometimes frank traumatic dislocation

Physical Examination:
Positive instability tests—anteriorly or posteriorly with sulcus sign; generalized hyperlaxity

Imaging:
Negative in many cases; patients with traumatic dislocations may have posterior or anterior Hill-Sachs lesions on x-ray, and corresponding labral pathology may be seen on magnetic resonance arthrography

Indications:
Persistent pain, loss of function, subluxation or dislocation despite appropriate rehabilitation

Contraindications:
Voluntary dislocators, poor compliance with prior rehabilitation efforts

Instrumentation and Sutures:
Spectrum instrument set used for direct insertion of #1 PDS or to pass nonabsorbable sutures (e.g., #2 braided suture) using a suture shuttle technique; careful suture management and secure knot tying are important

Evaluation under Anesthesia:
Anterior, inferior, and posterior instability testing at 0, 45, and 90 degrees of abduction to further define pathology is essential; sulcus sign that does not reduce when repeated with arm in external rotation suggests incompetent rotator interval

Portals:
Three portals for visualization, capsular advancement, and suture management
Posterior portal is slightly more lateral and inferior than standard for posterior plication
Anterosuperior lateral portal is used for suture management during anterior and inferior plication and for viewing posteriorly during posterior plication
Anteroinferior medial portal is the primary working portal for anterior and inferior plication, capsular split, and anchor placement and is used for suture management during posterior plication

Arthroscopic Findings:
Excessive laxity or redundancy indicated by deep capsular gutters; combinations of anterior, inferior, and posterior redundancy possible, with attenuated glenohumeral ligaments; though not typical, partial labral tears or complete labral detachments, along with Hill-Sachs lesions, may be found with traumatic dislocations

Continued

ARTHROSCOPIC REPAIR OF MULTIDIRECTIONAL SHOULDER INSTABILITY IN A NUTSHELL—cont'd

Plication Techniques:

Capsule lightly abraded to promote healing

1 to 1.5 cm of capsule captured and translated laterally and superiorly

Glenoid labrum pierced; suture passed and then tied for secure repair

Multiple sutures used to shift capsule and selectively reduce capsular volume inferiorly, and anteriorly and posteriorly as indicated

Capsular Split/Shift:

Used when a Bankart lesion is present

1-cm capsular split beginning at the inferior pole of the glenoid, advanced superiorly, shifts the capsule ~2 cm and tightens the axillary pouch

Cut the capsule using a narrow basket punch inserted through the anteroinferior medial portal

Interval Closure:

Perform when examination suggests or arthroscopic findings confirm excessive superior capsule and enlarged rotator interval

Insert one or two sutures through the superior capsule and into the middle glenohumeral ligament; tie inside of joint or on bursal side (for more tightening)

Postoperative Management:

Sling immobilization for 3+ weeks; internal rotation for primarily anterior repair, neutral rotation for primarily posterior repair; focus on range of motion initially and follow carefully, then add strengthening; light overhead sports activity at 4 months, progressing as able at 6 months; contact sports allowed at 8 months

---

Case Histories

Two cases are presented as examples of patients with glenohumeral instability who have failed a nonoperative physician-supervised treatment regimen and are candidates for an arthroscopic capsular plication or shift technique. As a general rule, these patients are young, active individuals with generalized hyperlaxity and symptomatic, recurrent glenohumeral instability in the anterior and inferior direction, the posterior and inferior direction, or all three directions.[14] Trauma may or may not be part of the history, although microtrauma is often involved in the injury pattern; these patients should not have a voluntary component. The degree of instability is often subluxation, as well as dislocation, without (case AB) and with (case FM) imaging evidence of traumatic capsulolabral pathology.

AB is a 19-year-old right-hand-dominant competitive swimmer who presented with left shoulder pain of 1-year duration. At about that time, she had increased her swimming regimen in an effort to improve her speed during competitions. Pain developed in her left shoulder that was not relieved with ice and a period of rest. AB was unable to resume swimming without pain that radiated to the lateral aspect of the arm, and she developed a "dead arm" sensation, though she denied any numbness in her hand. The complaints included pain at night, as well as pain in the overhead position. She reported that sometimes she felt her shoulder shift in and out of the joint. Nonsteroidal anti-inflammatory medication and a home exercise program resulted in minimal improvement. The addition of a physician-directed physical therapy program over a 4-month period was not success-

ful in eliminating her pain or allowing AB to resume swimming.

FM is an 18-year-old right-hand-dominant competitive skateboarder who presented after having multiple documented right shoulder dislocations and many episodes of subluxation with an accompanying "dead arm" sensation. This patient had also failed many attempts to resolve the problem through a nonoperative approach, including a physician-directed physical therapy program.

Physical Examination

In both cases, there was no evidence of swelling or atrophy, and the skin was intact. AB displayed generalized hyperlaxity, which was demonstrated by hyperextension of the elbows and knees and her thumbs touching the volar aspect of her forearm. She had a range of motion of 180 degrees of forward flexion, 90 degrees of external rotation, and internal rotation to T4 (fourth thoracic spinous process). In the supine position at 90 degrees of abduction, her external rotation was 135 degrees and internal rotation was 60 degrees. Instability testing was also performed, initially in the supine position. There was a positive anterior relocation sign and only minimal discomfort with the humeral head posteriorly directed. Anterior drawer testing revealed 1+ translation (humeral head shifts to the glenoid rim), with guarding; posterior drawer testing revealed 2+ translation (humeral head subluxes over the glenoid rim).[15] In the sitting position, there was a 2+ sulcus sign (2 cm inferior translation). No clicking was noted with instability testing or range of motion. Biceps active tests did not reveal any positive findings. As expected, there was greater tuberosity tenderness and a positive impingement sign. Other pertinent negative findings included no acromioclavicular tenderness, no scapular winging, a normal cervical spine examination, and an intact neurovascular examination. FM's physical examination was similar, except that he had less hyperlaxity but 2+ anterior translation of the humeral head while being more relaxed.

Imaging

Radiographs were obtained at the initial examination, including a true anteroposterior view, an axillary view, and a supraspinatus outlet view. One additional radiograph that is often obtained for patients with instability is the Stryker notch view. In AB's case, no abnormalities were identified on the radiographs. In particular, the glenohumeral joint was normal on the anteroposterior and axillary views, including the glenoid rim, and no Hill-Sachs lesion was found on the Stryker notch view. A closed magnetic resonance imaging study was available for review. Normal labral and capsular anatomy was appreciated, and no tendinous, cartilaginous, or bony pathology was identified. Additional cross-sectional imaging studies with arthrography were not considered necessary. In FM's case, there was a small posterior Hill-Sachs lesion noted on the plain radiograph. A magnetic resonance arthrogram also showed an anterior Bankart lesion.

Decision-Making Principles

The clinical diagnosis in both cases was primary multidirectional instability with secondary impingement. In the case of FM, consideration was given to an additional traumatic component—the anterior labral tear. Non-operative versus operative treatment was reviewed with each patient and his or her parents. Both had failed to improve with nonoperative treatment regimens in the past, and surgical intervention was offered. Open and arthroscopic approaches were reviewed pictorially. An arthroscopic capsular shift procedure was recommended in both cases for its ability to address all components of the instability pattern in a less invasive and more cosmetically pleasing manner. After the benefits were discussed, risks were reviewed with the patients, including but not limited to infection, recurrent instability, pain, stiffness, implant failure, functional limitations with regard to sports activity, and neurovascular compromise. Each patient was notified that additional procedures at the time of surgery might include a rotator interval closure or posterior plication; the need for these is often detected on the examination under anesthesia and during the diagnostic portion of the arthroscopy. Further, implants in the form of suture anchors might be used to supplement the repair or address any labral pathology encountered. The perioperative and postoperative courses were described. Each patient chose to proceed with the arthroscopic capsular shift technique.

Although not present in these cases, contraindications specific to this surgery include voluntary dislocators, patients with unacceptable psychological profiles, and those who were poorly compliant with the preoperative rehabilitation regimen.

Surgical Technique

The arthroscopic approach for glenohumeral instability repair allows a more accurate diagnosis of intra-articular pathology and enables the arthroscopic surgeon to address all aspects of the instability using techniques associated with less morbidity and often an easier recovery (Fig. 17-1). Certain instrumentation and specific skills, both of which can be attained by the surgeon, are essential for a successful outcome.

Positioning

The operation can be performed with the patient under general anesthesia in the lateral decubitus position or in the beach chair position under an interscalene block. When the lateral decubitus position is chosen, a beanbag is used to position the patient declined 20 degrees posteriorly. The arm is placed in a shoulder holder in 10 pounds of traction, and the shoulder is abducted 45 degrees and forward flexed 15 degrees. When using the beach chair position, a device such as the T-MAX Beach Chair Positioner (Tenet Medical Engineering, Calgary, Alberta, Canada) is advisable to ensure patient comfort and surgeon access. With the patient's hips and knees flexed comfortably, the head of the bed is brought to

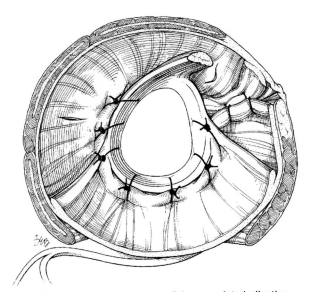

Figure 17–1 Schematic diagram of the completed plication technique for multidirectional glenohumeral instability that is primarily posterior and inferior, with closure of the rotator interval. (From Wolf EM, Pennington WT: Posterior shoulder instability: Arthroscopic management. In Imhoff AB, Ticker JB, Fu FH [eds]: An Atlas of Shoulder Arthroscopy. London, Martin Dunitz, 2003.)

approximately 70 degrees, and all down-facing surfaces are padded.

Examination under Anesthesia

Once anesthesia is administered, positioning is completed and the patient is secured on the operating room table. When muscle relaxation is achieved, an examination under anesthesia is performed to confirm the degree and direction of instability. Range of motion is assessed first and compared with the contralateral shoulder; then drawer testing of the shoulder is performed using a technique similar to that described by Altchek and coworkers.[2] This can be performed with anterior, posterior, and inferior drawer tests with the shoulder in three positions of abduction (0, 45, 90 degrees) and three positions of rotation (neutral, or midrange, and maximum internal and external rotation) to yield maximum information about laxity in both the inferior and superior portions of the anterior and posterior capsules. The anterior and posterior drawers are graded on a 0 to 3+ scale, where 0 = no increased translation compared with the contralateral side; 1+ = increased translation, with the humeral head translating to the glenoid rim; 2+ = actual subluxation of the humeral head over the glenoid rim that reduces after the anterior force is released; and 3+ = frank dislocation of the humeral head. The inferior drawer (sulcus sign) is also graded on a 0 to 3+ scale, with inferior translation perceived as separation between the humeral head and the acromion, such that $0 = \leq 1$ cm of inferior translation, $1+ = 1$ to 2 cm of inferior translation, $2+ = 2$ to 3 cm, and $3+ = \geq 3$ cm. Therefore, the magnitude of translation is used to help determine the location and amount of capsular laxity. For example, a 3+ inferior drawer (sulcus sign) with the arm adducted and in neutral rotation that decreases to 0 or 1+ at 90 degrees of abduction and neutral rotation suggests that the superior capsule is excessively lax compared with the inferior capsule. Conversely, a 2+ inferior drawer with the arm in abduction and external rotation suggests a significant component of inferior capsular laxity. A large sulcus sign with the arm adducted and in external rotation may indicate a pathologic rotator interval lesion.[15]

Three arthroscopic portals are used with these techniques. The posterior portal is usually placed in the soft spot of the infraspinatus, although this position can vary based on patient size and the planned procedure. If posterior plication is planned, it can be helpful to place the posterior portal slightly more lateral and inferior than the standard posterior portal to improve the approach to the capsule and posterior glenoid rim. An accessory posterior portal farther inferior and lateral is infrequently used. An anterosuperior lateral portal is used predominantly for suture management during anterior and inferior plication and for posterior viewing during posterior plication. This portal is located just anterior to the anterolateral corner of the acromion. From the glenohumeral perspective, this portal enters the joint just above or just anterior to the biceps tendon, anterior to the supraspinatus, at the lateral aspect of the rotator interval. This leaves enough room for a second portal, anteroinferior, which is placed lateral to the coracoid process and enters the joint above the subscapularis and lateral to the middle glenohumeral ligament. This portal is the primary working portal for anterior and inferior plication and is used for suture management during posterior plication. Accurate portal placement is important to permit adequate viewing and tissue repair. The anterior portals can be localized with a spinal needle to ensure correct placement. Cannulas that screw into place are helpful to maintain their position.

The operative extremity is now prepared and draped in the usual sterile fashion. Landmarks are outlined, including the acromion, scapular spine, clavicle, and coracoid. Lidocaine with epinephrine is injected into the planned portal sites. A spinal needle with a stylet is inserted into the glenohumeral from posterior, directed toward the tip of the coracoid process. Normal saline is injected into the joint to allow for distention, which can diminish the risk of articular damage when the arthroscope sheath is inserted. The posterior incision is made, and the blunt trocar and sheath are introduced into the joint, with backflow of fluid noted to confirm placement. The arthroscope is introduced, and the diagnostic portion of the arthroscopy is begun. The anterosuperior lateral portal is localized with a spinal needle, the skin incision is made, and a disposable cannula (at least 5.5 mm inner diameter) is introduced into the glenohumeral joint. Although this cannula is usually anterior to the biceps tendon, it can be introduced through the capsule in a direction posterior to the biceps tendon. This helps avoid cannula placement too inferior or medial in the anterior capsule, which would compromise placement of the second anterior cannula. The cannula is then brought anterior to the biceps, if it is not already there, and can be used for probing labral structures as needed.

Diagnostic Arthroscopy

Complete diagnostic arthroscopy, as described in Chapter 9, is performed. Specific arthroscopic findings for this pathology include excessive deep capsular gutters with an obvious drive-through sign. Attenuated glenohumeral ligaments, especially the inferior glenohumeral ligament, are common. An enlarged rotator interval may be noted, with a large volume anterosuperior to the biceps tendon. Less frequently, a complete labral tear is identified, although careful inspection might reveal small partial tears. Bony pathology is not common. At this point, the decision to place posterior sutures for plication can be made, based on the preoperative diagnosis and influenced by the examination under anesthesia and the arthroscopic findings.

Specific Surgical Steps

Posterior sutures are placed more often than not, although the number of sutures and therefore the amount of capsular plication vary, based on the instability pattern and the pathology identified. Posterior work is performed first, because this is more difficult to complete after the anterior structures have been tightened. If posterior plication is planned, which is often the case, the anteroinferior portal is established, and a disposable, screw-in cannula (at least 8.25-mm inner diameter) is inserted to accommodate larger instruments for capsular repair. At this point, only the inferior capsule is lightly abraded with a shaver, as access is easily achieved.

Switching sticks are then used to allow for a posterior working portal, and the anterosuperior lateral portal is used for posterior viewing. A disposable, screw-in cannula (at least 8.25-mm inner diameter) is inserted posteriorly, and the posterior capsule and remaining inferior capsule are lightly abraded with a shaver. The Spectrum tissue repair system (Linvatec, Largo, FL) is the primary instrument used for the reconstruction. This device allows the arthroscopic surgeon to pass a monofilament suture through soft tissue. The 45-degree left and right hooks and the crescent hooks are used most often. The plication can be achieved with a number 1 absorbable monofilament suture, such as PDS II (polydioxanone, Ethicon Inc., Piscataway, NJ); a number 2 braided, nonabsorbable polyester or nylon suture can also be used. A shuttle-relay suture passer (Linvatec), or simply a number 0 or 1 monofilament suture such as Prolene (polypropylene, Ethicon) with a half-hitch loop, is used to transport the nonabsorbable suture through the capsular tissue. A suture length of at least 30 inches, but preferably 36 inches, facilitates knot tying.

When working posteriorly or anteriorly, the object is to capture a sufficient amount of capsule more inferiorly and translate this tissue laterally and superiorly up to the labrum, which is used as the point of fixation. This creates a pleat of capsular tissue that folds onto itself, which is intended to scar together with the abrasion performed earlier. The capsule is often captured 1 to 1.5 cm from the glenoid, but the amount of tissue varies in each patient and with each plication stitch. If the labrum is deficient and cannot be used for fixation (which is uncommon), an anchor can be placed on the glenoid rim and its suture used for the plication at that position in the capsule.

When working posteriorly, as in the case of AB in the left shoulder, the right-angled hooks are best for capturing the capsule inferiorly (Fig. 17–2) and manipulating its tip to pass through the labrum (Fig. 17–3). If viewing is difficult when working on the most inferior stitch, lateral or slight inferior translation of the humeral head, with a positioning device or manually, can facilitate exposure. After passing through the capsule and labrum, the monofilament suture is advanced into the joint. If this suture is intended as the repair suture, such as with a PDS suture, most of it can be fed into the joint. The hook is removed from the labrum and capsule and then withdrawn back out the posterior cannula. The suture end that currently exits the posterior cannula will serve as the post limb for suture repair and can be marked with a clamp. The end of the suture in the joint is now retrieved through the posterior cannula. Alternatively, the suture end within the joint can be retrieved through the anterior cannula and clamped at its end while the hook is

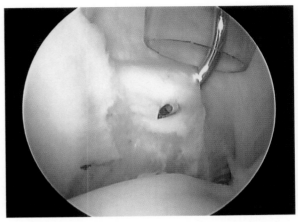

Figure 17–2   The tip of the angled hook pierces the capsule lateral and inferior to the glenoid rim.

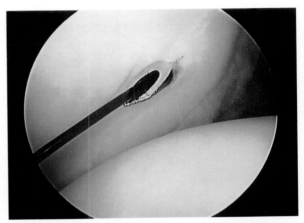

Figure 17–3   The angled hook with the capsule is translated superiorly to the glenoid rim, shifting the capsular tissue. The tip pierces the posterior labrum, creating the plication, or fold, in the capsule. The suture is then advanced into the joint.

withdrawn. After the suture is completely removed from the hook posteriorly, a suture retriever is used to grasp the anterior limb and deliver it posteriorly (Fig. 17–4). This extra step helps manage the sutures and can avoid suture tangling. (Further, as described later, this suture, which passes from a posterior direction through the capsule and labrum out the anterior cannula, can be used to shuttle a braided, nonabsorbable suture for the repair.) A secure knot of the arthroscopist's choice[7] that initially slides, such as the modified Roeder knot[3] or SMC knot[4] with alternating half hitches, is placed, firmly fixing the capsule up to the labrum (Fig. 17–5). Additional posterior sutures (up to two more) are placed as required, based on the surgeon's decision and the instability pattern. A crescent hook can be used for the more superior plication stitch, if desired.

Once the posterior plication is complete, switching sticks are used to place the arthroscope posteriorly and the disposable cannula back into the anterosuperior lateral portal to assist with suture management, but the anteroinferior medial portal is the primary portal used for the anterior and inferior repair. Two options are

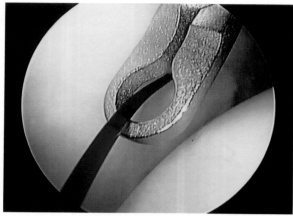

Figure 17–4 The suture is retrieved from the anteroinferior medial portal to bring this limb out the posterior portal for knot tying.

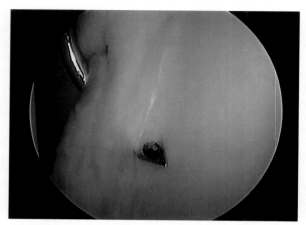

Figure 17–6 The hook tip, with a fold of inferior capsule, is passed through the anterior labrum.

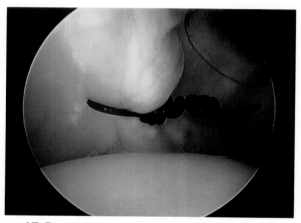

Figure 17–5 The knot secures the plication in this posterior region of capsule.

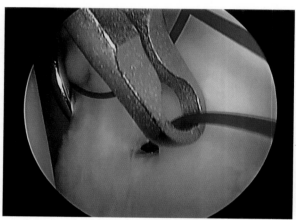

Figure 17–7 The suture retriever is brought from the anterosuperior lateral portal. Retrieving the suture directly at the hook tip decreases likelihood that the suture will tangle.

available to reduce the capsular volume. The capsule can be addressed as described earlier for the posterior capsule, where the tissue is plicated. The second option is to shift the capsule using the capsular split-shift technique. This approach is recommended when there is also a Bankart lesion, as in the case of FM, described later.

If plication is planned, light abrasion of the anterior and inferior capsule is completed. A well-developed inferior glenohumeral ligament, the primary anterior stabilizer,[14] is typically not identified. For a left shoulder, a left-angled hook is gently introduced through the anteroinferior medial cannula and manipulated inferiorly into the axillary pouch past the 6 o'clock position to capture the capsule, translate it to the labrum toward the 7 o'clock position, and pierce the labrum (Fig. 17–6) to advance a monofilament suture.

If this monofilament suture, such as Prolene, is serving to transport a braided suture or if a shuttle relay is used, it is advanced into the joint. A suture grasper is brought from the anterosuperior lateral portal, and the suture is withdrawn into this cannula (Fig. 17–7).

While this end is held securely, the hook is removed from the capsule and out the anteroinferior medial cannula. A half-hitch loop is created 6 to 8 cm from the end of the monofilament suture, and 6 to 8 cm of the end of the braided suture is placed into the loop, which is then tightened. If the shuttle relay is used, the wire loop at its midpoint is used to hold the end of the braided suture. The other end of the monofilament suture, or shuttle relay, exiting the anteroinferior medial cannula is pulled, drawing the suture loop with braided suture from the anterosuperior lateral cannula into the joint (Fig. 17–8), through the labrum and capsule (Fig. 17–9), and out the anteroinferior medial cannula (Fig. 17–10). This end of the braided suture, which is on the capsule side, is used for the posterior limb and is placed in the end of a single-lumen knot pusher for secure knot tying (Fig. 17–11). If the shuttle relay is used, once the braided suture passes through the labrum and capsule, it is no longer necessary to firmly pull it out of the cannula. If the shuttle relay is pulled too aggressively at this point, the plastic coating will tear, lengthening the loop, and

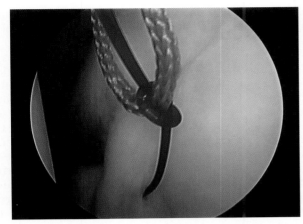

Figure 17–8 The braided suture, secured in the tightened loop of Prolene, is brought into the joint from the anterosuperior medial cannula by pulling on the other end of the Prolene suture at the anteroinferior medial cannula.

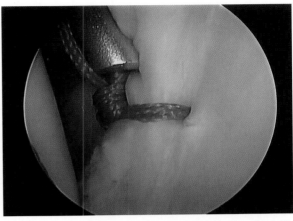

Figure 17–11 A sliding knot is placed and locked as the initial step in knot tying.

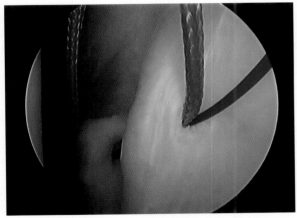

Figure 17–9 The shuttle construct is passed through the labrum and capsule.

the braided suture will be more difficult to remove from the loop.

Additional sutures are placed, advancing the capsule superiorly and plicating the capsule to the labrum (Fig. 17–12). A minimum of three sutures are placed anteriorly, each advancing more tissue superiorly and laterally to the labrum. A crescent hook can be used for the more superior plication stitch, if desired. The surgeon must be cautioned against accepting a thin "bite" of capsule or labrum, as this will compromise the suture fixation and repair. In addition, the middle glenohumeral ligament or the subscapularis should not be incorporated in this aspect of the repair to avoid incorrect tightening of the anteroinferior capsular tissue.

If there is an associated Bankart lesion, as in the case of FM, the capsular split-shift technique can be employed. The first step is to completely dissect the capsule off the glenoid neck if there is an anterior labroligamentous periosteal sleeve avulsion lesion or off the underlying subscapularis muscle if there is a Bankart lesion. The capsular split-shift procedure also advances

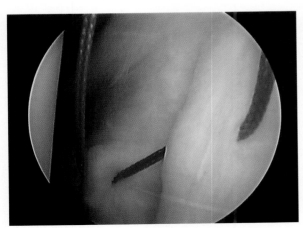

Figure 17–10 The braided suture is in position, with the fold of capsule evident.

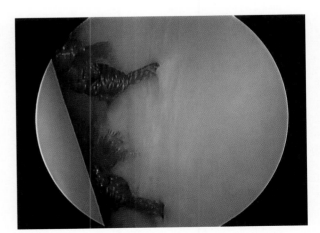

Figure 17–12 The plication is completed with additional sutures. Each knot is secured by locking the knot and tying alternating half hitches, with switching of the post.

the capsule superiorly. In the setting of a Bankart lesion, this shift retensions the capsule with minimal external rotation loss[10] and addresses the axillary pouch laxity associated with multidirectional instability. The inferior capsular split is made with a narrow-angled basket punch inserted from the anteroinferior medial portal (Fig. 17–13).

The capsule is divided from the inferior pole of the glenoid caudally into the axillary pouch. Care is taken to ensure that only capsular tissue is cut. Cadaveric dissection has shown that the axillary nerve is safe as long as the split does not extend closer than 1 cm from the capsular insertion on the humeral head.[13] The completed capsular division is diagrammed in Figure 17–14, with

point A at the intact posterior capsular attachment, point B representing the caudal extent of the split, and point C at the anterior origin of the split.

The length of the split should be half the desired capsular advancement. The usual split is 1 cm long. Superior tensioning of the capsule opens the split, bringing the caudal end of a 1-cm split (point B) 1 cm superiorly and anteriorly up the glenoid rim. The anterior corner of the capsule where the split originally began (point C) advances 2 cm up the glenoid rim. The capsule is then repaired back to the articular margin of the glenoid neck using three or four sutures secured to the glenoid rim with suture anchors. The choice of suture material and tools used to insert the sutures is based on surgeon preference and experience, but correct placement of sutures and anchors is critical to shifting the capsule.

The repair is diagrammed in Figure 17–15. The first suture should be placed just anterior to point B, with care being taken to capture only the capsule with the stitch. The first anchor should be placed on the articular margin of the glenoid 1 cm superior to the origin of the split. When the patient is in the lateral decubitus position, traction on the shoulder is reduced to 5 pounds, and the humeral head is reduced manually in the glenoid before tying the first suture. The second suture is placed at point C, and the second anchor is inserted 1 cm superior to the first anchor. This ensures that point C on the capsule is secured to the glenoid rim at the desired position (Fig. 17–16). One or two additional suture-anchor pairs are used to complete the repair of the capsule to the glenoid rim.

The final step, if required based on the examination under anesthesia and the arthroscopic findings, is rotator interval closure. This is well described in Chapter 14. The rotator interval closure can be performed using the same instruments used for the plication to approximate the superior capsule, including the supe-

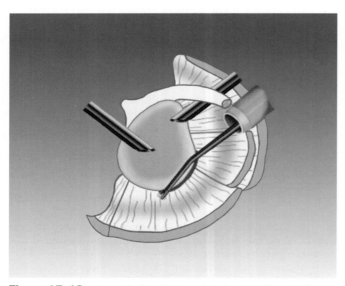

Figure 17–13 An angled basket punch is inserted through the low anterior portal to perform the split.

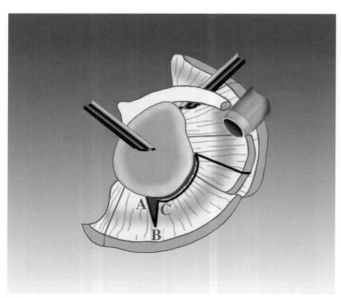

Figure 17–14 The completed capsular split. Point B is the caudal end of the split.

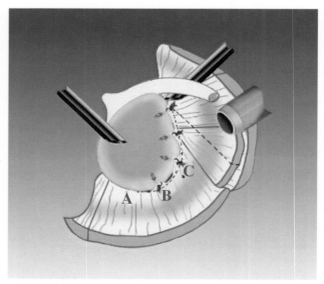

Figure 17–15 The capsule has now been shifted superiorly and repaired. For a 1-cm split, point B advances along the glenoid neck 1 cm, and point C advances 2 cm.

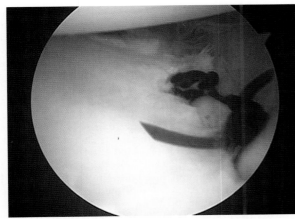

Figure 17-16 Arthroscopic view from the anterosuperior lateral portal of the split-shift repair on the anterior glenoid rim.

rior glenohumeral ligament, and the middle glenohumeral ligament. Two sutures are often used, although the more lateral stitch is often tied in a blind fashion with this inside technique and requires a closed-end suture cutter.

With the repair complete, the joint is irrigated and suctioned. The portals are closed using braided, absorbable sutures for the subcutaneous layer as necessary, and a sterile dressing is applied. Cryocompression can be employed, such as the Cryo-Cuff (Aircast, Inc., Summit, NJ), and a sling is applied. If this is primarily an anteroinferior procedure, a sling placing the forearm across the abdomen is sufficient. If the procedure is equally or primarily a posterior procedure, the sling must ensure that the arm is supported and placed toward a neutral position of rotation, using a small pillow attachment such as the UltraSling or UltraSling II (dj Orthopedics, Vista, CA).

Postoperative Management

The patient is discharged on the day of surgery. The arm is maintained in a sling for 3 weeks or longer, except when the patient showers or dresses. The sutures are removed 5 to 7 days after surgery, and radiographs are obtained at that time if anchors were placed. Range of motion to the elbow, wrist, and hand is encouraged immediately. Isometric strengthening is started for the biceps and triceps, external and internal rotators, and all three portions of the deltoid. Restricted range-of-motion exercises may be started after the first week, with limitations based on the patient and the direction of repair. The patient may use the arm for feeding and dressing after the second week. The sling is generally removed at 3 weeks, and range of motion is assessed by the surgeon. If the patient appears to have greater range of motion than anticipated, immobilization is considered for an additional week or more. In most cases, therapy begins, and active assisted range of motion is instituted, sometimes without any limitations, but this is dependent on the individual patient. At 6 weeks, active strengthening is

initiated, and range of motion is maximized. If motion greater than expected is appreciated on examination, stretching is deferred and reevaluated in 2 to 3 weeks. At 4 months postoperatively, the patient is permitted to begin tossing a ball or hitting ground strokes in tennis. A sport-specific reconditioning program is added as the patient progresses. At 6 months, the patient is permitted to begin throwing with more force or swinging a racket overhead. Contact sports are avoided until 8 months postoperatively.

Results

The results of arthroscopic plication techniques are reportedly 79% to 89 % successful.[1,6,17-19] These reports include anteroinferior and posteroinferior instability patterns involving subluxations and dislocations. These outcomes are certainly within the range reported for open instability repairs.[2,8,16] The results of the capsular split-shift procedure with a minimum 2-year follow-up were previously published; the overall recurrence rate for the modern suture anchor version of this repair was 6.9%.[11] The results at a minimum 5-year follow-up were presented more recently,[12] and this group had a redislocation rate of 7.2%. Ninety percent of athletic patients returned to their sport, but only 74% recovered to their preinjury level of competition.

Complications

In general, any complications that have been reported with other arthroscopic procedures may occur (see Chapter 9). Complications specific to arthroscopic glenohumeral instability surgery include recurrence of instability, loss of motion, and neurovascular injury.[5] These issues are reviewed in detail by Shaffer and Tibone.[9] An accurate diagnosis, cautious indications for the procedure, precise attention to the details of the technique to address the pathology, and a diligent supervised rehabilitation can help avoid these problems. In the capsular split-shift group of patients, there have been no axillary nerve injuries or other neurologic complications. However, all recurrences were caused by significant trauma, and approximately one third of the patients with recurrence had a significant Hill-Sachs lesion; it is believed that this lesion is, in part, related to recurrence. Arthroscopic bone grafting (using allograft osteoarticular bone plugs) is now being performed in patients with large Hill-Sachs lesions in an effort to further reduce recurrences.

References

1. Abrams JS: Arthroscopic suture capsulorrhaphy. In Imhoff AB, Ticker JB, Fu FH (eds): An Atlas of Shoulder Arthroscopy. London, Martin Dunitz, 2003, pp 159-165.
2. Altchek DW, Warren RF, Skyhar MJ, Ortiz G: T-plasty modification of the Bankart procedure for multidirec-

tional instability of the anterior and inferior types. J Bone Joint Surg Am 73:105-112, 1991.

3. Field MH, Edwards TB, Savoie FH: Technical note: A "new" arthroscopic sliding knot. Oper Tech Sports Med 8:250-251, 2000.

4. Kim SH, Ha KI: The SMC knot—a new slip knot with locking mechanism. Arthroscopy 16:563-565, 2000.

5. Lazarus MD, Guttmann D: Complications of instability surgery. In Iannotti JP, Williams GR (eds): Disorders of the Shoulder: Diagnosis and Management. Philadelphia, Lippincott Williams & Wilkins, 1999, pp 361-393.

6. Loren G, Snyder S, Karzel R, Wichman, M: Extended success of arthroscopic capsular plication for glenohumeral instability in the absence of a Bankart lesion. Paper presented at the 18th annual meeting of the Arthroscopy Association of North America, Apr 15-18, 1999, Vancouver, British Columbia, p 128.

7. McMillan ER, Caspari RB: Arthroscopic knot tying techniques. In Imhoff AB, Ticker JB, Fu FH (eds): An Atlas of Shoulder Arthroscopy. London, Martin Dunitz, 2003, pp 83-97.

8. Neer CS, Foster CR: Inferior capsular shift for involuntary inferior and multidirectional instability of the shoulder. J Bone Joint Surg Am 62:897-907, 1980.

9. Shaffer BS, Tibone JE: Arthroscopic shoulder instability surgery: Complications. Clin Sports Med 18:737-767, 1999.

10. Speer KP, Deng X, Torzilli PA, et al: Strategies for an anterior capsular shift of the shoulder: A biomechanical comparison. Am J sports Med 23:246-249, 1995.

11. Tauro JC: Arthroscopic inferior capsular split and advancement for anterior and inferior shoulder instability: Technique and results at 2 to 5 year follow-up. Arthroscopy 16:451-456, 2000.

12. Tauro JC: Long-term follow-up of the arthroscopic capsular split/shift. Paper presented at "Shoulder Surgery Controversies 2002," Oct 5, 2002, Costa Mesa, CA.

13. Tauro JC, Carter FM: Arthroscopic capsular advancement for anterior and anterior-inferior shoulder instability: A preliminary report. Arthroscopy 10:513-517, 1994.

14. Ticker JB, Fealy SF, Fu FH: Instability and impingement in the athlete's shoulder. Sports Med 19:418-426, 1995.

15. Ticker JB, Warner JJP: The selective capsular shift for anterior glenohumeral instability. In Fu FH, Ticker JB, Imhoff AB (eds): An Atlas of Shoulder Surgery. London, Martin Dunitz, 1998, pp 1-14.

16. Warner JJP, Johnson D, Miller M, Caborn DNM: Technique for selecting capsular tightness in repair of anterior-inferior shoulder instability. J Shoulder Elbow Surg 4:352-364, 1995.

17. Weber SC: Arthroscopic suture capsulorrhaphy in the management of type 2 and 3 impingement. Arthroscopy 16:430-431, 2000.

18. Wichman MT, Snyder SJ, Karzel RP, et al: Arthroscopic capsular plication for involuntary shoulder instability without a Bankart lesion. Arthroscopy 13:377, 1997.

19. Wolf EM, Eakin CL: Arthroscopic capsular plication for posterior shoulder instability. Arthroscopy 14:153-163, 1998.

Arthroscopic Repair of SLAP Lesions

NIKHIL N. VERMA, BRIAN J. COLE, AND ANTHONY A. ROMEO

ARTHROSCOPIC REPAIR OF SLAP LESIONS IN A NUTSHELL

History:
Traction injury or fall onto outstretched, abducted, and forward-flexed arm; pain in shoulder, often poorly localized; mechanical symptoms

Physical Examination:
Speed test, Yergason test, active compression (O'Brien) test, compression rotation test

Imaging:
True anteroposterior, scapular lateral, axillary radiographs; magnetic resonance imaging with or without contrast

Indications:
Persistent symptoms despite conservative management

Contraindications:
Minimal symptoms, incidental labral pathology on imaging

Surgical Technique:
Beach chair or lateral decubitus position; examination under anesthesia; standard portals; accessory anterior, lateral (trans–rotator cuff), posterolateral (portal of Wilmington), and accessory lateral portals
Type I: fraying treated with debridement
Type II: detachment of labrum and biceps treated with repair
Type III: superior labrum tear with intact biceps anchor treated with debridement or with repair if more than one third of labrum involved
Type IV: bucket handle tear of superior labrum extending into biceps treated with debridement, repair if more than one third of labrum involved, or biceps tenodesis for irreparable tear or revision

Postoperative Management:
Sling, early passive motion with advance to active motion and stretching; limit active flexion early with repair

Results:
Reduced pain and increased function in 80% to 90%

Complications:
Infection, stiffness, persistent pain, brachial plexus traction injury

Injuries to the superior glenoid labrum and biceps complex were initially described by Andrews et al.[1] in 1985 in a group of overhead throwing athletes. This injury pattern was reviewed and classified by Snyder et al.[28] in 1990 and given the name *superior labral anterior to posterior (SLAP) tear.* In a retrospective review of more than 700 cases of diagnostic shoulder arthroscopy, Snyder's group found that the incidence of superior labral pathology was 6%. Other studies have reported that the incidence of SLAP tears is between 6% and 12%.[15,21] In 1995, Maffet et al.[21] revised the classification system to include SLAP lesions associated with instability. The current classification system is illustrated in the nutshell table. Many different mechanisms of injury have been described for this lesion.[3,5,6,28] Some involve the repetitive overhead throwing motion in an athlete. Others include a fall on an outstretched, abducted, and forward-flexed arm or a single-event traction injury to the arm. The true natural history of this injury is unknown.

History

The presenting complaints of patients with SLAP lesions can be quite variable and are often similar to symptoms associated with other types of shoulder pathology. One key to diagnosis is maintaining a high index of suspicion if the patient's history matches one of the potential mechanisms of injury described earlier.

The most common presenting complaint of superior labral pathology is pain in the shoulder that is exacerbated with the arm in an abducted and forward-flexed position. This pain is often described as being deep within the shoulder and very poorly localized. Patients also describe "clicking," "popping," or "catching," often related to overhead activities. Care must be taken to exclude alternative diagnoses such as impingement, rotator cuff pathology, or acromioclavicular joint pathology; in addition, these conditions often coexist with SLAP lesions. When treating patients in whom shoulder pain persists despite appropriate rest and rehabilitation, a diagnosis of SLAP tear should be strongly considered.

Physical Examination

The initial examination of any patient with shoulder complaints should consist of inspection, range of motion, and strength testing. If the diagnosis of SLAP lesion is suspected, the physical examination should focus on stressing of the biceps anchor complex. The Speed test is performed with the arm elevated 90 degrees in the plane of the scapula, the elbow fully extended, and the forearm maximally supinated.[2] A downward pressure is then placed over the forearm, and pain in the anterior shoulder represents a positive test. The Yergason test is performed with the arm in a similar position, but with the forearm pronated and the examiner holding the wrist to resist active supination. Again, a positive test is defined as pain in the anterior shoulder–bicipital groove region.

Other tests have been described to specifically evaluate for the presence of SLAP lesions. The O'Brien test (active compression test) places the arm in a forward-flexed, adducted, and internally rotated (pronated) position (Fig. 18–1).[26] Downward pressure placed on the forearm by the examiner reproduces pain in the shoulder. Care must be taken to differentiate anterior shoulder pain, which may represent acromioclavicular joint pathology, and central shoulder pain, which is more consistent with a SLAP lesion. The forearm is then supinated, and downward pressure is reapplied to it. In this position, the pain in the shoulder should be reduced or eliminated.

The load-compression test places the arm in 90 degrees of abduction with the elbow flexed 90 degrees.[24] An axial load is applied to the shoulder while performing internal and external rotation. Reproduction of a painful clicking or popping in the shoulder is considered a positive test. Finally, the pain provocative test is performed with the patient in a sitting position, the arm abducted to 90 degrees, and the elbow flexed to 90 degrees.[22] The examiner then applies an external rotation force with the forearm in a pronated and then supinated position. Pain that is worse in a pronated position is consistent with a SLAP lesion.

Unfortunately, no single test can reliably establish the presence or absence of a SLAP lesion. Instead, one must use a combination of history and overall physical examination findings, along with a high clinical suspicion, to establish the diagnosis of a SLAP lesion. If a SLAP lesion is suspected, surgical arthroscopy is the gold standard for establishing a definitive diagnosis.

Imaging

Radiographic evaluation of a patient with shoulder pain should begin with plain radiographs, including an anteroposterior, scapular Y, and axillary lateral view. Additional films to evaluate for specific pathology, such as a Zanca or supraspinatus outlet view, may also be necessary. In patients with SLAP lesions, plain radiographs are usually normal. However, they can be very important in ruling out alternative diagnoses.

Currently, magnetic resonance imaging (MRI), with or without contrast arthrography, is recommended to evaluate for the presence of SLAP tears (Fig. 18–2). The majority of studies demonstrate about 90% sensitivity and specificity for the diagnosis of SLAP tears.[7,14,20,27] It is important, however, that the radiologist be familiar with the anatomy of the shoulder and its appearance on MRI. The surgeon should also make the radiologist aware of his or her level of suspicion of a SLAP tear. With the high degree of diagnostic accuracy achieved with plain MRI, use of contrast is generally not necessary.

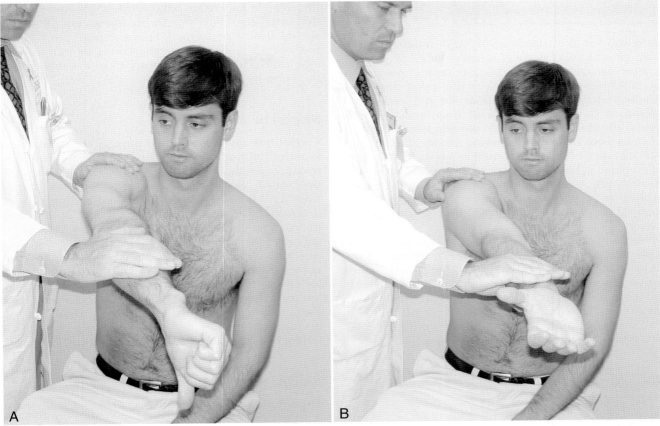

Figure 18–1   Active compression test. Deep anterior pain elicited with resisted downward force on the adducted, 90-degree forward elevated, and fully internally rotated arm *(A)* that is relieved with external rotation *(B)* is consistent with a **SLAP** tear. (From Miller MD, Cooper DE, Warner JJP: Review of Sports Medicine and Arthroscopy, 2nd ed. Philadelphia, WB Saunders, 2002, p 162.)

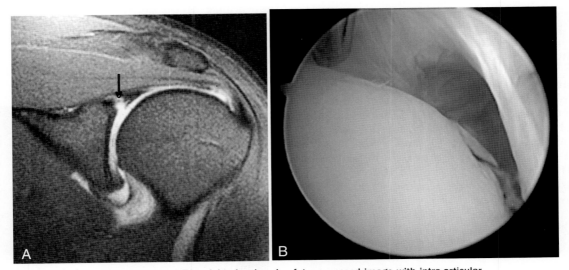

Figure 18–2   *A,* Oblique coronal, T1-weighted, spin-echo, fat-suppressed image with intra-articular administration of gadolinium demonstrates a type II SLAP lesion *(arrow)*. *B,* Arthroscopic view demonstrates detachment of the anterosuperior labrum and biceps anchor. (From Miller MD, Cooper DE, Warner JJP: Review of Sports Medicine and Arthroscopy, 2nd ed. Philadelphia, WB Saunders, 2002, p 199.)

Indications and Contraindications

Indications for the treatment of SLAP lesions include persistent symptoms despite adequate attempts at conservative management.[12,24,31] It is important to note again that SLAP lesions often coexist with other forms of pathology. Although SLAP lesions do not commonly respond to conservative forms of treatment, rest and physical therapy may help decrease symptoms. Physical therapy is directed toward achieving and maintaining full shoulder range of motion, strengthening the rotator cuff and scapular stabilizers, and treating other pathology. In patients with persistent symptoms despite adequate attempts at conservative management, arthroscopy is beneficial as both a diagnostic and a therapeutic modality.

Contraindications for the surgical treatment of SLAP lesions are fairly limited. Absolute contraindications include patients who are high-risk surgical candidates because of secondary medical conditions and those with local skin conditions or remote infections that could seed the joint. Relative contraindications include patients who are minimally symptomatic or those with incidental labral pathology found on imaging studies.

Surgical Technique

Positioning

Before induction of anesthesia, patients may receive an interscalene block to help with postoperative pain management. Patients are then anesthetized and placed in a sitting position to perform a thorough examination under anesthesia, as described later. The procedure itself can be performed in either the beach chair or the lateral decubitus position with the involved shoulder up. We prefer the lateral decubitus position in cases of suspected labral pathology because of the improved exposure with joint distraction. This can be especially helpful when working with the posterior labrum.

When using the lateral position, the patient should be tilted posteriorly approximately 20 to 30 degrees to place the glenoid parallel to the floor. The arm should be positioned in about 70 degrees of abduction and 20 to 30 degrees of forward flexion to maximize intra-articular visibility. Traction should be limited to 10 to 15 pounds to minimize the risk of postoperative brachial plexus neuropathy.[18,19] The beach chair position is described in Chapter 8, and no specific modifications are necessary for the treatment of SLAP lesions.

Examination under Anesthesia

Before diagnostic arthroscopy, a thorough examination under anesthesia is performed. The range of motion of the shoulder is assessed and recorded, paying specific attention to internal and external rotation with the arm in 90 degrees of abduction and external rotation with the arm at the side. Recently, much attention has focused on the possible association between SLAP lesions and shoulder instability,[10,17,18,23,26,30] so an assessment of stability should also be performed. Humeral head translation in the anterior and posterior directions, as well as sulcus sign testing, is performed, recorded, and compared with the opposite shoulder.

Diagnostic Arthroscopy

The arthroscope is introduced through the standard posterior portal, and the anterior portal is established. A systematic examination of the entire shoulder joint is then performed. Secondary pathology commonly coexists with SLAP lesions, and this should be identified before determining a specific treatment protocol. Specific areas to examine include the rotator cuff for evidence of partial and complete tears, as well as the rotator interval. Attention should also be focused on the anterior and posterior labrum below the level of the glenoid equator for evidence of detachment or fraying. Finally, the glenohumeral ligaments are examined for evidence of tears. Examination of the subacromial space should also be performed in selected patients with symptoms of impingement or acromioclavicular joint pathology.

Specific Surgical Steps

The surgical approach to the treatment of SLAP lesions is dependent on the tear pattern and classification.[4,12,24,28] The surgical steps are therefore presented based on the classification system proposed by Snyder et al.[28]

Type I

Type I tears involve a simple degenerative or frayed appearance of the superior labrum (Fig. 18–3). The biceps tendon anchor and the peripheral attachment of the superior labrum to the glenoid rim remain firmly

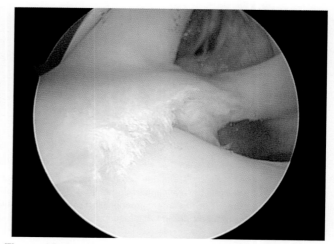

Figure 18–3 Arthroscopic view of a type I SLAP lesion. (From Gartsman GM: Shoulder Arthroscopy. Philadelphia, WB Saunders, 1993, p 120.)

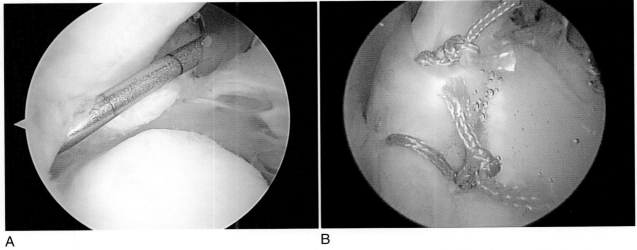

Figure 18–4 Arthroscopic view of a type II SLAP lesion *(A)* repaired with suture anchors *(B)*. (From Gartsman GM: Shoulder Arthroscopy. Philadelphia, WB Saunders, 1993, pp 120, 129.)

intact. Some authors debate the existence of these tears, claiming that they represent normal changes associated with the aging process.[12,21] If treatment is undertaken, simple debridement of the degenerative area is conducted using a motorized shaver. Extreme care must be taken to avoid detachment of the peripheral labrum or biceps anchor.

Type II

Type II tears are the most common type of SLAP lesion in most large series. This tear pattern results in detachment of both the superior labrum and the biceps anchor from the glenoid rim (Fig.18–4). The goal of surgical treatment is to firmly reattach the labrum–biceps anchor complex to the glenoid. Multiple techniques are currently available to perform this arthroscopic repair.[8,9,11,16,24,25,32]

The first step in assessing this type of tear is to confirm the detachment of the biceps from the glenoid. The presence of fraying on the inner portion of the labrum may be a clue to the underlying detachment. Direct examination with an arthroscopic probe should demonstrate laxity in the biceps anchor. A meniscoid-type labrum with only peripheral bony attachment may demonstrate some degree of laxity without true detachment and must be differentiated from a true SLAP lesion.[10,17] Surgical experience combined with the preoperative history, physical examination, and imaging findings can help confirm the diagnosis.

Once a type II tear has been confirmed, an accessory anterior portal is established. This portal is placed off the anterolateral edge of the acromion, just lateral to the biceps tendon, within the rotator interval. Recently, a trans–rotator cuff portal has also been described.[25] In either case, this portal is most easily created using an outside-in technique with spinal needle localization. Correct portal position is critical to the proper approach angle for suture anchor placement.

When the tear pattern extends along the posterior labrum, some authors advocate the placement of a posterior portal to perform the repair, given the difficulty of approaching the posterior glenoid at a proper angle for anchor placement from an anterior portal.[14] Most authors believe that a secure repair of the posterior labrum is absolutely necessary to eliminate anterior pseudolaxity that is present in conjunction with a posterior labral tear, demonstrated by the presence of a drive-through sign.[7,14] This laxity can lead to the development of a partial-thickness, inner-surface rotator cuff tear.[5,7,14,23] The posterolateral acromial portal (portal of Wilmington) is placed 1 cm anterior and 1 cm lateral to the posterolateral acromial angle (Fig. 18–5). The localization needle should then be directed toward the coracoid anteriorly. The goal is to allow placement of the anchor at a 45-degree angle to the glenoid surface.

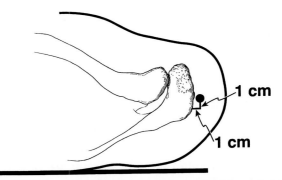

Figure 18–5 Position of the posterolateral acromial portal used to approach posterior type II SLAP lesions. It is located 1 cm lateral and 1 cm anterior to the posterior acromial angle. (From Burkhart SS, Morgan C: SLAP lesions in the overhead athlete. Orthop Clin North Am 32:431-441, 2001.)

Once the portals have been established, the superior glenoid and labrum are debrided using a 4.5-mm motorized shaver. This allows improved visualization of the glenoid rim for anchor placement. The bony bed is then further debrided manually with an arthroscopic rasp or with a power bur to provide a bleeding surface for healing. At this point, a suture anchor should be selected for use in the repair. Many anchor types are available commercially, including nonabsorbable anchors that are single- and double-loaded with suture (Fig.18–6) and absorbable anchors.

In this technique, a double-loaded suture anchor is used. A pilot hole is made for the anchor placement, proceeding percutaneously through the rotator cuff at an angle determined by targeting with an 18-gauge spinal needle. Alternatively, the hole can be placed directly through the anterior portal if the positioning is appropriate. This hole should be placed at the superior margin of the articular surface at the base of the biceps tendon. Care should be taken to achieve the proper angle of insertion to ensure stable bony purchase without disrupting the overlying cartilage surface. The anchor is then placed and seated to the appropriate depth. Depending on the system, a mark on the inserter may be required for correct positioning of the eyelet parallel to the biceps tendon.

Next, the two sutures are brought out through the anterior or posterior portal (portal 1) using a crochet hook. It may be helpful to use different colored sutures or to mark one suture so that they can be easily distinguished for proper suture management. To avoid suture entanglement, a switching stick can be used to isolate the sutures outside of portal 1. Only one limb of one suture should remain inside the portal. At this point, a shuttle relay with a crescent tip is passed through a second anterior accessory portal (portal 2) and under the labrum just anterior to the biceps anchor complex. The shuttle suture is brought out of portal 1, where it is tied to the suture limb from the suture anchor that was within the cannula. In this manner, the shuttle suture is pulled from portal 2, pulling one limb of the suture under the torn portion of the labrum and out portal 2. The corresponding second limb of this same suture is then isolated using a crochet hook and also brought out through portal 2. At this point, both ends of one suture are exiting the cannula within portal 2 and are securely looped around the torn portion of the labrum.

The next step is to isolate the suture limb that is on the superior, nonarticular margin of the labrum to be used as the post when tying an arthroscopic knot. This can be done using a knot pusher. This step is important for two reasons. First, it allows the knot to sit on the extra-articular side of the labrum. Second, it allows the knot to push the labrum down to the bony glenoid rim. An arthroscopic knot of the surgeon's choice is then tied to secure the knot. This process is repeated to secure the second suture around the torn labrum just posterior to the biceps anchor.

At this point, the quality of the repair is assessed through the arthroscope. The repair should be probed to ensure that it is secure. If necessary, additional anchors can be used to repair tears that extend anterior or posterior to the biceps anchor. In our experience, most repairs can be completed with one or two anchors, each with two sutures.

Type III

In type III SLAP lesions, the superior labrum is torn off the glenoid rim while the biceps anchor remains well fixed. In this case, there are two options available to the surgeon. The first is a simple debridement of the torn portion of the labrum. This can be performed with a motorized shaver or manually using arthroscopic instruments. Again, if debridement is chosen, care should be taken to avoid injury to or detachment of the biceps tendon anchor. Debridement is performed until only a stable rim of labrum remains intact.

If the tear involves more than one third the width labrum, a repair of the labrum can also be performed (Fig. 18–7).[4,13,24,28] This is done in the same manner described for the repair of type II lesions. Again, when debriding the superior glenoid surface in preparation for the repair, be careful not to detach the biceps tendon anchor. Usually the repair can be performed with one anchor placed adjacent to the biceps anchor, with one suture anterior and one suture posterior to the biceps tendon. Additional anchors can be used if needed.

Type IV

Type IV tears involve a bucket handle tear of the superior labrum associated with a tear extending up the biceps tendon. There are three options when dealing with this type of tear, depending on the size of the torn fragments. If the biceps tendon tear is less than one third the width of the tendon, it can be simply debrided using a mechanical shaver. The bucket handle tear of the superior labrum can then be treated in a similar fashion as described for a type III tear and either debrided or repaired.

If the torn portion of the biceps tendon is greater than one third the width of the tendon, an attempt at repair can be made (Fig. 18–8).[4,13,24,28] This is done using a single suture or by incorporating the torn portion of the biceps into a suture anchor. The labrum is then either debrided or repaired as described earlier.

The final option for type IV tears is to cut the biceps tendon and perform a biceps tenodesis.[4,13,24,28] A new all-arthroscopic technique for biceps tenodesis has been described, but it is beyond the scope of this chapter.[13] This option should be considered in cases in which the biceps tendon is deemed irreparable or in cases of revision with persistent symptoms or repair failure. Again, the superior labrum can be debrided or repaired as necessary.

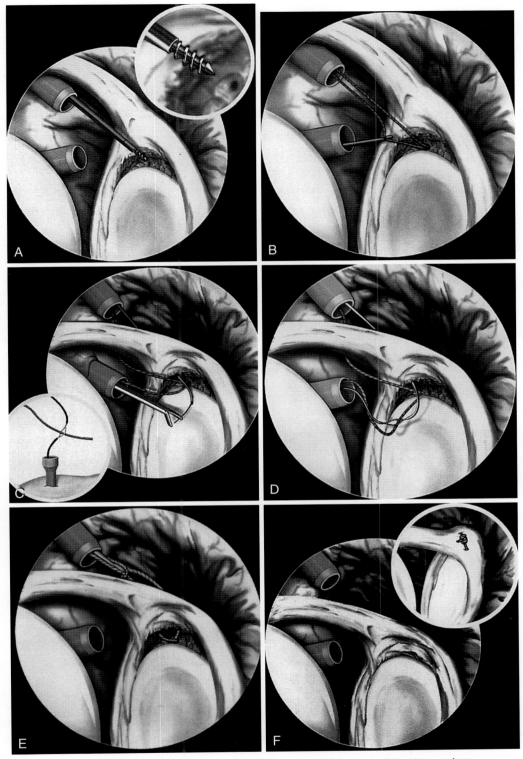

Figure 18–6   **Arthroscopic technique for the repair of type II SLAP lesions using suture anchors.**
(From Synder SJ, Banas MP, Belzer JP: Arthroscopic evaluation and treatment of injuries to the superior glenoid labrum. Instr Course Lect 45:65-70, 1996.)

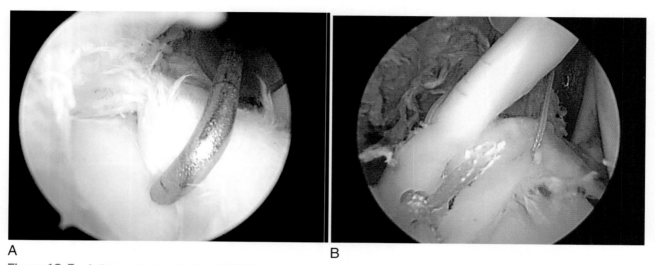

A B

Figure 18–7   Arthroscopic view of a type III SLAP lesion *(A)* repaired with suture anchors *(B)*. (From Gartsman GM: Shoulder Arthroscopy. Philadelphia, WB Saunders, 1993, pp 120, 131.)

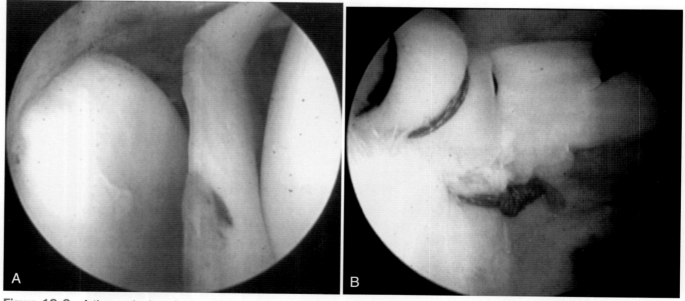

A B

Figure 18–8   Arthroscopic view of a type IV SLAP lesion *(A)* repaired with suture anchors and side-to-side repair of the biceps tendon split *(B)*. (From Miller MD, Cooper DE, Warner JJP: Review of Sports Medicine and Arthroscopy, 2nd ed. Philadelphia, WB Saunders, 2002, p 200.)

Postoperative Management

Postoperative management of repaired SLAP lesions is divided into three phases (Table 18–1). The initial phase consists of sling immobilization designed to limit swelling and inflammation. The second phase is mobilization. This phase begins with passive range of motion with the arm at the side and is slowly advanced to active range of motion with external rotation allowed in abduction. The final phase is stretching and strengthening. Stretching is performed in all directions, with an emphasis on posterior capsular stretching, and strengthening is concentrated on the rotator cuff, scapular stabilizers, and biceps muscles. Return to sports is permitted at 3 months, with overhead throwing delayed until 4 months. Patients undergoing debridement alone can resume immediate motion as tolerated.

Results

Other than the results following arthroscopic debridement, the results following superior labral repair are generally quite good, although there are few long-term follow-up studies.[28,29] Table 18–2 summarizes some of the current literature about the results of treatment of SLAP lesions.

Complications

Complications after the repair of SLAP lesions are relatively limited. Complications associated with shoulder arthroscopy include infection and brachial plexus neuropathy secondary to traction used during lateral position procedures. The most common complication specific to SLAP lesion repair is persistent pain and possible nonhealing of the repair. In these cases, repeat arthroscopy can be performed, with another attempt at repair. In our experience, these patients also obtain reliable pain relief from biceps tenodesis.

Table 18–1 **Rehabilitation Protocol after SLAP Lesion Repair**

Phase I	
Wk 1	Sling immobilization at all times
Phase II	
Wk 2–4	Passive ROM: FF to 90 degrees, ER to 40 degrees with arm at side
	No ER with arm abducted
	Codman exercises
	Sling between exercises
Wk 3–6	Discontinue sling
	Advance passive ROM as tolerated
	Begin limited ER in abduction
	Allow active ROM and use of arm for activities of daily living
Phase III	
Wk 6–16	Begin stretching and strengthening exercises involving rotator cuff and scapulothoracic and biceps muscles
	Advance active ROM as tolerated
3 mo	Allow return to sporting activities, with the exception of overhead throwing
4 mo	Begin light overhead throwing on level surface
	Continue stretching, with emphasis on posterior capsule
7 mo	Allow return to competitive throwing

ER, external rotation; FF, forward flexion; ROM, range of motion.
From Burkhart SS, Morgan C: SLAP lesions in the overhead athlete. Orthop Clin North Am 32:431-441, 2001.

Table 18–2

Results of Arthroscopic SLAP Lesion Repair

Author (Date)	No. of Patients	Surgical Procedure	Results
Cordasco et al. (1993)[9]	27	Debridement only	89% good or excellent results at 1-yr follow-up; 63% excellent results at 2-yr follow-up; only 44% RTC at 2-yr follow-up
Field and Savoie (1993)[11]	20	Arthroscopic suture repair	Average follow-up, 21 mo Rowe scale: 100% good or excellent results ASES scores: statistically significant increase in function score, decrease in pain score
Morgan et al. (1998)[23]	102	Arthroscopic suture repair	Average follow-up, 1 yr 97% good or excellent results 4% RTC among overhead throwers
Stetson et al. (1997)[29]	130	Multiple	Average follow-up, 3.2 yr 79% good or excellent results
O'Brien et al. (2002)[25]	31 patients (type II SLAP lesion)	Arthroscopic suture repair using transrotator cuff portal	Average follow-up, 3.7 yr 71% good or excellent, 19% fair results Average postop ASES score: 87.2

ASES, American Shoulder and Elbow Society; RTC, return to competition.

References

1. Andrews JR, Carson WG, McLeod WD: Glenoid labrum tears related to the long head of the biceps. Am J Sports Med 13:337-341, 1985.
2. Bennett WF: Specificity of the Speed's test: Arthroscopic technique for evaluating the biceps tendon at the level of the bicipital groove. Arthroscopy 14:789-796, 1998.
3. Bey MJ, Elders GJ, Huston LJ, et al: The mechanism of creation of superior labrum, anterior, and posterior lesions in a dynamic biomechanical model of the shoulder: The role of inferior subluxation. J Shoulder Elbow Surg 7:397-401, 1998.
4. Buford DA, Karzel RP, Snyder SJ: SLAP lesions: History, diagnosis, treatment and results. Tech Shoulder Elbow Surg 1:202-208, 2000.
5. Burkhart SS, Morgan CD: The peel-back mechanism: Its role in producing and extending posterior SLAP type II lesions and its effect on SLAP rehabilitation. Arthroscopy 14:637-640, 1998.
6. Burkhart SS, Morgan C: SLAP lesions in the overhead athlete. Orthop Clin North Am 32:431-441, 2001.
7. Chandnani VP, Yeager TD, DeBerardino T, et al: Glenoid labral tears: Prospective evaluation with MR imaging, MR arthrography, and CT Arthrography. Am J Radiol 161:1229-1235, 1993.
8. Conway JE: Arthroscopic repair of partial-thickness rotator cuff tears and SLAP lesions in professional baseball players. Orthop Clin North Am 32:443-456, 2001.
9. Cordasco FA, Steinmann S, Flatow EL, Bigliani LU: Arthroscopic treatment of glenoid labral tears. Am J Sports Med 21:425-431, 1993.
10. Detrisac DA, Johnson LL: Arthroscopic Shoulder Anatomy: Pathologic and Surgical Implications. Thorofare, NJ, Slack, 1986.
11. Field LD, Savoie FH: Arthroscopic suture repair of superior labral detachment lesions of the shoulder. Am J Sports Med 21:783-790, 1993.
12. Gartsman GM, Hammerman MD: Superior labrum, anterior and posterior lesions: When and how to treat them. Clin Sports Med 19:115-124, 2000.
13. Gartsman GM, Hammerman SM: Arthroscopic biceps tenodesis: Operative technique. Arthroscopy 16:550-552, 2000.
14. Gusmer PB, Potter HG, Schatz JA, et al: Labral injuries: Accuracy of detection with unenhanced MR imaging of the shoulder. Radiology 200:519-524, 1996.
15. Handleburg F, Willems S, Shahabpour M, et al: SLAP lesions: A retrospective multicenter study. Arthroscopy 14:856-862, 1998.
16. Hennrikus WL, Mapes RC, Bratton MW, Lapoint JM: Lateral traction during shoulder arthroscopy: Its effect on tissue perfusion measured by pulse oximetry. Am J Sports Med 23:444, 1995.
17. Ilahi OA, Labbe MR, Cosculluela BS: Variants of the anterosuperior glenoid labrum and associated pathology. Arthroscopy 18:882-886, 2002.
18. Jobe CM: Posterior superior glenoid impingement: Expanded spectrum. Arthroscopy 11:530-537, 1995.
19. Klein AH, France JC, Mutschler TA, Fu FH: Measurement of brachial plexus strain in arthroscopy of the shoulder. Arthroscopy 3:45, 1987.
20. Liu SH, Henry MH, Nuccion S, et al: Diagnosis of glenoid labral tears: A comparison between magnetic resonance imaging and clinical examinations. Am J Sports Med 24:149-154, 1996.
21. Maffet MW, Gartsman GM, Moseley B: Superior labrum–biceps tendon complex lesions of the shoulder. Am J Sports Med 23:93-98, 1995.
22. Mimori K, Muneta T, Nakagawa T, Shinomiya K: A new pain provocation test for superior labral tears of the shoulder. Am J Sports Med 27:137-142, 1999.
23. Morgan CD, Burkhart SS, Palmeri M, Gillespie M: Type II SLAP lesions: Three subtypes and their relationships to superior instability and rotator cuff tears. Arthroscopy 14:553-565, 1998.
24. Musgrave DS, Rodosky MW: SLAP lesions: Current concepts. Am J Orthop 30:29-38, 2001.
25. O'Brien SJ, Allen AA, Coleman SH, Drakos MC: The trans–rotator cuff approach to SLAP lesions: Technical aspects for repair and a clinical follow-up of 31 patients at a minimum of 2 years. Arthroscopy 18:372-377, 2002.
26. O'Brien SJ, Pagnani MJ, Fealy S, et al: The active compression test: A new and effective test for diagnosing labral tears and acromioclavicular joint abnormality. Am J Sports Med 26:610-613, 1998.
27. Palmer WE, Brown JH, Rosenthal DI: Labral-ligamentous complex of the shoulder: Evaluation with MR arthrography. Radiology 190:645-651, 1994.
28. Snyder SJ, Karzel RP, Del Pizzo W, et al: SLAP lesions of the shoulder. Arthroscopy 6:274-279, 1990.
29. Stetson WB, Karzel RP, Bana MP, et al: Long-term clinical follow-up of 140 patients with injury to the superior glenoid labrum. Arthroscopy 13:376, 1997.
30. Walch G, Boileau J, Noel E, et al: Impingement of the deep surface of the supraspinatus tendon on the posterior superior glenoid rim: An arthroscopic study. J Shoulder Elbow Surg 1:238-243, 1992.
31. Williams MM, Karzel RP, Snyder SJ: Shoulder Injuries in the Athlete: Surgical Repair and Rehabilitation. New York, Churchill Livingstone, 1996.
32. Yoneda M, Hiroaka A, Yamamoto T, et al: Arthroscopic stapling for detached superior glenoid labrum. J Bone Joint Surg Br 73:746-750, 1991.

Arthroscopic Subacromial Decompression

Andrew S. Rokito and Laith M. Jazrawi

ARTHROSCOPIC SUBACROMIAL DECOMPRESSION IN A NUTSHELL

History:
Anterolateral shoulder pain with overhead activities; night discomfort

Physical Examination:
Pain with forward elevation to 90 degrees (Neer sign); pain worsened with internal rotation and adduction (Hawkins sign); pain relieved with subacromial lidocaine injection

Imaging:
Plain radiographs (anteroposterior, axillary, and supraspinatus outlet view to determine acromial morphology); magnetic resonance imaging to rule out concomitant rotator cuff pathology

Indications:
Persistent symptoms refractory to conservative nonoperative treatment (relative rest, physical therapy, anti-inflammatory drugs, subacromial injections)

Contraindications:
Secondary causes of "impingement syndrome" that mimic primary impingement syndrome

Surgical Technique:
Beach chair or lateral decubitus position; three-portal (posterior, lateral, anterior) arthroscopy; begin with arthroscope posterior and shaver or bur lateral; switch to cutting-block technique, with arthroscope in lateral portal and shaver or bur in posterior portal to use scapular spine as resection guide

Postoperative Management:
Sling; progressive range of motion and strengthening, with resumption of activities when near-normal strength and range of motion are achieved and pain is minimal

Results:
70% to 90% good to excellent

Complications:
Failure to diagnose correctly, inadequate subacromial decompression, excessive acromial resection and fracture

Subacromial bursitis and rotator cuff tendinitis and tears have long been implicated as causes of pain, weakness, and functional limitations about the shoulder.[9,20] Before 1972, impingement syndrome was thought to occur by contact of the lateral edge of the acromion against the rotator cuff. Surgical treatment included lateral or total acromionectomy, which substantially weakened the deltoid and provided mixed functional results. Neer[20] advanced our understanding of shoulder impingement syndrome and implicated the anterior acromion and spur as culprits in subacromial impingement syndrome. He advocated an anterior acromioplasty rather than a lateral or total acromionectomy and reported consistently improved function and decreased pain.

The arthroscopic technique for subacromial decompression was first described in 1986.[17] As the procedure was described, the scope viewed from the posterior portal and the instruments entered from the lateral approach through a midlateral subacromial portal. In 1991, the "cutting-block" technique for acromioplasty was described.[22] This technique introduces the arthroscope through the lateral portal and uses the posterior half of the acromion as a guide for resection. The advantages of both these techniques versus open subacromial decompression include reduced deltoid morbidity, ability to assess intra-articular pathology, and improved cosmesis.

History

The diagnosis of impingement syndrome is based primarily on a careful history and physical examination. Patients may be involved in repetitive overhead activities, but symptoms can also occur following a traumatic event. Typically, patients complain of pain radiating over the anterolateral shoulder and upper arm that is exacerbated with overhead activities. Prolonged symptoms may lead to the compromise of lower level activities, including toileting and hygiene. In more advanced stages, complaints include night pain and pain while lying on the affected shoulder. Patients may have already had a course of physical therapy, anti-inflammatory drugs, and subacromial steroid injections, which often provide significant symptomatic relief, at least initially.

Physical Examination

The physical examination is guided by the basic principles of observation, palpation, assessment for range of motion, and provocative testing. Patients without rotator cuff pathology rarely demonstrate significant muscle atrophy, but they may demonstrate scapulothoracic dyskinesis as the scapula moves abnormally relative to the chest wall during active forward elevation. The anterior acromion, as well as the insertion of the supraspinatus tendon, may be tender to touch. Overlapping acromioclavicular pathology must be excluded clinically by palpating the acromioclavicular joint and performing a cross-arm adduction maneuver.

Commonly, pain is reproduced with forward elevation in the scapular plane (Neer impingement sign) above 90 degrees and is made worse with adduction and internal rotation (Hawkins sign). Selective lidocaine injection into the subacromial space (impingement test) often relieves these symptoms.

It is critical to remember that there are many causes of shoulder pain that result in symptoms generated secondarily from the subacromial space, and pain relief with the impingement test is not diagnostic of secondary impingement syndrome. Nonoutlet impingement, rotator cuff tears, unstable os acromiale, abnormalities in rotation, and shoulder instability can all generate pain that appears to be "impingement" related, and symptoms generated from the subacromial space are only secondary manifestations of these conditions. Therefore, treatment based solely on symptom relief following an injection into the subacromial space may fail to address the patient's underlying condition.

Imaging

Standard radiographs, including anteroposterior, axillary, supraspinatus outlet, and acromioclavicular joint views, are routinely obtained. The anteroposterior view allows assessment of the glenohumeral joint and acromiohumeral interval. The axillary view allows for the detection of os acromiale and assessment of the anterior acromion with respect to the distal clavicle. Acromial morphology is best evaluated on the supraspinatus outlet view (Fig. 19–1). The coracoacromial arch is formed by the acromion and the coracoacromial ligament. The acromion forms the osseous roof of the arch. The coracoacromial ligament, which extends from the lateral edge of the coracoid and inserts onto the undersurface of the acromion, forms the anterior extent of the arch. Recent studies suggest that acromial morphology may be related to rotator cuff disease, and individuals with a downward-sloping or hooked acromion may be more likely to develop subacromial impingement and rotator cuff tears.[14,15,21,25,26] Some studies, however, are based primarily on cadaveric specimens, and the impact of acromion slope and shape on cuff degeneration remains unclear.[15,21,25]

The acromioclavicular joint can also be a source of symptoms in patients with impingement. The joint itself can be painful due to degenerative changes alone. Osteophytes emanating from the undersurface of the medial acromion and distal clavicle can narrow the coracoacromial arch, further contributing to the impingement process. The joint should be evaluated both on physical examination and radiographically. This joint is most readily seen by angling the x-ray beam 15 degrees cephalad and reducing the voltage of the x-ray machine.

The integrity of the rotator cuff is confirmed by magnetic resonance imaging, arthrography, or ultrasonography. Magnetic resonance imaging is currently the study of choice for evaluating the rotator cuff. It allows assessment of the quality of the rotator cuff, size of the tear, and involvement of the biceps and labrum, and it can diagnose partial rotator cuff tears. Correlation between

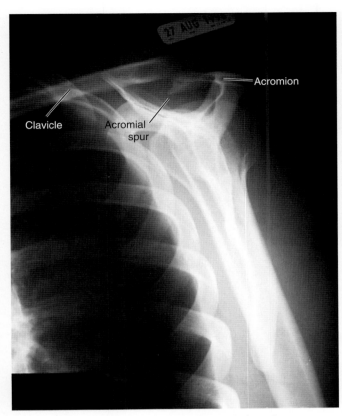

Figure 19–1   Standard outlet view demonstrating a large subacromial spur.

preoperative magnetic resonance imaging readings and intraoperative findings revealed a sensitivity of 100% and a specificity of 95% for full-thickness tears of the rotator cuff tendon.[16] Although arthrography provides accurate information regarding the existence of a cuff tear, it does not allow the assessment of partial-thickness tears, tear size, degree of retraction, and presence of muscle atrophy, nor does arthrography permit the detection of other sources of pain, including labral tears, loose bodies, and articular defects.

Ultrasonography has been shown to be useful for the identification of rotator cuff pathology.[6,8,18,19,24] The benefits of this imaging modality are that it is noninvasive and inexpensive. Unfortunately, the test is highly operator dependent, and the viewing area is constrained by the bony anatomy, limiting its usefulness. Because the acromial process cannot be penetrated, medial pathology at the joint line, such as a labral defect, is not well visualized.

Indications and Contraindications

The majority of patients with subacromial impingement can be treated successfully without surgery.[4] Nonoperative treatment involves rest from those activities that exacerbate the symptoms, stretching and strengthening exercises, nonsteroidal anti-inflammatory medications, and the judicious use of cortisone injections.[4] In general,

one to three injections over the course of 6 months to a year may be given. Indications for surgery include chronic stage II impingement, acute or chronic symptomatic full-thickness tears, and large partial-thickness (>50%) tears.

Surgical Technique

Anesthesia and Positioning

The procedure can be performed with the patient under general or regional anesthesia or a combination of both. The advantages of regional anesthesia include better postoperative pain control, the ability to begin range-of-motion exercises immediately, and the tendency for greater patient acceptance.[5,10] Ideally, shoulder arthroscopy should be performed under controlled hypotensive anesthesia.[7] The systolic blood pressure should be kept to less than 100 mm Hg whenever possible to control bleeding. This is especially critical during the subacromial decompression portion of the procedure, when visualization can be significantly compromised by bleeding.

The procedure is performed with the patient in either the beach chair or the lateral decubitus position (Fig. 19–2). Advantages of the beach chair position are relative ease of patient positioning, normal anatomic orientation of the shoulder, ability to manipulate the arm during the procedure, and lower risk of neurapraxia, which is associated with excessive traction in the lateral decubitus position. Many surgeons, however, prefer the lateral decubitus position; it is more familiar to them and allows for distraction, which facilitates work in the subacromial space.[2] With the patient in the lateral decubitus position, careful attention must be paid to protecting the bony prominences, as well as the brachial plexus and ulnar and peroneal nerves, with appropriate padding.

Examination under Anesthesia and Portal Placement

The procedure begins with a thorough, systematic examination under anesthesia. Range of motion in all planes is assessed first. Stability is then tested in the anterior, posterior, and inferior directions. If a manipulation under anesthesia is required to address any preoperative stiffness, this should be performed in a controlled, systematic fashion, always maintaining a short lever arm by grasping the humerus close to the axilla to avoid iatrogenic fracture. The shoulder is then gently manipulated in a slow, gradual fashion, assessing for audible or palpable lysis of adhesions. Manipulation is performed in all planes—elevation, abduction, adduction, and internal and external rotation—with the goal of achieving range of motion that is symmetrical with the contralateral side.

The bony landmarks and arthroscopic portals are carefully identified before beginning the procedure (Fig. 19–3) because this becomes difficult once fluid

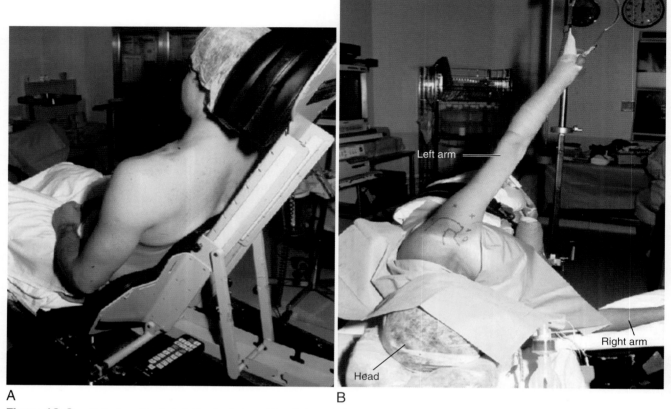

A   B

Figure 19–2 Patient positioning. *A,* Beach chair position. *B,* Lateral decubitus position. All bony prominences are well padded. The involved arm is suspended using 10 pounds of skin traction.

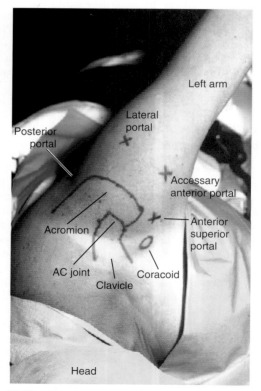

Figure 19–3 Bony landmarks, portal placement, and planned incision.

extravasation occurs. Three basic arthroscopic portals are used for this procedure. The posterior portal is located approximately 2 cm inferior and 1 cm medial to the posterolateral corner of the acromion. This portal allows adequate visualization of most of the glenohumeral joint and facilitates the placement of other portals. When establishing this portal, one hand is placed on top of the shoulder with the thumb palpating the "soft spot." The index finger of that same hand is used to palpate the coracoid process. Using a number 11 scalpel blade, a puncture is made through the skin only. The arthroscopic sheath and blunt-tipped trocar (Fig. 19–4) are then passed through the posterior deltoid and directed toward the coracoid process. The tip of the trocar is used to palpate the step-off between the posterior glenoid rim and the capsule. The sheath and trocar are then advanced between the humeral head and glenoid through the capsule. Precise placement of this portal is critical; if it is too medial or inferior, the suprascapular and axillary nerves, respectively, are at risk of injury.

The anterosuperior portal is used mainly for instrumentation. It is also used for better visualization of the posterior and anteroinferior portions of the joint when this is necessary. It is located approximately 1 cm inferior and medial to the anterolateral corner of the acromion, lateral to the coracoid process. When a distal clavicle excision is planned, it is helpful to place this portal more medially, in line with the acromioclavicular joint. The portal can be created with either an inside-out technique

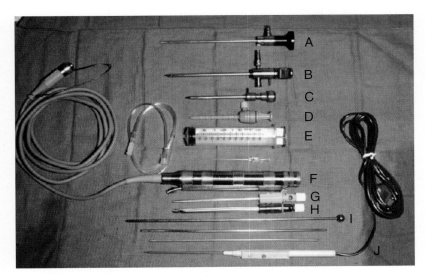

Figure 19–4 Basic instruments for shoulder arthroscopy. A, camera lens; B, arthroscopic trocar; C, arthroscopic cannula; D, disposable arthroscopic cannula; E, 60-mL syringe, flexible tubing, and 18-gauge spinal needle for joint insufflation; F, arthroscopic motorized shaver; G, arthroscopic full-radius resector; H, arthroscopic bur; I, switching sticks; J, arthroscopic Bovie.

2 Shoulder

using a Wissinger rod (i.e., switching stick) or an outside-in technique in which an 18-gauge spinal needle is used to confirm portal placement and direction.

The posterior portal, established initially for glenohumeral inspection, can also be used for initial visualization of the subacromial space. The arthroscopic sheath and trocar are simply redirected beneath the acromion. A lateral portal located 2 to 3 cm distal and parallel to the anterior margin of the acromion is used initially for instrumentation and then for visualization, as it provides an "outlet" view of the subacromial space. Excessively distal placement of this portal risks injury to the axillary nerve, which lies approximately 5 cm distal to the acromion.[6]

Diagnostic Arthroscopy

The procedure begins with a thorough, systematic arthroscopic evaluation of the glenohumeral joint. The articular surface of the rotator cuff is carefully inspected, and partial- or full-thickness tears are identified. A suture marker can be used to better assess the extent of a tear (Fig. 19–5). A monofilament suture is placed through a spinal needle passed percutaneously across the area in question. The end of the suture is then brought out through the anterosuperior portal using an arthroscopic grasping device. The suture is subsequently identified on the bursal surface of the cuff, and the questionable area is closely inspected.

Once the glenohumeral examination is completed and any associated intra-articular pathology has been addressed, attention is directed toward the subacromial space. If the patient is in the lateral decubitus position, the angle of traction is adjusted to maximize the acromiohumeral interval. This is achieved by less abduction of the arm (approximately 30 degrees) instead of the 50 to 70 degrees of abduction used with the intra-articular portion of the arthroscopy. Typically, 10 pounds of traction is sufficient. The arthroscopic sheath and trocar are directed beneath the acromion and swept laterally to clear bursal tissue and lyse adhesions. Avoidance

of the fat pad, which is located medially beneath the acromioclavicular joint, is important to prevent excessive bleeding.

Specific Surgical Steps

The subacromial space is distended, and the lateral portal is created. This portal is typically placed 2 to 3 cm distal and parallel to the anterior margin of the acromion. Placement of this portal slightly more posteriorly, in line with the posterior margin of the clavicle, may allow for better access and treatment of rotator cuff tears. A self-sealing arthroscopic cannula is used through this portal, and a motorized shaver or radiofrequency soft tissue ablation device is introduced to perform a partial bursectomy and to remove periosteum from the undersurface of the acromion.

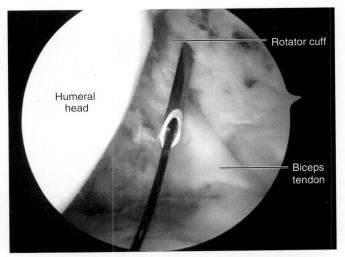

Rotator cuff

Humeral head

Biceps tendon

Figure 19–5 Suture marker technique. A monofilament suture is passed through a spinal needle placed through the area of suspected rotator cuff tear. The end of the suture is brought out through the anterior portal. The suture is subsequently identified on the bursal surface of the rotator cuffs.

The medial and lateral extents of the acromion are identified, along with the coracoacromial ligament. Using either an electrocautery or a radiofrequency device, the ligament is released from the undersurface of the acromion until the subdeltoid fascia is seen, avoiding injury to the overlying muscle. If the acromial branch of the thoracoacromial artery, which is located along the superomedial aspect of the coracoacromial ligament, is encountered, it should be cauterized to avoid excessive bleeding.

The acromioplasty is then performed using an arthroscopic bur. The anteroinferior acromion is approached first (Fig. 19–6). While viewing from the posterior portal, the bur is used to remove 5 to 8 mm of the inferior surface of the acromion, beginning at the anterolateral corner and proceeding medially. Additionally, the acromial osteophyte projecting anterior to the leading edge of the clavicle is removed.

The athroscope and bur are then interchanged to perform the posterior acromion resection (Fig. 19–7). This is done using a cutting-block technique.[22] While viewing from the lateral portal, the thickness and shape of the acromial arch are assessed. It is important to place the bur just underneath and parallel to the undersurface of the acromion. The spine of the scapula is used as a cutting block, and the bur is used to plane the undersurface of the acromion. Beginning at the low point of the acromion, the bur is swept from medial to lateral, proceeding to the anterior resection. This technique allows for the reproducible creation of a smooth, flat resection line. The resection should be assessed from both the lateral and posterior portals (Fig. 19–8). Final smoothing can be performed with an arthroscopic rasp if desired.

The acromioclavicular joint is left undisturbed unless there is pathology that warrants correction.

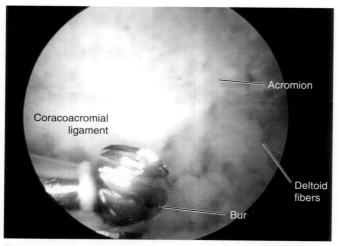

Figure 19–6 Anterior acromion resection. While viewing from the posterior portal, the bur is used to resect the anteroinferior aspect of the acromion.

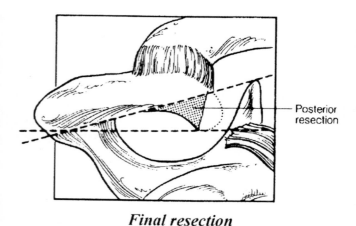

Final resection

Figure 19–7 Posterior acromion resection. While viewing from the lateral portal, the bur is used to plane the undersurface of the acromion, using the spine of the scapula as a cutting block.

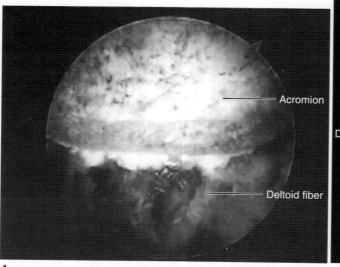

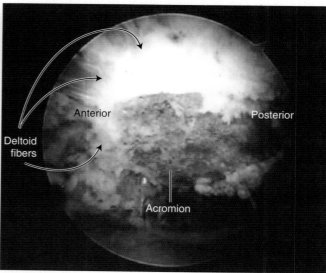

A   B

Figure 19–8 Final resection viewed from posterior (A) and lateral (B) portals.

This includes symptomatic acromioclavicular joint arthritis and inferior-projecting osteophytes contributing to impingement. The acromioclavicular joint is exposed by resecting the inferior capsule. The bur is then used to resect osteophytes emanating from the distal clavicle and medial acromion. The distal 7 to 10 mm of distal clavicle can be resected if clinically indicated. This is best accomplished with the arthroscope placed laterally and the bur anteriorly through an ancillary portal created in line with the acromioclavicular joint.

Once the acromioclavicular joint has been addressed, a rotator cuff tear, if present, can be dealt with. Tear size, morphology, and mobility are assessed through both the posterior and anterior portals. A traction suture or arthroscopic grasper can be used to assess the mobility of the tear. If desired, a soft tissue elevator can be used to release articular and bursa-sided adhesions. The tear is then repaired using a mini-open or all-arthroscopic technique.

Pearls and Pitfalls

1. Use controlled hypotensive anesthesia (systolic blood pressure <100 mm Hg).
2. Use appropriate padding of bony prominences, brachial plexus, and peroneal and ulnar nerves when employing the lateral decubitus position.
3. The trocar of the arthroscope is used to palpate the step-off between the posterior glenoid and the capsule before placement into the joint.
4. When a distal clavicle excision is planned, place the anterosuperior portal more medially, in line with the acromioclavicular joint. This allows the placement of instruments parallel to the distal clavicle.
5. The arthroscopic sheath and blunt-tipped trocar can be used to clear the subacromial space before placement of the arthroscope. A gentle sweeping motion helps clear the space of the often thickened bursal tissue, creating a window for initial visualization.
6. If a rotator cuff tear is present, the lateral working portal for the subacromial space should be placed slightly posterior to the anterior edge of the acromion. This permits better access to the tear.
7. A suture marker can be used to more closely inspect a specific region of the rotator cuff on both the articular and bursal surfaces.
8. When working in the subacromial space, avoidance of the fat pad, located medially beneath the acromioclavicular joint, is important to prevent excessive bleeding.
9. When using the cutting-block technique, it is important to place the bur parallel to and directly underneath the acromion. The bur is then swept along the undersurface of the acromion, being careful not to lever the hand. This creates a smooth, flat surface.
10. It is important not to disturb and potentially destabilize the acromioclavicular joint when performing an isolated acromioplasty. If, however, there are large osteophytes emanating from the undersurface of the acromion, these should be resected. The surgeon

may decide to perform a formal distal clavicle resection, if clinically indicated.

Postoperative Management

Physical therapy initially consists of range-of-motion exercises—passive, active, and assisted—with the goal of achieving full range of motion within 4 to 6 weeks following surgery. The type of physical therapy is based on the strength of the rotator cuff repair, tear size, and tissue quality. Classically, 6 weeks of passive motion, followed by an additional 4 to 6 weeks of active assisted motion, was used for all repair types. Today, however, physical therapy is usually individualized, with the early institution of active assisted motion depending on tear size, strength of repair, and tissue quality. Rotator cuff strengthening exercises are usually delayed until range of motion has been restored. Stretching exercises are continued throughout the strengthening phase of rehabilitation. Patients are usually able to resume heavy manual labor and sports participation at approximately 8 to 12 months following surgery.

Results

In general, arthroscopic subacromial decompression yields satisfactory results in patients with chronic stage II or III impingement. Since its introduction by Ellman in 1985,[11] several authors have documented successful outcomes with this procedure.[22-26] In 1991, Ellman and Kay[11] reported the results in 50 consecutive patients who underwent arthroscopic acromioplasty. An 88% satisfaction rate (excellent or good results) was found with follow-up of 1 to 3 years. Other investigators subsequently reported similar findings, with better results noted for patients without rotator cuff tears. Esch[12] reported 78% objective and 82% subjective success rates for patients undergoing arthroscopic subacromial decompression. Speer et al.[23] reported 88% good or excellent results following arthroscopic subacromial decompression in patients without rotator cuff tears. Similarly, Gartsman[13] found 88% satisfactory results in patients with intact rotator cuffs and 83% satisfactory results in patients with partial-thickness tears. Altchek and Carson[1] reported 73% excellent or good results in 40 patients who underwent arthroscopic acromioplasty.

Complications

In general, complications associated with arthroscopic subacromial decompression are relatively uncommon. The overall rate of infection is low and is no higher than that reported for other types of arthroscopic procedures. Neurovascular injury from aberrant portal placement is a rare occurrence. This can be avoided by marking the bony prominences at the start of the procedure before there is significant fluid extravasation, making their identification more difficult.

Error in diagnosis is probably the most common cause of persistent pain following this procedure. Conditions such as glenohumeral arthritis, acromioclavicular arthritis, labral tears, lesions of the biceps tendon, and subtle instability can result in continued shoulder pain if left untreated. A careful, detailed history and physical examination and appropriate diagnostic studies will minimize failure due to misdiagnosis.

Persistent pain can also result from insufficient supraspinatus outlet decompression. Retained bursal tissue can act as a space-occupying lesion, compromising the subacromial space. Incomplete release of the coracoacromial ligament can result in continued impingement. The ligament should be released from the entire undersurface of the acromion until the deltoid fascia is visualized. Surgical failure can also result from inadequate bone resection. Before completion of the procedure, the acromion should be viewed from both the posterior and lateral portals to ensure adequate bone resection.

Acromioclavicular joint osteophytes can cause persistent pain from impingement if they are not resected. This should be carried out carefully so as not to destabilize the joint.[3] Extensive capsular disruption has been associated with persistent acromioclavicular joint pain. A formal distal clavicle resection is reserved for those patients whose preoperative evaluation indicates pain emanating from this joint.

A rotator cuff defect, either partial or full thickness, can also cause continued pain following subacromial decompression. Extensive partial-thickness (>50%) and full-thickness tears should be repaired to avoid continued pain despite satisfactory decompression.

Conclusion

Impingement syndrome is a common source of pain and disability, and most patients can be treated effectively without surgery. Activity modification, physical therapy, anti-inflammatory drugs, and steroid injections are usually successful in resolving symptoms. When nonoperative treatment fails, arthroscopy and subacromial decompression are generally successful. It is critical to make the correct diagnosis, because several conditions can mimic the signs and symptoms of impingement syndrome. With postoperative physical therapy, a gradual return to activities as tolerated is the predictable outcome following an accurate diagnosis and a technically well-performed arthroscopic subacromial decompression.

References

1. Altchek DW, Carson EW: Arthroscopic acromioplasty: Current status. Orthop Clin North Am 28:157-168, 1997.
2. Baechler MF, Kim DH: Patient positioning for shoulder arthroscopy based on variability in lateral acromion morphology. Arthroscopy 18:547-549, 2002.
3. Barber FA: Coplaning of the acromioclavicular joint. Arthroscopy 17:913-917, 2001.
4. Blair B, Rokito AS, Cuomo F, et al: Efficacy of injections of corticosteroids for subacromial impingement syndrome. J Bone Joint Surg 78:1685-1689, 1996.
5. Brown AR, Weiss R, Greenberg C, et al: Interscalene block for shoulder arthroscopy: Comparison with general anesthesia. Arthroscopy 9:295-300, 1993.
6. Bryan WJ, Schauder K, Tullos HS: The axillary nerve and its relationship to common sports medicine shoulder procedures. Am J Sports Med 14:113-116, 1986.
7. Burkhart SS, Danaceau SM, Anthanasiou KA: Turbulence control as a factor in improving visualization during subacromial shoulder arthroscopy. Arthroscopy 17:209-212, 2001.
8. Chang CY, Wang SF, Chiou HJ, et al: Comparison of shoulder ultrasound and MR imaging in diagnosing full-thickness rotator cuff tears. Clin Imaging 26:50-54, 2002
9. Cofield RH: Rotator cuff disease of the shoulder. J Bone Joint Surg Am 67:974, 1985.
10. D'Alessio JG, Rosenblum M, Shea KP, Freitas DG: A retrospective comparison of interscalene block and general anesthesia for ambulatory shoulder arthroscopy. Reg Anesth 20:62-68, 1995.
11. Ellman H, Kay SP: Arthroscopic subacromial decompression for chronic impingement: Two- to five-year results. J Bone Joint Surg Br 73:395-398, 1991.
12. Esch JC: Arthroscopic subacromial decompression and postoperative management. Orthop Clin North Am 24:161-171, 1993.
13. Gartsman GM: Arthroscopic acromioplasty for lesions of the rotator cuff. J Bone Joint Surg Am 72:169-180, 1990.
14. Gill TJ, McIrvin E, Kocher MS, et al: The relative importance of acromial morphology and age with respect to rotator cuff pathology. J Shoulder Elbow Surg 11:327-330, 2002.
15. Gohlke F, Barthel T, Gandorfer A: The influence of variations of the coracoacromial arch on the development of rotator cuff tears. Arthroscopy 12:531-540, 1996.
16. Iannotti JP, Zlatkin MB, Esterhai JL, et al: Magnetic resonance imaging of the shoulder: Sensitivity, specificity, and predictive value. J Bone Joint Surg Am 73:17, 1991.
17. Johnson LL: Shoulder arthroscopy. In Johnson LL (ed): Arthroscopic Surgery: Principles and Practice. St. Louis, CV Mosby, 1986, pp 1371-1379.
18. Martin-Hervas C, Romero J, Navas-Acien A, et al: Ultrasonographic and magnetic resonance images of rotator cuff lesions compared with arthroscopy or open surgery findings. J Shoulder Elbow Surg 10:410-415, 2001.
19. Middleton WD, Reinus WR, Totty WG, et al: Ultrasonographic evaluation of the rotator cuff and biceps tendon. J Bone Joint Surg 68:440-450, 1986.
20. Neer CS II: Anterior acromioplasty for the chronic impingement syndrome in the shoulder: A preliminary report. J Bone Joint Surg Am 54:41, 1972.
21. Panni AS, Milano G, Lucania L, et al: Histological analysis of the coracoacromial arch: Correlation between age-related changes and rotator cuff tears. Arthroscopy 12:531-540, 1996.
22. Sampson TG, Nisber JK, Glick JM: Precision acromioplasty in arthroscopic subacromial decompression of the shoulder. Arthroscopy 7:301-307, 1991.
23. Speer KP, Lohnes J, Garrett WE Jr: Arthroscopic subacromial decompression: Results in advanced impingement syndrome. Arthroscopy 7:291-296, 1991.
24. Teefey SA, Hasan SA, Middleton WD, et al: Ultrasonography of the rotator cuff: A comparison of ultrasonographic and arthroscopic findings in one hundred consecutive cases. J Bone Joint Surg 82:498-504, 2000.
25. Toivonen DA, Tuite MJ, Orwin JF: Acromial structure and tears of the rotator cuff. J Shoulder Elbow Surg 4:376, 1995.
26. Wang JC, Shapiro MS: Changes in acromial morphology with age. J Shoulder Elbow Surg 6:55-59, 1997.

Acromioclavicular Joint Pathology

Gordon W. Nuber and David C. Flanigan

ACROMIOCLAVICULAR JOINT PATHOLOGY IN A NUTSHELL

History:
Direct trauma; pain and swelling over acromioclavicular (AC) joint

Physical Examination:
Tenderness to palpation over AC joint; positive cross-arm adduction, relieved with lidocaine injection into AC joint

Imaging:
Plain radiographs, including Zanca view with 15-degree cephalad orientation and reduction in power

Indications:
Persistent symptoms limiting activities and function

Contraindications:
Asymptomatic degenerative change or AC separation

Surgical Technique:
Positioning: beach chair or lateral decubitus
Arthroscopic portals: posterior, anterior, lateral, accessory
Arthroscopic procedure: subacromial decompression for visualization as needed; medial acromial resection; lateral clavicle excision, avoiding over- or underexcision

Postoperative Management:
Sling, immediate range of motion, rapid advance in strengthening, and return to sports following AC resection

Complications:
Under-resection, over-resection, instability, persistent pain

Injuries and degenerative conditions of the acromioclavicular (AC) joint that affect shoulder function are quite common. Most AC pathology is related to direct trauma, such as a fall onto the shoulder, or to repetitive use, such as weightlifting. Degenerative changes at the AC joint can lead to spur formation and secondary impingement of the rotator cuff. Most conditions affecting the AC joint can be treated conservatively, but chronic conditions that affect shoulder function, such as degenerative arthritis or osteolysis of the distal clavicle, may require operative treatment to eliminate pain and restore function. This chapter focuses on the pathomechanics of injury to the AC joint, along with the principles of diagnosis, the steps in treatment decision making, and the technical aspects of treating degenerative arthritis and osteolysis of the clavicle.

Anatomy

The AC joint is a diarthrodial joint formed by the distal clavicle and the medial facet of the acromion. The articular surface is covered by hyaline cartilage. The clavicle, along with the sternoclavicular and AC joints, forms the only bony connection between the upper extremity and the axial skeleton. Inclination of the AC joint is variable in both the sagittal and coronal planes. Interposed between the ends of the clavicle and the acromion is a cartilaginous disk of varying size and shape.[32] Disk degeneration is a natural process that occurs with age and may be present as early as the second decade of life.[13]

The AC joint is supported by a capsule reinforced by superior and inferior as well as anterior and posterior ligaments. The superior ligament is quite robust and is reinforced by attachments of fibers from the deltoid and trapezial fascia. The inferior AC ligament blends with fibers from the coracoacromial ligament. This AC ligament complex plays an important role in maintaining stability, primarily horizontal joint stability.[12,40] Anterior translation is restrained primarily by the inferior AC ligament.[24] Posterior translation is primarily a function of the superior and posterior ligaments.[21] The coracoclavicular ligaments comprise the trapezoid and the more medial conoid ligaments. They pass from the base of the coracoid to the inferior surface of the clavicle. These strong ligaments provide primarily vertical stability. Transection of the AC ligaments results in significant translation in the anteroposterior direction but not in the superior plane.[12] After injury to the AC ligaments, the coracoclavicular ligaments partially compensate for the injured capsule in restraining these forces, but their vertical orientation does not allow them to be an effective restraint to anteroposterior translation. This information implies that surgical reconstructions need to address both groups of ligaments.

The clavicle rotates as much as 45 degrees about its axis with arm motion. Most of this rotation occurs at the sternoclavicular joint. Motion at the AC joint is limited to 5 to 8 degrees owing to synchronous scapuloclavicular motion in which the scapula and clavicle move as a unit.[31]

Mechanism of Injury

Injury to the AC joint is the result of a combination of factors. First, its subcutaneous location makes it prone to injury due to direct or, infrequently, indirect trauma. Second, as a diarthrodial joint, it is predisposed to the same conditions affecting any joint in the body—degenerative conditions, infection, inflammatory arthritis, and crystalline disease. Third, because it is a small joint and must transmit the significant forces of the entire upper extremity across it, it is prone to changes related to repetitive stress.[11,34] Today's emphasis on athletic activity and weight training makes this joint particularly vulnerable to pathologic change.

Traumatic Injury

Most AC injuries are sustained as a result of direct trauma. Usually, the joint is injured by impact to the acromion with the arm in an adducted position, such as when falling off a bicycle or being run into the boards during an ice hockey match. The substantial stability of the sternoclavicular joint transmits the energy to the clavicle, coracoclavicular ligaments, and AC joint. The magnitude of the force determines the severity of the injury. Typically, the force is first transmitted to the AC joint, injuring the AC ligaments. If sufficient force is generated, the coracoclavicular ligaments and the deltotrapezial fascia are secondarily injured. Fractures of the distal clavicle may be associated with coracoclavicular ligament disruption.

Indirect trauma is a less common mechanism of injury. A fall onto the elbow or extended arm may transmit forces cephalad through the humerus up to the acromion. Injury is primarily to the AC ligaments, as the coracoclavicular ligaments are compressed via this mechanism of action.

Post-traumatic arthritic conditions are common after AC joint injuries owing to the frequency of injury to this joint. Studies have shown the late development of degenerative changes, particularly after grade I and II sprains of the AC joint.[5,38] Operative procedures that transfix the joint to preserve stability are more likely to result in degenerative conditions than are those that sacrifice the joint. Arthroscopic or open subacromial decompression and coplaning of the undersurface of the clavicle to eliminate spurs that impinge on the rotator cuff have not been associated with a greater incidence of postoperative degenerative changes and a subsequent increase of symptoms.[4,22]

Nontraumatic Conditions

Primary osteoarthritis of the shoulder is a relatively uncommon disorder. Primary involvement of the AC joint is more common than is degenerative arthritis of the glenohumeral joint. DePalma et al.[14] observed degenerative conditions in most AC joint specimens by the fourth decade of life. Others have noted similar findings, even in individuals who do not report a history of trauma or are asymptomatic.[8,35,36] Patients who are symptomatic from degenerative changes at the AC joint may localize pain and deformity to the joint or experience rotator cuff pathology due to secondary impingement in the subacromial space through inferior spur formation.[10]

Infection, crystalline disease, and inflammatory conditions of the AC joint are even more uncommon.

Repetitive Stress

Microtraumatic osteolysis of the distal clavicle is reported more frequently secondary to repetitive stressful activity, leading to subchondral stress fractures followed by a hypervascular response.[2,11,46] This entity is commonly found in weightlifters and is thought to be increasing owing to the popularity of weight training and its emphasis in fitness programs. Repetitive stresses to the subchondral bone are believed to lead to fatigue fractures, which initiate resorption of bone. Demineralization, subchondral cysts, osteopenia, and distal clavicle erosion ensue.[26,34]

History

Osteoarthritis is the most common cause in patients presenting with AC joint pain. The patient may have isolated symptoms localizing to the AC joint or may present with symptoms in conjunction with associated pathologic conditions, most notably, rotator cuff impingement. The pain may localize to the top of the shoulder, specifically to the AC joint, or to the anterolateral neck and upper arm. Injections of a hypertonic saline solution into the AC joint of volunteers produced pain over the joint itself and in the anterolateral neck, trapezius-supraspinatus region, and anterolateral deltoid. No pain was noted at the posterior aspect of the shoulder.[19] Pain may occur with daily activities and is usually most pronounced with cross-body adduction maneuvers. If there is associated rotator cuff pathology, typical impingement symptoms occur with overhead positions and abduction. Athletes involved in athletic training (typically, weightlifting) complain of pain with the bench press, incline press, and pushups.

Prominence of the AC joint compared with the asymptomatic side, along with an associated popping or grinding sensation, may be elicited. A prior history of trauma is important to determine any instability of the AC joint that may complicate treatment.

Injury to the AC joint should be suspected in anyone with pain after a traumatic event. Bike riders falling and landing directly on the top of the shoulder should arouse suspicion of an AC joint injury. Presence of an abrasion over the AC joint or localized prominence and pain should lead to further assessment.

Physical Examination

Inspection may reveal prominence of the end of the clavicle in relationship to the other AC joint. In acute traumatic injuries, displacement of the clavicle may also occur inferiorly or posteriorly, and evidence of a skin abrasion or contusion over the AC joint is likely. Motion of the arm and shoulder is likely to be restricted in the acutely injured. The AC joint is tender, and detection of instability is difficult because of splinting related to pain.

In patients who present without a history of trauma or with older injuries, inspection may reveal asymmetry or prominence of the joint. There is asymmetrical point tenderness over the AC joint, which is accentuated with forced cross-body adduction. Motion of the shoulder is seldom restricted. Assessment of instability of the distal clavicle is undertaken by grasping the clavicle between the thumb and forefinger while translating anteroposter-

iorly and superoinferiorly, with the other hand stabilizing the acromion. Crepitation of the joint may be felt with stability assessment or cross-body adduction. Tests for subacromial impingement should be undertaken to elicit rotator cuff involvement. If injection of lidocaine into the AC joint relieves symptoms, this confirms that the joint is the cause of the symptoms.

Imaging

Anatomy of the AC joint is frequently hard to evaluate on standard anteroposterior views of the shoulder due to overpenetration of the bony anatomy and overlap of the scapular spine. Zanca[45] described a modified anteroposterior examination angled 15 degrees cephalad that provides a clear and unobstructed view of the distal clavicle and AC joint. Reducing the voltage by half allows one to readily visualize the AC joint and judge intra-articular pathology and displacement. Patients with degenerative changes of the AC joint display joint narrowing, sclerosis, and osteophyte and cyst formation (Fig. 20–1). The hallmark of osteolysis of the distal clavicle is osteopenia, widening of the joint space, and actual loss of bony detail of the distal clavicle.

Axillary views of the shoulder are helpful to evaluate displacement of the distal clavicle posteriorly or intra-articular fractures. They are also beneficial in evaluating the adequacy of distal clavicle resection postoperatively. An axillary view is useful for evaluating the presence of an os acromion.

Outlet views of the shoulder with the beam of the x-ray shot down the scapular spine and angled 10 degrees caudad are excellent for imaging impingement. These views show acromial morphology along with compromise

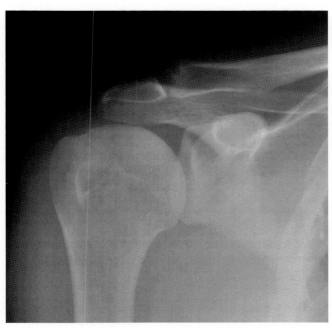

Figure 20–1   Radiograph of acromioclavicular joint demonstrating degenerative arthritis.

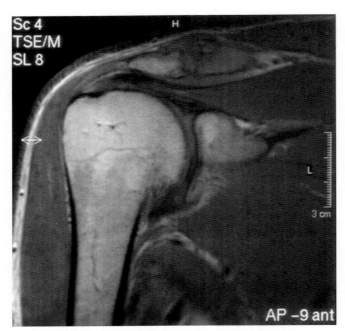

Figure 20–2 Magnetic resonance imaging scan of affected acromioclavicular joint showing degenerative changes.

of the subacromial outlet by clavicular spurs in individuals with clinical overlap of impingement and AC joint pathology.

Although weighted or stress views are still commonly ordered in emergency rooms, they are of little utility because we no longer make a distinction between the treatment of grade II and III sprains of the AC joint.[44]

Magnetic resonance imaging is very sensitive in detecting degenerative conditions of the AC joint, but these changes do not always correlate with symptoms (Fig. 20–2).[28] Magnetic resonance imaging is an excellent means of evaluating the rotator cuff and impingement symptoms and determining whether osteophytes from the AC joint may be a source of these symptoms. As a means of assessing isolated AC joint symptoms, however, this modality may be of little use. The presence of edema in the distal clavicle may have a correlation with symptoms. Bone scans are a sensitive test to show early degenerative changes or osteolysis of the AC joint not seen on routine radiologic studies, but they are too costly and impractical to use for the assessment of symptomatic joints.[11]

Classification of Traumatic Acromioclavicular Joint Injuries

Traumatic AC injuries are classified on the basis of the history and physical examination, along with the results of the radiologic examination. Injury types are based on the degree of injury to the AC ligaments, coracoclavicular ligaments, and deltotrapezial fascia. Allman[1] and Tossy et al.[39] described a three-type classification that

was later expanded to six types by Rockwood and Young[31]:

Type 1
    Sprain of AC ligament only
    No displacement
Type 2
    AC ligaments and joint capsule disrupted
    Coracoclavicular ligaments intact
    ≤50% vertical subluxation of clavicle
Type 3
    AC ligaments and capsule disrupted
    Coracoclavicular ligaments disrupted
    AC joint dislocated, with clavicle displaced superiorly and complete loss of contact between clavicle and acromion
Type 4
    AC ligaments and capsule disrupted
    Coracoclavicular ligaments disrupted
    AC joint dislocated, with clavicle displaced posteriorly into or through trapezius muscle
    Displacement confirmed on axillary radiograph
Type 5
    AC ligaments and capsule disrupted
    Coracoclavicular ligaments disrupted
    AC joint dislocated, with extreme superior elevation of clavicle (100% to 300% of normal)
    Complete detachment of deltoid and trapezius from distal clavicle
Type 6
    AC ligaments disrupted
    Coracoclavicular ligaments disrupted
    AC joint dislocated, with clavicle displaced inferior to acromion and coracoid process

Differential Diagnosis

The differential diagnosis of chronic AC joint problems includes a number of conditions specific to the AC joint and some that refer pain to the area, such as rotator cuff impingement or radicular pain from the cervical spine. The most common condition encountered is rotator cuff impingement. Because of the proximity of the AC joint and the likelihood that enlargement of the distal clavicle or osteophyte formation will lead to secondary impingement, treatment of rotator cuff problems frequently leads to treatment of the AC joint secondarily. History, physical examination, injection studies, and radiologic examination can help differentiate primary AC pathology and secondary involvement. Other primary shoulder problems that may have to be differentiated include calcific tendinitis, osteoarthritis of the glenohumeral joint, and adhesive capsulitis.

Common primary AC joint problems include osteoarthritis, osteolysis, and ligamentous sprains. Less common AC joint problems include rheumatoid arthritis, crystalline arthritis (gout and pseudogout), and septic arthritis. The least common problems affecting the AC joint are hyperparathyroidism and musculoskeletal tumors.

Treatment

Traumatic Injuries

Type 1 injuries lack evidence of instability and should be treated conservatively. Analgesics, cryotherapy, local wound care, and padding of the joint for contact sports are the only treatments required. Many of the chronic changes of the AC joint in athletes involved in contact sports may be due to old type 1 and 2 sprains.[5,38]

Type 2 injuries are treated similarly to type 1 injuries. These injuries may be more inclined to late degenerative changes of the AC joint because of its increased sagittal plane motion. Resection of an inadequate amount of distal clavicle may leave the patient with significant pain due to the increased anteroposterior translation.[7] A sling, analgesics, and cryotherapy aid the patient's comfort level. Return to athletic play after type 1 and 2 injuries is dependent on the athlete's ability to protect himself or herself and the restoration of motion and strength. Acutely, injections of anesthetic into the AC joint may provide comfort and allow a return to activity.

Most studies comparing operative and nonoperative treatment of type 3 injuries yield similar results.[3,23,38] A recent study of the natural history of type 3 injuries treated conservatively indicated that 20% of the patients considered their treatment suboptimal, although of the four suboptimal results, only one patient would have elected surgical treatment.[33] The only short-term strength deficit was with the bench press; long term, no deficit was noted between the involved and uninvolved extremities. Overhead athletes were not evaluated in this study.

Disagreement still exists regarding the acute treatment of type 3 injuries. Theoretically, adequate repair of the injured structures would require restoration of both the AC ligaments and the coracoclavicular ligaments. Currently, the preferred treatment of acute type 3 injuries is similar to the treatment of acute type 1 and 2 injuries. Rest, ice, sling, analgesics, and restoration of motion and strength when comfortable are appropriate. Surgical reconstructions are undertaken only if symptoms persist. A variation of the Weaver-Dunn procedure, with transfer of the coracoacromial ligament from the undersurface of the acromion to the resected end of the clavicle, is preferred.[41] This procedure can be performed early or late without compromising the results.

Other surgical procedures to restore AC joint integrity include dynamic muscle transfers[17]; primary AC joint fixation with pins, along with repair of the ligaments; and primary coracoclavicular ligament fixation, which requires augmentation with screws or bands between the coracoid and clavicle.[9] Recently, an arthroscopic technique to reconstruct and stabilize the AC joint was described.[42] An adequate study of type 3 injuries in overhead athletes has not been performed to determine whether repair or early reconstruction is necessary. We have treated three professional quarterbacks who sustained AC separations of the dominant extremity—one type 2 and two type 3 injuries. All returned to full function without surgical intervention. One went to the Pro-Bowl years after his injury.

Most authors agree that displacement of the distal clavicle through the trapezius leads to discomfort with motion. Type 4 injuries thus require some form of intervention. One option is closed reduction and conversion to a type 3 injury, followed by conservative treatment. The other option, which we prefer, is to surgically reduce the clavicle out of the trapezius and then resect the end of the clavicle and transfer the coracoacromial ligament into it. Closure of the deltotrapezial fascia over the clavicle augments the repair.

Type 5 AC injuries are thought to require surgical intervention because of the substantial deltotrapezial fascial stripping and potential for compromise of the overlying skin. In reality, many of these injuries are probably treated conservatively as type 3 injuries. Those that present with severe displacement and tenting of the skin probably warrant surgical intervention. The modified Weaver-Dunn procedure is preferred.

Type 6 injuries are rare. These injuries obviously require surgical reduction of the displaced clavicle. Excision of the end of the clavicle aids in this reduction.

Chronic Degenerative Disease

Nonoperative Treatment

Chronic conditions such as arthritis and osteolysis of the AC joint can be managed nonoperatively in most cases.[26,43] Obviously, the treatment has to be designed to fit the patient's pain level, dysfunction, level of activity, and expectations. Nonoperative treatment includes analgesics, nonsteroidal anti-inflammatory medications, injection with cortisone and anesthetics, and activity modification. Physical therapy may aid those with restricted motion and diminished strength. Most athletes involved in repetitive sports that cause symptoms are unwilling to modify their activity.

Operative Treatment

Resection of the distal clavicle is warranted in those unwilling to modify their activities or refractory to conservative care. Open resection of the distal end of the clavicle was described independently by Gurd[20] and Mumford[25] in 1941. This treatment has proved reliable in relieving pain due to AC pathology. With the advent of arthroscopy, methods of resecting the distal end of the clavicle were devised that were more cosmetically pleasing and less invasive to the soft tissue structures. These techniques were devised initially as an adjunct to resection of the osteophytes that contribute to impingement of the rotator cuff.[6,15,16] Resection can be accomplished indirectly in patients undergoing subacromial decompression for impingement or directly through a superior approach without violating the subacromial anatomy.[6,18]

Surgical Technique

An examination under anesthesia is performed to evaluate for underlying instability and restrictions in range of motion. The patient is positioned in the lateral decubitus position with the arm suspended from the boom in 50 degrees of abduction and 15 degrees of forward flexion with 10 pounds of weight (Fig. 20–3). Alternatively, a beach chair position can be used.

Arthroscopic portals are placed (Fig. 20–4). A posterior viewing portal is established one fingerbreadth inferior and medial to the posterior corner of the acromion. A second anterior portal is established between the coracoid and acromion, entering the joint between the biceps, superior edge of the subscapularis, and anterior labrum.

Complete diagnostic arthroscopy is completed before repositioning the arthroscope in the subacromial space. Once it is in the subacromial space, a third portal is established just lateral to the anterior third of the acromion and approximately 1 cm inferior to the inferior border of the acromion. This serves as the working portal initially. In cases in which impingement syndrome is believed to contribute to the patient's symptoms, a formal subacromial decompression is performed (Figs. 20–5 and 20–6). Alternatively, the subacromial space and acromion are not addressed other than to improve visualization of the AC joint.

We begin the acromioclavicular resection by removing the medial border of the acromion adjoining the clavicle for approximately 5 mm. This helps visualize the distal aspect of the clavicle. The electrocautery device is used to debride soft tissue around the distal clavicle inferiorly and obtain hemostasis. Typically, a significant "bleeder" exists on the posterior and inferior aspect of the distal clavicle. Resection of the distal clavicle begins through the lateral portal with a round-tipped bur. Further resection of the clavicle is undertaken using the initial anterior skin portal but redirecting the bur superiorly, so that it enters just under the AC joint. Resection of approximately 5 mm of the distal clavicle is all that is required to end up with a 7- to 10-mm gap between the acromion and clavicle (Fig. 20–7). Adequate visualization

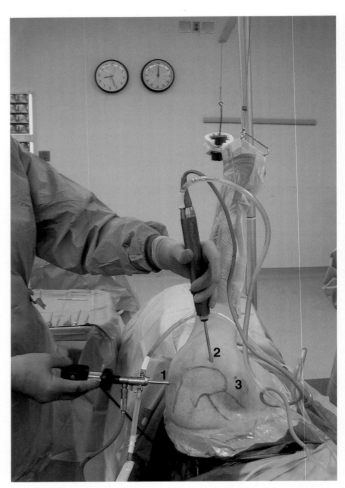

Figure 20–4　Arthroscopic portals. (1) Posterior viewing portal. (2) Anterior portal between the tip of the coracoid and the acromion. This portal can be used for both intra-articular assessment and resection of the clavicle. (3) Lateral portal for subacromial decompression.

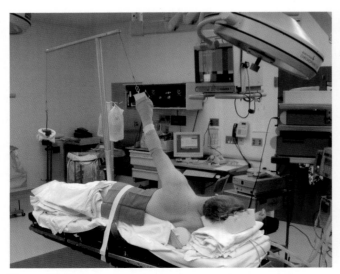

Figure 20–3　Lateral decubitus positioning for arthroscopy. Alternatively, the patient can be placed in the beach chair position.

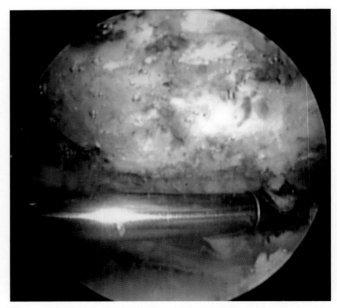

Figure 20–5　Arthroscopic view of the shoulder. Electrocautery is used to denude the undersurface of the acromion.

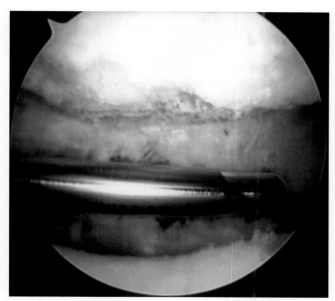

Figure 20–6   A full-radius shaver or bur may be used to resect the acromial hook.

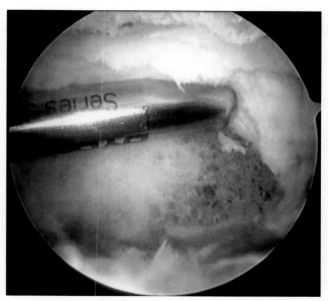

Figure 20–8   A full-radius synovial resector can be used to measure the amount of resection and the gap between the clavicle and acromion.

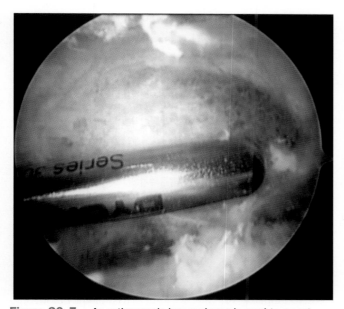

Figure 20–7   An arthroscopic bur or shaver is used to resect 5 mm of the medial aspect of the acromion and 5 mm of the lateral aspect of the clavicle.

of the entire clavicle circumferentially is necessary to ensure proper resection. As the clavicle is resected, it assumes a flatter or oval appearance, as opposed to the original circular shape. Adequate resection can be ensured by using the shaver or bur, which is approximately 5 mm wide, as a probe between the ends of bone (Fig. 20–8).

The arthroscope can also be positioned anterior and inferior to the joint while a calibrated probe is brought from the lateral portal to measure the amount of resec-

tion. After the resection is complete, the subacromial space is irrigated to remove "bone dust."

Postoperative Management

The patient is placed in a sling for comfort and until the scalene block wears off. The dressing is removed in 3 days. Steri-Strips are left in place until the patient is seen in the office at 7 to 10 days postoperatively. The patient is allowed to move the shoulder immediately as tolerated. After the first office visit, the patient starts physical therapy to restore range of motion and strength. Overhead sports are usually not resumed until 2 to 3 months postoperatively.

Results

Outcomes after arthroscopic resection have paralleled those of open procedures. Most athletes are able to return to athletic competition. The arthroscopic techniques also require less resection of bone, with 4 to 7 mm being sufficient to achieve satisfactory results.[46] Calcifications may occur after resection but have been shown to have no untoward affect on results.[37]

Complications

Complications can be related to either the AC joint injury itself or its treatment. Possible complications include resection of too much or not enough bone. Too much resection of the distal clavicle could result in instability, particularly in the sagittal plane. Inadequate resection could lead to persistent or recurrent symptoms. Most often, the posterior corner of the distal clavicle is not adequately resected. This can be avoided by adequate visualization of the entire end of the clavicle when performing arthroscopy. Other potential complications include thinning and fracture of the acromion or infection.

Associated fractures of the distal clavicle or coracoid need to be assessed and treated. Fractures of the coracoid are rare and are frequently missed when associated with AC strains. They are best seen on axillary radiographs. Calcification of the ligamentous structures are more common, particularly with injuries to the coracoclavicular ligament. These calcifications seem to be innocuous and may be present in up to half of AC injuries. They lead to no long-term consequences. Degenerative arthritis and osteolysis of the clavicle are common years after type 1 and 2 injuries[9] and can be dealt with as outlined previously in this chapter.

Additional complications related to the surgical treatment of AC instability can occur. The most severe is migration of pins from the AC joint. Smooth K-wires used to transfix the AC joint can break and migrate to the lungs, great vessels, or heart; thus, they should not be used. Infection of hardware or augmentation loops that hold the AC joint in place has also been reported. Using loops made of absorbable material or biologic substances avoids this complication.[27,29,30]

Conclusion

Injuries of a traumatic or degenerative nature are frequent at the AC joint and may affect shoulder function. These injuries can be divided into those related to direct or indirect trauma and those related to repetitive stress or degenerative conditions that affect virtually all diarthrodial joints. Most conditions affecting the AC joint can be treated conservatively, but chronic conditions affecting shoulder function and athletic activity may require operative intervention.

Open or arthroscopic techniques may be necessary to deal with AC joint displacement or the sequelae of displacement and late degenerative conditions. The results of such treatment are excellent, but attention to surgical technique is necessary to avoid complications.

References

1. Allman FL Jr: Fractures and ligamaentous injuries of the clavicle and its articulation. J Bone Joint Surg Am 49:774-784, 1967.
2. Auge WK, Fisher RA: Arthroscopic distal clavicle resection for isolated atraumatic osteolysis in weight lifters. Am J Sports Med. 26:189-192, 1998.
3. Bannister GC, Wallace WA, Stableforth PG, et al: The management of acute AC dislocation: A randomized, prospective, controlled trial. J Bone Joint Surg Br 71:848-850, 1989.
4. Barber FA: Coplaning of the AC joint. Arthroscopy 17:913-917, 2001.
5. Bergfield JA, Andrish JT, Clancy WG: Evaluation of the AC joint following first- and second-degree sprains. Am J Sports Med 6:153-159, 1978.
6. Bigliani LV, Nicholson GP, Flatow EL: Arthroscopic resection of the distal clavicle. Clin Orthop 24:133-141, 1993.
7. Blazar PE, Iannotti JP, Williams GR: Anteroposterior instability of the distal clavicle after distal clavicle resection. Clin Orthop 348:114-120, 1998.
8. Bonsell S, Pearsall AW IV, Heitman RJ, et al: The relationship of age, gender, and degenerative changes observed on radiographs of the shoulder in asymptomatic individuals. J Bone Joint Surg Br 82:1135-1139, 2000.
9. Bosworth BM: AC separation: New method of repair. Surg Gynecol Obstet 73:866-871, 1941.
10. Brown JN, Roberts SNJ, Hayes MG, Sales PS: Shoulder pathology associated with symptomatic AC joint degeneration. J Shoulder Elbow Surg 9:173-176, 2000.
11. Cahill BR: Osteolysis of the distal part of the clavicle in male athletes. J Bone Joint Surg Am 64:1053-1058, 1982.
12. Debski RE, Parsons IM IV, Woo SF, Freddic H: Effect of capsular injury on AC joint mechanics. J Bone Joint Surg Am 83:1344-1351, 2001.
13. DePalma AF: The role of the disks of the sternoclavicular and the AC joints. Clin Orthop 13:222-223, 1959.
14. DePalma AF, Callery G, Bennett GA: Variational anatomy and degenerative lesions of the shoulder joint. Instr Course Lect 6:255-281, 1949.
15. Ellman H: Arthroscopic subacromial decompression analysis of one- to three-year results. Arthroscopy 3:173-181, 1987.
16. Esch JC, Ozerkis LR, Helgager JA, et al: Arthroscopic subacromial decompression results according to the degree of rotator cuff tear. Arthroscopy 4:241-249, 1988.
17. Ferris BD, Bhamra M, Paton DF: Coracoid process transfer for AC dislocations: A report of 20 cases. Clin Orthop 242:184-194, 1989.
18. Flatow EL, Duralde XA, Nicholson GP, et al: Arthroscopic resection of the distal clavicle with a superior approach. J Shoulder Elbow Surg 4:41-50, 1995.
19. Gerber C, Galantay RV, Hersche O: The pattern of pain produced by irritation of the AC joint and the subacromial space. J Shoulder Elbow Surg 7:352-355, 1998.
20. Gurd FB: The treatment of complete dislocation of the outer end of the clavicle: A hitherto undescribed operation. Ann Surg 63:1094-1098, 1941.
21. Klimkiewicz JJ, Williams GR, Sher JJ, et al: The acromioclavicular capsule as a restraint to posterior translation of the clavicle: A biochemical analysis. J Shoulder Elbow Surg 8:119-124, 1999.
22. Kuster MS, Hales PF, Davis SJ: The effects of arthroscopic acromioplasty on the AC joint. J Shoulder Elbow Surg 7:140-143, 1998.
23. Larsen E, Bjerg-Nielsen A, Christensen P: Conservative or surgical treatment of AC dislocation: A prospective, controlled, randomized study. J Bone Joint Surg Am 68:552-555, 1986.
24. Lee KW, Debski RE, Chen, CH, et al: Functional evaluation of the ligaments at the AC joint during antero- and superoinferior translation. Am J Sports Med 25:858-862, 1997.
25. Mumford EB: AC dislocation: A new operative treatment. J Bone Joint Surg Am 23:799-801, 1941.
26. Murphy OB, Bellamy R, Wheeler W, Brower TD: Post traumatic osteolysis of the distal clavicle. Clin Orthop 109:108-114, 1975.
27. Neault MA, Nuber GW, Mary Mount JV: Infections after surgical repair of AC separations with nonabsorbable tape or suture. J Shoulder Elbow Surg 5:477-478, 1996.

28. Needell SD, Zlatkin MD, Sher JS, et al: MR injury of the rotator cuff peritendinous and bone abnormalities in an asymptomatic population. AJR Am J Roentgenol 166:863-867, 1996.

29. Nuber GW, Bowen MK: AC joint injuries and distal clavicle fractures. JAAOS 5:11-18, 1997.

30. Nuber GW, Bowen MK: Disorders of the acromioclaviculat joint: Pathophysiology, diagnosis and management. In Iannotti JP, Williams GR (eds): Disorders of the Shoulder: Diagnosis and Management. Philadelphia, Lippincott, Williams & Wilkins, 1999, pp 739-764.

31. Rockwood CA Jr, Young DC: Disorders of the AC joint. In Rokwood CA, Masten FA III (eds): The Shoulder, vol 1. Philadelphia, WB Saunders, 1990, pp 413-476.

32. Salter EG Jr, Nasca RJ, Shelley BS: Anatomical observation on the AC joint and supporting ligaments. Am J Sports Med 15:199-206, 1987.

33. Schlegel TF, Burks RT, Marcus RL, Dunn HK: A prospective evaluation of untreated acute grade III AC separations. Am J Sports Med 29:699-703, 2001.

34. Shaffer B: Painful condition of the AC joint. J Am Acad Orthop Surg 7:176-188, 1999.

35. Sher JS, Uribe JW, Posoda A, et al: Abnormal findings on magnetic resonance images of asymptomatic shoulders. J Bone Joint Surg Am 77:10-15, 1995.

36. Shubin S, Beth E, Wiater M, et al: Detection of AC joint pathology in asymptomatic shoulders with magnetic resonance imaging. J Shoulder Elbow Surg 10:204-208, 2001.

37. Snyder SJ, Banas MP, Karzel RP: The arthroscopic Mumford procedure: An analysis of results. Arthroscopy 11:157-164, 1995.

38. Taft TN, Wilson FC, Oglesby JW: Dislocation of the AC joint: An end-result study. J Bone Joint Surg Am 69:1045-1051, 1987.

39. Tossy JD, Mead NC, Sigmond HM: AC separations: Useful and practical classification for treatment. Clin Orthop 28:111-119, 1963.

40. Urist MR: Complete dislocations of the AC joint: The nature of the traumatic lesion and effective methods of treatment with an analysis of forty-one cases. J Bone Joint Surg 28:813-837, 1946.

41. Weaver JK, Dunn HK: Treatment of AC injuries, especially complete AC separation. J Bone Joint Surg Am 54:1187-1194, 1972.

42. Wolf EM, Pennington WT: Arthroscopic reconstruction for AC joint dislocation. Arthroscopy 17:558-563, 2001.

43. Worcester JN, Green DP: Osteoarthritis of the AC joint. Clin Orthop 58:69-73, 1968.

44. Yap JJL, Carl LA, Kvitne RS, McFarland EG: The value of weighted views of the AC joint: Results of a survey. Am J Sports Med 27:806-809, 1999.

45. Zanca P: Shoulder pain: Involvement of the AC joint (analysis of 1000 cases). AJR Am J Roentgenol 112:493-506, 1971.

46. Zawadsky M, Marra G, Wiater JM, et al: Osteolysis of the distal clavicle: Long-term results of arthroscopic resection. Arthroscopy 16:600-605, 2000.

Biceps Tendinitis

WARREN KUO, JAMES N. GLADSTONE,
AND EVAN L. FLATOW

BICEPS TENDINITIS IN A NUTSHELL

History:
Pain in bicipital groove, anterior shoulder pain; associated with rotator cuff pathology, chronic impingement syndrome, or acute traumatic events

Physical Examination:
Point tenderness; Speed and Yergason tests

Imaging:
Routine to rule out concomitant pathology; magnetic resonance imaging particularly helpful

Indications:
Failure of conservative management for at least 3 months

Contraindications:
Distorted anatomy (e.g., prior ulnar nerve transposition), ankylosed joint

Surgical Technique:
Decompression, tenotomy, tenodesis (open or arthroscopic)

Postoperative Management:
Sling, range of motion; protect tenodesis by avoiding active elbow flexion and supination for 6 weeks

Results:
Similar for tenotomy and tenodesis

Complications:
Infection, persistent pain

Significant controversy exists with regard to the functional role of the long head of the biceps and the appropriate procedures for its various pathologic conditions. Some consider it to have a merely vestigial function, whereas others believe that it plays a significant role as a shoulder stabilizer. As a result, treatment options have varied from preservation of the tendon[53,63] to tenotomy[27] or tenodesis.[18,26,48]

The difficulty lies in the fact that despite detailed descriptions of biceps anatomy and pathology,[69,9,16,34,44] its true role is not well understood. This chapter explores the current understanding of the biceps function and describes the treatment options available: decompression, tenotomy, and tenodesis. With advances in arthroscopic technology and improved arthroscopic skills, these procedures can now be performed arthroscopically with reduced morbidity.

Anatomy and Biomechanics

The biceps originates from two heads that form a conjoint tendon distally. The short head originates from the coracoid process. The intra-articular long head has a variable origin from both the labrum and the supraglenoid tubercle. Habermeyer et al.[30] described the long head originating from the posterosuperior labrum (50%), supraglenoid tubercle (20%), or both (30%). A cadaveric study by Vangsness et al.[69] found that in most cases the tendon was attached equally to both the labrum and the supraglenoid tubercle and that there were four types of biceps attachment to the labrum: type I, all posterior (22%); type II, mostly posterior with some anterior (33%); type III, equally anterior and posterior (37%); and type IV, all anterior (8%) (Fig. 21–1). From its labral attachment, the biceps tendon courses laterally and anteriorly to the bicipital groove, through the rotator cuff interval. The tendon is surrounded by a continuation of the synovial lining of the joint capsule, forming a sheath that ends as a blind pouch within the bicipital groove, making the tendon an intra-articular but extrasynovial structure (Fig. 21–2). The tendon passes deep to the coracohumeral ligament (thought to be a stabilizer of the tendon) and beneath the transverse humeral ligament into the bicipital groove formed by the lateral border of the lesser tuberosity and the medial (or anterior) border of the greater tuberosity. A recent histoanatomic study showed the superior glenohumeral ligament forming an anterior sling about the biceps tendon laterally but proximal to the groove. The supraspinatus provides fibers that intermingle with the posterior aspect of the roof of the sling. The subscapularis does not play a role in this slinglike structure and provides stability only at the level of the bicipital groove.[73] The long head and short head then meet as muscle bellies at the level of the deltoid insertion and insert as a single tendon into the bicipital tuberosity of the radius.

The function of the biceps tendon is debated. Studies implicating a stabilizing function have mostly been

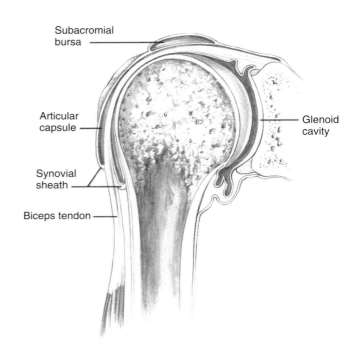

Figure 21–2   Depiction of the course of the biceps tendon from the labrum through the bicipital groove, demonstrating its intra-articular but extrasynovial position. (From Yamaguchi K, Bindra R: Disorders of the biceps tendon. In Iannotti JP, Williams GR [eds]: Disorders of the Shoulder: Diagnosis and Management. Philadelphia, Lippincott Williams & Wilkins, 1999, p 161.)

cadaveric, with simulated muscle loads; in vivo electromyographic studies usually show minimal activity and imply either no functional role or a static effect. Cadaveric studies have demonstrated that the biceps can function as an efficient stabilizer of the shoulder when the arm is elevated in the scapular plane in neutral rotation.[45] The biceps is able to decrease anterior, posterior,[36] and superior displacement[40] of the humeral head in the dependent position. It can also act as an anterior stabilizer with the arm abducted and externally rotated.[35] In a study that simulated superior labral tears, it was found that the biceps acts as a significant shoulder stabilizer[58] and is capable of reducing strain on the inferior glenohumeral ligament.[64] Electrical stimulation of the biceps during arthroscopic visualization produces glenohumeral compression,[1] which is one mechanism for controlling joint stability.[7,43]

A clinical study in patients with intact rotator cuffs but isolated ruptures of the long head of the biceps supported the joint stability concept, with an additional 2 to 6 mm of superior head translation in biceps-deficient patients compared with the opposite extremity.[72] Electromyographic studies of baseball pitchers with anterior instability revealed increased activity of the biceps, suggesting a compensatory role for lax ligaments. In addition, patients with rotator cuff tears and intact biceps were reported to have increased electromyographic activity in the biceps of the affected limb.[68] In contrast, other studies found no significant electroactivity of the long head of the biceps in response to isolated motion (with elbow and forearm position controlled), suggesting that

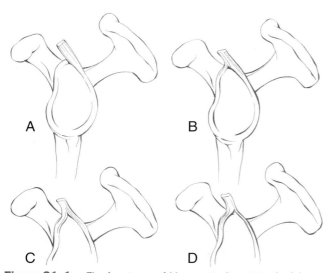

Figure 21–1   The four types of biceps attachment to the labrum. *A,* Type I, all posterior (22%). *B,* Type II, mostly posterior, with a small amount anterior (33%). *C,* Type III, equally anterior and posterior (37%). *D,* Type IV, all anterior (8%). (From Yamaguchi K, Bindra R: Disorders of the biceps tendon. In Iannotti JP, Williams GR [eds]: Disorders of the Shoulder: Diagnosis and Management. Philadelphia, Lippincott Williams & Wilkins, 1999, p 160.)

the long head acts passively or is active only in association with elbow and forearm activity.[42,74]

Historical Aspects

Historically, treatment has varied considerably. In the 1940s, tenodesis was advocated as the favored form of treatment.[18,26,48] By the 1970s, recommendations to preserve the tendon became popular because the tendon was thought to have a stabilizing role, particularly as part of the coracoacromial arch.[53,63] Recently, the pendulum has swung back toward releasing the tendon, either by simple tenotomy or by tenodesis, when it is implicated as the cause of pain. There remains wide debate as to the role of the tendon and the appropriate treatment for pathologic conditions.

Mechanism of Injury

Biceps pathology can be classified as degenerative or inflammatory, traumatic, or related to instability (Table 21–1).

Degenerative or Inflammatory

Biceps inflammation is usually secondary to pathology of the surrounding tissues. Neer[52] found that most cases of biceps degeneration were associated with subacromial impingement. Just as the rotator cuff can be abraded due to extrinsic factors such as a subacromial or distal clavicular spur, the biceps can be similarly affected.[56] Murthi et al.,[51] in a prospective trial of 200 patients undergoing arthroscopic surgery for subacromial decompression, found a strong association between biceps tendon disease and rotator cuff disease. Forty percent of these patients underwent tenodesis for biceps disease. Of these, 91% had an associated full-thickness rotator cuff tear.

The biceps tendon may exhibit intrinsic degeneration (tendinosis) or inflammation of the sheath (tendinitis), which is more accurately referred to as tenosynovitis.

Table 21–1
Classification of Biceps Pathology

Degenerative or Inflammatory

Associated with rotator cuff disease
Primary tendinitis and tendon degeneration (tendinosis)
Systemic or inflammatory disease

Traumatic

Overuse (muscle imbalance, glenohumeral laxity or instability)
Rupture (complete or partial)

Instability

Subluxation
Dislocation

Tendinosis may be diagnosed only after rupture or can manifest as fraying or partial tearing of the tendon (Fig. 21–3). Tenosynovitis is more obvious, with an inflamed or red and striated appearance to the tendon (Fig. 21–4).

Inflammation of the tendon within its groove, while the intra-articular portion remains unaffected, can be due to both mechanical and nonmechanical causes. Thickening of the synovium under the transverse humeral ligament in the bicipital groove may be seen, which is analogous to the tenosynovitis seen in de Quervain's disease.[17,18,44,48,61] A mechanical cause for

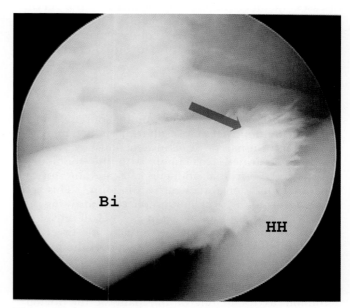

Figure 21–3 Partial tear (fraying) of biceps tendon *(arrow)*. Bi, biceps, HH, humeral head.

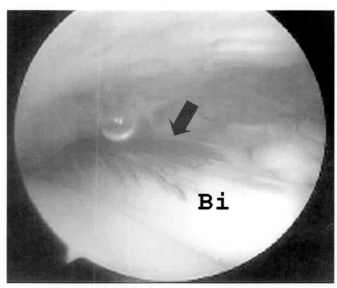

Figure 21–4 Inflammation of the biceps tenosynovium *(arrow)*. Bi, biceps.

both tendinitis and tendinosis may be degenerative changes in the bicipital groove. In a study by Pfahler et al.,[60] radiologic signs of groove degeneration correlated in 44% of patients with biceps disease on sonograms. Primary tendinitis is less common and refers to inflammation of the tendon without an identifiable cause. The role of hypoxia and hypovascularity as a cause of primary tendon degeneration remains unclear. Kannus and Jozsa[38] found hypoxic degenerative tendinopathy in many cases of long head rupture. Rathburn and MacNab[62] found diminished blood flow within the rotator cuff and biceps tendons with the arm in adduction, which improved with abduction. Systemic inflammatory disease can cause biceps tendinitis. These diseases include rheumatoid arthritis, lupus erythematosus, and crystalline arthropathies such as gout and pseudogout. The tendinitis is secondary to inflammation of the synovium, which may also involve other joints.

Traumatic

Overuse of the shoulder is a common source of microtraumatic tendinitis. It may result from sudden increased activity or unusual or repetitive actions by the arm. Overhead activities, particularly with the shoulder in flexion and horizontal adduction, create anterior and superior translation forces across the joint.[17] This activity, seen during the deceleration phase of throwing, may explain the risks of impingement in baseball pitchers. A tight posterior capsule can accentuate this by causing greater anterior and superior migration of the humeral head.[32] Weak periscapular muscles, especially the serratus anterior, can produce scapular dyskinesia, which can exacerbate impingement by not allowing the acromion to rotate out of the path of the forward-elevating humerus.[28] Jobe et al.[37] described an instability-impingement complex whereby repetitive overhead activity may eventually exceed the ability of the anterior constraints of the shoulder to compensate. This can fatigue the rotator cuff and biceps tendons and allow subtle anterior and superior migration of the humeral head, with subsequent impingement against the coracoacromial arch.[29]

Rupture of the long head of the biceps can occur in a normal tendon but often requires a significant trauma. A powerful supination force or the deceleration phase of a pitch can predispose the biceps to rupture.[1] More commonly, a rupture occurs in a degenerated tendon. In this case, the trauma may be minimal. Partial tears are often painful and can cause significant dysfunction. This is in contrast to complete ruptures, which often have acute but self-limited pain (in the anterior aspect of the upper arm) and can be associated with bruising down the anterior aspect of the arm.

Instability

Instability of the biceps tendon can vary from subluxation to frank dislocation. The major stabilizer of the tendon is the intact rotator cuff and the superior liga-

ments. Disruption to either the superior aspect of the subscapularis or the anterior aspect of the supraspinatus may allow the biceps tendon to dislocate medially.[9,13,14,31] In a cadaveric study, Petersson[59] found two types of medial dislocation. In four out of five cases, the biceps dislocated under a deep tear of the subscapularis; in the fifth case, the biceps slid over the top of the intact subscapularis tendon. Walch et al.[71] described changes to the biceps tendon associated with "hidden" lesions of the rotator interval. The hidden lesion, or the pulley complex formed by the coalescence of the coracohumeral and superior glenohumeral ligaments (as they insert onto the lesser tuberosity), was either absent or degenerated in cases of biceps instability. In the presence of a torn upper portion of the subscapularis, the biceps tendon can subluxate under the subscapularis tendon, because only the superficial fascia of the tendon is left intact.

Walch et al.[70] reported that it is unlikely for a biceps tendon to subluxate or dislocate unless there is an underlying cuff tear involving the rotator interval or subscapularis. There were only two cases of dislocation with an intact subscapularis, and 70% of dislocations were associated with massive rotator cuff tears involving both the supraspinatus and infraspinatus tendons.

History

A complete patient history is critical to directing the focus of the investigation. Important questions include the onset and nature of the pain, a history of any traumatic event, exacerbating activities, and sporting recreations (especially those involving repetitive throwing and overhead activities). Patients with biceps tendinitis often complain of pain at the bicipital groove, and occasionally an individual may present with spontaneous rupture. It is often difficult to distinguish this pain from that of impingement syndromes and rotator cuff tears. Biceps pain typically radiates anteriorly, whereas rotator cuff pain radiates toward the deltoid insertion. However, because biceps pathology is frequently associated with rotator cuff disease, both pain patterns may coexist. A functional history to assess any limitation of activities should also be obtained.

Physical Examination

The physical examination begins with inspection of muscular symmetry (specifically, evidence of proximal biceps tendon rupture), wasting, and any previous scars (Fig. 21–5). Palpation often reveals point tenderness at the bicipital groove. Assessment of the remainder of the joint, with attention to range of motion and strength (especially of the subscapularis), as well as provocative maneuvers such as impingement and apprehension tests, can assist in eliciting other coexisting diagnoses. Tests specifically assessing biceps pathology include the Speed test (resisted flexion of a supinated forearm results in pain at the bicipital groove)[54] and the

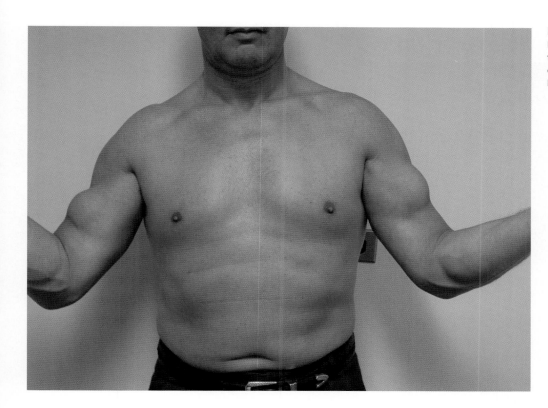

Figure 21–5 Rupture of the long head of the proximal biceps tendon. Note the distally contracted ("Popeye") muscle belly of the right upper arm.

Yergason test (resisted supination of the forearm with the elbow flexed to 90 degrees results in pain in the bicipital groove).[75] These tests are not pathognomonic, however.

Imaging

To date, no imaging modality accurately evaluates the biceps tendons. In part, this is due to the nonlinear course of the proximal part of the long head of the biceps. Therefore, the main purpose of diagnostic imaging is to rule out concomitant pathology. Any evaluation of the shoulder should start with radiographs before undertaking more advanced imaging studies.

Plain Radiography

Four views are taken as part of our standard shoulder series: an anteroposterior view with the humerus in neutral rotation, an anteroposterior view with the patient internally rotated 45 degrees to the x-ray beam, a supraspinatus outlet view, and an axillary view. These views may help identify any changes associated with rotator cuff disease, shoulder instability, previous fractures, acromial morphology, or disease of the glenohumeral and acromioclavicular joints.

The Cone (bicipital groove) view[16] assesses the size of the groove as well as any degenerative spurs or narrow-ing. It is obtained by directing the x-ray beam cephalad and 15 degrees medial to the long axis of the humerus with the cassette placed at the apex of the shoulder.

Arthrography

Arthrography has been used to assess biceps anatomy, changes to the groove, and any subluxation of the tendon. In addition, it is useful in the diagnosis of rotator cuff tears. However, arthrography is an invasive test, and filling of the biceps sheath can be unreliable. Filling of the sheath has been reported to be absent in up to 31% of arthrograms, especially in the presence of a full-thickness rotator cuff tear.[49,50]

Ultrasonography

Ultrasonography is a noninvasive, relatively inexpensive investigation that in some studies is equal to arthrography or magnetic resonance imaging (MRI).[49,65] However, it is operator dependent, and not all areas of the shoulder can be visualized owing to bony constraints.

Magnetic Resonance Imaging

MRI is our investigation of choice for assessing the rotator cuff and labrum. It has also become a highly favored modality for imaging the biceps.[11,12,20] MRI can

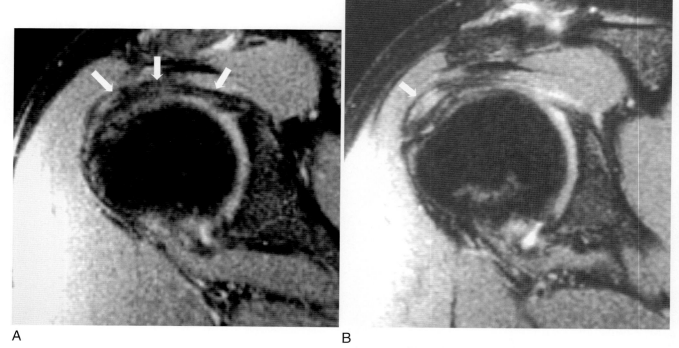

A   B

Figure 21–6   Magnetic resonance imaging biceps sequence. *A,* The biceps tendon courses over the humeral head and inserts on the labrum *(arrows). B,* Tendinosis in the tendon just proximal to the bicipital groove *(arrow).* (Courtesy of Sandra L. Moore, MD, New York, NY.)

determine the position of the biceps tendon within the groove and any effusion within the sheath (Fig. 21–6). Tendon subluxation can be seen in association with upper subscapularis deficiency and rotator interval lesions.

Injection of gadolinium contrast (magnetic resonance arthrography) provides greater sensitivity for subtle capsular derangements[47] and labral lesions (specifically, superior labral anterior to posterior [SLAP] lesions), but it makes the test invasive, and the increase in accuracy is debatable.[22] MRI has the disadvantage of being expensive, and its use it limited in claustrophobic patients and in those with certain metallic implants such as pacemakers or aneurysm clips.

Associated Injuries

Biceps tendinitis is most commonly associated with rotator cuff disease in the older population, whereas sports and repetitive overhead and throwing activities account for tendinitis in the younger population. Instability of the biceps tendon is invariably associated with tears in the rotator cuff (subscapularis or rotator interval) that allow the tendon to subluxate or dislocate medially. Glenohumeral instability may be a contributing factor in a young athlete presenting with bicipital tendinitis due to overload and should be evaluated in the examination. A history of trauma may accompany a patient with tendinitis, dislocation, or acute rupture of the biceps.

Treatment Options

Nonoperative

An athlete with acute tendinitis should be treated with rest and cessation of the exacerbating activity. In addition, modalities such as ice and ultrasonography should be directed to the shoulder. Patients without any contraindications may be started on a course of nonsteroidal anti-inflammatory medication. Spontaneous ruptures require only symptomatic treatment.[9,10] Mariani et al.[46] found that in patients with spontaneous rupture of the long head of the biceps, there was little difference in outcome between those treated operatively with tenodesis and those managed nonoperatively.

Injections of a local anesthetic agent mixed with corticosteroid may be of diagnostic and therapeutic value. Selective injections into the subacromial space and biceps sheath may assist in differentiating the source of pain.[39] It is important to avoid intratendinous injection of steroid; however, it can be difficult to inject the bicipital sheath with certainty. The injection is performed using a small-bore (22- or 25-gauge) needle. The point of maximal tenderness is elicited by palpation. It may be helpful to have the patient extend the arm at the side with the hand supinated. This rotates the bicipital groove more anteriorly. The needle is directed at the painful site and inserted until bone is touched. It is then slowly retracted while injecting until no or minimal resistance is felt. Resistance is usually felt if the needle is in the tendon, and a marked difference is noted once the needle is retracted into the sheath. If no relief is obtained from either a subacromial or a bicipital sheath injection, an intra-articular injection can be performed. However, relief from this injection is less specific because the pathology may be due to articular cartilage damage, an articular-sided partial rotator cuff tear, or a labral lesion. Even if no relief is obtained, the pathology may still be bicipital in origin, but in an extra-articular or extra-synovial region.

Once the acute symptoms have settled, patients should be started on a rehabilitation program. Physical therapy should be directed at any underlying pathology, restoring range of motion, and improving rotator cuff and periscapular muscle strength.[29] We do not believe that the biceps pathology itself can be addressed with physical therapy, but therapy may help treat associated conditions. An athlete's return to sporting activities should be increased gradually and in a methodical fashion.

Operative

Surgery is considered if 3 months of conservative treatment has failed to provide relief or if there is evidence of an irreversible condition such as subluxation or dislocation of the tendon. However, the appropriate operative treatment for the biceps tendon remains controversial. Options include decompression, tenotomy, or tenodesis (open or arthroscopic).

Decompression

One theory suggests that biceps pathology causes symptoms in a way analogous to de Quervain's stenosing tenosynovitis.[17,18,41,44,48,61] Therefore, an arthroscopic release of the tendon sheath may improve symptoms (M. Gross, personal communication, 2001). We consider this option only in a patient with minimal to moderate inflammation of an intact tendon. We have no long-term results using this procedure but believe that it has little risk and may be useful in specific situations.

Tenotomy

Tenotomy has become a popular option in the treatment of a diseased biceps tendon. Walch et al.[70] advocate its release in cases of subluxation and dislocation. Thomazeau et al.[66] reported favorable results of tenotomy of the biceps in association with rotator cuff tears. Gill et al.[27] obtained good results in the only study that has reported on isolated tenotomy. Eighty-seven percent of the patients were satisfied, and 97% returned to work an average of 1.9 weeks after surgery (range, 0 to 7 weeks). Only one patient complained of a cosmetic deformity and required a revision tenodesis.

Tenodesis

The most common association with biceps pathology is rotator cuff disease. Neviaser[55] found that patients had pathologic changes of tenosynovitis in the biceps tendon on arthrography. This was confirmed intraoperatively.[54]

He therefore recommended tenodesis as part of the treatment for impingement syndrome.[57]

Crenshaw and Kilgore[17] found that the 1-year results of patients treated with tenodesis were good to excellent in 87% of cases. Tenodesis was very effective for pain relief (obtained in 95% of patients by 3 months). Froimson[23] described an open technique for tenodesis that involved the placement of a knotted biceps tendon into a hole in the biceps groove shaped like a keyhole. He reported satisfactory results in all 11 patients (12 shoulders) at a follow-up of 24 months. The advantages of this procedure were avoidance of hardware, inherent stability (thereby allowing early movement of the shoulder and elbow), and removal of the remnant of the biceps from the joint to allow motion of the humeral head. Post and Benca[61] found excellent results with tenodesis without decompression. The Post technique involves placing the biceps tendon into a hole in the biceps groove. Sutures attached to the end of the tendon are brought out through smaller drill holes on either side but distal to the hole. These sutures are then passed back through the tendon and tied. Berlemann and Bayley,[3] in contrast, reported good results in only 9 of 15 shoulders undergoing isolated open tenodesis, with a long-term follow-up of 7 years. When comparing short-term to long-term follow-up, they found continued improvement in seven shoulders and deterioration in only two shoulders. Becker and Cofield[2] recommended biceps tenodesis in degenerated or unstable tendons but suggested that it should be accompanied by subacromial decompression.

Despite these good results, tenodesis of the biceps tendon need not be a routine procedure at the time of rotator cuff repair and subacromial decompression. Neer[53] found that acromioplasty alone relieved patients of their anterior shoulder pain despite a preoperative diagnosis of biceps tenosynovitis. Thus, he favored preserving the biceps tendon when possible to prevent the loss of the head depressor effect. In addition, many studies have shown good results with rotator cuff repair without tenodesis of the biceps tendon.[4-6,15,19,21,25,31,33,67]

More recently, a number of techniques have been described for arthroscopic tenodesis of the biceps. Gartsman and Hammerman[24] described tenodesis with sutures anchors, and Boileau[8] reported on arthroscopic tenodesis with an interference screw after pulling the tendon into the tunnel with sutures that have been delivered out the back of the shoulder by drilling through with pins.

Indications for Tenotomy or Tenodesis

We sacrifice the biceps when there is a partial tear or significant tenosynovitis (significant inflammation, atrophy, hypertrophy), subluxation, or dislocation of the tendon. The tendon is routinely sacrificed during total shoulder or humeral head replacement, especially in fracture cases.

The decision whether to perform tenodesis or tenotomy is based on the surgeon's personal preference and philosophy, as the clinical results are similar.[27] We perform tenotomy in elderly patients and in those for whom cosmesis is not a concern. Tenotomy is a relatively simple surgical procedure with easier rehabilitation. There may also be a role for tenotomy in providing pain relief from massive rotator cuff tears in the elderly. Tenodesis is performed on younger (typically younger than 50 years), more active patients, in those requiring upper extremity strength (such as manual laborers), and in those for whom cosmesis is of concern. Tenodesis tends to avoid the temporary ache or spasm that may accompany tenotomy, but active flexion must be temporarily limited following tenodesis.

Surgical Technique

Anesthesia and Positioning

All surgical procedures are performed in a routine manner. Once the patient has been brought into the operating room, anesthesia is administered in the form of an interscalene regional block. This may require augmentation with local anesthetic in the region of the portals, superiorly and medially along the acromioclavicular joint. The patient is placed upright in the beach chair position and secured to the table, and the arm is placed in an arm holder.

Diagnostic Arthroscopy

A standard posterior portal is created. The arthroscope is inserted, and the site for an anterior working portal is identified using a spinal needle placed lateral to the coracoid. The anterior portal enters the joint above the subscapularis tendon and below the biceps.

The biceps is carefully evaluated for evidence of pathology. A probe brought in through the anterior portal is positioned above the biceps tendon to pull it into the joint and allow visualization of the intertubercular segment (Fig. 21–7). The arthroscope should be advanced anteriorly and the view directed laterally to allow better visualization. Forward elevation of the arm may also assist visualization. Dragging the intertubercular segment of the biceps into the joint is particularly important to avoid missing otherwise unseen pathologic changes (Fig. 21–8). The remainder of the glenohumeral inspection identifies any other intra-articular pathology, especially of the rotator cuff.

Specific Surgical Steps

If there is a partial tear of the biceps or significant inflammation and a tenotomy is planned, it is performed at this point. An arthroscopic scissors or punch is introduced through the anterior working portal. The tendon is transected as laterally as possible to avoid an intra-articular fragment. The tendon is now able to retract distally into the bicipital groove. This can be aided by extending the elbow. The glenoid-sided remnant of the tendon is debrided back to the biceps anchor with a shaver.

If there is a partial tear of the biceps and a tenodesis is planned, a spinal needle is inserted percutaneously to

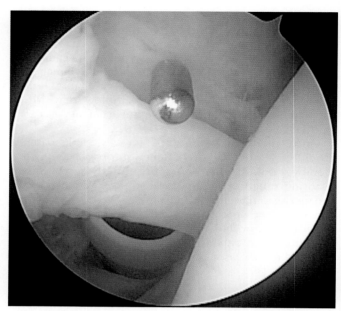

Figure 21–7 Probe through the anterior portal overlying the biceps tendon.

skewer the biceps tendon. Absorbable traction sutures (number 0 PDS) are introduced through the spinal needle and retrieved through the anterior cannula. The intra-articular portion of the biceps is then transected medially to maintain as much length as possible (Fig. 21–9).

If the portion of the tendon pulled into the joint from the groove is synovitic or constricted, and a release of the biceps sheath with debridement (tendon decompression) is planned, no further glenohumeral work is done, and the tendon is not released.

The arthroscope is removed from the glenohumeral joint. The blunt scope obturator is reinserted into the posterior portal and directed superiorly, aiming just inferior to the posterior edge of the acromion. The camera is inserted to visualize the subacromial space. A lateral portal is created two fingerbreadths lateral and about 1 cm posterior to the anterolateral corner of the acromion. The subacromial space is evaluated, and any concomitant pathology is addressed. In particular, a bursectomy and, if appropriate, an acromioplasty are performed. The bursectomy aids in visualization of the biceps sheath and should be taken far anteriorly and laterally. Good visualization is required to prevent injury to the underlying biceps tendon.

If a decompression or tenodesis is planned, the biceps is identified by rolling a probe over the sheath and feeling and seeing the underlying tendon bulge side to side. It can also be identified by shaving down anterolaterally until the pectoralis major tendon is identified. The biceps lies just medial to the pectoralis tendon and can be traced back up.

An additional anterolateral portal is placed over the bicipital groove. With the camera in the subacromial space, a spinal needle is used to localize the correct position and working angle of this portal. The anterior aspect

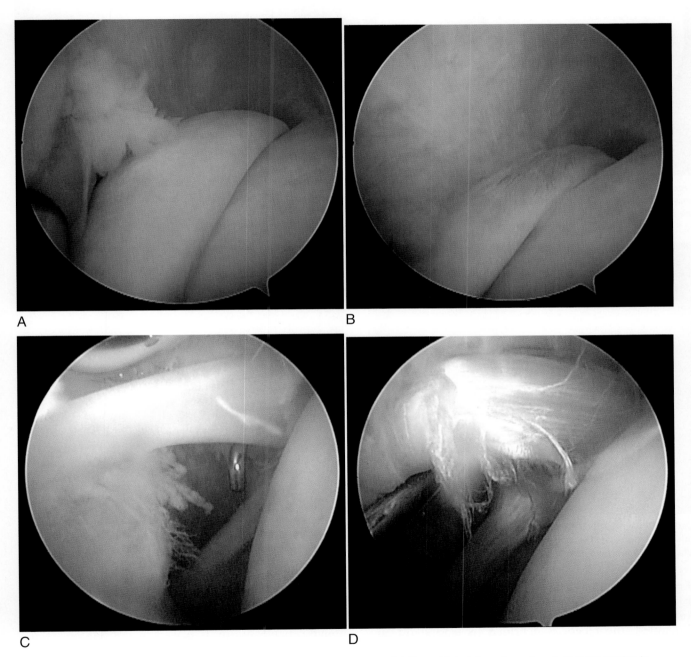

Figure 21–8 Pulling the biceps into the joint. *A*, Normal-appearing biceps. *B*, Inflamed intertubercular segment after the tendon is pulled into the joint. *C*, Normal-appearing tendon. *D*, Partial tear noted after the tendon has been pulled in with a grasper.

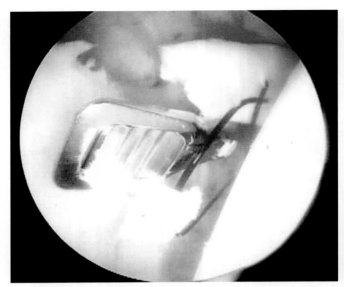

Figure 21–9 Release of the tendon should be as medial as possible to maintain length. Note the number 2 PDS stay suture in the lateral end.

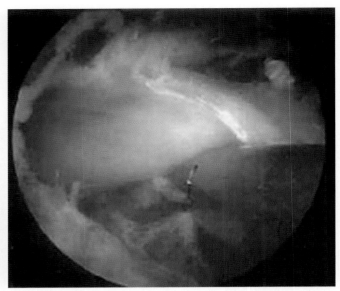

Figure 21–11 Biceps tendon visualized after complete sheath release.

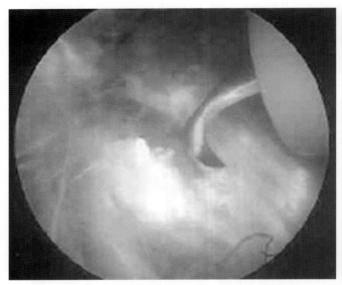

Figure 21–10 Bicipital sheath overlying the groove is released with a hook-tip bovie. The arthroscope and instruments are in the subacromial subdeltoid space.

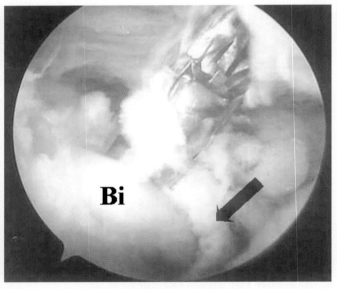

Figure 21–12 Tendon being retrieved from the groove with a grasper. Arrow indicates the released sheath. Bi, biceps.

of the sheath is then divided using an arthroscopic blade or hooked electrocautery device introduced through this portal (Figs. 21–10 and 21–11). If a decompression alone is planned, the biceps is debrided by teasing off any adherent synovium with a clamp or lightly with the shaver.

If a tenodesis is planned, the biceps is nudged out of the groove with a grasper (Fig. 21–12). The traction sutures are retrieved (Fig. 21–13), and the sutures and biceps are pulled up out of the groove through the anterolateral (biceps) portal after the cannula is removed (Fig. 21–14). The tendon is then shortened about 2 cm to create the appropriate muscle tension for the tenodesis. The tendon is sized using a sizing tunnel

(on the thumb-piece attachment to the Arthrex biotenodesis screwdriver [Arthrex, Inc., Naples, FL]) (Fig. 21–15). A baseball stitch or whipstitch, using number 2 nonabsorbable suture, is placed in the tendon, taking care to leave one end of the suture significantly longer than the other. The prepared biceps tendon in now pushed back down through the portal, leaving the free ends of the suture outside the skin. The cannula is reinserted into the biceps portal, and a guide pin is drilled into the anterior cortex of the biceps groove to a depth of 30 mm through this portal. A cannulated acorn reamer is inserted and drilled over this pin to the same depth. The size of the reamer corresponds to the width of the tendon (Fig. 21–16).

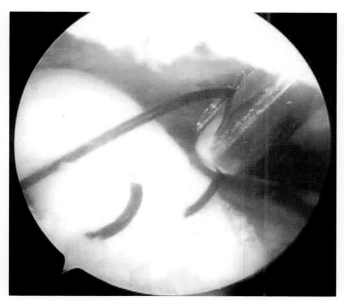

Figure 21–13 Stay suture from the end of the tendon being retrieved with a grasper.

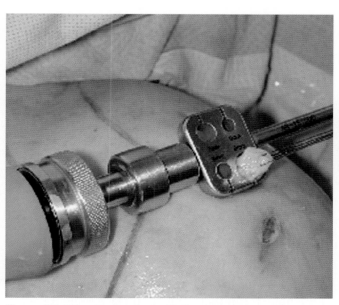

Figure 21–15 Tendon sized with the sizing device on the biotenodesis screwdriver.

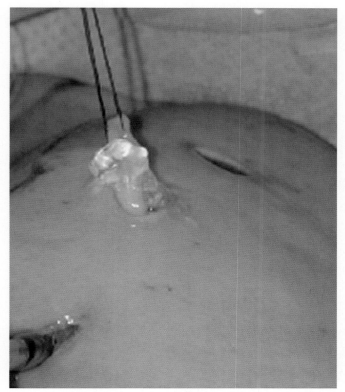

Figure 21–14 Biceps tendon delivered out of the anterolateral (biceps) portal after removal of the cannula.

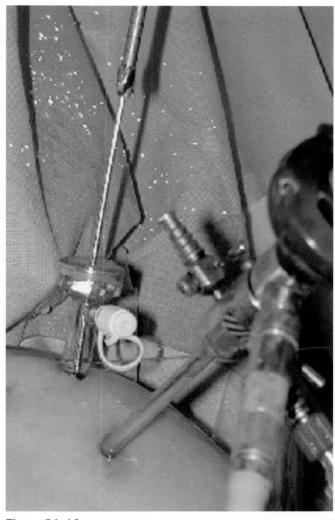

Figure 21–16 Cannulated reamer placed over a guidewire to drill a socket in the bicipital groove.

The biotenodesis interference screws are available in three sizes (7 by 23 mm, 8 by 23 mm, and 9 by 23 mm). A screw 1 mm larger than the width of the tendon is chosen. This is placed on the cannulated screwdriver. There is an additional cannulated thumb holder attachment that fits over the screwdriver but sits proximal to the screw. A flexible guidewire (with a distal loop) is passed through the screwdriver. The long free end of the suture is retrieved through the cannula and placed through the loop (Fig. 21–17), and the wire with the suture is pulled out the top end of the screwdriver. The screw, on the screwdriver, is then placed down the portal (Fig. 21–18). Tension is placed on the suture to control the tendon. The tendon is placed into the prepared hole, and the screw is slowly tightened. The thumb attachment holds the tendon down while it is being screwed in, thus preventing it from spinning. The screw is tightened until a good interference fit is achieved (Fig. 21–19). As a final step, the tendon is checked with a probe to ensure appropriate fixation.

If a "biotenodesis tray" is not available, a suture anchor can be used to shuttle the tendon into the hole and held while the interference screw is placed. A suture anchor is placed at the base of the drilled hole. One suture limb is whipstitched into the end of the tendon. By pulling on the other suture limb, the tendon is pulled to the base of the hole. It can then be held in place while the screw is inserted (Fig. 21–20).

The portals are closed with 4-0 Monocryl subcuticular sutures and Steri-strips. The wound is dressed with non-adhesive gauze and reinforced pads. The arm is placed in a padded foam sling, and the patient is discharged on oral analgesics.

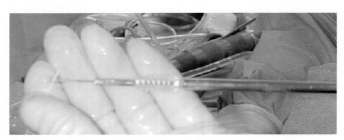

Figure 21–17   Number 2 suture placed through a wire loop to be threaded through the screwdriver. Note that the screw is already in place on the screwdriver.

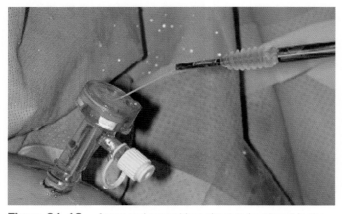

Figure 21–18   Screw and screwdriver about to be placed in the cannula.

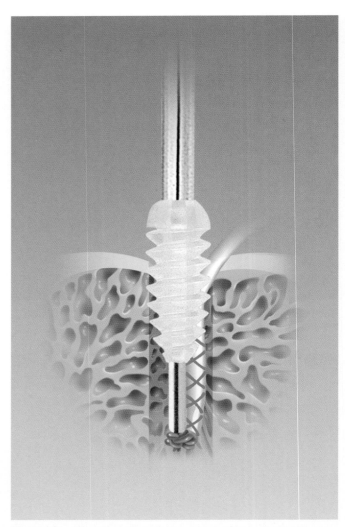

Figure 21–19   Illustration of the screw being inserted in the socket. The tendon is kept firmly seated at the base of the socket by the tip of the screwdriver, and the long end of the whipstitched suture passes through the cannulated screwdriver. (Courtesy of Arthrex, Inc., Naples, FL.)

Pearls and Pitfalls

1. It may be difficult to identify the biceps tendon and sheath. To help identify it, a thorough bursectomy should be performed. This includes following and removing the bursa anteriorly over the sheath. With the camera in the glenohumeral joint, a spinal needle can be used (inserted through the subacromial space) to spear the tendon and help locate it. Additionally, a suture can be passed through the tendon for identification. Also, the pectoralis major tendon serves as a landmark for the underlying biceps tendon.

2. If the tendon is too thin, it can be doubled over and sutured to itself. In this case, sufficient initial length must be maintained.

3. The whipstitch should have one long end and one short end. It is important to maintain one end as long as possible, because it has to fit up the entire length

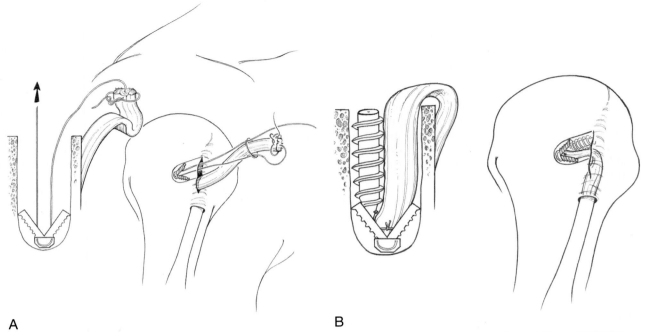

A   B

Figure 21–20   Illustration of suture anchor being used as a pulley system for interference screw tenodesis. *A,* Suture anchor at the base of the socket serves as a pulley to draw the tendon into the hole. *B,* The tendon is pulled tightly to the base of the socket and interference screw.

of the screwdriver. If this stitch is too short, it will be difficult to retrieve from the end of the screwdriver. Once it is delivered out the end of the screwdriver, a clamp should be placed on the end of the suture.

Open Technique

Open tenodesis techniques may still be required when an associated open shoulder procedure is being performed. This may be the case in some rotator cuff repair situations, such as revision surgery or for an athlete in whom the strongest possible repair is desirable. These repairs are achieved through a deltoid split. The biceps groove can be delivered into the wound by externally rotating the arm. The same technique described arthroscopically can then be performed as an open procedure.

Postoperative Management

Rehabilitation follows standard postoperative rotator cuff protocols and aims to control pain and inflammation, restore range of motion through stretching, and regain strength of the shoulder muscles. Because stiffness is not common following arthroscopy, achieving early motion (in the first 2 to 3 weeks) is not critical. Early passive elbow and wrist range-of-motion exercises are allowed, but active flexion of the elbow is restricted for 6 weeks to protect the tenodesis. Active extension of the elbow is permitted. After 6 to 8 weeks, active range-of-motion and strengthening exercises are commenced. Further rehabilitation depends on concomitant surgery, especially rotator cuff repair.

Results of Tenodesis

This is a relatively new technique, and although there are no long-term results to report, we have found the short-term results to be promising.

Complications

Wound infections are rare and usually superficial. A persistent deep infection requires immediate arthroscopic irrigation and debridement and a course of intravenous antibiotics. Extension of infection down the biceps sheath may require open debridement. Oozing and bleeding may require only dressing changes; however, infection is always suspected in a patient with prolonged drainage.

Persistent pain may follow tenodesis. It may be due to fixation devices, such as screws or suture knots, but it is usually self-limited. There is some anecdotal evidence that absorbable devices may incite an inflammatory reaction as they begin to resorb. Often ice, anti-inflammatory medication, and activity modification are sufficient to settle symptoms. There is always a risk of tenodesis failure, which may leave the patient with a cosmetic deformity.

Future Directions

Clearly, a better understanding of the functional role of the long head of the biceps is needed if we are to arrive at a consensus about the need for biceps preservation.

As science evolves, the ability to treat and heal the biceps in situ may develop, negating the need for tenodesis. Until then, critical evaluations of clinical outcomes must be collected to determine the most effective treatment options to relieve the pain caused by biceps disease. Some believe that the site for tenodesis should not be in the bicipital groove. It has been suggested that the groove may be part of the pathology and that tenodesis within the groove may not relieve symptoms. Tenodesis in an area away from the pathology, such as just distal to the pectoralis major tendon insertion, may be preferable (B. Cole, A. Romeo, personal communication, 2002).

Open tenodesis has demonstrated reliable results. As skills improve, arthroscopic techniques for tenodesis are becoming more popular. The development of instrumentation and devices has facilitated surgical techniques. Arthroscopic procedures reduce the morbidity of surgery, with less soft tissue dissection, and can be performed as outpatient procedures.

References

1. Andrews JR, Carson WG Jr, McLeod WD: Glenoid labrum tears related to the long head of the biceps. Am J Sports Med 13:337-341, 1985.
2. Becker DA, Cofield RH: Tenodesis of the long head of the biceps brachii for chronic bicipital tendonitis: Long-term results [see comments]. J Bone Joint Surg Am 71:376-381, 1989.
3. Berlemann U, Bayley I: Tenodesis of the long head of biceps brachii in the painful shoulder: Improving results in the long term. J Shoulder Elbow Surg 4:429-435, 1995.
4. Bigliani LU, Cordasco FA, McIlveen SJ, et al: Operative treatment of failed repairs of the rotator cuff. J Bone Joint Surg Am 74:1505-1515, 1992.
5. Bigliani LU, D'Alessandro DF, Duralde XA, et al: Anterior acromioplasty for subacromial impingement in patients younger than 40 years of age. Clin Orthop 246:111-116, 1989.
6. Bjorkenheim JM, Paavolainen P, Ahovuo J, et al: Surgical repair of the rotator cuff and surrounding tissues: Factors influencing the results. Clin Orthop 236:148-153, 1988.
7. Blasier RB, Guldberg RE, Rothman ED: Anterior shoulder stability: Contributions of rotator cuff forces and capsular ligaments in a cadaver model. J Shoulder Elbow Surg 1:140-150, 1992.
8. Boileau P: Arthroscopic biceps tenodesis: A new technique using bioabsorbable interference screw fixation. Tech Shoulder Elbow Sug 2:153-165, 2001.
9. Burkhead WZ Jr: The biceps tendon. In Rockwood CA Jr, Matsen FA III (eds): The Shoulder. Philadelphia, WB Saunders, 1990, pp 791-836.
10. Carroll RE, Hamilton LR: Rupture of biceps brachii: A conservative method of treatment. J Bone Joint Surg Am 49:1016, 1967.
11. Cervilla V Schweitzer ME, Ho C, et al: Medial dislocation of the biceps brachii tendon: Appearance at MR imaging. Radiology 180:523-526, 1991.
12. Chan TW, Dalinka MK, Kneeland JB, et al: Biceps tendon dislocation: Evaluation with MR imaging. Radiology 179:649-652, 1991.
13. Clark J, Sidles JA, Matsen FA: The relationship of the gleno-humeral joint capsule to the rotator cuff. Clin Orthop 254:29-34, 1990.
14. Clark JM, Harryman DT 2nd: Tendons, ligaments, and capsule of the rotator cuff: Gross and microscopic anatomy. J Bone Joint Surg Am 74:713-725, 1992.
15. Cofield RH: Tears of rotator cuff. Instr Course Lect 30:258-273, 1981.
16. Cone RO, Danzig L, Resnick D, et al: The bicipital groove: Radiographic, anatomic, and pathologic study. AJR Am J Roentgenol 141:781-788, 1983.
17. Crenshaw A, Kilgore W: Surgical treatment of bicipital tenosynovitis. J Bone Joint Surg Am 48:1496-1502, 1966.
18. DePalma A, Callery G: Bicipital tenosynovitis. Clin Orthop 3:69-85, 1954.
19. Ellman H, Hanker G, Bayer M: Repair of the rotator cuff: End-result study of factors influencing reconstruction. J Bone Joint Surg Am 68:1136-1144, 1986.
20. Erickson SJ, Fitzgerald SW, Quinn SF, et al: Long bicipital tendon of the shoulder: Normal anatomy and pathologic findings on MR imaging. AJR Am J Roentgenol 158:1091-1096, 1992.
21. Essman JA, Bell RH, Askew M: Full-thickness rotator-cuff tear: An analysis of results. Clin Orthop 265:170-177, 1991.
22. Flannigan B, Kursunoglu-Brahme S, Snyder S, et al: MR arthrography of the shoulder: Comparison with conventional MR imaging. AJR Am J Roentgenol 155:829-832, 1990.
23. Froimson AI: Keyhold tenodesis of biceps origin at the shoulder. Clin Orthop 112:245-249, 1975.
24. Gartsman GM, Hammerman SM: Arthroscopic biceps tenodesis: Operative technique. Arthroscopy 16:550-552, 2000.
25. Gazielly DF, Gleyze P, Montagnon C: Functional and anatomical results after rotator cuff repair. Clin Orthop 304:43-53, 1994.
26. Gilcreest E: Dislocation and elongation of the long head of the biceps brachii: An analysis of six cases. Ann Surg 104:118-138, 1936.
27. Gill TJ, McIrvin E, Mair SD, et al: Results of biceps tenotomy for treatment of pathology of the long head of the biceps brachii. J Shoulder Elbow Surg 10:247-249, 2001.
28. Glousman R, Jobe F, Tobine J, et al: Dynamic electromyographic analysis of the throwing shoulder with glenohumeral instability. J Bone Joint Surg Am 70:220-226, 1988.
29. Glousman RE: Instability versus impingement syndrome in the throwing athlete. Orthop Clin North Am 24:89-99, 1993.
30. Habermeyer P, Schmidt-Wiethoff R, Lehmann M: [Diagnosis and therapy of shoulder instability.] Wien Med Wochenschr 146:149-154, 1996.
31. Harryman DT, Mack LA, Wang KY, et al: Repairs of the rotator cuff. Correlation of functional results with integrity of the cuff. J Bone Joint Surg Am 73:982-989, 1991.
32. Harryman DT, Sidles JA, Clark JM, et al: Translation of the humeral head on the glenoid with passive glenohumeral motion. J Bone Joint Surg Am 72:1334-1343, 1990.
33. Hawkins RJ, Misamore GW, Hobeika PE: Surgery for full-thickness rotator-cuff tears. J Bone Joint Surg Am 67:1349-1355, 1985.
34. Hitchcock HH, Bechtol CO: Painful shoulder: Observations on the role of the tendon of the long head of the biceps brachii in its causation. J Bone Joint Surg Am 30:263-273, 1948.
35. Itoi E, Ruechle DK, Newman SR, et al: Stabilising function of the biceps in stable and unstable shoulders. J Bone Joint Surg Br 75:546-550, 1993; erratum in J Bone Joint Surg Br 76:170, 1994.

36. Itoi E, Motzkin NE, Morrey BK, et al: Stabilizing function of the long head of the biceps in the hanging arm position. J Shoulder Elbow Surg 3:135-142, 1994.

37. Jobe FW, Kvitne RS, Giangarra CE: Shoulder pain in the overhand or throwing athlete: The relationship of anterior instability and rotator cuff impingement. Orthop Rev 18:963-975, 1989; erratum in Orthop Rev 18:1268, 1989.

38. Kannus P, Jozsa L: Histopathological changes preceding spontaneous rupture of a tendon: A controlled study of 891 patients. J Bone Joint Surg Br 71:272-274, 1991.

39. Kennedy JC, Willis RB: The effects of local steroid injections on tendons: A biomechanical and microscopic correlative study. Am J Sports Med 4:11-21, 1976.

40. Kumar VP, Satku K, Balasubramaniam P: The role of the long head of biceps brachii in the stabilization of the head of the humerus. Clin Orthop 244:172-175, 1989.

41. Lapidus PW, Guidotti FP: Local injection of hydrocortisone in 495 orthopedic patients. Int Med Surg 26:234-244, 1957.

42. Levy AS, Kelly BT, Lintner SA, et al: Function of the long head of the biceps at the shoulder: Electromyographic analysis. J Shoulder Elbow Surg 10:250-255, 2001.

43. Lippitt SB, Vanderhooft J, Harris S, et al: Glenohumeral stability from concavity compression: A quantitative analysis. J Shoulder Elbow Surg 2:27-35, 1993.

44. Lippmann R: Bicipital tenosynovitis. N Y State J Med 44:2235-2240, 1944.

45. Malicky DM, Soslowsky LJ, Blasier RB, et al: Anterior glenohumeral stabilization factors: Progressive effects in a biomechanical model. J Orthop Res 14:282-288, 1996.

46. Mariani EM, Cofield RH, Askew LJ: Rupture of the tendon of the long head of the biceps brachii: Surgical versus nonsurgical treatment. Clin Orthop 228:233-239, 1988.

47. Massengill AD, Seeger LL, Yao L, et al: Labrocapsular ligamentous complex of the shoulder: Normal anatomy, anatomic variation, and pitfalls of MR imaging and MR arthrography. Radiographics 14:1211-1223, 1994.

48. Michele A: Bicipital tenosynovitis. Clin Orthop 18:261-267, 1960.

49. Middleton WD, Reinus WR, Totty WG, et al: Ultrasonographic evaluation of the rotator cuff and biceps tendon. J Bone Joint Surg Am 68:440-450, 1986.

50. Middleton WD, Reinus WR, Totty WG, et al: US of the biceps tendon apparatus. Radiology 157:211-215, 1985.

51. Murthi AM, Vosburgh CL, Neviaser TJ: The incidence of pathologic changes of the long head of the biceps tendon. J Shoulder Elbow Surg 9:382-385, 2000.

52. Neer CS II: Shoulder Reconstruction. Philadelphia, WB Saunders, 1990.

53. Neer CS: Anterior acromioplasty for the chronic impingement syndrome in the shoulder: A preliminary report. J Bone Joint Surg Am 54:41-50, 1972.

54. Neviaser RJ: Lesions of the biceps and tendonitis of the shoulder. Orthop Clin North Am 11:343-348, 1980.

55. Neviaser TJ: Arthrography of the shoulder. Orthop Clin North Am 11:205-217, 1980.

56. Neviaser TJ: The role of the biceps tendon in the impingement syndrome. Orthop Clin North Am 18:383-386, 1987.

57. Neviaser TJ, Neviaser RJ, Neviaser JS: The four-in-one arthroplasty for the painful arc syndrome. Clin Orthop 163:107-112, 1982.

58. Pagnani MJ, Deng XH, Warren RF, et al: Effect of lesions of the superior portion of the glenoid labrum on glenohumeral translation. J Bone Joint Surg Am 77:1003-1010, 1995.

59. Petersson CJ: Spontaneous medial dislocation of the tendon of the long biceps brachii: An anatomic study of prevalence and pathomechanics. Clin Orthop 211:224-227, 1986.

60. Pfahler M, Branner S, Refior HJ: The role of the bicipital groove in tendopathy of the long biceps tendon. J Shoulder Elbow Surg 8:419-424, 1999.

61. Post M, Benca P: Primary tendonitis of the long head of the biceps. Clin Orthop 246:117-125, 1989.

62. Rathburn J, MacNab I: The microvascular pattern of the rotator cuff. J Bone Joint Surg Br 52:540-553, 1970.

63. Rockwood CA, Lyons FR: Shoulder impingement syndrome: Diagnosis, radiographic evaluation, and treatment with a modified Neer acromioplasty [see comments]. J Bone Joint Surg Am 75:409-424, 1993.

64. Rodosky MW, Harner CD, Fu FH: The role of the long head of the biceps muscle and superior glenoid labrum in anterior stability of the shoulder. Am J Sports Med 22:121-130, 1994.

65. Teefey SA, Hasan SA, Middleton WD, et al: Ultrasonography of the rotator cuff: A comparison of ultrasonographic and arthroscopic findings in one hundred consecutive cases. J Bone Joint Surg Am 82:498-504, 2000.

66. Thomazeau H, Gleyze P, Frank A, et al: [Arthroscopic debridement of full-thickness tears of the rotator cuff: A retrospective multicenter study of 283 cases with 3-year follow-up.] Rev Chir Orthop Reparatrice Appar Mot 86:136-142, 2000.

67. Tibone JE, Elrod B, Jobe FW, et al: Surgical treatment of tears of the rotator cuff in athletes. J Bone Joint Surg Am 68:887-891, 1986.

68. Ting A, Jobe FW, Barto P, et al: An EMG analysis of the lateral biceps in shoulders with rotator cuff tears. Orthop Trans 11:237, 1987.

69. Vangsness CT Jr, Jorgenson SS, Watson T, et al: The origin of the long head of the biceps from the scapula and glenoid labrum: An anatomical study of 100 shoulders. J Bone Joint Surg Br 76:951-954, 1994.

70. Walch G, Nove-Josserand L, Boileau P, et al: Subluxations and dislocations of the tendon of the long head of the biceps. J Shoulder Elbow Surg 7:100-108, 1998.

71. Walch G, Nove-Josserand L, Levigne C, et al: Tears of the supraspinatus tendon associated with "hidden" lesions of the rotator interval. J Shoulder Elbow Surg 3:353-360, 1994.

72. Warner JJ, McMahon PJ: The role of the long head of the biceps brachii in superior stability of the glenohumeral joint. J Bone Joint Surg Am 77:366-372, 1995.

73. Werner A, Wuellar T, Boehm D, et al: The stabilizing sling for the long head of the biceps tendon in the rotator cuff interval: A histoanatomic study. Am J Sports Med 28:28-31, 2000.

74. Yamaguchi K, Riew RD, Galatz LM, et al: Biceps activity during shoulder motion: An electromyographic analysis. Clin Orthop 336:122-129, 1997.

75. Yergason R: Supination sign. J Bone Joint Surg 13:160, 1931.

CHAPTER

22

Rotator Cuff: Diagnosis and Decision Making

Ian K. Y. Lo and Stephen S. Burkhart

Rotator cuff disease has long been recognized as a common cause of shoulder pain in adults.[25,53,54,72,92,93,95] Despite recent advances in the arthroscopic treatment of rotator cuff disease, our knowledge of its cause and pathogenesis remains in its infancy.[5,25,53,54,92,93,95,96,103] The clinical severity of rotator cuff pathology may be regarded as a spectrum of disease from isolated bursitis and impingement to complete, irreparable rotator cuff tears.[*] The purpose of this chapter is to briefly review the assessment and treatment of full-thickness rotator cuff tears as they pertain to arthroscopic surgeons. The reader is referred to previous chapters for a complete discussion of impingement and impingement lesions.

◼ Anatomy, Pathoanatomy, and Biomechanics

The rotator cuff is formed from the tendinous insertions of the subscapularis, supraspinatus, infraspinatus, and teres minor muscles. Although these musculotendinous units have traditionally been described as discrete anatomic structures, the tendons of the rotator cuff fuse as one continuous band near their insertions into the tuberosities of the humerus.[26,44] This unique organization suggests that the muscles of the rotator cuff act in concert to provide the shoulder with normal joint kinematics.[26,44,96]

When observed from a glenohumeral arthroscopic view, the articular surface of the intact rotator cuff demonstrates an arching, cable-like thickening of the capsule surrounding a thinner crescent of tissue that inserts into the greater tuberosity of the humerus (Fig. 22–1).[13,22] This cable-like structure extends from its anterior attachment just posterior to the biceps tendon to the inferior border of the infraspinatus tendon posteriorly

(Fig. 22–2).[13,22] Similar to a load-bearing suspension bridge, the rotator cable transfers the stress from the supraspinatus and infraspinatus muscles by directing the force along the cable to its terminal insertions, effectively stress-shielding the thinner, weaker rotator crescent tissue.[10,20]

The primary mechanical function of the rotator cuff is to balance the force couples about the glenohumeral joint to provide a stable fulcrum of motion and functional glenohumeral kinematics.[9,10,14,24] Inman et al.[57] first described the coronal plane force couple as one in which the deltoid is balanced by the inferior portion of the rotator cuff (Fig. 22–3). However, more important clinically is the transverse plane force couple, where the anterior cuff (subscapularis) is balanced by the posterior cuff (infraspinatus and teres minor) (Fig. 22–4).[9,10,14,24] Rotator cuff tears involving most of the anterior cuff or most of the posterior rotator cuff may result in unstable kinematic patterns.[8] Thus, balancing both the transverse and coronal plane force couples is essential to provide a stable fulcrum for glenohumeral joint motion.[8-10,14,24,57]

Similar to the intact rotator cuff, a rotator cuff tear can also be likened to a suspension bridge, with the free margin of the tear corresponding to the cable, and the anterior and posterior attachments of the tear corresponding to the supports at each end of the cable's span (Fig. 22–5).[9,10,13,22] Such a model would predict that despite a tear of the supraspinatus tendon, the supraspinatus muscle can still exert a force on the humerus by means of its distributed load along the span of the suspension bridge configuration.[9,10,13,22] These observations, combined with our knowledge of the importance of balancing the force couples of the glenohumeral joint, explain why certain rotator cuff tears (termed *functional* rotator cuff tears), despite being massive in size, may demonstrate "normal" kinematic patterns[8] and why good results can be achieved after repair or partial repair even though a watertight

---

*See references 2, 5, 41, 53-55, 74, 92, 93, 95, 96, 103.

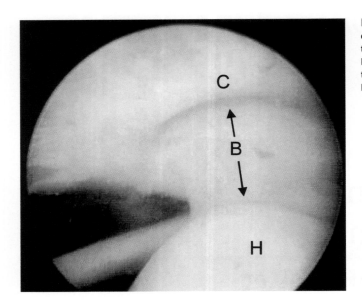

Figure 22–1 Arthroscopic view of a right shoulder demonstrating a cable-like thickening of the capsule surrounding a thinner crescent of tissue *(arrows)* that inserts into the greater tuberosity of the humerus. Note: The figure is oriented in the beach chair position, with the head of the patient toward the top. B, rotator crescent; C, rotator cable; H, humeral head.

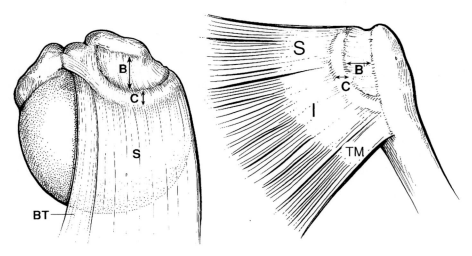

Figure 22–2 Superior and posterior projections of the rotator cable and crescent. The rotator cable extends from the biceps to the inferior margin of the infraspinatus, spanning the supraspinatus and infraspinatus insertions. B, mediolateral diameter of rotator crescent; BT, biceps tendon; C, width of rotator cable; I, infraspinatus; S, supraspinatus; TM, teres minor.

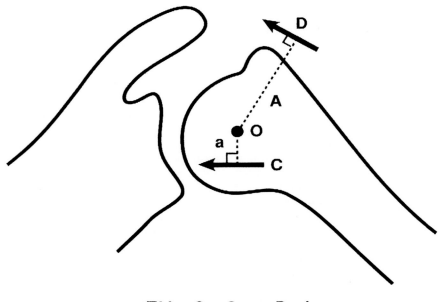

Figure 22–3 Coronal plane force couple. The inferior portion of the rotator cuff (below the center of rotation) creates a moment that must balance the deltoid moment. a, moment arm of the inferior portion of the rotator cuff; A, moment arm of the deltoid; C, resultant of rotator cuff forces; D, deltoid force; O, center of rotation.

$$\Sigma M_o = O = C \times a - D \times A$$
$$D \times A = C \times a$$

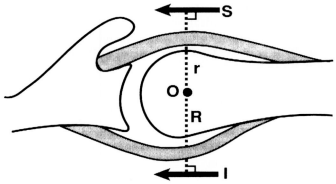

$$\Sigma M_O = O = IxR - Sxr$$
$$\therefore IxR = Sxr$$

Figure 22–4   Transverse plane force couple (axillary view). The subscapularis anteriorly is balanced against the infraspinatus and teres minor posteriorly. I, infraspinatus; O, center of rotation; r, moment arm of the subscapularis; R, moment arm of the infraspinatus and teres minor; S, subscapularis.

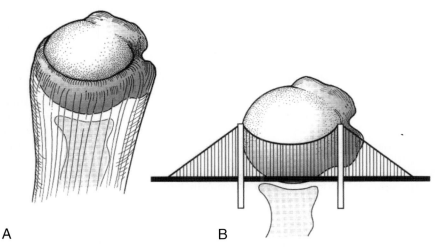

A   B

Figure 22–5   A rotator cuff tear *(A)* can be likened to a suspension bridge *(B)*. The free margin corresponds to the cable, and the anterior and posterior attachments of the tear correspond to the supports at each end of the cable's span.

closure is not obtained.[14,24,37,49,86,100] It should be emphasized, however, that complete closure and complete healing of the rotator cuff achieves functional results superior to those achieved with partial closure or partial healing of the rotator cuff with a persistent defect.[14,24,37,49,86,100]

Historical Aspects

The incidence of full-thickness tears of the rotator cuff has been reported to range from 5% to 40%.* Although there is an increasing incidence with age, the presence of a rotator cuff defect is not necessarily correlated with significant clinical symptoms. For example, magnetic resonance imaging (MRI) evidence of rotator cuff tears (full or partial thickness) may be found in up to 54% of asymptomatic individuals older than 60 years.[94] These

*See references 25, 27, 53, 54, 60, 61, 79, 83, 84, 89, 92, 93, 95, 103, 108.

results emphasize the fact that some individuals may demonstrate "normal" clinical function despite a rotator cuff tear, and they highlight the danger of basing clinical decisions on MRI evidence alone.

Why some individuals are able to "cope" with a rotator cuff tear and others are not is unclear. However, certain factors other than the presence of a defect in the rotator cuff may be responsible for the generation of symptoms. These include factors such as abnormal glenohumeral kinematics (as described earlier), abnormal scapular mechanics (e.g., SICK scapular syndrome [*s*capular malposition, *i*nferior medial border prominence, *c*oracoid pain and malposition, dys*k*ineses of scapular movement]), inflammation (e.g., synovitis, bursitis), compensatory muscular activation, and variations in pain tolerance.[8-10,62-65,92,93]

The previous gold standard of treatment for symptomatic full-thickness rotator cuff tears was open acromioplasty and rotator cuff repair.[1-3,25,29,32,52-55,81] Although satisfactory results were achieved in more than 80% of patients, a number of potential complications,[70,71,107] including infection, stiffness, and deltoid avulsion, led to the development of other, less invasive techniques for repair.

The advent of arthroscopy has greatly enhanced our understanding and treatment of rotator cuff disorders.[13] Whereas open rotator cuff surgery is largely restricted by an anterolateral incision, arthroscopy allows an expanded view of the rotator cuff through a number of different perspectives and treatment through multiple approaches.[13] Further, arthroscopy has the advantages of preservation of the deltoid origin, improved visualization, ability to treat multiple disorders simultaneously, and minimization of the complications of open surgery.

Many of the early reports on arthroscopic treatment of full-thickness rotator cuff tears focused on arthroscopic subacromial decompression and debridement of the rotator cuff. Although early results of debridement were generally good, these results deteriorated over the long term, particularly in young, active patients.[33,34,38] As repair techniques have evolved, arthroscopic rotator cuff repair has become achievable in almost all cases, including massive rotator cuff tears (>5 cm),[15-18] and debridement has generally fallen out of favor. In fact, the results of arthroscopic rotator cuff repair have been so promising that the use of open repair as the gold standard of treatment has been challenged.[21,40,77,98,109]

Mechanism of Injury

Many patients may describe a history of trauma initiating their symptoms, but in most cases, trauma is not the only factor involved in rotator cuff tearing. Both extrinsic (e.g., subacromial impingement, internal impingement, tensile overload, repetitive stress) and intrinsic (e.g., poor vascularity, changes in matrix composition and mechanical properties, aging) factors may be involved.[5,28,36,96,102,103] However, the relative contribution of these factors in the pathogenesis of rotator cuff disease and tearing remains unclear.

The two most commonly cited causes of rotator cuff tears are subacromial impingement and tendon degeneration. In 1972, Neer[78,80] implicated the shape of the coracoacromial arch in the pathogenesis of rotator cuff disease and proposed that the anterior third of the acromion, the coracoacromial ligament, and the acromioclavicular joint might compress and damage the rotator cuff. Bigliani et al.[4] classified the acromial morphology of 140 cadavers into three different types, based on the shape of the acromion on the supraspinatus outlet view: 17% of specimens were type I (flat acromion), 43% were type II (curved acromion), and 40% were type III (hooked acromion). In type II and III acromions, there was a significant increase in rotator cuff tears. Although the controversy continues to rage over whether these findings are primary causative factors or secondary changes, it appears that abnormal contact, whether primary or secondary, may aggravate an intact but dysfunctional rotator cuff and may also compromise repair.[69,73,83,84]

The degenerative changes associated with rotator cuff tears have been well documented. Various authors have demonstrated these pathologic changes (e.g., disruption, disorganization and thinning of collagen fascicles, dystrophic calcifications, formation of granulation tissue) and have correlated the presence of these findings with a significant decrease in the ultimate tensile strength of the supraspinatus tendon insertion.[*] Thus, in patients with a degenerative rotator cuff, trivial trauma (e.g., lifting a box) can lead to a complete tear.

Clinical Evaluation

Although the presentation of patients with rotator cuff disease may appear straightforward initially, in many cases, closer clinical evaluation reveals a confusing and complex problem. In many cases, several concomitant pathologies may exist in the same patient, making it imperative that the physician differentiate and diagnose each condition and determine which ones are symptomatic. Table 22–1 summarizes the common findings in patients with rotator cuff disease and other disorders that may occur concomitantly.

History

Most patients with rotator cuff tears recall a specific incidence or repetitive injury that initiated their symptoms. However, in many cases there is also a long-standing history of intermittent shoulder pain that has become progressively symptomatic. When presenting to the physician, most patients complain of anterolateral shoulder pain that is typically aggravated by repetitive use of the arm overhead. In severe cases, pain can be constant, with a significant component of night pain, and symptoms are usually prolonged, relentless, and functionally disabling.

Physical Examination

Depending on the size and chronicity of the tear, physical examination may demonstrate atrophy of the supraspinatus and infraspinatus muscles and palpable subacromial crepitus. In most cases, patients have tenderness along the anterolateral humerus, with positive impingement signs as described by Neer[78] and Hawkins and Kennedy.[51] Although passive range of motion is generally full, in larger tears, active range of motion is typically significantly limited, with many patients demonstrating only a shoulder "shrug." Strength may also be limited, particularly in external rotation, flexion, and abduction. In addition, specific tests such as the liftoff[42,43] and Napoleon[23,66,90] tests may be positive in cases of subscapularis tendon insufficiency.

---

*See references 27, 46, 58, 69, 82, 88, 89, 92, 93, 103, 104.

Table 22-1   **History and Physical Examination Features of Conditions Associated with and Commonly Confused with Rotator Cuff Tears**

	Rotator Cuff Tendinosis		AC Joint Derangement	SLAP Lesion	Primary Glenohumeral OA
	Impingement	Cuff Tear			
History					
Trauma	+/−	+/−	+/−	+	−
Pain	Anterior, superior, lateral ↑ with overhead use	Anterior, superior, lateral ↑ with overhead use	Superior ↑ with cross-body use	Posterior, superior ↑ with overhead, throwing	Anterior, posterior ↑ at extremes of motion
Disability	Overhead activities	Overhead activities, ADLs	Cross-body activities, weight lifting	Overhead activities, overhead sports	ADLs
Physical Examination					
Tenderness	Anterior, superior, lateral	Anterior, superior, lateral	Over AC joint	Posterior, superior	Anterior, posterior
Crepitus	Subacromial	Subacromial	Acromioclavicular	—	Glenohumeral
ROM	PROM = AROM May have ↓ IR	PROM > AROM May have ↓ IR AROM ↓ in ER and FE	PROM = AROM Full ROM	PROM = AROM Full ROM Overhead athletes may have ↑ ER and ↓ IR in abduction	PROM = AROM ↓ ROM, especially IR
Strength	Normal	Weakness in ER, FE	Normal	Normal, unless with spinoglenoid cyst	Normal
Special tests	+ Impingement signs + Painful arc + Impingement test	+ Impingement signs + Painful arc + Impingement test + Drop arm +/− Liftoff test +/− Napoleon test	+ Cross-body adduction	+ Jobe relocation test + O'Brien test + Biceps load test	

AC, acromioclavicular; ADLs, activities of daily living; AROM, active range of motion; ER, external rotation; FE, forward elevation; IR, internal rotation; OA, osteoarthritis; PROM, passive range of motion; ROM, range of motion; SLAP, superior labral anterior to posterior.

Imaging

Radiographic views of the shoulder (anteroposterior views in internal and external rotation, axillary view, outlet view, 30-degree caudal tilt view) should be obtained routinely. Radiographs may demonstrate sclerosis and spur formation on the undersurface of the acromion and sclerosis and cystic changes in the region of the greater tuberosity. The acromial morphology should be classified on the supraspinatus outlet view (Fig. 22–6), and the axillary view should be carefully evaluated for an os acromionale.

In massive tears, patients may demonstrate chronic proximal migration of the humerus. Although several authors[30,31,47,53] have correlated a decrease in the acromiohumeral distance (<7 mm) with the presence of rotator cuff tearing, proximal humeral migration is best evaluated by observing a break in the arch formed by the lower border of the humeral neck and the glenoid neck (Fig. 22–7). In some cases, patients may demonstrate congenital subacromial stenosis, with a decreased acromiohumeral distance but an intact glenohumeral arch (Fig. 22–8). These findings have been associated with an increased incidence of rotator cuff tearing.[11] Finally, radiographs should be evaluated for other associated disorders, including acromioclavicular arthritis and osteoarthritis.

To evaluate the integrity of the rotator cuff, several imaging modalities have been employed, including arthrography, ultrasonography, and MRI.[45,53,54,75,101] Although arthrography and ultrasonography have demonstrated accuracy in diagnosing complete rotator cuff tears, because of their invasiveness and operator-dependent nature, they have largely been supplanted by MRI in the general practice setting.[45,53,54,75,101] MRI has high specificity (95%) and sensitivity (100%) in diagnosing full-thickness rotator cuff tears.[56] However, the ability to detect partial tears is unclear.[75] MRI can provide information on tear size, tear configuration, tendon involvement, and tear chronicity (e.g., fatty infiltration, muscular atrophy), as well as suggest whether a massive rotator cuff tear is potentially repairable (Fig. 22–9). Careful evaluation of the axial views is necessary to identify subscapularis tendon involvement (Fig. 22–10). In addition to providing information on the rotator cuff, MRI can provide information on the bone pathology

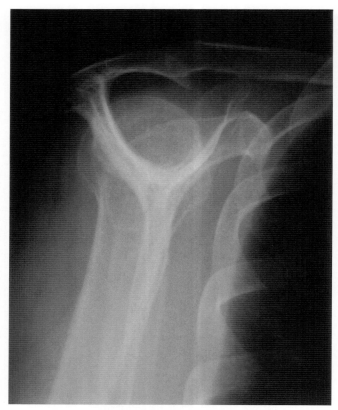

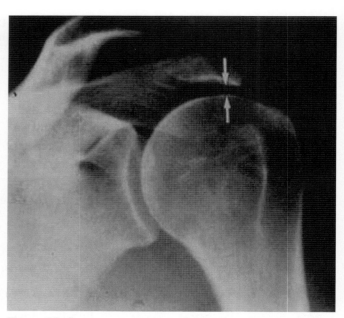

Figure 22–8 Anteroposterior radiograph demonstrating a case of congenital subacromial stenosis. Note that the inferior articular margins of the humerus and the glenoid are at the same level, implying that the narrowed acromiohumeral interval *(arrows)* is secondary to congenital subacromial stenosis.

Figure 22–6 Supraspinatus outlet radiograph demonstrating a type III acromion.

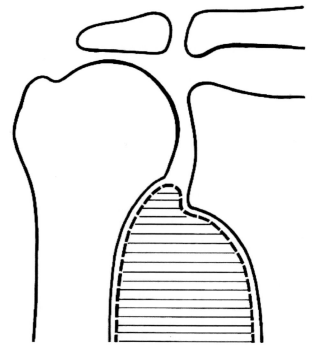

Figure 22–7 Diagrammatic representation of a true anteroposterior glenohumeral radiograph demonstrating a narrowed acromiohumeral distance with a "broken arch," signifying proximal humeral migration secondary to a rotator cuff tear.

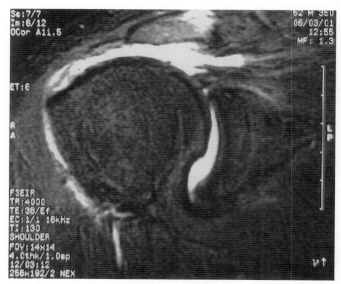

Figure 22–9 T2-weighted coronal magnetic resonance imaging scan of a right shoulder demonstrating a massive rotator cuff tear, with the rotator cuff tendon adjacent to the level of the glenoid.

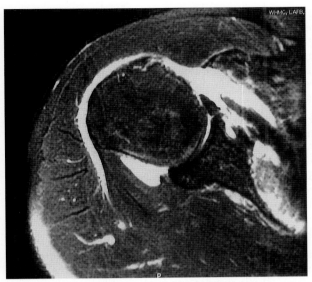

Figure 22–10 T2-weighted axial magnetic resonance imaging scan of a right shoulder demonstrating a complete tear of the subscapularis tendon.

the rotator cuff. Full-thickness rotator cuff tears (stage III impingement) can be further divided according to the tear pattern. The senior author has classified full-thickness rotator cuff tears into four major categories, according to the mobility of the margins of the rotator cuff tear (Fig. 22–11)[15-19]:

1. Crescent-shaped tears
2. U-shaped tears
3. L-shaped tears
4. Massive, contracted, immobile tears

It is critical that these tears be identified and classified during surgical repair; this allows almost all tears to be repaired arthroscopically in a tension-free manner. The reader is referred to Chapter 23 for a description of the repair of crescent-shaped, U-shaped, and L-shaped tears.

Associated Injuries

Many conditions may be associated with rotator cuff disease, including SLAP lesions, acromioclavicular joint arthritis, glenohumeral osteoarthritis, cuff tear arthropathy, and Bankart lesions.

(e.g., acromial shape), cartilage pathology (e.g., osteoarthritis), labral pathology (e.g., Bankart lesions, superior labral anterior to posterior [SLAP] lesions with or without spinoglenoid cyst), and ligamentous pathology (e.g., humeral avulsion of the glenohumeral ligament).

Treatment Options

Various treatment options exist for the management of rotator cuff tears, varying from nonoperative "benign neglect" to complex arthroscopic partial repair using an interval slide technique. Although satisfactory results may be obtained with many of these options, it should be remembered that few prospective, randomized trials exist comparing these treatments. Thus, controversy remains as to the absolute indications for each, and individual patient factors may significantly affect the final treatment decision.

Classification

Historically, Neer[79] proposed a three-stage classification of impingement syndrome and rotator cuff disease: stage I, reversible edema and hemorrhage of the rotator cuff; stage II, tendinitis and fibrosis; and stage III, tearing of

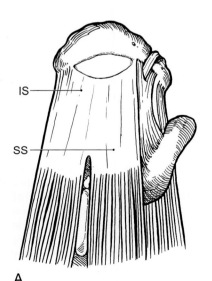
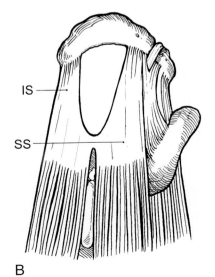
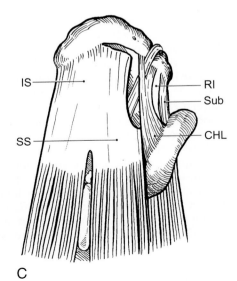

A   B   C

Figure 22–11 Superior views of various rotator cuff tear patterns. *A*, Crescent-shaped tear. *B*, U-shaped tear. *C*, L-shaped tear. CHL, coracohumeral ligament; IS, infraspinatus; RI, rotator interval; SS, supraspinatus; Sub, subscapularis.

Table 22–2	Nonoperative Modalities for the Treatment of Rotator Cuff Tears

Rest
Hot/cold therapy
Pain medications
Nonsteroidal anti-inflammatory drugs
Ultrasonography
Phonophoresis
Iontophoresis
Injection
Exercise

Nonoperative

In patients with full-thickness rotator cuff tears, particularly older, sedentary patients, a trial of nonoperative treatment may be indicated.* In a young, active patient who has suffered a traumatic tear with significant pain and functional disability, acute operative treatment should be seriously considered. Various nonoperative treatment modalities exist (Table 22–2) and should include a comprehensive exercise program (discussed later). The length of nonoperative treatment varies, depending on the degree of rotator cuff involvement and the patient's response to treatment. However, most authors agree that failure after 3 to 6 months of conservative treatment is an indication for operative intervention.†

Operative

For patients who have failed a comprehensive nonoperative treatment program or those with full-thickness rotator cuff tears who require strength for activities, operative treatment may be indicated. Since Neer's[78] description of impingement lesions in 1972, anterior acromioplasty combined with rotator cuff repair has been the foundation of treatment for full-thickness rotator cuff tears. Similarly, with the development of arthroscopic techniques, arthroscopic subacromial decompression-acromioplasty combined with arthroscopic rotator cuff repair can be considered the gold standard of treatment for full-thickness rotator cuff tears.[21,40,77,98,109] As stated previously, with proper tear pattern recognition, a tension-free rotator cuff repair to bone can be achieved arthroscopically.[21]

In rare cases, such as the so-called irreparable rotator cuff tear (i.e., a massive, contracted, immobile tear), a complete rotator cuff repair may not be achievable. In these tears, debridement of the rotator cuff was previously considered a valid treatment option.[9,10,39,85] However, with better understanding of the importance of the force couples about the shoulder, options such as partial rotator cuff repair combined with cuff mobiliza-

tion techniques (e.g., single- and double-interval slides) have yielded superior results.[13,14,24,67,99,100] In this situation, when a massive, dysfunctional, contracted, immobile rotator cuff tear is not completely repairable, the goal of partial rotator cuff repair is to achieve enough of a repair to regain overhead function. To do this, the rotator cuff repair must satisfy five biomechanical criteria[13,14,24,100]:

1. Force couples must be balanced in the coronal and transverse planes (see Figs. 22–3 and 22–4).
2. A stable fulcrum kinematic pattern must be reestablished.
3. The shoulder's "suspension bridge" must be reestablished (see Fig. 22–5).
4. The residual defect must occupy a minimal surface area.
5. The residual defect must possess edge stability.

This is achieved primarily by balancing the force couple between the anterior and posterior portions of the shoulder, which requires an intact subscapularis tendon anteriorly and an intact inferior half of the infraspinatus tendon posteriorly. Anatomically, this corresponds to the anterior and posterior attachments of the rotator cable (see Fig. 22–2).[22]

Obviously, a complete rotator cuff repair is preferable to a partial one. However, partial rotator cuff repair is a better option than tendon transfer, because partial repair respects and preserves the normal mechanics of the rotator cuff, whereas tendon transfers adversely affect shoulder mechanics.

Rehabilitation

Nonoperative

In addition to the nonoperative treatment modalities described earlier, a comprehensive exercise and rehabilitation program is essential for the success of nonoperative treatment. As described by Seltzer et al.[91] and Wirth et al.,[110] a comprehensive shoulder rehabilitation program can be divided into three distinct stages: stage I is designed to decrease inflammation while obtaining a full, painless range of motion; stage II is aimed at progressive strengthening of the rotator cuff, deltoid, and scapular stabilizers; and stage III is characterized by a progressive integration into normal unrestricted activities and sports (Table 22–3).

Operative

Rehabilitation following arthroscopic rotator cuff repair is as variable as the spectrum of repair techniques. Although some authors have implemented rotator cuff rehabilitation protocols similar to those for open repair,[40,77,98,109] because of the minimal risk of stiffness following arthroscopic repair, early range-of-motion exercises may be delayed, minimizing the risk of early postoperative repair failure.[21] In addition, in our experience, formal physical therapy is not usually required; a simple home therapy program is generally effective.[21] Table 22–4 summarizes the spectrum of rehabilitation

---

*See references 6, 50, 53, 54, 59, 76, 87, 91, 97, 101, 110.
†See references 6, 25, 50, 53, 54, 59, 76, 87, 91, 97, 101, 110.

Table 22–3	Comprehensive Exercise Rehabilitation Program for Patients with Rotator Cuff Tears	
Stage	Goal	Method
I	Decrease inflammation	Decrease inflammation using methods in Table 22–2
	Maintain range of motion	Stretching, range-of-motion exercises (pendulum exercises, rope and pulley, external rotation with stick, posterior capsular stretching)
II	Strengthening	Isotonic Theraband strengthening (deltoid, scapular stabilizers, rotator cuff, biceps, triceps)
III	Unrestricted activities	Progression to overhead activities and sports-specific exercises

Note: patients progress to the next stage once stage-specific goals have been achieved.

Table 22–4	Representative Early and Delayed Rehabilitation Protocols Following Arthroscopic Rotator Cuff Repair
Early Rehabilitation	Delayed Rehabilitation
Immobilizer for 3 wk	Immobilizer for 6 wk
Elbow/wrist ROM immediately	Elbow/wrist ROM immediately
Pendulum exercises immediately	Passive ER exercises with arm in adduction only
Shoulder shrugs immediately	
Active assisted ROM at 3-4 wk	Active and active assisted ROM at 6 wk
Pool exercises at 3-4 wk	Stretching at 6 wk
Formal physical therapy at 3-4 wk	
Rotator cuff strengthening at 7 wk	Strengthening at 12 wk (rotator cuff, deltoid, biceps, scapular stabilizers)
Deltoid strengthening after 12 wk	Consider formal physical therapy at 12 wk if necessary

ER, external rotation; ROM, range of motion.

programs following arthroscopic rotator cuff repair. The senior author uses a delayed rehabilitation program (see Table 22–4) to minimize the risk of disruption of the repair by early motion. Stiffness has not been a problem with this delayed program.

Results

Nonoperative

The overall success of nonoperative treatment of full-thickness rotator cuff tears has been reported to be as low as 32% and as high as 92%.[*] However, with longer follow-up, the results of nonoperative treatment deteriorate with time.[59] This wide disparity in satisfactory outcomes is due in part to different criteria used in determining a satisfactory outcome, different criteria used in diagnosing a rotator cuff tear, different nonoperative treatment programs and heterogenous patient populations. Various factors associated with the failure of conservative management include a delay in the initiation of nonsurgical treatment, patients with a type II or III acromion, patients >60 years of age, and patients with acromioclavicular joint symptoms.[2,3,5,87,91-98] Thus, when considering whether to initiate or continue nonoperative treatment it is important to individually assess the age, occupation, physical demands, mechanism of injury, disability, pain severity, tear morphology and tear size.

Operative

Several reports have now been published on arthroscopic subacromial decompression-acromioplasty and arthroscopic repair for full-thickness tears of the rotator cuff.[58-62] These studies demonstrated that satisfactory results were achieved in 85% to 95% of patients, with significant improvements in range motion, strength, and overall shoulder function. A recent review by the senior author[21] of 59 arthroscopic rotator cuff repairs at a mean of 3.5 years' follow-up demonstrated that good to excellent results were achieved in 95% of patients using the UCLA criteria. The results were particularly promising when considering massive rotator cuff repairs. Unlike previous reports of open rotator cuff repair, in which larger tears correlated with poorer outcomes,[49] the same percentages of good and excellent results were achieved in massive tears repaired arthroscopically as in smaller tears. The reason for superior arthroscopic results remains unclear, but it may be due in part to the ability to adequately assess the morphology and mobility of the tear pattern arthroscopically and to repair these tears according to their classification[21] (e.g., crescent-shaped vs. U-shaped). One can assume that decreased scarring and decreased deltoid morbidity with the arthroscopic approach also play a role.

Overall, the results of arthroscopic rotator cuff repair[21,40,77,98,109] are as good as, if not superior to, results in previous reports of open rotator cuff repair, with less morbidity and fewer complications. It should be remembered, however, that these reports are from expert arthroscopists, and the ability to generalize these results remains to be seen.

A 1993 report of arthroscopic debridement of massive, irreparable rotator cuff tears demonstrated improve-

---

[*]See references 6, 25, 50, 53, 54, 59, 76, 87, 91, 97, 101, 110.

ments in pain.[33] Despite improvements in range of motion, however, gains in strength and function were not achieved. In general, debridement was successful in cases in which the force couples were balanced in the transverse and coronal planes.[18,20,24] Alternatively, in patients with dysfunctional rotator cuff tears and unbalanced force couples, partial rotator cuff repair may be performed and has demonstrated significant improvements in pain, range of motion, and overall joint function.[14,24,100]

A recent review of 12 patients demonstrated that at a mean follow-up of 35.2 months after arthroscopic partial rotator cuff repair, the mean UCLA score improved from 8.9 to 31.7.[100] Good to excellent results were obtained in 83% of patients. The mean forward elevation increased to 160 degrees, with most patients obtaining overhead function. Seventeen percent of patients had fair or poor results. However, because of their poor preoperative status, even patients with fair results demonstrated significant improvements in pain and function.

Complications

The complications of arthroscopic rotator cuff repair can be divided into those related to general shoulder arthroscopy, those related to subacromial decompression, and those specifically related to arthroscopic rotator cuff repair.[105] Complications related to general shoulder arthroscopy (infection, fluid extravasation, neurovascular injury) and those related to subacromial space surgery (inadequate acromial resection, acromial fracture) have been summarized in previous chapters.

Because only a few reports have been published on arthroscopic rotator cuff repair, the data on complications are inadequate. Complications related specifically to arthroscopic rotator cuff repair have been limited to loose hardware, adhesive capsulitis, and failure of the repair.[21,40,77,98,105,109] At this point, only a few cases of each have been reported, so the incidence of each complication is unknown. However, it is clear that the rate of complications and secondary morbidity related to arthroscopic rotator cuff repair is significantly less than that associated with open repair.[21,40,70,71,77,98,105,107,109]

Loose hardware has been reported to occur in 0.75% of cases.[106] Usually, these cases can be identified intraoperatively during testing for anchor security,[77] and the incidence can be minimized by placing the anchor at an appropriate dead-man's angle.[12] Other possible hardware problems include suture breakage, anchor breakage, and knot-tying complications (e.g., suture entanglement, loose suture loops). Biodegradable poly-L-lactic acid or polyglycolic acid (PGA)–headed tacks that rely on the head of the device rather than suture for fixation of tendon to bone have a high failure rate and a significant rate of synovitis and are not recommended.[7,35,48] On the other hand, biodegradable poly-L-lactic acid suture anchors (Biocorkscrew, Arthrex, Inc., Naples, FL) with double-loaded sutures have worked very well for us and are our preferred means of fixation.

Adhesive capsulitis has been rarely reported following arthroscopic rotator cuff repair. Murray et al.[77] reported one case of adhesive capsulitis in 48 consecutive arthroscopic rotator cuff repairs, and this patient was treated nonoperatively with physical therapy.

Failure of arthroscopic rotator cuff repair has been reported to occur in 1.8% to 5.6% of cases.[21,40,77,98,109] In most instances, a persistent defect was diagnosed either clinically or during revision surgery.[21,40,77,98,109] Revision arthroscopic rotator cuff repair has been rarely reported; however, the results appear to be as good as those obtained with revision open repair.[68]

One aspect of arthroscopic rotator cuff repair that must be further defined is the presence of persistent asymptomatic defects of the rotator cuff. Similar to the results of open rotator cuff repair,[49] two studies reported a high incidence of persistent defects of the rotator cuff following arthroscopic repair.[37,86] However, excellent clinical results were still achieved, and the significance of such defects needs to be further elucidated.

Future Directions

The future of arthroscopic rotator cuff repair appears promising. Early and midterm results suggest that almost all rotator cuff tears are repairable arthroscopically and that arthroscopic rotator cuff repair is as good as, if not superior to, open rotator cuff repair. As techniques continue to evolve and progress, arthroscopic rotator cuff repair will increase in popularity and will likely extend from the hands of a few master arthroscopic surgeons to general orthopedic surgeons. Future studies will be required to determine whether these early promising results can be maintained long term and will be achievable in a general orthopedic practice.

Summary

- The primary function of the rotator cuff is to balance the force couples about the glenohumeral joint.
- Patients with shoulder pain must be carefully evaluated for rotator cuff disease and other associated pathologies.
- A trial of nonoperative treatment may be indicated in older, sedentary patients and in patients with minimal disability who do not require strength for activities.
- Arthroscopic subacromial decompression-acromioplasty combined with arthroscopic rotator cuff repair is the gold standard of treatment for repairable rotator cuff tears.
- If complete repair is not possible, partial rotator cuff repair should be considered.
- Arthroscopic rotator cuff repair is a technically demanding procedure.

References

1. Adamson GJ, Tibone JE: Ten-year assessment of primary rotator cuff repairs. J Shoulder Elbow Surg 2:57-63, 1993.

2. Arroyo JS, Flatow EL: Management of rotator cuff disease: Intact and repairable cuff. In Iannotti JP, Williams GR (eds): Disorders of the Shoulder. Diagnosis and Management. Philadelphia, Lippincott Williams & Wilkins, 1999, pp 31-56.

3. Bigliani L, Cordasco F, McIlveen S, et al: Operative repair of massive rotator cuff tears: Long term results. J Shoulder Elbow Surg 1:120-130, 1992.

4. Bigliani LU, Morrison DS, April EW: The morphology of the acromion and its relationship to rotator cuff tears. Orthop Trans 10:228, 1986.

5. Blevins FT, Djurasovic M, Flatow EL, et al: Biology of the rotator cuff tendon. Orthop Clin North Am 28:1-16, 1997.

6. Bokor DJ, Hawkins RJ, Huckell GH, et al: Results of non-operative management of full-thickness tears of the rotator cuff. Clin Orthop 294:103-110, 1993.

7. Burkart A, Imhoff AB, Roscher E: Foreign-body reaction to the bioabsorbable Suretac device. Arthroscopy 16:91-95, 2000.

8. Burkhart SS: Fluoroscopic comparison of kinematic patterns in massive rotator cuff tears: A suspension bridge model. Clin Orthop 284:144-152, 1992.

9. Burkhart SS: Arthroscopic debridement and decompression for selected rotator cuff tears: Clinical results, pathomechanics, and patient selection based on biomechanical parameters. Orthop Clin North Am 24:111-123, 1993.

10. Burkhart SS: Reconciling the paradox of rotator cuff repair versus debridement: A unified biomechanical rationale for the treatment of rotator cuff tears. Arthroscopy 10:4-19, 1994.

11. Burkhart SS: Congenital subacromial stenosis. Arthroscopy 11:63-68, 1995.

12. Burkhart SS: The deadman theory of suture anchors: Observations along a south Texas fence line. Arthroscopy 11:119-123, 1995.

13. Burkhart SS: Shoulder arthroscopy: New concepts. Clin Sports Med 15:635-653, 1996.

14. Burkhart SS: Partial repair of massive rotator cuff tears: The evolution of a concept. Orthop Clin North Am 28:125-132, 1997.

15. Burkhart SS: Arthroscopic rotator cuff repair: Indications and technique. Oper Tech Sports Med 5:204-214, 1997.

16. Burkhart SS: Arthroscopic repair of massive rotator cuff tears: Concept of margin convergence. Tech Shoulder Elbow Surg 1:232-239, 2000.

17. Burkhart SS: Current concepts: A stepwise approach to arthroscopic rotator cuff repair based on biomechanical principles. Arthroscopy 16:82-90, 2000.

18. Burkhart SS: Arthroscopic treatment of massive rotator cuff tears. Clin Orthop 390:107-118, 2001.

19. Burkhart SS, Athanasiou KA, Wirth MA: Margin convergence: A method of reducing strain in massive rotator cuff tears. Arthroscopy 12:335-338, 1996.

20. Burkhart SS, Cawley PW, Pflaster DS, et al: Symmetric tensile loading of the rotator cable: Demonstration of a stress-shielding effect on the rotator crescent. Unpublished data.

21. Burkhart SS, Danaceau SM, Pearce CE Jr: Arthroscopic rotator cuff repair: Analysis of results by tear size and by repair technique—margin convergence versus direct tendon-to-bone repair. Arthroscopy 17:905-912, 2001.

22. Burkhart SS, Esch JC, Jolson RC: The rotator crescent and rotator cable: An anatomic description of the shoulder's "suspension bridge." Arthroscopy 9:611-616, 1993.

23. Burkhart SS, Tehrany AM: Arthroscopic subscapularis tendon repair: Technique and preliminary results. Arthroscopy 18:454-463, 2002.

24. Burkhart SS, Wesley MN, Ogilvie-Harris DJ, et al: Partial repair of irreparable rotator cuff tears. Arthroscopy 10:363-370, 1994.

25. Burkhead WZ, Jr (ed): Rotator Cuff Disorders. Baltimore, Williams & Wilkins, 1996.

26. Clark JM, Harryman DT II: Tendons, ligaments, and capsule of the rotator cuff. J Bone Joint Surg Am 74:713-725, 1992.

27. Codman EA, Akerson TB: The pathology associated with rupture of the supraspinatus tendon. Ann Surg 93:348-359, 1931.

28. Cofield RH: Rotator cuff disease of the shoulder. J Bone Joint Surg Am 67:974-979, 1985.

29. Cofield RH, Parvizi J, Hoffmeyer PJ, et al: Surgical repair of chronic rotator cuff tears: A prospective long-term study. J Bone Joint Surg Am 83:71-77, 2001.

30. Cone RO III, Resnick D, Danzig L: Shoulder impingement syndrome: Radiographic evaluation. Radiology 150:29-33, 1984.

31. DeSmet AA, Ting YM: Diagnosis of rotator cuff tear on routine radiographs. J Can Assoc Radiol 28:54-57, 1977.

32. Ellman H, Hanker G, Bayer M: Repair of the rotator cuff: End-result study of factors influencing reconstruction. J Bone Joint Surg Am 63:1136-1144, 1986.

33. Ellman H, Kay SP, Wirth M: Arthroscopic treatment of full-thickness rotator cuff tears: 2- to 7- year follow-up study. Arthroscopy 9:195-200, 1993.

34. Esch JC, Ozerkis LR, Helgager JA, et al: Arthroscopic subacromial decompression to the degree of rotator cuff tear. Arthroscopy 4:241-249, 1988.

35. Freehill MQ, Harms D, Huber S, et al: PLLA tack synovitis following arthroscopic stabilization of the shoulder. Paper presented at the 69th annual meeting of the American Academy of Orthopaedic Surgeons, Feb 2002, Dallas, TX.

36. Fu FH, Harner CD, Klein AH: Shoulder impingement syndrome: A critical review, Clin Orthop 269:162-173, 1991.

37. Galatz LM, Ball CM, Teefey SA, et al: Complete arthroscopic repair of large and massive rotator cuff tears: Correlation of functional outcome with repair integrity. Paper presented at the 69th annual meeting of the American Academy of Orthopaedic Surgeons, Feb 2002, Dallas, TX.

38. Gartsman GM: Arthroscopic acromioplasty for lesions of the rotator cuff. J Bone Joint Surg Am 72:169-180, 1990.

39. Gartsman GM: Massive, irreparable tears of the rotator cuff: Results of operative debridement and subacromial decompression. J Bone Joint Surg Am 79:715-721, 1997.

40. Gartsman GM, Khan M, Hammerman SM: Arthroscopic repair of full-thickness tears of the rotator cuff. J Bone Joint Surg Am 80:832-840, 1998.

41. Gerber C: Massive rotator cuff tears. In Iannotti JP, Williams GR (eds): Disorders of the Shoulder: Diagnosis and Management. Philadelphia, Lippincott Williams & Wilkins, 1999, pp 57-92.

42. Gerber C, Hersche O, Farron A: Isolated rupture of the subscapularis tendon: Results of operative repair. J Bone Joint Surg Am 78:1015-1023, 1996.

43. Gerber C, Krushell RJ: Isolated rupture of the tendon of the subscapularis muscle: Clinical features in 16 cases. J Bone Joint Surg Br 73:389-394, 1991.

44. Gohlke F, Essigkrug B, Schmitz F: The pattern of the collagen fiber bundles of the capsule of the glenohumeral joint. J Shoulder Elbow Surg 3:111-128, 1994.

45. Greenway G, Fulmer JM: Imaging of the rotator cuff. In Burkhead WZ Jr (ed): Rotator Cuff Disorders. Baltimore, Williams & Wilkins, 1996, pp 73-99.

46. Hakagaki K, Ozaki J, Tomita Y, et al: Fatty muscle degeneration in the supraspinatus muscle after rotator cuff tear. J Shoulder Elbow Surg 5:194-200, 1996.

47. Hamada K, Fukuda H, Mikasa M, et al: Roentgenographic findings in massive rotator cuff tears: A long-term observation. Clin Orthop 259:92-96, 1990.

48. Harms D, Buss DD, Freehill MQ, et al: PLLA tack synovitis following arthroscopic stabilization of the shoulder. Paper presented at the 18th closed meeting of the American Shoulder and Elbow Society, 2001, Napa, CA.

49. Harryman DT II, Mach LA, Wang KY, et al: Repairs of the rotator cuff: Correlation of functional results with integrity of the cuff. J Bone Joint Surg Am 73:982-989, 1991.

50. Hawkins RH, Dunlop R: Nonoperative treatment of rotator cuff tears. Clin Orthop 321:178-188, 1995.

51. Hawkins RJ, Kennedy JC: Impingement syndrome in athletes. Am J Sports Med 8:151-158, 1980.

52. Hawkins RJ, Misamore GW, Hobeika PE: Surgery for full-thickness rotator-cuff tears. J Bone Joint Surg Am 67:1349-1355, 1985.

53. Iannotti JP (ed): Rotator Cuff Disorders: Evaluation and Treatment. Park Ridge, IL, American Academy of Orthopaedic Surgeons, 1991.

54. Iannotti JP (ed): The Rotator Cuff: Current Concepts and Complex Problems. Rosemont, IL, 1998, American Academy of Orthopaedic Surgeons, 1998.

55. Iannotti JP, Naranja RJ Jr, Gartsman GM: Surgical treatment of the intact and repairable cuff defect: Arthroscopic and open techniques. In Norris TR (ed): Orthopaedic Knowledge Update: Shoulder and Elbow. Rosemont, IL, American Academy of Orthopaedic Surgeons, 1997, pp 151-155.

56. Iannotti JP, Zlatkin MB, Esterhai JL, et al: Magnetic resonance imaging of the shoulder: Sensitivity, specificity, and predictive value. J Bone Joint Surg Am 73:17-29, 1991.

57. Inman VT, Saunders JB, Abbott LC: Observations on the function of the shoulder joint. J Bone Joint Surg Am 26:1-30, 1944.

58. Ishii H, Brunet JA, Welsh RP, et al: "Bursal reactions" in rotator cuff tearing, the impingement syndrome, and calcifying tendonitis. J Shoulder Elbow Surg 6:131-136, 1997.

59. Itoi E, Tabata S: Conservative treatment of rotator cuff tears. Clin Orthop 275:165-173, 1992.

60. Keyes EL: Observations on rupture of the supraspinatus tendon: Based upon a study of 73 cadavers. Ann Surg 97:840-856, 1933.

61. Keyes EL: Anatomical observations on senile changes in the shoulder. J Bone Joint Surg Am 17:935-960, 1935.

62. Kibler WB: Shoulder rehabilitation: Principles and practice. Med Sci Sports Exerc 30:S40-S50, 1998.

63. Kibler WB: The role of the scapula in athletic shoulder function. Am J Sports Med 26:325-337, 1998.

64. Kibler WB, Garrett WE Jr: Pathophysiologic alterations in shoulder injury. Instr Course Lect 46:3-6, 1997.

65. Kibler WB, Livingston B, Chandler TJ: Shoulder rehabilitation: Clinical application, evaluation, and rehabilitation protocols. Instr Course Lect 46:43-51, 1997.

66. Lo IK, Burkhart SS: Subscapularis tears: Arthroscopic repair of the forgotten rotator cuff tendon. Tech Shoulder Elbow Surg 3:282-291, 2002.

67. Lo IK, Burkhart SS: Arthroscopic repair of massive, contracted rotator cuff tears using single and double interval slides: Technique and preliminary results. Arthroscopy (in press).

68. Lo IK, Burkhart SS: Arthroscopic revision rotator cuff repair of failed repairs of the rotator cuff. Arthroscopy (in press).

69. Luo ZP, Hsu HC, Grabowski JJ, et al: Mechanical environment associated with rotator cuff tears. J Shoulder Elbow Surg 7:616-20, 1998.

70. Mansat P, Cofield RH, Kersten TE, et al: Complications of rotator cuff repair. Orthop Clin North Am 28:205-213, 1997.

71. Maranja RJ Jr, Iannotti JP, Gartsman GM: Complications of rotator cuff surgery. In Norris TR (ed): Orthopaedic Knowledge Update: Shoulder and Elbow. Rosemont, IL, American Academy of Orthopaedic Surgeons, 1997, pp 157-166.

72. Matsen FA III, Arntz CT, Lippitt SB: Rotator cuff. In Rockwood CA, Matsen FA III (eds): The Shoulder, 2nd ed. Philadelphia, WB Saunders, 1998, pp 755-839.

73. Miller MD, Flatow EL, Bigliani LU: Biomechanics of the coracoacromial arch and rotator cuff; kinematics and contact of the subacromial space. In Iannotti JP (ed): The Rotator Cuff: Current Concepts and Complex Problems. Rosemont, IL, American Academy of Orthopaedic Surgeons, 1998, pp 1-16.

74. Miniaci A: Massive rotator cuff tears. In Norris TR (ed): Orthopaedic Knowledge Update: Shoulder and Elbow. Rosemont, IL, American Academy of Orthopaedic Surgeons, 1997, pp 167-172.

75. Miniaci A, Salonen D: Rotator cuff evaluation: Imaging and diagnosis. Orthop Clin North Am 28:43-58, 1997.

76. Morrison DS: Conservative management of partial-thickness rotator cuff tears. In Burkhead WZ Jr (ed): Rotator Cuff Disorders. Baltimore, Williams & Wilkins, 1996, pp 249-257.

77. Murray TF, Lajtaj G, Mileski RM, et al: Arthroscopic repair of medium to large full-thickness rotator cuff tears: Outcome at 2- to 6-year follow-up. J Shoulder Elbow Surg 11:19-24, 2002.

78. Neer CS II: Anterior acromioplasty for chronic impingement in the shoulder: A preliminary report. J Bone Joint Surg Am 54:41-50, 1972.

79. Neer CS: Impingement lesions. Clin Orthop 173:70-77, 1983.

80. Neer CS II (ed): Cuff tears, biceps lesions and impingement. In Shoulder Reconstruction. Philadelphia, WB Saunders, 1990, pp 41-42.

81. Neer CS II, Flatow EL, Lech O: Tears of the rotator cuff: Long term results of anterior acromioplasty and repair. Orthop Trans 12:673-674, 1988.

82. Ogata S, Uhthoff HK: Acromial enthesopathy and rotator cuff tear: A radiologic and histologic postmortem investigation of the coracoacromial arch. Clin Orthop 254:39-48, 1990.

83. Ozaki J, Fujimoto S, Nakagawa Y, et al: Tears of the rotator cuff of the shoulder associated with pathologic changes in the acromion. J Bone Joint Surg Am 70:1224-1230, 1988.

84. Petersson CJ, Gentz CF: Ruptures of the supraspinatus tendon: The significance of distally pointing acromioclavicular osteophytes. Clin Orthop 174:143-148, 1983.

85. Rockwood CA Jr, Williams GR Jr, Burkhead WZ Jr: Debridement of degenerative, irreparable lesions of the rotator cuff. J Bone Joint Surg Am 77:857-866, 1995.

86. Romeo A: Personal communication, 2002.

87. Rowe CR: Ruptures of the rotator cuff: Selection of cases for conservative treatment. Surg Clin North Am 43:1531-1540, 1975.

88. Sano H, Uhthoff HK, Backman DS, et al: Structural disorders at the insertion of the supraspinatus tendon: Relation to tensile strength. J Bone Joint Surg Br 80:720-725, 1998.

89. Sarkar K, Uhthoff HK: Pathophysiology of rotator cuff degeneration, calcification, and repair. In Burkhead WZ

(ed): Rotator Cuff Disorders. Baltimore, Williams & Wilkins, 1996, pp 36-44.

90. Schwamborn T, Imhoff AB: Diagnostik and klassifikation der rotatorenmanschettenlasionen. In Imhoff AB, Konig U (eds): Schulterinstabilitat-Rotatorenmanschette. Darmstadt, Germany, Steinkopff Verlag, 1999, pp 193-195.

91. Seltzer DG, Kechele P, Basamania C, et al: Conservative management of rotator cuff tears. In Burkhead WZ Jr (ed): Rotator Cuff Disorders. Baltimore, Williams & Wilkins, 1996, pp 258-267.

92. Sher JS: Anatomy, function, pathogenesis and natural history of rotator cuff disorders. In Norris TR (ed): Orthopaedic Knowledge Update: Shoulder and Elbow. Rosemont, IL, American Academy of Orthopaedic Surgeons, 1997, pp 123-133.

93. Sher JS: Anatomy, biomechanics, and pathophysiology of rotator cuff disease. In Iannotti JP, Williams GR (eds): Disorders of the Shoulder: Diagnosis and Management. Philadelphia, Lippincott Williams & Wilkins, 1999, pp 3-29.

94. Sher JS, Uribe JW, Posada A, et al: Abnormal findings on magnetic resonance images of asymptomatic shoulders. J Bone Joint Surg Am 77:10-15, 1995.

95. Smith JG: Pathological appearances of seven cases of injury of the shoulder joint, with remarks. Lond Med Gaz 14:280, 1834.

96. Soslowsky LJ, Carpenter JE, Bucchieri JS, et al: Biomechanics of the rotator cuff. Orthop Clin North Am 28:17-30, 1997.

97. Takagishi N: Conservative treatment of ruptures of the rotator cuff. J Jpn Orthop Assoc 52:781-787, 1978.

98. Tauro JC: Arthroscopic rotator cuff repair: Analysis of technique and results at 2- and 3- year follow-up. Arthroscopy 14:45-51, 1998.

99. Tauro JC: Arthroscopic "interval slide" in the repair of large rotator cuff tears. Arthroscopy 15:527-530, 1999.

100. Tehrany AM, Burkhart SS: Massive rotator cuff tears: Results of arthroscopic partial repair. Paper presented at the 21st annual meeting of the Arthroscopy Association of North America, Apr 2002, Washington, DC.

101. Tifford CD, Plancher KD: Nonsurgical treatment of rotator cuff tears. In Norris TR (ed): Orthopaedic Knowledge Update: Shoulder and Elbow. Rosemont, IL, American Academy of Orthopaedic Surgeons, 1997, pp 135-149.

102. Uhthoff HK, Drummond DI, Sakar K, et al: The role of impingement syndrome: A clinical, radiological, and histological study. Int Orthop 12:97-104, 1988.

103. Uhthoff HK, Sano H: Pathology of failure of the rotator cuff tendon. Orthop Clin North Am 28:31-41, 1997.

104. Uhthoff HK, Sarkar K: Surgical repair of rotator cuff ruptures: The importance of the subacromial bursa. J Bone Joint Surg Br 73:399-401, 1991.

105. Weber SC, Abrams JS, Nottage WM: Complications associated with arthroscopic shoulder surgery. Arthroscopy 18(Suppl):88-95, 2002.

106. Weber SC, Sager R: All arthroscopic versus mini open repair in the management of tears of the rotator cuff. Proc Am Acad Orthop Surg 2:617, 2001.

107. Williams GR Jr: Complications of rotator cuff surgery. In Iannotti JP, Williams GR (eds): Disorders of the Shoulder: Diagnosis and Management. Philadelphia, Lippincott Williams & Wilkins, 1999, pp 93-127.

108. Wilson CL, Duff GL: Pathologic study of degeneration and rupture of the supraspinatus tendon. Arch Surg 47:121-135, 1943.

109. Wilson F, Hinov V, Adams G: Arthroscopic repair of full-thickness tears of the rotator cuff: 2- to 14- year follow-up. Arthroscopy 18:136-144, 2002.

110. Wirth MA, Basamania C, Rockwood CA Jr: Nonoperative management of full-thickness tears of the rotator cuff. Orthop Clin North Am 28:59-67, 1997.

CHAPTER

23

Arthroscopic Repair of Crescent-Shaped, U-Shaped, and L-Shaped Rotator Cuff Tears

Ian K. Y. Lo and Stephen S. Burkhart

ARTHROSCOPIC REPAIR OF CRESCENT-SHAPED, U-SHAPED, AND L-SHAPED ROTATOR CUFF TEARS IN A NUTSHELL

History:
    May have a history of trauma, age-related progression, or overuse

Physical Examination:
    Painful range of motion, weakness, impingement findings

Imaging:
    Standard shoulder series, magnetic resonance imaging, ultrasonography

Indications:
    Symptoms and impairment despite nonoperative management

Classification:
    Crescent-shaped, U-shaped, L-shaped, and massive contracted tears

Surgical Technique:
    Determine tear morphology; crescent-shaped tears require direct repair of lateral tendon edge to bone; U-shaped and
        L-shaped tears require initial side-to-side repair (margin convergence), multiple fixation points with double-loaded suture
        anchors placed at appropriate angle, placement of secure locked knots

Postoperative Management:
    Conservative, with protection of repair

Results:
    As good as or better than open repair

The advent of arthroscopy and arthroscopic repair techniques has advanced both our understanding and the treatment of the rotator cuff.[6] Whereas traditional open surgical procedures for rotator cuff disease are usually limited by an anterolateral exposure, arthroscopy is not restricted by spatial constraints. Rotator cuff tears can now be assessed and treated arthroscopically from several different angles, with minimal disruption to the overlying deltoid. This new perspective on evaluating and treating rotator cuff tears has led to the recognition of four major types of full-thickness rotator cuff tears[5,7-10]:

1. Crescent-shaped tears (Fig. 23–1*A*)
2. U-shaped tears (Fig. 23–2*A*)
3. L-shaped tears (Figs. 23–3*A* and 23–4*A*)
4. Massive, contracted, immobile tears

Crescent-shaped tears may be massive in size but do not typically retract medially (see Fig 23–1*A*). These tears demonstrate excellent mobility from a medial to lateral direction and may be repaired directly to bone with minimal tension (Fig 23–1*B*).

In contrast, U-shaped rotator cuff tears extend much farther medially than crescent-shaped tears, with the apex of the tear adjacent or medial to the glenoid rim (see Fig. 23–2*A*). Recognizing these tears is critical, because attempting to medially mobilize and repair the apex of the tear to a lateral bone bed will result in overwhelming tensile stresses in the middle of the repaired rotator cuff margin (i.e., tensile overload) and subsequent failure. Instead, these tears demonstrate significant mobility from an anterior to posterior direction and should initially be repaired in a side-to-side fashion using the biomechanical principle of margin convergence.[7] In such cases, sequential side-to-side suturing, from medial to lateral, of the anterior and posterior leaves of the tear causes the free margin of the rotator cuff to converge toward the bone bed on the humerus (Fig. 23–2*B*). The free margin of the rotator cuff can then be easily repaired to the bone bed in a tension-free manner (Fig.

23–2*C*). The technique of margin convergence not only allows the repair of seemingly irreparable tears but also minimizes strain at the repair site.[10] This theoretically decreases the risk of rerupture and subsequent failure of the rotator cuff repair.

Acute L-shaped tears demonstrate a longitudinal split along the fibers of the rotator cuff and a transverse limb along the insertion of the rotator cuff into the lateral bone bed (Fig. 23–3*A*). These tears should be repaired with side-to-side sutures along the longitudinal split (Fig. 23–3*B*); then the converged margin should be repaired to bone (Fig. 23–3*C*). In more chronic cases, the physiologic pull of the rotator cuff muscles posteriorly causes an L-shaped tear to assume a more U-shaped configuration (see Fig. 23–4*A*). However, one of the leaves (usually the posterior leaf) is more mobile than the other and can easily be brought to the bone bed and to the other leaf. In these cases, side-to-side suturing is first performed along the longitudinal split (Fig. 23–4*B*); then the converged margin is repaired to bone (Fig. 23–4*C*).

Rarely, tears may be classified as massive, contracted, and immobile. These tears represent less than 5% to 10% of massive rotator cuff tears. They demonstrate minimal mobility from a medial to lateral and an anterior to posterior direction, and they must be repaired using mobilization techniques such as an interval slide or double interval slide.[9,22,30]

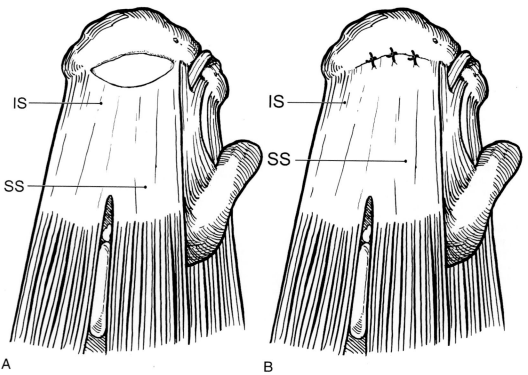

A   B

Figure 23–1 Crescent-shaped rotator cuff tear. *A,* Superior view of a crescent-shaped rotator cuff tear involving the supraspinatus (SS) and infraspinatus (IS) tendons. *B,* Crescent-shaped tears demonstrate excellent mobility from a medial to lateral direction and may be repaired directly to bone.

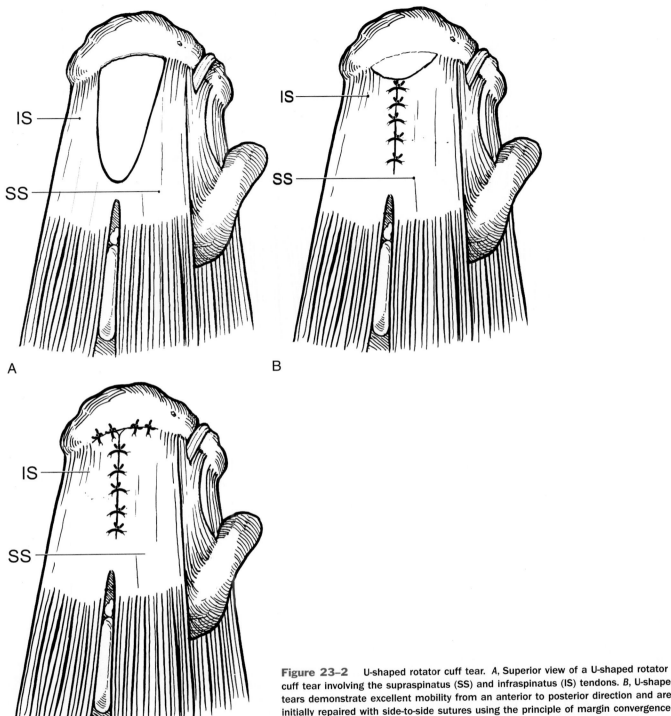

Figure 23–2   U-shaped rotator cuff tear. *A,* Superior view of a U-shaped rotator cuff tear involving the supraspinatus (SS) and infraspinatus (IS) tendons. *B,* U-shaped tears demonstrate excellent mobility from an anterior to posterior direction and are initially repaired with side-to-side sutures using the principle of margin convergence. *C,* The repaired margin is then repaired to bone in a tension-free manner.

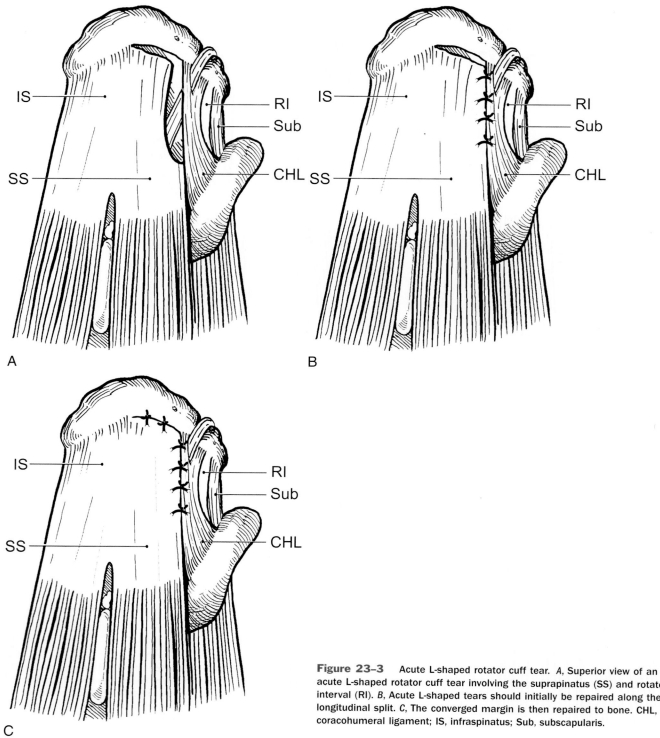

Figure 23–3 Acute L-shaped rotator cuff tear. *A*, Superior view of an acute L-shaped rotator cuff tear involving the suprapinatus (SS) and rotator interval (RI). *B*, Acute L-shaped tears should initially be repaired along their longitudinal split. *C*, The converged margin is then repaired to bone. CHL, coracohumeral ligament; IS, infraspinatus; Sub, subscapularis.

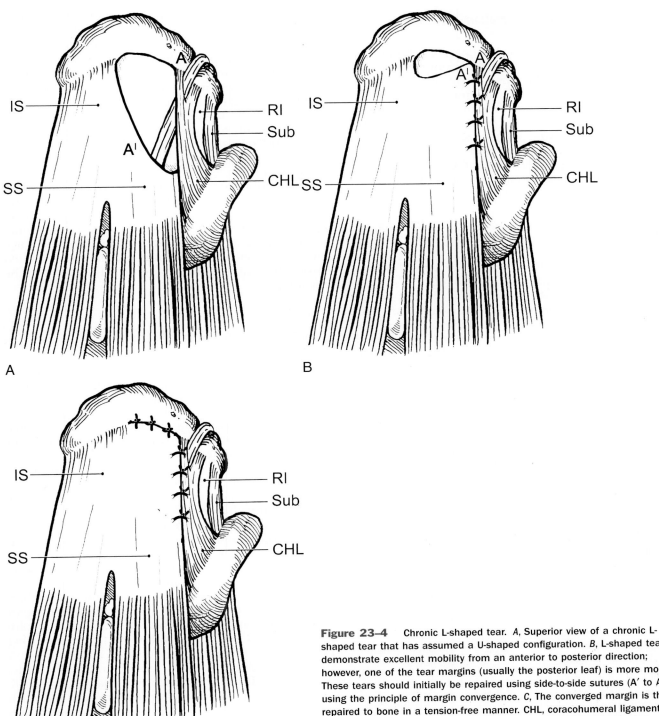

Figure 23–4   Chronic L-shaped tear. *A*, Superior view of a chronic L-shaped tear that has assumed a U-shaped configuration. *B*, L-shaped tears demonstrate excellent mobility from an anterior to posterior direction; however, one of the tear margins (usually the posterior leaf) is more mobile. These tears should initially be repaired using side-to-side sutures (A′ to A) using the principle of margin convergence. *C*, The converged margin is then repaired to bone in a tension-free manner. CHL, coracohumeral ligament; IS, infraspinatus; RI, rotator interval; SS, supraspinatus; Sub, subscapularis.

History and Physical Examination

The typical history and physical findings of patients who are appropriate candidates for arthroscopic rotator cuff repair are the same as for open repair and have been described in preceding chapters (summarized in Table 23–1). However, it is important to evaluate patients for subscapularis insufficiency, which can significantly increase the complexity of arthroscopic repair. This chapter focuses exclusively on posterosuperior rotator cuff tears; the reader is referred to other sources[13,21] and Chapter 24, Subscapularis Repair, for a complete description of arthroscopic subscapularis repair.

Imaging

Preoperatively, we routinely obtain five views—anteroposterior views in internal and external rotation, axillary view, outlet view, and 30-degree caudal tilt view—in all shoulder patients. Patients with rotator cuff tears typically demonstrate sclerosis of the undersurface of the acromion, sclerosis and cystic changes in the region of the greater tuberosity, and a type II or III acromion. In addition, careful attention is paid to the axillary view to evaluate for early glenohumeral arthritis or an os acromiale. Acromioclavicular joint arthritis may be variably present.

In massive tears, patients may demonstrate chronic proximal migration of the humerus, with a decrease in the acromiohumeral distance. We do not consider chronic proximal migration of the humerus a contraindication for rotator cuff repair and in some cases, the proximal migration may be reversed following repair (Fig. 23–5).

We routinely obtain a magnetic resonance imaging (MRI) scan in all preoperative shoulder patients. MRI can provide information on tear size, tear configuration, and tendon involvement, as well as suggest whether a massive rotator cuff tear is potentially repairable (Fig. 23–6). Careful evaluation of the axial views is necessary to identify subscapularis tendon involvement (Fig. 23–7). MRI may also demonstrate a spinoglenoid ganglion cyst, which can cause symptoms that mimic a rotator cuff tear.

We do not believe that long-standing tears, with their associated fatty degeneration or muscular atrophy, are a contraindication to surgical repair.[19,20] Although we agree with Gerber et al.[19] that rotator cuff repairs should be performed as soon as possible, in our experience patients can obtain significant improvement even when chronic tears are repaired more than 10 years after the initial injury.[12]

Indications and Contraindications

The indications for arthroscopic rotator cuff repair are the same as those for open rotator cuff repair. Thus, patients with persistent pain and disability following a course of nonoperative treatment, including anti-inflammatory medications, physical therapy, and subacromial cortisone injections, are considered candidates for arthroscopic rotator cuff repair.

The number-one contraindication to arthroscopic rotator cuff repair is related to the skills of the surgeon. Arthroscopic rotator cuff repair is a technically demanding procedure that requires an honest, critical assessment of one's surgical proficiency, the progress made during surgery, and the final repair construct. Conversion to an open or mini-open repair is recommended when the operative time is prolonged or when the security of the repair is suboptimal.

Otherwise, there are few contraindications for arthroscopic rotator cuff repair. In low-demand patients with preoperative *functional* rotator cuff tears, who require pain relief only and do not wish to participate in a long rehabilitation program, the surgeon may consider a subacromial decompression and debridement alone. Advanced cuff tear arthropathy is a relative contraindication to arthroscopic rotator cuff repair, and such patients may require a more extensive combined procedure (hemiarthroplasty with or without rotator cuff repair). In addition, patients with significant permanent neurologic deficits or medical conditions precluding surgery (including patients who are unable to tolerate the fluid load related to arthroscopic surgery) are not candidates for arthroscopic rotator cuff repair.

As stated earlier, we do not consider proximal humeral migration or fatty degeneration a contraindication to surgical repair.[19,20] Because we now understand how to repair massive rotator cuff tears using techniques such as margin convergence, we never perform open repairs. In our hands, arthroscopic techniques

Table 23–1	Typical History and Clinical Findings in Patients with Posterosuperior Rotator Cuff Tears

History	Physical Examination
History of trauma	Anterior, superior, lateral shoulder tenderness
Preceding history of intermittent "tendinitis" pain	Atrophy of the supraspinatus and infraspinatus
Anterior, superior, lateral shoulder pain	Subacromial crepitus
Pain exacerbated by overhead, lifting activities	Passive ROM > active ROM
Night pain, particularly when lying on shoulder	Full passive ROM
Subjective shoulder weakness and fatigue	Weakness in external rotation, flexion, abduction
Inability to raise arm overhead	Painful arc Positive impingement signs Positive impingement test

ROM, range of motion.

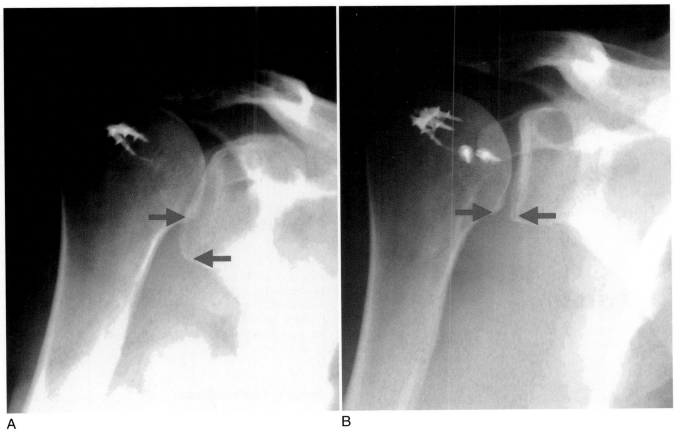

A   B

Figure 23–5   Anteroposterior glenohumeral joint radiographs of a right shoulder demonstrating reversal of proximal humeral migration. *A*, Proximal humeral migration is demonstrated preoperatively in this massive, recurrent rotator cuff tear. *B*, The proximal migration has been reversed following repair of the recurrent rotator cuff tear, which included a subscapularis tear. Note that the inferior articular margins of the proximal humerus and glenoid *(arrows)* are now at the same level.

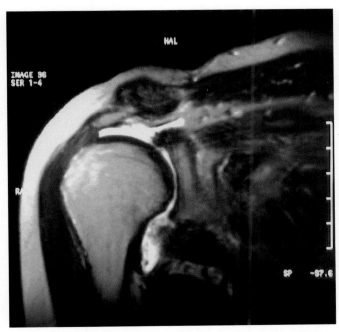

Figure 23–6   T2-weighted coronal magnetic resonance imaging scan demonstrating a massive tear of the posterosuperior rotator cuff, with its apex medially positioned above the superior glenoid margin.

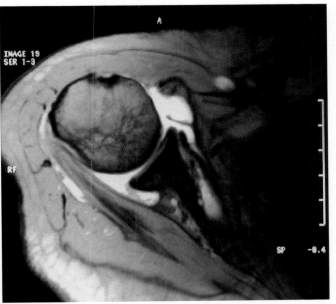

Figure 23–7   T2-weighted axial magnetic resonance imaging scan demonstrating a complete tear of the subscapularis tendon.

accomplish rotator cuff repairs that are as secure as open repairs, with less operative morbidity.[12]

Surgical Technique

Positioning and Examination under Anesthesia

Following induction of general anesthesia, an examination is performed documenting passive range of motion, glenohumeral translation, and general laxity. The patient is placed in the lateral decubitus position and is appropriately bolstered and padded. A warming blanket is applied to prevent hypothermia. Five to 10 pounds of balanced suspension is used with the arm in 20 to 30 degrees of abduction and 20 degrees of forward flexion (Star Sleeve Traction System, Arthrex, Inc., Naples, FL). By varying the amount of abduction and rotation, an assistant can maximize exposure and visualization.

Portal Placement

Three standard portals are used during arthroscopic rotator cuff repair (anterior, lateral subacromial, posterior) (Fig. 23–8). A posterior portal is established approximately 4 cm inferior and 4 cm medial to the posterolateral corner of the acromion; this portal is used for initial glenohumeral arthroscopy. The same skin puncture can be used for the posterior viewing portal and an instrument portal during subacromial bursoscopy and rotator cuff repair. An anterior glenohumeral portal is established using an outside-in technique just superior to the lateral half of the subscapularis tendon during diag-

nostic glenohumeral arthroscopy. This same skin puncture can be used for an anterior working portal and an inflow subacromial portal, and it can be used during distal clavicle resection, if indicated. The lateral subacromial portal is created approximately 3 cm lateral to the lateral aspect of the acromion, in line with the posterior border of the clavicle and parallel to the undersurface of the acromion. This portal serves as a viewing and working portal in the subacromial space. These three portals are the minimum number required during arthroscopic rotator cuff repair. Depending on the angle of approach, secondary accessory portals may be required.

Diagnostic Arthroscopy

Diagnostic glenohumeral arthroscopy is performed as described in previous chapters. All associated intra-articular pathologies (e.g., superior labral anterior to posterior [SLAP] lesions, chondromalacia) are treated as indicated. Diagnostic glenohumeral arthroscopy is performed to confirm the rotator cuff tear and to make an initial assessment of the size and extent of tearing (Fig. 23–9).

Specific Surgical Steps

Identification and Debridement of Tear Margins

After arthroscopic inspection and treatment of the glenohumeral joint, the arthroscope is introduced into the subacromial space through the posterior portal, and

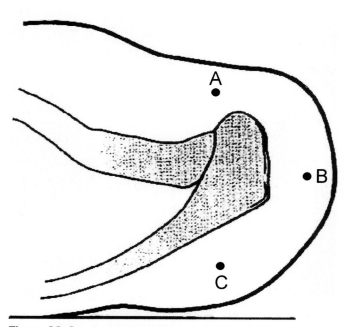

Figure 23-8 Portals for arthroscopic rotator cuff repair. A, The anterior portal is used as a working and inflow portal. B, The lateral portal is used as a working and viewing portal. C, The posterior portal is used as a working and viewing portal.

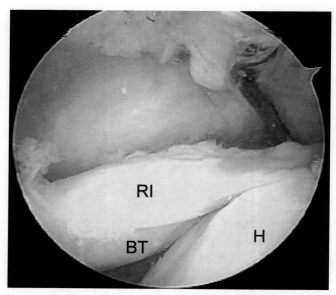

Figure 23-9 Arthroscopic view through a posterior glenohumeral portal of a massive recurrent rotator cuff tear in a right shoulder. Note that the subacromial space is visible through the tear. (All arthroscopic views are of right shoulders oriented in the beach chair position with the patient's head toward the top of the figure.) BT, biceps tendon; H, humeral head; RI, rotator interval.

a lateral subacromial portal is established as described earlier. An anterior portal is also established for inflow and as a working portal.

Before assessing and classifying the rotator cuff tear, all bursal and fibrofatty tissue must be debrided from the margins of the rotator cuff. Initially, the anterior and medial margins of the rotator cuff are debrided with the arthroscope posterior and the shaver (5-mm Resector, Stryker Endoscopy, Santa Clara, CA) lateral. However, to debride the posterior margin of the rotator cuff tear, it is easiest to view through the lateral portal and introduce the shaver through the posterior portal (Fig. 23–10). The true margin of the tear is commonly obscured by a synovialized "leader" of thickened bursal tissue. This tissue should be followed laterally, and if it is found to insert into deltoid fascia rather than bone, it is bursa and must be debrided until the tendon insertion into bone is clearly visualized. A judicious bursectomy or debridement is essential, because adventitial swelling during arthroscopic repair can obscure visualization.

Assessment of Rotator Cuff Mobility and Tear Pattern

The tear pattern can now be assessed by determining the mobility of the tear margins in the mediolateral and anteroposterior direction. To determine the mediolateral mobility of the rotator cuff tear, a tendon grasper (Arthrex, Inc., Naples, FL) is introduced through the lateral portal while viewing posteriorly. The medial margin of the tear is grasped and pulled laterally toward the bone bed (Fig. 23–11). If the tear can be brought to the bone bed easily, with minimal tension, the tear is

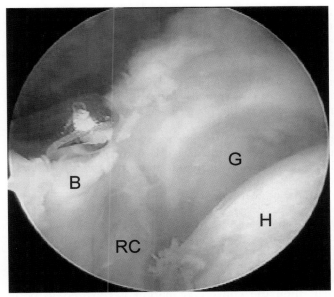

Figure 23–10   Arthroscopic debridement of the posterior margin of a rotator cuff tear through the posterior portal while viewing through the lateral portal. The overlying bursa (B) is debrided until the margin of the rotator cuff (RC) is exposed. G, glenoid; H, humeral head.

classified as crescent-shaped and can be directly repaired to bone (described later).

Tears that demonstrate minimal medial-to-lateral mobility are further assessed for anterior-to-posterior mobility. To determine this, the arthroscope is placed in the lateral portal, and the anteroposterior mobility of the

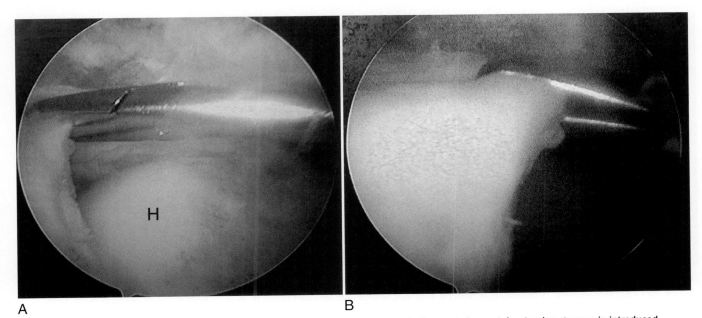

A   B

Figure 23–11   Assessment of medial to lateral mobility. With the arthroscope in the posterior portal, a tendon grasper is introduced through the lateral portal, grasps the margin of the rotator cuff tear (A), and pulls it laterally toward the bone bed (B). H, humeral head.

tear margins is assessed (Fig. 23–12). To test the posterior mobility of the anterior leaf of the rotator cuff tear, a tendon grasper is introduced through the posterior portal, and the anterior leaf of the tear is grasped and pulled posteriorly (see Fig. 23–12A). To test the anterior mobility of the posterior leaf of the rotator cuff tear, a tendon grasper is similarly introduced through the anterior portal, and the posterior leaf of the tear is grasped and pulled anteriorly (see Fig. 23-12B). If sufficient mobility is present to allow contact of the anterior and posterior leaves, the tear is a U-shaped tear and can be initially repaired with side-to-side sutures using the principle of margin convergence (described later).

L-shaped tears are similar to U-shaped tears; however, one of the leaves of the tear (usually the posterior leaf) has significantly more mobility than the other one. When assessed while viewing through the lateral portal, one leaf can easily be brought directly to the bone bed (Fig. 23–13). These tears should also be treated with side-to-side sutures along the longitudinal component of the tear; then the converged margin is repaired to bone (described later).

Tears without significant medial-to-lateral or anterior-to-posterior mobility are massive, contracted, immobile rotator cuff tears. Patients with such tears may be candidates for advanced mobilization techniques such as an interval slide.[9,22,30] Single or double interval slide techniques are beyond the scope of this chapter.

Subacromial Decompression

In the majority of repairable rotator cuff tears, a standard arthroscopic acromioplasty is performed using a cutting-block technique. However, if the tear is massive (>5 cm), even if it is completely repairable, a subacromial "smoothing" is performed as described by Matsen et al.[25] Subacromial decompression is accomplished by debriding the soft tissues on the undersurface of the acromion and resecting any small osseous irregularities. The coracoacromial ligament is preserved, because it is an essential restraint to anterosuperior migration of the humeral head if the rotator cuff repair fails or is nonfunctional.

Repair of Crescent-Shaped Tears

After identifying a crescent-shaped tear and performing a subacromial decompression, the bone bed on the humeral neck is prepared, just off the articular margin, using the 5-mm Resector shaver (Fig. 23–14). Decortication of bone should be avoided, because this can weaken anchor fixation. It has been shown that a bleeding bone surface rather than a bone trough is all that is required for satisfactory healing of tendon to bone.[28]

For fixation of the rotator cuff to bone, we prefer to use BioCorkscrew suture anchors (Arthrex, Inc., Naples, FL) double-loaded with number 2 Ethibond (Ethicon, Somerville, NJ) or number 2 Fiberwire (Arthrex). Although virtually all the current permanent and biodegradable suture anchors have adequate pullout strengths to resist physiologic loads,[1,2] the eyelet of the BioCorkscrew suture anchors consists of a flexible loop of number 4 polyester suture that is insert-molded into the body of the anchor (Fig. 23–15). This allows the suture to slide easily through the eyelet in any orientation and minimizes suture fouling and abrasion.[3,23]

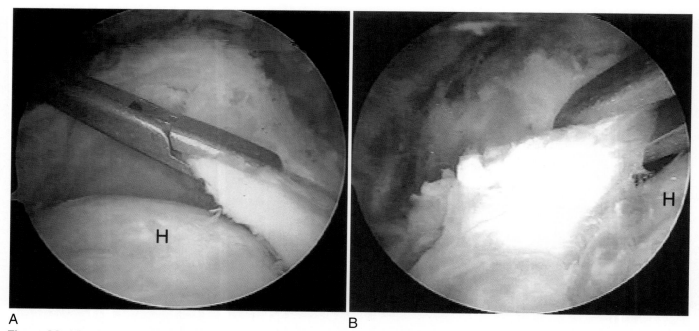

A   B

Figure 23–12 Assessment of mobility in a massive U-shaped rotator cuff tear. Arthroscopic view through a lateral portal in a recurrent massive rotator cuff tear. *A,* The posterior mobility of the anterior leaf is assessed by introducing a grasper through the posterior portal and pulling the anterior leaf posteriorly. *B,* The anterior mobility of the posterior leaf is assessed by introducing a grasper through the anterior portal and pulling the posterior leaf anteriorly. H, humeral head.

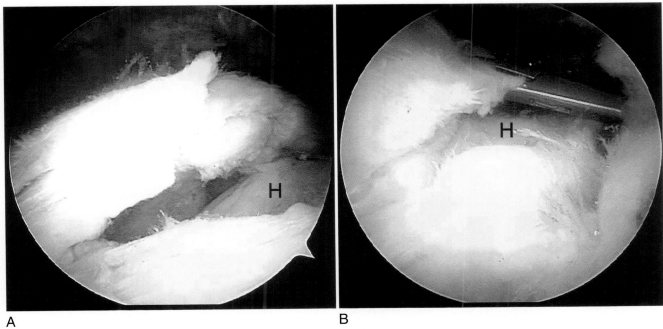

A   B

Figure 23–13   Assessment of mobility in an acute L-shaped tear. Arthroscopic view through a posterior portal. *A,* The rotator cuff tear can be seen with a longitudinal split posteriorly between the supraspinatus and infraspinatus tendons and a transverse component along its insertion into the greater tuberosity. *B,* A grasper has been introduced through a lateral portal, demonstrating reduction of the rotator cuff tear. H, humeral head.

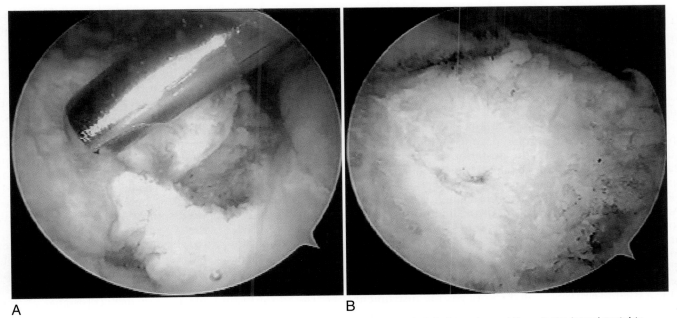

A   B

Figure 23–14   Bone bed preparation. Arthroscopic view through a posterior portal. *A,* A shaver is used through the lateral portal to initially debride the soft tissue remnants from the bone surface. *B,* Completed bone bed preparation.

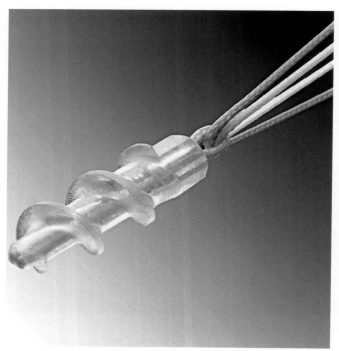

Figure 23–15 A 5-mm BioCorkscrew suture anchor (Arthrex, Inc., Naples, FL). Note that the suture eyelet can accommodate two sutures, and its flexibility minimizes suture fouling and friction.

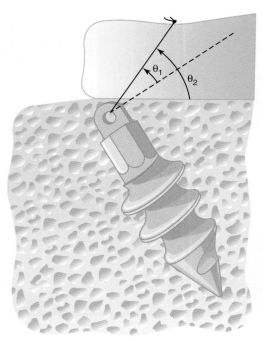

Figure 23–16 Representation of θ_1 and θ_2. θ_1 is the pullout angle for the anchor (i.e., the angle the suture makes with the perpendicular to the anchor), and θ_2 is the tension-reduction angle (i.e., the angle the suture makes with the direction of pull of the rotator cuff). Ideally, both θ_1 and θ_2 should be 45 degrees or less.

Anchors are inserted at 1-cm intervals, 4 to 5 mm off the articular surface and at an angle of approximately 45 degrees (i.e., dead-man's angle) to the bone surface to increase the anchor's resistance to pullout (Figs. 23–16 and 23–17).[4] With screw-in–type anchors (e.g., Bio-Corkscrew), the sutures are passed through the tendon after the anchor has been placed.

Standard suture-passing techniques are used, including retrograde or anterograde passing methods. For retrograde passage through the posterior rotator cuff, it is easiest to view through a lateral portal, obtaining a panoramic view of the suture passer, anchor, and sutures (Fig. 23–18). A suture-passing instrument (Penetrator, Arthrex, Inc., Naples, FL) is used to "line up the putt," so that the suture retriever ends up close to the suture and can easily capture it (see Fig. 23-18A). The Penetrator is then used to pierce the rotator cuff (see Fig. 23–18B), retrieve a suture (see Fig. 23–18C), and pull it back through the rotator cuff. For the anterior portion of the rotator cuff, an angled suture-passing instrument (45-degree BirdBeak, Arthrex, Inc., Naples, FL) provides a better angle of approach, but the same technique is used (Fig. 23–19). External rotation of the shoulder may improve the angle of approach.

For larger crescent-shaped tears, the central portion of the rotator cuff is best approached using a modified Neviaser portal, as described by Nord.[27] This portal is established in the "soft spot" bordered by the posterior clavicle, medial acromion, and scapular spine (Fig. 23–20A), and it is made large enough to just accommodate a suture-passing instrument (3 mm). A spinal needle is used to determine the proper location and angle of approach, and then a suture passer (usually the Penetrator) is "walked down"' the needle to ensure accurate placement (Fig. 23–20B). Sutures can then be passed in a similar retrograde fashion (Fig. 23–20C).

For anterograde suture passage, a special instrument such as the Viper suture passer (Arthrex, Inc., Naples, FL) is necessary; it is particularly useful for suture passage through the central portion of the rotator cuff. This invaluable instrument allows the surgeon to grasp the tissue, deliver the suture, and retrieve the suture in a single step. In addition, the tissue can be grasped and pulled toward the bone bed before stitch delivery to ensure that the proposed suture location is satisfactory (Fig. 23–21).

All sutures are passed through the rotator cuff before knot tying. A dedicated lateral portal is used for knot tying to minimize suture fouling. To maximize both loop security (maintenance of a tight suture loop around the enclosed soft tissue) and knot security (resistance of the knot to failure by slippage or breakage), stacked half hitches are tied with a double-diameter knot pusher (Surgeon's Sixth Finger, Arthrex, Inc., Naples, FL) (Fig. 23–22).[14,15,17] By using the Surgeon's Sixth Finger knot pusher, continuous tension can be maintained on the post limb as knots are tied; this prevents loosening of the soft tissue loop as sequential half hitches are thrown (i.e., loop security). Although several combinations of knots are possible, we prefer to initially stack three half hitches (base knot), followed by three consecutive half hitches

Text continued on p. 233

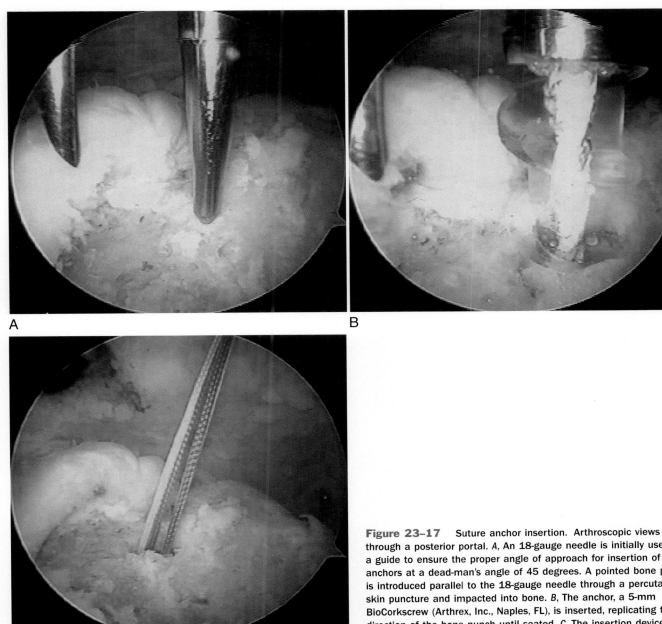

A

B

C

Figure 23–17   Suture anchor insertion. Arthroscopic views through a posterior portal. *A,* An 18-gauge needle is initially used as a guide to ensure the proper angle of approach for insertion of anchors at a dead-man's angle of 45 degrees. A pointed bone punch is introduced parallel to the 18-gauge needle through a percutaneous skin puncture and impacted into bone. *B,* The anchor, a 5-mm BioCorkscrew (Arthrex, Inc., Naples, FL), is inserted, replicating the direction of the bone punch until seated. *C,* The insertion device is removed, leaving the sutures protruding from the bone.

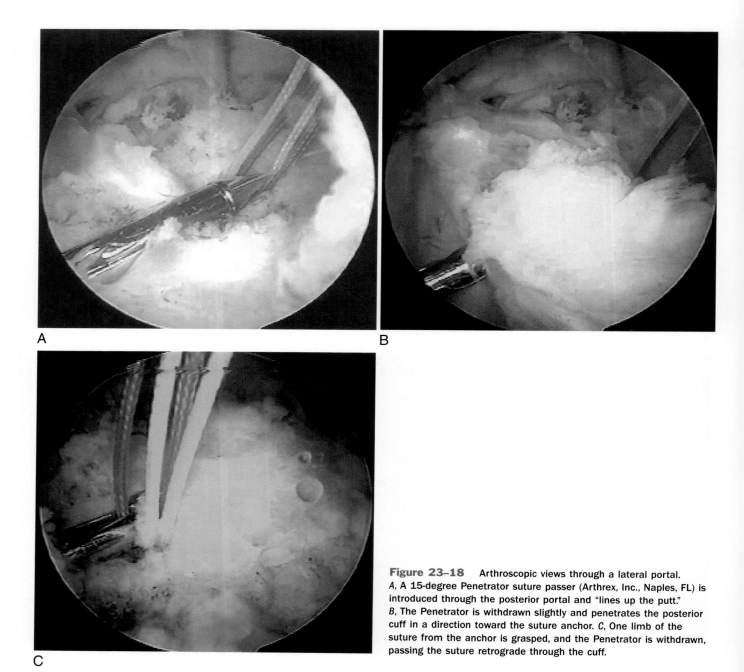

Figure 23–18 Arthroscopic views through a lateral portal. *A*, A 15-degree Penetrator suture passer (Arthrex, Inc., Naples, FL) is introduced through the posterior portal and "lines up the putt." *B*, The Penetrator is withdrawn slightly and penetrates the posterior cuff in a direction toward the suture anchor. *C*, One limb of the suture from the anchor is grasped, and the Penetrator is withdrawn, passing the suture retrograde through the cuff.

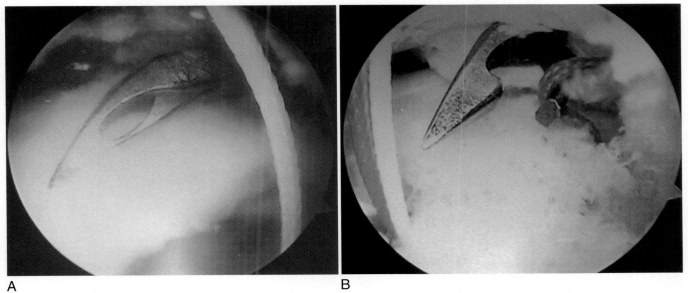

A   B

Figure 23–19   Anterior rotator cuff: retrograde passage. *A,* A 45-degree BirdBeak (Arthrex, Inc., Naples, FL) is introduced though the anterior portal and "lines up the putt." *B,* The BirdBeak is used to penetrate the anterior cuff, grasp one limb of the suture, and draw it through the rotator cuff in a retrograde fashion.

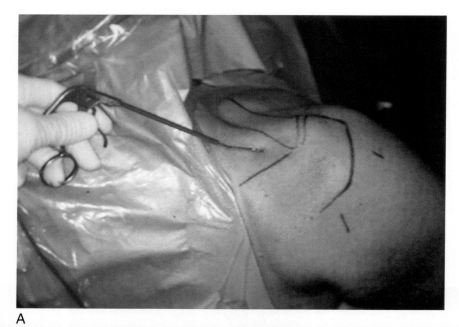

A

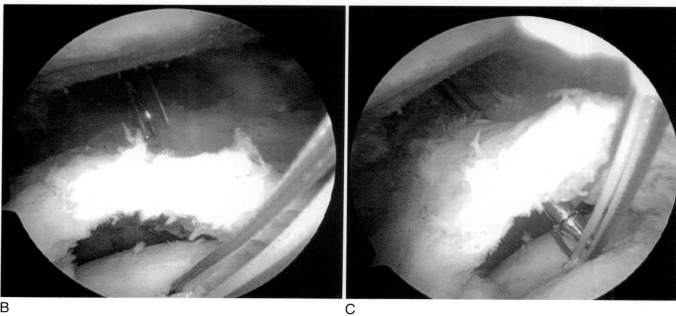

B   C

Figure 23–20   Central rotator cuff: retrograde passage. Arthroscopic views from a lateral portal. *A,* The modified Neviaser portal is created in the soft spot bordered by the posterior clavicle, medial acromion, and scapular spine. *B,* An 18-gauge spinal needle is used as a guide to determine the proper position of the portal to allow an adequate angle to the central rotator cuff. Using the needle as a guide, a Penetrator (Arthrex, Inc., Naples, FL) is "walked" down the spinal needle. *C,* The rotator cuff is penetrated and the suture grasped and passed in a retrograde fashion.

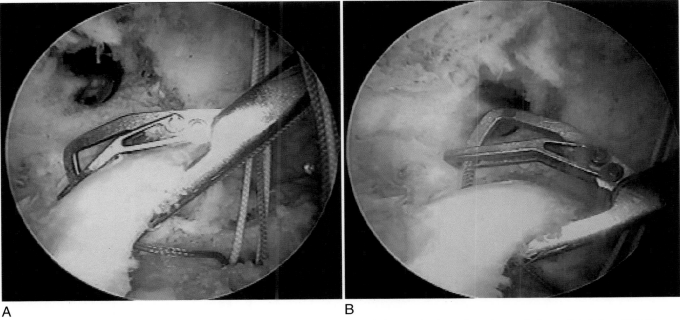

A   B

Figure 23–21 Anterograde suture passage using the Viper suture passer. Arthroscopic views through a posterior portal. *A,* A portion of the rotator cuff is grasped using the Viper suture passer (Arthrex, Inc., Naples, FL), and the proposed suture placement is assessed. *B,* Using a separate trigger on the instrument, the suture is passed to the upper jaw. The jaws are opened, passing the suture through the tendon.

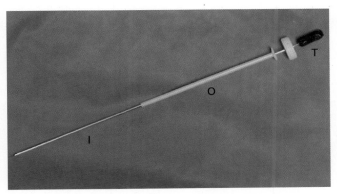

Figure 23–22 Double-diameter knot pusher. The double-diameter knot pusher (Surgeon's Sixth Finger, Arthrex, Inc., Naples, FL) consists of an inner (I) metallic tube with a sliding plastic outer (O) tube. A suture threader (T) is used to pass the suture limb through the inner metallic tube.

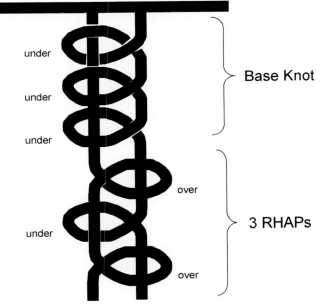

Figure 23–23 Arthroscopic surgeon's knot. A base knot of three half hitches in the same direction is tied, followed by three consecutive reversing half hitches on alternating posts (RHAPs).

on alternating posts (surgeon's knot; Fig. 23–23). This knot configuration has been demonstrated to have superior knot and loop security compared with commonly used arthroscopic sliding knots (e.g., Duncan loop, Tennessee slider).[24] In addition, this knot avoids the theoretical problem of suture abrasion as the suture slides through the anchor eyelet while a sliding knot is tied,[3,23] and it avoids damaging (or even cutting through) the rotator cuff tendon as the suture slides through the rotator cuff (the suture does not slide in this static knot configuration).

Posts are switched without rethreading the knot pusher. This is done by "flipping" the half hitch through differential tensioning of the suture limbs.[16] Because the post limb is always the limb under the most tension, the wrapping limb can be converted to the post limb by tensioning it to a greater degree than the original post limb, thereby "flipping" the post (Fig. 23–24). This not only is easy but also optimizes the strength of any knot.[16,17,24] Tissue indentation by the suture is a final indicator of good loop security (Fig. 23–25).

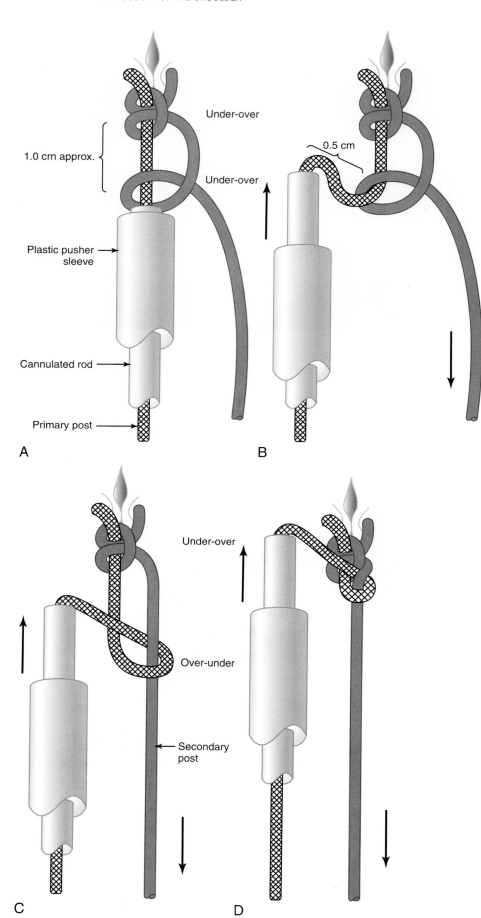

Under-over

1.0 crn approx.

Under-over

Plastic pusher sleeve

Cannulated rod

Primary post

A

0.5 cm

B

Under-over

Over-under

Secondary post

C

Under-over

D

Figure 23–24 Switching posts without rethreading. *A*, The half hitch is advanced with a double-diameter knot tier. *B*, The knot tier is backed off approximately 0.5 cm and then advanced past the half hitch. *C*, While advancing the knot tier, the secondary post is pulled, "flipping" the post. *D*, Past-pointing tightens the knot.

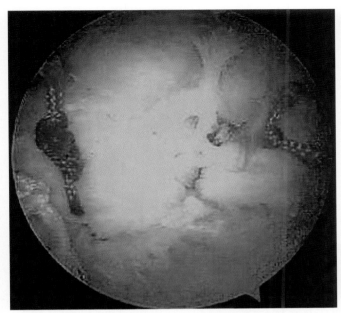

Figure 23–25   Arthroscopic view of a completed repair of a crescent-shaped rotator cuff tear.

Figure 23–26   Typical arthroscopic appearance, through the lateral portal, of a massive U-shaped rotator cuff tear with the apex above the level of the glenoid. BT, biceps tendon; H, humeral head.

Repair of U-Shaped Tears

After identifying a U-shaped rotator cuff tear, performing a subacromial decompression, and preparing the bone bed, the tear should initially be closed by margin convergence using side-to-side sutures. To best identify this tear configuration, the arthroscope is placed in the lateral portal, giving a "Grand Canyon" view of the massive tear (Fig. 23–26). Depending on the angle of approach and the availability of assistants, two methods are commonly used for passage of side-to-side sutures.

HAND-OFF TECHNIQUE

In this technique, a loaded (with number 2 Ethibond) suture passer (BirdBeak or Penetrator) is introduced through the posterior portal and penetrates the posterior leaf of the rotator cuff tear near the tear apex medially (Fig, 23–27*A*). A second empty suture passer is

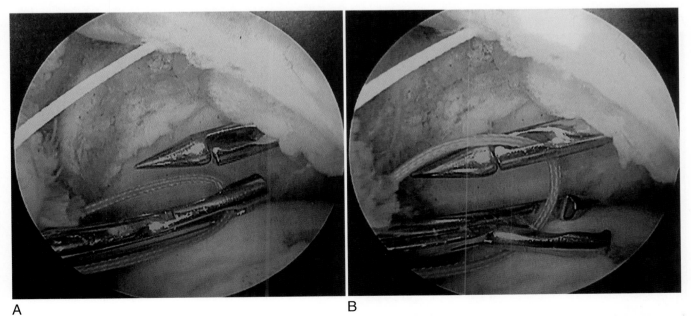

A   B

Figure 23–27   Side-to-side suturing using a hand-off technique. Arthroscopic view through the lateral portal. *A*, A loaded suture passer (Penetrator, Arthrex, Inc., Naples, FL) is introduced through the posterior portal and penetrates the posterior leaf of the rotator cuff tear. A second empty Penetrator is introduced through the anterior portal and penetrates the anterior leaf of the rotator cuff tear. *B*, The posterior suture passer "hands off" the suture to the anterior suture passer, which is withdrawn, passing the suture through the anterior leaf.

introduced through the anterior portal and penetrates the anterior leaf of the rotator cuff tear. A "hand-off" is performed from the posterior to the anterior suture passer (Fig. 23–27B), and the suture is withdrawn retrograde through the anterior leaf, effectively creating a side-to-side suture.

In a similar fashion, side-to-side sutures are sequentially placed at 5- to 10-mm intervals, progressing from medial to lateral. Ordinarily, four to five side-to-side sutures are required for massive U-shaped tears, with the most lateral suture abutting the medial portion of the bone bed. All side-to-side sutures are placed before knot tying to allow unobscured suture passage through the rotator cuff.

VIPER TECHNIQUE

In this technique, a loaded Viper suture passer is introduced through a posterior portal, and the suture is passed through the anterior leaf in an anterograde fashion (Fig. 23–28A). Successive sutures are then placed along the anterior tear margin (Fig. 23–28B). A Penetrator suture passer is introduced through the posterior portal, piercing the posterior rotator cuff medially and

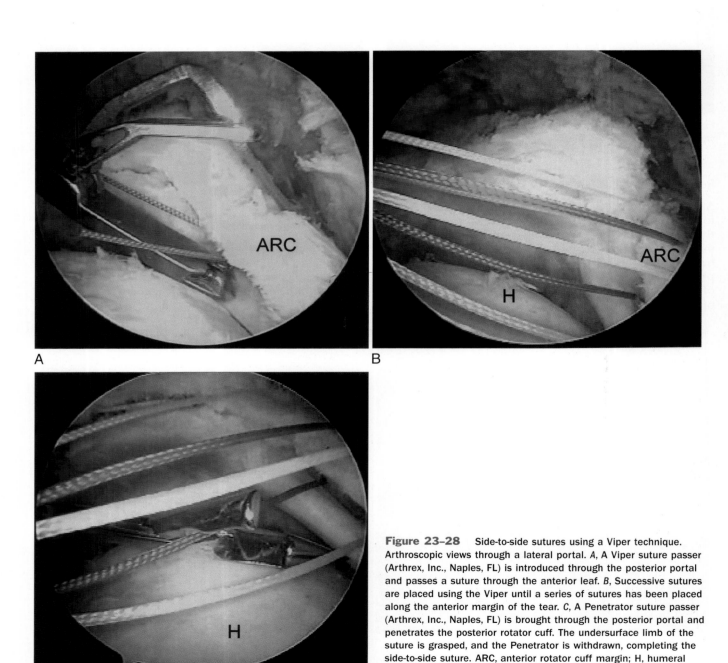

A

B

C

Figure 23–28 Side-to-side sutures using a Viper technique. Arthroscopic views through a lateral portal. *A*, A Viper suture passer (Arthrex, Inc., Naples, FL) is introduced through the posterior portal and passes a suture through the anterior leaf. *B*, Successive sutures are placed using the Viper until a series of sutures has been placed along the anterior margin of the tear. *C*, A Penetrator suture passer (Arthrex, Inc., Naples, FL) is brought through the posterior portal and penetrates the posterior rotator cuff. The undersurface limb of the suture is grasped, and the Penetrator is withdrawn, completing the side-to-side suture. ARC, anterior rotator cuff margin; H, humeral head.

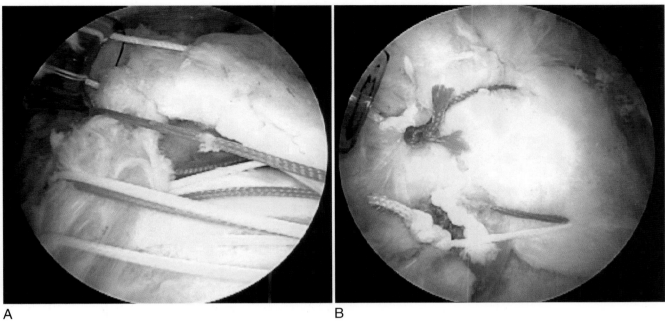

A   B

Figure 23–29   Arthroscopic views from a lateral portal following placement of side-to-side sutures *(A)* and after knot tying with convergence of the rotator cuff margin to the lateral bone bed *(B).*

grasping the undersurface limb of the medial suture (Fig. 23–28*C*). The Penetrator suture passer is then withdrawn, passing the undersurface suture limb retrograde through the posterior cuff, completing a side-to-side suture. This procedure is repeated, grasping each of the undersurface suture limbs in sequence while moving laterally with each successive suture.

Following the placement of side-to-side sutures, the sutures are tied in a sequential fashion from medial to lateral to effect margin convergence of the rotator cuff tear. Side-to-side sutures are tied as described earlier through a dedicated cannulated posterior portal. Knots are tied over the posterior leaf of the tear to avoid the theoretical problem of knot impingement on the undersurface of the anterior acromion.

As the sutures are tied from medial to lateral, the free margin of the rotator cuff converges laterally toward the bone bed (Fig. 23–29). After performing margin convergence with side-to-side suturing of the anterior and posterior leaves of the rotator cuff, the converged margin is secured to the bone bed. One suture anchor (Bio-Corkscrew) is placed for each leaf of the tear, similar to the technique described earlier. Anchors are placed approximately 1 cm from the rotator cuff margin to shift the leaves of the tear to the anchors as the knots are tied. This shift optimizes the force couple provided by the repaired rotator cuff muscles by maximizing the superior-to-inferior dimension of the bone attachments of the cuff.

Sutures are passed through the anterior and posterior leaves of the tear as described earlier using a Penetrator suture passer for the posterior leaf and a 45-degree BirdBeak suture passer for the anterior leaf. Knots are

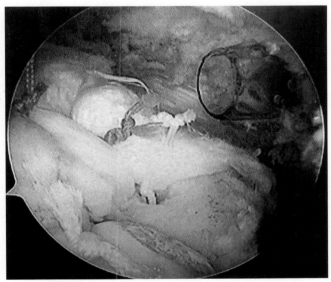

Figure 23–30   Arthroscopic view from a posterior portal of a completed U-shaped rotator cuff repair.

tied through a lateral portal while viewing through a posterior portal (Fig. 23–30).

Repair of L-Shaped Tears

After identifying an L-shaped rotator cuff tear (Fig. 23–31*A*), side-to-side sutures are similarly placed in a sequential fashion from medial to lateral. In these tears, it is important to determine which of the leaves is most

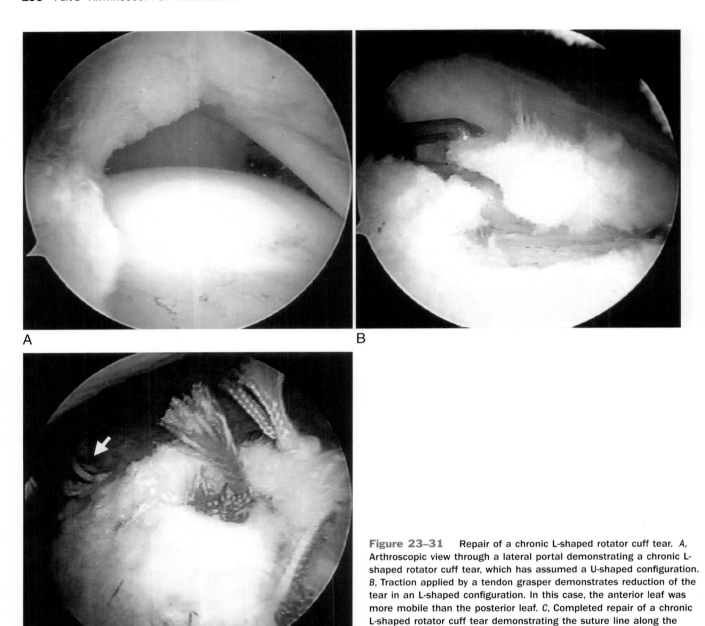

Figure 23–31 Repair of a chronic L-shaped rotator cuff tear. *A,* Arthroscopic view through a lateral portal demonstrating a chronic L-shaped rotator cuff tear, which has assumed a U-shaped configuration. *B,* Traction applied by a tendon grasper demonstrates reduction of the tear in an L-shaped configuration. In this case, the anterior leaf was more mobile than the posterior leaf. *C,* Completed repair of a chronic L-shaped rotator cuff tear demonstrating the suture line along the bone bed and margin convergence sutures along the longitudinal component of the tear *(arrow).*

mobile and to judge where sutures need to be placed. Further, the surgeon must determine (based on leaf mobility) which portion of the mobile leaf constitutes the "corner" of the L (Fig. 23–31*B*). Usually the posterior leaf is more mobile than the anterior leaf, and its lateral 2 to 3 cm can be brought directly to the bone bed. In these tears, side-to-side sutures are placed obliquely across the tear to shift the posterior leaf anteriorly and laterally. Alternatively, if the anterior leaf is more mobile, side-to-side sutures are placed obliquely across the tear to shift the anterior leaf posteriorly and laterally (see Fig. 23–31*B*). Side-to-side sutures are placed as described earlier, and sutures are tied to advance the posterior leaf toward the bone bed.

After shifting the more mobile leaf toward the bone bed, the cuff margin is secured to bone in a similar fashion as described earlier. Usually two to three anchors are required for secure tendon fixation to bone (Fig. 23–31*C*).

Pearls and Pitfalls

Turbulence Control

During arthroscopic shoulder surgery, particularly in the subacromial space, bleeding can obscure visualization and frustrate attempts to obtain an effective rotator cuff repair. In many cases, this is due to fluid leakage from noncannulated portals.[11] Fluid flow from these portals creates a suction effect by virtue of Bernoulli's principle and draws blood into the subacromial space. Simply blocking these portals using digital pressure facilitates a clear view by controlling turbulence within this closed system.

Double-Loading Suture Anchors

Double-loading suture anchors with number 2 Ethibond or number 2 Fiberwire allows two points of fixation for each anchor and provides an "extra" suture in case of suture breakage during knot tying.

Suture Passage

Passing all sutures through a crescent-shaped cuff tear before knot tying makes it easier to manipulate suture passers under the rotator cuff margin, because the cuff is not bound down by sutures that have already been tied. Although this may create a tangled suture mess, it can be easily remedied by sequentially grasping suture pairs proximal to the entanglement and retrieving them through a separate portal.

For U-shaped and L-shaped tears, we first pass all side-to-side sutures, then sequentially tie them from medial to lateral before placing suture anchors. The margin convergence achieved by side-to-side closure guides us in the precise placement of suture anchors and in the accurate passage of sutures from those anchors to achieve anatomic closure.

Postoperative Management

All arthroscopic rotator cuff repairs are performed on an outpatient basis. Following the procedure, the operated arm is placed at the side in a sling with a small pillow (Donjoy Ultrasling, DJ Orthopaedics, LLC, Vista, CA). The sling is worn continuously for 6 weeks, except during bathing and exercises.

Table 23–2 Rehabilitation Protocol Following Arthroscopic Rotator Cuff Repair

Time Period	Rehabilitation
0-6 wk	Immobilization: sling Elbow/wrist: active ROM Shoulder: passive external rotation in adduction only
6-12 wk	Shoulder: active ROM, avoid lateral abduction Stretching: forward flexion, internal rotation, external rotation
>12 wk	Strengthening: deltoid, biceps, triceps, rotator cuff, scapular stabilizers
>6 mo	Normal activities

ROM, range of motion.

The standard postoperative rehabilitation program is summarized in Table 23–2. However, if a subscapularis repair is performed, passive external rotation is limited to 0 degrees (i.e., straight ahead) for the first 6 weeks. In addition, terminal extension of the elbow is restricted if a biceps tenodesis was performed.

Results

The senior author recently reported the results of 59 arthroscopic rotator cuff repairs with a mean follow-up of 3.5 years.[12] Unlike previous reports, this study included a number of large and massive tears. Good and excellent results were achieved in 95% of patients using the UCLA criteria and were independent of tear size (i.e., large and massive tears fared as well as smaller tears). Importantly, U-shaped tears repaired by margin convergence had results comparable to those of crescent-shaped tears undergoing direct tendon-to-bone repair. This indirectly validates the process of classifying tears (crescent-shaped, U-shaped, L-shaped) and repairing them according to their classification (repair directly to bone, repair by margin convergence).

Table 23–3 Results of Arthroscopic Rotator Cuff Repair

Author (Date)	No. of Patients	Follow-up (yr)	Results	Comments
Burkhart et al. (2001)[12]	59	3.5	95% good/excellent	All tear sizes, including massive Good results in small and massive tears Good results in tears repaired by margin convergence or directly to bone
Wilson et al. (2002)[31]	100	5	88% good/excellent	Two techniques used (staple and suture anchor fixation) Second-look arthroscopy (staple group) showed watertight healing of 73% of tears
Murray et al. (2002)[26]	48	3.3	95% good/excellent	No massive tears, tears repaired directly to bone
Gartsman et al. (1998)[18]	73	2.5	84% good/excellent	Mostly smaller tears repaired directly to bone
Tauro (1998)[29]	53	>2	92% good/excellent	Mostly smaller tears repaired directly to bone

The results of arthroscopic rotator cuff repair in peer-reviewed journals is summarized in Table 23–3. Overall, these results suggest that arthroscopic rotator cuff repair achieves results that are superior to those obtained with traditional open surgical management.

Complications

No major intraoperative complications have been noted during arthroscopic rotator cuff repair. During prolonged procedures, however, the shoulder and particularly the deltoid can become quite swollen, impairing visualization and thereby increasing the difficulty of the procedure. Although compartment syndrome of the deltoid has not been reported in the published literature, we are aware of one case of deltoid necrosis presumably secondary to extravasation of fluid into the deltoid during a prolonged arthroscopic procedure. For this reason, we recommend that if visualization is impaired or the surgeon cannot easily complete the entire case within 2.5 hours, conversion to an open repair should be strongly considered.

Anchor pullout is a theoretical possibility, particularly in osteoporotic bone. However, inserting a corkscrew anchor at a dead-man's angle of 45 degrees or less maximizes anchor resistance to pullout.[4] We have not noted any fixation problems when anchors are inserted properly.

References

1. Barber FA, Herbert MA, Click JN: The ultimate strength of suture anchors. Arthroscopy 11:21-28, 1995.
2. Barber FA, Herbert MA, Click JN: Internal fixation strength of suture anchors: Update 1999. Arthroscopy 13:355-362, 1999.
3. Bardana DD, Burks RT, West JR: The effect of suture anchor design and orientation on suture abrasion: An in-vitro study. Arthroscopy (in press).
4. Burkhart SS: The deadman theory of suture anchors: Observations along a south Texas fence line. Arthroscopy 11:119-123, 1995.
5. Burkhart SS: Arthroscopic rotator cuff repair: Indications and techniques. Oper Tech Sports Med 5:204-214, 1997.
6. Burkhart SS: Shoulder arthroscopy: New concepts. Clinics Sports Med 15:635-653, 1996.
7. Burkhart SS: Arthroscopic repair of massive rotator cuff tears: Concept of margin convergence. Tech Shoulder Elbow Surg 1:232-239, 2000.
8. Burkhart SS: A stepwise approach to arthroscopic rotator cuff repair based on biomechanical principles. Arthroscopy 16:82-90, 2000.
9. Burkhart SS: Arthroscopic treatment of massive rotator cuff tears. Clin Orthop 390:107-118, 2001.
10. Burkhart SS, Athanasiou KA, Wirth MA: Margin convergence: A method of reducing strain in massive rotator cuff tears. Arthroscopy 12:335-338, 1996.
11. Burkhart SS, Danaceau SM, Athanasiou KA: Turbulence control as a factor in improving visualization during sub-acromial shoulder arthroscopy. Arthroscopy 17:209-212, 2001.
12. Burkhart SS, Danaceau SM, Pearce CE: Arthroscopic rotator cuff repair: Analysis of results by tear size and by repair technique—margin convergence versus direct tendon-to-bone repair. Arthroscopy 17:905-912, 2001.
13. Burkhart SS, Tehrany AM: Arthroscopic subscapularis repair: Technique and preliminary results. Arthroscopy 18:454-463, 2002.
14. Burkhart SS, Wirth MA, Simonich M, et al: Loop security as a determinant of tissue fixation security. Arthroscopy 14:773-776, 1998.
15. Burkhart SS, Wirth MA, Simonich M, et al: Knot security in simple sliding knots and its relationship to rotator cuff repair: How secure must the knot be? Arthroscopy 16:202-207, 2000.
16. Chan KC, Burkhart SS: How to switch posts without rethreading when tying half-hitches. Arthroscopy 15:444-450, 1999.
17. Chan KC, Burkhart SS, Thiagarajan P, et al: Optimization of stacked half-hitch knots for arthroscopic surgery. Arthroscopy 17:752-759, 2001.
18. Gartsman GM, Khan M, Hammerman SM: Arthroscopic repair of full-thickness tears of the rotator cuff. J Bone Joint Surg Am 80:832-840, 1998.
19. Gerber C, Fuchs B, Hodler J: The results of repair of massive tears of the rotator cuff. J Bone Joint Surg Am 82:505-515, 2000.
20. Goutallier D, Postel JM, Lavau L, et al: Fatty muscle degenerations in cuff ruptures. Clin Orthop 304:78-83, 1994.
21. Lo IK, Burkhart SS: Subscapularis tears: Arthroscopic repair of the forgotten rotator cuff tendon. Tech Shoulder Elbow Surg 3:282-291, 2002.
22. Lo IK, Burkhart SS: Arthroscopic repair of massive, contracted rotator cuff tears using single and double interval slides. Arthroscopy (in press).
23. Lo IK, Burkhart SS, Athanasiou KA: Abrasion resistance of two types of non-absorbable, braided sutures. Arthroscopy (in press).
24. Lo IK, Burkhart SS, Chan KC, et al: Arthroscopic knots: Determining the optimal balance of loop security and knot security. Arthroscopy (in press).
25. Matsen FA III, Arntz CT, Lippitt SB: Rotator cuff. In Rockwood CA Jr, Matsen FA III (eds): The Shoulder, 2nd ed. Philadelphia, WB Saunders, 1998, pp 755-839.
26. Murray TF, Lajtai G, Mileski RM, et al: Arthroscopic repair of medium to large full-thickness rotator cuff tears: outcome at 2- to 6-year follow-up. J Shoulder Elbow Surg 11:19-24, 2002.
27. Nord K: Modified Neviaser portal and subclavian portal in shoulder arthroscopy. Paper presented at the 19th annual meeting of the Arthroscopy Association of North America, Apr 14, 2000, Miami, FL.
28. St. Pierre P, Olson EJ, Elliott JJ, et al: Tendon-healing to cortical bone compared with healing to a cancellous trough: A biomechanical and histological evaluation in goats. J Bone Joint Surg Am 77:1858-1866, 1995.
29. Tauro JC: Arthroscopic rotator cuff repair: Analysis of technique and results at 2- and 3-year follow-up. Arthroscopy 14:45-51, 1998.
30. Tauro JC: Arthroscopic "interval slide" in the repair of large rotator cuff tears. Arthroscopy 15:527-530, 1999.
31. Wilson F, Hinov V, Adams G: Arthroscopic repair of full-thickness tears of the rotator cuff: 2- to 14-year follow-up. Arthroscopy 18:136-144, 2002.

Arthroscopic Subscapularis Repair

JEFF A. FOX, MAYO A. NOERDLINGER, LISA M. SASSO, AND ANTHONY A. ROMEO*

ARTHROSCOPIC SUBSCAPULARIS REPAIR IN A NUTSHELL

History:
Forceful external rotation against contracting subscapularis; forceful reaching

Physical Examination:
Positive liftoff, belly-press, and modified liftoff tests

Imaging:
Magnetic resonance imaging is most sensitive

Decision-Making Principles:
Large tears are not well tolerated and may result in poor shoulder function; small tears may be considered for nonoperative care

Surgical Technique:
Portals: anterior, posterior, accessory lateral
Debride lesser tuberosity, coracoidplasty
Place anchors
Shuttle suture, tie knots

Postoperative Management:
Passive range of motion, sling for first 6 weeks; active range of motion and strengthening thereafter

Subscapularis tears can be particularly disabling, especially in young, active patients who depend on normal shoulder strength and mobility. Unfortunately, many patients with subscapularis tears are initially misdiagnosed. A high index of suspicion based on the mechanism of injury and the physical examination findings can identify these tears before they become chronic, retracted, and otherwise difficult to manage. These injuries typically fall into two groups: those caused by a forceful external rotation moment against a contracting subscapularis muscle, and tendon failure following operative procedures involving detachment of the subscapularis muscle tendon unit. The focus of this chapter is the surgical technique used to manage subscapularis tears arthroscopically.

Case History

The patient is a 44-year-old, right-hand-dominant male pipe fitter. The injury occurred when he abruptly reached above his head to prevent a fall and noted the immediate onset of pain and weakness in the shoulder. He was treated initially with physical therapy and a subacromial corticosteroid injection, which failed to

*The senior author, Anthony A. Romeo, received research support from Arthrex International, Naples, Florida.

alleviate his symptoms. He ultimately underwent a magnetic resonance imaging (MRI) evaluation, and a subscapularis muscle tendon tear was diagnosed.

Physical Examination

The physical examination is critical to an accurate diagnosis of a subscapularis tear. Often patients present with anterior shoulder pain with a differential diagnosis that includes pain originating from the acromioclavicular joint, long head of the biceps, coracoid impingement, anterior capsulolabral damage, or fractures of the anterior glenoid rim or lesser tuberosity. Patients with large subscapularis tendon tears may have increased passive external rotation and weakness of active internal rotation. Owing to other powerful internal rotators, especially the pectoralis major, the shoulder must be placed in internal rotation to isolate and examine the subscapularis. Three tests—the belly-press test,[10] liftoff test,[11] and modified liftoff test[10]—improve our ability to examine the function of the subscapularis.

The belly-press test is performed by having the patient press his or her hand into the abdomen while keeping the elbow anterior to the midcoronal line of the body. If the patient cannot keep the elbow in that position, the subscapularis is not functioning, and this is a positive test (Fig. 24–1A). The liftoff test is performed with the arm internally rotated and the elbow flexed. This allows the dorsum of the hand to rest against the patient's back. This test requires the patient to reach behind the back and lift the hand posteriorly off the back. An inability to do so is a positive test for efficient function of the subscapularis (Fig. 24–1B). For the modified liftoff test, the arm is internally rotated behind the back with the hand positioned by the examiner 5 to 10 cm off the back; then the hand is released. If the patient is able to maintain the position of the hand in space as the subscapularis contracts, the test is negative. The test is positive when the patient is unable to maintain the position of the hand and it falls to the patient's back. This is also recognized as a subscapularis lag sign.[13]

Imaging

Plain radiographs should be obtained, including true anteroposterior, axillary lateral, and scapular lateral views. This series evaluates for arthritis and fractures. In cases of subscapularis insufficiency, anterior subluxation of the humeral head may be evident on the axillary lateral view.[19]

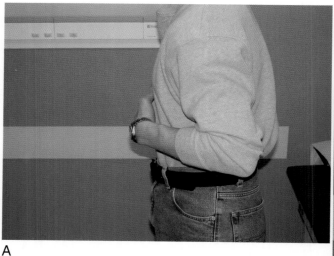

A

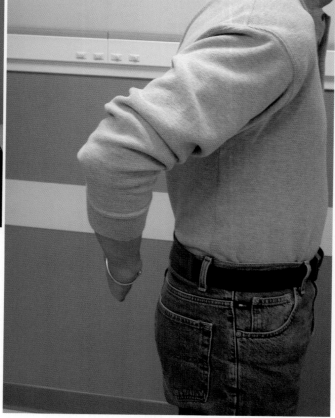

B

Figure 24–1   *A*, Patient with a positive belly-press test, unable to maintain his elbow in front of his trunk. *B*, Normal liftoff test. When the test is positive (abnormal), the patient cannot raise the hand off the back.

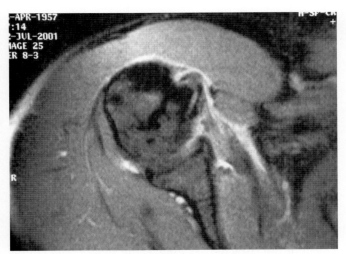

Figure 24–2 Magnetic resonance imaging scan of a torn subscapularis.

MRI is the most sensitive imaging modality to diagnose a subscapularis tear (Fig. 24–2). However, it is not uncommon for this tear to be missed.[7] Although we do not routinely use gadolinium enhancement to make the diagnosis, magnetic resonance arthrograms have an improved ability to detect subscapularis tears compared with routine MRI.[18,20] MRI also provides important clues to the status of the muscle, including the amount of fatty infiltration and atrophy. Subluxation or dislocation of the long head of the biceps tendon is readily assessed on MRI axial views. When displacement of the biceps tendon is seen on MRI, one should carefully evaluate the subscapularis tendon's insertion site. Subscapularis tears are associated with displacement of the biceps from the bicipital groove owing to the frequent disruption of the coracohumeral ligament's attachment on the humerus at the medial aspect of the bicipital groove.[21]

Decision-Making Principles

A tear of the subscapularis that leads to pain and functional deficit is best treated with operative repair. The decision to perform surgery when the subscapularis is torn is based on the patient's symptoms, as well as on the factors listed in Table 24–1. Tearing of the rotator cuff tendon leads to atrophy and fibrofatty degeneration of the muscle. Rotator cuff tears, including subscapularis tears, are best treated before they become irreparable[12] or the atrophic changes in the muscle are irreversible.

Surgical Technique

Instrumentation

Special instruments are required for arthroscopic repair of the subscapularis, including but not limited to a

Table 24–1

Surgery for Torn Subscapularis

Indications	Contraindications
Pain	Pain free, pseudoparalysis
Little atrophy on MRI	Severe atrophy on MRI
Fatty degeneration < Goutallier grade 3 on MRI	Fatty degeneration ≥ Goutallier grade 4 on MRI
Positive liftoff test, belly press, modified liftoff test	Rotator cuff arthropathy

crochet hook, single-hole knot pusher, suture-cutting device, and suture-passing and retrieval instrument.

Positioning

We prefer the beach chair position for arthroscopic repairs of the subscapularis. This position makes it simple for ancillary staff to set up the patient. The orientation of the shoulder is familiar to the surgeon, and the ability to move the arm and therefore the subscapularis insertion site easily during the procedure facilitates the surgical repair. Further, if the surgical procedure fails to achieve stable fixation, the beach chair position facilitates conversion to an open procedure.

Examination under Anesthesia

A thorough examination under anesthesia is performed before patient positioning. Preoperative shoulder crepitation, range of motion, and stability are documented and compared with the patient's contralateral shoulder. Our preferred method of anesthesia is a combination of an interscalene block and general endotracheal anesthesia. A long-acting interscalene block reduces the dosage of inhalation agents and narcotics necessary for effective general anesthesia, as well as provides postoperative pain relief throughout the day of surgery.[1] Using this method, more than 95% of our patients are discharged from the surgical facility within a few hours after completion of the arthroscopic repair.

Specific Surgical Steps

Portal Placement

Standard posterior and anterior portals are established. The anterior portal should be more medial (but still lateral to the coracoid) to prevent cannula crowding with the accessory anterolateral cannula. For isolated subscapularis repairs, the lateral portal routinely used for subacromial decompression is not needed. When there is also a rotator cuff tear involving the supraspinatus and posterior rotator cuff, this lateral portal is made 2 to 3 cm inferior to the lateral edge of the acromion and just anterior to a line that would bisect the anterior to posterior distance of the acromion. For all our subscapularis tendon repairs, an accessory anterolateral portal is created in the rotator interval just anterior and medial to the anterolateral corner of the acromion. This portal is typically 1 to 2 cm superior and 2 cm lateral to the standard anterior portal. The key to this portal is first localizing its intra-articular position with a spinal needle to ensure that it is placed optimally for the repair. The posterior cannula is introduced into the glenohumeral joint, and the arthroscope is placed through this cannula. The standard anterior portal is established using an inside-out technique. This establishes the portal within the lateral aspect of the rotator interval and below the biceps tendon. A systematic evaluation of the glenohumeral joint is performed. Arthroscopic evidence of abnormalities related to the glenoid rim, biceps tendon, or subscapularis tendon may alter the preoperative plan in 10% to 15% of patients undergoing rotator cuff surgery.[9]

A dynamic examination of the insertions of the subscapularis, supraspinatus, and infraspinatus is performed while viewing from the posterior portal. The subscapularis insertion can be visualized by advancing the arthroscope to the anterior aspect of the glenohumeral joint. The viewing lens is oriented laterally, and the arm is internally rotated. With complete subscapularis tears and subsequent retraction, the conjoined tendon and muscle of the short head of the biceps may be visible, and the tendon of the long head of the biceps is often displaced medially. In this situation, the subscapularis must be released from adhesions to the tendon. The axillary nerve is just anterior to the subscapularis tendon and can be visualized from the lateral portal when there is a complete rupture (Fig. 24–3).

Coracoidplasty

The effect of the coracoid on the subscapularis has been reported,[8,14] but it remains unclear whether there is any relationship between coracoid impingement and subscapularis tear. We systematically perform coracoidplasty as part of the treatment of subscapularis tears to avoid any pathologic mechanical process between the coracoid and the subscapularis repair. This process also provides more space for the technical steps related to the tendon repair.

Once the subscapularis tendon tear is identified, the capsule of the rotator interval is resected to visualize the coracoid process (Fig. 24–4). A shaver is used to debride the capsular tissue at the superior margin of the subscapularis tendon. Once the capsule has been cleared, a section of fatty tissue typically reveals itself at the inferior aspect of the coracoid. As long as the shaver stays lateral to the coracoid, there are no neurovascular structures in this interval, so it is safe to debride the fatty tissue until the coracoid is reached. An electrothermal device is used to clear the periosteum and soft tissue off the posterior aspect of the coracoid. A 4-mm bur is then used to remove bone from the posterior margin of the coracoid at an angle that takes more bone from the coracoid's posterolateral aspect (Fig. 24–5). By removing the bone, more space is created anterior to the subscapularis in a method analogous to subacromial decompression for supraspinatus pathology. When completed, there should be approximately 5 to 6 mm of space between the subscapularis and the coracoid tip.

Tendon Repair

The subscapularis tear is now formally addressed. Often, only part of the subscapularis is detached. Typically, the

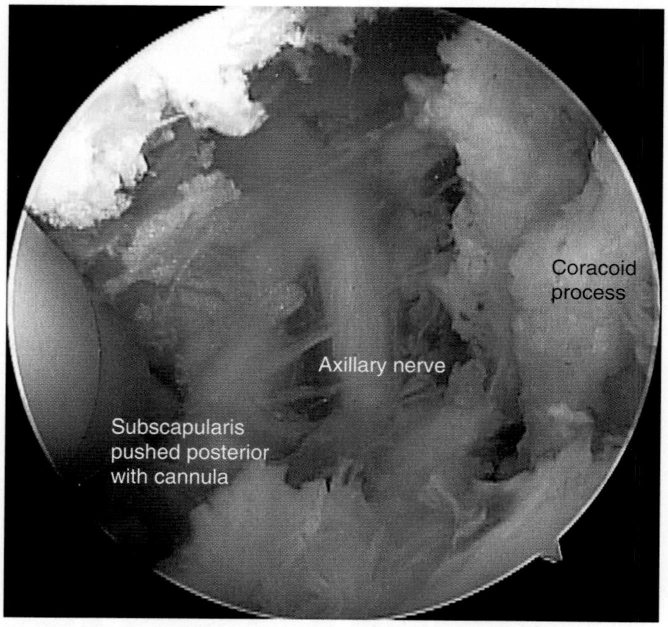

Figure 24–3 Arthroscopic image of the axillary nerve in a complete subscapularis tear, identified while freeing adhesions from the anterior aspect of the subscapularis tendon around the base of the coracoid process.

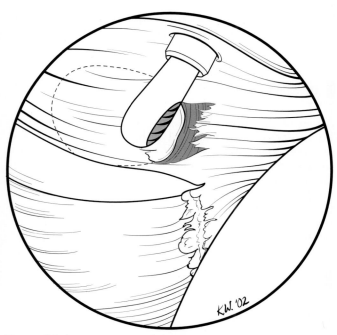

Figure 24–4 A shaver is used to clear soft tissue overlying the coracoid tip.

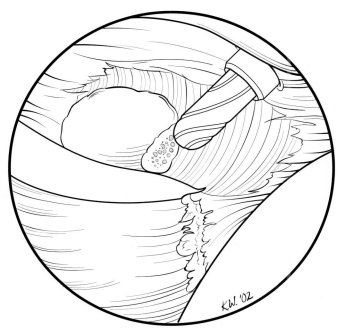

Figure 24–5 With the coracoid fully exposed, the bur is used to resect bone.

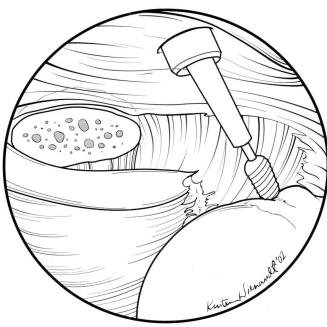

Figure 24–7 Preparation includes debriding soft tissue from the insertion site, followed by establishing a bleeding bone surface with a bur.

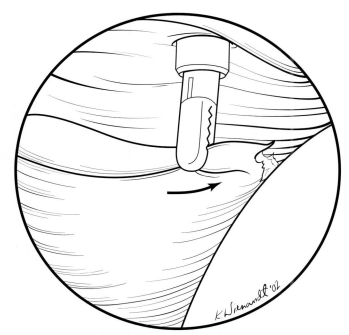

Figure 24–6 A grasper is used to assess the mobility of the subscapularis tendon.

superior one third to one half of the subscapularis is detached, while the inferior part remains attached to the lesser tuberosity. An arthroscopic grasper can be inserted through the anterior or anterolateral portal to grasp the subscapularis tissue and evaluate its mobility (Fig. 24–6).

Mobilization of the subscapularis tendon can be challenging. Meticulous dissection of the fibrous attachments to the coracoid, including release of the coracohumeral ligament structures and an anterior capsulotomy, should be accomplished. Medializing the insertion point of the subscapularis to the juxta-articular edge of the humerus is acceptable and does not adversely affect the clinical results in terms of pain relief, range of motion, and function.

A 5.0-mm shaver is inserted through the anterior portal, and all loose tissue is debrided. The tendon edge is "freshened" in a similar manner by removing frayed edges. Next, the middle glenohumeral ligament is identified. Because the ligament crosses at a 45-degree angle to the tendon, it is important to separate the ligament from the subscapularis to facilitate mobilization of the tendon. An electrothermal cutting device or shaver can be used to release the middle glenohumeral ligament from the subscapularis to improve lateral mobility.

The lesser tuberosity is prepared with a high-speed 4-mm bur through the anterior portal while the bur is visualized with the arthroscope in the posterior portal. The arm is rotated internally and abducted to deliver the tuberosity to the bur (Fig. 24–7).

After the initial debridement, the anterolateral accessory portal is established. First, localize the appropriate starting point and angle with an 18-gauge spinal needle. The angle should be from lateral and superior, centering on the prepared lesser tuberosity groove. It is important to avoid placing the cannula too close to the anterior cannula (Fig. 24–8).

Suture anchors designed for fixation in cancellous bone are critical for the success of arthroscopic tendon repairs. Rotator cuff repairs using suture anchors may be

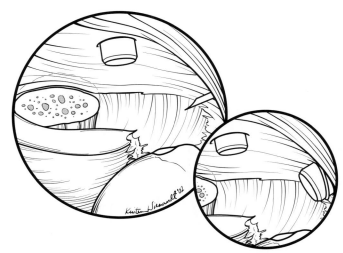

Figure 24–8 A spinal needle is used to identify the proper position of the accessory anterolateral portal.

less prone to failure with cyclic loading compared with tendon fixation using sutures through bone tunnels.[5] The anchors are inserted via the anterior portal; this allows them to be placed at a 45-degree angle to the bone, the so-called dead-man's angle.[2] The anchors are inserted 5 mm away from the articular surface to ensure that the tendon is approximated to the prepared bone and not to the articular surface. Each anchor is loaded with two sutures, which improves the ability to resist physiologic loads at the repair site.[5] The first anchor is placed at the most inferior aspect of the tear, with each subsequent anchor placed farther superiorly. This facilitates visualization as the procedure progresses. The final anchor is placed at the most superior aspect of the tendon insertion. The number of anchors used is determined by the size of the tear. Separating each double suture anchor by 5 to 8 mm, with a proportional distribution over the insertion site, affords enough points of fixation for repair security and avoids tension overload at any single fixation point.[3]

The first anchor is placed through the anterior cannula by sequentially using the punch (Fig. 24–9A) followed by the tap (Fig. 24–9B). The suture anchor is then screwed into place (Fig. 24–9C). To aid in suture management, a switching stick is placed in the cannula, and the cannula is removed. The sutures are then pulled outside of the cannula, and the cannula is slid back into the glenohumeral joint (Fig. 24–10). The sutures are held with a hemostat to aid in suture management. The next step is shuttling the suture through the subscapularis tendon. The suture limb that will be pulled through the subscapularis tendon is grasped with the crochet hook and pulled through the anterolateral portal (Fig. 24–11). A device such as the Suture Lasso or the Penetrator (both from Arthrex, Inc., Naples, FL) is pushed through the tendon via the anterior portal. The suture should be passed at an angle from lateral to medial through the entire tendon thickness, understanding that the articular side of the tendon will be more medial than the bursal side. Once the 30-degree Suture Lasso is

passed through the tendon (Fig. 24–12A), the loop is advanced. A crochet hook is used to grab the looped end of the Suture Lasso, and this is pulled through the anterolateral cannula (Fig. 24–12B).

The first suture limb is passed through the loop outside the anterolateral cannula, and the Lasso's loop is pulled back out through the tendon and the anterior portal, pulling the suture limb from the one anchor through the tendon (Fig. 24–13). The suture anchor should be visualized during this step to prevent unloading of the suture from the anchor. The suture should not be moving within the suture anchor.

The second limb of the suture (just pulled through the anterior cannula) is pulled through the anterolateral cannula with the crochet hook (Fig. 24–14). The Suture Lasso is passed back through the subscapularis tendon at a second site, with the intention of creating a mattress suture configuration (Fig. 24–15). The loop is grasped and pulled through the anterolateral cannula in a similar fashion as described for the first limb of the suture. The second limb is shuttled back through the tendon and out the anterior cannula. The two limbs of the suture are then pulled outside of the cannula using the switching stick technique described earlier, and a hemostat is used to secure them together (Fig. 24–16).

The second suture's two limbs are shuttled through the subscapularis with a similar technique, approximately 5 mm away from the first suture. Each suture should have independent paths through the rotator cuff tendon (Figs. 24–17 to 24–21).

To optimize suture management, secure the tendon one anchor at a time. After passing the two sutures from the first anchor, the sutures can be tied before moving on to the next anchor. Inevitably, however, more experience with arthroscopic repairs will reveal that it is more efficient to place the anchors and pass all the sutures required to repair the tendon before tying the suture knots. A second anchor is placed in a similar manner, but 5 to 8 mm more proximal on the insertion site. The

Text continued on p. 253

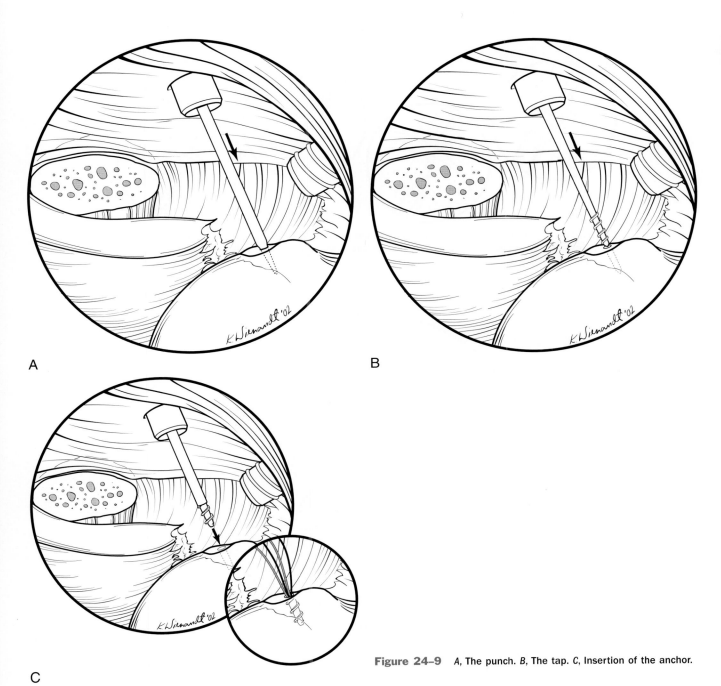

Figure 24–9   *A,* The punch. *B,* The tap. *C,* Insertion of the anchor.

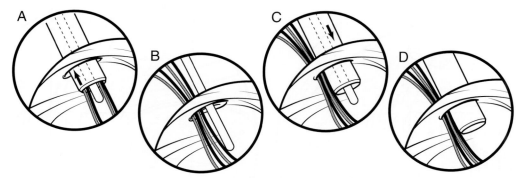

Figure 24–10 *A*, The switching stick is placed in the cannula, and the cannula is removed. *B*, Sutures are removed from the cannula. *C*, The cannula is reinserted. *D*, The switching stick is removed.

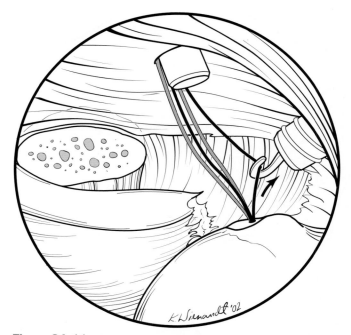

Figure 24–11 The suture that will be shuttled through the tendon is taken through the anterolateral portal.

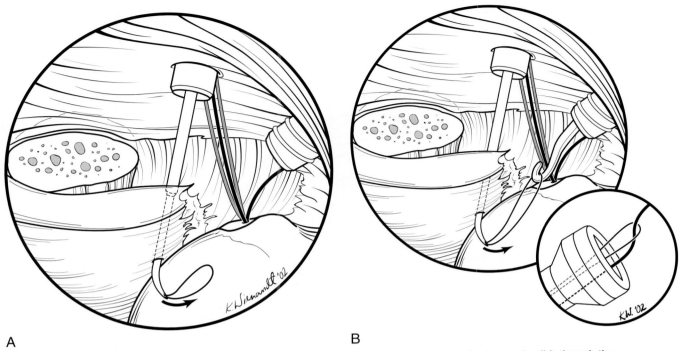

A   B

Figure 24–12   *A*, The loop of the Suture Lasso is advanced. *B*, A crochet hook is used to grasp the loop and pull it through the anterolateral portal. The suture limb is then passed through the loop of the Lasso suture.

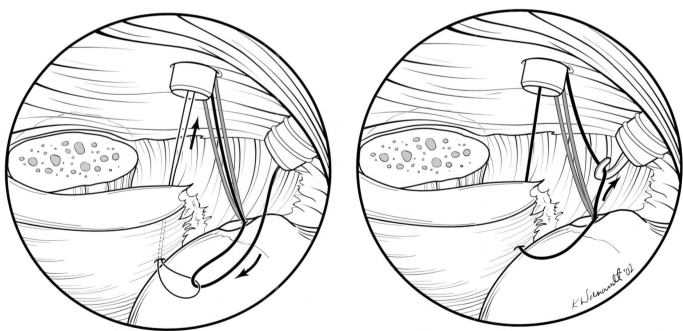

Figure 24–13   Shuttling the suture limb back through the tendon.

Figure 24–14   The second limb of the suture is pulled through the anterolateral portal.

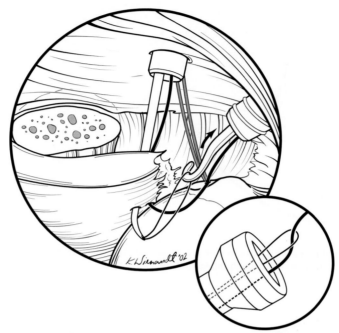

Figure 24–15 The Suture Lasso is passed back through the tendon, and the loop is retrieved and pulled through the anterolateral portal.

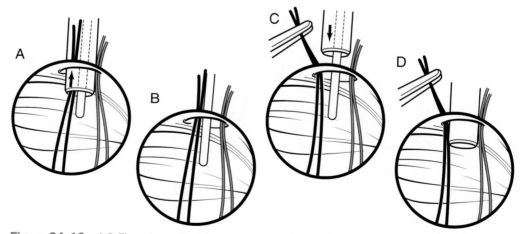

Figure 24–16 *A–D,* The suture, which was just shuttled through the tendon, is removed from the cannula to aid in suture management.

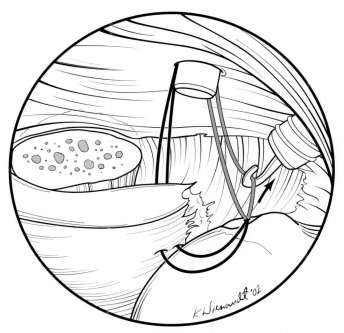

Figure 24–17   The second suture is shuttled through the tendon, beginning by pulling the suture to be shuttled through the anterolateral cannula.

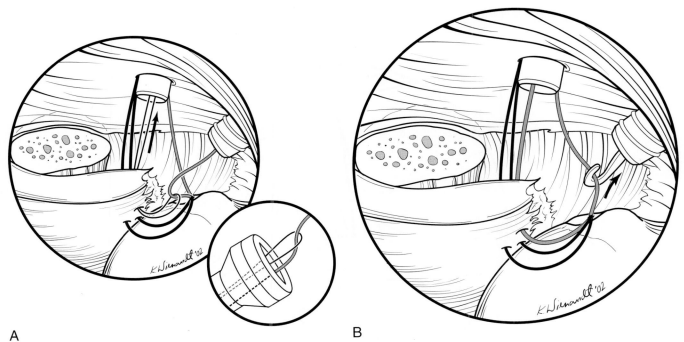

A   B

Figure 24–18   *A,* The Suture Lasso is passed through the tendon, and the suture loop is pulled through the anterolateral cannula. *B,* The second arm of the suture is pulled through the anterolateral cannula.

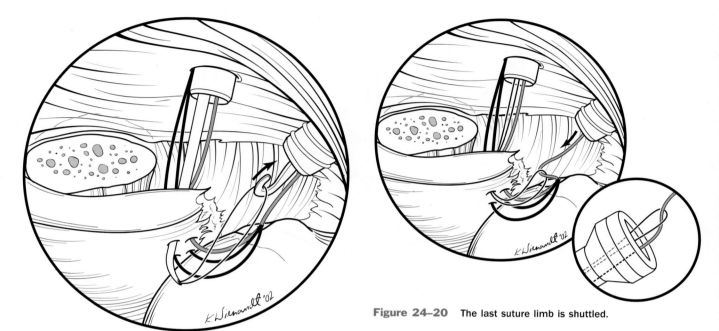

Figure 24–19 The Lasso loop is pulled.

Figure 24–20 The last suture limb is shuttled.

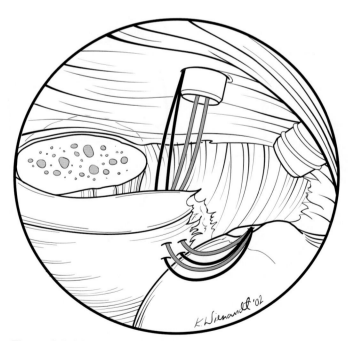

Figure 24–21 All four suture limbs are now through the tendon.

superior border of the subscapularis is then repaired to the most superior site of previous subscapularis tendon attachment. The most proximal anchor's last suture is placed over the top of the subscapularis, with only one limb of the tendon shuttled through the subscapularis belly (Fig. 24–22).

Either the anterolateral or the anterior portal can be used as the knot-tying portal. The anterolateral portal is most commonly used because of the ease of past-pointing suture limbs, which improves knot security. We use a clear, threaded 6-mm cannula for this portal, which is

ideal for knot tying. The most proximal suture anchor is tied first to set the ideal position of the entire subscapularis tendon (Fig. 24–23). The arm is rotated so that the suture, anchor, and cannula are in alignment before tying the knot. A crochet hook is used to grasp the two limbs of the most proximal suture and pull them through the anterolateral portal. When knots are tied, the patient's arm is internally rotated and forward flexed, which improves visualization of the knot. If tension is then placed on the suture limb in the tendon, while holding the other limb steady, the tendon is reduced to

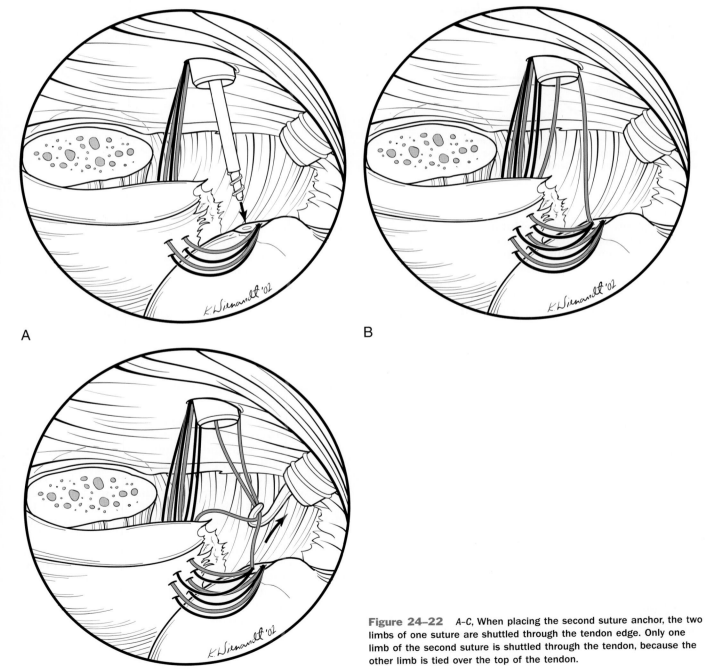

A

B

C

Figure 24–22 *A–C*, When placing the second suture anchor, the two limbs of one suture are shuttled through the tendon edge. Only one limb of the second suture is shuttled through the tendon, because the other limb is tied over the top of the tendon.

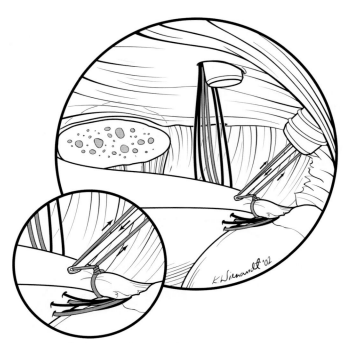

Figure 24–23 The first suture tied is the most superior one, with one limb over the top of the tendon to restore the anatomic location of the superior edge of the tendon.

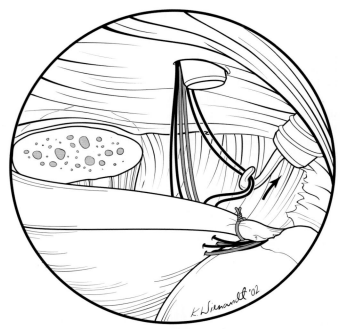

Figure 24–24 After the most proximal suture is tied, the next two sutures are pulled through the clear cannula and tied in position.

the tuberosity repair site. Multiple alternating half hitches with alternating posts are used to secure the suture knot; then the suture is cut. After the first suture is tied, the next two suture limbs from the same suture anchor are pulled out of the clear cannula with the crochet hook and tied (Fig. 24–24). The more medial limb of the two sutures is designated as the post to place the knot over the tendon.

Ideally, the knots should be placed over the tendon, not laterally over the tuberosity. A simple suture pattern is routinely used, which is adequate for maximal loading conditions of the tendon repair.[3,4] All knots are tied with a single-hole knot pusher. Each throw includes past-pointing the suture limbs to maximize loop security by reducing slack between the loops[6] (Fig. 24–25). A minimum of three alternating half hitches on alternating post limbs are included with every knot after a slip-knot or two half hitches are initially placed.[16] The sutures are cut at the end of the knot with a suture-cutting tool. The arm is then rotated to determine the security of the rotator cuff repair (Figs. 24–26 and 24–27). At the completion of the procedure, the portal sites are closed with interrupted monofilament sutures. The arm is protected with a padded sling that has an attached immobilization strap to avoid external rotation.

Pearls and Pitfalls

One must carefully evaluate the subscapularis tendon during routine arthroscopy, or symptomatic tears can be missed. If the biceps tendon is subluxated or dislocated out of its groove, a tenotomy or tenodesis of the biceps

tendon should be performed. The goal of the repair should be anatomic restoration with the superior edge of the subscapularis at the biceps groove. If the tear is complete, an extensive release is required. This entails approaching the region of the axillary nerve, which must be done with great care. As with any arthroscopic rotator cuff repair, suture management is important to the success of the procedure. The steps we have outlined should aid in this process.

Postoperative Management

The decreased surgical trauma with an arthroscopic repair compared with a deltopectoral interval approach results in less pain and narcotic use. Early range-of-motion exercises are instituted on the first postoperative day, but strengthening of the subscapularis is delayed 6 weeks to allow optimal healing of the tendon-bone interface. For the first 2 weeks, external rotation should be limited to 40 degrees to prevent stretching the repair site. The patient is allowed to forward elevate to 90 degrees and internally rotate to the abdomen. From 2 to 6 weeks, we allow the patient to gradually increase external rotation as tolerated, without manipulation by the therapist. Forward elevation is allowed to 140 degrees. This program may need to be adjusted for less secure repairs. The overall rehabilitation protocol is guided by several factors, including the size of the tendon tear, the quality of the repair, the surgeon's perception of the remaining tension on the repair, and patient-related variables such as chronic medical conditions.[22]

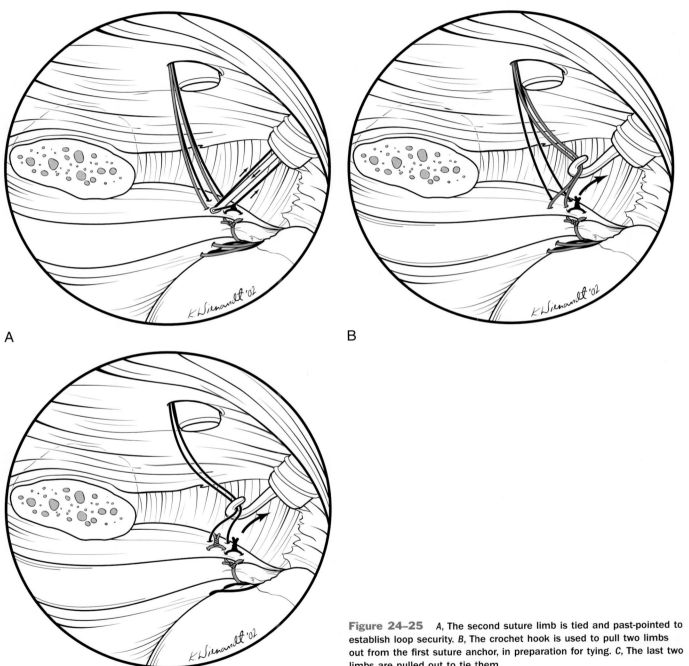

Figure 24–25   *A*, The second suture limb is tied and past-pointed to establish loop security. *B*, The crochet hook is used to pull two limbs out from the first suture anchor, in preparation for tying. *C*, The last two limbs are pulled out to tie them.

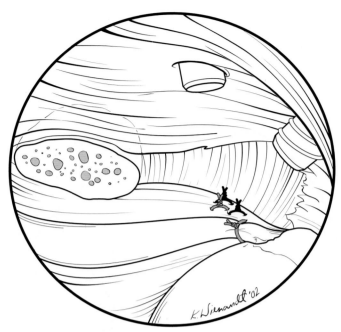

Figure 24–26 View from posterior cannula showing the final repair.

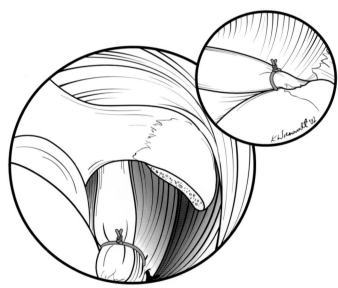

Figure 24–27 View from the anterolateral portal showing the tension set in the subscapularis tendon.

Results

Eighteen consecutive patients underwent arthroscopic subscapularis repair, with 14 patients available for follow-up longer than 1 year. The average age was 56 years (range, 32 to 85 years). Average follow-up was 27 months (range, 14 to 45 months). The tears were classified as type I, partial-thickness tear; type II, complete tear of upper 25% of tendon; type III, complete tear of upper 50% of tendon; and type IV, complete rupture of tendon.

A history of trauma was present for 71% of the tears. Delay in diagnosis ranged from 1 to 22 months after injury. In 64% of the cases, MRI interpretation failed to mention a subscapularis tear. Most of these films were reviewed by radiologists who did not specialize in musculoskeletal MRI. In three patients, an associated supraspinatus tear was identified by MRI and confirmed and repaired at the time of surgery. Four patients underwent a biceps tenodesis. One patient fell 2 weeks after surgery and required a second arthroscopic repair. There were no other complications.

Forward elevation improved from 138 to 161 degrees, and external rotation improved from 70 to 86 degrees. The ASES score increased from 46 to 82, and results of the simple shoulder test improved from 7 to 10 on a 12-question scale. The unadjusted Constant score (100-point absolute scale) was 75 for the operative side and 79 for the unaffected shoulder, suggesting a functional result similar to that of the unaffected shoulder. Seventy-nine percent of patients rated their function as good to excellent on the Rowe function subscale.

There are no published reports on the outcome of arthroscopic repair of the subscapularis tendon. Open repair of isolated subscapularis tendons has been reported in small case series, with acceptable results.[10,14,15,17] Our early results demonstrate successful pain relief and return of function. Further, our technique is safe, without a high risk of neurologic injury or other complications.

Complications

We have not experienced any neurovascular complications or infections. We have had one reruptured tendon in a patient who had another traumatic event.

References

1. Brown AR, Weiss R, Greenberg C, et al: Interscalene block for shoulder arthroscopy: Comparison with general anesthesia. Arthroscopy 9:295-300, 1993.
2. Burkhart SS: The deadman theory of suture anchors: Observations along a south Texas fence line. Arthroscopy 11:119-123, 1995.
3. Burkhart SS: A stepwise approach to arthroscopic rotator cuff repair based on biomechanical principles. Arthroscopy 16:82-90, 2000.
4. Burkhart SS, Fischer SP, Nottage WM, et al: Tissue fixation security in transosseous rotator cuff repairs: A mechanical comparison of simple versus mattress sutures. Arthroscopy 12:704-708, 1996.
5. Burkhart SS, Johnson TC, Wirth MA, Athanasiou KA: Cyclic loading of transosseous rotator cuff repairs: Tension overload as a possible cause of failure. Arthroscopy 13:172-176, 1997.
6. Burkhart SS, Wirth MA, Simonich M, et al: Knot security in simple sliding knots and its relationship to rotator cuff repair: How secure must the knot be? Arthroscopy 16:202-207, 2000.
7. Deutsch A, Altchek DW, Veltri DM, et al: Traumatic tears of the subscapularis tendon: Clinical diagnosis, magnetic

resonance imaging findings, and operative treatment. Am J Sports Med 25:13-22, 1997.

8. Ferrick MR: Coracoid impingement: A case report and review of the literature. Am J Sports Med 28:117-119, 2000.

9. Gartsman GM, Taverna E: The incidence of glenohumeral joint abnormalities associated with full-thickness, reparable rotator cuff tears. Arthroscopy 13:450-455, 1997.

10. Gerber C, Hersche O, Farron A: Isolated rupture of the subscapularis tendon. J Bone Joint Surg Am 78:1015-1023, 1996.

11. Gerber C, Krushell RJ: Isolated rupture of the tendon of the subscapularis muscle: Clinical features in 16 cases. J Bone Joint Surg Br 73:389-394, 1991.

12. Goutallier D, Postel JM, Bernageau J, et al: Fatty muscle degeneration in cuff ruptures: Pre- and postoperative evaluation by CT scan. Clin Orthop 304:78-83, 1994.

13. Hertel R, Ballmer FT, Lombert SM, Gerber C: Lag signs in the diagnosis of rotator cuff rupture. J Shoulder Elbow Surg 5:307-313, 1996.

14. Karnaugh RD, Sperling JW, Warren RF: Arthroscopic treatment of coracoid impingement. Arthroscopy 17:784-787, 2001.

15. Nerot C: Rotator cuff ruptures with predominant involvement of the subscapular tendon. Chirurgie 291:103-106, 1993-1994.

16. Nottage WM, Lieurance RK: Arthroscopic knot tying techniques. Arthroscopy 15:515-521, 1999.

17. Nove-Josserand L, Levigne C, Noel E, Walch G: [Isolated lesions of the subscapularis muscle: Apropos of 21 cases.] Rev Chir Orthop Reparatrice Appar Mot 80:595-601, 1994.

18. Pfirrmann CW, Zanetti M, Weishaupt D, et al: Subscapularis tendon tears: Detection and grading at MR arthrography. Radiology 213:709-714, 1999.

19. Ticker JB, Warner JJ: Single-tendon tears of the rotator cuff: Evaluation and treatment of subscapularis tears and principles of treatment for supraspinatus tears. Orthop Clin North Am 28:99-116, 1997.

20. Tung GA, Yoo DC, Levine SM, et al: Subscapularis tendon tear: Primary and associated signs on MRI. J Comput Assist Tomogr 25:417-424, 2001.

21. Walch G, Nove-Josserand L, Boileau P, Levigne C: Subluxations and dislocations of the tendon of the long head of the biceps. J Shoulder Elbow Surg 7:100-108, 1998.

22. Wilk KE: Rehabilitation after rotator cuff surgery. Tech Shoulder Elbow Surg 1:128-144, 2000.

2 Shoulder

Arthroscopic Management of Glenoid Arthritis

Scott P. Steinmann, Raymond M. Carroll,
and William N. Levine

ARTHROSCOPIC MANAGEMENT OF GLENOID ARTHRITIS IN A NUTSHELL

History:
Progressive pain with activities, night pain, mechanical symptoms, motion loss

Physical Examination:
Painful motion, motion loss, positive compression-rotation test, positive impingement signs

Imaging:
True anteroposterior (neutral, internal and external rotation), scapular lateral, axillary radiographs; magnetic resonance imaging for soft tissue pathology

Indications:
General: patients with glenohumeral arthritis without pain in the mid-arc of motion
Arthroscopic debridement: overlap symptoms of impingement or those that originate primarily from rotator cuff tears
Arthroscopic capsular release: motion loss in addition to arthritic change
Arthroscopic subacromial bursectomy: thickened bursa
Osteocapsular arthroplasty with glenoidplasty: capsular contractures and biconcave or posteriorly eroded glenoid

Contraindications:
Disease responsive to nonoperative treatment options; advanced disease likely to respond only to shoulder arthroplasty; unrealistic patient expectations

Surgical Technique:
Beach chair position, standard portals, thermal synovectomy, mechanical debridement, capsular release, osteophyte resection, glenoid recontouring

Postoperative Management:
Immediate unrestricted active range of motion, indwelling glenohumeral catheter, discontinue sling when comfortable

Results:
Initial pain relief from debridement, glenoidplasty with good short-term results

Complications:
Low complication rate equivalent to that of shoulder arthroscopy in general

Arthroscopic debridement of the glenohumeral joint for osteoarthritis (OA) is relatively uncommon owing to its limited indications. Historically, patients who have early OA and have failed conservative treatment are candidates for arthroscopic debridement. Unfortunately, the diagnosis of OA often is not made until the time of arthroscopic surgery, because the preoperative evaluation suggested other diagnoses.[2,4,13,21] Impingement syndrome is most commonly involved, although other preoperative diagnoses include rotator cuff tears, superior labral anterior to posterior (SLAP) lesions, instability, and adhesive capsulitis. The principal components of arthroscopic debridement include synovectomy, debridement of fraying cartilage and labrum, and removal of loose bodies. When adhesive capsulitis is present, appropriate capsular releases are indicated as well. Arthroscopic synovectomy for inflammatory conditions has been reported by a few authors and has had some success.[9-11,18,19] Synovial chondromatosis, although a rare condition in the shoulder, has also been treated successfully with arthroscopy.[1,21]

Many patients have concurrent procedures such as subacromial decompression, distal clavicle resection, and rotator cuff surgery, as indicated by the preoperative evaluation. Some authors consider subacromial bursectomy to be a primary component of the arthroscopic treatment of OA.[21] Patients with degenerative arthritis of the shoulder often have coexisting pathology, including loose bodies, labral tears, osteophytes, and articular cartilage defects. It seems likely that debridement of these lesions might provide some relief. There are currently few reports in the literature on the arthroscopic treatment of degenerative arthritis of the shoulder.[2,21] There are data suggesting that irrigation of the glenohumeral joint provides symptomatic relief by removing proteins and enzymes that contribute to the pathogenesis of OA. The goal of arthroscopic debridement is not to reverse or halt the progression of OA but to provide a period of symptomatic relief. Arthroplasty remains the gold standard for the treatment of severe arthritic changes of the glenohumeral joint.

History

The typical history for patients with OA is progressive pain with activity over time. Early in the disease process, the pain is related to strenuous or exertional activities. Over time, however, the pain occurs with activities of daily living. In later stages, patients may have pain at rest and at night. Early in the disease, when patients are symptomatic but have good motion, the pain may be mistaken for impingement syndrome or rotator cuff disease. With progression of the disease, the shoulder may develop secondary capsular and muscular contractures, with loss of active and passive motion. In addition to complaints of pain, patients often report mechanical symptoms such as catching or grinding with use of the shoulder. In many instances, OA is diagnosed at the time of arthroscopic surgery for another diagnosis.

Physical Examination

The hallmark finding of glenohumeral OA is loss of motion of the shoulder. In early stages of the disease, however, there is often painful motion but no loss of motion. When loss of motion is evident, the examiner must document the loss of both active and passive motion. Loss of active and passive motion is consistent with soft tissue contractures.. In OA, this finding is termed *secondary adhesive capsulitis*. In patients who have preserved passive motion but loss of active motion, rotator cuff pathology should be ruled out. The presence of lag signs is confirmatory for rotator cuff tearing. The compression-rotation test has been described to identify glenohumeral OA.[4] The patient is positioned in the lateral decubitus position, with the symptomatic shoulder up. The examiner presses firmly on the proximal humerus to "load" the glenohumeral joint. The patient then actively internally and externally rotates the arm. A positive test is one that produces pain or crepitus with this maneuver. At best, this test is only a screening tool, as there is no published report of its sensitivity or specificity in diagnosing OA. Many patients who are ultimately diagnosed with OA were noted to have positive impingement signs preoperatively, but whether these signs were related to the OA or to subacromial pathology is unclear. In many cases, a subacromial decompression was performed concurrently with the arthroscopic debridement. Patients with early OA may have positive impingement signs. These findings may be related to the location of the articular lesions in the glenohumeral joint or, more likely, to the synovitis in the joint. Some authors have noted chronic bursa-sided changes in the subacromial space of these patients.[4,21]

Imaging

A standard shoulder series including a true anteroposterior view in the scapular plane, with neutral and internal and external rotation views; a scapular lateral view; and an axillary view should be obtained on all patients before surgical intervention (Figs. 25–1 and 25–2). The classic findings of glenohumeral OA are joint space narrowing, osteophyte formation, subchondral sclerosis, and subchondral cyst formation. Poor technique in obtaining the anteroposterior or axillary view can obscure the subtle clues of early OA. On the axillary view, posterior wear of the glenoid is often noted in later stages of the disease. Unfortunately, significant articular cartilage damage (grade IV) is often unrecognized on plain films. A magnetic resonance imaging (MRI) scan may be helpful if the diagnosis is uncertain. Although false-negatives have been reported, MRI is more sensitive in diagnosing early-stage OA than are plain radiographs. MRI is clearly superior in diagnosing concurrent soft tissue pathology (Fig. 25–3). Twenty-eight of 61 patients (45%) in the Cameron et al. study[2] of grade IV chondral lesions had no radiographic (MRI or x-ray) evidence of OA on preoperative imaging. In the Ellman et al. study,[4] preoperative radiographs were negative in 14 of 18

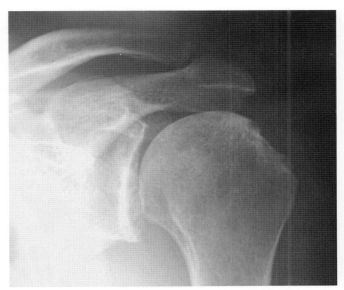

Figure 25–1 Anteroposterior radiograph shows subchondral sclerosis, loss of joint space, and early osteophyte formation.

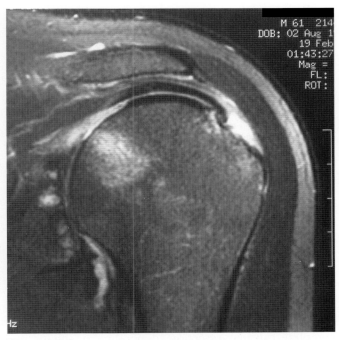

Figure 25–3 Coronal, oblique, T2-weighted magnetic resonance imaging scan shows loss of articular cartilage, subchondral cyst formation of the glenoid, and a full-thickness rotator cuff tear.

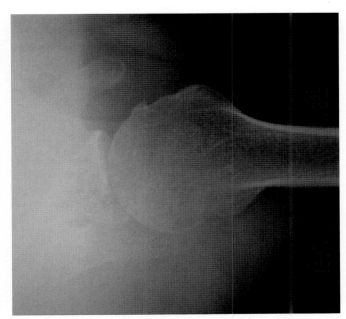

Figure 25–2 Axillary lateral radiograph reveals complete loss of joint space and posterior wear.

patients. Five of 11 (45%) MRI scans failed to diagnose OA preoperatively, although the pathology was correctly identified on MRI in 4 patients whose radiographs were negative. Weinstein et al.[20] reported that preoperative radiographs were normal in 5 of 25 (20%) shoulders with arthroscopic diagnoses of OA.

Treatment Options and Indications

In exploring the arthroscopic treatment options in a patient with degenerative disease of the shoulder, there

are basically four avenues of approach. First, a simple debridement of the glenohumeral joint can be performed. This includes removal of loose bodies, resection of labral tears, and shaving of articular cartilage defects. This has been shown to result in pain relief and patient satisfaction.[2,4,11,21] An advantage of arthroscopy includes the ability to confirm the clinical diagnosis. This was shown initially by Ellman et al.,[4] who, in a series of patients with impingement syndrome, found several patients with evidence of intra-articular glenohumeral degenerative changes. It is important to recognize, however, as Ellman and others have pointed out, that if the surgeon is confident of the clinical diagnosis, he or she should treat the impingement syndrome or rotator cuff tear and, in addition, perform debridement for the glenohumeral degenerative changes.[2,4] The finding of glenohumeral arthrosis in addition to a rotator cuff tear should not change the initial operative plan. If the surgeon believes that the patient's main symptoms originate from the rotator cuff, that should be addressed primarily at surgery, in addition to debridement of the glenohumeral joint. Today, the common use of MRI and the careful examination of radiographs allow early identification of arthritic changes in the shoulder.[17]

Arthroscopy gives the surgeon the opportunity to examine the glenohumeral joint. If degenerative changes are present, the lesions can be debrided and the patient informed afterward of the additional pathology encountered. Even in young persons with primary dislocation of the shoulder, osteochondral injury may occur in almost one half of patients.[16]

A second, more extensive operative approach is to perform a capsular release in addition to glenohumeral joint debridement. This is an option for patients with limited motion preoperatively in addition to arthritic changes in the shoulder joint. Release of the capsule might involve a gentle manipulation under anesthesia as a first step. If minor adhesions of the capsule exist, this is a simple way to gain additional motion. An examination under anesthesia also allows the surgeon to ascertain the area of tightness and determine which portion of the capsule needs the greatest attention. In particular, gentle manipulation in forward elevation might release adhesions in the inferior capsular area, which is near the axillary nerve. If motion is gained with manipulation under anesthesia, extensive arthroscopic surgery in the area of the axillary nerve may be avoided. The surgeon should be particularly careful in patients with osteoporosis to avoid stress that might induce a fracture. Forceful external rotation is most often associated with a higher risk of iatrogenic fracture. If the examination under anesthesia determines a need for capsular release—typically a loss of 15 to 20 degrees of motion in any plane—preparation for arthroscopic capsular release can be made. The surgeon has the option of performing either selective capsular release of only the tight area or complete capsular resection, depending on his or her experience and skill.

A third option to consider in patients with glenohumeral arthrosis is to explore the subacromial space and perform an inspection and debridement. It has been noted that patients with glenohumeral arthritis may have a thickened subacromial bursa, and when this is debrided, it allows increased joint motion and reduces pain.[21] In addition, viewing of the subacromial space allows adequate evaluation of the rotator cuff to determine the possible existence of associated rotator cuff tears. A bony subacromial decompression is not typically performed in the setting of shoulder arthritis, but if a bony spur is encountered, it can be removed; the coracoacromial ligament should be preserved.

A fourth option is to attempt to reconstruct a more normal bony architecture of the glenohumeral joint. This involves aggressive resection of osteophytes and recontouring of the glenoid if significant posterior or anterior wear has occurred. This technique also typically involves release of a significant portion of the joint capsule. This surgical procedure has been termed an *osteocapsular arthroplasty*.[8] When the glenoid is recontoured with arthroscopic instruments, this is termed a *glenoidplasty*.[8] If there is significant posterior subluxation, with posterior wear of the glenoid, the anterior glenoid is leveled and the typical biconcavity is removed in an attempt to re-form the normal curve of the native glenoid surface. This extensive procedure requires a high level of familiarity with arthroscopic techniques in the shoulder. Because it is a new procedure, there are few long-term data on the ability of recontouring to change the natural history of glenohumeral arthritis.

Choosing which of these four options to perform on an arthritic shoulder depends on the skill, philosophy, and experience of the surgeon and on the degree of arthritis. Some authors, for example, do not recommend arthroscopy in advanced arthritic conditions.[21] Although better results might be expected in patients with less arthritic change, there have not been enough studies done to help orthopedic surgeons determine which patients should not be candidates for arthroscopic treatment.

When treating patients who might be candidates for arthroscopic techniques, one should first explore standard nonoperative modalities, such as nonsteroidal anti-inflammatory medications, steroid injections, and physical therapy. In older geriatric patients, total shoulder arthroplasty remains the standard treatment against which arthroscopy should be measured. There are, however, some patients for whom total shoulder arthroplasty might not be a suitable option, such as those who are young or very active. Hemiarthroplasty has often been offered to younger patients with glenohumeral arthritis, but in patients with significant posterior wear and subluxation, this is not a good option.

The type of pain that a patient has is also a consideration. The pain of shoulder arthrosis can be divided into three types. First is pain at the extremes of motion. This is usually due to osteophytes and stretching of the inflamed capsule and synovium. Second is pain at rest, which is thought to be due to synovitis. Pain at night is not the same as pain at rest. Night pain may be due to synovitis, but it can also be due to awkward positions or increased pressure on the joint. Third is pain in the mid-arc of motion; this is usually accompanied by crepitus and typically represents articular surface damage. Some patients have crepitus that is almost painless; it may be noted by the patient but is not a major focus of pain.

The first two types of pain (at extremes of motion and at rest) may be helped by an arthroscopic procedure, but pain during the mid-arc of motion is a potentially poor prognostic indication and requires closer examination. The patient's glenohumeral joint should be compressed while moving through a mid-arc of motion. If this causes significant discomfort, the articular surfaces might be damaged to such an extent that arthroscopy will not offer significant pain relief.

Limitation of motion can also be related to pain and has several causes. Impinging osteophytes can abut, limit movement, and result in pain. Congruous incongruity, with a biconcavity of the glenoid, can also result in loss of motion. Capsular contracture from prior injury or surgery might increase joint contact forces and result in pain. A pseudocontracture can also occur if there is significant posterior subluxation or large loose bodies.

Surgical Technique

The patient is placed in the beach chair position after regional anesthesia (interscalene block) is obtained (Fig. 25–4). A standard posterior arthroscopic portal is made in the usual fashion. Under direct arthroscopic vision, an anterior portal is made using an 18-gauge spinal needle to locate the position. Typical findings include synovitis, especially on the undersurface of the rotator cuff; fraying of the labrum; and articular cartilage changes (Figs. 25–5 and 25–6). The status of the articular surfaces must be

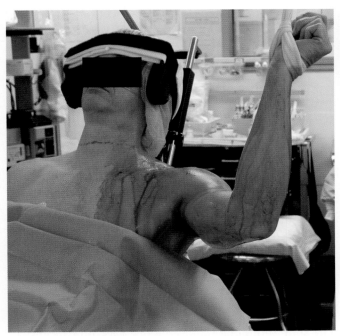

Figure 25–4   Patient prepped in the beach chair position.

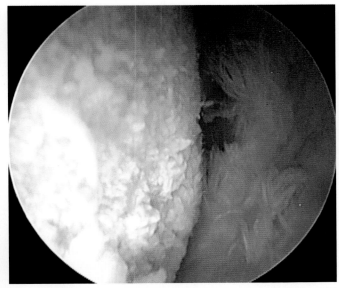

Figure 25–6   The humeral head reveals areas of grades III and IV changes *(left)*. Fraying of the anterior labrum is also noted *(right)*.

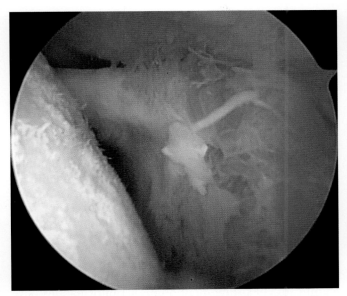

Figure 25–5   Typical synovitis on the undersurface of the cuff involving the biceps anchor and superior labrum.

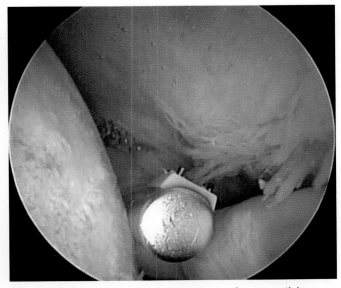

Figure 25–7   A thermal wand is used to perform a partial synovectomy on the undersurface of the rotator cuff.

documented to guide future treatment, should it become necessary. Once the diagnosis has been established, debridement is performed. Arthroscopic thermal devices are especially helpful for performing the partial synovectomy when synovitis is present (Fig. 25–7) because they minimize bleeding. A full-radius shaver is used to debride the fraying labrum and loose bodies. It is useful to keep the suction on to maximize the flow of saline through the shoulder joint and the flow of debris into the shaver. If there is restricted passive range of motion consistent with adhesive capsulitis (not motion loss due

to osteoarthritic bony constraints), it is important to perform the appropriate capsular or interval releases to regain passive motion. If the patient has extensive OA with capsular contraction and osteophyte formation, capsular resection may be required in addition to osteophyte removal to improve postoperative range of motion. Typically, the shoulder capsule is removed from the rotator interval, extending into the posteroinferior axillary recess at the back of the joint.

Once impinging osteophytes have been removed, labral tears debrided, and any capsular contracture addressed, the condition of the glenoid surface can be inspected. If there is a biconcave glenoid from posterior wear, recontouring of the surface (glenoidplasty) may be performed. The procedure involves converting the biconcave glenoid into a single concavity (Fig. 25–8). This can potentially restore the position of the humeral head, reducing the posterior subluxation. Restoration of a single concavity might also increase the surface area of the glenohumeral articulation, decreasing joint pressure. A reversal of the posterior subluxation might help relax contracted anterior soft tissues as well. At present, there are no long-term studies of the effect of this technique.

The procedure is performed with an anterior and a posterior portal. Viewing is alternated from front to back, and large and small burs are used to remove the remaining cartilage from the anterior glenoid facet; then the central vertical bony ridge is resected. Once a single concave surface is established, a large rasp can be used to smooth the surface. This is similar to the technique of reaming the anterior portion of the glenoid during total shoulder arthroplasty to restore the native version of the glenoid. Because a portion of subchondral bone is removed by this technique, long-term follow-up is needed to determine whether any medial migration of the humeral head occurs as a consequence of the procedure.

Some authors believe that, at a minimum, soft tissue decompression of the subacromial space should be part of the arthroscopic treatment for OA.[21] They have documented the presence of a thickened bursa, consistent with chronic bursitis, and believe that bursectomy is always indicated in these patients. However, we recommend a formal subacromial decompression only when the preoperative evaluation and intraoperative arthroscopic findings implicate the subacromial space as a source of pain. Ellman et al.[4] performed subacromial decompression in 15 of 18 (83.3%) patients. Their indication for this procedure was chronic bursal thickening in patients with Bigliani type II (curved) and III (hooked) acromions. We believe that the bleeding

undersurface of the acromion is a risk for subacromial fibrosis and loss of motion; therefore, we do not recommend routine subacromial decompression.

Postoperative Management

We institute full, unrestricted active range of motion on postoperative day 1. The physical therapy prescription is for full passive, active assisted, and active range of motion. Patients undergoing capsular release for adhesive capsulitis stay in the hospital overnight with an indwelling glenohumeral catheter for postoperative analgesia and begin full passive range of motion, with the goal of maintaining the motion gained at surgery during the postoperative healing phase. Patients should be allowed to go back to work as soon as they are comfortable. Most patients benefit from a structured therapy program under the guidance of a trained therapist, who can encourage the patient to maintain the range of motion achieved in the operating room. There are no limits, and full passive and active motion are allowed. The sling should be removed a few days after surgery to encourage a greater arc of motion.

Once the initial postoperative phase is over, rotator cuff rehabilitation is started.

Results

There are currently few studies examining the benefit of arthroscopic debridement of the shoulder for degenerative arthritis. Some studies have shown a benefit of synovectomy of the glenohumeral joint in cases of rheumatoid arthritis.[5,9,10,13-15,18,19] The outcome of arthroscopic debridement in OA has been addressed in only a small number of reports. Ellman et al.[4] demonstrated the benefit of debridement of the glenohumeral joint in patients undergoing surgery for impingement syndrome. That study showed the advantage of arthroscopy over open surgery in detecting coexisting pathology in patients with impingement syndrome. Similarly, Gartsman and Taverna[6] showed that coexisting intra-articular pathology occurred in 60% of patients undergoing arthroscopic repair for a full-thickness rotator cuff tear. Significant coexisting glenohumeral abnormalities have been noted by others during arthroscopic shoulder surgery.[2,12,21] Cofield[3] and others[7,13] demonstrated relief of symptoms in patients undergoing arthroscopic lavage of the glenohumeral joint.

In two series of patients undergoing debridement for glenohumeral degeneration, a high percentage of patients in both studies reported initial pain relief (100% and 88%).[2,21] The mechanism of pain relief is unclear, but it may involve the removal of painful synovium or the dilution of degenerative debris. Of note, in neither study was pain relief related to the radiographic stage of arthritis. In the study by Cameron et al.,[2] pain level was not correlated with the location of the lesion. Return of pain and failure, however, were associated with osteochondral lesions greater than 2 cm in diameter. Although it

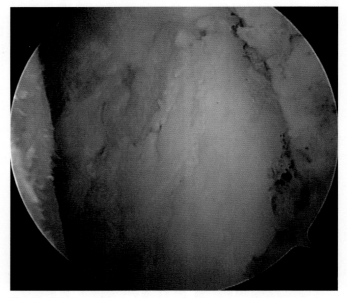

Figure 25–8 Arthroscopic view of a biconcave glenoid treated arthroscopically.

appears that arthroscopic debridement of the gleno-humeral joint for arthritis may offer some patient satisfaction, it is still unclear whether there is a certain amount of arthritis for which the procedure will prove to be ineffective.

To date, the results of glenoidplasty, the most extensive form of debridement of the glenohumeral joint, has been reported in only one article.[8] That study looked at 14 patients whose average age was 50 years, 12 of whom had severe glenohumeral arthritis. Motion was restricted in all patients. At an early follow-up of 3 years, active motion had increased in the majority, and 86% thought that they were either significantly improved or improved by the procedure; 92% strongly agreed that the surgery was worthwhile. There were no complications and no evidence of medial migration of the humerus on the axillary view.

Importantly, whether simple debridement of the glenohumeral joint or a more advanced glenoidplasty is done, future potential surgery, including total shoulder arthroplasty, is not jeopardized. Overall, positive prognostic indicators in a patient with degenerative arthritis include impingement pain at the end of motion, rest pain, painless crepitus, no pain with glenohumeral compression or rotation, and large inferior osteophytes or loose bodies. Negative prognostic indicators include pain at the midrange of motion, painful crepitus, pain with glenohumeral compression or rotation, and minimal osteophytes or loose bodies.

Arthroscopic debridement of the glenohumeral joint appears to be useful for short-term pain relief, with a large majority of patients believing that the procedure is worthwhile. Age does not appear to be a factor, but range of motion may not improve significantly after the procedure. Patients with minimal to severe arthritis may benefit from the procedure. In patients with severe arthritis, significant improvements are unlikely unless extensive debridement, such as a glenoidplasty, is performed. Although total shoulder replacement is the gold standard against which to measure results, in active patients in whom a replacement is either unsuitable or undesirable, arthroscopic treatment may be of benefit.

Complications

None of the previously published series reported any complications with this technique. Ogilvie-Harris and Wiley[13] reported 15 complications in 439 patients (3%) undergoing arthroscopic surgery. The reported complication rate for shoulder arthroscopy is very low in general.

References

1. Buess E, Friedrich B: Synovial chondromatosis of the glenohumeral joint: A rare condition. Arch Orthop Trauma Surg 121:109-111, 2001.
2. Cameron BD, Galatz LM, Ramsey ML, et al: Non-prosthetic management of grade IV osteochondral lesions of the glenohumeral joint. J Shoulder Elbow Surg 11:25-32, 2002.
3. Cofield R: Arthroscopy of the shoulder. Mayo Clin Proc 58:501-508, 1983.
4. Ellman H, Harris E, Kay SP: Early degenerative joint disease simulating impingement syndrome: Arthroscopic findings. Arthroscopy 8:482-487, 1992.
5. Gachter A, Gubler M: [Shoulder arthroscopy in degenerative and inflammatory diseases.] Orthopade 21:236-240, 1992.
6. Gartsman GM, Taverna E: The incidence of glenohumeral joint abnormalities associated with full-thickness, reparable rotator cuff tears. Arthroscopy 13:450-455, 1997.
7. Johnson LL: The shoulder joint: An arthroscopic perspective of anatomy and pathology. Clin Orthop 223:113-125, 1987.
8. Kelly E, O'Driscoll S, Steinmann S: Arthroscopic glenoidplasty and osteocapsular arthroplasty for advanced glenohumeral arthritis. Paper presented at the Annual Open Meeting of the American Shoulder and Elbow Surgeons, 2001.
9. Matthews LS, LaBudde JK: Arthroscopic treatment of synovial diseases of the shoulder. Orthop Clin North Am 24:101-109, 1993.
10. Midorikawa K: The short term results of shoulder arthroscopic synovectomy in rheumatoid patients. Kyusyu RA 8:53-56, 1989.
11. Midorikawa K, Hara M, Emoto G, et al: Arthroscopic debridement for dialysis shoulders. Arthroscopy 17:685-693, 2001.
12. Miller C, Savoie FH: Glenohumeral abnormalities associated with full-thickness tears of the rotator cuff. Orthop Rev 23:159-162, 1994.
13. Ogilvie-Harris DJ, Wiley AM: Arthroscopic surgery of the shoulder. J Bone Joint Surg Br 60:201-207, 1986.
14. Pahle JA, Kvarnes L: Shoulder synovectomy. Ann Chir Gynaecol 198:37-39, 1985.
15. Petersson C: Shoulder surgery in rheumatoid arthritis. Acta Scand 57:222-226, 1986.
16. Taylor DC, Arciero RA: Pathologic changes associated with shoulder dislocations: Arthroscopic and physical examination findings in first-time, traumatic anterior dislocations. Am J Sports Med 25:306-311, 1997.
17. Umans HR, Pavlov H, Berkowitz M, et al: Correlation of radiographic and arthroscopic findings with rotator cuff tears and degenerative joint disease. J Shoulder Elbow Surg 10:428-433, 2001.
18. Wakitani S, Imoto K, Saito M, et al: Evaluation of surgeries for rheumatoid shoulder based on the destruction pattern. J Rheumatol 26:41-46, 1999.
19. Weber A, Bell S: Arthroscopic subacromial surgery in inflammatory arthritis of the shoulder. Rheumatology 40:384-386, 2001.
20. Weinstein DM, Bucchieri JS, Pollock RG, et al: Arthroscopic debridement of the shoulder for osteoarthritis. Arthroscopy 16:471-476, 2000.
21. Witwity T, Uhlmann R, Nagy MH, et al: Shoulder rheumatoid arthritis associated with chondromatosis, treated by arthroscopy. Arthroscopy 7:233-236, 1991.

Arthroscopic Management of Shoulder Stiffness

GARY M. GARTSMAN

ARTHROSCOPIC MANAGEMENT OF SHOULDER STIFFNESS IN A NUTSHELL

History:
  Possibly prior trauma, diabetes, or thyroid dysfunction; painful limited range of motion

Physical Examination:
  Reduction in passive and active glenohumeral motion; scapulothoracic substitution of motion

Imaging:
  Standard radiographs; magnetic resonance imaging as needed

Indications:
  Pain and stiffness despite 6 months of nonoperative treatment

Contraindications:
  Postoperative and post-traumatic stiffness, which may require open release; malunited fractures associated with stiffness; patients in the inflammatory or contracting phase of idiopathic adhesive capsulitis

Surgical Technique:
  Interscalene block, examination under anesthesia, gentle manipulation; joint entry at superior margin of glenoid, rotator interval release, anterior capsule release, subscapularis delineation, subacromial bursectomy (if needed)

Postoperative Management:
  Intravenous hydrocortisone, subacromial hydrocortisone, steroid dose pack, pillow (not sling) under axilla, continuous passive motion for 2 weeks, physical therapy

Results:
  Reduced pain and increased motion and strength in the majority of patients

---

There are four basic conditions that produce shoulder stiffness and are amenable to arthroscopic treatment: idiopathic adhesive capsulitis, the diabetic stiff shoulder, post-traumatic stiffness, and postoperative stiffness.[1,5,6,10] Idiopathic adhesive capsulitis is widely believed to be a painful but self-limited condition that resolves after 1 to 2 years.[1] Reports suggest that although many patients improve, they have significant limitations of movement

and function. Additionally, many patients suffering from disabling pain are unwilling to wait for their condition to resolve and inquire about operative treatment.

Shoulder stiffness in patients with diabetes seems to cause greater pain and is more refractory to nonoperative treatment than is idiopathic stiffness.[5,6] The impairment from post-traumatic stiffness is related directly to the severity of the trauma. Postoperative stiffness can be

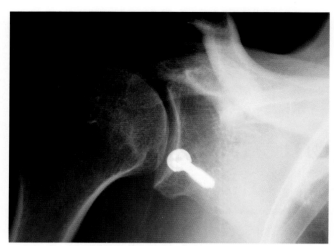

Figure 26-1   Postsurgical stiffness after a Bristow procedure. (From Gartsman GM: Shoulder Arthroscopy. Philadelphia, WB Saunders, 2003, p 144.)

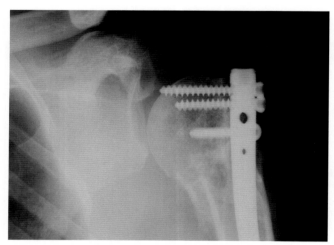

Figure 26-2   Post-traumatic and postsurgical stiffness after open reduction and internal fixation. (From Gartsman GM: Shoulder Arthroscopy. Philadelphia, WB Saunders, 2003, p 144.)

the result of excessive scarring in the area of surgical treatment (subacromial adhesions after rotator cuff repair, anterior glenohumeral capsular contracture after a Bankart procedure),[10] but profound glenohumeral joint contractures can occur after surgical treatment that does not violate the capsule (Figs. 26–1 and 26–2).[8]

Arthroscopy is advantageous in that it enables the surgeon to release intra-articular, subacromial, and subdeltoid adhesions without dividing the subscapularis.[2,4] Postoperatively, active range of motion can be started immediately without concern for tendon dehiscence.

History

A thorough history that ascertains prior trauma or shoulder difficulties is important. Patients should be queried about diabetes and thyroid dysfunction. Most patients either recall a trivial antecedent injury or cannot recall

an inciting event. Patients with all types of adhesive capsulitis present with painful, limited shoulder motion.[9] Pain at night interferes with sleep, and routine activities of daily living that require reaching overhead or behind the back are difficult and painful. Rapid movements in particular may cause severe pain. Patients demonstrate restricted passive and active motion, such that the motion is usually less than 50% that of the contralateral shoulder.

Physical Examination

Passive range of motion in elevation, abduction, and external rotation (in adduction with the patient's arm at the side and in maximum allowable abduction) is recorded. Internal rotation is measured at the vertebral level to which the patient can reach with the extended thumb. Behind-the-back internal rotation is usually decreased; occasionally, however, it may be close to normal because internal rotation measured in this manner includes not only glenohumeral movement but also scapulothoracic motion. With prolonged shoulder stiffness, scapulothoracic motion may be increased to compensate for the loss of glenohumeral rotation. For this reason, stabilizing the scapula with one hand while the arm is maximally abducted to eliminate scapulothoracic motion during external and internal rotation provides a more accurate measure of glenohumeral rotation. Muscle strength in elevation and external rotation is also assessed.

Imaging

Radiographs are typically normal, but mild osteopenia from disuse may be present. Standard anteroposterior, axillary, and supraspinatus (scapular) outlet radiographs are obtained. Magnetic resonance imaging is helpful when rotator cuff or labral pathology is suspected.

Differential Diagnosis

Numerous other shoulder conditions produce painful limited motion, but these are eliminated by patient history, physical examination, and radiographic evaluation. Patients with rotator cuff tears present with passive motion greater than active motion, weakness evident on manual muscle testing, and abnormal magnetic resonance imaging scans or arthrograms. Patients with osteoarthrosis have plain radiographs depicting loss of glenohumeral joint space (Fig. 26–3). Patients with post-traumatic stiffness may have malunited fractures, and those with postoperative stiffness may have internal fixation interfering with motion.

Indications and Contraindications

Surgical intervention is considered if the patient has persistent pain and stiffness after 6 months of appropriate

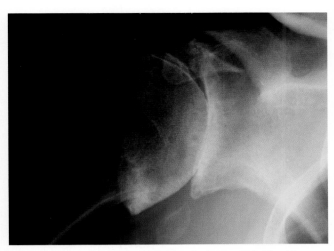

Figure 26–3   Osteoarthrosis. (From Gartsman GM: Shoulder Arthroscopy. Philadelphia, WB Saunders, 2003, p 144.)

nonoperative care. Severe stiffness is defined as 0 degrees of external rotation and less than 30 degrees of abduction. Moderate stiffness is defined as a decrease of 30 degrees in either plane compared with the contralateral shoulder. Although loss of internal rotation is clinically significant to the patient, by itself, it is not considered an indication for arthroscopic release. One exception is the throwing athlete. In these patients, posterior contracture and decreased internal rotation may be the only problems, and these patients may be candidates for arthroscopic release while addressing all intra-articular pathology. If stiffness persists at 6 months but pain has diminished, nonoperative care is continued for an additional 2 months, with the hope that the decrease in pain indicates that the stiffness is about to resolve, or "thaw," spontaneously. If there is no improvement in the range of motion 2 months later, surgery is considered. If at 4 to 6 months after the start of nonoperative treatment external rotation remains at neutral or worse, operative intervention is recommended, because a response to further nonoperative care is unlikely.

Contraindications for arthroscopic treatment exist mainly in patients with postoperative and post-traumatic stiffness. Patients who have had surgical procedures for instability with subscapularis takedown or shortening may develop profound soft tissue contractures. The contracture in these patients is typically extra-articular between the subscapularis and the conjoined tendon. Open release is often necessary, in addition to arthroscopic glenohumeral joint release. Patients with mildly malunited greater tuberosity or proximal humerus fractures can be treated arthroscopically, but patients with badly malunited fractures or internal fixation require open release, removal of hardware, and fracture osteotomy, as indicated. Patients in the inflammatory or contracting phase of idiopathic adhesive capsulitis should not undergo surgery, because the procedure may accelerate the contracture.

Surgical Technique

Examination under Anesthesia

After induction of anesthesia, both shoulders are examined for range of motion in elevation, abduction, and external rotation in adduction. The affected shoulder is placed in maximal abduction, and internal and external rotation are measured.

Manipulation

Before arthroscopic treatment, gentle closed manipulation is performed. It is difficult to quantify the term *gentle*, but only a small amount of force is applied to the shoulder in abduction and then in elevation. If the shoulder responds to closed manipulation, it will move with minimal force. If motion improves with abduction and elevation, the arm is placed in external rotation. This is performed with the shoulder in maximal abduction and then in adduction. If motion continues to improve, internal rotation stretching begins by internally rotating the shoulder in maximal abduction. If motion improves, the shoulder is stretched in cross-body adduction and finally in behind-the-back internal rotation. If the shoulder does not respond to abduction and elevation, no additional attempts at external or internal rotation are made, owing to torsional stresses associated with excessive external and internal rotation. In this scenario, proceeding directly to arthroscopy is indicated. If the shoulder responds to manipulation but full movement is not achieved, arthroscopy and release of the remaining adhesions are indicated. If full range of motion is obtained after manipulation, the arthroscope is inserted to confirm that the capsule is released completely. Some shoulders with full range of motion after manipulation have persistent capsular contracture because the manipulation may be releasing only extra-articular adhesions.

Specific Surgical Steps

Joint Entry

Entry into the stiff shoulder is always difficult because, by definition, the joint volume is reduced. Forceful entry may damage the articular surfaces. The tight, thickened posterior capsule makes spinal needle entry difficult, and the generalized capsular stiffness limits the amount of fluid that can be injected. A standard metal cannula and a rounded trocar may be helpful, as they are larger and stiffer than the spinal needle, and palpation of the posterior glenohumeral joint is easier.

The entry position is critical. Joint entry through the traditional "soft spot" (located at the level of the glenoid equator) increases the risk of cartilage surface damage. At this level, the glenohumeral joint space is narrowest, making trocar entry difficult. Entering the joint superiorly relative to the glenoid, the rotator cuff, and the humeral head is safer and easier, because the joint is widest in that location (Fig. 26–4). The skin is incised, and the cannula and trocar are inserted until bone is palpated. The shoulder is internally and externally rotated to determine whether the trocar tip rests on the humeral head (movement detected) or the glenoid (no movement). Lowering the hand holding the trocar elevates the trocar tip in an effort to palpate the superior glenoid rim. At this point, joint entry is attempted (Fig. 26–5).

Once the arthroscope is in the glenohumeral joint, it is directed at the rotator interval. Percutaneous placement of a spinal needle positioned lateral to the coracoid process is performed to target the entrance point for a 5-mm cannula and trocar.

Rotator Interval Release

The first step in the operation is to release the rotator interval (Figs. 26–6 and 26–7). This can be accomplished with a motorized soft tissue resector. The resector is inserted through the cannula into the joint; then the cannula is backed out of the joint, leaving the resector tip in the rotator interval. Soft tissue is excised from an area bounded by the biceps tendon medially, the superior border of the subscapularis tendon inferiorly, and the humeral head laterally. Before removing the resector, the cannula is reintroduced into the joint. The arthroscope is withdrawn from the posterior cannula, leaving an indwelling cannula. A closed manipulation is attempted, as described earlier. If full range of motion is obtained, the arthroscope is reintroduced posteriorly to verify that the capsule is divided and that the humeral head is properly located. If full range of motion is not achieved, or if motion has improved but the capsule is not completely divided, the anterior capsule is released.

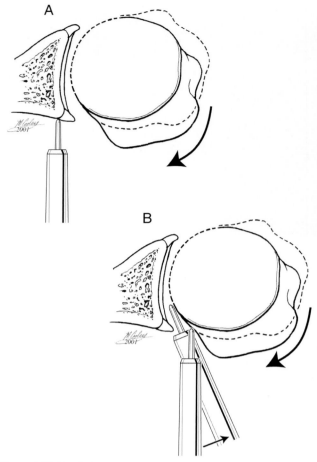

Figure 26–5   Palpate bone to determine the entry point. *A*, Palpate the glenoid. The trocar is too medial. *B*, Move the trocar laterally to enter the joint. (From Gartsman GM: Shoulder Arthroscopy. Philadelphia, WB Saunders, 2003, p 146.)

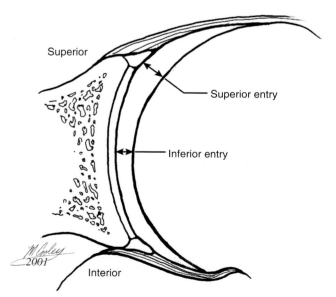

Figure 26–4   Location of joint entry. (From Gartsman GM: Shoulder Arthroscopy. Philadelphia, WB Saunders, 2003, p 146.)

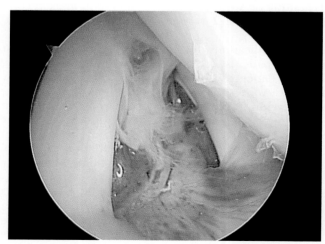

Figure 26–6   Contracted rotator interval. (From Gartsman GM: Shoulder Arthroscopy. Philadelphia, WB Saunders, 2003, p 146.)

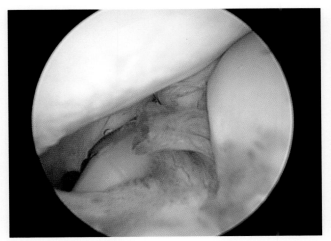

Figure 26–7   Synovitis in the rotator interval. (From Gartsman GM: Shoulder Arthroscopy. Philadelphia, WB Saunders, 2003, p 146.)

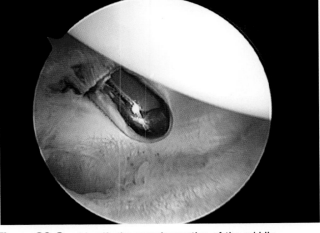

Figure 26–9   **Identify the superior portion of the middle glenohumeral ligament.**   (From Gartsman GM: Shoulder Arthroscopy. Philadelphia, WB Saunders, 2003, p 147.)

Anterior Capsule Release

The point where the middle glenohumeral ligament crosses the subscapularis tendon is identified (Fig. 26–8). It is important to separate the subscapularis tendon from the middle glenohumeral ligament, which is facilitated by an electrocautery device. It is helpful to divide fibers of the middle glenohumeral ligament gradually until the tendinous portion of the superior subscapularis is visualized. A blunt dissector is inserted anterior to the middle glenohumeral ligament to separate the two structures. A Harryman soft tissue punch (Smith and Nephew Endoscopy, Andover, MA) is helpful to remove a 5- to 10-mm strip of anterior capsule. This includes the middle glenohumeral ligament and the superior portion of the anteroinferior glenohumeral ligament. Alternatively, electrocautery may be used for this portion of the procedure (Figs. 26–9 to 26–16).

Usually, a small amount of increased lateral humeral head displacement results after these steps, allowing the

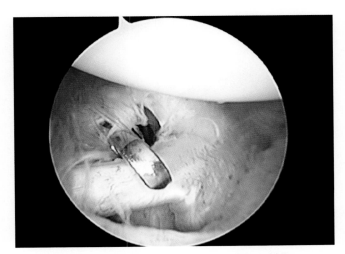

Figure 26–10   **Divide the superior portion of the middle glenohumeral ligament.** (From Gartsman GM: Shoulder Arthroscopy. Philadelphia, WB Saunders, 2003, p 147.)

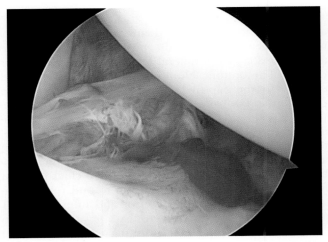

Figure 26–8   **Contracted anterior capsule.** (From Gartsman GM: Shoulder Arthroscopy. Philadelphia, WB Saunders, 2003, p 147.)

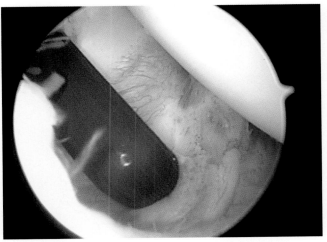

Figure 26–11   **Apply cautery to the middle glenohumeral ligament covering the subscapularis.** (From Gartsman GM: Shoulder Arthroscopy. Philadelphia, WB Saunders, 2003, p 147.)

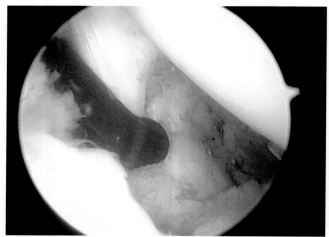

Figure 26–12   Apply cautery to the middle glenohumeral ligament covering the subscapularis. (From Gartsman GM: Shoulder Arthroscopy. Philadelphia, WB Saunders, 2003, p 148.)

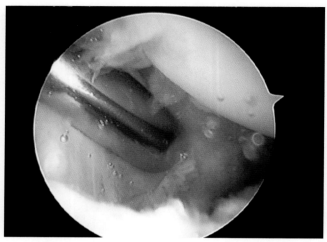

Figure 26–15   Use a blunt dissector anterior to the subscapularis. (From Gartsman GM: Shoulder Arthroscopy. Philadelphia, WB Saunders, 2003, p 148.)

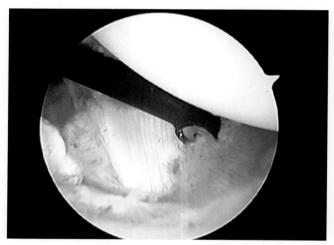

Figure 26–13   Apply cautery to the middle glenohumeral ligament covering the subscapularis. (From Gartsman GM: Shoulder Arthroscopy. Philadelphia, WB Saunders, 2003, p 148.)

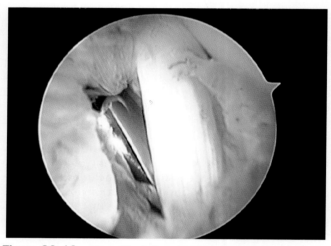

Figure 26–16   Use a blunt dissector posterior to the subscapularis. (From Gartsman GM: Shoulder Arthroscopy. Philadelphia, WB Saunders, 2003, p 148.)

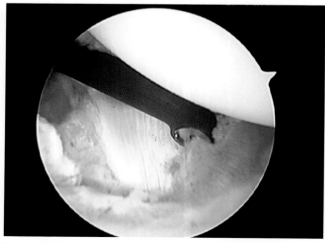

Figure 26–14   Apply cautery to the middle glenohumeral ligament covering the subscapularis. (From Gartsman GM: Shoulder Arthroscopy. Philadelphia, WB Saunders, 2003, p 148.)

arthroscope to be advanced anteriorly and inferiorly to more clearly visualize the posterior portion of the anteroinferior glenohumeral ligament and the inferior capsule. The bottom, blunt jaw of the punch is placed exterior to the capsule to divide it from anterior to posterior as far from the glenoid labrum as possible (Figs. 26–17 and 26–18). The extent of this release depends on the amount of axillary pouch contracture, which may limit the degree of advancement of the punch without applying excessive distraction to the glenohumeral joint. This is usually about the 5-o'clock position for a right shoulder. To gain access to and release the axillary pouch safely, the posterior and inferoposterior areas of the capsule are treated next.

The soft tissue punch and cannula are removed from the anterior portal and exchanged for a metal cannula and trocar. The arthroscope is removed from the posterior portal and inserted anteriorly. Under direct vision,

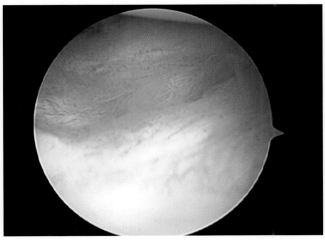

Figure 26–17   **Contracted inferior capsule.** (From Gartsman GM: Shoulder Arthroscopy. Philadelphia, WB Saunders, 2003, p 148.)

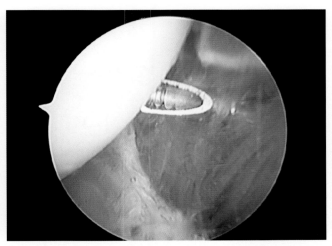

Figure 26–19   **A shaver is used to resect the posterior capsule.** (From Gartsman GM: Shoulder Arthroscopy. Philadelphia, WB Saunders, 2003, p 149.)

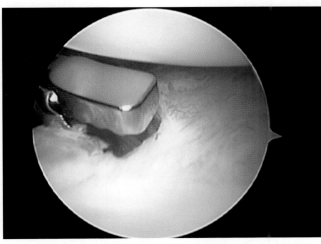

Figure 26–18   **Capsular punch in the anteroinferior capsule.** (From Gartsman GM: Shoulder Arthroscopy. Philadelphia, WB Saunders, 2003, p 149.)

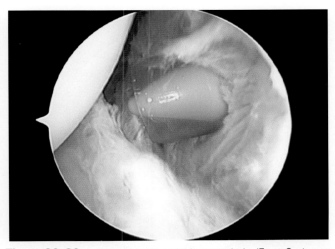

Figure 26–20   **Insert a large cannula posteriorly.** (From Gartsman GM: Shoulder Arthroscopy. Philadelphia, WB Saunders, 2003, p 149.)

the small plastic cannula and trocar are placed posteriorly. The glenohumeral joint is usually too tightly contracted to allow insertion of a larger diameter cannula. A motorized shaver is used to resect 5 to 10 mm of posterior capsule, beginning superiorly and moving inferiorly (Fig. 26–19). Once the posterior capsule has been resected, a large-diameter cannula is inserted that will accommodate the capsular resection punch (Figs. 26–20 and 26–21).

The punch is used to resect a 10-mm strip of the posteroinferior capsule beginning 5 to 10 mm from the glenoid labrum to avoid any labral damage. The last step in the intra-articular portion of the procedure is complete release of the inferior capsule. Often, surgical division is not necessary because the last portion of the capsule can be released through manipulation, which avoids placing instruments near the axillary nerve.

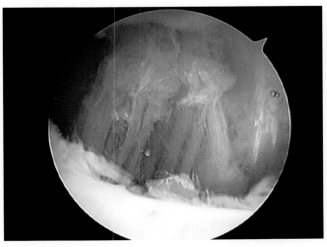

Figure 26–21   **Complete the posterior capsular resection with a punch.** (From Gartsman GM: Shoulder Arthroscopy. Philadelphia, WB Saunders, 2003, p 149.)

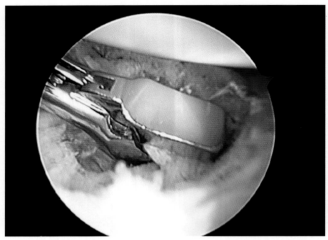

Figure 26–22 Return the arthroscope to the posterior portal and complete the inferior capsular resection. (From Gartsman GM: Shoulder Arthroscopy. Philadelphia, WB Saunders, 2003, p 150.)

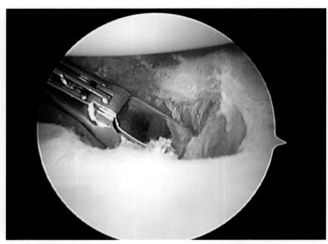

Figure 26–24 Inferior capsular resection. (From Gartsman GM: Shoulder Arthroscopy. Philadelphia, WB Saunders, 2003, p 150.)

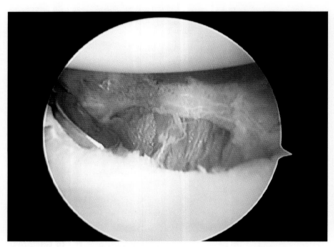

Figure 26–23 Inferior capsular resection. (From Gartsman GM: Shoulder Arthroscopy. Philadelphia, WB Saunders, 2003, p 150.)

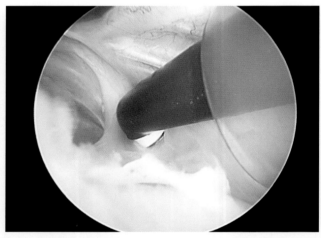

Figure 26–25 Remove subacromial adhesions, if present. (From Gartsman GM: Shoulder Arthroscopy. Philadelphia, WB Saunders, 2003, p 150.)

Following manipulation, the arthroscope is inserted to inspect the gap between the resected edges of the capsule and to confirm that the humeral head is normally located. If full range of motion is not obtained with manipulation, the arthroscope is inserted posteriorly and the cannula and punch anteriorly, and the inferior capsule is resected (Figs. 26–22 to 26–24).

Subscapularis Delineation

A blunt dissector is used to release any adhesions anterior and posterior to the subscapularis. To achieve full passive range of motion, it is generally safe to resect the superior tendinous border of the subscapularis.

Subacromial Bursectomy

The arthroscope is introduced into the subacromial space. If the subacromial space is not clearly seen, a motorized soft tissue resector is used to remove bursa and adhesions (Fig. 26–25).

An acromioplasty is not performed even if there is arthroscopic evidence of impingement, such as rotator cuff or coracoacromial ligament fraying. By definition, a patient with adhesive capsulitis cannot move the shoulder into the positions consistent with the clinical diagnosis of impingement. The raw acromial bone surface produced after acromioplasty creates the opportunity for postoperative adhesions and should be avoided.

Postoperative Management

To reduce postoperative inflammation and adhesion formation, the following protocol is used. Following arthroscopic confirmation of shoulder stiffness resulting from capsular contracture, but before soft tissue resection, the anesthesiologist gives the patient 100 mg of hydrocortisone intravenously. Intra-articular cortisone is not given at the conclusion of the procedure, because resection of the capsule causes the steroid to extravasate and lose its effectiveness. In patients with post-traumatic or postsurgical stiffness and with subacromial adhesions requiring release, 1 mg of hydrocortisone (Solu-Cortef) is injected into the subacromial space at the conclusion of the operation. Postoperatively, the patient is placed on a methylprednisolone (Medrol) dose pack. Steroids are not used in patients with diabetes.

A sling or immobilizer is not used. Instead, a pillow is placed under the axilla to keep the arm away from the chest, and the patient is encouraged to avoid placing the arm in internal rotation. The patient is admitted to the hospital overnight. A continuous passive motion chair is used to maintain the full range of motion gained during the surgical procedure. Continuous passive motion begins the afternoon of the operation. It is extremely helpful to visit the patient on the afternoon of the surgical procedure and to demonstrate that the patient now has full range of motion. This is easily done, because the patient's shoulder is still anesthetized from the interscalene block. This visual demonstration of full movement impresses on the patient that the operation was successful. One should emphasize to the patient that complete recovery depends on adherence to the postoperative rehabilitation program. On discharge from the hospital, the patient uses the chair four times daily for 1 hour each session. This regimen continues for 2 weeks. At that time, the patient is seen in the clinic, and if movement is satisfactory, the continuous passive motion chair is discontinued.

Passive elevation while the patient is supine and external rotation with the aid of a dowel or pulley are continued. The patient is encouraged to use the arm for all activities and motions that are comfortable. The patient is seen again at 6 weeks, 3 months, and 6 months postoperatively.

If the patient has not achieved full range of motion by 3 months, a repeat contracture release is recommended. At this point, however, usually only gentle closed manipulation is necessary.

Results

Ogilvie-Harris, Harryman, and Warner and their colleagues have published landmark articles describing their results.[2-5,7-10] Arthroscopic treatment is generally successful, with the degree of improvement depending on the patient's underlying condition. Warner et al.[9] reported on 23 patients with idiopathic adhesive capsulitis treated with arthroscopic release. In that study, the Constant score improved an average of 48 points. Flexion improved a mean of 49 degrees, external rotation 45 degrees, and internal rotation by eight spinous processes. Harryman[2-4] documented improved patient satisfaction, function, and pain relief in a population of patients with diabetes, although the range-of-motion improvement was not as great as that seen in patients with idiopathic adhesive capsulitis.

References

1. Griggs SM, Ahn A, Green A: Idiopathic adhesive capsulitis: A prospective functional outcome study of nonoperative treatment. J Bone Joint Surg 82:1398-1407, 2000.
2. Harryman DT II: Shoulders: Frozen and stiff. Instr Course Lect 42:247-257, 1993.
3. Harryman DT II: Arthroscopic management of shoulder stiffness. Oper Tech Sports Med 5:264-274, 1997.
4. Harryman DT II, Matsen FA III, Sidles JA: Arthroscopic management of refractory shoulder stiffness. Arthroscopy 13:133-147, 1997.
5. Ogilvie-Harris DJ, Myerthall S: The diabetic frozen shoulder: Arthroscopic release. Arthroscopy 13:1-8, 1997.
6. Scarlat MM, Harryman DT II: Management of the diabetic stiff shoulder. Instr Course Lect 49:283-293, 2000.
7. Warner JJP: Frozen shoulder: Diagnosis and management. J Am Acad Orthop Surg 5:130-140, 1997.
8. Warner JJP, Allen AA, Marks PH, Wong P: Arthroscopic release of postoperative capsular contracture of the shoulder. J Bone Joint Surg Am 79:1151-1158, 1997.
9. Warner JJP, Answorth A, Marks PH, Wong P: Arthroscopic release for chronic refractory adhesive capsulitis of the shoulder. J Bone Joint Surg Am 78:1808-1816, 1996.
10. Warner JJP, Greis PE: The treatment of stiffness of the shoulder after repair of the rotator cuff. J Bone Joint Surg Am 79:1260-1269, 1997.

Arthroscopic Management of Scapulothoracic Disorders

JAMES D. O'HOLLERAN, PETER J. MILLETT, AND JON J. P. WARNER

ARTHROSCOPIC MANAGEMENT OF SCAPULOTHORACIC DISORDERS IN A NUTSHELL

History:
Posteromedial shoulder pain with crepitus

Physical Examination:
Point tenderness over superomedial angle or inferior pole of scapula with painful range of motion with or without audible or palpable crepitus; diagnostic injection helpful

Imaging:
Tangential scapular radiographs (rule out osteochondroma), computed tomography with or without three-dimensional reconstruction, magnetic resonance imaging

Indications:
Failure to respond to conservative treatment, including rest, nonsteroidal anti-inflammatory drugs, activity modification, physical therapy, and corticosteroid injections

Contraindications:
Asymptomatic crepitus and unfamiliarity with regional anatomy (arthroscopic contraindication)

Surgical Technique:
Patient positioned prone; arm in extension and internal rotation
Initial portal: 2 cm medial to medial scapular edge at level of spine
Working portal: spinal needle target 4 cm inferior to first portal
Expose superomedial angle and excise bone using bur

Postoperative Management:
Sling; early range of motion; progressive strengthening, including rotator cuff and scapular stabilizers

Results:
Small case series with encouraging results comparable to those of open resection

Complications:
Pneumothorax, neurovascular injury, incomplete resection

Symptomatic scapulothoracic bursitis and crepitus are difficult and often poorly understood disorders of the scapulothoracic articulation, and little has been written about arthroscopic or open solutions for refractory pain from this region.[2-6,8,13,14,17-20,23] The first step in understanding bursitis and crepitus, as described by Kuhn et al.,[10] is to recognize the subtle differences between these two related but distinct entities. Historically, several terms have been used to describe elements of these disorders, including snapping scapula, scapulothoracic syndrome, washboard syndrome, and rolling scapula.[9] Boinet[1] is generally credited with the first description of scapulothoracic crepitus in 1867, and in 1904, Mauclaire[12] described three subclasses: *froissement,* a gentle physiologic friction sound; *frottement,* a louder grating sound that is usually pathologic; and *craquement,* a consistently pathologic loud snapping sound. Milch[14] later added to the understanding by differentiating scapulothoracic crepitus into two categories: a loud, usually painful grating sound caused by a bony lesion, and a less intense sound caused by a soft tissue lesion such as bursitis. Kuhn et al.[9,10] extrapolated from Milch and proposed that frottement may represent a soft tissue lesion or bursitis, whereas craquement represents an osseous lesion as the source of the painful scapulothoracic crepitus. Precise distinction, if possible, is often made radiographically or surgically, and it is crucial to understand that clinically symptomatic bursitis may exist without an audible sound or palpable crepitus. Further, isolated crepitus in the absence of pain may be physiologic. Nevertheless, the timing of conservative versus operative treatment is often influenced by the cause and nature of the symptoms, and an understanding of these two entities will assist the clinician in appropriate diagnosis and treatment.

Anatomy and Biomechanics

Understanding the anatomy and biomechanics of the scapulothoracic articulation is important when treating these problems.[3,5,7,9,10,18,21] Kuhn et al.[9,10] described the two major and four minor, or adventitial, bursae in the scapulothoracic articulation (Fig. 27–1). The first major bursa, the infraserratus bursa, is located between the serratus anterior muscle and the chest wall. The second, the supraserratus bursa, is found between the subscapularis and the serratus anterior muscles. The anatomic consistency of these bursae is well documented. In addition,

four minor bursae have been identified; however, they have not been found consistently in cadaveric or clinical studies. These bursae have been postulated to be adventitial in nature, arising in response to abnormal biomechanics of the scapulothoracic articulation.[19] Two have been described at the superomedial angle of the scapula, and historical accounts identify the location to be either infraserratus or supraserratus. A third site of pathology is at the inferior angle of the scapula, thought to be an infraserratus bursa. The fourth location, the trapezoid bursa, is at the medial base of the spine of the scapula, underlying the trapezius muscle. Usually, the bursa in the region of the superior angle of the scapula is the symptomatic one. The scapular noises encountered in crepitus arise from anatomic changes in the soft tissues in the articulation or from bony incongruity due to anatomic anomalies of the bones themselves.

Differential Diagnosis

The differential diagnosis of scapulothoracic bursitis includes soft tissue lesions such as atrophied muscle, fibrotic muscle, anomalous muscle insertions, and elastofibroma, which is a rare but benign soft tissue tumor located on the chest wall and elevating the scapula.[3,9-11,16,18,19] The differential diagnosis of scapulothoracic crepitus is expansive[3,9,10] and includes several anatomic anomalies located between the scapula and the chest wall. Osteochondromas can arise from the undersurface of the scapula or the posterior aspect of the ribs. Luschka's tubercle is a prominence of bone at the superomedial aspect of the scapula, and that same region can have an excessively hooked surface that alters scapulothoracic dynamics (Fig. 27–2). Malunited fractures of the scapula or the ribs can lead to crepitus. Reactive bone spurs can form from repetitive microtrauma of the

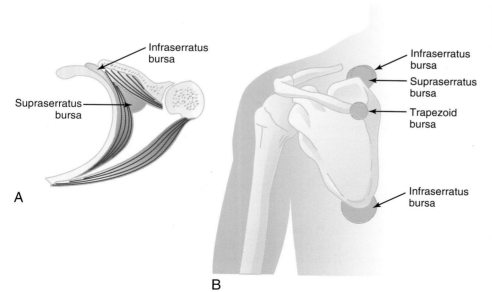

Figure 27–1 Two major bursae *(A)* and four minor, or adventitial, bursae *(B)* have been described in the scapulothoracic articulation.

Infraserratus bursa

Supraserratus bursa

A

Infraserratus bursa

Supraserratus bursa

Trapezoid bursa

Infraserratus bursa

B

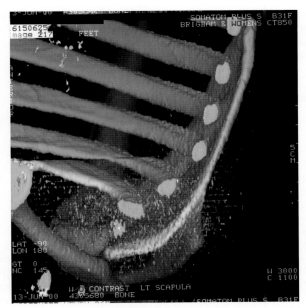

Figure 27–2 Three-dimensional computed tomography of the scapulothoracic articulation showing the prominent superomedial angle, often referred to as Luschka's tubercle.

periscapular musculature. Infectious causes such as tuberculosis or syphilis can lead to pathologic changes in the soft tissues. Additionally, incongruity of the articulation can exist secondary to scoliosis or thoracic kyphosis, leading to altered biomechanics and crepitus. Last, the differential diagnosis of all forms of scapulothoracic pathology must include unrelated disorders such as cervical spondylosis and radiculopathy, glenohumeral pathology, and periscapular muscle strain.

Clinical Evaluation

Clinical evaluation of scapulothoracic bursitis and crepitus begins with a thorough history and physical examination.

History

The history of the problem is similar in both disorders. Patients with bursitis report pain with overhead activity, often with a history of trauma or repetitive overuse in work or recreation. This constant motion irritates the soft tissues, leading to inflammation and a cycle of chronic bursitis and scarring. This tough, fibrotic bursal tissue can lead to mechanical impingement and pain with motion and hence further inflammation. Audible or palpable crepitus may accompany the bursitis, but the lesion is one of the soft tissues. Patients with scapulothoracic crepitus may additionally report a family history,[9] and it is occasionally bilateral.

Physical Examination

The physical findings of bursitis include localized tenderness over the inflamed area. The superomedial border of the scapula is the most common location, but the inferior pole is also a site of pathology. A mild fullness can be palpated, and audible or palpable crepitus may be present. Physical findings in patients with crepitus include point tenderness as well, but visual inspection may reveal a fullness or pseudowinging (not neurologic in nature) due to compensation of scapular mechanics from painful bursitis. A mass may be palpable. The scapula grates as the shoulder is put through a range of motion, but crucial to differentiating crepitus from true winging is the presence of a normal neuromuscular examination with overall normal scapulothoracic motion. In some patients with the appearance of winging, this may be secondary to pain from the scapulothoracic articulation, and motor examination of the serratus anterior and trapezius demonstrates normal function of these muscles. Again, crepitus alone in the absence of pain may be physiologic and may not warrant treatment.

Injection of a corticosteroid and local anesthetic is helpful to confirm the diagnosis. If this injection is accurately placed into the symptomatic scapulothoracic bursa and the patient notes significant pain relief, this confirms the diagnosis and points to the anatomic location of the bursa in question. The steroid may also have an antiinflammatory effect that facilitates a physical therapy program, as noted later.

Imaging

Radiographs should include tangential scapular views to identify bony anomalies. The role of computed tomography, with or without three-dimensional reconstruction, is still debated[15,22] (see Fig. 27–2), but in patients with suspected osseous lesions and normal radiographs, this additional imaging is often helpful. Magnetic resonance imaging can identify the size and location of bursal inflammation, but its usefulness is also debated.

Treatment Options

Nonoperative

Once the diagnosis of scapulothoracic bursitis or crepitus has been made, the initial treatment is nonoperative management. Rest, nonsteroidal anti-inflammatory drugs, and activity modification are used, and physical therapy is initiated. Therapy should emphasize various local modalities and periscapular muscle strengthening, particularly in adding physical bulk to the subscapularis and serratus anterior to elevate the scapula off the chest wall.[13,23] Additionally, postural training and a figure-of-eight harness can minimize thoracic kyphosis, which may be an aggravating factor. Subtle weakness of the serratus anterior muscle may allow the scapula to tilt forward so that its upper border "washboards" over the ribs and irritates the bursa. Therefore, strengthening of this muscle is very important, as it may resolve pain by restoring normal scapular mechanics. As noted previously, injection of a corticosteroid and a local anesthetic can assist in treatment as well as in diagnosis. When considering the duration of conservative management, the underlying diagnosis is important. Scapulothoracic bursal inflammation secondary to overuse and repetitive strain is treated quite successfully with the aforementioned measures. In contrast, true crepitus, especially due to a structural anatomic lesion such as an osteochondroma, is unlikely to benefit from conservative measures alone.[14] In such cases, a trial of conservative management should be attempted, but the threshold for progression to operative management should be significantly lower.

Operative

The vast majority of patients improve with conservative measures; for those who fail, many surgical procedures have been described. For bursitis, open bursectomy of the involved region, either the superomedial angle or the inferior pole, has been performed with success.[12,13,17,23] Likewise, crepitus has been successfully treated with open excision of the superomedial border of the scapula itself (Figs. 27–3 and 27–4).[14,20] Although variations in the techniques are numerous and beyond the scope of this chapter, the essential steps involve a fairly large exposure and subperiosteal elevation of the medial periscapular musculature, with identification of the pathologic tissue and excision of the inflamed bursa, irregular or pathologic bone, or both. The elevated muscle layers are sutured back to bone through drill holes, and the skin is often closed over a drain. Success has been good, and rehabilitation, though varied, generally follows a course of early passive motion, active motion by 4 weeks, and strengthening by 8 to 12 weeks.

As in other areas of the body, arthroscopic treatment of scapulothoracic disorders has been proposed as an alternative to open surgery in an attempt to minimize the morbidity of the exposure, with its muscle takedown, and to facilitate early rehabilitation and return to preoperative function.

Case History

EW is a 33-year-old woman with a 6-month history of superomedial scapular pain with occasional crepitus, exacerbated by overhead activity. Although no specific antecedent event can be identified, she reported a history of repetitive overhead use, including playing tennis and filing papers on a high shelf. She denied a positive family history or bilateral complaints.

Physical Examination

Physical examination revealed her cervical spine and shoulder to be free from pathology. The superomedial

angle of the scapula had a doughy fullness, and local palpation to that area elicited tenderness and re-created her pain patterns. Range of motion of the scapulothoracic articulation revealed mild crepitus on palpation.

Imaging

Imaging included tangential scapular view radiographs to rule out bony anomalies. Three-dimensional computed tomography was not performed because EW's history, physical examination, and radiographs suggested scapulothoracic bursitis and not crepitus from a discrete bony lesion.

Decision-Making Principles

In EW's case, conservative therapy consisting of rest, activity modification, and physical therapy for periscapular muscle strengthening has failed. Localized injection of corticosteroid and anesthetic to the area of tenderness at the superomedial angle of the scapula provided immediate relief and therefore confirmed the diagnosis.

After a thorough discussion of the risks and benefits of operative versus continued conservative therapy, the patient wished to proceed with surgical excision. She elected to undergo arthroscopic bursal debridement to minimize the morbidity and rehabilitation associated with a full open approach. This was a reasonable decision, given the absence of evidence of a large bony or discrete soft tissue lesion that might require open excision.

Surgical Technique

Positioning

Arthroscopic scapulothoracic bursectomy is performed with the patient in the prone position, with the arm placed behind the back in extension and internal rotation (the so-called chicken wing position) to assume an attitude of winging off the posterior thorax (Fig. 27–5). This position results in scapular protraction and facilitates entry of the arthroscopic instruments into the bursal space.

Specific Surgical Steps

The standard arthroscopic portals are used (Fig. 27–6). The initial "safe" portal is placed 2 cm medial to the medial scapular edge at the level of the scapular spine, between the serratus anterior and the posterior thoracic wall. This avoids the dorsal scapular nerve and artery, which course along the medial border of the scapula. The space is localized with a spinal needle and distended with approximately 30 mL of saline, and the portal is created. A blunt obturator is inserted into the subserratus space. Care must be taken to avoid overpenetration through the chest wall or, more commonly, through the serratus anterior into the subscapular (axillary) space. The 30-degree arthroscope is inserted, and fluid is

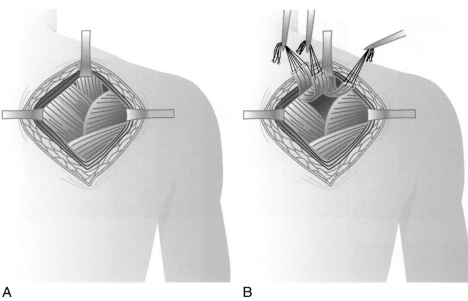

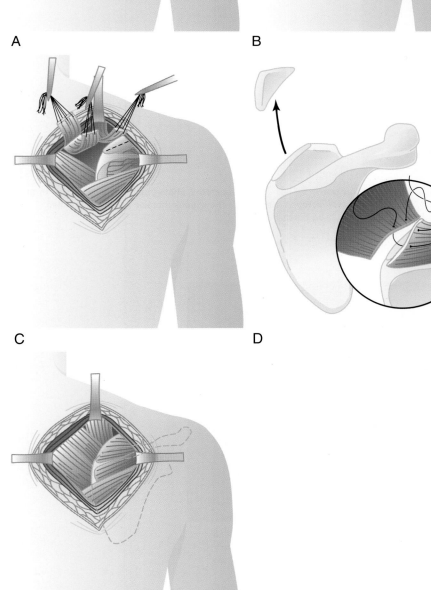

A

B

C

D

E

2 Shoulder

Figure 27–3   Open excision of the superomedial border of the scapula. *A*, The superomedial border of the scapula is exposed by elevating the trapezius muscle from the spine of the scapula. *B*, The supraspinatus, rhomboids, and levator scapulae muscles are subperiosteally dissected from the superomedial scapula and tagged. *C*, The superomedial angle is excised with an oscillating saw. *D* and *E*, The previously tagged muscles are repaired back to bone through drill holes.

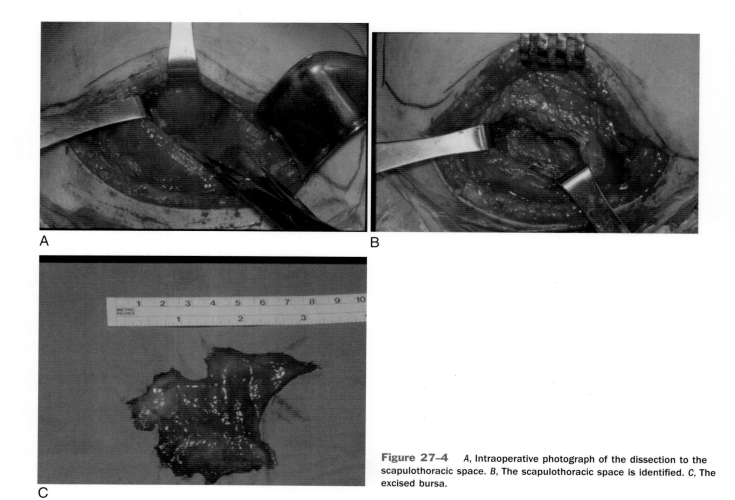

A

B

C

Figure 27–4 *A,* Intraoperative photograph of the dissection to the scapulothoracic space. *B,* The scapulothoracic space is identified. *C,* The excised bursa.

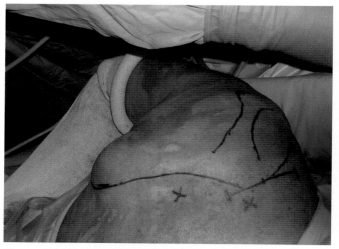

Figure 27–5 The patient is positioned prone in the so-called chicken wing position to assume an attitude of winging off the posterior thorax. Note the markings for the standard arthroscopy portals.

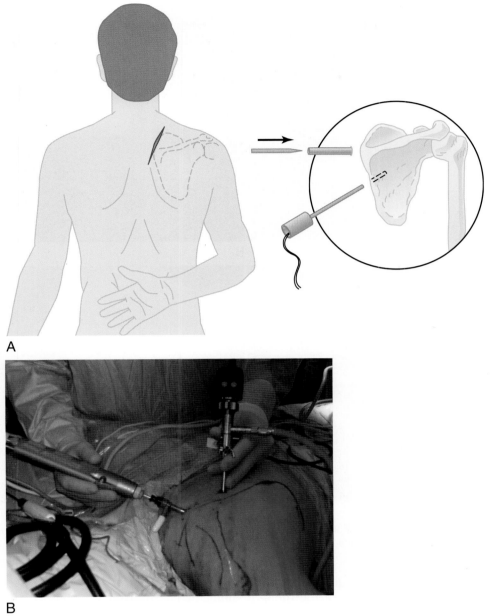

Figure 27–6 *A,* Placement of the two standard portals used for arthroscopic resection of the scapulothoracic bursa. *B,* The patient in the prone position with the portals established.

infiltrated to distend the subserratus space. We prefer to use an arthroscopy pump but keep the pressure low (30 mm Hg) to minimize fluid extravasation or dissection of fluid into the axilla. The second "working" portal can then be localized under direct visualization using a spinal needle. This is placed approximately 4 cm inferior to the first portal. A 6-mm cannula is inserted through the lower portal, and a motorized shaver and bipolar radiofrequency device are used to resect the bursal tissue (Fig. 27–7). The radiofrequency device is particularly useful to minimize bleeding in the vascular, inflamed tissue. Because there are minimal anatomic landmarks for resection, a methodic approach is essential, ablating from medial to lateral and then from inferior to supe-

rior. To facilitate visualization, the surgeon should be prepared to switch viewing portals as needed and to have a 70-degree arthroscope readily available. Spinal needles can be used to help outline the medial border of the scapula, and a probe can be used to palpate the ribs and intercostal muscles anteriorly and the scapula and serratus anterior posteriorly. If necessary, an additional portal can be placed superiorly, as described by Chan et al.,[5] although portals superior to the spine of the scapula may put the dorsal scapular neurovascular structures, accessory spinal nerve, and transverse cervical artery at risk.

The superomedial angle of the scapula is identified by palpation through the skin. The radiofrequency device

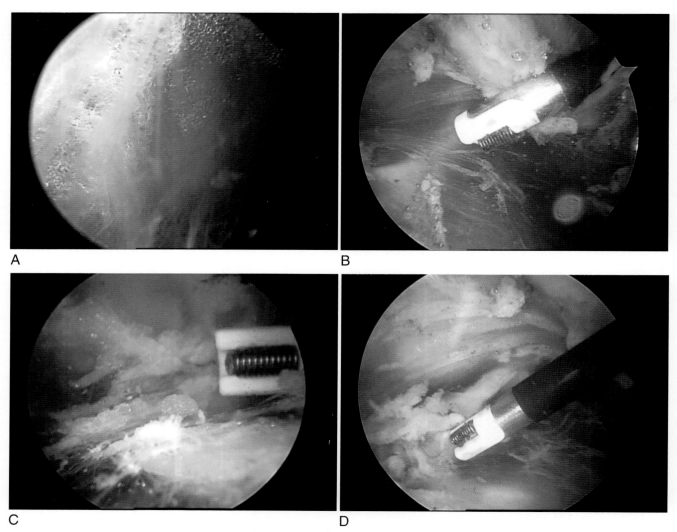

Figure 27–7 *A*, The bursal tissue is evident in the scapulothoracic space. *B*, The electrocautery device is visualized in the scapulothoracic space. *C* and *D*, The bursal tissue is excised using the cautery.

is used to detach the conjoined insertion of the rhomboids, levator scapulae, and supraspinatus from the bone subperiosteally. A partial scapulectomy is then performed using a motorized shaver and a bur. The periosteal sleeve is not repaired and is allowed to heal through scarring. It may be difficult to fully define the superior scapular angle owing to swelling from arthroscopic fluid, and in such cases, a small incision allows exposure of the angle and its resection. The trapezius muscle is split, and the rhomboids and serratus muscles are dissected from the scapula. The superior angle is resected, and then the rhomboids and serratus are repaired through drill holes to the superior scapula.

Postoperative Management

Postoperatively, the patient is placed in a sling for comfort only, as opposed to the 4 weeks required for an open approach. Gentle passive motion is initiated immediately to avoid stiffness. At 4 weeks, active and active assisted range of motion is begun, together with isometric exercises. After 8 weeks, strengthening of the periscapular muscles begins.

Results

Cuillo and Jones[6] introduced the concept of arthroscopic debridement of the scapulothoracic articulation in 1992, and Harper et al.[8] reported on the first series of arthroscopic bony debridements of the superomedial angle of the scapula in 1999. The arthroscopic anatomy was thoroughly described by Ruland et al.,[21] and an alternative arthroscopic portal was introduced by Chan et al.[5] in 2002. Early results of arthroscopic treatment seem promising, with minimal morbidity and an early return to function. Nevertheless, no large series has been published, and it must be emphasized that this technique is used primarily by experienced arthroscopists.

Complications

Complications of arthroscopic resection include pneumothorax, neurologic or vascular injury, and failure to resect all pathologic tissue. To our knowledge, there are no published reports of these complications, but the experience is still in its infancy.

References

1. Boinet: Snapping scapula. Societe Imperiale de Chirurugie (2nd ser) 8:458, 1867.
2. Bristow WR: A case of snapping shoulder. J Bone Joint Surg 6:53-55, 1924.
3. Butters K: The scapula. In Rockwood CA, Matsen FA (eds): The Shoulder, 2nd ed. Philadelphia, WB Saunders, 1998, pp 391-427.
4. Carlson HL, Haig AJ, Stewart DC: Snapping scapula syndrome: Three cases and an analysis of the literature. Arch Phys Med Rehabil 78:506-511, 1997.
5. Chan BK, Chakrabarti AJ, Bell SN: An alternative portal for scapulothoracic arthroscopy. J Shoulder Elbow Surg 11:235-238, 2002.
6. Cuillo JV, Jones E: Subscapular bursitis: Conservative and endoscopic treatment of "snapping scapula" or "washboard syndrome." Orthop Trans 16:740, 1992-1993.
7. Edelson JG: Variations in the anatomy of the scapula with reference to the snapping scapula. Clin Orthop 322:111-115, 1996.
8. Harper GD, McIlroy S, Bayley JI, Calvert PT: Arthroscopic partial resection of the scapula for snapping scapula: A new technique. J Shoulder Elbow Surg 8:53-57, 1999.
9. Kuhn JE: The scapulothoracic articulation: Anatomy, biomechanics, pathophysiology, and management. In Iannotti JP, Williams GE (eds): Disorders of the Shoulder: Diagnosis and Management. Philadelphia, Lippincott Williams & Wilkins, 1999, pp 817-845.
10. Kuhn JE, Plancher KD, Hawkins RJ: Symptomatic scapulothoracic crepitus and bursitis. J Am Acad Orthop Surg 6:267-273, 1998.
11. Majo J, Gracia I, Doncel A, et al: Elastofibroma dorsi as a cause of shoulder pain or snapping scapula. Clin Orthop 388:200-204, 2001.
12. Mauclaire M: Craquements sous-scapulaires pathologiques traits par l'interposition musculaire interscapulothoracique. Bull Mem Soc Chir Paris 30:164-168, 1904.
13. McClusky GM III, Bigliani LU: Surgical management of refractory scapulothoracic bursitis. Orthop Trans 15:801, 1991.
14. Milch H: Partial scapulectomy for snapping in the scapula. J Bone Joint Surg Am 32:561-566, 1950.
15. Mozes G, Bickels J, Ovadia D, Dekel S: The use of three-dimensional computed tomography in evaluating snapping scapula syndrome. Orthopedics 22:1029-1033, 1999.
16. Neilsen T, Sneppen O, Myhre-Jensen O, et al: Subscapular elastofibroma: A reactive pseudotumor. J Shoulder Elbow Surg 5:209-213, 1996.
17. Nicholson GP, Duckworth MA: Scapulothoracic bursectomy for snapping scapula syndrome. J Shoulder Elbow Surg 11:80-85, 2002.
18. Parsons TA: The snapping scapula and scapular exostoses. J Bone Joint Surg Br 55:345-349, 1973.
19. Percy EC, Birbrager D, Pitt MJ: Snapping scapula: A review of the literature and presentation of 14 patients. Can J Surg 31:248-250, 1988.
20. Richards RR, McKee MD: Treatment of painful scapulothoracic crepitus by resection of the superomedial angle of the scapula: A report of three cases. Clin Orthop 247:111-116, 1989.
21. Ruland LJ, Ruland CM, Matthews LS: Scapulothoracic anatomy for the arthroscopist. Arthroscopy 11:52-56, 1995.
22. Sans N, Jarlaud T, Sarrouy P, et al: Snapping scapula: The value of 3D imaging. J Radiol 80:379-381, 1999.
23. Sisto DJ, Jobe FW: The operative treatment of scapulothoracic bursitis in professional pitchers. Am J Sports Med 14:192-194, 1986.

ARTHROSCOPY OF THE ELBOW

Elbow: Anesthesia, Patient Positioning, Portal Placement, Normal Arthroscopic Anatomy, and Diagnostic Arthroscopy

Jim C. Hsu and Ken Yamaguchi

Elbow arthroscopy is a technically demanding surgical procedure that requires precise knowledge of the elbow anatomy. The proximity of neurovascular structures to the joint, the complex joint anatomy, the unfamiliar orientations of the elbow in various positions, and the premium placed on surgical speed to avoid tissue edema all add to the challenge. Although these concerns are substantial, surgeons experienced in elbow arthroscopy can treat an ever-expanding range of disorders with minimal risk of morbidity and complications. Much of our increased ability to treat the elbow arthroscopically can be traced to fundamental improvements in our understanding of surgical anatomy and in the basic surgical setup.

Anesthesia

Anesthesia options for elbow arthroscopy include general anesthesia or regional blocks. General anesthesia is the most popular choice because it provides complete muscle relaxation and flexibility in the prone or lateral decubitus position, which may be poorly tolerated in awake patients.[10] General anesthesia without regional block also allows immediate postoperative neurologic examination to verify that no nerve injury has occurred. Additionally, periodic neurologic examinations are possible in the perioperative period to allow the early detection of avoidable complications such as compartment syndrome or overly compressive dressings.

If the patient cannot tolerate general anesthesia, scalene, axillary, or regional intravenous (Bier) blocks are the options. Regional blocks may also be used in combination with general anesthesia for postoperative pain control; however, several disadvantages limit the utility of regional block as the primary method of anesthesia for elbow arthroscopy. Axillary block is not always successful in providing complete anesthesia about the elbow. Patients may not tolerate the prone or lateral decubitus position if they are not under general anesthesia. Pain from tourniquet tightness or the subsidence of anesthetic effect can limit the available operative time when using regional block anesthesia. If conversion to an open procedure is required, the patient may need to undergo general anesthesia to allow additional operative time, and the patient may have to be turned supine for intubation if he or she was initially in the prone or lateral decubitus position.

Perioperative Use of Antibiotics

In elbow arthroscopy, the skin surfaces of many portal sites are millimeters away from the joint capsule and joint space. In a recent review of 473 consecutive elbow arthroscopies, Kelly et al.[7] noted 34 cases (7.1%) of infection, with 1 elbow joint infection and 33 superficial portal site infections. Because of this, prophylactic use of perioperative antibiotics is strongly recommended in elbow arthroscopy. Postoperative oral antibiotic coverage until the portal incisions have healed should also be considered.

Positioning

In 1985, Andrews and Carson[3] first reported on supine positioning with a traction device for elbow arthroscopy. Morrey[13] described supine positioning without a traction device in 1986, using instead an assistant to secure the extremity during the procedure. Poehling et al.[21] reported on elbow arthroscopy in the prone position in 1989. O'Driscoll and Morrey[16] described the lateral decubitus position for elbow arthroscopy in 1992. The prone position has become the most widely preferred position. The surgeon should be familiar with the strengths and limitations of each option and should choose a position that allows adequate anterior and posterior exposure, sufficient range of motion, and conversion to an open procedure if necessary.

Supine Position

The supine position allows the most flexibility in the choice of anesthesia. It facilitates the use of regional block anesthesia for elbow arthroscopy, because patients often do not tolerate the prone or lateral decubitus position if awake. The supine position also allows safe conversion from regional to general anesthesia if necessary, without repositioning or redraping.[11] The supine position facilitates airway maintenance in general anesthesia.

For the surgeon, the supine position presents the patient's elbow joint in a more familiar anatomic orientation, with the anterior compartment facing up and the posterior compartment down. This allows easier conceptualization of the intra-articular anatomy. Although the reversed anatomic orientation as seen in the prone or lateral decubitus position can become familiar with experience, the complexity of the elbow joint anatomy presents abundant inherent challenges to arthroscopy, and the standard anatomic reference provided by the supine position may initially facilitate the procedure.

The significant disadvantage of supine positioning stems mostly from the limited posterior access and arm instability. Additionally, the suspension device is costly to acquire and time-consuming to set up. A second device or a scrubbed assistant is also needed to stabilize the arm during arthroscopy because the arm is suspended on a traction rope and would swing freely without a stabilizing force. Manipulation of the elbow during arthroscopy can be limited with the arm in traction. In addition, posterior compartment access and visualization may be compromised because elbow extension is more difficult to achieve and sustain; with the instruments and operative field above the hands of the surgeon, extensive procedures in the posterior compartment can lead to the surgeon's fatigue and difficulty in maintaining the instruments' position.

Prone Position

The prone position was developed to address the shortcomings of the supine position. The setup for the upper extremity is simple compared with that of the supine position: a stationary arm bolster or arm board is used to hold the upper arm parallel to the floor, and the elbow rests in 90 degrees of flexion as the forearm hangs freely off the end. No additional equipment or personnel is required to provide stability during the procedure; the arm rests securely on the arm bolster. Because the hand is not attached to the suspension device, manipulation of the elbow is possible from near full flexion to full extension. Posterior compartment access and visualization are improved, and maintenance of equipment positioning is easier with the operative field below the hands of the surgeon. Because the anterior compartment is on the inferior aspect of the elbow in the prone position, gravity allows the neurovascular structures along the anterior aspect of the antecubital fossa to fall away from the joint space, providing an additional margin of safety during portal placement and the arthroscopic procedure. Conversion to an open procedure, if necessary, is facilitated by the prone position, especially for open procedures through a posterior midline approach.

Disadvantages of the prone position arise mostly from the anesthetic and logistic considerations related to the patient's being face-down. The reversed position (relative to the more conventional orientation of the supine position) requires familiarization and proficiency in anatomic conceptualization. Chest rolls, padded face and head holders, knee pads, and pillows need to be placed strategically to protect the prominent areas vulnerable to pressure sores during the procedure. Although regional anesthesia is possible, patients rarely tolerate the prone position for the duration of the procedure. If patient discomfort or anxiety demands conversion to general anesthesia, the prone position makes intubation difficult if not impossible, and repositioning and redraping are needed. Although general anesthesia is preferable with the prone position, it also presents additional concerns. For example, the inherent difficulty of ventilating the patient in the chest-down position may raise the risk of respiratory compromise in those with poor pulmonary function or large body habitus. Finally, the prone position may not be feasible in patients with shoulder pathology such as glenohumeral arthritis or adhesive capsulitis, because the shoulder may not allow enough abduction for positioning and external and internal rotation during the procedure.

Lateral Decubitus Position

The lateral decubitus position, first described by O'Driscoll and Morrey,[16] combines the advantages and avoids the pitfalls of the supine and prone positions. Because the operative arm is set up over an arm bolster, as in the prone position, the lateral decubitus position offers all the benefits of the prone position over the supine position: less complicated setup, inherent stability of the elbow, and easy access to the posterior compartment. Like the supine position, the lateral decubitus position also avoids the major drawbacks of the prone position: increased risk of respiratory compromise and reliance on general anesthesia. Patients tolerate lying on their side much better than lying prone, and the use of regional anesthesia is more feasible if the need to convert to general anesthesia is less of a concern. Patients with decreased pulmonary reserves also avoid the risk of increased respiratory compromise. Should intraoperative conversion to general anesthesia become necessary owing to regional block failure or positional discomfort, placement of a laryngeal mask airway or endotracheal tube is much more feasible with the patient in the lateral decubitus position than prone.

Fluid Infusion Pump

Distention of the elbow joint with pressurized inflow of fluid facilitates visualization of the operative field by increasing the available space and controlling blood loss, which can significantly obscure the view. Most important, joint distention also displaces neurovascular structures away from the working space within the joint, providing an additional margin of safety during portal placement. With joint distention, the distance from the anterolateral portal to the radial nerve increases from 4 to 11 mm, the distance from the anteromedial portal to the median nerve increases from 4 to 14 mm, and the distance from same portal to the brachial artery increases from 9 to 17 mm.[9]

Although joint distention is important in preventing neurovascular injury, two caveats should be noted. First, the recommended position of elbow flexion during portal placement may be as important as joint insufflation in protecting anterior neurovascular structures, because elbow extension eliminates the protective benefit of joint distention and brings the nerves closer to bone.[12] Second, joint distention does not significantly increase the distance between the neurovascular structures and the capsule and therefore does not decrease the risk of an "inside-out" injury during arthroscopy. This is especially relevant during procedures such as synovectomy and capsular release, in which excision of soft tissue occurs immediately deep to the neurovascular structures at risk.[12]

As reported by O'Driscoll et al.,[17] capsular rupture in fresh frozen cadaver elbows occurs at approximately 80 mm Hg. Care should be taken not to overdistend the joint during the procedure, because joint capsule rupture, fluid extravasation, and periarticular tissue edema can render elbow arthroscopy extremely difficult to perform.

Arthroscopic Equipment

The vast majority of elbow arthroscopy procedures can be performed with the standard 4-mm large-joint arthroscope. The larger arthroscope provides a wider field of vision, and the cannula's larger caliber allows improved inflow and outflow of fluid. Some have advocated the use of the 2.7-mm small-joint arthroscope for difficult situations, such as accessing a tight compartment or in small patients. Mixing large and small arthroscopic equipment during a case should be approached with caution, for the caliber and length mismatches of the arthroscopes, cannulas, and sheaths may make it impossible to switch the arthroscope among the various portals without cumbersome maneuvers to change the cannula.

Arthroscopic Portals

Although numerous portals have been described for elbow arthroscopy, there are nine portals of established utility, and these can be grouped by anatomic location: lateral, medial, and posterior. A thorough knowledge of the three-dimensional relationships between surface landmarks and neurovascular anatomy is required for the surgeon to operate effectively while avoiding damage to neurovascular structures.

Lateral Portals

The lateral portals allow access to the anterior elbow compartment. In general, three lateral portals have been described: anterolateral, midanterolateral, and proximal anterolateral (Fig. 28–1). The radial nerve and its important continuation, the posterior interosseous nerve, are the primary structures at risk; other superficial structures that may be injured include the posterior branch of the lateral antebrachial cutaneous nerve and the posterior antebrachial cutaneous nerve. The radial nerve courses in a posterior to anterior direction, piercing the lateral intermuscular septum approximately 10 cm proximal to the lateral humeral epicondyle with the radial collateral artery, and proceeds distally between the brachialis and brachioradialis.[14] The radial nerve then divides into the superficial branch and the posterior interosseous nerve,

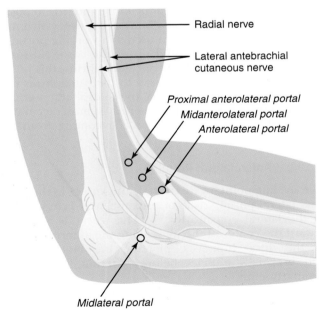

Figure 28–1   Lateral portals. Proximal anterolateral, midanterolateral, and anterolateral portals. The lateral portals are perhaps the most dangerous because of their proximity to nerves. The posterior branch of the lateral antebrachial cutaneous nerve, the radial nerve, and the posterior interosseous nerve are the main structures at risk, especially during placement of the anterolateral portal. As illustrated, more proximally oriented portals are safer because they are farther away from the radial nerve. (The midlateral portal is shown to illustrate its location at the center of the triangle formed by the radial head, lateral epicondyle, and olecranon.)

which courses just superficial to the anterolateral joint capsule before entering the supinator muscle.

Anterolateral Portal

As first described by Andrews and Carson[3] in 1985, the anterolateral portal starts 3 cm distal and 1 cm anterior to the lateral epicondyle.[2] The blunt trocar is advanced toward the center of the joint, through the extensor carpi radialis brevis and anterolateral joint capsule. If a previous medial portal has been established, the inside-out technique can be used to establish this portal.[10]

The anterolateral portal allows an excellent view of the medial aspect of the anterior elbow joint, including the medial aspects of the radial head, coronoid process, trochlea, and coronoid fossa. It also functions well as a working portal with the arthroscope in the medial portals.[10]

The path of the anterolateral portal is near the radial nerve, within 4.9 to 9.1 mm when the elbow is in 90 degrees of flexion and distended with fluid.[4,10] Some anatomic studies have also found this portal to be within 2 mm of the posterior antebrachial cutaneous nerve.[9] For these reasons, the anterolateral portal has become less popular, and most advocate a more proximal starting point.

Midanterolateral Portal

This portal is located just anterior to the radiocapitellar joint. It is more proximal than the anterolateral portal and is best located by topping the radiocapitellar joint when the arm is supinated and pronated. This portal offers the advantage of a slightly more anterior to posterior approach to the anterior bony structures, which may be more advantageous when used as a working portal to debride either the coronoid tip or the coronoid fossa. Additionally, in cases of severe osteoarthritis, this portal allows entry into the joint distal to the osteophytes that are often present just proximal to the capitellum on the lateral condylar ridge. This portal is most accurately placed with an inside-out approach coming from the medial side.

Proximal Anterolateral Portal

The starting point for this portal, also known as the proximal lateral portal,[23] is 2 cm proximal and 1 cm anterior to the lateral epicondyle.[4,10,11] The trocar is advanced toward the center of the joint along the anterior surface of the distal humerus, piercing the brachioradialis and brachialis muscles before entering the anterior compartment.[10]

The proximal anterolateral portal can be used as the initial portal and provides excellent, complete visualization of the anterior compartment, including the anterior and lateral radial head, capitellum, lateral gutter, anterior ulnohumeral joint, and anterior elbow capsular margin.[10,22]

The proximal anterolateral portal was developed as an alternative to the anterolateral portal to avoid possible injury to the radial nerve. In an anatomic study, the radial nerve was found to be an average distance of 3.8 mm in extension and 7.2 mm in 90 degrees of flexion from the distal anterolateral portal; in contrast, it was 7.9 mm in extension and 13.7 mm in flexion from the proximal anterolateral portal.[6] The posterior branch of the lateral antebrachial cutaneous nerve lies 6.1 mm from this portal, compared with 2 mm from the anterolateral portal.[4,9]

Medial Portals

Like the lateral portals, the medial portals allow access to the anterior compartment of the elbow joint. Two principal portals have been described: anteromedial and proximal anteromedial (Fig. 28–2).[8] The ulnar nerve, median nerve, brachial artery, and medial antebrachial cutaneous nerve are the main structures at risk in medial portal placement. Because medial portal placement relies on the medial intermuscular septum and the medial epicondyle to protect the ulnar nerve posteriorly, extreme care should be exercised in patients with anterior subluxation of the ulnar nerve during elbow flexion. Prior ulnar nerve transposition is a relative contraindication; medial portal placement should be avoided unless the nerve can be unequivocally palpated (as in some cases after subcutaneous transposition) and its course clearly avoided.[15]

Anteromedial Portal

First described by Andrews and Carson,[3] the anteromedial portal starts 2 cm anterior and 2 cm distal to the medial epicondyle. Aiming for the center of the joint, the portal passes through the flexor-pronator origin and

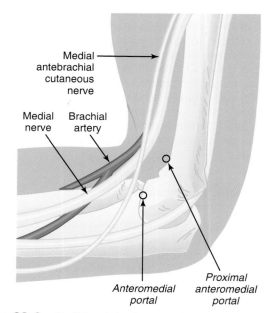

Figure 28–2 Medial portals. Anteromedial and proximal anteromedial portals. The ulnar nerve is protected by the medial intermuscular septum anteriorly. The median nerve, brachial artery, and medial antebrachial cutaneous nerve are the main structures at risk. Similar to the lateral side, more proximal portals are safer than distal portals.

the brachialis muscle before entering the joint anterior to the medial collateral ligament.[10] The anteromedial portal allows visualization of the entire anterior compartment of the elbow joint and can be useful for instrumentation of the medial gutter.[11] The primary structure at risk during placement of this portal is the medial antebrachial cutaneous nerve, which lies an average of 1 mm from the starting point.[4] The median nerve also lies in proximity to this portal, on average 7 to 14 mm away. By staying on the anterior cortex of the humerus during trocar advancement, the portal stays deep to the brachialis, which protects the median nerve and the brachial artery. Because both the starting point and the course of the anteromedial portal are anterior to the medial epicondyle, a nontransposed and nonsubluxating ulnar nerve is at minimal risk if the portal is placed properly.

Proximal Anteromedial Portal

Poehling et al.[21] first reported on this portal in 1989. The starting point is 2 cm proximal to the medial epicondyle and just anterior to the medial intermuscular septum; it is approximately 6 mm from the medial antebrachial cutaneous nerve.[1] The medial intermuscular septum is palpated, and the portal is established anterior to the septum as the trocar is introduced, aiming for the radial head and avoiding the ulnar nerve, which lies immediately posterior to the septum, 3 to 4 mm away.[1] Anterior to the portal, the brachialis muscle protects the median nerve and the brachial artery. The path of the proximal anteromedial portal is, on average, 22 mm away from the median nerve.[8] The path aims more distally and courses more parallel to the median nerve, instead of coursing perpendicular to and aiming directly at the nerve, as in the anteromedial portal.

Posterior Portals

For access to the posterior compartment of the elbow joint, four portals are available: proximal posterolateral, distal posterolateral, midlateral, and direct posterior (Fig. 28–3). The course of the ulnar nerve along the

posteromedial aspect of the distal arm precludes the safe establishment of posteromedial portals.

Proximal Posterolateral Portal

The starting point for the proximal posterolateral portal is 3 cm proximal to the olecranon and along the lateral border of the triceps tendon. The elbow is held at 45 degrees as a blunt trocar is advanced toward the center of the olecranon fossa to pierce the posterolateral capsule and enter the joint.[4] This portal allows visualization of the olecranon tip, olecranon fossa, and posterior trochlea, as well as the medial and lateral gutters. The primary structure at risk is the lateral triceps tendon; the risk of injury can be minimized by staying close to the posterior humeral cortex during portal establishment.[11] The medial antebrachial cutaneous nerve and the posterior antebrachial cutaneous nerve lie, on average, 20 and 25 mm away from the portal, respectively.[9] During examination and instrumentation of the medial gutter, care should be taken to avoid injury to the ulnar nerve, which lies just superficial to the medial capsule and posterior bundle of the medial collateral ligament.[18,21]

Distal Posterolateral Portal

The posterolateral elbow can be accessed anywhere along the lateral border of the triceps tendon, from the standard proximal spot 3 cm proximal to the olecranon to the straight lateral "soft spot." A useful portal is located directly lateral to the olecranon tip or slightly proximal or distal, as needed. Through this portal, the posterior radiocapitellar joint, olecranon tip, and olecranon fossa can be visualized, and excision of a lateral olecranon spur, resection of a posterolateral plica, and debridement of the radial aspect of the ulnohumeral joint can be performed. The primary structures at risk through this portal are the ulnohumeral joint cartilage and the tendon of the lateral triceps.[22]

Midlateral Portal

Also known as the direct lateral or soft-spot portal, the midlateral portal is located at the center of the triangle

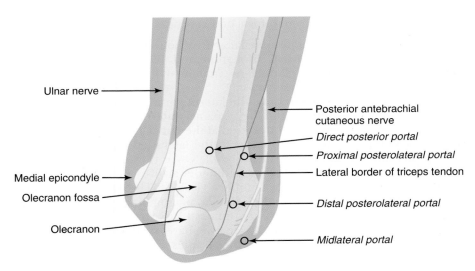

Figure 28–3 Posterior portals. Midlateral, proximal posterolateral, distal posterolateral, and direct posterior portals. Superficially, the posterior antebrachial cutaneous nerve is at risk. The ulnar nerve is at risk posteromedially; with the nerve separated from the joint space by only the capsule and the posterior bundle of the medial collateral ligament, inside-out injury can occur. (See also Figure 28–1 for the midlateral portal location.)

Ulnar nerve

Medial epicondyle

Olecranon fossa

Olecranon

Posterior antebrachial cutaneous nerve

Direct posterior portal

Proximal posterolateral portal

Lateral border of triceps tendon

Distal posterolateral portal

Midlateral portal

3 Elbow

defined by the radial head, lateral humeral epicondyle, and olecranon. The trocar passes through the anconeus muscle and the joint capsule into the joint space. Through this portal, the inferior portions of the radial head and the capitellum, as well as the ulnohumeral articulation, are in view. This portal is useful for the visualization of these structures and as an initial entry point for joint insufflation; its use as a portal for instrumentation is limited. The main structure at risk for injury in the midlateral portal is the posterior antebrachial cutaneous nerve, an average of 7 mm away.[1] Because leakage of fluid into the surrounding soft tissues is common, it may be prudent to use this portal at or near the end of the arthroscopic procedure.[4,19,21]

Direct Posterior Portal

The direct posterior portal is located midline and 3 cm proximal to the olecranon tip.[19,20] The blunt trocar is advanced toward the olecranon fossa, through the triceps tendon and posterior capsule, into the posterior compartment. This portal allows visualization of the entire posterior compartment.[10] With visualization through the posterolateral portal, the direct posterior portal is useful for instrumentation in olecranon osteophyte excision and posterior loose body removal.[10,15] This portal also facilitates the transhumeral approach to the anterior compartment during the arthroscopic Outerbridge-Kashwagi procedure, in which the bone between the olecranon and coronoid fossa is removed with a bur.[18] The posterior antebrachial cutaneous nerve and the ulnar nerve are 23 and 25 mm away from the direct posterior portal, respectively.[5]

Diagnostic Arthroscopy

A careful preoperative history should be obtained, and a physical examination should be performed. A prior history of surgery to the elbow region should be elicited, especially ulnar nerve transposition; if the ulnar nerve has been transposed, one should palpate, percuss for the nerve, and note its course, if possible. Alternatively, the nerve can be located and marked preoperatively with ultrasonography. During the physical examination, the following should be noted: neurovascular function distal to the joint, elbow range of motion, joint stability, anterior subluxation or dislocation of the ulnar nerve during elbow flexion, and specific location of pain or tenderness. Anterior subluxation or dislocation of the ulnar nerve during elbow flexion is another important finding. If the course of the ulnar nerve is difficult to ascertain owing to subluxation or prior transposition, medial portals may need to be modified or avoided.

Preoperative intravenous antibiotics are given. Setup and anesthesia are based on the surgeon's preference. We routinely set up the patient in the lateral decubitus position using a padded arm bolster (Fig. 28–4). As mentioned earlier, the lateral decubitus position allows the same positioning of the arm, elbow, and forearm as the prone position, without its associated disadvantages such as risk of respiratory compromise. The setup is also somewhat intuitive, as it resembles knee arthroscopy. The

elbow should be positioned and draped so that the arm is supported by the bolster at the proximal upper arm, the elbow rests at 90 degrees, and the antecubital fossa is free from contact with the bolster. General anesthesia is preferred; use of regional anesthesia makes the immediate postoperative motor and sensory examination difficult to perform and interpret. The video monitor is set on the opposite side of the patient.

An examination under anesthesia is performed to determine elbow range of motion and stability. A nonsterile tourniquet is placed on the upper arm. Once the area is prepared and draped, surface landmarks and prior incisions, if any, are marked (Fig. 28–5). It is important to outline and mark the landmarks before joint distention. The medial epicondyle, lateral epicondyle, and ulnar nerve are outlined; in addition to portal localization, these markings provide a visual reminder of the medial and lateral orientation during the procedure. After the landmarks have been identified and marked on the skin, the lateral soft-spot portal location is identified, and 20 to 30 mL of saline is injected into the elbow joint space (Fig. 28–6). A successful intra-articular injection is often accompanied by slight elbow extension as the joint space is filled, and there is backflow out of the needle as the syringe is removed.

Unless prior ulnar nerve transposition or severe ulnar nerve subluxation precludes it, the preferred initial portal is the proximal anteromedial portal. The starting point is 2 cm proximal to the medial epicondyle and just anterior to the medial intermuscular septum. A number 11 blade is used to incise the skin only. This minimizes the risk of injury to the medial antebrachial cutaneous nerve. Next, the blunt trocar and cannula for the 4-mm (or, rarely, 2.7-mm, for small patients) arthroscope are introduced toward the radial head, once again feeling the intermuscular septum (which protects the ulnar nerve) and maintaining contact with the anterior cortex of the humerus (the brachialis muscle anterior to the trocar protects the median nerve and brachial artery).

The anterior compartment of the elbow joint is examined at this time. Using a 4-mm, 30-degree arthroscope, the following structures are examined (Fig. 28–7):

- Capitellum and radial head
- Anterior and lateral joint capsule
- Coronoid fossa and coronoid process

The radiocapitellar articulation should be examined with the arm in pronation and in supination. The joint capsule should be examined for thickening, scarring, and inflammation.

At this time, the lateral portal can be established. We prefer to use the proximal anterolateral portal. A spinal needle is introduced at the starting point, 2 cm proximal and 1 cm anterior to the lateral epicondyle, aiming for the center of the joint. Once the proper position and course are identified under arthroscopic view, the skin is incised with a number 11 blade. The trocar is then introduced with the cannula, maintaining contact with anterior cortex of the humerus to avoid injury to the radial nerve. Alternatively, we have used a portal expander system (Arthrex, Inc., Naples, FL), whereby a thin guide

Text continued on p. 300

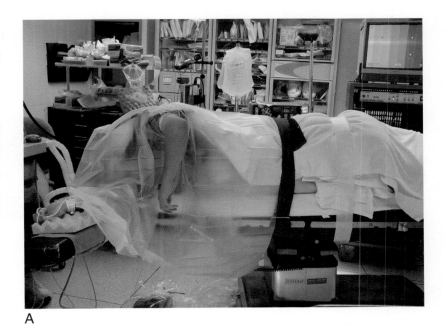

A

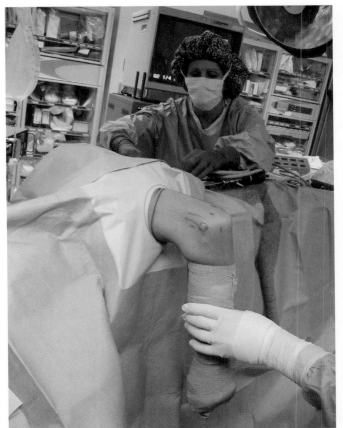

B

Figure 28–4   Lateral decubitus position. *A*, The patient is positioned with the operative side up. A tourniquet is applied to the operative arm, which rests over a bolster. *B*, It is important to ensure that the antecubital fossa area is not obstructed by the bolster or drape; this allows the anterior neurovascular structures to fall away from the center of the joint and provides a margin of safety from inside-out injury.

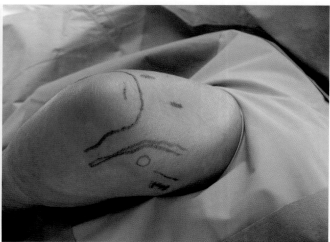

B

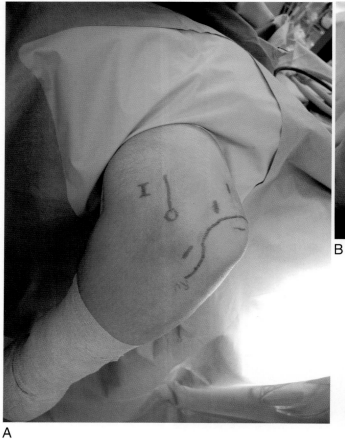

A

Figure 28–5 Surface landmarks. The following landmarks are drawn on the arm before joint insufflation: olecranon, lateral epicondyle, medial epicondyle, and ulnar nerve. *A,* Lateral view: lateral epicondyle and olecranon. *B,* Medial view: medial epicondyle, olecranon, and ulnar nerve.

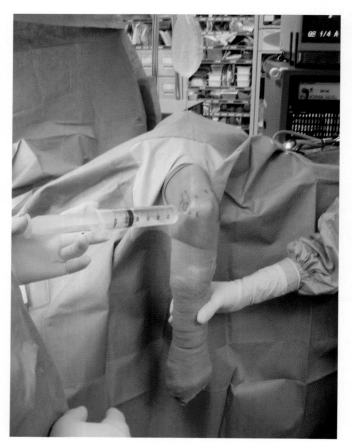

Figure 28–6 Joint insufflation. After landmarks are drawn, 20 to 30 mL of saline is injected into the elbow joint through the midlateral portal, located at the center of the triangle formed by the lateral epicondyle, olecranon, and radial head. Successful intra-articular injection is confirmed by the observation of slight elbow extension as the joint is distended and by the backflow of fluid through the needle.

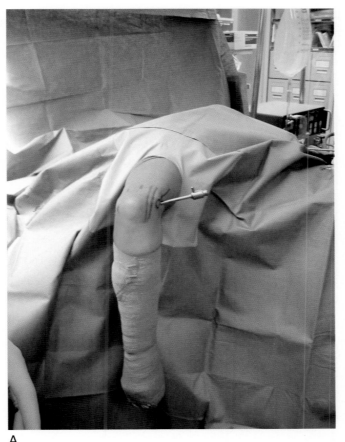

A

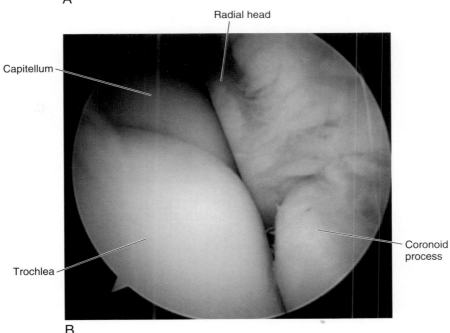

Radial head

Capitellum

Coronoid
process

Trochlea

B

Figure 28–7   Proximal anteromedial portal. This is the preferred starting portal unless
prior medial elbow surgery or injury precludes its safe placement. *A*, Trocar and cannula
are inserted through the proximal anteromedial portal. *B*, Principal structures are the
coronoid process, trochlea, radial head, and capitellum.

Continued

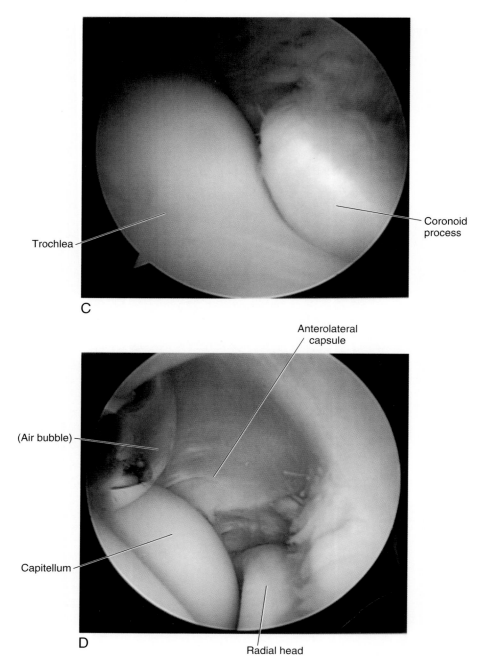

Figure 28–7, cont'd. *C,* Coronoid process and trochlea. *D,* Radial head, capitellum, and anterolateral capsule.

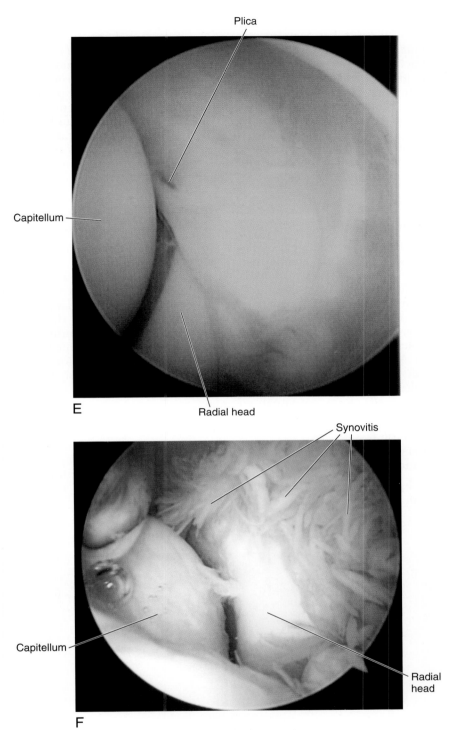

Figure 28–7, cont'd. *E,* Radiocapitellar joint interposed by plica. *F,* Radial head surrounded by synovitis.

pin is introduced after the starting point has been localized with a spinal needle and the skin has been incised; cannulated expanders of increasing girth are introduced over the wire until the tract for the portal is well established (Fig. 28–8). This gradual enlargement of the tunnel lessens soft tissue tearing from plunging of the trocar and facilitates the reintroduction of arthroscopic instruments, often making the portal cannula unnecessary.

With the help of a switching stick, the 30-degree arthroscope is introduced through the lateral portal, and the following structures are examined (Fig. 28–9):

● Medial joint capsule
● Trochlea
● Coronoid fossa and coronoid process

The lateral portal has also been used to evaluate ulnohumeral joint instability, as described by Timmerman et al.[24]

After the anterior compartment has been examined, the posterior compartment is accessed. The standard proximal posterolateral portal is established with the elbow in 45 degrees of flexion. The entry point is 3 cm proximal to the tip of the olecranon and along the lateral edge of the triceps tendon. Again, only the skin is incised with the number 11 blade. The blunt trocar is introduced, aiming for the olecranon fossa. With the 30-degree camera, the following structures are visualized (Fig. 28–10):

● Olecranon tip and olecranon fossa
● Medial and lateral gutters
● Posterior aspect of the radiocapitellar joint

If desired, arthroscope insertion through the midlateral portal can provide enhanced views of the posterior radial head, capitellum, and ulnohumeral articulation. The olecranon fossa should be carefully examined for loose bodies (Fig. 28–11). During examination of the medial gutter, care should be taken to avoid injury to the ulnar nerve, which runs immediately superficial to the joint capsule and the posterior bundle of the medial collateral ligament.[16] If instrumentation is needed, the direct posterior portal can be established after confirming the location with a spinal needle.

At the end of the procedure, the incisions are closed with nylon sutures. A compressive dressing with an anterior splint is applied to keep the elbow in extension.

Postoperative Management

In the recovery area, after the patient has regained alertness and orientation, a neurovascular examination is repeated to ensure that no neurovascular compromise has occurred. The splint is generally removed on postoperative day 1. An exercise program for active and active assisted range of motion (flexion, extension, pronation, and supination) is demonstrated for the patient to continue at home. We routinely prescribe a course of oral antibiotics until the incisions have become dry, usually at the first postoperative visit approximately 1 week later.

Conclusion

Our understanding of the clinical anatomy as it relates to portal placement during elbow arthroscopy allows the interested and skilled arthroscopist to treat a variety of intra-articular problems of the elbow joint. Owing to

Text continued on p. 306

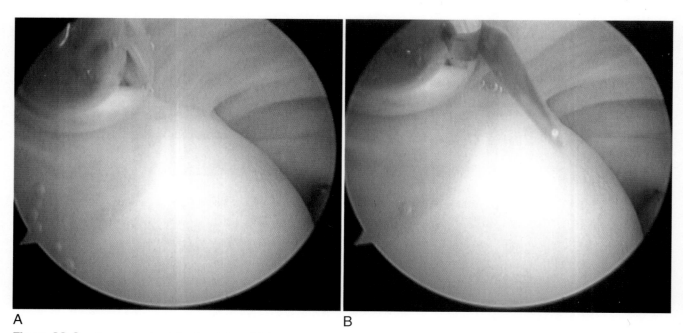

A   B

Figure 28–8   Proximal anterolateral portal establishment using the portal expander system. *A,* Anterolateral capsule and capitellum, seen through the medial portal. *B,* The starting point and trajectory are confirmed using a spinal needle.

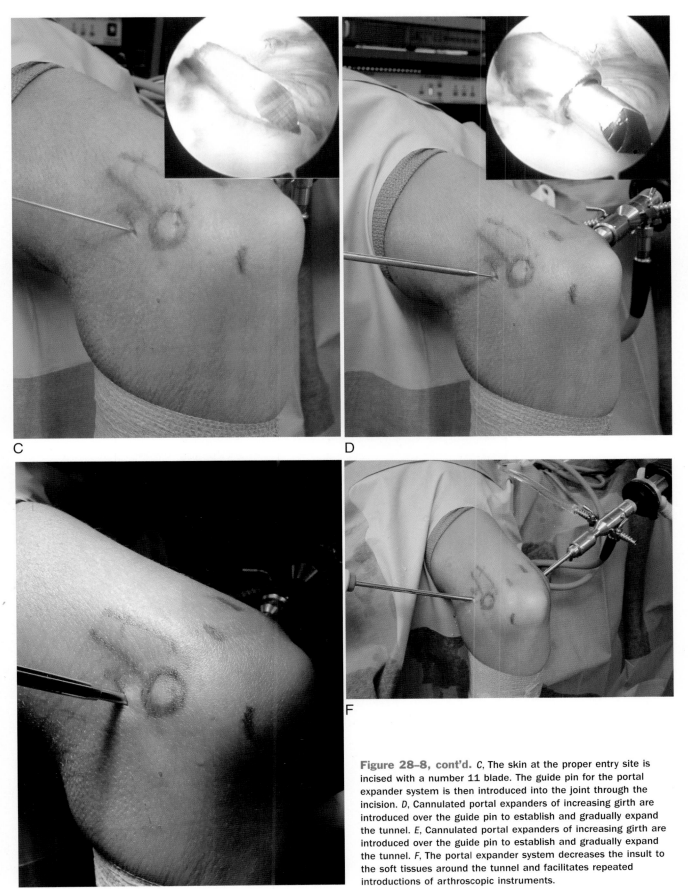

Figure 28–8, cont'd. *C*, The skin at the proper entry site is incised with a number 11 blade. The guide pin for the portal expander system is then introduced into the joint through the incision. *D*, Cannulated portal expanders of increasing girth are introduced over the guide pin to establish and gradually expand the tunnel. *E*, Cannulated portal expanders of increasing girth are introduced over the guide pin to establish and gradually expand the tunnel. *F*, The portal expander system decreases the insult to the soft tissues around the tunnel and facilitates repeated introductions of arthroscopic instruments.

3 Elbow

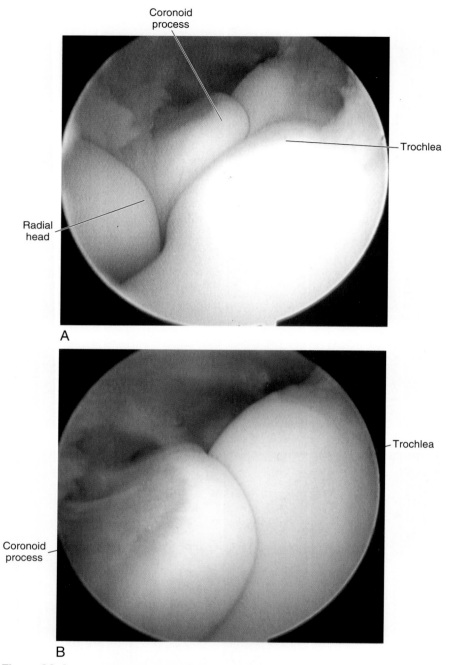

Figure 28–9 Proximal anterolateral portal. *A,* Initial view: radial head, coronoid process, and trochlea. *B,* Coronoid process and trochlea.

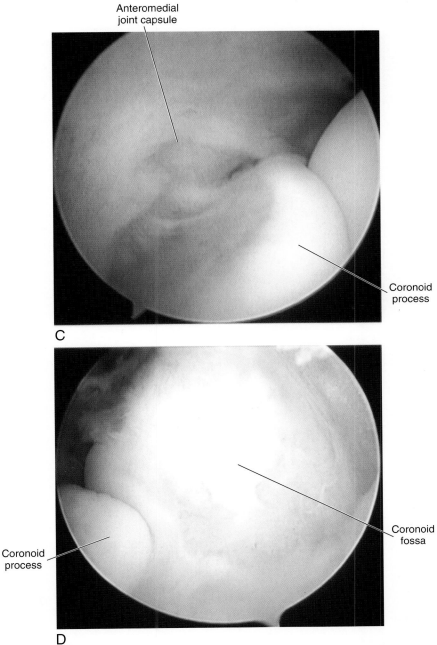

Figure 28–9, cont'd. *C*, Coronoid process and anteromedial joint capsule. *D*, Coronoid fossa and coronoid process.

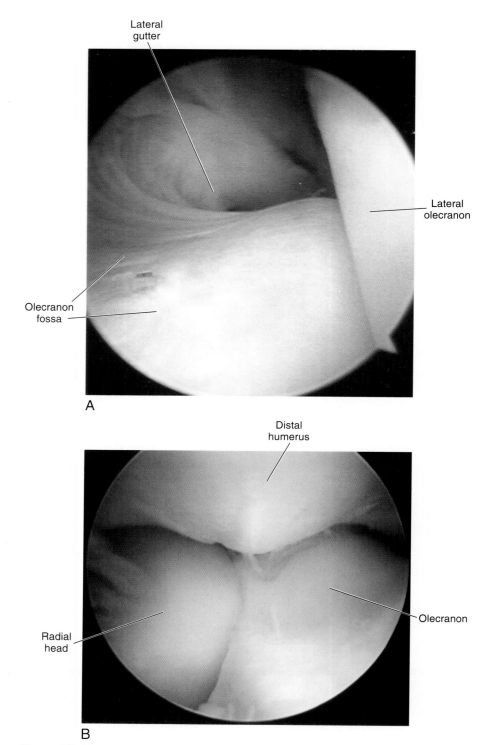

Figure 28–10 Posterior compartment. *A,* Proximal posterolateral portal: lateral gutter, lateral aspect of the olecranon fossa, and lateral olecranon. *B,* Proximal posterolateral portal: posterior aspects of the radial head and capitellum, proximal radioulnar articulation, and ulnohumeral articulation.

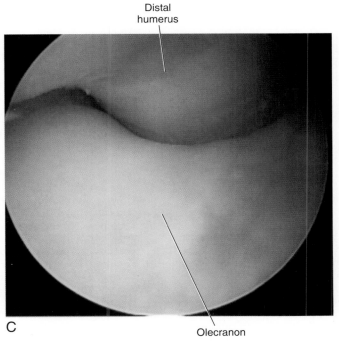

Figure 28–10, cont'd. *C*, Midlateral portal: ulnohumeral articulation.

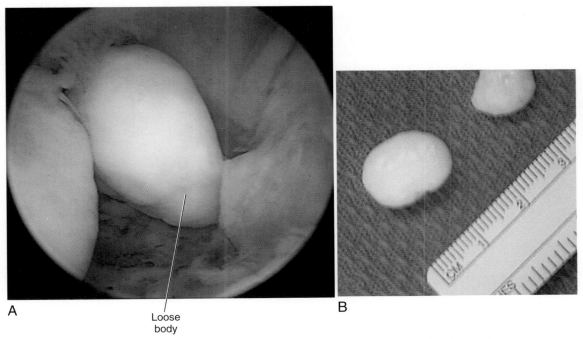

Figure 28–11   Loose bodies in posterior elbow compartment. This patient had posterior elbow pain and intermittent block to motion at the end of extension. *A*, A loose body is seen in the olecranon fossa. *B*, The loose bodies are removed with a grasper through an enlarged direct posterior portal.

the variety of patient positions and portals available, the surgeon must establish a familiar and comfortable routine that minimizes the chance of neurovascular complications. Once the requisite skills are mastered, elbow arthroscopy can be a particularly gratifying procedure for both patient and surgeon.

References

1. Adolfsson L: Arthroscopy of the elbow joint: A cadaveric study of portal placement. J Shoulder Elbow Surg 3:53-61, 1994.
2. Andrews JR, Baumgarten TE: Arthroscopic anatomy of the elbow. Orthop Clin North Am 26:671-677, 1995.
3. Andrews JR, Carson WG: Arthroscopy of the elbow. Arthroscopy 1:97-107, 1985.
4. Andrews JR, St Pierre RK, Carson WG Jr: Arthroscopy of the elbow. Clin Sports Med 5:653-662, 1986.
5. Baker CL, Brooks AA: Arthroscopy of the elbow. Clin Sports Med 15:261-281, 1996.
6. Field LD, Altchek DW, Warren RF, et al: Arthroscopic anatomy of the lateral elbow: A comparison of three portals. Arthroscopy 10:602-607, 1994.
7. Kelly EW, Morrey BF, O'Driscoll SW: Complications of elbow arthroscopy. J Bone Joint Surg Am 83:25-34, 2001.
8. Lindenfeld TN: Medial approach in elbow arthroscopy. Am J Sports Med 18:413-417, 1990.
9. Lynch GJ, Meyers JF, Whipple TL, et al: Neurovascular anatomy and elbow arthroscopy: Inherent risks. Arthroscopy 2:191-197, 1986.
10. Lyons TR, Field LD, Savoie FH: Basics of elbow arthroscopy. In Price CT (ed): Instructional Course Lectures, vol 49. Rosemont, IL, American Academy of Orthopaedic Surgeons, 2000, pp 239-246.
11. McKenzie PJ: Supine position. In Savoie FH, Field LD (eds): Arthroscopy of the Elbow. New York, Churchill Livingstone, 1996, pp 35-39.
12. Miller CD, Jobe CM, Wright MH: Neuroanatomy in elbow arthroscopy. J Shoulder Elbow Surg 4:168-174, 1995.
13. Morrey BF: Arthroscopy of the elbow. In Anderson LD (ed): Instructional Course Lectures, vol 35. Rosemont, IL, American Academy of Orthopaedic Surgeons, 1986, pp 102-107.
14. Narakas AO: Compression and traction neuropathies about the shoulder and arm. In Gelberman RH (ed): Operative Nerve Repair and Reconstruction, Philadelphia, JB Lippincott, 1991, pp 1147-1175.
15. O'Driscoll SW: Operative elbow arthroscopy. Part 1. Loose bodies and synovial conditions. In Green DP, Hotchkiss RN, Pederson WC (eds): Operative Hand Surgery, 4th ed. New York, Churchill Livingstone, 1999, pp 235-249.
16. O'Driscoll SW, Morrey BF: Arthroscopy of the elbow: Diagnostic and therapeutic benefits and hazards. J Bone Joint Surg Am 74:84-94, 1992.
17. O'Driscoll SW, Morrey BF, An KN: Intraarticular pressure and capacity of the elbow. Arthroscopy 6:100-103, 1990.
18. Plancher KD, Peterson RK, Brezenoff L: Diagnostic arthroscopy of the elbow: Set-up, portals, and technique. Oper Tech Sports Med 6:2-10, 1998.
19. Poehling GG, Ekman EF: Arthroscopy of the elbow. In Jackson DW (ed): Instructional Course Lectures, vol 44. Rosemont, IL, American Academy of Orthopaedic Surgeons, 1995, pp 217-228.
20. Poehling GG, Ekman EF, Ruch DS: Elbow arthroscopy: Introduction and overview. In McGinty JB, Caspari RB, Jackson RW, Poehling GG (eds): Operative Arthroscopy, 2nd ed. Philadelphia, Lippincott-Raven, 1996, pp 821-828.
21. Poehling GG, Whipple TL, Sisco L: Elbow arthroscopy: A new technique. Arthroscopy 5:222-224, 1989.
22. Savoie FH, Field, LD: Anatomy. In Savoie FH, Field LD (eds): Arthroscopy of the Elbow. New York, Churchill Livingstone, 1996, pp 3-24.
23. Stothers K, Day B, Regan WR: Arthroscopy of the elbow: Anatomy, portal sites, and a description of the proximal lateral portal. Arthroscopy 11:449-457, 1995.
24. Timmerman LA, Schwartz ML, Andrews JR: Preoperative evaluation of the ulnar collateral ligament by magnetic resonance imaging and computed tomography arthrography. Am J Sports Med 22:26-31, 1994.

CHAPTER

29

Arthroscopic Management of Osteochondritis Dissecans of the Elbow

RICHARD J. THOMAS AND A. BOBBY CHHABRA

ARTHROSCOPIC MANAGEMENT OF OSTEOCHONDRITIS DISSECANS OF THE ELBOW IN A NUTSHELL

History:
Dominant arm in adolescent athlete, complaints of lateral elbow pain, extension loss, mechanical symptoms

Physical Examination:
Radiocapitellar compression test (supination and pronation in extension), clicking or mechanical symptoms with range of motion

Imaging:
Standard radiographs with rim of sclerotic bone, flattening; magnetic resonance imaging

Indications:
Failure of conservative management and painful mechanical symptoms

Contraindications:
Asymptomatic patient with radiographic evidence of disease

Surgical Technique:
Routine arthroscopy portals, drilling (intact), debridement or abrasion (fibrillation or fissuring), fragment removal or abrasion (exposed bone or loose fragment), fixation (large fragment)

Postoperative Management:
Sling, range of motion, protection of repair; throwing 4 to 5 months postoperatively

Results:
Improved range of motion, alleviation of pain

Complications:
Neurovascular, arthrofibrosis, hematoma, compartment syndrome, infection

Osteochondritis dissecans (OCD) of the elbow most often affects adolescent throwing athletes and gymnasts. OCD is defined as separation of a portion of articular cartilage. The most common site of OCD in the elbow is the capitellum. These lesions often produce loose bodies that ultimately can cause painful mechanical symptoms in the elbow. The cause of OCD is unclear, although overuse, microtrauma, and ischemia caused by repetitive valgus loading of the radiocapitellar joint have been described as possible causes.[13,18,19] If it is diagnosed early,

treatment consists of conservative management with avoidance of activities, bracing, and physical therapy.[21] However, if the condition progresses, more aggressive management is necessary. Current treatment options include joint debridement, abrasion chondroplasty, removal of loose bodies, drilling of lesions, and fixation of large OCD fragments. Elbow arthroscopy allows for grading and definitive treatment of OCD lesions and is an attractive alternative to open management of this difficult problem.[2,18,21]

History

OCD of the elbow is most commonly diagnosed in the dominant arm of adolescents[19] (13 to 16 years old) who participate in throwing sports, gymnastics, racquet sports, or weightlifting. The patient typically presents with progressive lateral elbow pain associated with activity without a history of trauma. Common complaints include pain, loss of extension, and popping or locking of the elbow if an unstable fragment or loose body is present.[21] However, these findings are not specific for OCD, and other causes should be considered. Panner's disease (osteochondrosis of the elbow) has similar symptoms but can be differentiated from OCD by the younger age of the patient, its self-limited nature, full range of motion, and radiographic findings (Table 29–1).

Physical Examination

The entire upper extremity should be examined, and any swelling or loss of motion should be noted. The radiocapitellar compression test is performed with the elbow in maximum extension. Supination and pronation loads the radiocapitellar joint and can reproduce symptoms if an OCD lesion is present.[2] Clicking or popping with motion may be a sign of a loose body and should be documented.

Imaging

Standard anteroposterior and lateral radiographs can be diagnostic in the evaluation of OCD lesions (Fig. 29–1). OCD of the elbow appears as a radiolucent lesion most commonly in the capitellum. Flattening of the articular surface may also be evident. A rim of sclerotic bone often surrounds the radiolucent region. In capitellar involvement, radial head irregularity may be present. However, early in the disease, plain films may be normal.[21] In these cases, computed tomography or magnetic resonance imaging may be useful in evaluating the extent of a lesion and detecting any loose bodies (Fig. 29–2).[21]

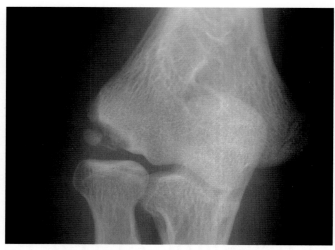

Figure 29–1 Anteroposterior radiograph of the right elbow of a 15-year-old boy reveals an osteochondritis dissecans lesion that has separated from the articular surface.

Takahara et al.[22] described using magnetic resonance imaging for the early detection of OCD in the elbows of young baseball players. An OCD lesion that is still attached to the subchondral bone presents as low signal intensity in the superficial capitellum. High signal between the osteochondral fragment and the remainder of the capitellum on T2-weighted images is consistent with a detached fragment.

Indications and Contraindications

Failure of conservative management and painful mechanical symptoms are the major indications for the arthroscopic treatment of OCD of the elbow (Table 29–2).[5,16,21]

Baumgarten et al.[3] established a classification system for OCD lesions of the elbow to help guide treatment (Table 29–3).

Surgical Technique

Positioning

Baumgarten et al.[3] described placing the patient supine for arthroscopic treatment. An overhead traction frame is used to hold the arm in position. Micheli et al.[12] also

Table 29–1 Differentiating Panner's Disease from Osteochondritis Dissecans

Panner's Disease	Osteochondritis Dissecans
Self-limited	Progressive; can be associated with permanent joint
Ages 4-8 yr	Adolescents
Primarily affects capitellum	Also affects capitellum
Involves entire ossific nucleus of capitellum on radiograph	Involves only portion of capitellum on radiograph
Treat with rest, activity modification	Often requires operative intervention

Table 29–2 Indications for Operative Management of Osteochondritis Dissecans

Failure to respond to conservative treatment
Mechanical symptoms with elbow motion
Loose bodies present without arthritis
Evidence of fracture of articular cartilage surface

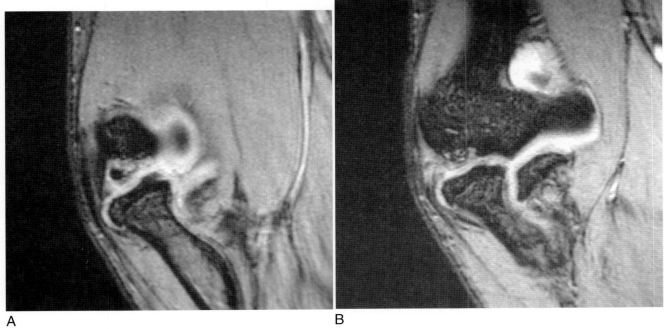

A   B

Figure 29–2   *A* and *B*, Sequential magnetic resonance imaging scans of an osteochondritis dissecans lesion of the capitellum.

Table 29–3	**Grading System for Osteochondritis Dissecans of the Elbow**	
Grade	Description	Treatment
I	Smooth but soft, ballotable cartilage	Drilling of lesion if symptomatic
II	Fibrillations or fissuring of articular cartilage	Removal of all cartilage back to stable rim and abrasion chondroplasty
III	Exposed bone with fixed osteochondral fragment	Removal of osteochondral fragment and abrasion chondroplasty
IV	Loose but undisplaced fragment	Removal of osteochondral fragment and abrasion chondroplasty
V	Displaced fragment with resultant loose bodies	Abrasion chondroplasty of exposed bone, removal of loose bodies

From Baumgarten TE, Andrews JR, Satterwhite YE: The arthroscopic classification and treatment of osteochondritis dissecans of the capitellum. Am J Sports Med 26:520-523, 1998.

prefer to place the patient supine for ease of transition to an open arthrotomy, if necessary, for the removal of large loose bodies or the fixation of large fragments. Day[6] described placing the patient in the prone position for good limb control and easier access to the posterior and anterior compartments. In the prone position, gravity aids in displacing the neurovascular structures away from the surgical area. For the removal of loose bodies, O'Driscoll[14] places his patients in the lateral decubitus

position with the involved side up, the elbow flexed at 90 degrees, and the arm supported by a padded bolster.

Diagnostic Arthroscopy

Routine elbow arthroscopic portals are used. Portals are placed carefully so that neurovascular injury is avoided. Baumgarten et al.[3] routinely use a direct lateral portal for visualization so that an OCD lesion is not missed. Byrd and Jones[5] recommend the use of anterolateral and anteromedial portals for inspection of the anterior compartment and anterior capitellum while the lateral and ancillary lateral portals are used for inspection of the posterior radiocapitellar region. The posterior and posterolateral portals are used for access to the posterior compartment.

There is debate over which size arthroscope is best for the evaluation and treatment of elbow OCD. Baumgarten et al.[3] prefer the 2.7-mm scope for better mobility and visualization in tight spaces. However, this scope has a reduced field of view compared with a 4.5-mm arthroscope. A 4.5-mm scope, however, places the neurovascular structures of the elbow at greater risk for injury and is more difficult to maneuver in the elbow joint.

Specific Surgical Steps

Once the portals have been established, the scope introduced, and the joint examined, osteophytes and synovium should be debrided and loose bodies removed to improve visualization before initiating treatment of the OCD lesion.[3] The anterior, lateral, and posterior compartments are explored to avoid missing loose bodies.[16] The entire joint is explored using a systematic approach, and all articular surfaces are probed for soft areas, fissures, or loose flaps of cartilage. Once the OCD lesion is visualized and examined, appropriate treatment is determined. Symptomatic grade I lesions are treated with drilling. Grade II lesions are treated with debridement of the loose cartilage back to a stable rim with an arthroscopic shaver. An arthroscopic bur is then used to abrade the underlying subchondral bone until it bleeds (abrasion chondroplasty).[3,17] Grade III and IV lesions are treated by removal of the osteochondral fragment and abrasion chondroplasty. Again, the bone is burred back to bleeding cancellous bone. A probe or osteotome may be required to lever the fragment away from the capitellum.[3] Grade V lesions are treated with abrasion chondroplasty and removal of loose bodies.

Although most OCD lesions of the elbow are not amenable to fixation, if the fragment is large, one may consider fixation. Kuwahata and Goro[10] described using Herbert screws for fixation with an open lateral approach. The fragment is removed first, and the underlying bed is curetted. Cancellous bone graft from the iliac crest or lateral humeral condyle is packed into the crater, and the articular cartilage is replaced and secured with a Herbert screw advanced beneath the articular surface. Other methods of fixation include Kirschner wires[20] and cancellous screws.[8] Most studies, however, show that there is little to be gained by the fixation of these fragments.[4,11,20,22] Research is limited in the use of arthroscopy for the fixation of OCD lesions in the elbow.

Postoperative Management

Recommendations for postoperative management following arthroscopic debridement of OCD lesions of the elbow vary widely from surgeon to surgeon and depend on the procedure performed. Baumgarten et al.[3] recommend physical therapy immediately after surgery, with a program consisting of active range of motion, isometrics, and pain and swelling control. Progressive resistance exercises are initiated as pain diminishes. Byrd and Jones[5] prefer to regain range of motion initially and then begin gentle resistance exercises at 3 months, with full resistance at 4 months. In throwing athletes, a throwing program is initiated at 4 to 5 months postoperatively.

Results

Results of arthroscopic treatment of OCD of the elbow are limited to studies with an average follow-up of 3.5 years (Table 29–4).[3,5,15,17] Baumgarten et al.[3] reported an improvement in elbow flexion by 14 degrees and in extension by 6 degrees; the majority of their OCD patients returned to preoperative activities following

Table 29–4

Results of Surgical Treatment of Osteochondritis Dissecans (OCD)

Author (Date)	Type of Study	Patient Population	Type of Surgery	Follow-up Time	Results
Baumgarten et al. (1998)[3]	Retrospective	16 adolescents, 17 elbows	Arthroscopic abrasion chondroplasty and/or loose body removal	Average, 48 mo; minimum, 24 mo	Average flexion contracture decreased by 14 degrees, extension contracture by by 6 degrees; all but 3 returned to preoperative level of activity
O'Driscoll and Morrey (1992)[15]	Retrospective	24 elbows with loose bodies, adults and adolescents; 4 patients had OCD	Arthroscopic removal of loose bodies		18 of 24 elbows improved in range of motion and symptoms; all 4 patients with OCD improved
Byrd and Jones (2002)[5]	Retrospective	10 baseball players, average age 13.8 yr	Arthroscopic synovectomy, abrasion chondroplasty, and/or loose body removal	Average, 3.9 yr	Excellent results in pain, swelling, mechanical symptoms, activity limitation, range of motion; grade of lesion correlated poorly with outcome
Ruch et al. (1998)[17]	Retrospective	12 adolescents, average age 14.5 yr	Arthroscopic debridement and/or loose body removal	Average, 3.2 yr	11 patients reported excellent pain relief and no limitations of activities
Bauer et al. (1992)[1]	Retrospective	7 children younger than 16 yr, 23 adults older than 16 yr	23 loose body removal or removal of undisplaced lesion by open arthrotomy	Average, 23 yr	Impaired motion and pain in half of elbows; degenerative joint disease in more than half

arthroscopic abrasion chondroplasty and removal of loose bodies. O'Driscoll and Morrey[15] reported good results following arthroscopic removal of loose bodies. Byrd and Jones[5] reported excellent results in adolescent baseball players following treatment of OCD. They found that the grade of the lesion correlated poorly with the duration and character of the symptoms. There was no correlation between advanced stage of the disease and poor outcome. However, they reported a poor prognosis if the lesion extended into the lateral border of the capitellum. Ruch et al.[17] described a "lateral capsular sign," which is a lateral bony fragment found on postoperative films but not during the arthroscopy. This finding correlated with a worse prognosis.

Although most studies on the arthroscopic treatment of elbow OCD are short term, Bauer et al.[1] reported an average 23-year follow-up after open treatment of OCD elbow lesions. Of the 31 patients, 23 were treated by removal of loose bodies or debridement of one undisplaced lesion. All procedures were done with an open arthrotomy technique. More than half the elbows had pain symptoms, decreased range of motion, and radiographic changes of degenerative joint disease at follow-up. Long-term studies are needed to determine the benefits of arthroscopic treatment of OCD of the elbow.

Complications

The major risk of arthroscopic elbow surgery is injury to the many neurovascular structures that exist in a relatively small area (Table 29–5). Care must always be taken in the placement of portals. The anterior portals place the radial and posterior interosseous nerves at risk on the lateral side; medially, the median nerve is at risk. A posteromedial portal places the ulnar nerve at risk and is not recommended.[7] Nerve palsies following arthroscopic elbow surgery are usually transient and result from local anesthetic, the tourniquet, or blunt injury.[9] Other complications of treatment include arthrofibrosis, hematoma, and compartment syndrome. Joint space or deep wound infections are rare. Superficial wound infections and prolonged drainage from portal sites are more common.[9]

Table 29–5   Complications of Arthroscopic Treatment of Osteochondritis Dissecans

Neurovascular injury
Arthrofibrosis
Compartment syndrome
Rare joint space or deep wound infection
Superficial infection
Prolonged drainage from portal sites
Retained loose bodies
Degenerative joint disease

References

1. Bauer M, Jonsson K, Josefsson PO, et al: Osteochondritis dissecans of the elbow: A long-term follow-up study. Clin Orthop 284:156-160, 1992.
2. Baumgarten TE: Osteochondritis dissecans of the capitellum. Sports Med Arthrosc Rev 3:219-223, 1995.
3. Baumgarten TE, Andrews JR, Satterwhite YE: The arthroscopic classification and treatment of osteochondritis dissecans of the capitellum. Am J Sports Med 26:520-523, 1998.
4. Brown R, Blazina ME, Kerlan RK, et al: Osteochondritis of the capitellum. J Sports Med 2:27-46, 1974.
5. Byrd JWT, Jones KS: Arthroscopic surgery for isolated capitellar osteochondritis dissecans in adolescent baseball players: Minimum three-year follow-up. Am J Sports Med 30: 474-478, 2002.
6. Day B: Elbow arthroscopy in the athlete. Clin Sports Med 15:785-797, 1996.
7. Jerosch J, Schroder M, Schneider T: Good and relative indications for elbow arthroscopy: A retrospective study on 103 patients. Arch Orthop Trauma Surg 117:246-249, 1998.
8. Johnson LL (ed): Arthroscopic Surgery: Principles and Practice, vol 2, 3rd ed. St Louis, CV Mosby, 1986, pp 1446-1477.
9. Kelly EW, Morrey BF, O'Driscoll SW: Complications of elbow arthroscopy. J Bone Joint Surg Am 83: 25-34, 2001.
10. Kuwahata Y, Goro I: Osteochondritis dissecans of the elbow managed by Herbert screw fixation. Orthopedics 21: 449-451, 1998.
11. McManama GB Jr, Micheli LJ, Berry MV, et al: The surgical treatment of osteochondritis dissecans of the capitellum. Am J Sports Med 13:11-21, 1985.
12. Micheli LJ, Luke AC, Mintzer CM, Waters PM: Elbow arthroscopy in the pediatric and adolescent population. Arthroscopy 17:694-699, 2001.
13. Nagura S: The so-called osteochondritis dissecans of Konig. Clin Orthop 18:100-122, 1960.
14. O'Driscoll SW: Elbow arthroscopy for loose bodies. Orthopedics 15:855-859, 1992.
15. O'Driscoll SW, Morrey BF: Arthroscopy of the elbow: Diagnostic benefits and hazards. J Bone Joint Surg Am 74:84-94, 1992.
16. Reddy AS, Kvitne RS, Yocum LA, et al.: Arthroscopy of the elbow: A long-term clinical review. Arthroscopy 16:588-594, 2000.
17. Ruch DS, Cory JW, Poehling GG: The arthroscopic management of osteochondritis dissecans of the adolescent elbow. Arthroscopy 14:797-803, 1998.
18. Ruch DS, Poehling GG: Arthroscopic treatment of Panner's disease. Clin Sports Med 10:629-636, 1991.
19. Schenck RC Jr, Goodnight JM: Osteochondritis dissecans. J Bone Joint Surg Am 78:439-456, 1996.
20. Singer KM, Roy SP: Osteochondrosis of the humeral capitellum. Am J Sports Med 12:351-360, 1984.
21. Stubbs MJ, Field LD, Savoie FH: Osteochondritis dissecans of the elbow. Clin Sports Med 20:1-9, 2001.
22. Takahara M, Shundo M, Kondo M, et al: Early detection of osteochondritis dissecans of the capitellum in young baseball players: Report of three cases. J Bone Joint Surg Am 80:892-897, 1998.

3 Elbow

Arthroscopic Synovectomy of the Elbow

JAMES A. TOM AND MARK D. MILLER

ARTHROSCOPIC SYNOVECTOMY OF THE ELBOW IN A NUTSHELL

History:
Pain and swelling; loss of motion; crepitation

Physical Examination:
Warmth, tenderness, and swelling; crepitus; limitation of motion from pain; soft tissue laxity; rule out malalignment

Imaging:
Plain radiographs (anteroposterior, lateral, and axial views); magnetic resonance imaging to assess for concomitant pathology

Indications:
Persistent symptoms with minimal articular degeneration, refractory to conservative nonoperative therapy

Contraindications:
Fibrous capsular contracture, joint ankylosis, previous ulnar nerve transposition, post-traumatic deformity, congenital anomalies

Surgical Technique:
Examination under anesthesia: range of motion, stability, and alignment; topographic landmarks (radial head, medial and lateral humeral epicondyles, tip of olecranon)

Patient position: prone with shoulder in 90 degrees of abduction, elbow in 90 degrees of flexion, and forearm pointed toward floor

Operating room setup: primary surgeon directly lateral to flexed elbow; surgical assistant and scrub nurse with instruments on same side as primary surgeon; viewing monitor and infusion pump on opposite side of patient; anesthesiologist at head of table

Arthroscopic portals: proximal anteromedial, proximal anterolateral, posterolateral, straight posterior; direct lateral as alternative to straight posterior

Diagnostic arthroscopy: perform systematic examination; evaluate and biopsy proliferative synovium; assess for concomitant pathology (capsular contracture, loose bodies, chondral defects, osteophytes)

Arthroscopic synovectomy, with systematic resection of proliferative synovium:
Anterior compartment: radiocapitellar articulation, coronoid process, ulnohumeral articulation, medial and lateral gutters
Posterior compartment: olecranon fossa, trochlear groove, medial and lateral gutters

Postoperative Management:
Ice application, elevation with arm sling, analgesia; strengthening and range of motion of shoulder, elbow, and wrist immediately after procedure and for 4 to 6 weeks; increase level of activity as tolerated

Complications:
Neurovascular injury, forearm compartment syndrome, superficial wound infection, hematoma formation, iatrogenic cartilage damage, tourniquet problems, instrument breakage, loss of motion, synovial fistula formation with persistent drainage

Synovitis of the elbow can occur as localized disease, such as an inflamed lateral synovial plica,[12] or, more commonly, as proliferative and generalized disease, such as rheumatoid arthritis.[6,13,17,19,20,24,29-31] Other conditions in which diffuse synovitis may affect the elbow include synovial chondromatosis,[11,16] pigmented villonodular synovitis,[14,16] and hemophilic synovitis.[38]

Early synovitis of the elbow causes pain and associated motion loss. Continued progression of the disease leads to articular cartilage deterioration, periarticular soft tissue attenuation and compromise, and eventually subchondral bone erosion and loss.[19,29,37] The loss of bone and soft tissue about the elbow results in obliteration of the normal joint contour and subsequent instability.[1,13,29]

Synovitis of the elbow is often amenable to conservative nonoperative treatment, which may include medications, splinting, physiotherapy, and, occasionally, steroid injections.[6,24,37] However, if the synovitis causes persistent symptoms and becomes chronic, with no response to medical management, open or arthroscopic synovectomy may provide significant pain relief and functional improvement.[6,15,17,20,24,29,37] In addition, synovectomy may help prevent advanced joint destruction if it is performed during the early stages of rheumatoid arthritis.[13,22,34]

Open synovectomy of the elbow is a generally accepted procedure for inflammatory diseases such as rheumatoid arthritis.[15,17,19,29-31,36] A lateral Kocher approach, which provides adequate joint exposure, is used most commonly.[17,29,30,40,46] A posterior Bryan-Morrey triceps-splitting approach,[9] a combined medial and lateral approach,[29] and a transolecranon approach[20,29] have also been described. Synovectomy with concomitant excision of the radial head for rheumatoid arthritis remains controversial.[29,30,37,40]

Compared with open synovectomy, arthroscopic synovectomy of the elbow is technically demanding, with a higher risk of neurovascular injury.[19,24,29] However, arthroscopic synovectomy has several advantages, including superior joint visualization,[10,24,29,37] decreased postoperative pain from smaller incisions,[10,19,29] and earlier rehabilitation.[19,29,37] Thus, arthroscopic synovectomy can be a valuable adjunct in the management of synovitis of the elbow in select patients who have not responded to conservative treatment.

History

Patients with early synovitis of the elbow often complain of pain and swelling. They also describe loss of motion that is associated with pain and occasionally crepitation. Concurrent with disease progression, elbow mechanics are compromised as a result of articular destruction, soft tissue attenuation, and joint incongruity. Subsequently, patients report loss of motion that is accompanied by mechanical symptoms, such as locking or catching. Patients also may complain of elbow instability.[1,13,29]

Extra-articular pain or discomfort is caused by extension of synovitis beyond the elbow joint.[29] Uncontrolled extension of synovitis can result in compression of adjoining neural structures, such as the posterior interosseous nerve[21] and the ulnar nerve.[23] Subsequently, patients describe associated symptoms of neuritis. Finally, because the olecranon bursa often communicates with the elbow joint in rheumatoid arthritis, patients may present with concomitant pain and swelling over the olecranon that is consistent with olecranon bursitis.[29]

Physical Examination

Physical examination of an elbow afflicted by early synovitis reveals warmth, tenderness, and swelling. Synovitis may be palpable over a lateral triangle defined by the radial head, lateral humeral epicondyle, and tip of the olecranon.[6,29] Motion, which is restricted by pain, is characterized by limitation of flexion-extension and pronation-supination. Mild flexion contracture of the elbow may be present.

As synovitis becomes progressive, limitation of motion is accompanied by intra-articular crepitus, which may reflect articular destruction and joint incongruity. Laxity from soft tissue attenuation of the collateral ligaments can be demonstrated by varus and valgus stress. Malalignment from previous injury or advanced joint degeneration may be present. Resolution of early synovitis often improves pain and function; however, mild flexion contracture of the elbow may persist.[29]

Imaging

Plain radiographs of the elbow consisting of standard anteroposterior, lateral, and axial views should be evaluated for joint degeneration and congruity, malalignment, and osseous abnormalities such as loose bodies and osteophytes. Stress radiographs may be obtained to assess for laxity.[6] In synovitis of the elbow from rheumatoid arthritis, plain radiographs are helpful to determine the stage and extent of disease based on one of two classification schemes—the Mayo classification[28] or the modified Steinbrocker classification.[42] Magnetic resonance imaging of the elbow may be a valuable adjunct to evaluate osteochondral lesions and soft tissue integrity.

Indications and Contraindications

Arthroscopic elbow synovectomy is indicated in patients who have persistent symptoms associated with elbow synovitis, despite nonoperative management, and minimal articular degeneration.[4,29,37] In patients with rheumatoid arthritis, synovectomy during early stages of the disease can improve pain and function and prevent joint destruction.[8,17,22,29,36,46,47] Synovectomy with concomitant resection of the radial head for rheumatoid arthritis is controversial.[29,30,37,40]

Arthroscopic synovectomy is contraindicated in patients with significant distortion of normal bony or soft tissue anatomy, which may hinder the safe creation of arthroscopic portals.[6,37,45] For example, fibrous capsular contracture or joint ankylosis may prevent adequate joint distention, which is important for displacement of neurovascular structures away from the arthroscopic portals.[6,37,45] Other distortions of the normal anatomy include previous ulnar nerve transposition,[6,37] post-traumatic deformity,[37] and congenital anomalies.[37]

Surgical Technique

Arthroscopic synovectomy of the elbow has been described previously.[19,24,30,31,44] Here, our preferred surgical technique is reviewed.

Positioning

Arthroscopic synovectomy can be performed with the patient in the supine,[3,26,30] lateral decubitus,[19,26,30,31,37] or prone[26,30,35] position. Each position has distinct advantages and disadvantages. We prefer the prone position, as described by Poehling et al.,[35] because it allows improved elbow manipulation, easier access to the posterior aspect of the elbow, and a more stable elbow position. No traction is required because gravity distracts and helps distend the elbow joint, displacing neurovascular structures away from the arthroscopic portals.[6,7] The prone position also facilitates conversion from an arthroscopic to an open procedure if necessary.[6,7,26,35]

For the prone position, the patient is carefully logrolled onto the operating table, with cushioned supports beneath the chest, abdomen, and bony prominences to avoid compression. A pneumatic tourniquet is placed on the arm at the midhumeral level. A sandbag is placed under the shoulder to increase mobility. An arm board is attached parallel to the operating table at the level of the arm. The arm is allowed to hang over the arm board with the shoulder in 90 degrees of abduction, the elbow in 90 degrees of flexion, and the forearm pointed toward the floor.

Examination under Anesthesia

After induction of general anesthesia, the elbow is examined to confirm range of motion, stability, and alignment. Because topographic landmarks can be difficult to localize after joint distention, the elbow is carefully palpated to identify and demarcate the radial head, medial and lateral humeral epicondyles, and tip of the olecranon. These landmarks are outlined on the skin before joint distention. A clear understanding of the topographic anatomy of the elbow can decrease the risk of injury to neurovascular structures.

Operating Room Setup

The primary surgeon stands or sits directly lateral to the flexed elbow (Fig. 30–1). The surgical assistant and scrub nurse, with the Mayo stand for instruments, are positioned on the same side as the primary surgeon. The stand that contains the video monitor, camera, recording equipment, and infusion pump and the stand for the irrigation bags are located on the opposite side of the patient. An infusion pump is set at 35 mm Hg to maintain joint distention. The anesthesiologist is situated at the head of the table.

Specific Surgical Steps

The arm is prepared and draped free to allow for intraoperative manipulation. A Coban bandage is applied from the fingers to the proximal forearm just below the region of the arthroscopic portals to minimize fluid extravasation into the forearm. The arm is exsanguinated by elevation and use of an Esmarch bandage before the pneumatic tourniquet is inflated to 200 mm Hg.

Topographic landmarks and arthroscopic portals on the elbow are carefully reviewed and outlined before joint distention. Joint distention is achieved by placing an 18-gauge spinal needle into the joint through the

Figure 30–1 Operating room setup for elbow arthroscopy with the patient in the prone position. The locations of the primary surgeon, operating room personnel, and equipment are shown.

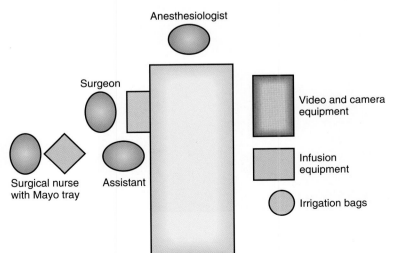

Anesthesiologist

Surgeon

Surgical nurse with Mayo tray

Assistant

Video and camera equipment

Infusion equipment

Irrigation bags

anconeal triangle (a lateral soft spot bordered by the radial head, lateral epicondyle, and tip of the olecranon process) and injecting 15 to 25 mL of saline solution. Joint distention with more than 15 to 25 mL of fluid increases the risk of capsular disruption and fluid extravasation.[32,37] Backflow of fluid through the spinal needle verifies proper entry into the joint.

Four arthroscopic portals are commonly used: proximal anteromedial (proximal medial),[35] proximal anterolateral (proximal lateral),[18,41,43] posterolateral,[5,6] and straight posterior (posterocentral).[5-7,26,34] Alternatively, a direct lateral (midlateral) portal may be used instead of a straight posterior portal. A mixture of 0.25% bupivacaine and 1:100,000 epinephrine solution is injected around the portal sites to reduce bleeding as the arthroscopic portals are created.

The proximal medial portal, as described by Poehling et al.,[35] is initially established with the elbow in 90 degrees of flexion. The portal is located 2 cm proximal to the medial epicondyle and just anterior to the medial intermuscular septum to avoid injury to the ulnar nerve. The portal is placed by directing an 18-gauge spinal needle along the anterior aspect of the humerus into the joint. Return of fluid through the spinal needle indicates proper entry into the joint. The spinal needle is withdrawn, the overlying skin is carefully incised with a number 11 scalpel blade to avoid injury to the medial antebrachial cutaneous nerve, and a hemostat is used for blunt dissection along the same trajectory as the spinal needle to the medial joint capsule.

Following blunt dissection with a hemostat, a blunt trocar is advanced, staying anterior to the medial intermuscular septum and directed toward the radial head while maintaining contact with the anterior aspect of humerus, to avoid injury to the median nerve and brachial artery.[6,25,26,35] The trocar penetrates the flexor-pronator tendon and medial capsule before entering the joint. Return of fluid through the cannula confirms

intra-articular placement. The cannula remains in the joint for the entire procedure.

After the proximal medial portal is established, a 4-mm, 30-degree arthroscope is inserted through the cannula to examine the anterior compartment, which includes the anterior and lateral capsule, radiocapitellar articulation, coronoid process, ulnohumeral articulation, and medial and lateral gutters (Fig. 30–2). This portal is used interchangeably with the proximal lateral portal for visualization and instrumentation during arthroscopic synovectomy of the anterior compartment.

The proximal lateral portal, as described by Stothers et al.,[43] Field et al.,[18] and Savoie and Field,[41] is then established with the elbow in 90 degrees of flexion. The portal is located 2 cm proximal and 1 cm anterior to the lateral epicondyle to avoid injury to the radial nerve. Portal placement is determined by guiding a spinal needle just anterior to the radiocapitellar articulation into the joint. The spinal needle is withdrawn, the overlying skin is carefully incised to avoid injury to the posterior antebrachial cutaneous nerve, and a hemostat is used for blunt dissection to the lateral joint capsule.

Following blunt dissection with a hemostat, a blunt trocar is advanced toward the center of the joint while maintaining contact with the anterior aspect of the humerus. The trocar is carefully directed toward the capsule lateral to the radial head rather than anterior to it to avoid injury to the radial nerve. The trocar penetrates the brachioradialis and brachialis muscles, as well as the lateral capsule, and is advanced into the joint under direct visualization.

The proximal lateral portal can also be created using an inside-out technique. In this technique, the arthroscope in the proximal medial portal is positioned on the capsule lateral to the radial head and then replaced by a Wissinger rod, which tents the overlying skin. The overlying skin is incised, and a cannula is placed over the

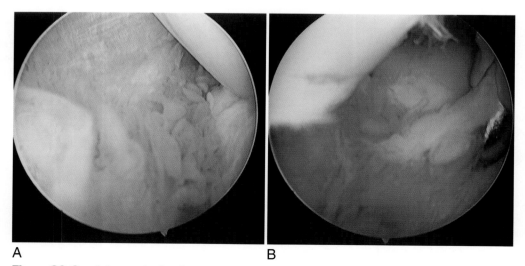

A   **B**

Figure 30–2 Arthroscopic view from the proximal medial portal shows involvement of the ulnohumeral articulation *(A)* and the radiocapitellar articulation *(B)* with diffuse synovitis. (Instrumentation is placed through the proximal lateral portal.)

Wissinger rod into the joint. The cannula remains in the joint for the entire procedure. The proximal lateral portal also allows for instrumentation and visualization of the anterior compartment.

After the proximal lateral portal is established, a probe is inserted through the cannula to examine the anterior compartment for other conditions that may be associated with synovitis, such as loose bodies, chondral defects, and osteophytes. In patients with rheumatoid arthritis, the synovium should be evaluated to determine the stage and extent of disease; if indicated, a biopsy of the proliferative synovium is obtained.

Arthroscopic synovectomy in the anterior compartment of the elbow is performed by using the proximal medial portal for visualization and the proximal lateral portal for instrumentation with probes, grasping forceps,

synovial resectors, and burs. Excision of proliferative synovium is completed in a systematic manner from the lateral and medial aspects of the anterior compartment (Fig. 30–3). Manipulation of the forearm in pronation and supination is important to resect proliferative synovium around the radial neck (Fig. 30–4). Both the proximal medial and proximal lateral portals are used interchangeably for visualization and instrumentation to facilitate excision of proliferative synovium.

Following arthroscopic synovectomy in the anterior compartment, the posterolateral portal is established with the elbow in 45 degrees of flexion. The portal is located 3 cm proximal to the tip of the olecranon at the lateral border of the triceps tendon.[5,6,26,37] After demarcating the portal, a skin incision is carefully made to avoid injury to the medial and posterior antebrachial

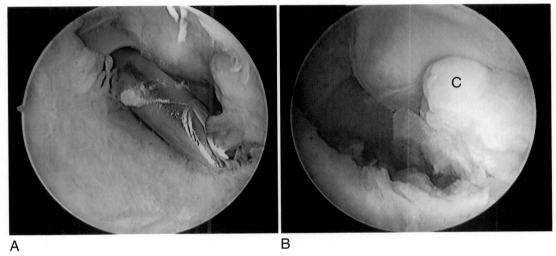

A   B

Figure 30–3 Arthroscopic view from the proximal medial portal shows the ulnohumeral articulation during *(A)* and after *(B)* debridement of proliferative synovium from the base of the coronoid (C). (Instrumentation is placed through the proximal lateral portal.)

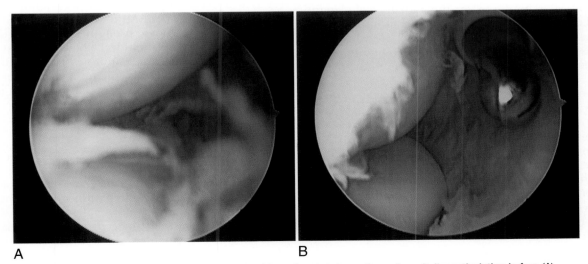

A   B

Figure 30–4 Arthroscopic view from the proximal lateral portal shows the radiocapitellar articulation before *(A)* and after *(B)* debridement of proliferative synovium. (Instrumentation is placed through the proximal medial portal.)

cutaneous nerves, and blunt dissection is carried out to the posterolateral joint capsule. A blunt trocar is directed along the lateral border of the triceps tendon toward the olecranon fossa. The blunt trocar penetrates the posterolateral capsule before entering the joint. Return of fluid through the cannula verifies intra-articular placement. The posterolateral portal allows for instrumentation and visualization of the posterior compartment.

After the posterolateral portal is created, a 4-mm, 30-degree arthrosope is inserted through the cannula to examine the posterior compartment, which includes the tip of the olecranon, posterior trochlea, olecranon fossa, and medial and lateral gutters. Caution is required when evaluating the medial gutter because the ulnar nerve is located just superficial to the medial capsule.[2,26,33] A 4-mm, 70-degree arthroscope is used to visualize the posterior portion of the ulnar collateral ligament.[6] Occasionally, a 2.7-mm, 30-degree arthroscope may be needed to examine the posterior compartment in small patients.

The straight posterior portal is then established with the elbow in 45 degrees of flexion. The portal is located 3 cm proximal to the tip of the olecranon in the midline.[5-7,26,34] As long as the portal is in the midline, the posterior antebrachial cutaneous nerve and the ulnar nerve are not at risk of injury. The portal is placed under direct visualization from the posterolateral portal by directing a spinal needle through the triceps tendon into the olecranon fossa. The spinal needle is withdrawn, the overlying skin is incised, and a hemostat is used for blunt dissection to the posterior capsule.

Following blunt dissection with the hemostat, a blunt trocar is advanced through the tendon of the triceps muscle and posterior capsule into the joint. The straight posterior portal is used primarily for instrumentation but can be used interchangeably with the posterolateral portal for visualization of and complete access to the posterior compartment, which includes the olecranon fossa, posterior trochlea, and medial and lateral gutters.

Alternatively, a direct lateral portal can be established as an accessory portal to the posterior compartment. The portal is located in the anconeal triangle, which is a lateral soft spot bordered by the radial head, lateral humeral epicondyle, and tip of the olecranon. To create the portal, the skin is incised over the site where the spinal needle had been placed for initial joint distention, and a hemostat is used for blunt dissection to the lateral capsule.

Following blunt dissection with a hemostat, a blunt trocar is advanced through the lateral soft spot and directed through the anconeus muscle to access the radiocapitellar articulation or between the anconeus and triceps muscles to access the posterior compartment. In the posterior compartment, the portal is used primarily for visualization but is interchangeable with the posterolateral portal for instrumentation to facilitate arthroscopic synovectomy. However, the portal has limited access to the medial gutter[17] and has been associated with early fluid extravasation into the soft tissues.[26]

Arthroscopic synovectomy in the posterior compartment is routinely performed using the posterolateral portal for visualization and the straight posterior portal for instrumentation with probes, grasping forceps, synovial resectors, and burs. Excision of proliferative synovium is achieved in a systematic manner from the olecranon fossa, trochlear groove, and medial and lateral gutters of the posterior compartment. The posterolateral portal and the straight posterior portal can be used interchangeably, if necessary, to facilitate a complete synovectomy in the posterior compartment. Related arthroscopic procedures such as osteophyte excision, loose body extrication, and contracture release are performed concurrently with synovectomy when indicated.

After completion of the procedure, swelling about the elbow is decreased by gentle manual compression and passive range of motion in flexion and extension. If necessary, Hemovac suction drains can be placed in the anterior and posterior compartments. Local anesthetics can be injected into the joint to provide postoperative pain relief and to facilitate early motion of the elbow. The wounds are closed with 3-0 nylon suture and covered with sterile dressings. Finally, the elbow is lightly wrapped in an elastic bandage for compression and placed in an arm sling for support and elevation. The tourniquet is deflated after an average operative time of 25 to 40 minutes.

Postoperative Management

Immediately after the procedure, ice is applied to the elbow, the operative extremity is elevated with an arm sling, and analgesia is provided as needed. Patients are given home physical therapy exercises for grip strengthening and gentle active and active assisted range of motion involving the shoulder, elbow, and wrist. They are instructed to increase their level of activity using the elbow as tolerated. Patients are routinely discharged on the same day after removal of the Hemovac suction drains (when present) and neurovascular examination of the operative upper extremity.

Continuous passive motion may be used at home for 1 to 3 weeks in patients who need additional assistance for rehabilitation. An outpatient physical therapy program that includes strengthening and range of motion involving the shoulder, elbow, and wrist is initiated after 24 hours and continues for 4 to 6 weeks. If range of motion is difficult to achieve after 2 to 3 weeks, flexion and extension static splints may be considered.

Results

Favorable results with significant relief of pain have been described after arthroscopic synovectomy of the elbow for localized and proliferative inflammatory disorders such as lateral synovial fringe or plica,[12] synovial chondromatosis,[11,16] pigmented villonodular synovitis,[16] and rheumatoid arthritis[19,24,44] (Table 30-1). However, many of the results reported in the literature are based on individual case studies or small numbers of patients and do

Table 30-1

Results Following Elbow Arthroscopy

Author (Date)	Diagnosis	No. of Patients	No. of Elbows	Mean Follow-up (mo)	Significant Improvement	Excellent or Good Results (%)
Clarke (1988)[12]	Lateral synovial plica	3	3	N/A	Yes	
Byrd (2000)[11]	Synovial chondromatosis	2	2	48	Yes	
Ekman et al. (1997)[16]	Pigmented villonodular synovitis	1	1	66	Yes	
	Synovial chondromatosis	1	1	N/A	Yes	
Lee and Morrey (1997)[24]	Rheumatoid arthritis	11	14	3		93
		11	14	42		57
Thal (1996)[44]	Rheumatoid arthritis	46	46	60	Yes	
Horiuchi et al. (2002)[19]	Rheumatoid arthritis	20	21	24		71
		20	21	42		43

N/A, not available.

not include long-term follow-up. No results have been found in the literature for arthroscopic synovectomy in the management of hemophilic synovitis.

Clarke[12] reported a series of three patients who presented with lateral elbow pain that was associated with a catching or popping sensation. Elbow arthroscopy revealed a fibrotic lateral synovial fringe or plica that impinged between the radial head and capitellum during flexion and extension of the elbow with the forearm in pronation. All three patients underwent arthroscopic excision of the lateral synovial plica, resulting in improvement in pain and associated symptoms.

Byrd[11] described two patients with synovial chondromatosis of the elbow that was diagnosed and managed by elbow arthroscopy. Arthroscopic debridement of synovial proliferation and removal of multiple loose bodies were performed. Both patients continued to have relief of pain and mechanical symptoms 4 years postoperatively.

Ekman et al.[16] reported a case involving a patient with pigmented villonodular synovitis and synovial chondromatosis that developed 6 years apart in the same elbow. Both disorders were diagnosed by characteristic findings during elbow arthroscopy. The patient was successfully treated for both disorders by arthroscopic synovectomy and, for synovial chondromatosis, by the removal of loose bodies.

In elbow synovitis caused by rheumatoid arthritis, open synovectomy of the elbow has been found to provide pain relief in 70% to 90% of patients up to 3 years postoperatively.[8,15,17,36,46,47] Porter et al.[36] reported pain relief at least 6 years after open synovectomy. Lee and Morrey,[24] Thal,[44] and Horiuchi et al.[19] described comparable results with short-term follow-up after arthroscopic synovectomy of the elbow in patients with rheumatoid arthritis. However, long-term results of arthroscopic synovectomy remain unclear.

Lee and Morrey[24] reported a series of 14 elbows in 11 patients who underwent arthroscopic synovectomy for refractory elbow pain and associated loss of motion caused by rheumatoid arthritis. Based on the Mayo

elbow performance score, excellent or good results were achieved in 93% of 14 elbows at 3 months postoperatively. However, only 57% maintained excellent or good results after an average of 42 months postoperatively. Thal[44] presented a review of 46 patients who underwent arthroscopic synovectomy of the elbow for inflammatory arthritis. All patients had decreased pain and improved motion over a 5-year period postoperatively.

Horiuchi et al.[19] reported a series of 21 elbows in 20 patients who underwent arthroscopic synovectomy for refractory elbow pain or swelling caused by rheumatoid arthritis. Based on the Mayo elbow performance score, excellent or good results were obtained in 71% of 21 elbows at 2 years postoperatively. Excellent or good results were maintained in 43% after final evaluation at a minimum of 42 months postoperatively. However, 76% of the 21 elbows were only mildly painful or not painful after final evaluation, which is comparable to results obtained after open synovectomy.

The rate of recurrent elbow synovitis after arthroscopic synovectomy in patients with rheumatoid arthritis is comparable to that after open synovectomy. Recurrent synovitis has been observed in 16% to 43% of elbows after open synovectomy.[8,36,47] Horiuchi et al.[19] found recurrent synovitis in 24% of 21 elbows after arthroscopic synovectomy.

Complications

Arthroscopic synovectomy of the elbow requires a concise preoperative plan, knowledge and clear understanding of elbow anatomy, and familiarity with the procedure to avoid technical difficulties and decrease the risk of complications. For example, repeated placement of a cannula through the joint capsule causes rapid fluid extravasation into the soft tissues, which can obstruct visualization, impede manipulation of arthroscopic instruments, and, if excessive, lead to a forearm compartment syndrome.

Neurovascular injury may occur as a result of imprudent skin incisions, aberrant placement of arthroscopic portals with blunt trocars, overaggressive fluid distention, or inadvertent violation of the joint capsule with the synovial resector.[3,25-27,34,39] Other potential complications include superficial wound infection, hematoma formation, iatrogenic cartilage damage, tourniquet problems, instrument breakage, loss of motion, and synovial fistula formation with persistent drainage.

Conclusion

Synovitis of the elbow can occur as a result of localized or proliferative inflammatory diseases such as lateral synovial plica, synovial chondromatosis, pigmented villonodular synovitis, hemophilic synovitis, and rheumatoid arthritis. Arthroscopic synovectomy of the elbow can be an important diagnostic and therapeutic modality in select patients with synovitis of the elbow that is not responsive to conservative nonoperative management. Arthroscopic synovectomy of the elbow requires a concise preoperative plan, thorough understanding of the anatomic relationships around the elbow, and familiarity with the technique and instrumentation so that the procedure can be performed quickly and efficiently, without complications and with minimal risk of neurovascular injury.

References

1. Amis AA, Hughes SJ, Wright V: A functional study of the rheumatoid elbow. Rheum Rehab 21:151-156, 1982.
2. Andrews JR, Baumgarten TE: Arthroscopic anatomy of the elbow. Orthop Clin North Am 26:671-677, 1995.
3. Andrews JR, Carson WG: Arthroscopy of the elbow. Arthroscopy 1:97-107, 1985.
4. Angelo RL: Advances in elbow arthroscopy. Orthopedics 16:1037-1046, 1993.
5. Baker CL, Brooks AA: Arthroscopy of the elbow. Clin Sports Med 15:261-281, 1996.
6. Baker CL Jr, Jones GL: Arthroscopy of the elbow. Am J Sports Med 27:251-264, 1999.
7. Baker CL, Shalvoy RM: The prone position for elbow arthroscopy. Clin Sports Med 10:623-628, 1991.
8. Brumfield RH Jr, Resnick CT: Synovectomy of the elbow in rheumatoid arthritis. J Bone Joint Surg Am 67:16-20, 1985.
9. Bryan RS, Morrey BF: Extensive posterior exposure of the elbow: A triceps-sparing approach. Clin Orthop 166:188-192, 1982.
10. Bynum CK, Tasto J: Arthroscopic treatment of synovial disorders in the shoulder, elbow, and ankle. Am J Knee Surg 15:57-59, 2002.
11. Byrd JWT: Arthroscopy of the elbow for synovial chondromatosis. J South Orthop Assoc 9:119-124, 2000.
12. Clarke RP: Symptomatic, lateral synovial fringe (plica) of the elbow joint. Arthroscopy 4:112-116, 1988.
13. Day B: Arthroscopic management of elbow disorders: Osteochondritis dissecans, loose bodies, synovitis, arthritis, and fracture fixation. In Chow JCY (ed): Advanced Arthroscopy. New York, Springer-Verlag, 2001, pp 193-202.
14. DiCaprio MR, Damron TA, Stadnick M, Fuller C: Pigmented villonodular synovitis of the elbow: A case report and literature review. J Hand Surg [Am] 24:386-391, 1999.
15. Eichenblat M, Hass A, Kessler I: Synovectomy of the elbow in rheumatoid arthritis. J Bone Joint Surg Am 64:1074-1078, 1982.
16. Ekman EF, Cory JW, Poehling GG, et al: Pigmented villonodular synovitis and synovial chondromatosis arthroscopically diagnosed and treated in the same elbow. Arthroscopy 13:114-116, 1997.
17. Ferlic DC, Patchett CE, Clayton ML, Freeman AC: Elbow synovectomy in rheumatoid arthritis: Long-term results. Clin Orthop 220:119-125, 1987.
18. Field LD, Altchek DW, Warren RF, et al: Arthroscopic anatomy of the lateral elbow: A comparison of three portals. Arthroscopy 10:602-607, 1994.
19. Horiuchi K, Momohara S, Tomatsu T, et al: Arthroscopic synovectomy of the elbow in rheumatoid arthritis. J Bone Joint Surg Am 84:342-347, 2002.
20. Inglis AE, Ranawat CS, Straub LR: Synovectomy and debridement of the elbow in rheumatoid arthritis. J Bone Joint Surg Am 53:652-662, 1971.
21. Ishikawa H, Hirohata K: Posterior interosseous nerve syndrome associated with rheumatoid synovial cysts of the elbow joint. Clin Orthop 254:134-139, 1990.
22. Jerosch J, Schroder M, Schneider T: Good and relative indications for elbow arthroscopy: A retrospective study on 103 patients. Arch Orthop Trauma Surg 117:246-249, 1998.
23. Keret D, Porter KM: Synovial cyst and ulnar nerve entrapment: A case report. Clin Orthop 188, 213-216, 1984.
24. Lee BP, Morrey BF: Arthroscopic synovectomy of the elbow for rheumatoid arthritis: A prospective study. J Bone Joint Surg Br 79:770-772, 1997.
25. Lindenfeld TN: Medial approach in elbow arthroscopy. Am J Sports Med 18:413-417, 1990.
26. Lyons TR, Field LD, Savoie FH III: Basics of elbow arthroscopy. Instr Course Lect 49:239-246, 2000.
27. Miller CD, Jobe CM, Wright MH: Neuroanatomy in elbow arthroscopy. J Shoulder Elbow Surg 4:168-174, 1995.
28. Morrey BF, Adams RA: Semiconstrained arthroplasty for the treatment of rheumatoid arthritis of the elbow. J Bone Joint Surg Am 74:479-490, 1992.
29. Nestor BJ: Surgical treatment of the rheumatoid elbow: An overview. Rheum Dis Clin 24:83-99, 1998.
30. Norberg FB, Savoie FH III, Field LD: Arthroscopic treatment of arthritis of the elbow. Instr Course Lect 49:247-253, 2000.
31. O'Driscoll SW, Morrey BF: Arthroscopy of the elbow: Diagnostic and therapeutic benefits and hazards. J Bone Joint Surg Am 74:84-94, 1992.
32. O'Driscoll SW, Morrey BF, An KN: Intraarticular pressure and capacity of the elbow. Arthroscopy 6:100-103, 1990.
33. Plancher KD, Peterson RK, Brezenoff L: Diagnostic arthroscopy of the elbow: Set-up, portals, and technique. Oper Tech Sports Med 6:2-10, 1998.
34. Poehling GG, Ekman EF: Arthroscopy of the elbow. Instr Course Lect 44:217-223, 1995.
35. Poehling GG, Whipple TL, Sisco L, et al: Elbow arthroscopy: A new technique. Arthroscopy 5:222-224, 1989.
36. Porter BB, Richardson C, Vainio K: Rheumatoid arthritis of the elbow: The results of synovectomy. J Bone Joint Surg Br 56:427-437, 1974.
37. Ramsey ML: Elbow arthroscopy: Basic setup and treatment of arthritis. Instr Course Lect 51:69-72, 2002.
38. Rodriguez-Merchan EC, Magallon M, Galindo E, et al: Hemophilic synovitis of the knee and the elbow. Clin Orthop 343:47-53, 1997.

39. Ruch DS, Poehling GC: Anterior interosseous nerve injury following elbow arthroscopy. Arthroscopy 13:756-758, 1997.

40. Rymaszewski LA, Mackay I, Amis AA, et al: Long-term effects of excision of the radial head in rheumatoid arthritis. J Bone Joint Surg Br 66:109-113, 1984.

41. Savoie FH III, Field LD: Anatomy. In Savoie FH III, Field LD (eds): Arthroscopy of the Elbow. New York, Churchill Livingstone, 1996, pp 3-24.

42. Steinbrocker O, Traeger CH, Batterman RC: Therapeutic criteria in rheumatoid arthritis. JAMA 140:659-665, 1949.

43. Stothers K, Day B, Regan WR: Arthroscopy of the elbow: Anatomy, portal sites, and a description of the proximal lateral portal. Arthroscopy 11:449-457, 1995.

44. Thal R: Arthritis. In Savoie FH III, Field LD (eds): Arthroscopy of the Elbow. New York, Churchill Livingstone, 1996, pp 103-116.

45. Timmerman LA: Arthroscopic treatment of the elbow. In Chapman MW (ed): Chapman's Orthopaedic Surgery. Philadelphia, Lippincott Williams & Wilkins, 2001, pp 2233-2246.

46. Tulp NJ, Winia WP: Synovectomy of the elbow in rheumatoid arthritis: Long-term results. J Bone Joint Surg Br 71:664-666, 1989.

47. Vahvanen V, Eskola A, Peltonen J: Results of elbow synovectomy in rheumatoid arthritis. Arch Orthop Trauma Surg 110:151-154, 1991.

Arthroscopic Management of Soft Tissue Impingement in the Elbow

DANIEL J. GURLEY, LARRY D. FIELD,
AND FELIX H. SAVOIE III

ARTHROSCOPIC MANAGEMENT OF SOFT TISSUE IMPINGEMENT IN THE ELBOW IN A NUTSHELL

History:	Painful locking or catching of the elbow that can be resolved with gentle manipulation; lateral elbow pain at 90 to 110 degrees of flexion
Physical Examination:	Painful band over radiocapitellar joint; lateral elbow tenderness; snapping with passive pronation and flexion
Imaging:	Radiographs; magnetic resonance imaging (generally to rule out other pathology, such as posterolateral rotatory instability, loose bodies)
Indications:	Painful snapping plica and as an adjunct to other arthroscopic procedures (e.g., treatment of lateral epicondylitis)
Contraindications:	Distorted anatomy (edema, swelling, prior ulnar nerve transposition) preventing safe arthroscopy
Surgical Technique:	Prone position with tourniquet; diagnostic arthroscopy; view from anteromedial portal to assess radial head; view from posterolateral portal to visualize plica in lateral gutter; excise plica from soft-spot working portal
Postoperative Management:	Sling, soft dressing, early range of motion, early progression to activities as tolerated
Results:	Excellent with accurate diagnosis
Complications:	Neurovascular, extravasation, stiffness

Elbow snapping caused by a synovial plica was initially described by Clarke[4] in 1988. Since that time, the presence of a synovial band, or plica, adjacent to the radiocapitellar joint has become an accepted explanation for the cause of such snapping.[1,3,5,6,11] Little, however, has been published on the topic. Antuna and O'Driscoll[2] presented a case series of snapping plicae that represented 8.7% of their arthroscopic elbow procedures performed during a given period. Moore,[7] Nirschl and Pettrone,[8] and Stack and Hunt[12] have all described a synovial fringe excision as part of the operative treatment of lateral epicondylitis. Clarke[4] suggested that a symptomatic synovial plica should be included in the differential diagnosis of tennis elbow or lateral elbow pain. He also suggested that some diagnoses of loose bodies are actually symptomatic plicae.

History

Patients with elbow soft tissue impingement present with a spectrum of symptoms, the most dramatic of which is a painful locking or catching of the elbow that can be resolved with gentle manipulation. These symptoms can easily be confused with those of a loose body, except that the pain is fairly reproducible over the radiocapitellar joint. More subtle presentations are often difficult to distinguish from lateral epicondylitis or tennis elbow. A painful plica tends to be more symptomatic with elbow flexion and extension and not as painful with wrist extension and gripping. Many patients have had extensive treatment for lateral epicondylitis with recalcitrant symptoms.

Physical Examination

Often a band is palpable over the lateral aspect of the radiocapitellar joint. This point is slightly more distal than is typical lateral epicondylitis pain. A "flexion-pronation" test has been described that reproduces symptoms and often snapping as well. The forearm is maximally pronated and passively flexed to 90 to 110 degrees. Snapping can be felt during flexion from 90 to 110 degrees.[2] Other causes of lateral elbow pain include posterolateral rotatory instability (PLRI), which is characterized by pain with supination while under a valgus load at a flexion angle of about 40 degrees.[9]

Imaging

Radiographs, tomograms, and magnetic resonance imaging scans do not contribute positively to the diagnosis of soft tissue impingement or symptomatic elbow plica. However, imaging studies may have a role in the workup of other possibilities in the differential diagnosis. PLRI can occasionally be diagnosed with magnetic resonance imaging. Loose bodies may be seen with any of these modalities.

Indications and Contraindications

The most satisfying indication is a palpable, painful, snapping plica. However, because many surgeons advocate elbow arthroscopy for the treatment of lateral epicondylitis, PLRI, and excision of loose bodies, this allows for direct inspection at the time of surgery. No specific contraindication exists, but one must consider general contraindications to elbow arthroscopy, as discussed elsewhere in this text.

Surgical Technique

Positioning

We prefer the prone position for all elbow arthroscopy (Fig. 31–1). We routinely use a pneumatic tourniquet

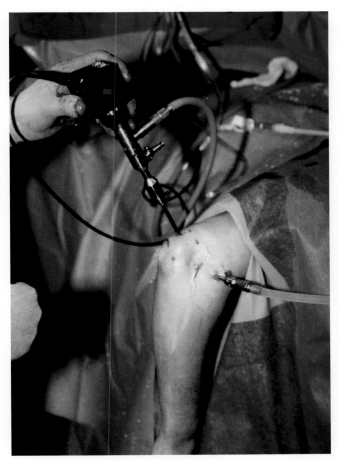

Figure 31–1   Patient in prone position for elbow arthroscopy.

and a prone arm holder. The supine and lateral decubitus positions are reasonable alternatives.

Examination under Anesthesia

The PLRI test is performed to evaluate the radioulnohumeral ligament. Additionally, the flexion-pronation test may be helpful to palpate the snapping plica.

Diagnostic Arthroscopy

A systematic assessment of the entire elbow joint is important to avoid missing associated lesions or loose bodies. The plica can be identified by viewing from an anteromedial portal, but it is most easily seen in the posterolateral gutter as viewed from a posterolateral portal (Figs. 31–2 and 31–3). The lesion varies from a synovial fold to an almost meniscoid-type tissue impinging on the articular surface of the radial head.

Specific Surgical Steps

Several portals are essential for the successful diagnosis and treatment of these synovial plicae. A proximal anteromedial portal is used for viewing the

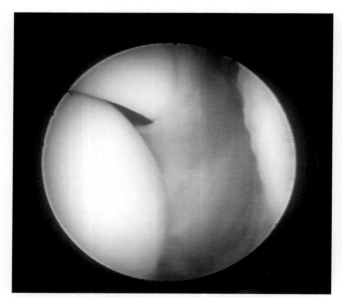

Figure 31-2   View of plica from anteromedial portal.

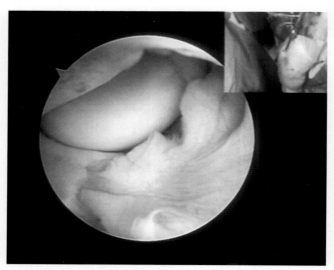

Figure 31-4   Plica excised.

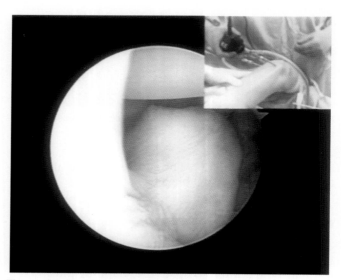

Figure 31-3   View of plica from posterolateral portal.

radiocapitellar joint and assessing for plicae. A lateral working portal can be created in a safely established proximal anterolateral position to start the excision anteriorly. The posterolateral portal affords an excellent view of the plica and the radial head. The radial head should be carefully inspected for chondromalacia from an abrading plica. A soft-spot portal is then established to excise the lateral plica with a motorized resector (Fig. 31-4).

Pearls and Pitfalls

1. Take care to avoid damaging the articular surface of the radiocapitellar joint.

2. Take care to avoid damaging the lateral collateral ligament complex during arthroscopic plica resection.

3. A plica is occasionally seen in conjunction with lateral epicondylitis. Diagnostic arthroscopy before open or arthroscopic lateral epicondylar debridement often reveals a plica that may be causing continued unexplained symptoms.

Postoperative Management

The elbow is placed in a soft dressing and sling for comfort. Activities are started in the first week. Formal physical therapy is generally not needed unless the patient has difficulty regaining range of motion. Our experience is that simple plica excision does not cause excessive stiffness.

Results

In the Mayo Clinic series, 12 of 14 patients had complete relief following surgery.[2] One of the two failures had untreated PLRI. The other patient had two subsequent arthroscopies without improvement after an initial 4-year period of no symptoms. Clarke[4] reported on three patients, all of whom recovered completely.

Complications

Other than the usual potential complications of elbow arthroscopy, this procedure does not significantly increase patient risk.[10] No complications have been reported, and we have not experienced any complications associated with plica removal.

References

1. Akagi M, Nakamura T: Snapping elbow caused by the synovial fold in the radiohumeral joint. J Shoulder Elbow Surg 7:427-429, 1998.
2. Antuna SA, O'Driscoll SW: Snapping plicae associated with radiocapitellar chondromalacia. Arthroscopy 17:491-495, 2001.
3. Caputo AE, Hartford CT, Proia AD, Urbaniak JR: The radiocapitellar meniscal complex: An anatomical and histological analysis. Paper presented at the annual meeting of the American Society for Surgery of the Hand, Sept 1999, Boston.
4. Clarke R: Symptomatic, lateral synovial fringe (plica) of the elbow joint. Arthroscopy 4:112-116, 1988.
5. Commandre FA, Taillan B, Benezis C, et al: Plica synovialis (synovial fold) of the elbow: Report on one case. J Sports Med Phys Fitness 28:209-210, 1988.
6. Jackson RW, Patel D: Synovial lesions: Plicae. In McGinty JB, Caspari RB, Jackson RW, Poehling GG (eds): Operative Arthroscopy. New York, Lippincott-Raven, 1996, pp 447-458.
7. Moore M Jr: Radiohumeral synovitis: A cause of persistent elbow pain. Surg Clin North Am 33:1363-1371, 1953.
8. Nirschl RP, Pettrone FA: Tennis elbow. J Bone Joint Surg Am 61:832-839, 1979.
9. O'Driscoll SW, Bell DF, Morrey BF: Posterolateral rotatory instability of the elbow. J Bone Joint Surg Am 73:440-446, 1991.
10. O'Driscoll SW, Morrey BF: Arthroscopy of the elbow: Diagnostic and therapeutic benefits and hazards. J Bone Joint Surg Am 74:84-94, 1992.
11. Ogilvie WH: Discussion on minor injuries of the elbow joint. Proc R Soc Med 23:306-322, 1929.
12. Stack JK, Hunt WS: Radio-humeral synovitis. Q Bull Northwestern Univ 20:394-397, 1946.

3 Elbow

Arthroscopic Management of Valgus Extension Overload of the Elbow

DANIEL J. GURLEY, LARRY D. FIELD, AND FELIX H. SAVOIE III

ARTHROSCOPIC MANAGEMENT OF VALGUS EXTENSION OVERLOAD OF THE ELBOW IN A NUTSHELL

History:
Throwing athlete with extension loss and posterior or posteromedial elbow pain while throwing

Physical Examination:
Rule out concomitant medial collateral ligament insufficiency

Imaging:
Radiographs demonstrating posterior olecranon osteophyte on lateral view; magnetic resonance imaging to evaluate medial collateral ligament

Indications:
Throwing athlete with isolated posteromedial pain in extension with no identifiable valgus instability

Contraindications:
Distorted anatomy (edema, swelling, prior ulnar nerve transposition) preventing safe arthroscopy; associated valgus instability without medial collateral ligament reconstruction

Surgical Technique:
Prone position with tourniquet; diagnostic arthroscopy; arthroscopic valgus instability test; excise posteromedial olecranon spur; assess olecranon fossa for hypertrophy and need for deepening or fenestration; repeat arthroscopic valgus instability test

Postoperative Management:
Sling, soft dressing, early range of motion; early progression to activities as tolerated, including throwing within 3 months

Results:
Excellent with accurate diagnosis

Complications:
Neurovascular, extravasation, stiffness, unrecognized medial collateral ligament insufficiency leading to onset of valgus instability

Valgus extension overload is a condition of the elbow commonly seen in throwing athletes. The excessive valgus force applied to the thrower's elbow can cause impingement of the posteromedial olecranon into the olecranon fossa during extension. Over time, this repetitive action can lead to chondromalacia and osteophyte formation and can cause loose bodies to develop. This overload often occurs as part of the complex of medial elbow instability, in which case both the overload and the instability must be addressed for treatment to be successful. However, isolated, symptomatic posteromedial impingement frequently occurs. King et al.[4] were the first to recognize that medial olecranon impingement can be caused by hypertrophy of the olecranon fossa and humerus in combination with cubitus valgus. Wilson et al.[7] described the entity and offered a treatment protocol. They noted that although conservative rehabilitation can benefit overhand throwers, the presence of a spur on radiographs almost always requires surgical excision for a successful outcome. We believe that this condition can be treated effectively with arthroscopic assessment and debridement.

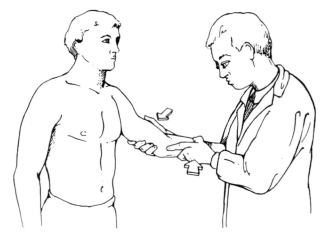

Figure 32–1   Physical examination may yield a flexion contracture, tenderness posteriorly or posteromedially along the olecranon, and evidence of concomitant medial collateral ligament insufficiency.

History

Patients with valgus extension overload typically complain of a loss of extension with posterior or posteromedial pain. A detailed determination of the pitching phase in which the pain occurs is important. Most patients with valgus extension overload report pain during the acceleration and follow-through phases. It is critical to question the patient carefully about the location and character of the pain. A good history and physical examination help differentiate isolated valgus extension overload from medial collateral ligament (MCL) insufficiency, flexor-pronator damage, olecranon stress fracture, or lateral elbow injury. A detailed history also helps exclude neurologic injury, shoulder symptoms, and triceps tendinitis.

Physical Examination

Along with a good history, a complete physical examination is vital in diagnosing valgus extension overload. Valgus stability must be assessed when considering valgus extension overload (Fig. 32–1). Additionally, medial elbow instability, if not addressed when treating valgus extension overload, may lead to treatment failure. MCL instability can be subtle, with ligament sectioning studies indicating a 3-degree difference when the anterior band of the MCL is cut.[2]

Posterior olecranon impingement can be elicited by elbow extension that produces posterior pain. Palpation of the posteromedial olecranon may exhibit tenderness. Locking or catching of the elbow as well as crepitus during range of motion may suggest loose bodies, chondromalacia, or osteophyte formation. A flexion contracture may be present with either osteophyte impingement or anterior capsular contracture.

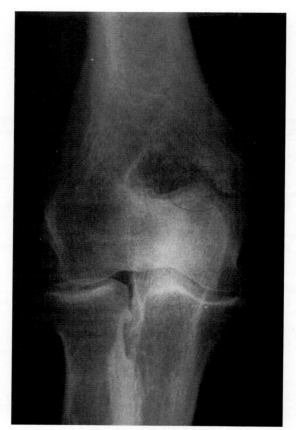

Figure 32–2   Anteroposterior radiograph demonstrating spur formation along the posteromedial olecranon.

Imaging

Radiographs frequently reveal a posterior olecranon osteophyte on routine lateral or anteroposterior views (Fig. 32–2). Some authors advocate olecranon axial views to demonstrate the presence of medial olecranon osteophytes.[7] However, because radiographs are unable to predict chondral lesions and soft tissue injuries, and because of the frequent underestimation of loose bodies by conventional radiographs, computed tomography and magnetic resonance imaging are frequently employed. Magnetic resonance imaging can also be important in investigating a potential MCL tear.[5]

Indications and Contraindications

The most important contraindication for debridement of valgus extension overload spurs is gross valgus instability. The best indication for debridement is in a throwing athlete with isolated posteromedial pain in extension with no identifiable valgus instability. It is often helpful to obtain a magnetic resonance imaging scan of the MCL to confirm its status. Success can be expected in patients with no instability. However, in patients with significant valgus instability, simply removing the posteromedial spurs might destabilize the elbow and worsen the patient's symptoms. It is important to discuss with the patient that if significant valgus instability is identified during surgery, MCL reconstruction may be necessary.

Surgical Technique

Positioning

We prefer the prone position for all elbow arthroscopy (Fig. 32–3). Posteromedial olecranon spur excision is especially facilitated by the prone position. We routinely use a pneumatic tourniquet and a prone arm holder.

Examination under Anesthesia

Examination under anesthesia is essential to develop a feel for the character and cause of any extension block. A bony block has a hard, sudden stop and a feeling of bony impingement. Anterior capsular contracture often has a slightly softer feel at terminal extension. Valgus instability testing throughout the range of motion helps assess the status of the MCL.

Diagnostic Arthroscopy

Diagnostic arthroscopy must include a complete inspection and evaluation of the elbow. An arthroscopic valgus instability test should be performed, and medial stability should be documented (Fig. 32–4).[3] Examination of the olecranon–olecranon fossa articulation shows osteophyte formation on the posteromedial olecranon. Additionally, the olecranon fossa of the humerus may show chondromalacia or spur formation. Loose body formation is common, and a systematic examination of the entire elbow is necessary to identify and remove any loose bodies present.

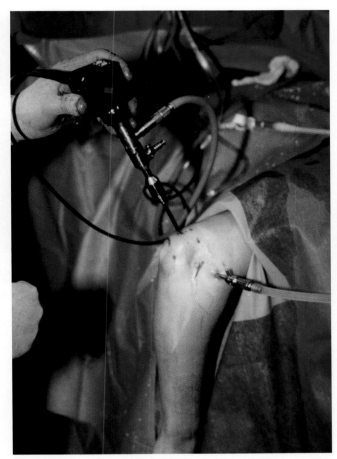

Figure 32–3   Intraoperative photograph demonstrating prone positioning for elbow arthroscopy.

Specific Surgical Steps

After complete diagnostic arthroscopy and identification of a posteromedial olecranon spur, resection is carried out. First, a viewing portal is established through a posterolateral portal. Next, a direct posterior or triceps-splitting portal is established for access of the motorized resector or bur. After clearing out the olecranon fossa, the articular cartilage is carefully inspected. Areas of chondromalacia can be treated by the surgeon's choice of microfracture, abrasion chondroplasty, or benign neglect. The posteromedial spur is then resected (Fig. 32–5). It is extremely important to be mindful of the ulnar nerve's close relationship to the medial olecranon. Previous reports of open excision emphasized a biplanar spur excision. It is important to follow this recommendation while working with the arthroscope. Besides removing the posterior spur, the medial aspect of the spur must also be excised. While working medially, use a hooded bur, and always keep the hooded part toward the ulnar nerve. Occasionally, hypertrophy of the olecranon fossa necessitates a deepening or fenestration of the olecranon fossa (Fig. 32–6). This can easily be performed using the identical instruments and positioning. When the resection is complete, always assess elbow extension and valgus

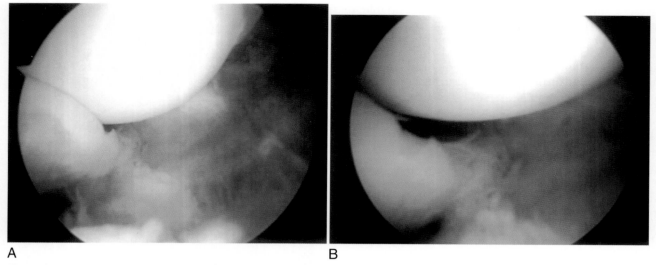

A   B

Figure 32–4   The arthroscopic valgus instability test is performed to assess for significant opening in the ulnohumeral articulation, which is consistent with medial instability. *A,* Reduced position. *B,* Notable diastasis in the medial ulnar and distal humeral articulation.

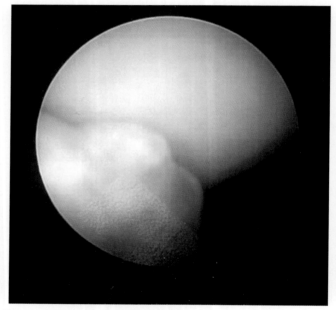

Figure 32–5   Arthroscopic view of posteromedial bone spur.

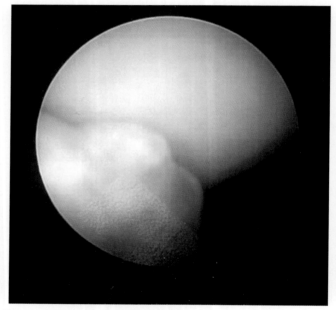

Figure 32–6   Hypertrophy may necessitate a deepening or fenestration of the olecranon fossa, as seen here arthroscopically.

instability with a repeat arthroscopic valgus instability test (Table 32–1).

Pearls and Pitfalls

Elbow arthroscopy has one of the highest propensities for neurologic injuries. In addition to the usual worries about safe portal placement, using a motorized resector or bur in close proximity to the ulnar nerve is risky. Use of a hooded shaver always pointed away from the ulnar nerve provides only a small margin for error. A careful arthroscopic valgus instability test before and after spur excision helps prevent unrecognized MCL instability.

Table 32–1   Specific Surgical Steps for Arthroscopic Treatment of Valgus Extension Overload
Examination under anesthesia for valgus instability, extension block
Diagnostic arthroscopy
Arthroscopic valgus instability test
Excision of loose bodies (if present)
Excision of posterior olecranon spur
Excision of medial olecranon spur
Evaluation of olecranon fossa for hypertrophy
Deepening or fenestration of olecranon fossa if necessary
Repeat arthroscopic valgus instability test

Postoperative Management

Patients with valgus extension overload undergoing isolated spur excision are moved rapidly through the rehabilitation process. A sling is used sparingly for comfort for the first 7 to 10 days. After the first week, patients are encouraged to use the elbow normally for activities of daily living, and they can begin strengthening and range-of-motion exercises. We include flexor-pronator mass strengthening to help improve dynamic valgus stability. When patients reach a pain-free plateau, they can be advanced through an interval throwing program.[6] This throwing program typically begins at 6 weeks. A target date for return to competitive pitching is 3 to 4 months.

Results

The initial report by Wilson et al.[7] included five patients treated with open biplanar spur excision. One reoperation (20%) was required in a patient with severe chondromalacia of the olecranon articular surface. Bartz et al.[1] reported on their results following "mini-open" decompression. In this mini-open group, 19 of 24 baseball pitchers obtained complete relief. These 19 were able to return to their previous level of competition with equal or greater throwing velocity compared with preoperative measurements. However, two patients required reoperation for MCL reconstruction.

Complications

Although it has not been reported for this diagnosis and procedure, ulnar nerve injury is the most devastating and important potential complication when using a motorized resector adjacent to the medial gutter. Also, as noted earlier, unrecognized MCL instability has been a cause of reoperation. It is difficult to diagnose this condition in the early postoperative period, and it may become apparent only when the athlete is unable to regain pitching velocity and control. Recognition of this entity preoperatively or at least intraoperatively is essential for optimal treatment of these patients.

References

1. Bartz RL, Bryan WJ, Lowe W: Posterior elbow impingement. Oper Tech Sports Med 9:245-252, 2001.
2. Callaway GH, Field LD, Deng XH, et al: Biomechanical evaluation of the medial collateral ligament of the elbow. J Bone Joint Surg Am 79:1223-1231, 1997.
3. Field LD, Altchek DW: Evaluation of the arthroscopic valgus instability test of the elbow. Am J Sports Med 24:177-181, 1996.
4. King JW, Brelsford HJ, Tullos HS: Analysis of the pitching arm of the professional baseball pitcher. Clin Orthop 67:116-123, 1969.
5. Ward WG, Belbhobek GH, Anderson TE: Arthroscopic elbow findings: Correlation with preoperative radiographic studies. Arthroscopy 8:498-502, 1992.
6. Wilk KE, Arrigo C, Andrews JR: Rehabilitation of the elbow in the throwing athlete. J Orthop Sports Phys Ther 17:305-317, 1993.
7. Wilson FD, Andrews JR, Blackburn TA, et al: Valgus extension overload in the pitching elbow. Am J Sports Med 11:83-88, 1993.

3 Elbow

33

Arthroscopic Management of Degenerative Joint Disease in the Elbow

ETHAN R. WIESLER AND GARY G. POEHLING

ARTHROSCOPIC MANAGEMENT OF DEGENERATIVE JOINT DISEASE IN THE ELBOW IN A NUTSHELL

History:
Pain and swelling, mechanical symptoms, motion loss

Physical Examination:
Decreased range of motion, crepitus

Imaging:
Plain radiographs (anteroposterior, lateral, and axial views); radial head views, contralateral elbow

Indications:
Pain, elbow contracture, radiographic degenerative joint disease

Contraindications:
Joint ankylosis, previous ulnar nerve transposition, reflex sympathetic dystrophy, soft tissue compromise, excessive heterotopic ossification

Surgical Technique:
Position: lateral with armrest
Arthroscopic portals: proximal anteromedial, proximal anterolateral, midlateral, posterolateral, straight posterior
Diagnostic arthroscopy: perform systematic examination, debridement, loose body removal, radial head and osteophyte removal as needed

Postoperative Management:
Early range of motion, strengthening, dynamic splinting, continuous passive motion

Results:
60% to 90% satisfaction

Complications:
Neurovascular injury, heterotopic ossification, compartment syndrome, infection, instrument failure, reflex sympathetic dystrophy, cartilage damage, synovial fistula

Recent advances in the techniques and instrumentation of elbow arthroscopy have enabled surgeons to expand the indications for this procedure and the treatment options available. Thorough knowledge of elbow anatomy and surrounding neurovascular structures is paramount. In addition, as surgeons have gained experience with arthroscopy of the elbow, the results have improved. There are limitations, however, when using elbow arthroscopy to treat advanced degenerative joint disease (DJD).

History

The use of arthroscopy as a diagnostic tool for elbow disorders should not replace a careful clinical examination and patient history. As with all elbow injuries, the history, including timing, onset, and nature of symptoms, is important. The patient's age, participation in sports, and past injuries and surgery should also be noted. A careful medical history should focus on the presence of inflammatory arthritis, because monoarticular inflammatory arthropathy may be confused with isolated DJD.

Physical Examination

The physical examination consists of range-of-motion assessment (flexion, extension, pronation-supination), neurovascular examination, location of symptoms, and comparison to the contralateral side. Mechanical symptoms such as clicking, locking, or popping suggest loose bodies or an articular defect such as osteochondritis dissecans.

Imaging

The routine radiographic evaluation consists of anteroposterior and lateral plain radiographs. Adjunctive views include radial head and contralateral views, which are especially helpful in adolescents or those with posttraumatic conditions and in the differentiation of inflammatory versus degenerative disease. Computed tomography typically provides little additional information, except in the evaluation of concurrent heterotopic ossification. Likewise, magnetic resonance imaging has little to offer and is not used routinely.

Indications and Contraindications

Table 33–1 lists our current indications and contraindications for elbow arthroscopy. A progressive joint contracture, unresolving symptoms following conservative treatment, or a fixed contracture greater than 10 degrees, with elbow symptoms of pain when compared with the contralateral side, are our indications for arthroscopic evaluation.

Surgical Technique

For arthroscopy, the patient is placed in the lateral position, with the affected elbow on an arm holder (Fig. 33–1). Range-of-motion assessment is done preoperatively with the patient under anesthesia. The initial approach to the anterior joint is done after capsular distention with sterile normal saline in the anatomic soft spot. A proximal anteromedial portal is established, allowing visualization of the anterior radiocapitellar joint, coronoid process, and any loose bodies or

Table 33–1 Indications and Contraindications for Elbow Arthroscopy

Indications[2,3,7,10,20]

Loose bodies
Osteochondritis dissecans
Rheumatoid arthritis—synovectomy
Contracture, arthrofibrosis
Degenerative joint disease (mild to moderate)
Pigmented villonodular synovitis
Lateral epicondylitis
Radial head fracture
Radial head resection
Synovial chondromatosis
Infection, septic arthritis
Posterolateral instability (?)

Contraindications

Degenerative joint disease (advanced)
Previously transposed ulnar nerve (prevents any medial approach)
Excessive heterotopic bone
Reflex sympathetic dystrophy
Soft tissue compromise

osteophytes in the anterior joint (Fig. 33–2). An inside-out portal is created for instrumentation in the anterior joint, through the standard anterolateral portal. We use a 4.5-mm shaver introduced through a cannula in the anterolateral portal to debride the anterior radiocapitellar joint (Fig. 33–3). Leaving the patient's hand free in this operating position also facilitates manipulation of the forearm into pronation-supination to provide access to the entire radial head.

Depending on the size of the patient, a 2.7-mm arthroscope and instrumentation are used for the posterior elbow joint and posterior radiocapitellar joint. Initial placement of the 2.7-mm camera in the midlateral portal allows inspection of the posterior surface of the capitellum, proximal radioulnar joint, and ulnohumeral joint (Fig. 33–4); based on preoperative studies, it also allows for the evaluation and location of any loose bodies. If a simple debridement is performed, instruments are inserted into the adjacent or posterolateral portal (Fig. 33–5).

Loose bodies are often found in the posterior joint, and accessory portals are made as needed through separate incisions (straight posterior or posterolateral). When the radial head is involved, as it may be in later stages of the disease, an arthroscopic radial head excision may be done (Fig. 33–6). The camera is kept in the proximal medial portal, and a 5-mm bur is placed in the anterior or direct lateral portal for excision. Similarly, simple excision of marginal osteophytes, followed by an evaluation of range of motion (ROM) in the operating room, may be helpful. Our current practice is to make a small lateral arthrotomy extension of the straight lateral portal to facilitate removal of a hypertrophic radial head.

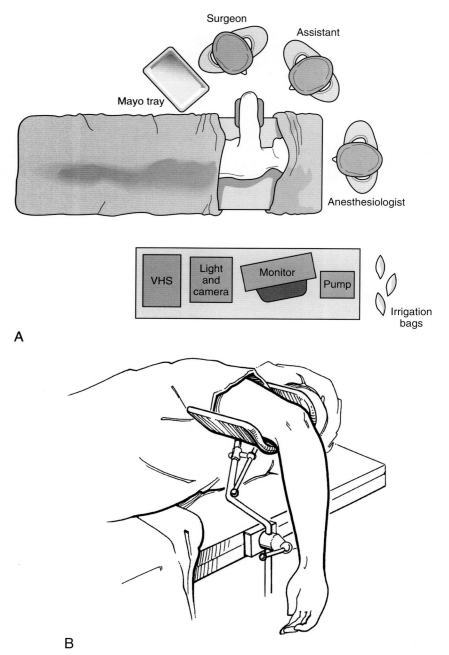

Figure 33–1   *A*, Operating room setup. *B*, Lateral position.

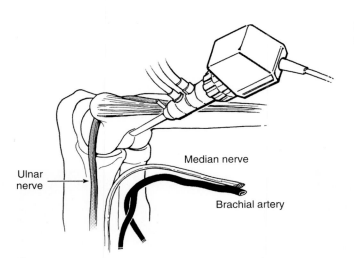

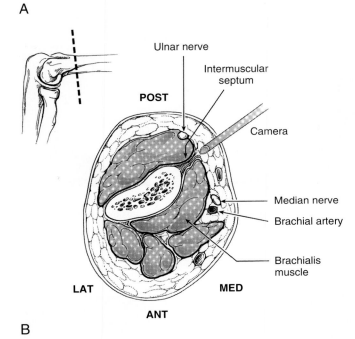

Figure 33–2 *A,* Proximal medial portal placement. *B,* Cross section of proximal medial portal.

Ulnar nerve

Median nerve

Brachial artery

A

Ulnar nerve

Intermuscular septum

POST

Camera

Median nerve

Brachial artery

Brachialis muscle

LAT

MED

ANT

B

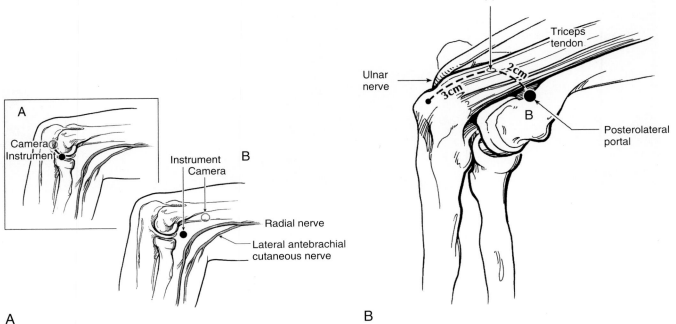

A

Camera
Instrument

B

Instrument
Camera

Radial nerve

Lateral antebrachial cutaneous nerve

A

A

Triceps tendon

Ulnar nerve

2cm

3cm

B

Posterolateral portal

B

Figure 33–3 *A,* Location of lateral (A) and adjacent lateral (B) portal placement. *B,* Straight posterior (A) and posterolateral (B) portal placement.

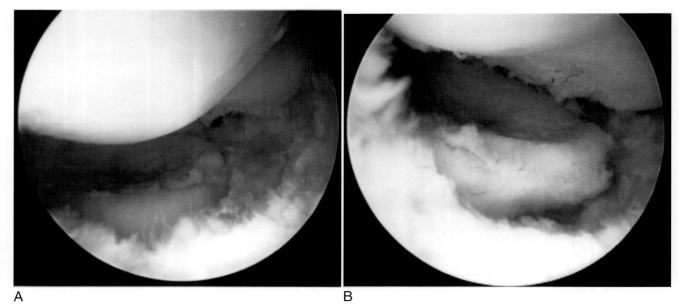

A   B

Figure 33–4   *A* and *B*, Arthroscopic views of moderate radiocapitellar degenerative joint disease (seen from the proximal medial portal).

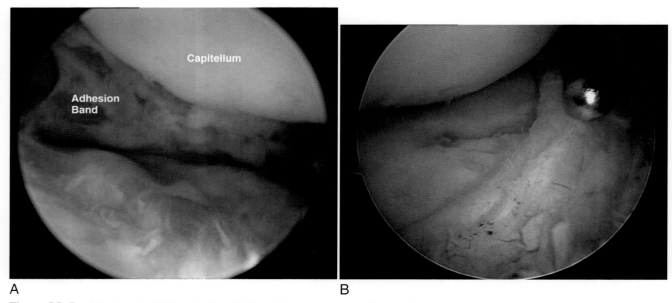

A   B

Figure 33–5   Adhesion band *(A)* and early radial head degenerative joint disease *(B)*.

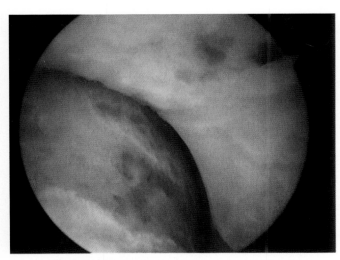

Figure 33–6 Moderate ulnohumeral degenerative joint disease (seen from the adjacent lateral portal).

Arthroscopic fenestration of the olecranon fossa, combined with olecranon tip osteotomy, is also used for flexion contractures with posterior compartment involvement.

Postoperative Management

Our postoperative regimen consists of unrestricted motion as pain allows. Formal physical therapy is begun 3 days postoperatively. Active and passive ROM is used, and continuous passive motion or serial static or dynamic splinting may be used, depending on individual patient goals. Continuous passive motion may be used for significant associated arthrofibrosis, although its efficacy is unclear.

If a simple debridement or radial head excision was performed arthroscopically, the patient is instructed to begin range-of-motion exercises immediately. We have not seen heterotopic ossification as a complication of elbow arthroscopy for this condition and therefore do not prescribe any prophylaxis.

Results

In 1992, O'Driscoll and Morrey[16] reported on 71 arthroscopic elbow procedures for various indications, including for diagnostic purposes. Although their indications did not specifically include DJD, there were diagnoses of pain, limited ROM, and loose bodies. They reported a 73% benefit in patients overall, but a 62% benefit for patients who had the operation for diagnostic purposes only.

Redden and Stanley[17] reported in 1993 on 12 patients undergoing olecranon fossa fenestration for the treatment of DJD. At 16 months, all patients had diminished pain and relief of elbow locking. ROM was not significantly improved, and one patient lost 30 degrees of extension.

In 1994, Schneider et al.[19] reported long-term (5.8 years) results in 67 patients, approximately one third of whom had a diagnosis of DJD. ROM, Figgie scores, and job function improved in this subset of patients. However, patients with symptoms of more than 2 years' duration and advanced DJD were unimproved. Additionally, the procedure had to be interrupted in three patients with advanced arthrosis due to technical problems.

Moskal et al.[13] reported anecdotally on 13 of 14 patients with DJD who had improved ROM, decreased pain, and 93% satisfaction with elbow arthroscopy at 1 to 5 years' follow-up. They also advocated olecranon fossa fenestration rather than olecranon tip osteotomy to restore extension, and radial head excision for radiocapitellar disease.

O'Driscoll[15] advocated the use of arthroscopy in the early stages of DJD for osteophyte excision and supported previous investigators who had warned of the procedure's difficulty in cases of advanced arthritis and arthrosis secondary to diminished joint compliance, with a resultant greater proximity to crucial neurovascular structures.

Kim and Shin[9] also reported increased ROM, with a total 44-degree increase in arc of motion; 92% of patients (n = 63) achieved overall improvement. Longer than 1 year after surgery, however, there were no further improvements. Jerosch et al.[7] found very little improvement in patients with severe DJD (n = 40).

Ward and Anderson[21] reported 90% improved function in 35 adult athletes who underwent arthroscopy for loose body removal or osteophyte excision.

Complications

Complications following elbow arthroscopy are listed in Table 33–2. Morrey[12] succinctly pointed out that because multiple portals may be necessary to perform satisfactory osteophyte excision in patients with DJD, all three nerves at the elbow are vulnerable to injury. Hahn and Grossman,[6] Andrews and Carson,[1] Ruch and Poehling,[18] and Kelly et. al.[8] all reported limited, single nerve injuries from elbow arthroscopy. The consensus is that although all the nerves at the elbow may be at risk, the following principles provide a margin of safety:

Table 33–2
Complications Following Elbow Arthroscopy
Neurovascular injury
Arthrofibrosis
Compartment syndrome
Infection
Complex regional pain syndrome
Cartilage damage
Tourniquet-related problems
Instrument failure or breakage
Synovial fistula

3 Elbow

1. Proximal portals are safer than distal ones.
2. Use of an inside-out portal on the lateral side of the elbow decreases the risk of radial nerve injury.
3. Joint distention diminishes but does not eliminate the risk of nerve injury.
4. The radial nerve at the anterolateral portal is most at risk.
5. Elbow flexion to 90 degrees aids in portal placement.
6. Posteromedial and direct anterior portals should be avoided.
7. Capsular laxity and compliance are diminished in advanced DJD.[4]

Gofton and King[5] submitted a case report of heterotopic ossification following elbow arthroscopy. The overall complication rate in several series is approximately 6% to 12%, including neurovascular injury, transient nerve palsy, and various other complications.[11] Stiffness following arthroscopy for DJD is exceedingly rare (<1%).

With advances and experience, the rate of complications following elbow arthroscopy has decreased significantly.

Conclusion

Although most authors include DJD as an indication for arthroscopy, especially when accompanied by loose bodies, progressive loss of motion, or increasing pain, the stage of DJD at which arthroscopy is beneficial remains unclear.[2,3,7,10,14,16] Advanced joint arthrosis reduces joint compliance, putting vital neurovascular structures at significantly greater risk. Further, the technical aspects of gaining joint access with standard instruments make the procedure more difficult.

Our current indications for elbow arthroscopy for DJD, whether primary or secondary, are mild to moderate disease, clinical or radiographic evidence of loose bodies, progressive pain, and limited ROM. We also support other authors' findings of the benefits of either radial head excision or posterior joint osteotomy through olecranon osteotomy or distal humeral fenestration, based on clinical examination and intraoperative findings.

References

1. Andrews JR, Carson WG: Arthroscopy of the elbow. Arthroscopy 1:97-107, 1985.
2. Baker CL, Brooks AA: Arthroscopy of the elbow. Clin Sports Med 15:261-281, 1996.
3. Ekman EF, Poehling G: Arthroscopy of the elbow. Hand Clin 10:453-460, 1994.
4. Gallay SH, Richards RR, O'Driscoll SW: Intraarticular capacity and compliance of stiff and normal elbows. Arthroscopy 9:9-13, 1993.
5. Gofton WT, King JW: Heterotopic ossification following elbow arthroscopy. Arthroscopy 17:1-5, 2001.
6. Hahn M, Grossman JA: Ulnar nerve laceration as a result of elbow arthroscopy. J Hand Surg [Br] 23:109, 1998.
7. Jerosch J, Schroder M, Schneider T: Good and relative indications for elbow arthroscopy. Arch Orthop Trauma Surg 117:246-249, 1998.
8. Kelly EW, Morrey BF, O'Driscoll SW: Complications of elbow arthroscopy. J Bone Joint Surg Am 83:25-34, 2001.
9. Kim SJ, Shin SJ: Arthroscopic treatment for limitation of motion of the elbow. Clin Orthop 375:140-148, 2000.
10. Lyons TR, Field LD, Savoie FH III: Basics of elbow arthroscopy. Instr Course Lect 49:239-246, 2000.
11. Marshall PD, Fairclough JA, Johnson SR, Evans EJ: Avoiding nerve damage during elbow arthroscopy. J Bone Joint Surg Br 75:129-131, 1993.
12. Morrey BF: Complications of elbow arthroscopy. Instr Course Lect 49:255-257, 2000.
13. Moskal MJ, Savoie FH III, Field LD: Elbow arthroscopy in trauma and reconstruction. Orthop Clin North Am 30:163-177, 1999.
14. Nowici KD, Shall LM: Arthroscopic release of a posttraumatic flexion contracture in the elbow: A case report and review of the literature. Arthroscopy 8:544-547, 1992.
15. O'Driscoll SW: Operative treatment of elbow arthritis. Curr Opin Rheumatol 7:103-106, 1995.
16. O'Driscoll SW, Morrey BF: Arthroscopy of the elbow. J Bone Joint Surg Am 74:84-93, 1992.
17. Redden JF, Stanley D: Arthroscopic fenestration of the olecranon fossa in the treatment of osteoarthritis of the elbow. Arthroscopy 9:14-16, 1993.
18. Ruch DS, Poehling GG: Anterior interosseous nerve injury following elbow arthroscopy. Arthroscopy 13:756-758, 1993.
19. Schneider T, Hoffstetter I, Fink B, Jerosch J: Long-term results of elbow arthroscopy in 67 patients. Acta Orthop Belg 60:378-383, 1994.
20. Tedder JL, Andrews JR: Elbow arthroscopy. Orthop Rev 21:1047-1053, 1992.
21. Ward WG, Anderson TE: Elbow arthroscopy in a mostly athletic population. J Hand Surg [Am] 18:220-224, 1993.

Arthroscopic Management of Elbow Stiffness

CRAIG M. BALL, LEESA M. GALATZ, AND KEN YAMAGUCHI

ARTHROSCOPIC MANAGEMENT OF ELBOW STIFFNESS IN A NUTSHELL

History:
Painful motion loss with history of trauma; extension loss and difficulty with activities of daily living

Physical Examination:
Decreased active and passive motion

Imaging:
Plain radiographs (anteroposterior, lateral, and radiocapitellar oblique); computed tomography for heterotopic ossification

Indications:
Failed nonoperative treatment; pain or elbow contracture that interferes with activities of daily living; >30-degree flexion contracture and <130 degrees of flexion

Contraindications:
Altered neurovascular anatomy, extra-articular heterotopic bone, significant bony deformity, infection, unrealistic expectations

Surgical Technique:
Position: lateral decubitus with arm holder
Arthroscopic portals: proximal medial, proximal lateral, accessory lateral, posterolateral, direct posterior
Surgical procedure: anterior compartment adhesion release; loose body removal; arthroscopic basket to incise or resect anterior capsule from lateral to medial to visualize brachialis fibers; posterior compartment debridement; posterior capsule and medial and lateral gutter debridement or release

Postoperative Management:
Extension splint, ice, nonsteroidal anti-inflammatory drugs, active and active assisted range of motion, static splinting as needed

Results:
High satisfaction with significant return of motion

Complications:
Neurovascular injury, progressive motion loss, heterotopic ossification, compartment syndrome, infection, instrument failure, reflex sympathetic dystrophy, cartilage damage, synovial fistula

Loss of motion of the elbow is a common complication that most often occurs as a result of trauma. Arthritic conditions, burns, congenital abnormalities, and various types of cerebral injury can also cause elbow stiffness.[9,22,31,35,36] These conditions have generally been divided into those with intrinsic or extrinsic causes.[22] Intrinsic contractures have an intra-articular cause of motion loss, whereas extrinsic contractures typically spare the joint space. In practice, many stiff elbows have both intrinsic and extrinsic components, and

all contributing pathology must be addressed during treatment.

When severe, elbow stiffness is poorly tolerated and can significantly interfere with the ability to perform activities of daily living.[22] The aim of treatment in these cases is to restore a pain-free functional range of motion to the joint. Surgery is generally reserved for those cases refractory to an extended period of nonoperative treatment. This consists of both active and passive physical therapy programs that may be coupled with dynamic or static splinting.[5,13] Manipulation of the elbow under anesthesia has also been described.[6] Nonoperative treatment is most effective in contractures of short duration and with little evidence of intra-articular damage. In established elbow contractures, the results have generally been disappointing.[3,11]

Many different surgical procedures have been used to treat the stiff elbow, and most authors have used an open approach.[10,12,15,21,22,38,39] Satisfactory results have generally been reported with these techniques.[12,15,21,38-40] However, open contracture release may result in additional soft tissue trauma, which can increase the risk of recurrence and restrict early physical therapy secondary to pain. In addition, open techniques may not allow complete assessment and treatment of associated intra-articular pathology.

Arthroscopic treatment of the stiff elbow is an alternative strategy with the potential benefits of improved joint visualization, decreased postoperative morbidity, and a more rapid functional recovery. Although not all elbow contractures are amenable to arthroscopic treatment, certain contractures with intrinsic and extrinsic (capsular) causes can be treated arthroscopically. However, this is a technically demanding procedure, and extensive experience with elbow arthroscopy is required if satisfactory results are to be achieved and complications avoided.

History

The diagnosis of elbow contracture is usually not difficult, and the cause is often clear from the history. Post-traumatic contracture can occur at any age but typically involves young, active patients. The specific components of a post-traumatic contracture vary, depending on the mechanism of injury. Often the most limiting element to motion is the elbow joint capsule, which can become thickened and fibrotic. However, motion loss may also be secondary to intra-articular causes. Osteoarthritis typically does not develop until the mid or late fifth decade. The osteophyte formation characteristic of elbow osteoarthritis produces articular incongruity, limiting motion. In these patients, flexion contracture develops insidiously and progressively, with pain in terminal extension being the most common complaint.

Important elements of the history include the severity and duration of motion loss and the response to previous treatment, including physical therapy, splinting, and surgery. Extrinsic (extra-articular) causes of elbow stiffness are typically not painful; this includes many cases of post-traumatic contracture. Pain often implies some type of intra-articular (intrinsic) derangement, such as that seen with arthritis, impingement, or loose bodies. The functional impact of the contracture on the patient is also important when deciding on treatment. Terminal flexion is more important in performing activities of daily living than is terminal extension,[24] although loss of elbow extension is usually the most common complaint. Patient age and level of function, coexistent upper extremity pathology, and the presence of medical comor-bidities also need to be considered. Finally, the treating physician should assess the treatment expectations of the patient and the potential for compliance with a postoperative rehabilitation program.

Physical Examination

The physical examination includes a detailed assessment of the entire upper extremity. The skin and surrounding soft tissues of the elbow should be evaluated for areas of fibrosis, previous incisions, skin grafts, or areas of wound instability. Regardless of cause, an adequate soft tissue envelope is critical when considering arthroscopic contracture release. Active and passive range of motion should be measured using a goniometer. This determines the primary direction of motion loss and current level of functional limitation. It also allows one to assess the response to subsequent treatment modalities.

Dynamic strength and stability of the elbow are essential for a successful result and should be carefully assessed. An elbow with inadequate motor strength is unlikely to maintain motion gains after arthroscopic release, and an elbow that is unstable generally requires ligament reconstruction. A complete neurologic examination is also important, especially in a patient with a history of previous trauma or surgery to the elbow. Special attention should be paid to the ulnar nerve, which may require decompression or transposition at the time of surgery. Transposition of the nerve may also be indicated in the presence of significant flexion loss (<100 degrees). Finally, the remaining joints of the upper extremity should be evaluated.

Imaging

Anteroposterior, lateral, and radiocapitellar oblique radiographs usually provide most of the necessary information regarding the cause of an elbow contracture (Fig. 34-1). Intra-articular involvement, including the status of fracture healing, articular congruity, and extent of degenerative change, can be assessed, in addition to identifying retained hardware and the presence of heterotopic ossification. In patients who have significant loss of supination and pronation, radiographs of the forearm and wrist should also be obtained. Computed tomography can be useful to map out areas of heterotopic ossification but is typically not required. This is because extrinsic causes of contracture that cannot safely be reached from within the joint are not amenable to arthroscopic treatment (Fig. 34-2). The use of magnetic resonance imaging has been reported in the assessment of post-traumatic flexion contractures,[7] but it has little role in our practice.

Indications and Contraindications

Selecting appropriate candidates for arthroscopic contracture release is difficult and requires assessment of

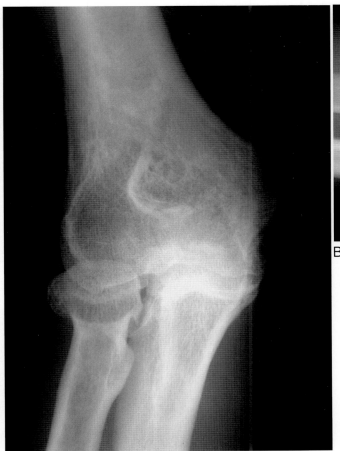

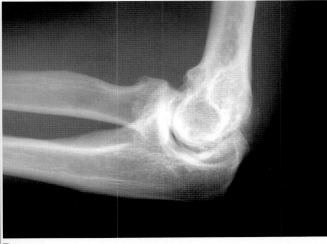

A

B

Figure 34–1 *A* and *B*, Plain radiographs of the elbow usually provide most of the information needed about the cause of motion loss.

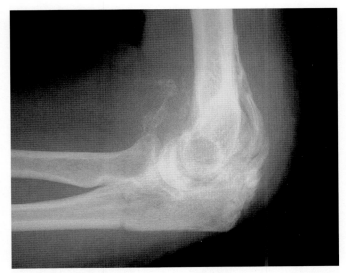

Figure 34–2 Extrinsic causes of contracture that cannot safely be reached from within the joint require open surgical correction.

both the pathologic process and the patient. It is generally recommended that all patients with elbow stiffness be given a trial of nonoperative treatment before surgery is considered, particularly in contractures of short duration and when there is no significant intra-articular

involvement. Surgical treatment is indicated when restricted elbow motion interferes with activities of daily living and fails to improve despite nonoperative measures. Patients with a flexion contracture of more than 30 degrees or flexion less than 130 degrees are candidates for arthroscopic treatment. Certain patients with lesser degrees of flexion contracture but symptoms of intra-articular pathology (pain, popping, locking) may also be considered.

Contraindications to arthroscopic treatment of elbow stiffness include previous surgical procedures that may have altered the neurovascular anatomy around the elbow (medial elbow approaches, ulnar nerve transposition). Certain conditions that result in significant extra-articular deformity are also contraindications for arthroscopic release. Extrinsic causes of contracture that cannot safely be reached from within the joint (heterotopic ossification) require open surgical correction. Conditions that produce significant disruption of the normal ulnohumeral architecture (displaced fracture, chronic dislocation, end-stage degenerative or inflammatory arthritis) are also not amenable to arthroscopic treatment. Active joint infection and unrealistic patient expectations are additional contraindications.

A relative contraindication is limited experience with elbow arthroscopy. The arthroscopic assessment and treatment of elbow stiffness can be extremely challenging, and the surgeon must have extensive experience to achieve a successful result.[33] Involvement in a child is also a relative contraindication, unless the contracture is extensive.

Surgical Technique

All surgery is performed with the patient under general endotracheal anesthesia and in the lateral decubitus position. A well-padded high arm tourniquet is used, which is inflated after exsanguination of the limb. The arm is supported in an arm holder, allowing free access to both sides of the elbow joint. Bony landmarks and the course of the ulnar nerve are outlined with a sterile marking pen following skin preparation. Care is taken to ensure that the nerve cannot be subluxated or placed in an anteriorly transposed position. When draping, the forearm and hand are wrapped firmly in a compression bandage to decrease the space available for fluid extravasation during the procedure. This also allows space for dispersion of the fluid at the completion of the case.

The joint is initially distended with up to 20 mL of sterile saline. This is injected through the "soft spot" at the site of the direct lateral portal. A 4.5-mm, 30-degree arthroscope is used for the procedure, along with the standard camera and video recording equipment. The arthroscope is inserted via the proximal medial portal, which is located 2 cm proximal to the medial epicondyle, just anterior to the medial intermuscular septum. Following skin incision, a blunt trocar is used to palpate the intermuscular septum. The trocar is then directed anterior to this structure to penetrate the capsule of the elbow joint. A proximal lateral "working" portal is established under direct vision using spinal needle localization. This portal is located 2 cm proximal to the lateral epicondyle, just anterior to the lateral supracondylar ridge. A blunt trocar is initially used through this portal to break down intra-articular adhesions and elevate the capsule from the anterior aspect of the distal humerus (Fig. 34–3). This allows a working space to be established.

Synovectomy and debridement of adhesions are then undertaken using a 4.5-mm oscillating shaver. This is done with the elbow in both pronation and supination to allow complete debridement of the anterior radiocapitellar joint. All loose bodies are removed, and any osteophytes are debrided using a 4-mm oscillating bur. Anterior capsular release is initiated only after complete debridement of the anterior compartment has been accomplished (Fig. 34–4).

Sharp release of the anterior capsule begins from the proximal lateral portal. This is performed under direct arthroscopic vision using a 15-degree up-cutting basket resector. Initially the plane between the brachialis and anterior capsule is identified and developed by blunt dissection. Then, progressing from lateral to medial, the capsule is incised directly (Fig. 34–5). It is helpful during this portion of the procedure to establish an accessory lateral portal and use the blunt trocar as a retractor (Fig.

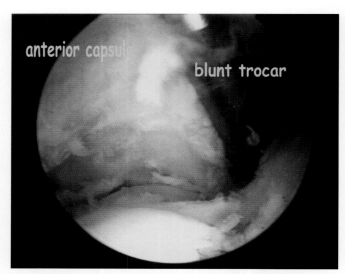

Figure 34–3　A blunt trocar is used to elevate the anterior capsule from the distal humerus, creating an initial working space.

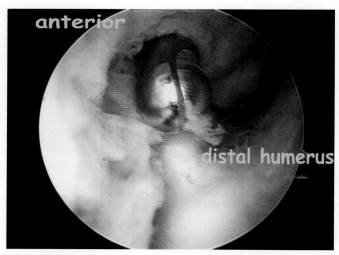

Figure 34–4　Complete debridement of the anterior joint space is required before capsular release.

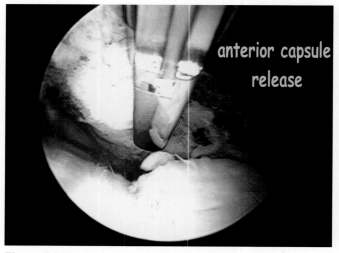

Figure 34–5　Starting laterally, anterior capsular release is performed under direct arthroscopic vision using a 15-degree up-cutting resector.

34–6). The arthroscope is then transferred to the proximal lateral portal using a switching stick, and the release is completed from the medial side (Fig. 34–7). Extreme care is required during the initial part of the release from the lateral side because of the proximity of the radial nerve.

Release of the capsule is continued until the brachialis muscle fibers are visible from medial to lateral (Fig. 34–8). Resection of the proximal portion of the released capsule can then be undertaken safely. Visualization within the joint space is maintained by the use of retractors; use of a suction device, such as the oscillating shaver, is avoided. This enables a greater degree of control during this portion of the procedure. At all times one must ensure that both the arthroscope and the instruments are within the joint. In addition, it is impor-

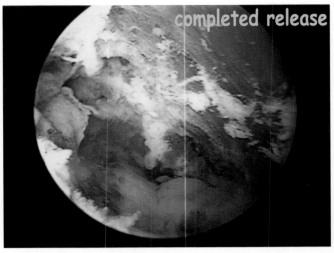

Figure 34–8 The exposed fibers of the brachialis muscle form the endpoint of the release.

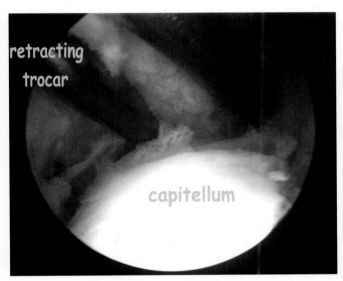

Figure 34–6 A blunt trocar is inserted through an accessory lateral portal. This is used as a retractor to maintain visualization during the release.

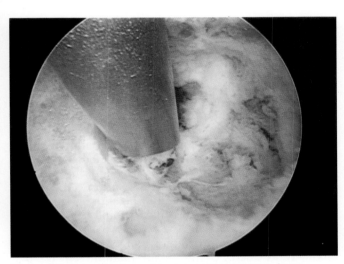

Figure 34–9 A bur is used to deepen the olecranon fossa.

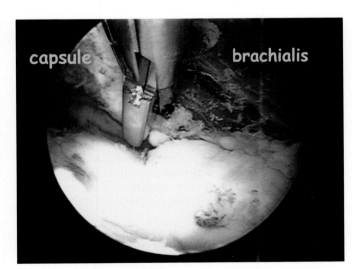

Figure 34–7 The release progresses from lateral to medial across the anterior joint space. The arthroscope and resector are then switched to complete the release from the medial side.

tant that no dissection occurs superficial to the undersurface of the brachialis muscle belly.

A posterolateral and a direct posterior portal are used to perform the posterior joint debridement. The arthroscope is initially inserted via the posterolateral portal. Through the direct posterior portal, a blunt trocar is used to break down adhesions and elevate the capsule from the posterior aspect of the distal humerus. This creates a working space. Scar tissue and adhesions are then resected from the olecranon fossa using the 4.5-mm oscillating shaver. Loose bodies are removed, and osteophytes are debrided from the olecranon and the humerus. If necessary, a bur can be used to deepen the olecranon fossa (Fig. 34–9).[23,29] Alternatively, complete fenestration can be performed. The importance of these procedures in the posterior compartment to restore range of motion to the elbow is well recognized.[27]

The final portion of the procedure involves debridement of the posterior capsule, including release of the

3 Elbow

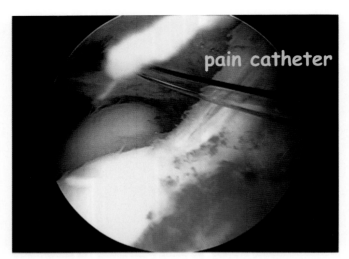

Figure 34–10 An epidural pain catheter placed in the joint at completion of the procedure provides excellent postoperative pain control.

medial and lateral gutters. Excision of adhesions in the lateral gutter is started proximally and continued distally. With the arthroscope in the posterolateral portal, a mid-lateral or soft-spot portal is usually necessary to adequately debride the posterior radiocapitellar joint. The arthroscope can be maintained in this portal, and the shaver can be switched to the direct posterior portal for debridement of the medial gutter. To avoid injury to the ulnar nerve, a fully hooded shaver should be used. Release of the posterior bundle of the medial collateral ligament is not performed, which may limit the extent to which a significant flexion loss can be improved. Because the ulnar nerve may also need to be addressed in these patients, this part of the procedure should be performed open.

At the end of the procedure, range of motion of the elbow is assessed. Gentle manipulation can be performed, if necessary, to release any remaining capsular contracture. An epidural catheter connected to a patient-controlled pain pump (BREG Pain Care 2000, BREG Inc., Vista, CA) filled with local anesthetic (bupivacaine [Marcaine] 0.5% without epinephrine) is placed in the joint (Fig. 34–10). This provides excellent pain control during the early postoperative period. A continuous axillary block can be used as an alternative. The portal sites are closed with interrupted nylon sutures, and a padded dressing is applied. The elbow is placed in full extension and held in this position by application of an anterior splint.

Postoperative Management

The arm is maintained in the extension splint and vertically elevated for 24 to 36 hours. Ice and anti-inflammatory medications are used during this period to control edema. The splint is then removed, and active and active assisted range-of-motion exercises are commenced. Control of inflammation and swelling is critical during this stage. The patient remains in the hospital for 2 to 3 days, depending on progress. Upon discharge, a home exercise program of active and active assisted range-of-motion exercises is continued. Static splints can be used at night and during rest as needed, in either flexion or extension, depending on which motion has been more difficult to achieve. These are usually discontinued at 3 to 4 weeks, once adequate range of motion has been maintained. Continuous passive motion is not routinely used, nor do we routinely use prophylaxis for heterotopic ossification.

If, after 4 to 6 weeks, progress with conventional therapy remains unsatisfactory, dynamic splinting can be employed. In general, however, we have not found this necessary. Patients are allowed to return to light duties once pain and swelling subside, which is usually by 3 to 4 weeks. For those who require more physical use of their upper extremity, return to work is delayed for 6 to 8 weeks, or until they can perform their duties without pain.

Results

Arthroscopic treatment of the stiff elbow was first reported by Nowicki and Shall[25] in 1992. The following year, Jones and Savoie[16] reported improved motion and decreased pain in 12 patients with flexion contractures of the elbow treated by arthroscopic debridement. Mean flexion contracture improved from 38 degrees to 3 degrees in their series, although one patient sustained a permanent posterior interosseous nerve palsy. In 1994, Byrd[4] reported on the results of arthroscopic treatment of arthrofibrosis after type I radial head fractures. His patients gained an average of 30 degrees of extension and 14 degrees of flexion. The same year, Timmerman and Andrews[37] reported good to excellent results in 79% of 19 patients with post-traumatic stiffness treated by arthroscopic debridement and manipulation. Extension improved from a mean of 29 degrees to 11 degrees; flexion improved from a mean of 123 degrees to 134 degrees.

In 1996, Savoie and Jones[33] reported on their experience with 53 capsular release procedures in 53 patients. The average preoperative range of motion in these patients was from 46 degrees of extension to 96 degrees of flexion. This improved to 5 degrees and 138 degrees, respectively, following surgery, with significant increases in pronation and supination observed as well. Savoie et al.[34] also reported on the arthroscopic management of painful restriction of motion due to elbow arthritis. In a series of 24 patients, flexion contracture improved from an average of 40 degrees preoperatively to 8 degrees postoperatively, and elbow flexion improved from an average of 90 degrees to 139 degrees. All patients had a significant decrease in pain.

Both post-traumatic and degenerative causes of arthrofibrosis were included in the study by Phillips and Strasburger.[28] They reported increased motion and decreased pain in 25 patients at an average of 18 months after arthroscopic treatment of arthrofibrosis of the elbow, with an average 41-degree improvement in total arc of motion. Patients with post-traumatic arthritis had more severe flexion contractures preoperatively than did those with degenerative arthritis, but they had more improvement postoperatively. Kim and Shin[19] also observed that patients with post-traumatic stiffness had more marked limitation of extension and a lower total range of motion preoperatively (73 degrees) than did those with degenerative stiffness (86 degrees). However, no significant difference existed in postoperative range of motion, with 92% of 63 patients obtaining significant improvement in range of motion following arthroscopic treatment.

We have looked specifically at patient outcome following arthroscopic treatment of post-traumatic elbow contractures.[2] In our series of 14 consecutive patients, elbow extension improved from a mean of 35.4 degrees to 9.3 degrees postoperatively, and flexion improved from a mean of 117.5 degrees to 132.9 degrees. This improvement in motion was highly significant. All patients had improved function after the procedure, with an average self-reported functional ability score of 28.3 out of 30. Patient satisfaction was high, although pain relief was less predictable than the expected gains in range of motion and function. One patient developed a superficial portal site infection that resolved. There were no other complications.

Complications

Arthroscopic treatment of the stiff elbow is a technically demanding procedure, and significant complications have been reported. Neural and vascular structures appear to be most at risk,[20,26] and the reduced capsular compliance of the stiff elbow increases the potential for injury.[8] Both transient[18] and permanent[16] nerve injuries have been reported, including one case of complete transection of the median and radial nerves.[14] The normal anatomic relationships of the nerves can become distorted by an elbow contracture. Meticulous attention to detail is therefore required during surgery. Despite these concerns about nerve injury, the risk appears to be relatively low for surgeons with extensive experience in elbow arthroscopy.[17,30]

Other potential complications of the procedure are the same as those reported for routine elbow arthroscopy. These include infection,[30] hematoma formation, articular cartilage damage, breakage of arthroscopic instruments,[18] and persistent drainage from the portal sites.[26] The overall complication rate following elbow arthroscopy has been reported to be between 0 and 15%.[1,17,20,26,32] Temporary or minor complications are more common than serious or permanent ones, although the risk increases for more complex procedures.

Progressive loss of motion obtained at the time of surgery may cause the procedure to fail. Failure to comply with the postoperative physical therapy program is usually the cause, but results may deteriorate despite compliance. Poor skin quality, weakened muscles, and extensive scarring can all be contributing factors. An inadequately performed debridement and capsular release will not improve range of motion. In addition, failure to adequately address elbow osteophytes and loose bodies can result in persistent pain. If the surgeon has inadequate visualization or other concerns about the procedure, he or she should abandon the arthroscopic surgery and complete the procedure in an open fashion.

Conclusion

Arthroscopic treatment of the stiff elbow can reliably improve range of motion and offers a high degree of patient satisfaction, with significant improvements in function. The ability to treat elbow stiffness arthroscopically offers significant advantages over traditional open procedures. The limited skin incisions and reduced soft tissue dissection decrease soft tissue scarring and the chance of recurrent contracture. In addition, the improved visualization allows better definition of involved structures and more precise treatment of them, reducing patient morbidity and allowing accelerated postoperative rehabilitation. Arthroscopic treatment of the stiff elbow is technically demanding, and extensive experience in elbow arthroscopy is required. Complications do occur, and pain relief is generally less predictable than the expected improvements in range of motion and function. However, with meticulous attention to detail and proper patient selection, excellent results can generally be expected.

References

1. Andrews JR, Carson WG: Arthroscopy of the elbow. Arthroscopy 1:97-107, 1985.
2. Ball CM, Meunier M, Galatz LM, et al: Arthroscopic treatment of post-traumatic elbow contracture. J Shoulder Elbow Surg 11:624-629, 2002.
3. Bonutti PM, Windau JE, Ables BA, et al: Static progressive stretch to reestablish elbow range of motion. Clin Orthop 303:128-134, 1994.
4. Byrd JWT: Elbow arthroscopy for arthrofibrosis after type I radial head fractures. Arthroscopy 10:162-165, 1994.
5. Dickson RA: Reverse dynamic slings: A new concept in the treatment of post-traumatic elbow flexion contractures. Injury 8:35-38, 1976.
6. Duke JB, Tessler RH, Dell PC: Manipulation of the stiff elbow with patient under anaesthesia. J Hand Surg [Am] 16:19-24, 1991.
7. Fortier MV, Forster BB, Pinney S, et al: MR assessment of posttraumatic flexion contracture of the elbow. J Magn Reson Imaging 5:473-477, 1995.
8. Gallay SH, Richards RR, O'Driscoll SW: Intraarticular capacity and compliance of stiff and normal elbows. Arthroscopy 9:9-13, 1993.
9. Garland DE, O'Hallarin RM: Fractures and dislocations about the elbow in the head injured adult. Clin Orthop 168:38-41, 1982.
10. Gates HS III, Sullivan FL, Urbaniak JR: Anterior capsulotomy and continuous passive motion in the treatment of post-traumatic flexion contracture of the elbow. J Bone Joint Surg Am 74:1229-1234, 1992.

11. Gelinas JJ, Faber KJ, Patterson SD, King GJW: The effectiveness of turnbuckle splinting for elbow contractures. J Bone Joint Surg Br 82:74-78, 2000.

12. Glynn JJ, Niebauer JJ: Flexion and extension contracture of the elbow: Surgical management. Clin Orthop 117:289-291, 1976.

13. Green DP, McCoy H: Turnbuckle orthotic correction of elbow flexion contractures after acute injuries. J Bone Joint Surg Am 61:1092-1095, 1979.

14. Haapaniemi T, Berggren M, Adolfsson L: Complete transection of the median and radial nerves during arthroscopic release of post-traumatic elbow contracture. Arthroscopy 15:784-787, 1999.

15. Husband JB, Hastings H: The lateral approach for operative release of post-traumatic contracture of the elbow. J Bone Joint Surg Am 72:1353-1358, 1990.

16. Jones GS, Savoie FH III: Arthroscopic capsular release of flexion contractures (arthrofibrosis) of the elbow. Arthroscopy 9:277-283, 1993.

17. Kelly EW, Morrey BF, O'Driscoll SW: Complications of elbow arthroscopy. J Bone Joint Surg Am 83:25-34, 2001.

18. Kim SJ, Kim HK, Lee JW: Arthroscopy for limitation of motion of the elbow. Arthroscopy 11:680-683, 1995.

19. Kim SJ, Shin SJ: Arthroscopic treatment for limitation of motion of the elbow. Clin Orthop 375:140-148, 2000.

20. Lynch GJ, Meyers JF, Whipple TL, et al: Neurovascular anatomy and elbow arthroscopy: Inherent risks. Arthroscopy 2:190-197, 1986.

21. Mansat P, Morrey BF: The column procedure: A limited lateral approach for extrinsic contracture of the elbow. J Bone Joint Surg Am 80:1603-1615, 1998.

22. Morrey BF: Post-traumatic contracture of the elbow: Operative treatment, including distraction arthroplasty. J Bone Joint Surg Am 72:601-618, 1990.

23. Morrey BF: Primary degenerative arthritis of the elbow: Treatment by ulnohumeral arthroplasty. J Bone Joint Surg Br 74:409-413, 1992.

24. Morrey BF, Askew LJ, An KN, Chao EY: A biomechanical study of normal functional elbow motion. J Bone Joint Surg Am 63:872-877, 1981.

25. Nowicki KD, Shall LM: Arthroscopic release of a post-traumatic flexion contracture in the elbow: A case report and review of the literature. Arthroscopy 8:544-547, 1992.

26. O'Driscoll SW, Morrey BF: Arthroscopy of the elbow: Diagnostic and therapeutic benefits and hazards. J Bone Joint Surg Am 74:84-94, 1992.

27. Ogilvie-Harris DT, Gordon R, Mackay M: Arthroscopic treatment for posterior impingement in degenerative arthritis of the elbow. Arthroscopy 11:437-443, 1995.

28. Phillips BB, Strasburger S: Arthroscopic treatment of arthrofibrosis of the elbow joint. Arthroscopy 14:38-44, 1998.

29. Redden JF, Stanley D: Arthroscopic fenestration of the olecranon fossa in the treatment of osteoarthritis of the elbow. Arthroscopy 9:14-16, 1993.

30. Reddy AS, Kvitne RS, Yocum LA, et al: Arthroscopy of the elbow: A long-term clinical review. Arthroscopy 16:588-594, 2000.

31. Roberts PH, Pankratz FG: The surgical treatment of heterotopic ossification at the elbow following long-term coma. J Bone Joint Surg Am 61:760-763, 1979.

32. Rupp S, Tempelhof S: Arthroscopic surgery of the elbow: Therapeutic benefits and hazards. Clin Orthop 313:140-145, 1995.

33. Savoie FH III, Jones GS: Arthroscopic management of arthrofibrosis of the elbow. In McGinty JB, Caspari RB, Jackson RW, Poehling GG (eds): Operative Arthroscopy, 2nd ed. Philadelphia, Lippincott-Raven, 1996, pp 887-896.

34. Savoie FH III, Pierce ND, Field LD: Arthroscopic management of the arthritic elbow: Indications, technique, and results. J Shoulder Elbow Surg 8:214-219, 1999.

35. Seth MK, Khurana JK: Bony ankylosis of the elbow after burns. J Bone Joint Surg Br 67:747-749, 1985.

36. Sherk HH: Treatment of severe rigid contractures of cerebral palsied upper limbs. Clin Orthop 125:151-155, 1977.

37. Timmerman LA, Andrews JR: Arthroscopic treatment of post-traumatic elbow pain and stiffness. Am J Sports Med 22:230-235, 1994.

38. Urbaniak JR, Hansen PE, Beissinger SF, Aitken MS: Correction of post-traumatic flexion contracture of the elbow by anterior capsulotomy. J Bone Joint Surg Am 67:1160-1164, 1985.

39. Wilner P: Anterior capsulectomy for contractures of the elbow. J Int Coll Surg 11:359-361, 1948.

40. Wilson PP: Capsulectomy for the relief of flexion contractures of the elbow following fracture. J Bone Joint Surg Br 26:71-86, 1944.

Arthroscopic Fracture Management in the Elbow

Michael D. Feldman and Jonathan A. Gastel

ARTHROSCOPIC FRACTURE MANAGEMENT IN THE ELBOW IN A NUTSHELL

Physical Examination:
Inspection, palpation, neurovascular evaluation

Imaging:
Routine orthogonal radiographs; computed tomography and magnetic resonance imaging as needed

Indications:
Displaced intra-articular fractures with limited metaphyseal involvement

Contraindications:
Distorted anatomy (edema, swelling, malalignment)

Surgical Technique:
Patient positioned prone or supine; C-arm assistance, gravity inflow, joint distention as needed; establish proximal medial portal first, anterolateral portal second; irrigation, debridement, inspection, open reduction and internal fixation of larger fragments; remove smaller fragments, open when necessary

Postoperative Management:
Sling, early range of motion; progress based on fracture stability and rigidity of fixation

Complications:
Inadequate reduction or fixation, neurovascular, severe swelling due to fluid extravasation

With recent improvements in arthroscopic equipment and surgical skills, the indications for elbow arthroscopy are rapidly expanding. Initially used only as a diagnostic tool, elbow arthroscopy is now widely used to treat various soft tissue and osteochondral lesions. One area that has received little attention to date but shows great promise is the treatment of intra-articular fractures of the elbow. Fracture problems can be divided into two categories: acute fractures, and chronic fractures and post-fracture complications. Most of the literature discusses the treatment results of chronic fractures (more than 3 months since the injury)[3,4]; few articles discuss the treatment of acute fractures.[1,2]

History

Elbow fractures are generally categorized as either intra-articular or extra-articular; both types have similar incidences in young individuals with good-quality bone and in older patients with osteoporotic bone. The patient history is usually straightforward, except in the case of multitrauma patients, in whom other injuries or mental status may mask a closed elbow fracture with no clinical deformity. Inadequate fracture management of intra- or extra-articular fractures is well known to result in poor elbow function that translates into significantly compromised use of the upper extremity. Such fractures can be the result of high-energy trauma and may be associated with other skeletal or nonskeletal injuries, or they can result from a low-energy fall on the outstretched hand. In any situation, expedient fracture management—with the goal of allowing quick return of elbow motion—is the primary issue in the treatment of these relatively common orthopedic injuries.

Physical Examination

The physical examination must always include inspection, palpation, range of motion, neurologic testing of the wrist and hand, and evaluation of adjoining joints (shoulder girdle, wrist, hand). Typically, patients present with significant pain, swelling, ecchymoses, and gross deformity of the elbow, especially when a fracture is associated with a dislocation. Ligament instability may also be present and must be assessed by placing a varus or valgus stress on the elbow in varying degrees of flexion. Range of motion is generally quite painful, especially in the acute setting. Pre- and postreduction neurovascular examinations are critical to document neurologic or vascular changes from baseline following reduction maneuvers.

Imaging

Thoughtful preoperative planning is essential to optimize the postoperative outcome. Satisfactory anteroposterior and lateral radiographs of the elbow should be obtained and studied before surgery (Fig. 35–1). Some fractures may also require preoperative computed tomography or magnetic resonance imaging scans to better define the fracture configuration (Fig. 35–2). Electrodiagnostic testing may be necessary when nerve injury around the elbow is diagnosed preoperatively. Ultrasonography and bone scanning have little role in the treatment of operative fractures of the elbow. Potential locations for hardware (interfragmentary screws) and proposed incisions should be identified, with special consideration given to zones of soft tissue trauma and previous scars.

Indications and Contraindications

The indications for arthroscopy of acute elbow fractures include displaced intra-articular fractures with limited metaphyseal involvement. Intra-articular fractures such as lateral condylar, capitellar, radial head, and simple

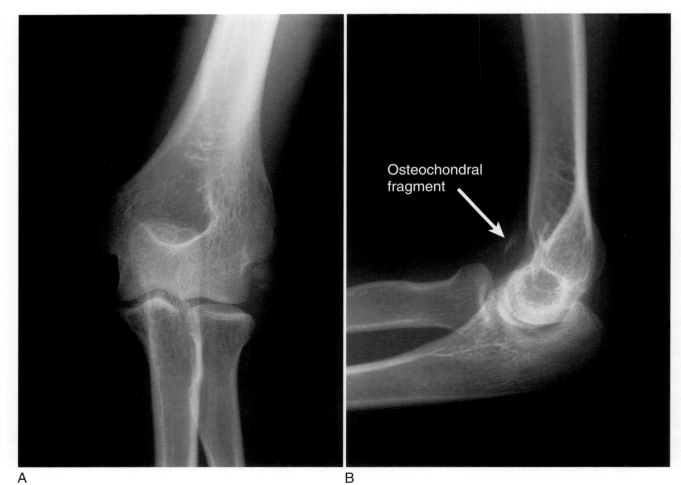

Osteochondral fragment

A

B

Figure 35–1 *A,* Anteroposterior radiograph of a type II capitellar fracture. *B,* Lateral radiograph of a type II capitellar fracture.

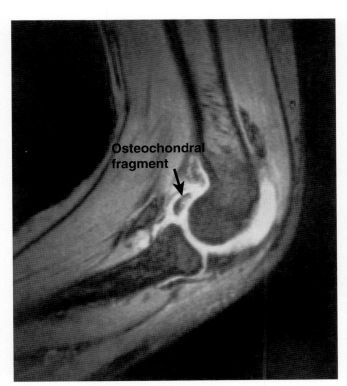

Figure 35–2 Magnetic resonance imaging scan of a type II capitellar fracture, sagittal view.

intercondylar fractures may be amenable to arthroscopic or arthroscopically assisted reduction and internal fixation. In addition to the intra-articular fracture lines seen on preoperative radiographs, it is common to see additional fracture lines or loose osteochondral fragments during arthroscopy, which can also be treated.

Absolute contraindications to arthroscopy of acute elbow fractures are the same as those for arthroscopy in general—localized infection, gross soft tissue contamination, neurovascular injury, and severe edema or swelling that precludes palpation of anatomic landmarks. Relative contraindications include fractures or fracture-dislocations that cause significant distortion of elbow anatomy. Additionally, in these cases, complications secondary to severe localized soft tissue swelling due to fluid extravasation are possible. Some would say that open fractures are a relative contraindication to arthroscopy, although in grade I and selected grade II open fractures, arthroscopy may provide improved irrigation and debridement while minimizing further soft tissue trauma compared with conventional open techniques.

Surgical Technique

Positioning and Examination under Anesthesia

Under adequate anesthesia, the patient is placed prone or supine—depending on surgeon preference—on the operating room table. The operative extremity is placed

in an elbow arthroscopy holder (Smith and Nephew Endoscopy, Andover, MA, or Instrument Makar, East Lansing, MI) as far proximal as possible. After the extremity is appropriately prepared and draped, a sterile tourniquet is applied. Anatomic landmarks and proposed incisions are marked, and the tourniquet is inflated. A mini C-arm is also draped sterile for use. Owing to the risk of excessive soft tissue swelling secondary to fluid extravasation, gravity inflow rather than pump inflow is recommended.

Usually, in acute fractures, distention due to hemarthrosis is already present, and joint distention with saline is not necessary. However, if there is no effusion, injection of the joint with 10 to 15 mL of saline through the posterolateral soft spot is recommended. The proximal medial portal is usually established first using a double-port cannula, and intra-articular placement is confirmed by extravasation of fluid from one of the ports. Upon entering the joint, visualization can be difficult secondary to hemarthrosis and fibrinous debris. The double-port cannula is extremely useful at this point, as it allows for both inflow and outflow, which aids in irrigating the joint. An anterolateral portal is made under direct visualization, and a 3.5-mm full-radius shaver is inserted to remove the remaining blood and debris from the joint.

Diagnostic Arthroscopy

A thorough arthroscopic examination is performed. Posterior portals are also created to visualize the olecranon fossa and the medial and lateral gutters. Articular surfaces are evaluated for chondral defects and fracture lines, recesses are checked for loose osteochondral fragments, and the medial ligamentous complex is evaluated for disruption. In some instances, the joint capsule is torn, and this is documented as well. After determination of the intra-articular pathology, loose fragments are removed, chondral lesions are debrided to a stable rim, and the fracture is treated.

Specific Surgical Steps

When intra-articular fracture fragments are present, a determination is made whether to fix or excise the fragments. Fragments that have healthy articular cartilage with adequate subchondral bone should be repaired; fragments with comminuted or damaged cartilage with little attached bone should be excised (Fig. 35–3). Fracture reduction can be performed with either a probe or a grasper; occasionally, a reduction tenaculum can be used. Once an acceptable reduction is obtained, provisional fixation is maintained with Kirschner wires placed perpendicular to the fracture line, if possible. The mini C-arm is used to confirm the reduction, and final fixation is performed using cannulated screws, headless screws, or absorbable pins, depending on the fracture configuration.

Certain fracture patterns, such as noncomminuted intercondylar fractures, may require both an open and an arthroscopic approach. In these cases, the arthro-

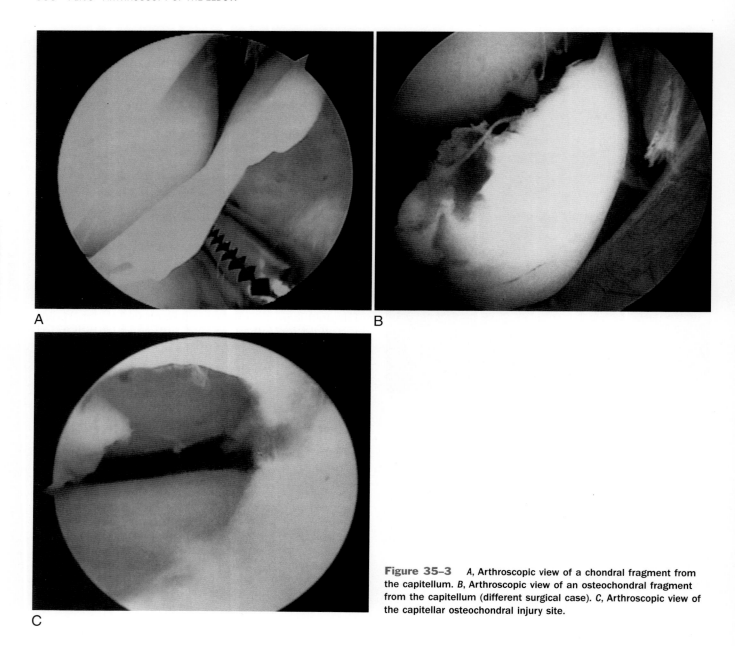

Figure 35–3 *A*, Arthroscopic view of a chondral fragment from the capitellum. *B*, Arthroscopic view of an osteochondral fragment from the capitellum (different surgical case). *C*, Arthroscopic view of the capitellar osteochondral injury site.

scopic approach is used to aid in reduction of the articular surface, and conventional incisions are used to view and fix the extra-articular components. Limited incisions, ligamentotaxis, and other indirect reduction maneuvers are helpful at this point to minimize further soft tissue injury. Even if the intra-articular fractures cannot be reduced arthroscopically, the arthroscope can still be used in a dry fashion to aid in visualization when using limited incisions.

After fracture fixation has been performed, arthroscopic visualization is used to confirm satisfactory articular congruency, and fluoroscopy is used to confirm acceptable placement of the hardware. Generally, fracture fixation should be as rigid as possible to allow early range of motion. Finally, incisions are closed, and a bulky dressing posterior splint, placing the elbow at 90 degrees, is applied.

Pearls and Pitfalls

Because arthroscopy of acute fractures involves working on an acutely traumatized joint, complications are more likely. Soft tissue swelling may distort and disguise anatomic landmarks, making portal placement more difficult. An 18-gauge spinal needle with or without fluoroscopy can be extremely helpful in locating proper portal positions. In arthroscopically assisted reductions, proposed incisions occasionally fall over portal sites. In these cases, the incision is made first to protect neurovascular structures and to locate the capsule before creating the portal.

Fluid inflow and outflow must be monitored closely during arthroscopy of acute fractures. Although the arthroscopic pump is commonly used for elbow arthroscopy, it is not recommended for acute fractures because the capsule may be torn, leading to significant fluid extravasation. Maintaining high flow and low pressure during the case avoids potential complications due to excessive soft tissue swelling, such as compartment syndrome and vascular compromise. A separate outflow cannula may be necessary to improve arthroscopic visualization.

Inadequate reduction and inadequate fixation are two potential pitfalls that deserve special attention. Although arthroscopy of acute fractures may aid in visualizing the fracture lines, it is still technically demanding to reduce the fragments through limited incisions or indirect reduction techniques. More demanding still is providing rigid fixation through these limited incisions. In cases in which the reduction or fixation is tenuous, it is better to revert to conventional open techniques so that the principles of fracture treatment (i.e., anatomic reduction and rigid fixation) are maintained.

Postoperative Management

Postoperatively, gentle range-of-motion exercises are begun as soon as wound stability is ascertained; with stable internal fixation or in cases of fragment excision, this may be within 2 days of surgery. However, progression of therapy is dictated by both the fracture pattern and the rigidity of fixation and is individualized for each patient.

Complications

Complications can be subdivided into two categories—those related to elbow arthroscopy in general, and those specifically related to arthroscopy of acute fractures. Examples of the former include neurovascular damage during portal placement, iatrogenic articular injury due to scuffing, and postoperative fistula formation at the portal sites. Most of these complications can be prevented with careful attention to anatomy and the principles of portal placement, as discussed elsewhere.

Postoperative wound complications may be slightly higher in elbow arthroscopy for acute fractures than in elbow arthroscopy in general due to the traumatized soft tissue envelope and the prolonged surgical time. Severe swelling denotes significant soft tissue injury, and surgery should be delayed. Superficial and deep infections can be prevented by administering preoperative antibiotics and gentle handling of the skin and soft tissues. Finally, wound problems can be minimized by placing portals and incisions in appropriate locations so that instruments do not put excess tension on the skin.

Conclusion

Arthroscopic management of elbow fractures, though still in its formative stages, offers an exciting and less invasive alternative to standard open fracture management. As the skilled arthroscopist's experience increases, and as more specific instrumentation is developed, the utility and indications for its use will likely expand. Outcome data, which now consist mainly of case reports, will be expanded in the future to help surgeons select the most efficacious intervention for each subcategory of elbow fracture.

Arthroscopy of acute elbow fractures is gaining acceptance as a valuable tool in the identification, treatment, and prevention of intra-articular pathology. Arthroscopy allows for minimally invasive surgical exposure and little soft tissue trauma while providing excellent visualization of fracture fragments and associated injuries in the joint. Although the procedure is technically demanding, decreased soft tissue dissection and improved articular reduction should minimize postoperative complications. Thorough arthroscopic debridement of organized hematoma and fibrinous debris may also decrease postoperative adhesions and improve elbow range of motion. Identification of additional intra-articular pathology not seen on preoperative imaging studies may prove valuable in providing a more accurate prognosis for these injuries. With many potential benefits and minimally increased risk, arthroscopy of acute elbow fractures should be considered in operative cases.

References

1. Feldman MD: Arthroscopic excision of type II capitellar fractures. Arthroscopy 13:743-748, 1997.
2. Hardy P, Menguy F, Guillot S: Arthroscopic treatment of capitellum fractures of the humerus. Arthroscopy 18:422-426, 2002.
3. Menth-Chiari WA, Poehling GG, Ruch DS: Arthroscopic resection of the radial head. Arthroscopy 15:226-230, 1999.
4. Menth-Chiari WA, Ruch DS, Poehling GG: Arthroscopic excision of the radial head: Clinical outcome in 12 patients with post-traumatic arthritis after fracture of the radial head or rheumatoid arthritis. Arthroscopy 17:918-923, 2001.

3 Elbow

Arthroscopic Management of Lateral Epicondylitis

KEVIN P. MURPHY AND RONALD A. LEHMAN, JR.

ARTHROSCOPIC MANAGEMENT OF LATERAL EPICONDYLITIS IN A NUTSHELL
History: Traumatic or repetitive cause; lateral-sided elbow pain; pain with elbow motion, wrist extension
Physical Examination: Tenderness over lateral epicondyle; pain with resisted wrist dorsiflexion; resisted middle finger extension; "chair test" with elbow in full extension, forearm pronated, and wrist dorsiflexed; diminished grip strength
Imaging: Standard radiographs with rim of sclerotic bone, flattening; magnetic resonance imaging
Indications: Failure of conservative management for at least 3 to 6 months
Contraindications: Distorted anatomy (e.g., prior ulnar nerve transposition), ankylosed joint
Surgical Technique: Patient positioned prone; elbow distention; routine arthroscopy portals; debride capsule, extensor carpi radialis brevis, and lateral epicondyle with shaver or bur
Postoperative Management: Sling, early range of motion, control of inflammation
Results: More than 80% achieve significant improvement
Complications: Neurovascular, failure to improve, stiffness

Lateral epicondylitis—also known as tennis elbow because of its early association with lawn tennis[32]—is a common musculoskeletal problem that may result from minor trauma or as an overuse phenomenon. It was first described by Runge[52] in 1873 as a painful condition of the wrist and finger extensors on the lateral side of the elbow. Since then, various causes have been reported, including bursitis, synovitis, ligament inflammation, periostitis, extensor tendon tears, and microscopic rupture with formation of reparative tissue in the extensor carpi radialis brevis (ECRB) origin on the lateral epicondyle.[8,19,20,39,52]

The hallmark of care is nonoperative treatment, although approximately 5% to 10% of patients develop chronic symptoms and may eventually require surgical intervention.[11,13,16,18,29,39] Various open,[2,15,16,20,39] percutaneous,[10,60] and endoscopic[22] surgical techniques have been described for recalcitrant cases. It appears that the percutaneous method is associated with less morbidity than are open techniques; however, inadequate resection and the inability to address intra-articular pathology are significant drawbacks.[4,38,42,43] This may be particularly important because concurrent intra-articular pathology has been reported to occur in 11% to 19% of cases.[38,44] In two recent series, we found that at 2-year follow-up, patients treated with arthroscopic ECRB release subjectively reported feeling "much better" to "better" in 83% to 95% of cases.[9,44]

History

Several variables are important in the evaluation of patients with lateral epicondylitis. First, the nature and character of the patient's symptoms must be elicited. This includes whether the pain began after a single traumatic event or repetitive episodes. Also, one should inquire about the character and location of the pain and the presence or absence of catching, clicking, or locking, which may indicate loose intra-articular bodies.

Second, the patient should be asked about provocative maneuvers or insults that exacerbate the symptoms. For instance, a throwing athlete who reports a decrease in pitch velocity or an inability to "let the ball go" may have pain on forced extension, which could be a sign of posterior olecranon impingement.[8] Posterior interosseous nerve (PIN) entrapment must also be differentiated from lateral epicondylitis. Pain in the extensor mass (distal to the radial head), weakness with wrist or finger extension, and pain with percussion over the course of the nerve points to PIN entrapment as the diagnosis. However, many authors believe that this diagnosis requires positive electromyographic testing changes in the PIN.[38] Radiocapitellar degenerative changes should also be considered and can be ruled out by physical examination and plain radiographs.[46] Patients with radiocapitellar pathology usually have pain and clicking with elbow motion and episodes of intermittent locking. Other causes of lateral elbow pain include C7 radiculitis, anconeus muscle compartment syndrome,[1] and posterolateral rotatory instability.[41] These conditions must be considered and thoroughly evaluated.

Third, the patient's preoperative history is needed to assess previous surgical procedures and their possible role in a subluxating ulnar nerve or other associated problem. Less commonly, compression of the musculocutaneous nerve or a symptomatic posterolateral plica has been implicated as a cause of lateral elbow pain.

Finally, the patient should be asked about demographic data and age, hand dominance, occupation, length of conservative treatment, number of corticosteroid injections, and duration and magnitude of symptoms.

Physical Examination

All compartments about the elbow should be evaluated and carefully examined. In particular, the lateral epicondyle and extensor mass should be palpated for point tenderness consistent with lateral epicondylitis or other tendinopathies. Tenderness about the lateral epicondyle, most commonly 5 mm distal and anterior to the lateral epicondyle,[46] is present in nearly all patients with lateral epicondylitis. Patients usually exhibit pain with resisted wrist dorsiflexion with the elbow extended. Resisted extension of the middle finger also occurs in up to 78% of patients, and this can be confused with a PIN syndrome. Pain with resisted supination is also present in 51% of patients.[58] In addition, pain with handshaking and turning doorknobs is quite common. The "chair test," which involves asking the patient to lift the back of a chair with the elbow in full extension, the forearm pronated, and the wrist dorsiflexed, generates apprehension before the attempt.[46] Grip strength is diminished in up to 78% of patients.[58]

Imaging

Plain Radiographs

Routine diagnostic radiographs, including an anteroposterior view with the elbow in full extension and a lateral view with the elbow at 90 degrees of flexion, may be helpful if there is a history of trauma of if one suspects intra-articular pathology. Unfortunately, loose bodies located in the posterior compartment are often difficult to visualize with plain radiographs.[8,12,22,40,59] Ward et al.[59] reported a 75% accuracy rate for radiographs, in comparison to arthrograms, which have an accuracy rate of 89% with 100% sensitivity. Calcification of the ECRB secondary to long-standing lateral epicondylitis with significant degenerative tissue can be visualized on plain films in up to 25% of cases.[39] Finally, an axial view may help outline the olecranon and its articulations.[8]

Magnetic Resonance Imaging

Although not routinely recommended, magnetic resonance imaging may be useful for the evaluation of osteochondral lesions and loose bodies, especially in the radiocapitellar joint and posterior compartments, respectively.[24,55] It may also show enhancement of the degenerative tissue of the ECRB or injuries to the soft tissues, especially the lateral collateral ligament complex. Magnetic resonance arthrography with saline or gadolinium further increases the sensitivity for detecting undersurface tears.

Indications and Contraindications

Historically, indications for elbow arthroscopy included diagnosis of elbow pain, removal of loose bodies, excision of osteophytes, synovectomy, lysis of adhesions, and debridement of osteochondritis dissecans lesions of the capitellum and chondromalacia of the radial head.[*] Additional indications include the release of elbow contractures secondary to trauma or degenerative arthritis, tennis elbow release, olecranon bursectomy, radial head excision, and fracture treatment.[†] Specific indications for arthroscopic release include persistent pain of greater than 3 to 6 months' duration that is resistant to treatment with nonsteroidal anti-inflammatory drugs, physical therapy, rest, activity modification, ice, stretching, strengthening, counterforce band therapy, and injections.

Contraindications to elbow arthroscopy include any significant distortion of normal bony or soft tissue anatomy that precludes safe entry of the arthroscope into the joint, previous surgery or hardware (including previous ulnar nerve transposition) that may interfere with medial portal placement, a severely ankylosed joint, and local soft tissue infection or osteomyelitis.[6,8]

Surgical Technique

Positioning and Examination under Anesthesia

The patient is placed in the prone position, and the arm is positioned with the olecranon superior and the elbow at 90 degrees of flexion to gravity (Fig. 36–1).[48] The surgeon is seated.

Ligamentous examination is performed for varus and valgus instability, as well as for posterolateral subluxation, before preparing and draping.[41] Range of motion is also noted. Because the patient is often apprehensive while being examined in the clinic, these examinations are best performed in the operating room under anesthesia. The posterolateral instability examination is performed with the extremity placed over the patient's head with the shoulder in full external rotation. A valgus, supination, and axial compression load is applied to the fully extended elbow. When the elbow is flexed to 20 to 40 degrees, subluxation or dislocation of the radiohumeral joint occurs. This produces an obvious deformity proximal to the radial head (sulcus sign). Range of motion is

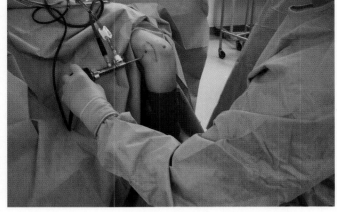

Figure 36–1   Patient in the prone position with the surgeon seated. A 2.7-mm arthroscope is in the proximal medial portal.

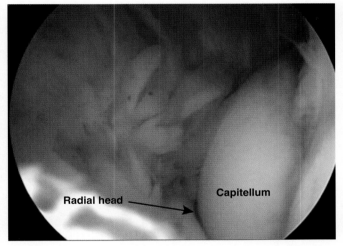

Radial head   Capitellum

Figure 36–2   Arthroscopic image showing synovitis and fraying of the capsule—a type I lesion.

also evaluated in flexion and extension and compared with the contralateral elbow.

Diagnostic Arthroscopy

Diagnostic arthroscopy is performed to determine the presence and extent of concomitant intra-articular pathology. In addition, the nature and extent of the ECRB complex are classified.[7,8,37] Type I lesions are characterized by fraying of the capsule and tendon undersurface without a distinct tear (Fig. 36–2). Type II lesions have linear tears along the undersurface of the capsule and ECRB tendon (Fig. 36–3). Type III lesions consist of minimally retracted partial avulsion or complete avulsion of the tendon (Fig. 36–4).

Specific Surgical Steps

After positioning, the anatomic landmarks about the elbow are palpated and outlined with a skin marker

[*]See references 3,5,14,17,21,24,25,34,47,51,55.
[†]See references 7,22,27,28,30,31,35,40,45,48,49,57.

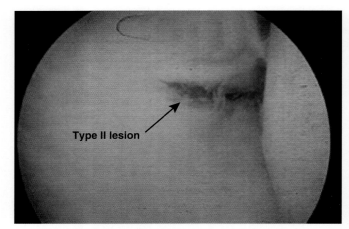

Figure 36–3 Type II lesion showing a linear tear along the undersurface of the capsule and extensor carpi radialis brevis (ECRB) tendon.

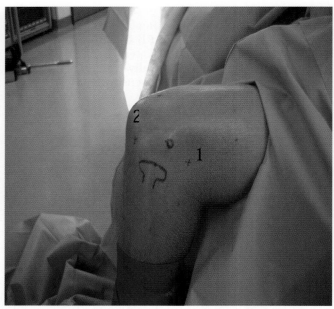

Figure 36–5 Proximal lateral (1) and direct lateral (2) portals.

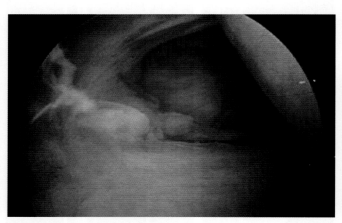

Figure 36–4 Arthroscopic image of a type III lesion with retraction and avulsion of the tendon.

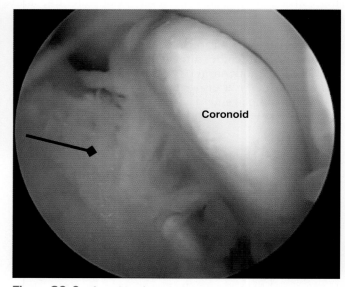

Figure 36–6 Synovitis of the anterior compartment *(arrow).*

(Fig. 36–5). This should be completed before distention of the joint with fluid or subsequent extravasation. First, the elbow joint is distended with 20 mL of saline injected with an 18-gauge spinal needle through a direct lateral approach. This also serves to displace the neurovascular structures anteriorly.[29] Next, the proximal medial portal (which is the standard viewing portal) is established approximately 2 cm proximal and 2 cm anterior to the intermuscular septum of the medial epicondyle through a 2-mm skin incision using a number 11 scalpel blade. The septum is palpated, and the subcutaneous tissue is spread bluntly with a small hemostat. This "nick and spread" technique protects the cutaneous nerves in the area. A blunt trocar is then introduced into the joint, followed by either a 2.7- or a 4-mm, 30-degree arthroscope. Care must be taken when inserting the cannula to ensure that the instruments remain anterior to the intermuscular septum and in direct contact with the anterior surface of the humerus. The joint is distended using a fluid pump with 40 mm Hg pressure, the anterior compartment of the elbow is thoroughly inspected, and any existing intra-articular pathology is noted and addressed

(Fig. 36–6). In particular, the radiocapitellar joint and the lateral portion of the capsule are examined for abnormalities and classified. The proximal lateral portal is then established approximately 2 cm proximal and 2 cm anterior to the lateral epicondyle under direct visualization using a spinal needle, followed by a similar skin incision and cannula insertion technique.

With visualization obtained through the proximal medial portal, the lateral capsule and undersurface of the ECRB tendon are easily visualized and evaluated. To visualize the undersurface of the ECRB tendon, the arthroscope is advanced past the radial head. This places the tendon directly in front of the camera, where it can be followed directly to its origin on the lateral

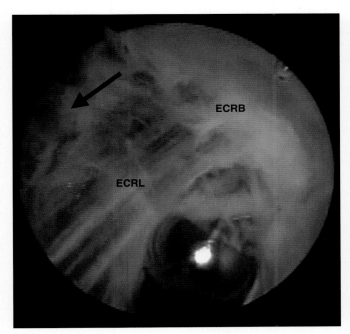

Figure 36–7 Fatty degenerative changes *(black arrow)* in the extensor carpi radialis brevis (ECRB) tendon overlying the extensor carpi radialis longus (ECRL).

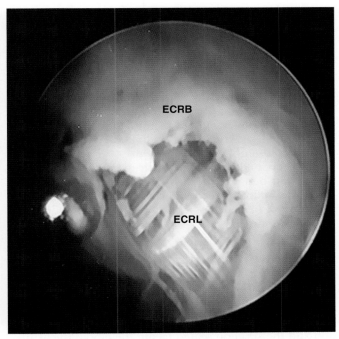

Figure 36–9 A 4.5-mm incisor is used to debride the extensor carpi radialis brevis (ECRB) tendon insertion on the lateral epicondyle. ECRL, extensor carpi radialis longus.

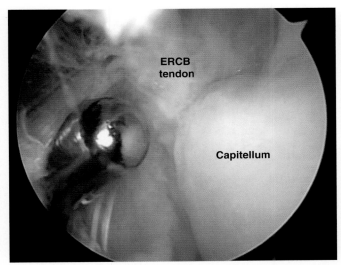

Figure 36–8 A 4.5-mm incisor is used to begin debridement of the extensor carpi radialis brevis (ECRB) tendon.

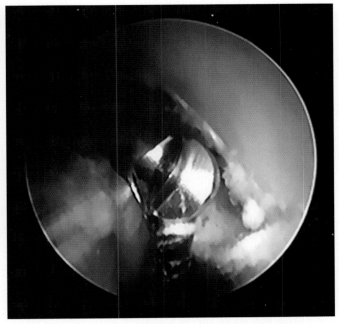

Figure 36–10 A 4.0-mm abrader is used to decorticate the lateral epicondyle. Extensor carpi radialis brevis (ECRB) release is completed.

epicondyle. The capsule adheres to the undersurface of the ECRB tendon and is often torn or may be thin and translucent. A 4.5-mm synovial resector is then introduced through the proximal lateral portal. The abnormal tissue appears grossly degenerative, with discolored tissue and varying degrees of fibrous changes and tears (Fig. 36–7). If the capsule is present, it is debrided to reveal the undersurface of the ECRB (Fig. 36–8). Release of the ECRB tendon is begun at the site of pathology (either degenerative tissue or tear) and is continued back to its origin on the lateral epicondyle (Fig. 36–9). Care

must be taken to avoid damage to the corresponding articular surface. After release of the visible ECRB origin, a 4.5-mm rounded bur is used to decorticate the lateral epicondyle and the distal portion of the lateral condylar ridge in the area of the ECRB origin (Fig. 36–10). The

3 Elbow

cadaveric study by Kuklo et al.[29] showed that this release removes an average of 23 mm of the ECRB tendon. The 30-degree arthroscope provides adequate release (if taken to the limit of the visualization) while protecting the lateral collateral ligaments that are more posterior.[29]

If needed, a direct lateral portal can be made with the elbow in 90 degrees of flexion.[54] The elbow is then extended, and the arthroscopic cannula is inserted into the posterior compartment of the elbow. The posterior compartment is visualized, and if any synovitis, loose bodies, or osteophytes are present, a straight posterior portal is created through the triceps tendon at a point equidistant between the medial and lateral epicondyles. This portal allows excellent access to the posterior joint without risk of neurologic injury. After completion, the portals are closed with 3-0 nylon and a soft dressing is applied.

Pearls and Pitfalls

Arthroscopic release of the ECRB tendon is technically challenging. With the patient placed in the prone position and the surgeon seated facing the elbow, the arthroscopic movements are not intuitive and take some time to perfect. When draping the patient, the surgeon takes a seated position with the arthroscopy drape across his or her thighs. By flexing the patient's wrist and placing the dorsal aspect of the wrist on the surgeon's thigh, elbow flexion and extension are easily controlled by simply raising and lowering the operating table. This is particularly helpful when visualizing the posterior compartment with the elbow in extension.

When establishing the portals, the "nick and spread" technique is particularly helpful to avoid injury to the sensory cutaneous nerves and the PIN.[50] The tip of the number 11 blade is placed through the skin, and the skin is pulled distally to create a small incision. A hemostat is then used to spread open the skin and mobilize the nerves away from the path of the cannula. The smaller 2.7-mm arthroscope is easily passed into the distended joint capsule, providing a distinct advantage over the 4-mm arthroscope. If a 4-mm arthroscope is desired, it can be placed over a switching stick after establishment of the portals. It is difficult to penetrate the capsule with either size arthroscope.

The ECRB tendon attaches along the distal and anterolateral aspect of the lateral epicondyle, covering an area of approximately 1.5 cm. When addressing the ECRB tendon insertion, it is imperative to carry the debridement up the lateral flare of the epicondyle until the entire insertion site is removed from bone. Decortication of the epicondyle may stimulate a healing response, but it also aids the surgeon by ensuring that the entire ECRB tendon has been released. Proper use of the abrader flattens this ridge and removes the last remaining fibers off the ECRB tendon. After releasing the ECRB tendon, the extensor carpi radialis longus tendon is easily visualized as it travels proximally toward its insertion site.

Decortication should not be extended posterior to the epicondyle, as this may disrupt the lateral collateral ligament complex. Use of a 30-degree arthroscope prevents compromise of the lateral collateral ligaments because it does not allow significant posterior visualization. A 70-degree arthroscope provides better posterior visualization, which may actually allow the surgeon to access the posterior structures.

A postoperative intra-articular injection for pain relief is not recommended. The injection may extravasate and result in a transient radial nerve palsy, making both the patient and the surgeon uncomfortable until it resolves.

Postoperative Management

The elbow is placed in a soft dressing, and motion is encouraged immediately postoperatively. Patients should have met with a physical therapist preoperatively to discuss the following:

- Restoration of full active range of motion (ROM)
- Strengthening in pain-free ROM
- Proper use of a sling, icing, and hand gripping
- Ergonomic education
- Importance of protocol compliance to ensure the best functional outcome

Exercises begin as soon as symptoms subside, and patients progress through three phases of rehabilitation.

Acute Phase (Postoperative Days 1 to 7)

- Sling for comfort
- Ice for 20 to 30 minutes several times a day
- Active and active assisted ROM for elbow and wrist in all planes to tolerance
- Passive modalities as necessary

Subacute Phase (Weeks 1 to 4)

- Continue active and active assisted ROM and neural glides
- Progressive isotonic exercises to tolerance
- Friction massage to portal sites as they heal
- Ice and passive modalities as necessary

Return to Activity Phase (Week 4+)

- Address ergonomic issues for work and home
- Functional progression to work and sports activities
- Continue active ROM and strengthening exercises
- Ice and passive modalities as necessary
- Return to work and sports pain free

Results

Since 1994, arthroscopy has been used routinely when surgical intervention is indicated for lateral epicondylitis. In a series by the senior author (KPM), 16 patients were treated for recalcitrant lateral epicondylitis after an average of 31.7 months of conservative treatment (including rest, activity modification, ice, nonsteroidal anti-inflammatory drugs, corticosteroid injections, and physical therapy).[36] On physical examination, patients consistently had point tenderness over the lateral epicondyle, as well as pain on resisted wrist dorsiflexion with the elbow extended. All patients underwent diagnostic arthroscopy and arthroscopic release of the origin of the ECRB tendon with decortication of the lateral epicondyle, as described earlier. All 16 elbows in the series had lesions on the undersurface of the ECRB tendon. There were five type I lesions, five type II lesions, and six type III lesions as classified by Baker et al.,[7,8] with associated pathology found in 18.8% of the elbows. All patients were followed for a minimum of 1 year, with four being lost to subsequent follow-up secondary to military reassignment. Twelve of the 16 patients (75%) were followed for an average of 24.1 months (range, 15 to 33 months). There were no complications and no need for additional procedures; the average return to unrestricted work was 6 days. Ten of the 12 patients (83.3%) reported feeling much better as a result of their surgery, 2 reported feeling better, and none reported feeling the same or worse. Using a pain analog scale (0 to 10, with 10 being the worst pain), the average pain at rest was 0.58 (range, 0 to 3), the average pain with activities of daily living was 1.58 (range, 0 to 5), and the average pain with sports and work was 3.25 (range, 0 to 8).

In the only other clinical study involving arthroscopic release of the ECRB, we assessed the clinical utility of 42 releases in 40 patients with an average follow-up of 2.8 years.[9] In this series, 95% of the elbows were rated as either "much better" or "better" by the patients. Using a pain analog scale, the average pain score at rest was 0.87 (range, 0 to 8), the average pain score with activities of daily living was 1.5 (range, 0 to 10), and the average pain score with sports or work was 1.9 (range, 0 to 8). The average functional score was 11.1 points out of a possible 12 (range, 6 to 12 points). Among the patients who were working at the time of surgery (36 elbows), the average return to work was 2.2 weeks (range, 1 to 6 weeks). Most of the patients (62%) were pain free; however, 10% still had some pain with activities of daily living. This is consistent with published reports on open procedures. These early findings indicate that arthroscopic release for recalcitrant lateral epicondylitis is a safe and reliable procedure. It also provides several distinct advantages, including the ability to address concomitant intra-articular pathology, preservation of the common extensor origin,[7] accelerated rehabilitation, and early return to work. In a comparative study of open procedures, only 8 of 44 patients who were employed returned to work by 6 weeks after surgery, with 13 patients not returning until 12 weeks postoperatively.[58] In addition, Nirschl and Pettrone[39] found that tennis players took more than 6 months to return to competitive play and an average of 2.6 months to be symptom free.

Thus, the arthroscopic approach may best balance the positive aspects of both open and percutaneous procedures. This treatment allows an earlier return to work and may be more anatomically compatible with the elbow musculature, with minimal degradation of grip strength.[9,58]

Complications

Elbow arthroscopy is fraught with potentially hazardous complications. The most frequent complications involve the neurovascular structures; however, complications are unusual.

When nerve injuries do occur, they are usually transient, but permanent injuries have been reported. Nonetheless, Marshall et al.[33] recommended placing the forearm in pronation to move the PIN farther from the portal site.

With the anteromedial and anterolateral portals, the radial and posterior interosseous nerves are at risk on the lateral side, whereas the posterior antebrachial cutaneous nerve is most at risk medially. A study by Kuklo et al.[29] showed that the distance from portals to neurovascular structures averaged 5.4 mm for the radial nerve and 26.1 mm for the lateral antebrachial cutaneous nerve using the proximal lateral portal. For the proximal medial portal, the posterior antebrachial cutaneous nerve was 8 mm from the portal on average, and the ulnar nerve averaged 30.3 mm from the portal. In independent studies, Guhl[23] and Rupp and Tempelhof[53] reported injury to the radial nerve sensory branch, and Jones and Savoie[26] and Thomas et al.[56] described damage to the PIN. The posteromedial portal is not recommended because of the proximity to the ulnar nerve. In a separate series, O'Driscoll and Morrey[41] reported seven complications: three episodes of transient radial nerve palsy (attributed to extravasation of local anesthetic) and four episodes of persistent drainage.

References

1. Abrahamsson SO, Sollerman C, Soderberg T: Lateral elbow pain caused by anconeus compartment syndrome: A case report. Acta Orthop Scand 58:589-591, 1987.
2. Almquist EE, Necking L, Bach AW: Epicondylar resection with anconeus muscle transfer for chronic lateral epicondylitis. J Hand Surg [Am] 23:723-731, 1998.
3. Andrews JR, Carson WG: Arthroscopy of the elbow. Arthroscopy 1:97-107, 1985.
4. Andrews JR, Craven WM: Lesions of the posterior compartment of the elbow. Clin Sports Med 10:637-652, 1986.
5. Andrews JR, St Pierre RK, Carson WG Jr: Arthroscopy of the elbow. Clin Sports Med 5:653-662, 1986.
6. Baker CL, Brooks AA: Arthroscopy of the elbow. Clin Sports Med 15:261-281, 1996.
7. Baker CL, Cummings PD: Arthroscopic management of miscellaneous elbow disorders. Oper Tech Sports Med 6:16-21, 1998.
8. Baker CL, Jones GL: Current concepts: Arthroscopy of the elbow. Am J Sports Med 27:251-264, 1999.
9. Baker CL, Murphy KP, Gottlob CA, Curd DT: Arthroscopic classification and treatment of lateral epicondylitis: Two-year clinical results. J Shoulder Elbow Surg 9:475-482, 2000.
10. Baumgard SH, Schwartz DR: Percutaneous release of the epicondylar muscle for humeral epicondylitis. Am J Sports Med 0:223-226, 1982.

11. Boyd HB, McLeod AC: Tennis elbow. J Bone Joint Surg Am 55:1183-1187, 1973.

12. Brooks AA, Baker CL: Arthroscopy of the elbow. In Stanley D, Kay N (eds): Surgery of the Elbow: Scientific and Practical Aspects. London, Edward Arnold Limited, 1998, pp 71-81.

13. Calvert PT, Allum RL, Macpherson IS, Bentley G: Simple lateral release in treatment of tennis elbow. J R Soc Med 78:912-915, 1985.

14. Clarke RP: Symptomatic, lateral synovial fringe (plica) of the elbow joint. Arthroscopy 4:112-116, 1988.

15. Coonrad RW, Hooper WR: Tennis elbow: Its course, natural history, conservative and surgical management. J Bone Joint Surg Am 55:1177-1182, 1973.

16. Cyriax JH: The pathology and treatment of tennis elbow. J Bone Joint Surg 18:921-940, 1936.

17. Day B: Elbow arthroscopy in the athlete. Clin Sports Med 15:785-797, 1996.

18. Gardner RC: Tennis elbow: Diagnosis, pathology, and treatment. Nine severe cases treated by a new reconstructive operation. Clin Orthop 72:248-253, 1970.

19. Goldberg EJ, Abraham E, Siegal I: The surgical treatment of chronic lateral humeral epicondylitis by common extensor release. Clin Orthop 233:208-212, 1988.

20. Goldie I: Epicondylitis lateralis humeri (epicondylalgia or tennis elbow): A pathological study. Acta Chir Scand Suppl 339, 1964.

21. Greis PE, Halbrecht J, Plancher KD: Arthroscopic removal of loose bodies of the elbow. Orthop Clin North Am 26:679-689, 1995.

22. Grifka J, Boenke S, Kramer J: Endoscopic therapy in epicondylitis radialis humeri. Arthroscopy 11:743-748, 1995.

23. Guhl JF: Arthroscopy and arthroscopic surgery of the elbow. Orthopedics 8:1290-1296, 1985.

24. Janarv PM, Hesser U, Hirsch G: Osteochondral lesions in the radiocapitellar joint in the skeletally immature: Radiographic MRI, and arthroscopic findings in 13 consecutive cases. J Pediatr Orthop 17:311-314, 1997.

25. Jerosch J, Schroder M, Schneider T: Good and relative indications for elbow arthroscopy: A retrospective study on 103 patients. Arch Orthop Trauma Surg 117:246-249, 1998.

26. Jones GS, Savoie FH: Arthroscopic capsular release of flexion contractures (arthrofibrosis) of the elbow. Arthroscopy 9:277-283, 1993.

27. Kerr DR: Prepatellar and olecranon arthroscopic bursectomy. Clin Sports Med 12:137-142, 1993.

28. Kim SJ, Kim HK, Lee JW: Arthroscopy for limitation of motion of the elbow. Arthroscopy 11:680-683, 1995.

29. Kuklo TR, Taylor KR, Murphy KP, et al: Arthroscopic release for lateral epicondylitis: A cadaveric model. Arthroscopy 15:259-264, 1999.

30. Lee BPH, Morrey BF: Arthroscopic synovectomy of the elbow for rheumatoid arthritis: A prospective study. J Bone Joint Surg Br 79:770-772, 1997.

31. Lo IKY, King GJW: Arthroscopic radial head excision [case report]. Arthroscopy 10:689-694, 1994.

32. Major HP: Lawn-tennis elbow. BMJ 2:557, 1883.

33. Marshall PD, Fairclough JA, Johnson SR, et al: Avoiding nerve damage during elbow arthroscopy. J Bone Joint Surg Br 75:129-133, 1993.

34. Morrey BF: Arthroscopy of the elbow. Instr Course Lect 35:102-107, 1986.

35. Morrey BF: Acute and chronic instability of the elbow J Am Acad Orthop Surg 4:117-128, 1996.

36. Murphy KP, Baker CL: Arthroscopic findings associated with lateral epicondylitis. Orthop Trans 22:1305, 1998.

37. Murphy KP, Kuklo TR, Baker CL: Arthroscopic findings associated with lateral epicondylitis. Orthop Trans 21:222, 1997.

38. Nirschl RP: Tennis elbow. Orthop Clin North Am 4:787-800, 1973.

39. Nirschl RP, Pettrone FA: Tennis elbow: The surgical treatment of lateral epicondylitis. J Bone Joint Surg Am 61:832-839, 1979.

40. Nowicki KD, Shali LM: Arthroscopic release of a posttraumatic flexion contracture in the elbow: A case report and review of the literature. Arthroscopy 8:544-547, 1992.

41. O'Driscoll SW, Morrey BF: Arthroscopy of the elbow. J Bone Joint Surg Am 74:84-94, 1992.

42. Ogilvie-Harris DJ, Schemitsch E. Arthroscopy of the elbow for removal of loose bodies. Arthroscopy 9:5-8, 1993.

43. Organ SW, Nirschl RP, Kraushaar BS, Guidi EJ: Salvage surgery for lateral elbow. Am J Sports Med 25:746-750, 1997.

44. Owens BD, Murphy KP, Kuklo TR: Arthroscopic release for lateral epicondylitis. Arthroscopy 17:582-587, 2001.

45. Phillips BB, Strasburger S: Arthroscopic treatment of arthrofibrosis of the elbow joint. Arthroscopy 14:38-44, 1998.

46. Plancher KD, Halbrecht J, Lourie GM: Medial and lateral epicondylitis in the athlete. Clin Sports Med 15:283-305, 1996.

47. Poehling GG, Ekman EF: Arthroscopy of the elbow. Instr Course Lect 44:217-223, 1995.

48. Poehling GG, Whipple TL, Sisco L, Goldman B: Elbow arthroscopy: A new technique. Arthroscopy 5:222-224, 1989.

49. Redden JF, Stanley D: Arthroscopic fenestration of the olecranon fossa in the treatment of osteoarthritis of the elbow. Arthroscopy 9:14-16, 1993.

50. Rodeo SA, Forster RA, Weiland AJ: Neurological complications due to arthroscopy. J Bone Joint Surg Am 75:917-926, 1993.

51. Ruch DS, Poehling GG: Arthroscopic surgery of the elbow: Therapeutic benefits and hazards. Clin Orthop 313:140-145, 1995.

52. Runge F: Zur Genese und Behandlung des Schreibekrampfes. Berl Klin Wochenschr 10:245-248, 1873.

53. Rupp S, Tempelhof S: Arthroscopic surgery of the elbow: Therapeutic benefits and hazards. Clin Orthop 313:140-145, 1995.

54. Stothers K, Day B, Regan WR: Arthroscopy of the elbow: Anatomy, portal sites, and a description of the proximal lateral portal. Arthroscopy 11:449-457, 1995.

55. Takahara M, Shundo M, Kondo M, et al: Early detection of osteochondritis dissecans of the capitellum in young baseball players: Report of three cases. J Bone Joint Surg Am 80:892-897, 1998.

56. Thomas MA, Fast A, Shapiro D: Radial nerve damage as a complication of elbow arthroscopy. Clin Orthop 215:130-131, 1987.

57. Timmerman LA, Andrews JR: Arthroscopic treatment of posttraumatic elbow pain and stiffness. Am J Sports Med 22:230-235, 1994.

58. Verhaar J, Walenkamp G, Kester A, et al: Lateral extensor release for tennis elbow: A prospective long-term follow-up study. J Bone Joint Surg Am 75:1034-1043, 1993.

59. Ward WG, Belhobek GH, Anderson TE: Arthroscopic elbow findings: Correlation with preoperative radiographic studies. Arthroscopy 8:498-502, 1992.

60. Yerger B, Turner T: Percutaneous extensor tenotomy for chronic tennis elbow: An office procedure. Orthopedics 8:1261-1263, 1985.

Arthroscopic Management of Olecranon Bursitis

MICHAEL H. HANDY

ARTHROSCOPIC MANAGEMENT OF OLECRANON BURSITIS IN A NUTSHELL

History:
  Traumatically induced; complaints of swelling, pain, and, rarely, signs and symptoms of infection

Physical Examination:
  Circumscribed swelling over the olecranon, usually with minimal tenderness, erythema, and edema; significant tenderness, erythema, or edema suggests infection

Imaging:
  Plain films screen for bone and joint abnormalities and soft tissue deposits

Indications:
  Failure of conservative treatment (chronic, recurrent, or refractory bursitis) and septic olecranon bursitis

Contraindications:
  Inadequate trial of nonoperative treatment

Surgical Technique:
  Position the patient supine, with the elbow across the chest
  Use regional or general anesthesia with a tourniquet
  Tunnel the proximal central, distal central, and lateral portals from 1 cm away
  Insufflate the bursa
  Using a 4.5-mm shaver, systematically excise the bursa, beginning with the subcutaneous portion
  Using the bur, remove olecranon spurs when present
  Remove loose bodies when present
  Average operative time: 30 to 40 minutes

Postoperative Management:
  Compressive dressing, early motion, long-term protective padding

Pearls and Pitfalls:
  Leaving small amounts of peripheral bursa has not been shown to affect outcome or recurrence
  Surgical treatment of patients with rheumatoid arthritis and connective tissue disorders should be approached cautiously because of increased complications and lower success rates

Results:
  One recurrence in 41 published cases; lower wound complication rate compared with open treatment

Complications:
  Persistent tenderness, recurrence, infection

Olecranon bursitis is a common condition of the elbow that only rarely requires surgical intervention. Open bursectomy has been the procedure of choice after failure of nonoperative treatment, but reports of incision-related complications have led surgeons to apply arthroscopic techniques to reduce patient morbidity. Although there is a general scarcity of literature on the natural history and results of conservative and surgical treatment, arthroscopic bursectomy has been well described in recent literature and has been shown to produce reliable results with minimal morbidity.

History

Clinical evidence strongly implicates repetitive trauma against the bony prominence of the olecranon as the cause of olecranon bursitis. This would account for the increased incidence in males, laborers whose work involves leaning on their elbows, wrestlers, and athletes who wear protective elbow gear.[1] Recognized predisposing conditions include gout, rheumatoid arthritis, infection, and CREST syndrome (calcinosis, Raynaud phenomenon, esophageal dysmotility, sclerodactyly, and telangiectasia).[6] Patients present with acute or chronic swelling over the olecranon. Significant pain or tenderness is worrisome and could indicate infection.[11]

At the cellular level, mucoid or myxomatous degeneration of fibrous tissue occurs between the skin and underlying bone. An adventitious border, rather than the endothelial lining seen in true bursae, forms around the periphery. Its walls consist of fibroblasts and collagen fibrils with infiltrations of lymphocytes, macrophages, and plasma cells.[3] The bursa initially distends with mucoid, hemorrhagic fluid that subsequently turns brown and granular. The fluid can serve as a site of urate crystal or calcified body deposition, as well as infection.[6]

Physical Examination

Findings include circumscribed swelling over the olecranon, usually with minimal tenderness, erythema, and edema. Significant tenderness, erythema, or edema suggests infection.

Imaging

Plain radiographs should be obtained to screen for bone and joint abnormalities and soft tissue deposits.

Indications and Contraindications

Acute treatment is nonoperative and consists of a compression dressing, brief immobilization, nonsteroidal anti-inflammatory drugs, and long-term padding to minimize further trauma to the bursa.[3] Aspiration and long-acting corticosteroid injections are also effective treatments.[9] The aspirate should be sent for Gram stain, culture, and crystal analysis. Temporary placement of an indwelling angiocatheter has also been described.[2,10] These measures resolve olecranon bursitis in most cases. In the rare case of chronic, recurrent, refractory, or septic olecranon bursitis, surgical treatment is indicated (Fig. 37-1).

Surgical Technique

Positioning and Anesthesia

The patient is positioned supine, with the arm draped across a pillow placed on the chest. This enables the elbow to be in 45 degrees of flexion, where visualization of the bursa is maximal.[5] Lateral or prone positioning is also technically feasible.

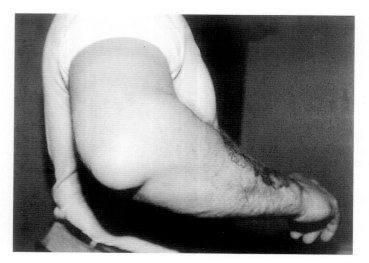

Figure 37-1 This patient's olecranon bursitis was refractory to conservative treatment. (From Baker CL, Cummings PD: Arthroscopic management of miscellaneous elbow disorders. Oper Tech Sports Med 6:16-21, 1998.)

The procedure can be performed with the patient under local anesthesia, but general or regional anesthesia is preferred to facilitate tourniquet use.[3] Inflow pumps set at a low pressure (35 mm Hg) help maintain bursal distention while using the suction-resection tip.[5] Gravity drain alone can also be sufficient.[3] Extravasation has not been a problem with either technique.[3]

Specific Surgical Steps

Although Kerr and Carpenter[4] initially described three portals at equal intervals (120 degrees) around the perimeter of the bursa, later authors advocated avoiding the medial portal to reduce the risk of ulnar nerve injury. Instead, proximal central, distal central, and lateral portals have been recommended.[1,7] Portal sites and the bursa are first injected with 1% lidocaine (Xylocaine) or 0.25% bupivacaine and 1:100,000 epinephrine solution to reduce bleeding.[3] Alternatively, the bursa can be injected with saline.[5] Portals should be tunneled from 1 cm away, rather than being made directly through the skin overlying the bursa, to prevent collapse.[1,5] After

insufflation of the bursa, a sharp obturator, arthroscopic knife, or basket forceps is used to make clean punctures through which instruments can be advanced into the bursa (Fig. 37–2).[3,5]

Using a 4.5-mm shaver, the bursa is systematically excised. Resection begins with the subcutaneous portion of the bursa, being careful not to damage the skin or subcutaneous fat.[3,5] Transillumination confirms complete excision of the superficial bursa.[2,5] Next, attention is turned to the deep portion of the bursa, where resection continues until the fibers of the triceps can be seen (Fig. 37–3). Instruments are shifted from portal to portal to complete the resection.[3] A curved, flexible shaver can assist with removal of the peripheral bursa (Fig. 37–4). However, allowing small amounts of peripheral bursa to remain has not been associated with recurrence.[3] Small olecranon spurs, when seen, are removed with the arthroscopic bur while trying to avoid penetration of the triceps tendon itself (Fig. 37–5).[2,5] The shaver tip, basket forceps, and grasper remove loose bodies without the need for separate procedures (Fig. 37–6).[2,5] Average operative time ranges from 30 to 40 minutes.[3,5]

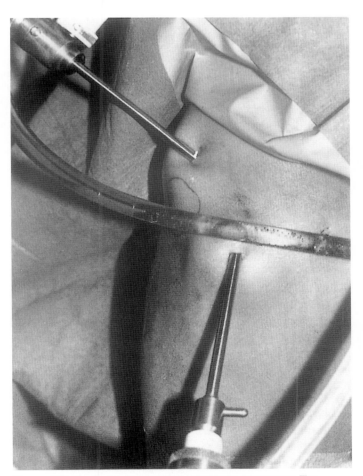

Figure 37–2 Portal placement for olecranon bursectomy. The arthroscope is in the proximal central portal, and the shaver is in the lateral portal. (From Baker CL, Cummings PD: Arthroscopic management of miscellaneous elbow disorders. Oper Tech Sports Med 6:16-21, 1998.)

3 Elbow

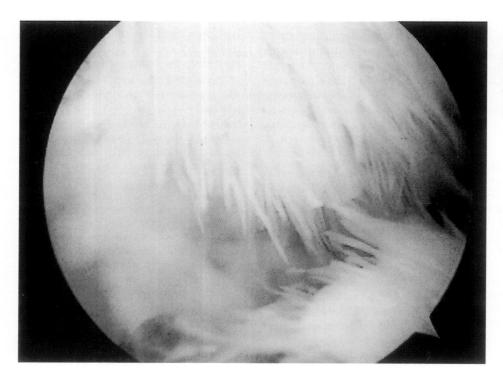

Figure 37–3   Arthroscopic view of the olecranon bursa showing the subcutaneous tissue above and the bursal covering of the triceps tendon below. (From Savoie FH: Miscellaneous disorders. In Savoie FH, Field LD [eds]: Elbow Arthroscopy. New York, Churchill Livingstone, 1996, pp 145-149.)

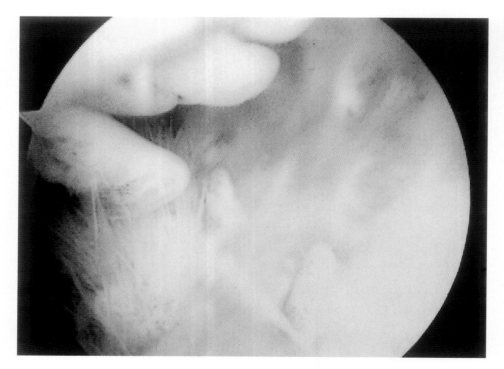

Figure 37–4   Gouty tophi within the olecranon bursa. (From Savoie FH: Miscellaneous disorders. In Savoie FH, Field LD [eds]: Elbow Arthroscopy. New York, Churchill Livingstone, 1996, pp 145-149.)

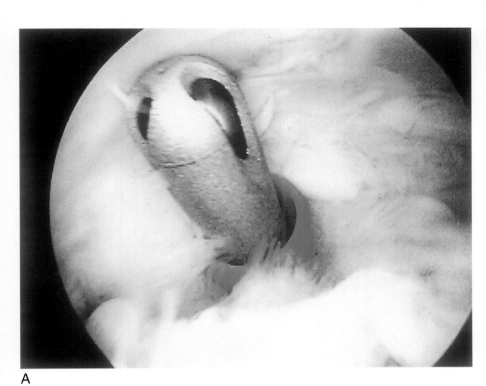

A

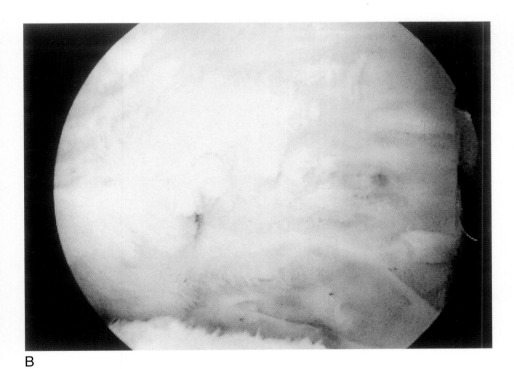

B

Figure 37–5   *A,* Distal central view of arthroscropic debridement being performed with the shaver through the proximal central portal. *B,* Postexcision view from the same portal. (From Savoie FH: Miscellaneous disorders. In Savoie FH, Field LD [eds]: Elbow Arthroscopy. New York, Churchill Livingstone, 1996, pp 145-149.)

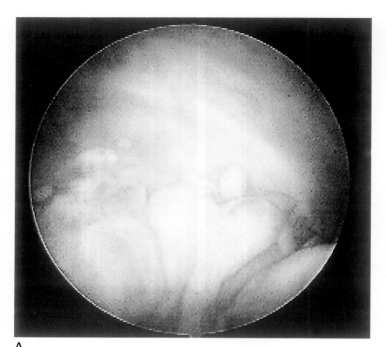

A

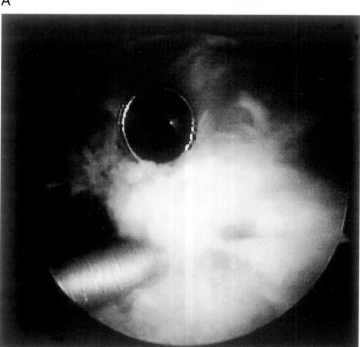

B

Figure 37–6 *A*, Olecranon spur protruding through the triceps tendon. *B*, Spur resection with the arthroscopic bur in the same patient. (From Savoie FH: Miscellaneous disorders. In Savoie FH, Field LD [eds]: Elbow Arthroscopy. New York, Churchill Livingstone, 1996, pp 145-149.)

Postoperative Management

After wound closure, a compressive dressing is applied, and elbow motion is started immediately.[2,3,5] The dressing and sutures are removed at 10 days, and resumption of activities progresses as tolerated. Protective padding is worn for several months during sports participation and other activities that risk elbow aggravation.

Results and Complications

Open Surgery

According to our literature review (summarized in Table 37–1), two primary open techniques have been clinically evaluated. Quayle and Robinson[6] proposed excision of the olecranon prominence through a midlateral incision

Table 37–1

Surgical Treatment of Olecranon Bursitis

Author (Date)	No. of Patients	Treatment	Average Follow-up (mo)	Recurrences	Other Complications (No. of Patients)	Remarks
Quayle and Robinson (1978)[6]	11	Open partial olecranonectomy ± windowing of deep bursal wall	36	0	Elbow tenderness (most) Hypesthesia (2) Tender and adherent scars (2)	
Stewart (1997)[10]	21	Open complete bursal excision	62	3	Hematoma (1) Stitch abscess (1) Persistent symptoms (1)	Recurrences in patients with RA (2) and CREST-like disorder (1)
Kerr (1990, 1993)[3,4]	4	Arthroscopic partial bursal excision	7.6	0	Infection (1)	Infection in patient with gout and immunosuppression
Savoie (1996)[7]	6	Arthroscopic total bursal excision	NA	0	Draining bursal fistula	
Ogilvie-Harris and Gilbart (2000)[5]	31	Arthroscopic total bursal excision	31	1	Persistent tenderness (4)	Recurrence in patient with RA and bursal-synovial fistula
Schulze et al. (2000)[8]	9	Arthroscopic total bursal excision				Earlier return to work compared with open bursectomy (10 vs. 18 days)

CREST, calcinosis, Raynaud phenomenon, esophageal dysmotility, sclerodactyly, and telangiectasia; NA, not available; RA, rheumatoid arthritis.

and longitudinal split of the triceps tendon. The bursa's deep wall was windowed in cases of excessive distention; otherwise, it was left intact. There were no recurrences in their 11 cases, and all patients returned to work within 6 weeks (average follow-up, 3 years). Complications included elbow tenderness for 3 months in "most" patients; transient hypesthesia in two patients; and tender, adherent scars in two patients.

The second technique, total olecranon bursectomy with or without partial osseous resection was evaluated retrospectively in a study of 21 patients with aseptic olecranon bursitis.[10] Thirteen patients underwent bursectomy alone, and eight had bursectomy with partial osseous resection. Successful resolution of symptoms occurred in 15 of 16 patients (94%) without rheumatoid arthritis and in 2 of 5 patients (40%) with rheumatoid arthritis. Complications in the nonrheumatoid group included one hematoma, one stitch abscess, and one recurrence at 2 years. The patient with recurrence was subsequently diagnosed with a connective tissue disorder most consistent with CREST syndrome. The one patient with gout had a successful outcome without complications. Unsatisfactory results in the rheumatoid group were symptom persistence for 7 months in one patient and recurrence requiring repeat bursectomy in two patients (at 1 and 6 years). Failure to perform partial excision of the olecranon was not implicated as a cause of failure in any patient. The authors concluded by recommending a lateral incision, complete bursectomy,

removal of osteophytes when present, meticulous closure, and a compressive dressing. They also cautioned surgeons about the rates of recurrence and long-term symptom relief when considering operative treatment for rheumatoid patients.

Arthroscopic Surgery

In an attempt to reduce wound complications associated with open treatment, Kerr[3,4] investigated techniques for arthroscopic olecranon and prepatellar bursectomy. Four patients with olecranon bursitis were included in his expanded study of 11 patients. All had failed conservative treatment. The cause of the bursitis was traumatic in two cases, inflammatory (gout) in one, and infectious in one. Following arthroscopic bursectomy, there were no recurrences and one complication. The patient with gout, who was also taking immunosuppressive medications, developed a postoperative infection that resolved with irrigation, debridement, and intravenous antibiotics. No problems with wound healing, hypesthesia, or tenderness occurred.

Subsequent studies have also reported favorable results. In Savoie's[7] six arthroscopically treated cases of refractory olecranon bursitis, there were no recurrences and one complication. A draining bursal fistula developed from the lateral portal in one patient and resolved uneventfully with packing.

3 Elbow

The largest study, performed by Ogilvie-Harris and Gilbart,[5] followed the outcomes of 31 consecutive cases of refractory olecranon bursitis treated arthroscopically. Patient age ranged from 19 to 57 years (average, 31 years), and duration of symptoms ranged from 3 months to 4 years (average, 1.1 years). All patients had undergone aspiration and cortisone injection at least once. Preoperatively, 29 of 31 patients (94%) complained of tenderness. Postoperatively, 4 of those 29 patients (14%) had persistent tenderness. One bursa re-formed at 6 months in a 22-year-old rheumatoid arthritis patient; subsequent workup demonstrated communication of the bursa with the elbow joint. Because of this case, the authors suggested caution when considering bursectomy in rheumatoid patients.

A Swiss study that compared nine arthroscopically treated patients with openly treated controls found an equivalent level of satisfaction by the Morrey scale and a significantly earlier return to work—10 days versus 18 days ($P = 0.041$)—in those treated arthroscopically.[8]

Conclusion

Arthroscopic bursectomy is well described and is effective in treating refractory olecranon bursitis in most cases, with results and complications comparable to those of open excision. The potential benefits of arthroscopic bursectomy—fewer wound complications and earlier return to work—should be weighed against the possibility of longer operative time and increased equipment needs. The possibility of increased complication rates and unsatisfactory outcomes should be considered before suggesting surgical treatment in patients with rheumatoid arthritis.

References

1. Baker CL, Cummings PD: Arthroscopic management of miscellaneous elbow disorders. Oper Tech Sports Med 6:16-21, 1998.
2. Baker CL Jr, Jones GL: Arthroscopy of the elbow. Am J Sports Med 27:251-264, 1999.
3. Kerr DR: Prepatellar and olecranon arthroscopic bursectomy. Clin Orthop 12:137-142, 1993.
4. Kerr DR, Carpenter CW: Arthroscopic resection of olecranon and prepatellar bursae. Arthroscopy 6:86-88, 1990.
5. Ogilvie-Harris DJ, Gilbart M: Endoscopic bursal resection: The olecranon bursa and prepatellar bursa. Arthroscopy 16:249-253, 2000.
6. Quayle JB, Robinson MP: A useful procedure in the treatment of chronic olecranon bursitis. Injury 9:299-302, 1978.
7. Savoie FH: Miscellaneous disorders. In Savoie FH, Field LD (eds): Elbow Arthroscopy. New York, Churchill Livingstone, 1996, pp 145-149.
8. Schulze J, Czaja S, Linder PE: Comparative results after endoscopic synovectomy and open bursectomy in chronic bursitis olecrani. Swiss Surg 6:323-327, 2000.
9. Smith DL, McAfee JH, Lucas LM, et al: Treatment of nonseptic olecranon bursitis: A controlled, blinded prospective trial. Arch Intern Med 149:2527-2530, 1989.
10. Stewart NJ: Surgical treatment of aseptic olecranon bursitis. J Shoulder Elbow Surg 6:49-54, 1997.
11. Viggiano DA, Garret JC, Clayton ML: Septic arthritis presenting as olecranon bursitis in patients with rheumatoid arthritis. J Bone Joint Surg 62:1011-1012, 1980.

ARTHROSCOPY OF
THE WRIST AND HAND

Wrist and Hand: Patient Positioning, Portal Placement, Normal Arthroscopic Anatomy, and Diagnostic Arthroscopy

LEONID I. KATOLIK AND JOHN J. FERNANDEZ

WRIST AND HAND ARTHROSCOPY IN A NUTSHELL

Indications:
Wrist pain unresponsive to treatment, adjunct to diagnostic evaluation and staging of wrist pathology, management of intra-articular pathology

Contraindications:
Complex regional pain, severe degenerative arthritis, fixed or distorted anatomy

Surgical Technique:
Patient positioned supine with traction; standard portal placement

Establish 3-4 portal; establish outflow and ulnar 4-5 or 6-R portal; examine radiocarpal and ulnocarpal joint; switch to 4-5 or 6-R portal to examine triangular fibrocartilage complex and ulnar structures; establish midcarpal portals and examine midcarpal joint; perform dynamic examination of scapholunate and lunotriquetral ligaments through midcarpal and radiocarpal portals

Postoperative Management:
Pathology dependent

Results:
Pathology dependent

Complications:
Related to positioning, setup, portal placement; infection, fluid extravasation, equipment failure

Arthroscopic surgery of the wrist and hand is a relatively new and rapidly evolving discipline. Chen reported on diagnostic arthroscopy of the wrist in 1979.[3] By the late 1980s, Roth et al. began to elucidate the role and efficacy of wrist arthroscopy.[7] Throughout the 1990s, new techniques and technology began to emerge, demonstrating the utility of wrist arthroscopy as a powerful diagnostic and staging tool and, for the skilled arthroscopist, a valuable treatment modality.[6]

Successful application of arthroscopy relies on mastery of the anatomy of the dorsal wrist to allow safe and efficacious portal placement. Proper visualization of the radiocarpal, midcarpal, and distal radioulnar joints is required. Finally, in order to appreciate subtle findings with the arthroscope, the surgeon must be able to distinguish between normal anatomy and abnormal pathology.[4]

Indications

The utility of arthroscopic surgery of the wrist is threefold: as a diagnostic adjunct, as a staging device, and as an operative alternative to arthrotomy for the treatment of intra-articular pathology. As such, it is indicated for (1) diagnosis of unexplained wrist pain despite 3 months of nonoperative management; (2) debridement of chondral lesions, removal of loose bodies, or synovectomy; (3) excision of dorsal wrist ganglia; (4) treatment of mechanical symptoms secondary to interosseous ligament pathology or triangular fibrocartilage complex (TFCC) pathology; (5) adjunctive visualization for reduction and fixation of articular fractures; (6) evaluation and treatment of carpal instability; and (7) treatment of ulnar impaction syndrome, including debridement of the TFCC and lunotriquetral ligament, and distal ulna resection.

Contraindications

Wrist arthroscopy is relatively contraindicated in patients with complex regional pain syndrome. This includes patients demonstrating symptoms of constant, burning pain that is worsened with the slightest activity, associated vasomotor changes, sensitivity to coldness, and dysesthesias and paresthesias of the hand. In addition, although the indications for arthroscopic management of arthritic conditions of the wrist are expanding, severe degenerative arthritis, particularly with associated fixed deformity, remains a relative contraindication.

Surgical Technique

Positioning and Setup

Wrist arthroscopy is generally performed as an outpatient procedure. General anesthesia or preferably regional block anesthesia is used. Regional blocks include axillary, supraclavicular, and scalene blocks. Bier block anesthesia should be avoided because it may limit the time available for the procedure. The patient is positioned supine on the operating table with the operative extremity placed on an arm table. A single dose of appropriate antibiotic is given preoperatively. The upper extremity is prepared to the axilla and draped using sterile technique. A padded sterile tourniquet is placed around the upper arm.

The arthroscopic equipment that will be used should be prepared, positioned, checked, and calibrated. The video equipment, arthroscopic fluid system, and other needed equipment is placed adjacent to the foot of the bed directly facing the surgeon, who is standing adjacent to the head of the bed across the arm table (Fig. 38–1). The assistant can stand adjacent to or across from the surgeon, depending on preferences and the requirements of the procedure.

Traction needs to be applied across the wrist to facilitate atraumatic portal placement and instrumentation of the wrist. Before application of a traction device, the upper extremity should be exsanguinated and the tourniquet inflated. Traction can be applied by a variety of methods. A commercially available "traction tower" is recommended because it applies effective traction, isolated across the wrist (Fig. 38–2). It also facilitates positioning and allows for comfortable access to the wrist from the dorsum for the surgeon and the assistant.

Keys to positioning include the following:

1. A firm, stable surface for the traction tower. If a padded table is used, place the plastic lid from the traction tower tray on the padded table to provide a more stable surface. The shoulder is abducted 90 degrees, and the elbow is flexed 90 degrees and rests on the tower base. Velcro straps secure the upper arm to the base and the forearm to the tower itself.
2. Padding of skin contact areas. Areas of exposed skin can be burned by thermal exposure to the traction tower if it has recently been sterilized, or by electrical current if cautery is used with a malfunctioning

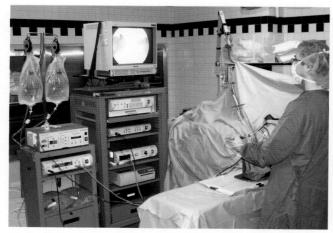

Figure 38–1 Positioning and preparation. The video monitor and other equipment are placed across from the surgeon at the foot of the table. The surgeon is at the head of the bed at the dorsal surface of the wrist.

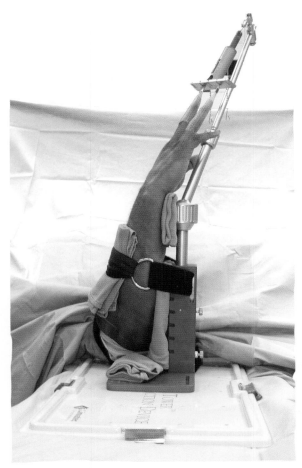

Figure 38–2 Traction tower. Apply 10 to 15 pounds of traction across the digits with finger traps. All the skin must be insulated from the metal parts of the traction tower. A firm surface should be placed beneath the base of the tower. If a padded arm board is used, the lid of the traction tower box can be used as support.

grounding pad. All contact areas should be padded with towels. A folded sterile towel is placed under the elbow on the base of the tower, another is placed between the volar forearm and the tower itself, another is used between the volar wrist and the

ball-and-socket articulation of the tower, and one is placed on the dorsal forearm beneath the Velcro strap.

3. Proper height adjustment of the ball-and-socket articulation of the tower. This should be adjusted so that the wrist flexion crease is just distal to the articulation. This allows the wrist to be placed in 10 to 15 degrees of flexion. It also allows ulnar and radial deviation of the wrist to facilitate access.

4. The use of finger traps. Traction should be applied across the middle and ring fingers, with additional traps added to minimize shear stress on fragile skin if necessary. Metal finger traps are preferred because they seem to be more effective in holding the digits. Nylon disposable traps are also available but tend to slip more often than the metal traps. Approximately 10 to 15 pounds of traction is applied. This should be checked throughout the procedure, as stress-relaxation of the tissues will cause the tension to decrease.

A 2.5- or 3-mm short-barreled arthroscope with a 30-degree angle provides ample visualization (Fig. 38–3). Smaller arthroscopes have a more limited field of view, and larger arthroscopes are too bulky for most wrists. Additional equipment for wrist arthroscopy includes an arthroscopic hook probe, small basket forceps, small grasping forceps, and small powered resectors for debridement of tissue (Fig. 38–4).

Fluid inflow systems include gravity and pump-assisted devices. A pump-assisted system is preferred for its effectiveness. The pressure should be set to 30 to 40 mm Hg. Inflow is through the sheath of the arthroscope, and outflow is through an 18-gauge catheter placed in the 6-U or 6-R portal. Care should be used in fracture cases owing to increased fluid extravasation, which could lead to compartment syndrome or acute carpal tunnel syndrome. To date, no cases of compartment syndrome following wrist arthroscopy have been reported.

Portal Placement

All portals are defined by their relationship to the extensor compartments of the wrist (Fig. 38–5). This anatomy

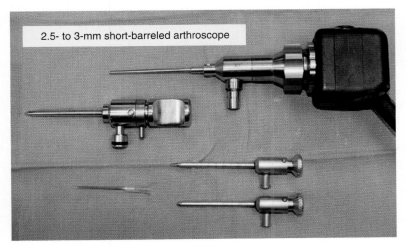

2.5- to 3-mm short-barreled arthroscope

Figure 38–3 Wrist arthroscopy equipment. A 2.5- or 3-mm arthroscope with a short barrel and 30-degree angle should be used. The sleeves and trocars are of similar size and configuration.

4 Wrist and Hand

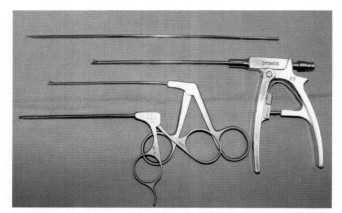

Figure 38–4 Wrist arthroscopy equipment. A small hook probe is important for probing structures. Small suction punches and graspers are also necessary. A small-joint tissue resector assists in debriding tissues.

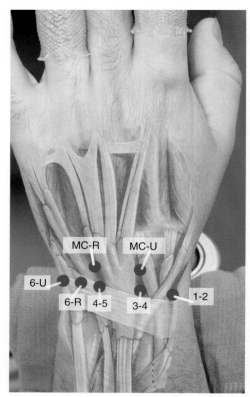

Figure 38–6 Wrist anatomy. A thorough knowledge of the local anatomy is important. This allows effective positioning of portals using local landmarks. MC, midcarpal; R, radial; U, ulnar.

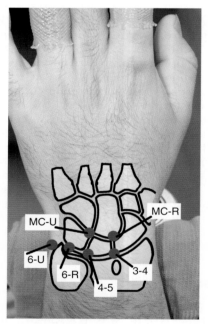

Figure 38–5 Wrist portals. The names of the portals are based on their relative position to the local anatomy. MC, midcarpal; R, radial; U, ulnar.

should be carefully studied and committed to memory (Fig. 38–6). Landmarks are drawn on the skin before portal placement and should include the distal radius, Lister's tubercle, distal ulna and ulnar styloid, extensor carpi ulnaris (ECU) tendon, extensor pollicis longus tendon, and midcarpal joint (Fig. 38–7).

The 1-2 portal is seldom used. It lies at the radiocarpal joint level between the tendons of the extensor pollicis brevis and extensor carpi radialis longus. Its utility is limited by the risks associated with its close proximity (<3 mm) to the radial artery and radial sensory nerve. This portal may allow additional visualization of the distal scaphoid, radial styloid, and radial-sided ligaments not

provided by the 3-4 portal. This may be clinically useful in the treatment of fractures of the scaphoid and radial styloid.

The 3-4 portal is the principal working portal. It lies at the radiocarpal joint level between the extensor pollicis longus tendon and the tendons of the extensor digitorum communis. The portal is approximately 1 cm distal to Lister's tubercle, just proximal and dorsal to the scapholunate joint interval. There is minimal risk to neurovascular structures. This portal effectively allows visualization of the scaphoid and lunate fossa of the distal radius, scapholunate ligament, ligaments of Testut and Kuenz, radioscaphocapitate ligament complex, radiolunate ligaments, proximal scaphoid, lunate, and radial attachment of the articular disk of the TFCC. Depending on the individual anatomy and laxity of the wrist, large portions of the TFCC itself may also be examined

The 4-5 portal is made at the radiocarpal joint level between the extensor digitorum communis and the extensor digiti minimi tendons. This portal allows excellent visualization of the articular disk of the TFCC and the lunotriquetral ligament. It is also a good working portal for the insertion of instruments.

The 6-U portal lies just ulnar to the ECU tendon at the ulnocarpal joint level. It is in very close proximity to the dorsal ulnar nerve. There is a high risk of injury to these nerve branches when using this portal. This portal should be avoided if possible, but it can be used as a fluid

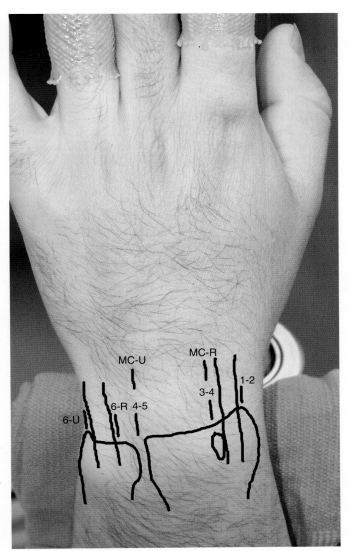

Figure 38–7   Anatomy landmarks. The important landmarks include the bone boundaries of the radial and ulnar styloids, the boundaries of the extensor carpi ulnaris and extensor carpi radialis brevis tendons, and the prominence of Lister's tubercle. The portals are placed relative to these landmarks as shown. MC, midcarpal; R, radial; U, ulnar.

articulation as well as the proximal pole of the capitate and the distal pole of the scaphoid. Dynamic testing of the scapholunate ligament should be performed while using this portal to assess the integrity of the scapholunate ligament.

The midcarpal-ulnar (MC-U) portal is placed 1 cm distal to the 4-5 portal in line with the fourth metacarpal. Entry places the arthroscope between the point just distal to the lunotriquetral articulation below and the capitohamate articulation above. The hamate facet of the lunate, when present, can be visualized in up to 65% of patients.[9] The lunotriquetral ligament can be assessed through this portal.

Additional portals may be added at the scaphotrapeziotrapezoid joint and the distal radioulnar joint. These are generally reserved for advanced procedures.

Diagnostic Arthrosocopy

The small confines of the wrist mandate a concise rubric for visualization.[2] In contradistinction to large-joint arthroscopy, small-joint arthroscopy relies primarily on rotation of the arthroscope's camera lens for visualization, rather than large movements of the arthroscope itself. Only very small movements are necessary when advancing or retracting the scope. Common errors include "overshooting" the joint and placing the scope into the capsular tissues, thereby disorienting the surgeon. Also because of the limited space, the placement of portals and instruments is critical. This is particularly true when trying to visualize and work with instruments in the same area. The arthroscope and instruments interfere with each other and compete for the same space, often displacing each other and blocking access to the area. The principles of triangulation are important and can help avoid this problem. These unique obstacles make wrist arthroscopy challenging.

The arm and wrist are exsanguinated and positioned in the traction tower as described previously. Anatomy landmarks are palpated and the portals marked. A 1.5-inch, 22-gauge needle is used to enter the radiocarpal joint at the 3-4 portal site. The joint is insufflated with 10 mL of normal saline solution. Ease of inflow and free egress of fluid confirm appropriate joint entry. Skin incisions are made only through the dermis, taking care to keep the sharp edge of the blade facing distally and not overpenetrate the deeper tissues. A small curved hemostat is used to spread through the subcutaneous tissues to the wrist capsule before placing the cannula. The hemostat can be used to penetrate the capsule, but great care should be used. The curved portion should be facing toward the proximal joint surface with the tips pointing up. This way, the curved part of the hemostat parallels the joint surface. Firm but gentle force is applied. If excessive force is used, the cartilage surface can easily be injured. Once the hemostat has penetrated the capsule, a small gush of fluid will be seen, confirming placement in the joint. The hemostats are gently spread to open the capsular portal slightly.

The 3-4 portal is created first. The blunt, rounded trocar is used to palpate the scaphoid distally and the

outflow portal or for additional instrument access if its size is limited.

The 6-R portal is just radial to the ECU at the ulnocarpal joint level. Similar to the 4-5 portal, it allows visualization of the palmar and ulnar insertion of the TFCC as well as the TFCC itself. It is also a good working portal for outflow and insertion of instruments. The prestyloid recess may be visualized palmarly and is distinguished from a TFCC detachment by its synovial lining and the taut nature of the TFCC.

The midcarpal-radial (MC-R) portal is placed 1 cm distal to the 3-4 portal at the midcarpal joint level, just on the ulnar side of the extensor carpi radialis brevis tendon. The somewhat restricted access of this joint can make it difficult to enter, so care should be used. This portal allows visualization of the scapholunate radius proximally. With a firm twisting motion, it is advanced into the radiocarpal joint through the portal. As with all portals, care must be exercised to avoid inadvertent, forceful overpenetration of the joint, which can lead to chondral injury. The cannula and trocar can then be advanced dorsally and ulnarly over the surface of the carpus. The cannula is now pointing ulnarly and is lying dorsal to the carpus at the radiocarpal joint level. This effectively holds the cannula in place, allowing for easy exchange of the trocar and placement of the arthroscopic camera. The obturator should be removed gently to allow the sheath to fill with fluid and to allow any trapped air pockets to escape. Any remaining bubbles can be evacuated by selective positioning of the outflow cannula.

The arthroscope is inserted into the cannula, and inflow is established. Attention is first directed ulnarly to establish outflow. The joint line is transilluminated (Fig. 38–8), allowing visualization of the ECU, superficial veins, and, occasionally, sensory nerve branches. Under direct visualization, an 18-gauge needle is placed radial to the ECU, and outflow is established. In a similar fashion, the 4-5 portal is established under direct visualization, and a small hook probe is inserted into the wrist.

The small hook probe is invaluable for this procedure. It is used to probe the integrity of the ligaments and TFCC. It is also a useful gauge for assessing the size of lesions. In addition, it can assist in pushing or pulling structures that obstruct the field of view and in performing procedures such as TFCC repairs and arthroscopically assisted fracture reductions.

The arthroscope is slowly retracted into the "straight-ahead" position with the scope pointing directly palmarly and perpendicular to the surface of the dorsal wrist. The scope is rotated so that the lens points radially and inferiorly.

The distal articular surface of the distal radius is examined first. The radial styloid surface and scaphoid fossa are examined (Fig. 38–9). The scope is minimally advanced palmarly, and the radioscaphocapitate ligament complex can be examined (Fig. 38–10). The ligaments of Kuenz and Testut can be examined along the palmar aspect adjacent to the radioscaphocapitate ligament complex, attaching to the volar aspect of the scapholunate ligament (Fig. 38–11).

The lens is rotated clockwise so that the sagittal ridge comes into view, followed by the lunate fossa of the radius. As the scope is advanced ulnarly, the lunate fossa and the radial insertion of the TFCC are inspected (Fig. 38–12).

The scope is again retracted to the straight-ahead position. The lens is rotated superiorly, and the scope is tilted inferiorly. This allows visualization of the carpal bones themselves, as well as the intercarpal ligaments. The examination begins by looking at the proximal scaphoid, then advancing ulnarly to the scapholunate ligament (Fig. 38–13). One must be sure to advance distally and dorsally on the scapholunate ligament to examine it entirely. The examination continues ulnarly to the lunate surface and then the lunotriquetral ligament and interval. The lunotriquetral ligament may be difficult if not impossible to see from the 3-4 portal. This ligament is sometimes part of the capsular tissue and is confluent with the articular cartilage. Unless there is some pathology in the ligament, it may not be visualized.

For better visualization of the ulnar side of the wrist, the arthroscope is placed in the 4-5 portal and the probe is switched to the 3-4 portal. As the scope is advanced distally and the optic rotated ulnarly and distally, the lunotriquetral ligament can be visualized (Fig. 38–14). The radiolunate ligaments and ulnocarpal complex may be visualized palmarly (Fig. 38–15). Proceeding ulnarly, the pisotriquetral recess may be seen, covered by a thin

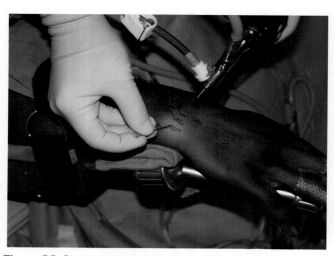

Figure 38–8 Transillumination. The light from the arthroscope can help outline its relative position. Sometimes, it can also show structures beneath the skin such as veins and nerves, which are important to avoid during portal placement.

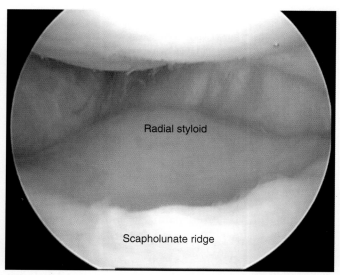

Figure 38–9 View from the 3-4 portal looking radially. The radial styloid and scaphoid fossa are examined. The scapholunate ridge defines the border between the scaphoid fossa and lunate fossa. It is also a good landmark for the scapholunate interval and ligament above.

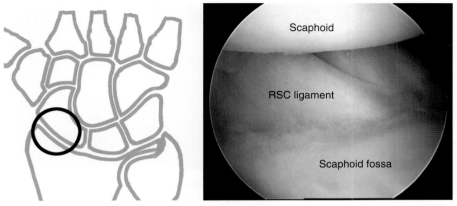

Figure 38–10   View from the 3-4 portal looking radially and palmarly. The radioscaphocapitate (RSC) ligament extends from the volar lip of the distal radius across the waist of the scaphoid, attaching to the waist of the capitate. The long radiolunate ligament can be seen ulnarly.

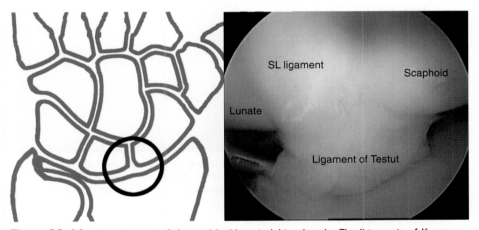

Figure 38–11   View from the 3-4 portal looking straight palmarly. The ligaments of Kuenz and Testut are seen as a tuft of synovial tissue at the base of the scapholunate (SL) interval and ligament. It is a neurovascular conduit and has no structural importance.

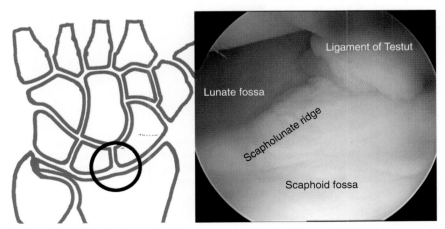

Figure 38–12   View from the 3-4 portal looking ulnarly. The scapholunate ridge again comes into view, and the lunate fossa can be examined. The radiolunate and ulnocarpal ligaments start to come into view.

4   Wrist and Hand

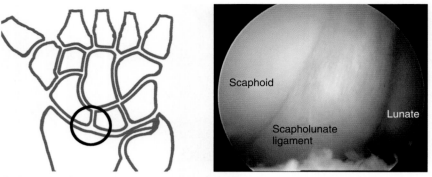

Figure 38–13 View from the 3-4 portal looking superiorly and dorsally. The scapholunate ligament can be seen between the scaphoid and the lunate. The ligament can be probed for defects. Stress testing can be done while looking at the ligament to test for instability.

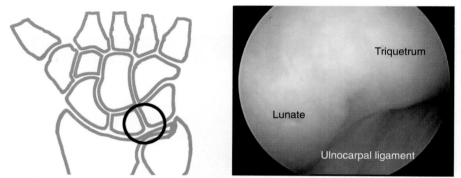

Figure 38–14 View from the 6-R portal looking ulnarly and dorsally. The lunotriquetral ligament can be difficult to see if it is normal. It is confluent with the articular cartilage and sometimes is part of the capsular tissue. The ligament should be probed to evaluate its integrity.

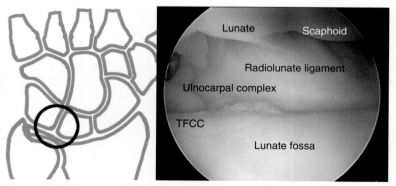

Figure 38–15 View from the 6-R portal looking palmarly. The ulnocarpal ligament complex stretches from the distal radius and triangular fibrocartilage complex (TFCC) to the lunate and triquetrum palmarly. The palmar portion of the TFCC can also be visualized through this portal.

synovium (Fig. 38–16). The scope is withdrawn slightly, and the prestyloid recess and the entire extent of the TFCC are inspected. The TFCC has a broad attachment radially across the ulnar border of the radius, with the ulnocarpal ligament located volarly, the base of the ulnar styloid ulnarly, and the ECU tendon sheath dorsally (Fig. 38–17).

Probing of the TFCC is important to assess its integrity. Applying pressure to the surface of the TFCC with a probe depresses it slightly. If the TFCC is normal, the resting tension allows the articular disk to spring back when pressure is removed. This "trampoline" effect, or ballottement, is lost when there is a tear of the TFCC (Fig. 38–18).

It is important to inspect the midcarpal joint.[1] This is a more confined area, and a 1.7- or 1.9-mm arthroscope, if available, is preferred. The MC-R and MC-U portals are created, with outflow in the MC-U portal. The arthroscope is inserted in the MC-R portal and the lens rotated radially and superiorly, thus sweeping across the concave surface of the scaphoid to the scaphotrapeziotrapezoid joint. Rotation of the arthroscope allows visualization and dynamic inspection of the scapholunate ligament and interval (Fig. 38–19). The arthroscope is withdrawn slightly, and the entirety of the radial midcarpal joint is visualized.

The scope is then placed in the MC-U portal. The lunotriquetral joint is seen below, with the capitohamate joint above. The lunotriquetral ligament can be inspected and assessed dynamically (Fig. 38–20). This allows further inspection of the articular surface of the capitate. One should also take time to assess the lunatohamate articulation, if present. In some cases, there is chondromalacia at the tip of the hamate, causing dorsal

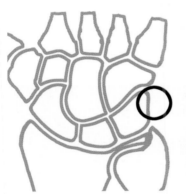
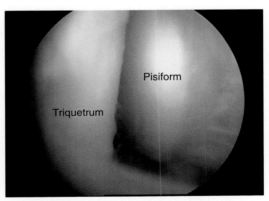

Figure 38–16 View from the 6-R portal looking palmarly and ulnarly. If the triquetrum is followed palmarly and ulnarly, the pisiform will come into view. Sometimes synovial tissue blocks this path, making this view inaccessible.

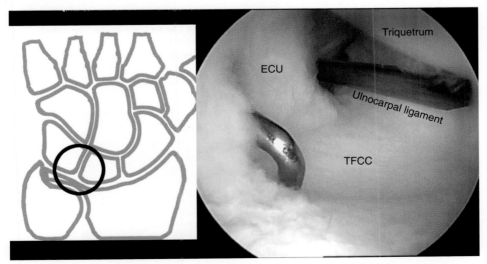

Figure 38–17 View from the 4-5 portal looking ulnarly. The outflow is through an 18-gauge needle in the 6-U portal. The probe is in the 6-R portal to examine the triangular fibrocartilage complex (TFCC). The TFCC attaches along the radial margin of the distal radius at the lunate fossa. The dorsal attachment is the capsule next to the extensor carpi ulnaris (ECU) tendon.

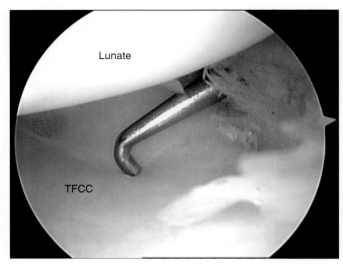

Figure 38–18 View from the 4-5 portal looking ulnarly. The triangular fibrocartilage complex (TFCC) is being palpated with the small hook probe. The "trampoline test" demonstrates the TFCC resisting the pressure of the probe. If the TFCC were torn, the normal tension would be lost and the TFCC would be flaccid when pushed with the probe.

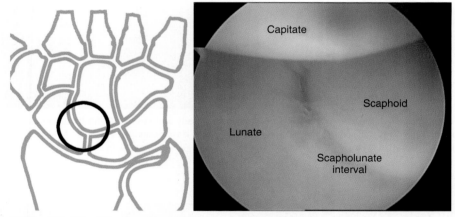

Figure 38–19 View from the MC-R portal. The capitate can be seen above. The lunate and scaphoid articulate with a very narrow gap. The ligament itself is not seen from this view. If there were significant scapholunate ligament incompetence, this gap would be larger or would open under stress.

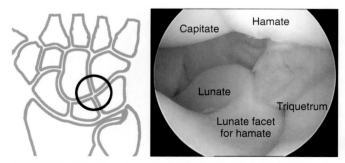

Figure 38–20 View from the MC-U portal. The lunate and triquetrum articulate with a small gap. The lunate can have a small facet for articulation with the hamate. This facet can be the source of early chondromalacia and a possible source of ulnar wrist pain.

wrist pain. As the wrist is extended and the lens directed dorsoulnarly, the attachment of the wrist capsule to the distal carpal row can be inspected.

Pearls and Pitfalls

Proper setup, positioning, and traction are critical. This part of the procedure is often relegated to a junior individual or assistant, but it is one of the most critical components of arthroscopy. It should be performed carefully, because poor positioning or poor traction can limit the procedure and increase its difficulty.

The biggest pitfall is poor portal placement. Placing the ulnar portals under direct vision and assessing access with a 22-gauge needle before committing to portal placement can avoid this complication.

If there is synovitis and capsular thickening dorsally, a local synovectomy and debridement will facilitate visualization. This may require switching between the 3-4 portal and 4-5 portal with the arthroscope and small-joint tissue resector several times.

Each arthroscopic examination should be performed consistently and systematically as outlined here to avoid overlooking possible sources of pathology. This includes examination of the midcarpal joint.

Postoperative Management

After arthroscopy, the portals are closed with simple or horizontal mattress interrupted nylon sutures and infiltrated with 0.25% bupivacaine (Marcaine). A gently compressive dressing is applied to the wrist with fluffed gauze and 3-inch Webril padding. A palmar splint is applied with the wrist in 10 to 20 degrees of extension, allowing the digits unencumbered extension and flexion. If there is TFCC pathology, and particularly if there has been repair or debridement, a long arm splint should be used, with the forearm in slight supination and the elbow at 90 degrees of flexion.

The patient is instructed to maintain strict elevation, with active range of motion to the digits every hour for 10 minutes. Ice may be applied dorsally at the wrist and hand. After 4 to 5 days, the splint and dressings can be removed. The wounds can be cleansed with soap and water and covered with small adhesive bandages. A removable splint can be used for comfort, but the patient should be encouraged to discontinue use of the splint as soon as the wrist allows.

Postoperative pain control can be achieved with mild narcotics and nonsteroidal anti-inflammatory drugs. Early return to work in a light or sedentary capacity is encouraged, with full-duty use within 4 weeks, depending on the intraoperative findings and treatment.

No supervised therapy is necessary for the first month. A home-based program is followed, including range of motion with gentle stretching, strengthening with putty, and scar modalities with deep tissue massage. If, after 4 to 6 weeks, there are continued deficits or complaints, supervised therapy may be recommended to fit the needs of the patient and to address any remaining limitations.

Results

Wrist arthroscopy has proved to be a valuable tool for the diagnosis of wrist pathology. It also serves as a powerful tool to stage the severity of known lesions. Nagle and Benson[6] retrospectively reviewed the results of 84 wrist arthroscopies. In 98% of arthroscopies performed for diagnostic purposes, the procedure helped establish the exact nature of the wrist pathology and ended a prolonged workup. Similarly, for 96% of patients undergoing arthroscopy for purposes of staging, arthroscopy was helpful in guiding further treatment. As wrist arthroscopy matures as a discipline, its utility as a definitive operative modality will be clarified.

Complications

Owing to the relatively small number of reported cases, the complication rate of wrist arthroscopy is not known, but it is estimated at 2% to 3%.[6] Potential complications can be divided into four categories: complications associated with arm positioning or traction, complications related to portal placement, complications specific to a procedure, and miscellaneous surgical complications.[10]

Attention to setup may reduce complications associated with positioning. Care must be taken to pad the elbow, particularly when it is secured to the traction tower. This avoids direct pressure on the ulnar nerve. Traction time should be kept to a minimum. The least amount of traction necessary to facilitate arthroscopic exposure should be used; rarely is more than 10 pounds of traction beneficial. This may minimize traction injuries to peripheral nerves in the anesthetized arm. Additionally, finger traps may place undue strain on friable skin. Finally, prolonged traction may injure the ligaments of the metacarpal phalangeal joints, which may manifest as postoperative edema and stiffness.[11]

Complications related to portal placement and instrumentation are minimized by a thorough knowledge of the anatomy of the dorsal wrist.[1] Forceful insertion of cannulas and instruments should be avoided. The 1-2 portal risks injury to both the radial artery and the sensory branches of the radial nerve. The 6-U and, to a lesser extent, the 6-R portals risk injury to the dorsal sensory branch of the ulnar nerve. The 3-4 and 4-5 portals are relatively safe. The scaphotrapeziotrapezoid portal may jeopardize the radial artery. Although not previously described, radiocarpal portals may jeopardize the arborization of the posterior interosseous nerve in the dorsal wrist capsule, potentially leading to the development of a painful neuroma. Injury to surface tendons can be minimized by careful palpation and marking before the creation of portals. In addition, sharp dissection should be carried out only through the dermis and the soft tissues, then spread with a blunt hemostat. Late rupture of the extensor pollicis longus has been reported following wrist arthroscopy.[5] This is indicative of injury at the time of arthroscopy, followed by later attritional changes.

Fluid extravasation is a potential complication, particularly in a recently injured patient. Using gravity-controlled inflow and limiting use of a pressure-controlled inflow device to brief durations when visualization is unduly compromised may minimize this potential complication. The forearm is checked periodically during the procedure to evaluate forearm distention. Additionally, a light Coban wrap (3M, Minneapolis, MN) can be applied to the forearm to minimize the effects of extravasation.

Infection poses a theoretical risk, although no cases of infection following wrist arthroscopy were reported in a multicenter survey conducted by the Arthroscopy Association of North America.[8] In nearly 400,000 arthroscopic procedures of all joints, the infection rate was 0.07%. Staphyloccocal species accounted for 76% of these infections.

Finally, wrist arthroscopy is an equipment-dependent procedure. Because few instruments can effectively substitute for the small tools designed for use in the wrist, premature termination of an arthroscopic procedure may be necessary due to equipment failure.

References

1. Abrams RA, Petersen M, Botte MJ, et al: Arthroscopic portals of the wrist: An anatomic study. J Hand Surg [Am] 19:940-944, 1994.
2. Berger RA: Arthroscopic anatomy of the wrist and distal radioulnar joint. Hand Clin 15:393-413, 1999.
3. Chen YC: Arthroscopy of the wrist and finger joints. Orthoped Clin N Am 10:723-733, 1979.
4. Dennison D, Weiss AP: Diagnostic imaging and arthroscopy for wrist pain. Hand Clin 15:415-421, 1999.
5. Fortems Y, Mawhinney I, Lawrence T, et al: Late rupture of extensor pollicis longus after wrist arthroscopy. Arthroscopy 11:322-323, 1995.
6. Nagle DJ, Benson LS: Wrist arthroscopy: Indications and results. Arthroscopy 8:198-203, 1992.
7. Roth JH, Poehling GG, Whipple TL: Arthroscopic Surgery of the wrist. Instr Course Lect 37:183-194, 1988.
8. Small NC: Complications in arthroscopy: The knee and other joints. Arthroscopy 2:253-258, 1986.
9. Viegas SF: Midcarpal arthroscopy: Anatomy and technique. Arthroscopy 8:385-390, 1992.
10. Warhold LG, Ruth RM: Complications of wrist arthroscopy and how to prevent them. Hand Clin 11:81-89, 1995.
11. Whipple TL: Precautions for arthroscopy of the wrist. Arthroscopy 6:3-4, 1990.

CHAPTER

39

Arthroscopic Management of Scapholunate Injury

JOHN J. FERNANDEZ AND LEONID I. KATOLIK

Dorsal Carpal Ganglia

Dorsal carpal ganglia and occult dorsal carpal ganglia generally present as a mass centered over the radiocarpal joint region at the scapholunate interval between the extensor digitorum communis and extensor pollicis longus. The origin of the cyst is most commonly the dorsal distal region of the scapholunate ligament but can include the scaphotrapeziotrapezoid joint. Patients are typically in the second to fifth decade of life, and there is a female-to-male preponderance of 2 to 4:1. Spontaneous resolution with time may occur in 30% to 60% of cases. Recurrence following treatment with observation, aspiration, or open surgery may be as high as 50%.[9] Additionally, open treatment may be complicated by postoperative stiffness and an unsightly scar.

Differential diagnosis for a dorsal wrist mass should include extensor tenosynovitis, inclusion cyst, foreign body granuloma, lipoma, and infectious granuloma. A history of inflammatory arthritis raises the possibility of synovitis, tenosynovitis, rheumatoid nodule, or joint effusion.

History

Patients seek medical attention for complaints of pain, cosmetic deformity, or the presence of an enlarging mass. They typically describe a weak grip and pain that is worse with extension-type activities. Ganglia may appear suddenly or develop slowly over time. Periodic activity-related changes in size are common.

Physical Examination

Dorsal carpal ganglia may present as an obvious mass or may be apparent only with wrist flexion. Occult ganglia are not clinically apparent or palpable but present with symptomatic dorsal wrist pain, possibly due to compression of the terminal branches of the posterior interosseous nerve.

Imaging

Routine radiographs, although part of a thorough workup of dorsal wrist pain, do not generally contribute significant information in terms of guiding treatment unless there is underlying degenerative or inflammatory arthritis causing the deformity or cyst. Additional studies, including magnetic resonance imaging (MRI) and ultrasonography, may be performed if the history and physical examination warrant but are not routinely used.

Indications and Contraindications

No definitive studies exist to elucidate the efficacy of arthroscopic ganglion resection. Surgical treatment is indicated following failure of nonoperative modalities. Excision is warranted if the ganglion is cosmetically unacceptable or if it is painful and interferes with function. Relative contraindications include the presence of neighboring infections, open wounds, or chronically contaminated inflammatory skin conditions. Additionally, previous open dorsal wrist surgery that may make portal placement and visualization difficult is a relative contraindication.

Surgical Technique

A standard wrist arthroscopy setup is used. Contrary to the sequence in standard wrist arthroscopy, the 6-R portal is established first. This allows examination of the proximal carpal row and the intrinsic ligaments for concurrent pathology without disrupting the ganglion stalk. When looking from the 6-R portal across the dorsum of the carpus, the scaphoid and lunate can be seen in profile (Fig. 39–1). The arthroscope is directed dorsally to the scapholunate ligament, where ganglia usually originate. Gentle pressure over the ganglia may help identify the stalk. There is often some synovitis surrounding the stalk (Fig. 39–2).[2]

The 3-4 portal is then established with an 18-gauge needle directly through the ganglion, sometimes rupturing it into the joint. A full-radius resector is inserted into the 3-4 portal and used to resect the ganglion and its base, as well as a 1-cm segment of the dorsal capsule surrounding the 3-4 portal (Fig. 39–3). Care is taken to preserve the integrity of the scapholunate ligament. Midcarpal arthroscopy is then performed to rule out the

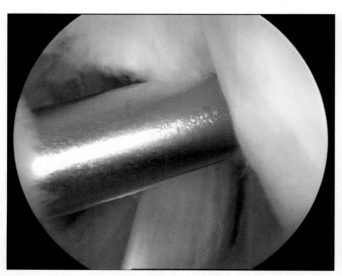

Figure 39–3 Resecting the cyst. A small-joint tissue resector is inserted through the 3-4 portal and through the substance of the ganglion. The resector is used to excise the ganglion and the capsule surrounding the 3-4 portal.

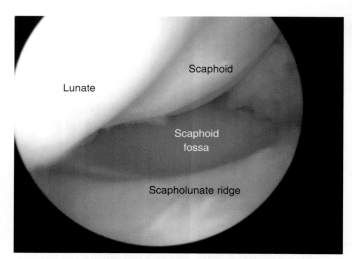

Figure 39–1 View from the 6-R portal looking radially and dorsally. The scaphoid and lunate can be seen in profile. The reflection of the dorsal capsule is distal and dorsal. This is where the stalk of the cyst is found. There may be synovitis in this area.

presence of a dual stalk. Secondary stalks may be disrupted by placement of the MC-R and MC-U portals. At the completion of arthroscopy, the dorsal wrist is reexamined. If the ganglion is not flat, the 3-4 portal is enlarged, and the ganglion sac is pulled out.

Pearls and Pitfalls

Recurrence is minimized by excising a dorsal capsular window 1 cm^2 around the stalk of the ganglion. It is helpful to resect the capsule until the ulnar border of the extensor carpi radialis brevis tendon is seen from the inside of the joint. Further capsule resection can then be extended distally and ulnarly. Usually, the extensor pollicis longus tendon can also be seen at the base of the resection site (Fig. 39–4). Visualization through the midcarpal portal is necessary, because some ganglia have dual stalks.

Postoperative Management

A dorsal soft compressive dressing is applied with a volar wrist splint holding the wrist in 10 to 20 degrees of extension. At 1 week, dressings and sutures are removed, and patients may begin gentle active and active assisted range-of-motion exercises. A prefabricated wrist splint is used for comfort for 4 to 6 weeks. Patients should avoid forceful activity with the hand and wrist for 6 weeks. Formal therapy is instituted after 4 to 6 weeks if there are deficits in range of motion or strength or hypertrophic scarring.

Results

Unpublished data from Singh and Osterman et al. described only one recurrence in more than 80

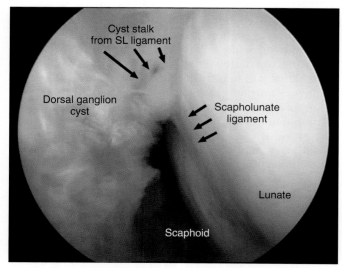

Figure 39–2 View from the 6-R portal looking radially and dorsally. The stalk of the cyst can be seen entering the scapholunate ligament (SL) complex at its distal margin.

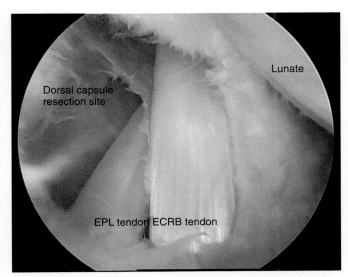

Figure 39–4 Resection margins. After resection of the capsule, the extensor carpi radialis brevis (ECRB) and extensor pollicis longus (EPL) tendons should be visible. Sometimes the extensor digitorum communis tendons from the fourth compartment can be seen.

patients.[14] Luchetti et al.[8] demonstrated recurrence in 2 of 34 resections and residual dorsal wrist pain in 3 of 34 patients.

Complications

Recurrence, although not a true complication of surgery, is a risk. Scapholunate ligament injury with subsequent instability can occur but is not specific to arthroscopic treatment. Conversion to an open procedure is necessary if a technical or anatomic difficulty precludes adequate visualization.

Intercarpal Ligament Injuries

Intercarpal ligament injuries amenable to arthroscopic treatment include but are not limited to scapholunate ligament tears and lunotriquetral ligament tears.

Scapholunate Ligament Tears

The role of the scapholunate ligament complex in wrist kinematics is well established. Stability of the scapholunate articulation requires competence of both intrinsic and extrinsic wrist ligaments. Although scapholunate ligament injury alone may not produce a dorsal intercalated segment instability pattern, it may, with future attenuation of extrinsic structures, lead to such instability. Persistent scapholunate dissociation leads to extension of the lunate, which unloads its articulation with the radius and increases contact forces at the radioscaphoid articulation and dorsal capitolunate joint. This leads to progressive arthrosis, pain, and impairment over time.

History

Typically, scapholunate ligament injuries result from a hyperextension force to the wrist with forearm pronation and intercarpal supination.

Physical Examination

Examination reveals tenderness over the scapholunate interval. The scaphoid stress test or Watson maneuver evaluates abnormal motion of the scaphoid with radial and ulnar deviation of the wrist. Scapholunate dissociation results in subluxation of the proximal pole of the scaphoid over the dorsal lip of the distal radius. Occasionally, a palpable clunk may be felt as the subluxed scaphoid relocates.

Imaging

In addition to posteroanterior (PA) and lateral views of the wrist, radial and ulnar deviation and clenched fist views may demonstrate scapholunate dissociation. The PA view should demonstrate three smooth radiographic arcs defining normal carpal relationships. Discontinuity of any of these arcs suggests intercarpal instability. A scapholunate gap greater than 5 mm ("Terry Thomas sign") is diagnostic of scapholunate dissociation. The "scaphoid ring sign" may appear as the scaphoid collapses into flexion and demonstrates a foreshortened appearance. The scapholunate angle is normally 30 to 60 degrees (average, 47 degrees). Angles greater than 80 degrees are indicative of pathology.

If the initial evaluation is inconclusive, immobilization for 5 to 7 days and reevaluation are appropriate. Arthrography and MRI are reserved for patients who are still symptomatic at 6 weeks despite normal radiographs. Although arthrography is a sensitive study for the detection of scapholunate ligament injury, it does not quantitate the extent of the injury or the status of the extrinsic ligaments.[17] MRI may emerge as the diagnostic modality of choice, but it requires a strong magnet, dedicated extremity coils, and an experienced radiologist. The gold standard for the diagnosis of wrist pathology is still wrist arthroscopy.

Indications and Contraindications

Arthroscopic treatment of a scapholunate ligament injury may be diagnostic, therapeutic, or salvage. Arthroscopy is indicated in the acute setting for the diagnosis of injury, debridement of partial tears, and arthroscopic reduction and internal fixation of associated fractures. For chronic scapholunate ligament disruptions, arthroscopy can help in staging the injury and in performing debridement, synovectomy, and radial styloidectomy as adjunctive measures. Associated carpal injuries, including fractures, remain relative contraindications to arthroscopic management. Table 39–1 describes the arthroscopic classification of scapholunate ligament injuries.[4]

Surgical Technique

A standard wrist arthroscopy setup is used. With the arthroscope in the 3-4 portal and a probe in the 4-5

| Table 39–1 | Arthroscopic Classification of Scapholunate Ligament Injury | |

Grade	Description	Treatment
I	Attenuation or hemorrhage without incongruency	Immobilization
II	Incongruency of carpal space, with gap less than width of probe	Arthroscopic reduction and pinning
III	Incongruency of carpal space, with probe easily passing between scaphoid and lunate	Arthroscopic or open reduction and pinning
IV	Incongruency of carpal space, with 2.7-mm arthroscope passing between scaphoid and lunate	Open reduction and repair or capsulodesis

From Geissler WB, Freeland AE: Arthroscopically assisted reduction of intraarticular distal radial fractures. Clin Orthop 327:125-134, 1996.

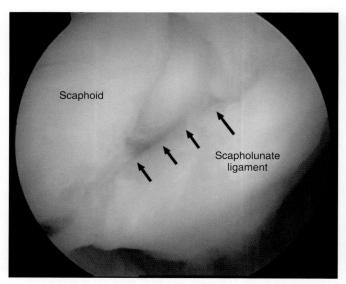

Figure 39–5 View from the 3-4 portal looking dorsally. A partial tear of the scapholunate ligament can be seen. There is a small gap, but it is less than 3 mm. The resector is used to debride the unstable portions of the ligament.

portal, the scapholunate ligament complex is examined. The long radiolunate and radioscaphocapitate ligaments are visualized and probed. The scapholunate ligament, which usually tears from the scaphoid, is visualized and probed from dorsal to volar, and any damage is staged (see Table 39–1). Widening of the scapholunate articulation is often better assessed through the midcarpal portals, where the articulation is not obstructed by a ligamentous fold obscuring the view of the joint.[7]

A partial scapholunate ligament injury, usually involving the central or membranous portion of the ligament, is a stable injury. Similarly, a complete scapholunate ligament tear that spares the dorsal capsular insertions and results in no gapping is also deemed stable. A shaver may be used to resect any frayed ligament that impinges on the radiocarpal joint. The scapholunate articulation should then be reassessed for subtle instability that would warrant percutaneous pinning to maintain alignment and allow for ligament healing.[12]

A complete scapholunate ligament tear that is reducible (grade II or III), without gross widening (<3 mm), and without dorsal intercalated segment instability can be treated by arthroscopic reduction and internal fixation. The scapholunate ligament tear can be visualized and debrided through the 3-4 portal (Fig. 39–5). Two 0.045-inch Kirschner wires (K-wires) placed dorsally into the scaphoid and lunate are used as joysticks to aid reduction. The arthroscope is placed into the midcarpal space, and reduction of the scapholunate articulation is performed under direct visualization. When reduction is satisfactory, three or four K-wires are placed across the scapholunate and scaphocapitate joints (Fig. 39–6).[5]

Grade IV acute injuries with marked widening of the scapholunate joint require open reconstruction with capsulodesis. The avulsed scapholunate ligament is generally repaired to the scaphoid with bone anchors.

Chronic tears of the scapholunate ligament lose their intrinsic ability to heal and require either open reconstruction and capsulodesis, if the articular surfaces are

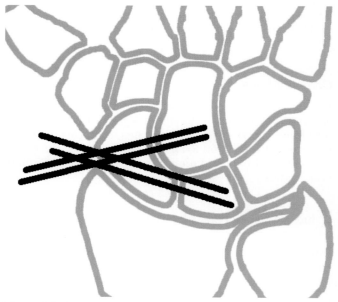

Figure 39–6 Pinning of the scapholunate interval. K-wires (0.045 inch) are used to cross both the scapholunate and scaphocapitate articulations. The scaphoid must be extended relative to the lunate, and the gap must be reduced as much as possible.

intact, or scaphoid excision and four-corner fusion, if there is early arthrosis. Arthroscopy is useful for the evaluation of chondral injury and for articular debridement and radial styloidectomy in early scapholunate advanced collapse.

Postoperative Management

Following simple debridement of the scapholunate ligament, patients are placed in a short arm splint for 7 to

10 days. Sutures are removed at that point, a removable short arm splint is placed, and gentle range-of-motion exercises are begun. Grip strengthening does not begin for 6 weeks.

Following scapholunate pinning, a short arm splint is applied for 1 week, after which a short arm cast is placed for 8 weeks. Finger range of motion is begun immediately. The pins are removed at 10 to 12 weeks, and a removable short arm splint is placed. Wrist range of motion and grip strengthening begin at 3 months.

Results

Debridement of partial scapholunate ligament injuries has been shown to resolve symptoms in 85% of patients.[13] Debridement of complete tears results in symptom resolution in only 67% of patients. For complete tears, arthroscopic reduction and internal fixation were more efficacious in maintaining reduction and relieving symptoms in tears less than 3 months old. Tears older than 3 months have a worse prognosis.[21]

Complications

The main complication of arthroscopic treatment of scapholunate ligament injuries is inadequate relief of symptoms due to pain and instability. Open treatment is generally recommended to address persistent incompetence of the scapholunate ligament and instability.

Lunotriquetral Ligament Tears

Lunotriquetral ligament tears may be traumatic or degenerative. They typically occur as a result of forced pronation, as in a fall on an outstretched arm. Degenerative injuries may be associated with ulnar impaction or may occur as a late complication of scapholunate ligament or triangular fibrocartilage complex (TFCC) injury. These injuries often occur as part of a spectrum of injury involving the extensor carpi ulnaris, TFCC, distal radioulnar joint (DRUJ), ulnocarpal ligaments, and chondral surfaces. As such, the role of isolated lunotriquetral ligament injury is unclear. Similarly, evaluation of the results of treatment is difficult, because treatment of associated injuries may alter lunotriquetral symptoms.[12]

History

Patients may describe ulnar-sided wrist pain that is worse with pronation and ulnar deviation (power grip).

Physical Examination

Examination seeks to distinguish lunotriquetral injuries from the spectrum of injuries that usually accompany them. Palpation of the lunotriquetral ligament dorsally may elicit pain and crepitation. Lateral pressure over the ulnar snuffbox between the extensor carpi ulnaris and flexor carpi ulnaris distal to the ulnar head may reproduce the patient's symptoms and could suggest lunotriquetral ligament injury but may also signify injury to the TFCC. The examiner may attempt to reproduce the

patient's pain by stabilizing the lunate with one hand and applying a translating force to the triquetrum with the other (lunotriquetral shuck or shear test). Relief of pain by injection of local anesthetic into the lunotriquetral joint heightens suspicion for lunotriquetral ligament injury.[11]

Imaging

In addition to PA and lateral views of the wrist, radial and ulnar deviation and clenched fist views may demonstrate lunotriquetral instability. Widening of the lunotriquetral interval, volar flexion of the lunate, increase in the capitolunate angle, and decrease in the scapholunate angle may be noted. However, even with large tears of the lunotriquetral ligament, radiographs may be normal. Arthrography has a very high false-negative rate but demonstrates lunotriquetral tears best by midcarpal injection. MRI has limited utility.[11]

Indications and Contraindications

Arthroscopy allows excellent visualization of lunotriquetral pathology for diagnosis and staging and may also aid in the dynamic examination of the lunotriquetral articulation. Relative contraindications include any factor that would hamper portal placement or render visualization inadequate.

Surgical Technique

A standard wrist arthroscopy setup is used. The 4-5 or 6-R portal is used to visualize ulnocarpal structures, including the TFCC and lunotriquetral interval. The probe is used to assess the dorsal and palmar portions of the ligament, as well as the attachments of the lunate and triquetrum to the TFCC and wrist capsule. A resector may be used to excise any synovium and debris that impairs visualization. The lunotriquetral articulation is sometimes best evaluated through the midcarpal portals. Large tears can often lead to a gap seen arthroscopically but not radiographically (Fig. 39–7). The ability to pass an arthroscope through the lunotriquetral interval into the radiocarpal space indicates severe instability. Even if arthroscopic treatment is not possible, arthroscopy can aid in decision making and planning for the repair or reconstruction of associated injuries.

Partial lunotriquetral injury with an intact dorsal capsuloligamentous complex is a stable lesion. With the arthroscope in the 4-5 portal and a shaver in the 6-R portal, the lunotriquetral ligament is carefully debrided to a stable rim of tissue. Complete injury to the lunotriquetral ligament and dorsal capsuloligamentous complex can lead to palmar flexion of a destabilized lunate and volar intercalated segment instability. Stabilization can require open dorsal capsulodesis with suture anchors in the lunate and triquetrum, followed by pinning of the lunotriquetral articulation.[18]

An advanced arthroscopic alternative to open surgery is ulnocarpal plication with lunotriquetral pinning. This effectively forms a capsulodesis of the lunotriquetral joint. While viewing from the 3-4 portal, an 18-gauge needle is passed through the 6-U portal. Two 2-0 PDS

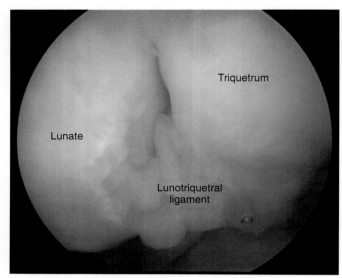

Figure 39–7 View from the 4-5 portal looking dorsally. A complete tear of the lunotriquetral ligament is appreciated. There is also early gapping at the interval. This tissue is debrided with a small-joint resector.

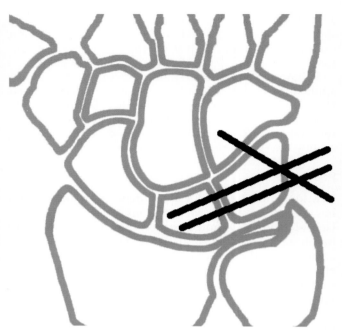

Figure 39–8 Pinning of the lunotriquetral interval. Similar to scapholunate pinning, several K-wires are inserted to hold the lunotriquetral joint and midcarpal joint reduced.

sutures are passed into the joint and retrieved with a wire loop suture retriever through the 6-R portal. The goal is to surround the ulnolunate and ulnotriquetral ligaments. Suture anchors can also be placed in the lunate and triquetrum dorsally. Tension on these sutures and manual pressure on the lunate facilitate reduction of the lunotriquetral joint, which can then be pinned under fluoroscopic guidance (Fig. 39–8). Traction is released from the tower, and the plicating sutures are tied beneath the skin at the 6-U portal, after which the suture anchors can also be tied.[12]

Postoperative Management

After simple debridement, patients are splinted for 1 week, followed by the use of a prefabricated wrist splint for comfort for an additional 4 weeks. Gentle range-of-motion exercises begin at 1 week, and strenuous activity with the hand and wrist is avoided for 6 weeks. Formal therapy can begin in 4 to 6 weeks if there are continued deficits in motion or strength.

After arthroscopic capsulodesis, patients are immobilized in a long arm splint for 1 week and then casted in neutral rotation for 8 weeks, after which the pins are removed. A removable splint is placed, and patients begin gentle range-of-motion exercises. Immobilization is discontinued at 12 weeks, and therapy proceeds to include forearm rotation as well as strengthening.

Results

Limited data exist to support arthroscopic reduction and internal fixation of the lunotriquetral joint with arthroscopic plication of the ulnolunate and ulnotriquetral ligaments. Debridement alone for partial lunotriquetral ligament tears was found to provide good pain relief.[19] Debridement alone for complete lunotriquetral liga-

ment tears gives mixed results.[16] Four-corner arthrodesis with scaphoid excision remains a salvage alternative for patients who have failed prior treatment.

Complications

The main complication of arthroscopic treatment of lunotriquetral injuries is inadequate relief of symptoms due to pain and instability. Advanced arthroscopic treatment, relying on the 6-U portal, risks injury to branches of the dorsal ulnar sensory nerves.

Distal Radius Fractures

Eighty percent of the load borne by the carpus is transferred to the distal radius. Articular incongruity of as little as 1 to 2 mm at the radiocarpal joint following intraarticular distal radius fracture may result in degenerative wrist pain and stiffness. Further, as radial height is lost due to fracture subsidence, more load is transferred to the ulna, resulting in increased stress on ulnar-sided structures. The imperative to restore articular congruity is tempered by the postoperative stiffness that generally results from the capsular and ligamentous dissection necessary for the visualization of fracture fragments.

Arthroscopically assisted reduction of distal radius fractures seeks to achieve anatomic restoration with limited soft tissue dissection.[22] The benefits of arthroscopy may be combined with proven principles of external fixation and percutaneous pinning or limited internal fixation in the management of these injuries. Associated injuries to the intercarpal ligaments and the TFCC can be present in up to 66% of distal radius fractures. Fracture debris can be removed, and associated carpal ligament injuries and TFCC tears can be assessed.

History

Distal radius fractures typically occur as a result of a high-energy injury that drives the carpus into the distal radius. Patients present with marked pain, swelling, and deformity of the wrist.

Physical Examination

The entire extremity should be examined for associated injuries. Distal neurovascular integrity should be documented both before and after reduction.

Imaging

High-quality PA, lateral, and oblique views of the wrist are essential for operative planning. Prereduction images show the direction and extent of initial displacement of fragments. Traction views assist in discerning intra-articular from extra-articular fractures. Computed tomography allows assessment of displacement or characterization of fracture pattern when this is unclear.

Indications and Contraindications

Arthroscopically assisted treatment of intra-articular distal radius fractures is best for simple fractures with large, well-defined fragments (e.g., radial styloid fracture, isolated die-punch fracture, central depression fracture, dorsal or volar Barton fracture). Intervention is indicated for an articular step-off greater than 2 mm following closed reduction (Fig. 39–9). Signs of a complicating carpal injury (disruption of Gilula lines) or suspected DRUJ injury are also indications for arthroscopy. Concomitant injury that precludes positioning for arthroscopy is a relative contraindication.

Arthroscopy has no major advantage in patients with open fractures, compartment syndrome, or massive soft tissue injury.

Surgical Technique

Distal radius fractures are treated 2 to 7 days after injury. This delay minimizes bleeding from the fracture site, which can obscure the field of view. A standard wrist arthroscopy setup is used. Alternatively, a horizontal setup may be used, whereby the pronated arm is placed on a hand table, with traction applied through finger traps and weights hung off the end of the table. The operating room is arranged so that fluoroscopy can be performed concurrently. To minimize fluid extravasation, one should wrap the arm in a compressive dressing, maintain a separate outflow, and use lactated Ringer's solution, which is rapidly absorbed from soft tissues.

The normal landmarks are often distorted due to swelling. The intersection of a line drawn down the radial aspect of the long finger and a horizontal line at the level of the ulnar styloid approximates the 3-4 portal. The midaxis of the ring finger approximates the 4-5 portal. A needle placed into the joint with aspiration of hemarthrosis confirms proper placement. The cannula is placed, and gravity-assisted lavage is begun with outflow through the 6-R portal. The arthroscope can now be placed. A resector through the 4-5 portal can assist in evacuating clots and debris. When visualization is satisfactory, diagnostic arthroscopy is begun to assess the fracture as well as any associated injuries.[3]

Reduction may be accomplished by traction alone. Often the fragments need to be mobilized with the probe in the joint or with an elevator through a separate skin incision over the fracture. Depressed fragments may additionally be elevated by intrafocal manipulation with a K-wire or probe (Fig. 39–10).

Once the distal articular fracture fragments are reduced and stabilized, the main bodies of the distal fragments are fixed to the proximal shaft using addition wires, external fixator, or volar plates.

4 Wrist and Hand

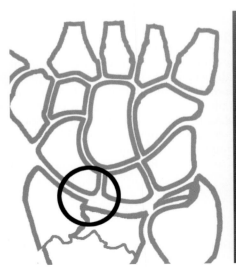
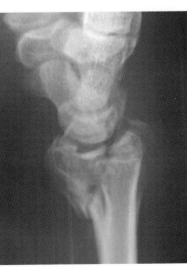

Figure 39–9 A displaced intra-articular fracture of the distal radius is best assessed arthroscopically. Even when radiographs show an acceptable reduction, arthroscopy often reveals residual displacement.

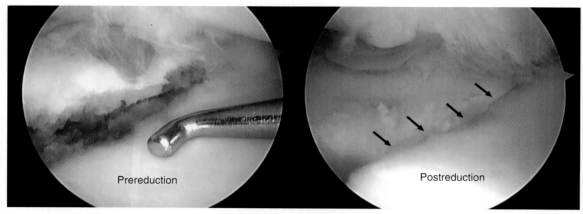

Figure 39–10 Displaced distal radius fracture. The pre- and postreduction pictures reveal the efficacy of the arthroscopic reduction. The probe is used to assist in the reduction and later to assess the stability of fixation.

Specific Fracture Management Techniques

RADIAL STYLOID FRACTURE

A 0.045-inch K-wire is placed into the radial styloid and used as a joystick to achieve reduction under arthroscopic visualization. The wire is then driven across the fracture site. A cannulated screw can be placed over the wire to compress the fracture site, or additional K-wires can be placed adjacently. Special attention should be paid to possible injury of the scapholunate ligament because of the high association with radial styloid fractures.

BARTON FRACTURE

Barton fractures should be plated volarly as classically described, but without violating the wrist capsule. Articular reduction and any associated intra-articular soft tissue pathology are evaluated arthroscopically.

Postoperative Management

Edema control, pin care, and mobilization of the digits are the early focus. Elastic wraps may help minimize edema. Dressings are removed at 1 week, and pin care is performed twice daily with hydrogen peroxide. Therapy is prescribed for active and active assisted metacarpophalangeal and proximal interphalangeal joint motion. The patient is followed radiographically for the first 3 weeks. The wrist is protected in either a cast or a fracture splint. K-wires may be removed at 6 to 8 weeks. At this point, therapy aimed at recovering wrist and forearm motion is begun. At 12 weeks, strength and conditioning are begun, based on the radiographic appearance of the fracture.

Results

Many authors have found arthroscopy to be a valuable adjunct in the treatment of intra-articular distal radius fractures.[1] Anatomic reduction and early recognition

and treatment of associated soft tissue injuries should have a positive effect on outcome.

Complications

The complications of these techniques are similar to those encountered in any limited approach to fixation of the wrist. Secondary fracture displacement, extensor tendon rupture, complex regional pain syndrome, and injury to the superficial branch of the radial nerve have all been reported. The risk of injury to the contents of the anatomic snuffbox are minimized if wires enter more palmarly and proximally in the snuffbox. A thorough knowledge of dorsal wrist anatomy, fixation principles, and fracture type is mandatory for successful arthroscopically assisted treatment of distal radius fractures.

Scaphoid Fractures

Fractures of the scaphoid account for 70% of carpal fractures. Forced wrist hyperextension and pronation drive the scaphoid into the distal radius. This injury typically occurs in young adult males and is a common athletic injury. For nondisplaced fractures, acute cast immobilization may result in successful union in 90% to 95% of cases. Union rates decrease as time to treatment increases and as displacement increases. Further, the duration of cast immobilization is typically longer with more proximal scaphoid fractures. The goals of arthroscopically assisted fixation for fractures of the scaphoid include providing secure fixation until solid union is achieved, minimizing extremity immobilization and soft tissue dissection, and identifying concomitant wrist injuries.[6]

History

Patients typically present with radial-sided wrist pain after a fall on an outstretched arm.

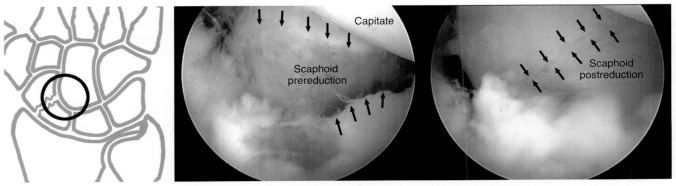

Figure 39–11 Displaced scaphoid fracture. Similar to distal radius fractures, scaphoid fractures can be assessed and reduced arthroscopically. Because of the geometric shape and configuration of the scaphoid, radiographs alone are unreliable. Fluoroscopy and arthroscopy are more sensitive and specific in assessing the quality of the fracture reduction.

Physical Examination

There is palpable tenderness in the anatomic snuffbox.

Imaging

Zero-rotation PA and lateral radiographs of the wrist should be obtained. If these fail to demonstrate a fracture, PA views in radial and ulnar deviation may allow better visualization of the scaphoid margins. Clenched fist views may help identify scapholunate ligament disruption as the cause of pain. A bone scan or MRI scan is useful to identify occult fractures. A negative scan at 3 to 5 days after injury rules out a scaphoid fracture. Computed tomography best defines cortical integrity and fracture pattern and may help identify a humpback deformity from palmar comminution of the scaphoid.

Indications and Contraindications

Fixation of scaphoid fractures is indicated for nondisplaced unstable fractures (vertical oblique), displaced (>1-mm step-off and 15-degree angulation) but reducible fractures, fractures with a delayed presentation, proximal pole fractures, fibrous nonunions, and fractures associated with other wrist injuries. Arthroscopic reduction with internal fixation avoids disruption of the scaphoid's blood supply or dissection of the strong radioscaphocapitate ligament. Contraindications include associated soft tissue compromise.

Surgical Technique

A diagnostic arthroscopy is performed using the standard arthroscopy setup. Care is taken to evacuate fracture hematoma. The fracture is well visualized via the MC-U portal. The fracture can be manipulated manually or with K-wire joysticks inserted into the dorsal proximal and distal fragments of the scaphoid to allow for reduction. Once the fracture is reduced arthroscopically (Fig. 39–11), radiographs are taken to confirm the general alignment of the scaphoid.

The fracture can be fixed with percutaneous pins or a percutaneous screw. It can be pinned percutaneously by inserting three or four 0.045- or 0.035-inch K-wires antegrade from the proximal pole of the scaphoid next to the lunate and advancing them distally into the distal scaphoid. The pins are then pulled back until they clear the articular surface of the proximal scaphoid and are left prominent at the scaphoid tubercle. If a percutaneous screw is used, the K-wire is advanced through the proximal pole of the scaphoid across the fracture and through the tubercle palmarly. A headless compression screw can then be placed antegrade from proximal to distal within the scaphoid. A Herbert-Whipple or Acutrak screw can be used in this setting (Fig. 39–12).

If desired, the Herbert-Whipple compression jig can be used in the more conventional application, with placement of a retrograde screw from the scaphoid tubercle into the proximal pole of the scaphoid. The hand is removed from traction, and an incision is made radial to the flexor carpi radialis centered on the scaphotrapeziotrapezoid joint. Blunt dissection avoids injury to the palmar cutaneous nerve and the radial artery. Access to the distal pole of the scaphoid is improved by excision of the volar tubercle of the trapezium. The hand is then replaced in traction. The arthroscope is placed in the

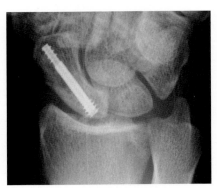

Figure 39–12 Headless compression screw fixation. A headless screw can be placed antegrade or retrograde across the fracture after it is reduced arthroscopically.

4-5 portal. A 1-2 portal is created under direct visualization, and the target hook of the compression jig is introduced and centered on the dorsal proximal scaphoid. The guide barrel is placed on the exposed volar distal scaphoid, and the jig is compressed. A guide pin can now be placed, with a second pin added to control rotation. A drill and tap are placed over the central pin, and an appropriately sized screw is placed across the fracture. Reduction is confirmed arthroscopically and fluoroscopically.[10,15]

Postoperative Management

Patients are immobilized in a splint for 7 to 10 days. At that point, dressings and sutures are removed, and the patient is placed in a forearm-based thumb spica splint. Early protected active range of motion is begun at 2 to 3 weeks. Full resumption of forceful or athletic activities is allowed only after confirmation of fracture healing by computed tomography scan. This usually takes a minimum of 3 to 4 months.

Results

Percutaneous screw fixation of the scaphoid has been shown to lead to more rapid union and faster return to activities than immobilization alone.[1] Whipple[20] originally reported uncomplicated union of 19 of 20 arthroscopically treated scaphoid fractures at 1 year.

Complications

Complications generally involve injury to the radial artery and superficial branch of the radial nerve during placement of the 1-2 portal. Careful patient selection and attention to reduction and the details of fracture fixation can avoid these risks.

References

1. Auge WK 2nd, Velazquez PA: The application of indirect reduction techniques in the distal radius: The role of adjuvant arthroscopy. Arthroscopy 16:830-835, 2000.
2. Bienz T, Raphael JS: Arthroscopic resection of the dorsal ganglia of the wrist. Hand Clin 15:429-434, 1999.
3. Geissler WB: Arthroscopic treatment of intra-articular distal radius fractures. Atlas Hand Clin 2:97-124, 1997.
4. Geissler WB, Freeland AE: Arthroscopically assisted reduction of intraarticular distal radial fractures. Clin Orthop 327:125-134, 1996.
5. Geissler WB, Haley T: Arthroscopic management of scapholunate instability. Atlas Hand Clin 6:253-274, 2001.
6. Geissler WB, Hammit MD: Arthroscopic aided fixation of scaphoid fractures. Hand Clin 17:575-588, 2001.
7. Kozin SH: The role of arthroscopy in scapholunate instability. Hand Clin 15:435-444, 1999.
8. Luchetti R, Badia A, Alfarano M: Arthroscopic resections of dorsal wrist ganglia and treatment of recurrences. J Hand Surg [Am] 25:38-40, 2000.
9. Osterman AL, Raphael JS: Arthroscopic resection of dorsal ganglion of the wrist. Hand Clin 11:7-12, 1995.
10. Plancher KD: Arthroscopic reduction internal fixation of the scaphoid. Atlas Hand Clin 6:325-332, 2001.
11. Ritter MR, Chang DS, Ruch DS: The role of arthroscopy in the treatment of lunotriquetral ligament injuries. Hand Clin 15:445-454, 1999.
12. Ruch DS, Bowling J: Arthroscopic assessment of carpal instability. Arthroscopy 14:675-681, 1998.
13. Ruch DS, Poehling GG: Arthroscopic management of partial scapholunate and lunotriquetral injuries of the wrist. J Hand Surg [Am] 21:412-417, 1996.
14. Singh D, Osterman AL: Arthroscopic ganglion resection. Atlas Hand Clin 6:359-369, 2001.
15. Taras JS, Sweet S, Shum W, et al: Percutaneous and arthroscopic screw fixation of scaphoid fractures in the athlete. Hand Clin 15:467-473, 1999.
16. Tolan S, Savoie FH 3rd, Field LD: Arthroscopic management of lunotriquetral instability. Atlas Hand Clin 6:275-283, 2001.
17. Weiss AP, Akelman E, Lambiase R: Comparison of the findings of triple-injection cinearthrography of the wrist with those of arthroscopy. J Bone Joint Surg Am 78:348-356, 1996.
18. Weiss AP, Sachar K, Glowacki KA: Arthroscopic debridement alone for intercarpal ligament tears. J Hand Surg [Am] 22:344-349, 1997.
19. Westkaemper JG, Mitsionis G, Giannakopoulos PN, Sotereanos DG: Wrist arthroscopy for the treatment of ligament and triangular fibrocartilage complex injuries. Arthroscopy 14:479-483, 1998.
20. Whipple TL: The role of arthroscopy in the treatment of intra-articular wrist fractures. Hand Clin 11:13-18, 1995.
21. Whipple TL: The role of arthroscopy in the treatment of scapholunate instability. Hand Clin 11:37-40, 1995.
22. Wolfe SW, Easterling KJ, Yoo HH: Arthroscopic-assisted reduction of distal radius fractures. Arthroscopy 11:706-714, 1995.

Endoscopic Carpal Tunnel Release

CHARLOTTE SHUM AND ANDREW J. WEILAND

ENDOSCOPIC CARPAL TUNNEL RELEASE IN A NUTSHELL

History:
Pain and paresthesias along median nerve distribution at night and with repetitive activities; numbness and tingling in palmar radial three and a half digits

Physical Examination:
Tinel sign (tapping over volar wrist leads to paresthesias); Phalen sign (60 seconds of wrist flexion leads to paresthesias); decreased sensation and thenar atrophy

Electrodiagnostic Testing:
Abnormal sensory latency greater than 3.5 msec; motor latency greater than 4.5 msec; asymmetry between hands greater than 0.5 msec for sensory conduction or 1 msec for motor conduction

Indications:
Persistent symptoms failing conservative treatment (nonsteroidal anti-inflammatory drugs, injections, splinting); axonal loss as noted by electrodiagnostic testing or by physical exam findings—constant numbness, persistent or progressive symptoms for more than 1 year, loss of sensibility, weakness or thenar atrophy

Contraindications:
Inflammatory synovitis or arthritis, bony deformity, anatomic abnormalities, carpal canal masses, median nerve lesions, small hands, tight canals, stiff wrists, recurrent carpal tunnel syndrome

Surgical Technique:
One- or two-portal technique

Postoperative Management:
Volar splint for 7 days; immediate finger flexion and extension, wrist flexion and digital flexion; scar desensitization

Results:
Similar to open surgery, but with less early postoperative pain and morbidity, less pillar pain

Complications:
Nerve injury, neurapraxia, pillar pain, incomplete release

In 1854, Paget described a patient with an enlarged median nerve at the entrance of the carpal canal and associated adhesions; this patient was managed with amputation of the arm because of unrelenting pain and sensory dysfunction secondary to a fracture of the distal radius.[3,27,29,34] Putnam[42] in 1880 and Pierre Marie and Foix[41] in 1913 described the clinical picture of carpal tunnel syndrome, and Brain et al.[7] in 1947 detailed the surgical treatment of the condition in six patients. The surgical treatment of carpal tunnel syndrome, however, was not generally accepted until the publication of a series of articles by Phalen[35-40] beginning in 1950.

Currently, carpal tunnel syndrome is recognized as the most common entrapment neuropathy,[33] affecting an estimated 1% of the adult population and 5% of the working population in the United States.[20,31] Carpal tunnel release is the most commonly performed operation in the field of hand surgery and is also one of the most successful. A study in Maine revealed this procedure to be the sixth most common outpatient ambulatory surgery procedure, translating to about 400,000 carpal tunnel releases in the United States each year.[23] The estimated economic costs exceed $2 billion a year.[30]

History

The diagnosis of carpal tunnel syndrome can be strongly suggested by the patient's history. Carpal tunnel syndrome is a symptom complex resulting from compression of the median nerve within the carpal tunnel at the level of the wrist (Fig. 40–1). It is characterized by pain and paresthesias along the median nerve distribution during the night and also during repetitive activities. Numbness and tingling are experienced in the palmar radial three and a half digits, although some patients may complain of numbness extending to the ulnar digits or radiating proximal to the wrist as well.[47,48,53] Weakness and clumsiness of the hand are frequently reported.

In the past, the typical carpal tunnel patient was a postmenopausal woman; however, more recently, a younger population of patients has emerged. The sex distribution in this group is equal, and their symptoms emerge during manual labor and resolve with rest. Their jobs often consist of repetitive tasks requiring wrist flexion or gripping with exposure to vibration.[50]

In the workup of carpal tunnel syndrome, thoracic outlet syndrome, cervical pathology, pronator syndrome, and other possible causes of median nerve compression must be considered and ruled out.

Physical Examination

Physical examination findings confirm the patient's symptoms. Provocative tests assist in the diagnosis by producing paresthesias in the median nerve distribution. The Tinel sign is present if light tapping at the volar wrist elicits paresthesias in the median nerve–innervated digits. The Phalen test is positive if pain or paresthesias develop after 60 seconds when the wrists are dropped into a flexed position while the elbows rest on a table with the forearms vertical. A Tinel sign at the wrist is specific for carpal tunnel syndrome in patients with positive Phalen tests.[21,22] The Durkan median nerve compression test, which is both sensitive and specific for carpal tunnel syndrome, is positive if symptoms arise after 30 seconds of sustained direct pressure applied by the examiner's thumbs over the median nerve just proximal to the distal wrist crease.[9]

Tests for sensory and motor loss also aid in the diagnosis. Decreased sensation in the median nerve

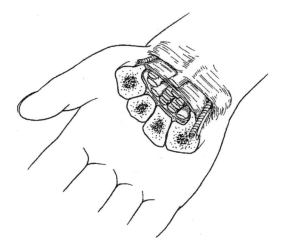

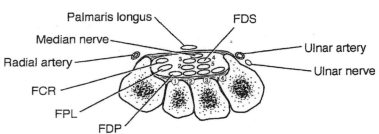

Figure 40–1 Cross section of wrist anatomy. The median nerve lies under the transverse carpal ligament, which bridges radially from the scaphoid tuberosity and trapezial beak to the pisiform and hook of the hamate ulnarly. FCR, flexor carpi radialis; FDP, flexor digitorum profundus; FDS, flexor digitorum superficialis; FPL, flexor pollicis longus.

distribution and thenar atrophy occur in the later stages of carpal tunnel syndrome. Testing sensibility to light touch by stroking the fingers with a piece of cotton and comparing one to another reveals hypesthesia in the median (not ulnar) distribution.[4,25] Sensation in the palm and thenar eminence remains normal because innervation is provided by the palmar cutaneous branch of the median nerve. Threshold testing, including Semmes-Weinstein monofilaments or vibrometry, is sensitive in evaluating compression neuropathies because these tests can detect gradual changes in nerve function as more nerve fibers are lost. Innervation-density tests, such as static and moving two-point discrimination tests, are more appropriate for the assessment of nerve regeneration after nerve repair; results are often normal in mild to moderate cases of carpal tunnel syndrome.[4,6]

Motor weakness is more subjective and more difficult to assess. Flattening of the thenar eminence indicates atrophy of the median nerve–innervated abductor pollicis brevis. The strength of the abductor pollicis brevis, the most superficial muscle of the thenar eminence, is examined by palpation during active opposition or resisted palmar abduction of the thumb against the examiner's finger.

In questionable cases, a steroid injection is often diagnostic as well as therapeutic.[19] Green[19] also found that improvement after injection was correlated with a good response to surgery in 94% of patients. A 2-mL equal-part mixture of 1 mL corticosteroid and 1 mL of lidocaine (Xylocaine) can be injected with a 25-gauge needle inserted at a 45-degree angle proximal to the distal wrist crease and ulnar to the palmaris longus, taking care to redirect the needle if paresthesias are experienced. Poor response to injection, however, did not correlate with poor response to surgery.

Electrodiagnostic Testing

Electrodiagnostic testing is considered the gold standard and can provide objective evidence of median nerve pathology.[24,33] It can be used to confirm the diagnosis as well as to provide information about prognosis.[25] The electromyogram is most useful when trying to differentiate carpal tunnel syndrome from cervical radiculopathy or thoracic outlet syndrome.[49] Positive nerve conduction velocities demonstrate increased latencies and are up to 90% sensitive and 60% specific.[51] Sensory conduction studies are more likely to show early abnormality. Abnormal values include distal sensory latencies greater than 3.5 msec, distal motor latencies greater than 4.5 msec, and asymmetry between hands of more than 0.5 msec for sensory conduction and more than 1 msec for motor conduction.[18] False-negative results can occur in younger patients as well as in patients with mild or exertion-related cases of carpal tunnel syndrome. A negative electrodiagnosic test does not rule out carpal tunnel syndrome in the presence of clinical signs and symptoms. Moreover, if a patient has a history and physical examination consistent with carpal tunnel syndrome, it is not necessary to order electrical studies.[25]

Imaging

Radiographic imaging is of limited value in the evaluation of upper extremity neuropathies. Wrist radiographs may be taken to evaluate for malunion, Kienböck disease, and arthritis in patients with a relevant history.[5] If carpal tunnel release is to be performed endoscopically, radiographs are recommended to look for bony abnormalities. Patients with radicular symptoms warrant radiographic workup of the cervical spine. If there is concern about brachial plexus pathology or a Pancoast tumor, a chest radiograph may be of help.

Treatment

Nonoperative management should be initiated in all patients except those with severe disease. Treatment includes anti-inflammatory medication and wrist splinting in the neutral position at night and during symptom-provoking activities. Modification of activities and of the work environment can also be beneficial.[16] Steroid injection provides transitory relief in up to 80% of patients, although only 22% remain symptom free after 18 months (Fig. 40–2).[15,16]

Surgical management should be undertaken when conservative measures fail or when patients present with

4 Wrist and Hand

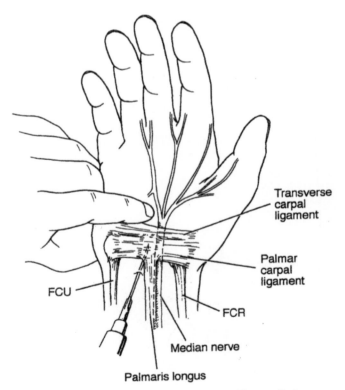

Figure 40–2 Carpal tunnel steroid injection. The needle is inserted at a 45-degree angle from proximal to distal, just proximal to the distal wrist crease and ulnar to the palmaris longus. The needle should be redirected if paresthesias are elicited. FCR, flexor carpi radialis; FCU, flexor carpi ulnaris.

findings consistent with axonal loss—constant numbness, persistent or progressive symptoms for longer than 1 year, loss of sensibility, and weakness or thenar atrophy.[22] Moreover, a recent study by Gerritsen et al.[17] comparing splinting with surgery for relief of carpal tunnel syndrome reinforced previous findings that although splinting can effectively manage early symptoms, it is ineffective for long-term treatment. The patients treated with carpal tunnel release had better long-term outcomes than did those treated with splinting alone.

Surgery can be performed using either open or endoscopic release techniques. Although open carpal tunnel release has been the preferred method, it is associated with prolonged scar tenderness, weakness of grip, and pillar pain in the first 6 months postoperatively.[26,46] Endoscopic carpal tunnel release was introduced to reduce the postoperative morbidity reported with open release. Its potential advantages include decreased postoperative pain, less scarring, and decreased loss of grip strength allowing an earlier return to work.[11,12] Disadvantages include a higher risk of injury to the median nerve, superficial palmar arch, and tendons.[22,28]

The use of endoscopic techniques requires comprehensive knowledge of the relevant anatomy as well as specialized training.[43] A laboratory bioskills course with cadaveric specimens is strongly advised. Ideal candidates for endoscopic treatment have a diagnosis of *idiopathic* carpal tunnel syndrome. Contraindications include patients with inflammatory synovitis or arthritis or bony deformity secondary to fracture or dislocation. Patients with congenital anatomic abnormalities (e.g., abnormal hook of the hamate), carpal canal masses, median nerve lesions, small hands, very tight carpal canals, stiff wrists, or recurrent carpal tunnel syndrome after release are also contraindicated. Patients should give consent for both endoscopic and open carpal tunnel release, and the surgeon should be prepared to convert to an open procedure if visualization problems are encountered secondary to fogging, equipment malfunction, inability to remove synovium from the transverse carpal ligament (TCL), or atypical anatomy.

There are two methods of endoscopic carpal tunnel release: a one-portal technique developed by Agee,[1] and a two-portal technique developed by Chow.[10]

Surgical Technique

Agee Single-Portal Technique

This surgery can be performed with the patient under regional or general anesthesia, although more experienced surgeons may perform it using local anesthesia. If local anesthesia is used, approximately 4 mL of 1% lidocaine without epinephrine is injected subcutaneously in line with the proximal wrist crease extending from the flexor carpi ulnaris to the flexor carpi radialis. Injecting deep to the forearm fascia is not recommended because the anesthetic will fill the carpal canal and possibly compromise the endoscopic view of the TCL.

A tourniquet is used. Before tourniquet elevation, surgical landmarks should be marked. These include the flexor carpi ulnaris, flexor carpi radialis, and palmaris longus tendons, as well as the pisiform and hook of the hamate (Fig. 40–3A). A 1.5- to 2-cm transverse incision is marked in line with the proximal wrist crease between the flexor carpi ulnaris and flexor carpi radialis, centered over the palmaris longus if present (Fig. 40–3B). A longitudinal line should also be drawn from the center of the wrist flexion crease (over the proposed incision) to

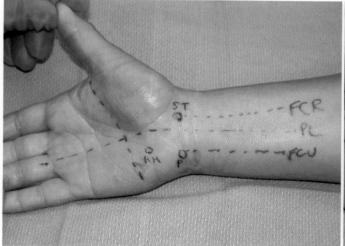
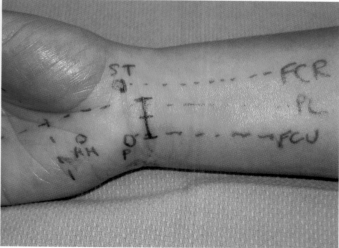

A   B

Figure 40–3 *A,* Surgical landmarks, including the flexor carpi ulnaris (FCU), flexor carpi radialis (FCR), palmaris longus (PL), pisiform (P), and hook of the hamate (HH), as well as a longitudinal dotted line in line with the base of the ring finger and a transverse line along the distal border of the fully abducted thumb (Kaplan's cardinal line). *B,* A 15- to 20-mm transverse incision is marked in the proximal wrist crease between the FCU and FCR, centered over the PL if present. (Courtesy of Kawaljit S. Gill, MD.)

the palmar base of the ring finger. This is the trajectory for the instrument and should lie radial to the hook of the hamate.

The MicroAire Carpal Tunnel Release System includes the handpiece and disposable blade assembly, eyepiece endoscope, synovial elevator, and small and standard hamate finders (Fig. 40–4). The sterile field should also include two double-pronged skin hooks, two Ragnell right-angle retractors, Adson tissue forceps, tenotomy scissors, and a number 15 blade.

An Esmarch is used to exsanguinate the limb, and the tourniquet is inflated to 250 mm Hg. The incision is made as previously marked, centered over the volar wrist between the flexor carpi ulnaris and flexor carpi radialis, through skin only. The subcutaneous tissues are bluntly dissected down to the antebrachial fascia, taking care to preserve cutaneous nerves by spreading longitudinally. The palmaris longus is retracted radially to protect the palmar cutaneous branch of the median nerve. A U-shaped incision is made in the forearm fascia to create a 10- by 10-mm distally based flap that is retracted distally with a skin hook to expose the underlying median nerve (Fig. 40–5).[44] A tenotomy scissors is then used to gently spread and separate the fascia from the underlying ulnar bursae. The synovial elevator is inserted in line with the base of the ring finger and is used to separate the synovium from the undersurface of the TCL. A "washboard effect" is felt as the transverse fibers of the TCL are rasped across with the elevator.

With the wrist slightly extended, the hamate finders are sequentially passed distally, aiming at the base of the ring finger, to create a space for the blade assembly (Fig. 40–6). The hamate finder is passed along the ulnar aspect of the tunnel, hugging the radial aspect of the hook of the hamate, until it can be palpated subcutaneously distal to the TCL. Care is taken not to pass distal to the Kaplan cardinal line to protect the superficial

palmar arch, which is located about 2 to 2.5 cm distal to the hook of the hamate.[44]

After creation of a passageway for the blade assembly with one or two passes of the hamate finders, the device can be inserted into the carpal tunnel. With the non-scope hand, the wrist is held in slight extension, with the surgeon's thumb placed in the palm to palpate the distal extent of the TCL as well as the tip of the blade assembly. The device is then introduced and advanced while aiming at the base of the ring finger, hugging the hook of the hamate, and pressing the viewing window tightly against the underside of the TCL to protect the median nerve (Fig. 40–7). The fibers of the TCL are visualized immediately upon introduction. If the fibers are not apparent, the surgeon should clear synovium from the ligament again. The surgeon must confirm and plainly visualize the location of the TCL or else convert to an open release.

The device is inserted until its tip is just distal to the distal end of the TCL (Fig. 40–8). A Ragnell retractor is used to protect the skin distal to the incision during ligament release. The blade is then elevated, and the device is pulled back proximally to divide the TCL under direct visualization (Fig. 40–9). More than one pass may be required to divide the ligament (Fig. 40–10). Partial blade elevation can be useful during subsequent passes for ligament division while protecting more palmar structures. Elevation of the blade distal to the Kaplan cardinal line may injure the superficial palmar arch or the common digital nerve to the ring and long fingers. The device should be reinserted to inspect ligament division. A U-shaped defect with wide separation of the cut edges indicates complete ligament transection. A V-shaped defect indicates remaining intact fibers of the TCL.

After complete release, the device is removed, and the antebrachial fascia proximal to the skin incision is divided approximately 2 to 3 cm with tenotomy scissors

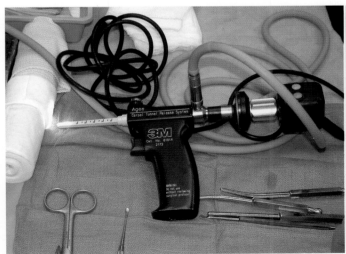
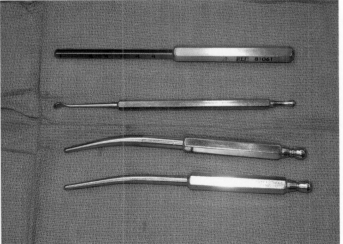

A   B

Figure 40–4 *A,* MicroAire Carpal Tunnel Release System. The handpiece, blade assembly, and endoscope are fully assembled and checked for correct operation, which includes blade elevation and retraction and clear video image. *B,* MicroAire instruments. From top to bottom: blade-shaped hamate finder, synovium elevator, standard hamate finder, and small hamate finder. (Courtesy of Kawaljit S. Gill, MD.)

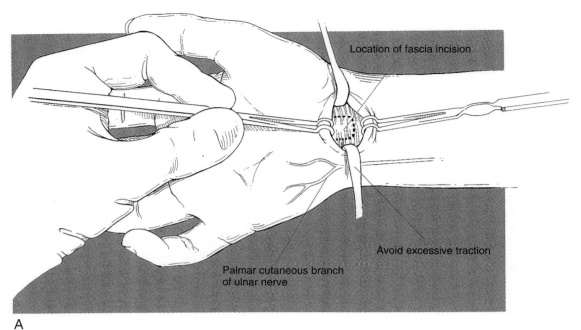

Location of fascia incision

Avoid excessive traction

Palmar cutaneous branch
of ulnar nerve

A

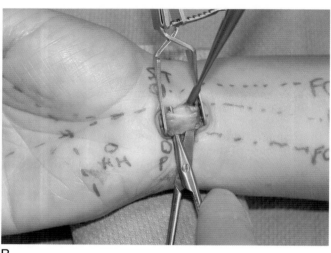

B

Figure 40–5 *A*, A U-shaped incision is made in the forearm fascia to create a distally based flap. *B*, The forearm fascia is elevated longitudinally before making a transverse incision. (Courtesy of Kawaljit S. Gill, MD.)

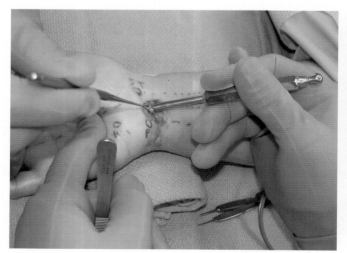

Figure 40–6 The hamate finder dilates the carpal canal and creates a path for the endoscopic device. (Courtesy of Kawaljit S. Gill, MD.)

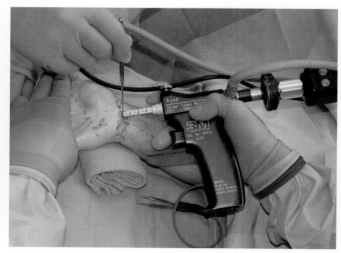

Figure 40–7 The endoscopic device is inserted and held snugly against the underside of the transverse carpal ligament, aiming at the base of the ring finger and hugging the hook of the hamate. (Courtesy of Kawaljit S. Gill, MD.)

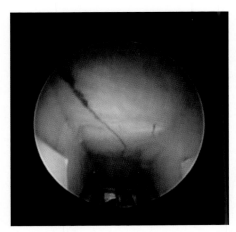

Figure 40–8   The distal end of the transverse carpal ligament is visualized before blade elevation. (Courtesy of Kawaljit S. Gill, MD.)

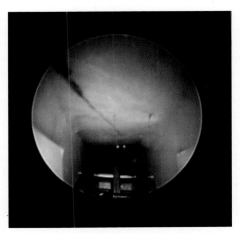

Figure 40–9   With no intervening structures between the device and the ligament, the blade is elevated and pulled proximally to divide the ligament. (Courtesy of Kawaljit S. Gill, MD.)

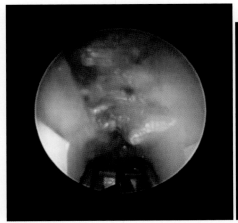

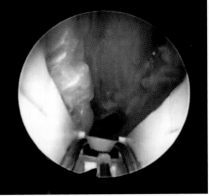

A   B

Figure 40–10   *A*, First pass, with incomplete release. More than one pass may be required to divide the ligament. *B*, Complete release. The two cut edges of the ligament have retracted beyond the width of the blade assembly. (Courtesy of Kawaljit S. Gill, MD.)

4 Wrist and Hand

under direct vision (Fig. 40–11). The device is reinserted into the carpal tunnel distal to the ligament to look for arterial bleeders. The tourniquet is deflated, and the device is slowly withdrawn. After hemostasis is obtained, the skin is closed with 5-0 nylon or a running subcuticular stitch. A sterile dressing is placed, and a volar splint is applied, keeping the fingers free for motion.

Chow Two-Portal Extrabursal Technique

This procedure is performed with a tourniquet, intravenous sedation, and local anesthesia (1% lidocaine without epinephrine) administered subcutaneously proximal to the entry portal.[14] A 4-mm, 30-degree rigid endoscope with a light bar situated on the same side as the direction of view is required. A slotted cannula houses the camera and holds the instrument in the carpal canal during the procedure. A curved synovial elevator-dissector and a ridged obturator trocar tip are additional instruments designed by Chow and available from Smith and Nephew Dyonics. There is also a synovial

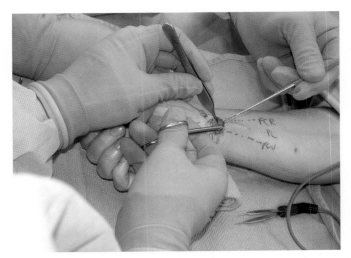

Figure 40–11   Release of the forearm fascia. (Courtesy of Kawaljit S. Gill, MD.)

elevator-like tip for the ridged trocar that allows one to clear the canal and place the trocar in one step. Three disposable knives (probe knife, triangle knife, and hook knife) are used to divide the ligament through the slotted cannula. A hand-holder device stabilizes the wrist in extension during the procedure. A superficial palmar arch depressor, the "Chow catcher," is used to depress the superficial arch in the palm while passing the trocar tip past the arch.

The entry portal is located ulnar to the median nerve and radial to the ulnar neurovascular bundle (Fig. 40–12). The pisiform is palpated, and a 10- to 12-mm transverse line is drawn from the midpoint of the pisiform perpendicular to the long axis of the forearm. A second 5-mm line is drawn from the radial terminus of the first line perpendicular to the first line and directed proximally. A third line measuring 10 to 12 mm is drawn from the proximal terminus of the second line perpendicular to both the second line and the long axis of the forearm directed radially. This transverse third line is the entry portal, and it should be in line with the radial border of the fourth ray, ulnar to the palmaris longus.

The incision is made through skin only. Subcutaneous veins are retracted or coagulated. The flexor retinaculum is identified and divided in line with the incision. A Ragnell retractor or skin hook is used to elevate the distal edge of the retinaculum (Fig. 40–13). The curved synovial elevator is then passed radial to the hook of the hamate and used to clear the synovium away from the undersurface of the TCL. Passing the tip of the dissector along the undersurface of the TCL produces the "washboard effect" as the transverse fibers are rasped. This ensures proper placement, because scraping Guyon's canal or the subcutaneous space would not produce this effect. Alternatively, the curved dissector-obturator and slotted cannula assembly can be introduced and used to push synovium from the underside of the TCL.

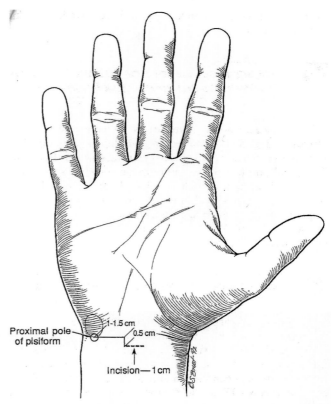

Figure 40–12 Chow two-portal endoscopic technique. The entry portal is located by drawing a 10- to 12-mm transverse line radially from the pisiform and a second 5-mm line proximally and longitudinally from the end of the first line. A third line (the entry portal), measuring 10 to 12 mm directed transversely, is drawn radially from the end of the second line.

Figure 40–13 A Ragnell retractor is used to elevate the distal edge of the flexor retinaculum.

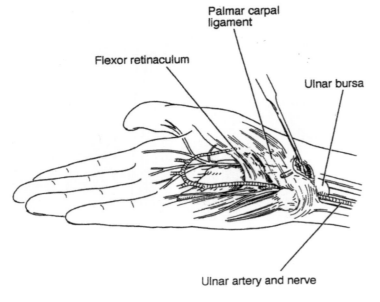

The slotted cannula–ridged trocar assembly is inserted into the proximal portal and advanced distally, hugging the hook of the hamate with the nose of the device against the undersurface of the TCL. The surgeon must be mindful not to force the tip of the trocar through the forearm fascia or the TCL.

The exit portal is established first by drawing the Kaplan cardinal line (distal border of the fully abducted thumb) and a longitudinal line from the third web space (Fig. 40–14). A line that bisects the angle formed by these two lines is then drawn and extended proximally and ulnarly 1 cm. A small 5-mm incision is made at this site, and the slotted cannula–trocar assembly is passed through the incision.

The wrist and metacarpophalangeal joints are now extended and strapped to the hand holder. The assembly device lies parallel to the fourth ray. The trocar tip should be passed superficial to the superficial palmar arch. Placing the palmar arch depressor distal to the exit portal and using it to depress the soft tissues while the trocar is passed can be helpful (Fig. 40–15). This also protects the surgeon's thumb from injury by the tip of the trocar. The ridged obturator trocar is then removed, and the endoscope is inserted proximally to visualize the TCL (Fig. 40–16). If there are intervening tissues that obscure the fibers of the TCL, the scope is withdrawn, and the ridged trocar is replaced. The slotted sheath or

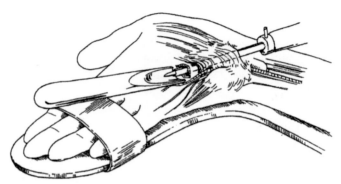

Figure 40–15   The slotted cannula–ridged trocar assembly is advanced distally under the transverse carpal ligament, hugging the hook of the hamate in line with the fourth ray. A superficial palmar arch depressor is used to depress the palmar arch as the trocar is passed through the exit portal.

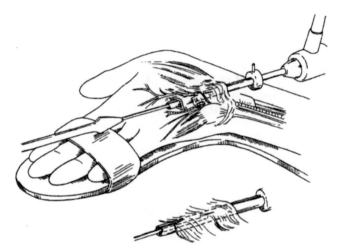

Figure 40–16   With the hand placed in hyperextension by hand-holder device, the endoscope is placed in the slotted cannula through the proximal portal. The probe knife is inserted in the distal portal for forward cutting of the distal edge of the transverse carpal ligament, after making sure that there are no intervening tissues obscuring visualization of the ligament.

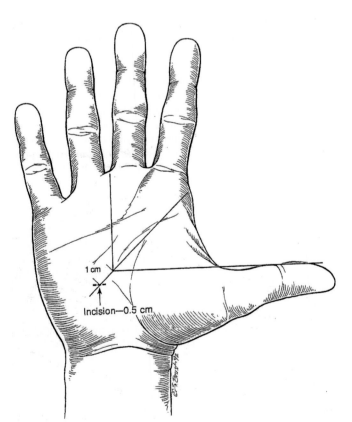

Figure 40–14   The exit portal is established by drawing a line that bisects the angle formed by the distal border of the fully abducted thumb and the third web space, about 10 mm proximally and ulnarly.

assembly device can be rotated 5 to 10 degrees ulnarly; if this approach fails, the device should be removed, and synovial elevation with subsequent trocar–slotted cannula insertion can be repeated. If, after a second attempt, visualization is still not successful, conversion to an open procedure is recommended.

With the endoscope inserted in the entry portal, the distal edge of the TCL is identified for division. The probe knife is inserted through the distal portal to palpate the TCL and to cut the distal 5 to 6 mm of the ligament with its forward-cutting blade. The triangle knife replaces the probe knife in the exit portal and is used to make a fenestration in the middle of the TCL. It is subsequently turned ulnarly and withdrawn. All blades are inserted with the tip turned toward the ulnar aspect of the canal. The tip is then rotated toward the ligament and is visible through the slotted cannula. Last, a hook or retrograde knife, which has a blunt tip to avoid injury

4 Wrist and Hand

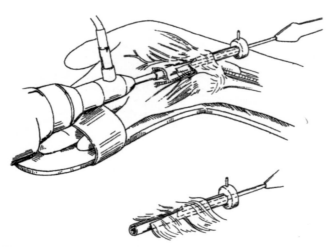

Figure 40-17 After releasing the distal half of the ligament, the endoscope is moved to the distal portal, and the retrograde knife is used to release the proximal half of the ligament from the proximal portal.

to blood vessels in the subcutaneous space, is passed. This knife is inserted into the fenestration and is pulled distally (cutting proximal to distal) to release the distal TCL. The scope is then placed in the distal (exit) portal of the slotted cannula, and the hook knife is inserted into the entry portal and used to release the remaining TCL from distal to proximal (Fig. 40-17).

The retrograde knife is removed, and a probe is placed to check under direct vision the complete release of the TCL. A gap between the cut edges of the TCL indicates complete division. The endoscope can then be removed from the exit portal, placed back into the proximal portal, advanced to the distal end of the slotted cannula, and withdrawn proximally as a unit while viewing the cut edges of the ligament and the intervening gap. A retractor can be placed into the proximal portal, and complete release can be visualized directly under loupe magnification.

The tourniquet is released, and hemostasis is obtained with electrocautery. The wound is irrigated by squirting fluid from the entry portal, which egresses from the distal portal. Simple sutures of 5-0 nylon are used to close the incisions.

Postoperative Management

There is no single correct method of managing patients postoperatively. A volar splint may be applied, with encouragement of digital range of motion during the first week. Finger flexion and extension allow for nerve gliding and prevent nerve entrapment in the scar. The patient can then remove the dressing, cover the wound with an adhesive bandage, and begin wrist range of motion. Simultaneous wrist flexion and digital flexion are avoided initially to prevent bowstringing of tendons at the wrist. Scar massage for desensitization is begun by the patient after 2 weeks. Heavy lifting and pushing with the palm are avoided for the first 3 weeks.

Results

The advantages of endoscopic surgery are achieved by avoiding an incision through the palmar skin, cutaneous neurovascular structures, palmar fascia, and palmaris brevis. Patients have decreased scar tenderness, pillar pain, weakness, and bowstringing, and they return to work earlier.

In 1992, Agee et al.[2] reported a randomized, prospective trial with a 6-month follow-up. Patients with single-portal endoscopic release returned to work a median of 21 days sooner than did open-release patients. Although early postoperative pain and morbidity were diminished, at 6 weeks postoperatively, the results were comparable to those of standard open carpal tunnel release. Two patients required additional open release; one of these had an initial incomplete release. Two patients also had transient ulnar nerve neurapraxia.

In 1993, Brown et al.[8] published a prospective, randomized study with an 84-day follow-up. They reported less scar tenderness and earlier return to work (median 14 days versus 28 days) after two-portal endoscopic carpal tunnel release compared with open release. Four complications occurred: one partial transection of the superficial palmar arch, one digital nerve contusion, one ulnar nerve neurapraxia, and one wound hematoma.

The same year, Palmer et al.[31] compared single- and double-portal endoscopic carpal tunnel release with open release in a prospective, nonrandomized study with a 6-month follow-up. Endoscopic release patients had a faster recovery of strength and range of motion and less midpalm scar tenderness. In this study, patients returned to work sooner with endoscopic release and soonest after Agee release.

In the most recent randomized, prospective study, published by Trumble et al.[52] in 2002, endoscopic release resulted in greater symptom relief, function improvement, and patient satisfaction in the first 3 months after surgery. Patients also returned to work earlier. No complications with endoscopic release occurred in this study.

Complications

Major injuries to the median and ulnar nerves, flexor tendons, and superficial palmar arch have been reported with endoscopic release.[28] However, since their initial introduction, both single- and double-portal endoscopic techniques have been modified, resulting in much safer procedures today. Injury to both the median and ulnar nerves has occurred with all carpal tunnel release techniques (including open release). Most injuries, however, are neurapraxias that resolve. Although pillar pain and palmar tenderness have been reduced, they have not been eliminated with endoscopic release. Cadaver studies demonstrated incomplete release of the TCL in up to 50% of the specimens,[45] although clinically, patients may still get symptomatic relief.

The learning curve for endoscopic carpal tunnel release is steep, and experience decreases the risk of complications. Endoscopic carpal tunnel release is safest when performed by a surgeon who is trained in the technique and performs the procedure frequently.[13]

References

1. Agee JM, McCarroll HR, North ER: Endoscopic carpal tunnel release using the single proximal incision technique. Hand Clin 10:647-659, 1994.
2. Agee JM, McCarroll HR Jr, Tortosa RD, et al: Endoscopic release of the carpal tunnel: A randomized prospective multicenter study. J Hand Surg [Am] 17:987-995, 1992.
3. Akelman E, Weiss AP: The etiology of and surgical options for carpal tunnel syndrome. Curr Opin Orthop 5:8-15, 1994.
4. Bell-Krotoski J, Weinstein S, Weinstein C: Testing sensibility, including touch-pressure, two-point discrimination, point localization, and vibration. J Hand Ther 6:114-123, 1993.
5. Bindra RR, Evanoff BA, Chough LY, et al: The use of routine wrist radiography in the evaluation of patients with carpal tunnel syndrome. J Hand Surg [Am] 22:115-119, 1997.
6. Borg K, Lindblom U: Diagnostic value of quantitative sensory testing (QST) in carpal tunnel syndrome. Acta Neurol Scand 78:537-541, 1988.
7. Brain WR, Wright AD, Wilkinson M: Spontaneous compression of both median nerves in the carpal tunnel: Six cases treated surgically. Lancet 1:277-282, 1947.
8. Brown RA, Gelberman RH, Seiler JG 3rd, et al: Carpal tunnel release: A prospective, randomized assessment of open and endoscopic methods. J Bone Joint Surg Am 75:1265-1275, 1993.
9. Bruske J, Bednarski M, Grzelec H, Zyluk A: The usefulness of the Phalen test and the Hoffmann-Tinel sign in the diagnosis of carpal tunnel syndrome. Acta Orthop Belg 68:141-145, 2002.
10. Chow JC: Endoscopic carpal tunnel release: Two-portal technique. Hand Clin 10:637-646, 1994.
11. Chow JC: Endoscopic carpal tunnel release. Clin Sports Med 15:769-784, 1996.
12. Delaere O, Bouffioux N, Hoang P: Endoscopic treatment of the carpal tunnel syndrome: Review of the recent literature. Acta Chir Belg 100:54-57, 2000.
13. Einhorn N, Leddy JP: Pitfalls of endoscopic carpal tunnel release. Orthop Clin North Am 27:373-380, 1996.
14. Fischer TJ, Hastings H 2nd: Endoscopic carpal tunnel release: Chow technique. Hand Clin 12:285-297, 1996.
15. Gelberman RH, Aronson D, Weisman MH: Carpal-tunnel syndrome: Results of a prospective trial of steroid injection and splinting. J Bone Joint Surg Am 62:1181-1184, 1980.
16. Gerritsen AA, de Krom MC, Struijs MA, et al: Conservative treatment options for carpal tunnel syndrome: A systematic review of randomised controlled trials. J Neurol 249:272-280, 2002.
17. Gerritsen AA, de Vet HC, Scholten RJ, et al: Splinting vs surgery in the treatment of carpal tunnel syndrome: A randomized controlled trial. JAMA 288:1245-1251, 2002.
18. Glowacki KA, Breen CJ, Sachar K, Weiss AP: Electrodiagnostic testing and carpal tunnel release outcome. J Hand Surg [Am] 21:117-121, 1996.
19. Green DP: Diagnostic and therapeutic value of carpal tunnel injection. J Hand Surg [Am] 9:850-854, 1984.
20. Hulsizer DL, Staebler MP, Weiss AP, Akelman E: The results of revision carpal tunnel release following previous open versus endoscopic surgery. J Hand Surg [Am] 23:865-869, 1998.
21. Kanaan N, Sawaya RA: Carpal tunnel syndrome: Modern diagnostic and management techniques. Br J Gen Pract 51:311-314, 2001.
22. Katz JN, Simmons BP: Clinical practice: Carpal tunnel syndrome. N Engl J Med 346:1807-1812, 2002.
23. Keller RB, Largay AM, Soule DN, Katz JN: Maine Carpal Tunnel Study: Small area variations. J Hand Surg [Am] 23:692-696, 1998.
24. Kilmer DD, Davis BA: Electrodiagnosis in carpal tunnel syndrome. Hand Clin 18:243-255, 2002.
25. Kulick RG: Carpal tunnel syndrome. Orthop Clin North Am 27:345-354, 1996.
26. Kuschner SH, Brien WW, Johnson D, Gellman H: Complications associated with carpal tunnel release. Orthop Rev 20:346-352, 1991.
27. Lin R, Lin E, Engel J, Bubis JJ: Histo-mechanical aspects of carpal tunnel syndrome. Hand 15:305-309, 1983.
28. Muller LP, Rudig L, Degreif J, Rommens PM: Endoscopic carpal tunnel release: Results with special consideration to possible complications. Knee Surg Sports Traumatol Arthrosc 8:166-172, 2000.
29. Paget J: Lectures on Surgical Pathology. Philadelphia, Lindsey & Blakiston, 1854, p 40.
30. Palmer DH, Hanrahan LP: Social and economic costs of carpal tunnel surgery. Instr Course Lect 44:167-172, 1995.
31. Palmer DH, Paulson JC, Lane-Larsen CL, et al: Endoscopic carpal tunnel release: A comparison of two techniques with open release. Arthroscopy 9:498-508, 1993.
32. Palumbo CF, Szabo R: M. Examination of patients for carpal tunnel syndrome sensibility, provocative, and motor testing. Hand Clin 18:269-277, 2002.
33. Patiala H, Rokkanen P, Kruuna O, et al: Carpal tunnel syndrome: Anatomical and clinical investigation. Arch Orthop Trauma Surg 104:69-73, 1985.
34. Pfeffer GB, Gelberman RH, Boyes JH, Rydevik B: The history of carpal tunnel syndrome. J Hand Surg [Br] 13:28-34, 1988.
35. Phalen GS: The carpal-tunnel syndrome: Seventeen years' experience in diagnosis and treatment of six hundred fifty-four hands. J Bone Joint Surg Am 48:211-228, 1966.
36. Phalen GS: The diagnosis of carpal tunnel syndrome. Cleve Clin Q 35:1-6, 1968.
37. Phalen GS: Reflections on 21 years' experience with the carpal-tunnel syndrome. JAMA 212:1365-1367, 1970.
38. Phalen GS: The carpal-tunnel syndrome: Clinical evaluation of 598 hands. Clin Orthop 83:29-40, 1972.
39. Phalen GS: The birth of a syndrome, or carpal tunnel revisited. J Hand Surg [Am] 6:109-110, 1981.
40. Phalen GS, Gardner WR, La'Londe AA: Neuropathy of the median nerve due to compression beneath the transverse carpal ligament. J Bone Joint Surg Am 30:109-112, 1950.
41. Pierre Marie M, Foix C: Atrophie isolee de l'eminence thenar d'origine nevritique. Role du ligament annulaire anterieur du carpe dans la pathogenie de la lesion. Rev Neurol 26:647-649, 1913.
42. Putnam J: A series of cases of paraesthesia—mainly of the hand—of periodic occurrence and possibly of vasomotor origin. Arch Med 4:147, 1880.
43. Rotman MB, Donovan JP: Practical anatomy of the carpal tunnel. Hand Clin 18:219-230, 2002.
44. Ruch DS, Poehling GG: Endoscopic carpal tunnel release: The Agee technique. Hand Clin 12:299-303, 1996.
45. Seiler JG 3rd, Barnes K, Gelberman RH, Chalidapong P: Endoscopic carpal tunnel release: An anatomic study of the two-incision method in human cadavers. J Hand Surg [Am] 17:996-1002, 1992.
46. Seradge H, Seradge E: Piso-triquetral pain syndrome after carpal tunnel release. J Hand Surg [Am] 14:858-862, 1989.

4 Wrist and Hand

47. Shum C, Parisien M, Strauch RJ, Rosenwasser MP: The role of flexor tenosynovectomy in the operative treatment of carpal tunnel syndrome. J Bone Joint Surg Am 84:221-225, 2002.
48. Slater RR Jr: Carpal tunnel syndrome: Current concepts. J South Orthop Assoc 8:203-213, 1999.
49. Slater RR Jr, Bynum DK: Diagnosis and treatment of carpal tunnel syndrome. Orthop Rev 22:1095-1105, 1993.
50. Szabo RM: Carpal tunnel syndrome as a repetitive motion disorder. Clin Orthop 351:78-89, 1998.
51. Szabo RM, Slater RR Jr: Diagnostic testing in carpal tunnel syndrome. J Hand Surg [Am] 25:184, 2000.
52. Trumble TE, Diao E, Abrams RA, Gilbert-Anderson MM: Single-portal endoscopic carpal tunnel release compared with open release: A prospective, randomized trial. J Bone Joint Surg Am 84:1107-1115, 2002.
53. Werner RA, Andary M: Carpal tunnel syndrome: Pathophysiology and clinical neurophysiology. Clin Neurophysiol 113:1373-1381, 2002.

Arthroscopy of the First Carpometacarpal Joint

BASSEM T. ELHASSAN AND MARK H. GONZALEZ

ARTHROSCOPY OF THE FIRST CARPOMETACARPAL JOINT IN A NUTSHELL

History:
Documented progressive pain at the base of the first carpometacarpal (CMC) joint exacerbated by grasping, pinching, and thumb motion

Physical Examination:
Loss of abduction of the CMC joint and compensatory metacarpophalangeal joint hyperextension; reproduction of pain with the grind test (simultaneous passive compression and rotation of the CMC joint)

Imaging:
Anteroposterior, lateral, oblique, and stress views of the CMC joint
Robert view—taken with the forearm fully pronated, the shoulder internally rotated, and the thumb abducted—shows a true anteroposterior view of the CMC joint articulation

Indications:
Early osteoarthritis, post-traumatic degeneration of the CMC joint, Bennett fracture

Contraindications:
Cellulitis about the hand and thumb, complete ankylosis of the CMC joint, previous surgery about the joint

Surgical Technique:
Diagnostic arthroscopy: evaluate the articular surface of the joint and the joint ligament, and look for loose bodies; in case of fracture, intra-articular involvement and degree of displacement can be ascertained
Arthroscopic debridement: synovectomy and washing of the trapeziometacarpal (TM) joint, as well as removal of loose bodies
Capsular shrinkage: using an electrothermal probe, the capsule and the ligaments of the TM joint can be painted to effect capsular shrinkage
Reduction of intra-articular fracture: the joint is visualized, and fracture reduction is checked after applying 5 to 7 pounds of traction; K-wires can be used as joysticks to align fragments and to pin the reduction
Arthroscopic trapeziectomy: partial or complete resection or the trapezium is performed with a power bur
Interposition arthroplasty: flexor carpi radialis or palmaris longus autograft is interposed in the CMC joint after resection of the trapezium; an absorbable suture is tied to one end of the tendon graft, and the tendon is pulled inside the joint with the use of a large curved needle and then packed

Postoperative Management:
Simple debridement: early postoperative range of motion
Trapeziectomy and interposition arthroplasty: immobilization in a thumb spica for 3 weeks, then range of motion and strengthening of the thumb
Fracture fixation: immobilization in a thumb spica for 6 weeks, then range of motion and strengthening of the thumb

The thumb is one of the most important parts of the hand and plays a pivotal role in its complex function. It has adapted to support and serve each finger individually in grasping and precise manipulation. It imparted power and strength to the hand, which is why it was titled "pollis" by Charles Bell in 1833.[10] It made the human hand highly complex by allowing great mobility and prehensile activities. This high level of functioning necessitated the sacrifice of bony stability for mobility. Added to this are the high compression forces transmitted from the tip through the length of the thumb and magnified across the basal joint, which makes this joint highly prone to develop arthritis.

Besides arthritis, many other problems can affect the thumb basal joint, including instability, fracture, and dislocation, which may compromise the thumb's function and result in significant impairment. Surgical intervention, including arthrotomy, is required in many of these conditions. However, arthrotomy of the first carpometacarpal (CMC) joint may result in significant morbidity because of the need to perform extensile approaches for exposure, with the risk of disrupting the surrounding ligaments.

Arthroscopy of the thumb CMC joint was introduced by Menon[23] in 1996. Since that time, only a few surgical procedures have been performed arthroscopically on the thumb CMC joint with good results reported for the management of CMC arthritis.

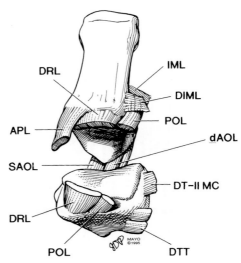

Figure 41–1 The first carpometacarpal (CMC) joint, open from the dorsum to show the deep anterior oblique ligament (dAOL), or beak ligament, lying within the joint ulnar to the volar tubercle of the metacarpal. The rest of the ligaments are the dorsotrapeziotrapezoid (DTT), superficial anterior oblique (SAOL), dorsoradial (DRL), posterior oblique (POL), intermetacarpal (IML), dorsal intermetacarpal (DIML), dorsal trapezio-II metacarpal (DT-II MC), and abductor pollicis longus (APL) tendon. (From Bettinger P, Linscheid R, Berger R, et al: An anatomic study of the stabilizing ligaments of the trapezium and trapeziometacarpal joint. J Hand Surg [Am] 24:786-798, 1999.)

Anatomy and Biomechanics

As the human hand climbed the evolutionary ladder, the stability of the base of the thumb was compromised in the interest of mobility and the refinement of a dominant prehensile digit.[27] The trapeziometacarpal (TM) joint of the human's simian ancestors functioned as a single-axis hinge, allowing only flexion-extension of the thumb in the plane of the palm. This may explain why there was no evidence of degenerative arthritis upon dissecting these joints. The acquisition of a functional universal joint in the TM articulation, along with muscles to provide active apposition, completed the development of the human thumb. The thumb TM joint is reciprocally biconcave, with the dorsoradial articular facet having significantly less depth than the ulnar-volar facet, leading to substantially more dependence on capsular stability (Fig. 41–1).[10]

The thumb is positioned in approximately 80 degrees of pronation relative to the plane of the hand.[19] The combination of this position of the thumb and the bony anatomy of the TM and metacarpophalangeal joints allows apposition—a combined motion of extension, abduction, and rotation.

The anatomic relationships and position of the structures superficial to the capsule of the TM joint are as follow (Fig. 41–2). The tendons of the first and third compartments pass superficial to the joint dorsoradially and dorsally, respectively. In addition, two or three branches of the superficial radial nerve and the radial artery pass superficial to the TM joint.[14]

There are 16 deep ligaments that stabilize the trapezium and the TM joint. Seven of these ligaments are direct stabilizers of the TM joint, and the remaining nine ligaments stabilize the trapezium itself, as reported by Berger and Bettinger.[3] The trapezium is located at the radial aspect of the wrist, with no bony radial stabilizers, and it lacks a fixed axial base of support because of a mobile scaphoid, which makes it inherently unstable. The ligaments surrounding the trapezium are essential stabilizers of this bone, which sustains high axial and cantilever bending loads during pinch and grasp (Figs. 41–3 and 41–4).[4,7,11,22,25]

From a geometric point of view, the TM joint is also inherently unstable because the width of the thumb metacarpal is 34% greater than the width of the trapezium, and the ligaments surrounding the joint are essential in providing a stable, mobile joint.[3] The seven ligaments that stabilize the TM joint are the superficial anterior oblique ligament (SAOL), deep anterior oblique ligament (DAOL), dorsoradial ligament (DRL), posterior oblique ligament (POL), ulnar collateral ligament (UCL), intermetacarpal ligament (IML), and dorsal intermetacarpal ligament (DIML).[5,8,15,18,21,24,26,30]

The SAOL is a capsular ligament that originates from the volar tubercle of the trapezium, 0.5 mm proximal to the articular surface, and inserts broadly across the volar-ulnar aspect of the first metacarpal, distal to the articular margin of the volar styloid process (Fig. 41–5; see Fig. 41–1). The SAOL is superficial to the DAOL. Its anatomic position neither stabilizes the TM joint in flexion nor prevents dorsal metacarpal

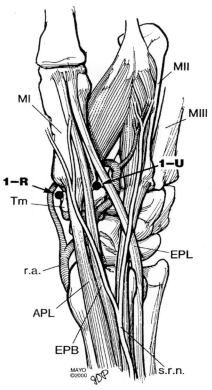

Figure 41-2 The anatomic relationships and position of the structures superficial to the capsule of the trapeziometacarpal joint. 1-R and 1-U are the radial and ulnar portals for the first carpometacarpal joint, respectively. APL, abductor pollicis longus; EPB, extensor pollicis brevis; EPL, extensor pollicis longus; MI, II, and III, first, second, and third metacarpals; r.a., radial artery; s.r.n., branches of the superficial radial nerve; Tm, trapezium. (Copyright Mayo Clinic, 2000.)

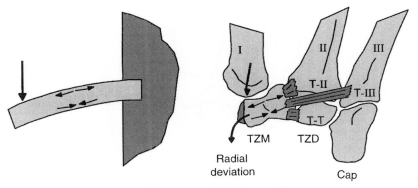

Figure 41-3 The principle of cantilever bending. The trapezium (TZM) is fixed on its ulnar aspect to the carpus and second and third metacarpals and is loaded in a dorsoradial direction by the first metacarpal. This is similar to a diving board that is fixed at one end and loaded at the opposite end. The dorsal and volar trapezio-II and -III metacarpals (T-II and T-III) function as tension bands to support the trapezium against the cantilever bending forces. Cap, capitate; T-T, trapeziotrapezoid; TZD, trapezoid. (From Bettinger P, Linscheid R, Berger R, et al: An anatomic study of the stabilizing ligaments of the trapezium and trapeziometacarpal joint. J Hand Surg [Am] 24:786-798, 1999.)

4 Wrist and Hand

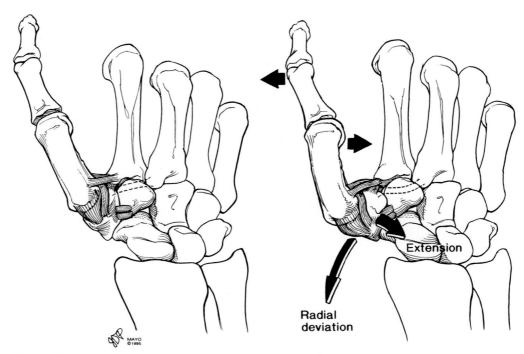

Figure 41–4 Ligamentous laxity of the ligaments restraining the trapezium and first carpometacarpal joint leads to extension and radial deviation of the trapezium due to cantilever bending forces. (From Bettinger P, Linscheid R, Berger R, et al: An anatomic study of the stabilizing ligaments of the trapezium and trapeziometacarpal joint. J Hand Surg [Am] 24:786-798, 1999.)

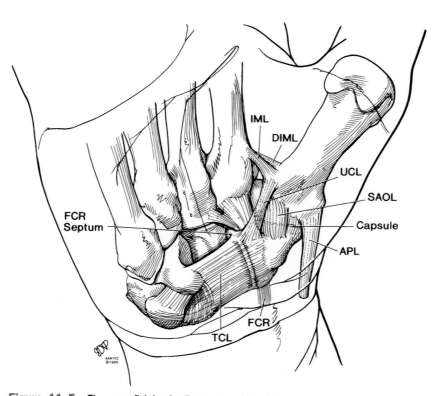

Figure 41–5 The superficial volar ligaments of the first carpometacarpal joint and the trapezium. APL, abductor pollicis longus tendon; DIML, dorsal intermetacarpal ligament; FCR, flexor carpi radialis tendon; IML, intermetacarpal ligament; SAOL, superficial oblique anterior ligament; TCL, transverse carpal ligament; UCL, ulnar collateral ligament. (From Bettinger P, Linscheid R, Berger R, et al: An anatomic study of the stabilizing ligaments of the trapezium and trapeziometacarpal joint. J Hand Surg [Am] 24:786-798, 1999.)

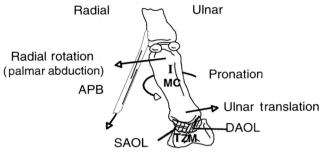

Figure 41–6 The deep anterior oblique ligament (DAOL) serves as a pivot point for the first carpometacarpal joint and plays a role in first metacarpal (I MC) pronation. The abductor pollicis brevis (APB) abducts the thumb. SAOL, superficial anterior oblique ligament; TZM, trapezium. (From Bettinger P, Linscheid R, Berger R, et al: An anatomic study of the stabilizing ligaments of the trapezium and trapeziometacarpal joint. J Hand Surg [Am] 24:786-798, 1999.)

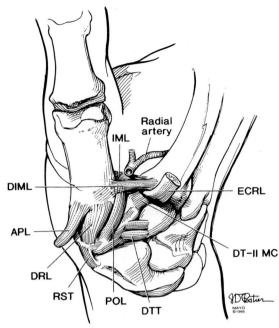

Figure 41–7 The first carpometacarpal joint and trapezial ligaments seen from a dorsoradial view. APL, abductor pollicis longus tendon; DIML, dorsal intermetacarpal ligament; DRL, dorsoradial ligament; DT-II MC, dorsal trapezio-II metacarpal ligament; DTT, dorsal trapeziotrapezoid; ECRL, extensor carpi radialis longus; IML, intermetacarpal ligament; POL, posterior oblique ligament; RST, radial scaphotrapezial. (From Bettinger P, Linscheid R, Berger R, et al: An anatomic study of the stabilizing ligaments of the trapezium and trapeziometacarpal joint. J Hand Surg [Am] 24:786-798, 1999.)

subluxation. Its laxity allows a significant amount of rotation before acting as a constraint. In flexion, it limits only pronation; in extension, it limits both pronation and supination.

The DAOL, or beak ligament, is an intra-articular ligament located deep to the SAOL (see Fig. 41–1). It originates from the base of the first metacarpal (beak), just ulnar to the volar styloid, and inserts onto the volar central apex of the trapezium, just ulnar to the ulnar edge of the trapezoid ridge. The DAOL shares responsibility with the SAOL for stabilizing the volar metacarpal against subluxation. It serves as a pivot for rotation, especially pronation, to produce apposition (Fig. 41–6). Moreover, it prevents ulnar subluxation of the base of the thumb metacarpal toward the index metacarpal with continued abduction loading (see Fig. 41–3).

The DRL is the second thickest and widest ligament (after the transcarpal ligament) attaching to the trapezium. It is the shortest ligament spanning the TM joint (Fig. 41–7; see Fig. 41–1). It is capsular and fan shaped, originating from the dorsoradial tubercle of the trapezium, and inserts onto the dorsal edge of the base of the thumb metacarpal. It merges with the POL at its ulnar margin. The DRL becomes taut with supination and pronation when the TM joint is flexed and with dorsal or dorsoradial subluxating forces in all TM positions except full extension.

The POL is a capsular ligament that originates on the dorsoulnar side of the trapezium and inserts onto the dorsoulnar aspect of the thumb metacarpal and the palmar-ulnar tubercle, along with the IML (see Figs. 41–1 and 41–7). It is taut in wide apposition, abduction, and supination and resists ulnar translation of the metacarpal base during apposition and abduction.

The UCL is an extracapsular ligament that typically overlaps the SAOL by 2 to 3 mm. It originates from the distal margin of the transcarpal ligament, on the trapezoid ridge, and inserts onto the palmar-ulnar tubercle of the thumb metacarpal along with the IML, superficial and ulnar to the SAOL (see Fig. 41–5). The UCL is taut in abduction, pronation, and extension, and it limits volar subluxation of the thumb metacarpal.

The IML is an extracapsular ligament that originates from the dorsoradial aspect of the index metacarpal, radial to the extensor carpi radialis longus insertion, and inserts onto the palmar-ulnar tubercle of the base of the thumb, along with the UCL and POL (see Figs. 41–5 and 41–7). It is taut in supination, abduction, and opposition and stabilizes the metacarpal against radiovolar translation of its base.

The DIML is an extracapsular ligament that originates from the dorsoradial tubercle of the index metacarpal, superficial to the extensor carpi radialis longus insertion, and inserts onto the dorsoulnar corner of the thumb metacarpal (see Fig. 41–7). It functions primarily as a constraint against metacarpal pronation.

First Carpometacarpal Joint Diseases

The TM joint is an incongruent, semiconstrained saddle joint with biconcavoconvex articulation, with the axis of the saddles perpendicular to each other.[1,6,21] This articulation allows flexion-extension, abduction-adduction, and apposition-circumduction.

Many disease entities may affect the first CMC joint, including idiopathic arthritis, post-traumatic arthritis resulting from chronic ligamentous instability or malunited fractures, rheumatoid arthritis, fracture, dislocation, instability, infection, and tumor.[9,21] The most common disease entity that affects the first CMC joint is idiopathic arthritis that involves mostly postmenopausal women.

As suggested by Linscheid,[22] the cantilever bending forces on the trapezium may increase the tangential dorsoradial subluxating force, contributing to cartilage erosion and degeneration (see Fig. 41–4). Several authors[16,20,31] have reported that the essential lesion contributing to progressive deterioration of the TM joint cartilage in idiopathic arthritis is attenuation of the DAOL.

Classification of Osteoarthritis of the First Carpometacarpal Joint

Various classifications based on clinical instability and radiographic findings have been described.[5,12] Eaton and Littler[12] described four stages, based on radiographic findings:

Stage I: Normal joint contours and less than one-third joint subluxation.
Stage II: Arthritis with small bone or calcific fragments smaller than 2 mm; greater than one-third joint subluxation.
Stages III and IV: Advanced arthritis.

Another classification reported by Burton[5] is based on findings from the clinical examination and plain radiographs:

Stage I: Joint laxity and pain with heavy or repetitive use. The joint is hypermobile on physical examination. Radiographs show minimal change.
Stage II: Crepitance and instability on physical examination. Radiographs show cartilage loss, especially in the volar compartment of the TM joint.
Stages III and IV: Similar to Eaton and Littler's classification, representing advanced stages of arthritis.

History

Patients with first CMC joint arthritis typically present with pain localized to the base of the thumb exacerbated by pinching and repetitive motion of the involved thumb. An accurate diagnosis of first CMC joint arthritis is important when considering treatment options, because there are many other painful conditions that cause pain at the base of the thumb or on the radial side of the wrist. These conditions include carpal tunnel syndrome, de Quervain tenosynovitis, scaphoid fracture or nonunion, and radioscaphoid and scaphotrapezial arthritis.[10,28]

Physical Examination

The physical examination is characterized by pain over the radiovolar aspect of the TM joint, with laxity and exacerbation of pain upon radial or sometimes dorsal stress. Abduction may be limited or painful; otherwise, the range of motion is functional. The grind test, consisting of compression and passive motion of the TM joint, might be positive, and there is usually mild crepitance with reproduction of the pain. Many patients with first CMC joint arthritis experience a compensatory metacarpophalangeal motion, so this joint should be examined for a hyperextension deformity.[13]

Imaging

The radiographic evaluation of the first CMC joint should include anteroposterior, lateral, and oblique views. Arthritic changes, including spurs, osteophytes, and joint damage, are useful to diagnose for operative planning. The Robert view is a special view taken with the forearm fully pronated, the shoulder internally rotated, and the thumb abducted; it shows a true anteroposterior view of the CMC joint articulation.

In the normal thumb, the longitudinal axis of the metacarpal approximately bisects the trapezium. With laxity, the longitudinal axis shifts radially and may even sit outside the radial margin of the trapezium, especially if the thumb is stressed. Stress views are sometimes indicated and are performed by stressing the joint radially with an ulnarly directed pressure. This view demonstrates the radial subluxation of the thumb metacarpal out of the trapezial saddle with laxity.[10]

Treatment Options

Similar to the treatment of other arthritic joints, the first line of treatment for first CMC joint arthritis consists of anti-inflammatory medications, intra-articular steroid injections, and immobilization with a thumb spica splint. Most patients respond to this modality. For patients who fail to respond adequately, surgical management is indicated. Open surgical procedures include ligament reconstruction, as described by Eaton and Littler,[12] with transfer of the flexor carpi radialis tendon for patients with ligamentous laxity and early arthritic changes. Other surgical procedures include trapeziectomy and hematoma arthroplasty,[17] osteotomy of the first metacarpal,[29] and trapeziometacarpal fusion for young, high-demand patients.

Arthroscopic evaluation and management of TM joint arthritis was introduced by Menon[23] and Berger.[2] It is an exciting alternative to surgical management for patients with stage I or II arthritis. Exploration, debridement, and synovectomy can be accomplished arthroscopically. Arthroscopy addresses both the inflammatory and the ligamentous components of the problem. Radiofrequency energy can be used for capsular shrinkage. Partial and complete trapeziectomy, depending on the arthroscopic appearance of the scaphotrapeziotrapezoid joint, can also be performed arthroscopically in patients with advanced osteoarthritis.[23]

Indications

1. Post-traumatic arthritis
2. Idiopathic arthritis—stages I and II
3. Idiopathic arthritis—end stage
4. Intra-articular (Bennett) fracture, which can be managed with arthroscopically assisted reduction and internal fixation

Contraindications

1. Ehlers-Danlos syndrome or collagen disease
2. Metacarpophalangeal joint hyperextension
3. TM joint overlying skin cellulitis
4. Raynaud syndrome

Surgical Technique

The operating room setup is similar to that for elective wrist arthroscopy. The patient is placed in the supine position with the affected arm at a right angle to the body. A light and power source, television monitor, video tape recorder, and power shaver should be positioned separately on the table opposite the surgeon. A tourniquet is placed on the upper arm and is preset to 250 mm Hg. Anesthesia is administered in the same manner as for other upper extremity arthroscopic procedures and is currently limited to either regional or general anesthesia. A single dose of antibiotics is generally administered immediately before the procedure.

The arm is scrubbed and draped in the usual manner. Using a sterile Chinese finger trap, 5 pounds of traction is applied to the thumb (Fig. 41–8A). The landmarks for the arthroscopic portals are determined by palpating and marking the TM joint, the proximal posterior edge of the base of the first metacarpal, the radial artery, and the tendons of the abductor pollicis longus and extensor pollicis brevis. The tourniquet is inflated to 250 mm Hg. Then the joint is entered through two portals: the 1-R (radial) and the 1-U (ulnar) portals (Fig. 41–8B).

According to the anatomic study by Gonzalez et al.,[14] creation of the entry sites is safer if one makes a 4- to 5-mm longitudinal incision just palmar and radial to the abductor pollicis longus tendon and a second incision just ulnar to the extensor pollicis brevis tendon (see Figs.

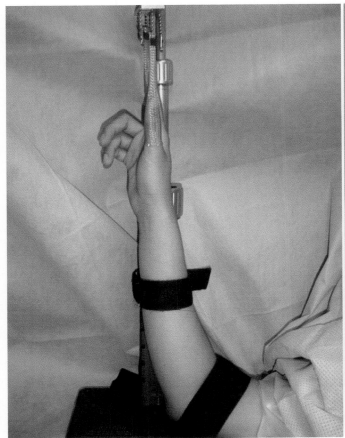 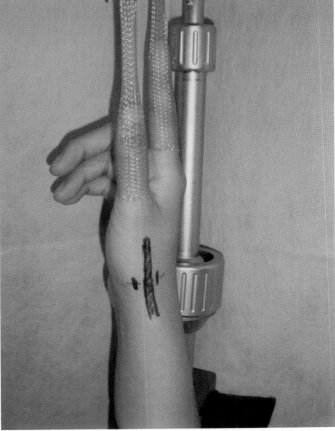

A B

Figure 41–8 The hand is mounted on a special hand tower, with Chinese finger traps used to pull on the thumb and index finger. Weight is added as needed, usually 5 pounds. *A,* The setup. *B,* Landmarks for the portals. The first extensor compartment is marked, and the two portals are located radial (**1-R**) and ulnar (**1-U**) to it.

4 Wrist and Hand

41–2 and 41–8*B;* Figs. 41–9 through 41–11). Blunt subcutaneous dissection exposes the capsule to protect nearby neurovascular structures. The arthroscopic portal is usually the ulnar portal, and the working portal is the volar portal, but either one can be used to visualize the different TM joint ligaments. The 1-U portal is preferred to visualize the DRL, POL, and UCL[31] (Fig. 41–12).

To estimate the angle of entry, a 20-gauge needle is advanced into the joint, demonstrating the level of the base of the first metacarpal through the planned portal site. The joint is then distended with 0.9% NaCl (normal saline). A skin incision is made over the markings with a number 11 blade. Blunt dissection using a small hemostat, particularly on the dorsal side, is performed to protect the sensory branch of the radial nerve and the dorsal branch of the radial artery. Once the joint capsule is encountered, a blunt obturator and cannula are used to enter the joint, followed by a 2-mm arthroscope.

The joint is continuously irrigated through the arthroscope using normal saline and a small joint pump. Initially, it is difficult to achieve good visualization because of the arthritic changes in the joint. A 1.9-mm synovial resector is introduced, and the hypertrophied synovium is removed to gain better visualization.

The surgeon then systematically inspects the joint, interchanging the portals to inspect the entire joint. The base of the first metacarpal is identified by moving the thumb. The trapezium is inspected from ulnar to radial, followed by the oblique ligament, which is identified on the volar aspect. The dorsal ligaments can be inspected on the dorsoradial aspect of the joint. Using a probe, the integrity of the different ligaments is determined. Any loose body can be easily removed using an arthroscopic grasper. Debridement and drilling can be performed for mild stage I or II arthritis of the joint.

If the arthritis affecting the joint is advanced, with the majority of the articular surface eburnated, at least half of the distal trapezium is resected from medial to lateral using a 2.9-mm round bur. Care is taken not to damage the volar oblique ligament. Sufficient bone, usually 3 or 4 mm, is removed to expose the cancellous subchondral region. All loose fragments are removed by continuous irrigation and suction.

Fascia lata allograft, a Gore-Tex cardiovascular patch, or autogenous tendons (flexor carpi radialis or palmaris longus) can be used as interposition material, as described by Menon.[23] The surgical steps are the same, regardless of the interposition material. Gore-Tex is usually folded to form a 5- by 15-mm tape.

The palmaris longus tendon, or three quarters of the flexor carpi radialis tendon, is procured by multiple transverse incisions. An absorbable suture is tied to one end of the tendon graft. The other end of the suture is swaged onto a large, curved needle. The dorsal portal is enlarged using skin hooks. The large needle is passed through the opening in the dorsal capsule and brought through the joint. The volar capsule and thenar musculature are pierced, and the needle is pulled over the thenar eminence. By pulling on the suture, one can introduce the end of the tendon into the joint. The

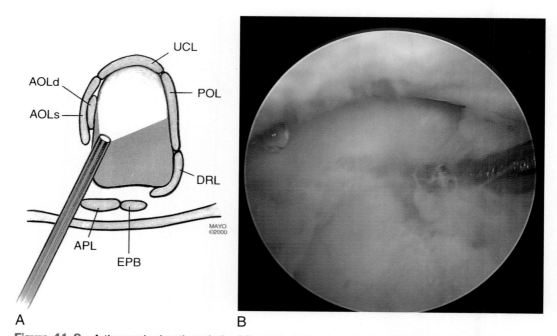

Figure 41–9 Arthroscopic view through the 1-R portal. A, Drawing of an intra-articular view of the first carpometacarpal joint and ligament. The light area represents the ligaments that are well visualized through this portal. B, The same view seen through an arthroscope. AOLd, deep anterior oblique ligament; AOLs, superficial anterior oblique ligament; APL, abductor pollicis longus; DRL, dorsoradial ligament; EPB, extensor pollicis brevis; POL, posterior oblique ligament; UCL, ulnar collateral ligament. (A from Bettinger P, Berger R: Functional ligamentous anatomy of the trapezium and trapeziometacarpal joint [gross and arthroscopic]. Hand Clin 17:151-168, 2001.)

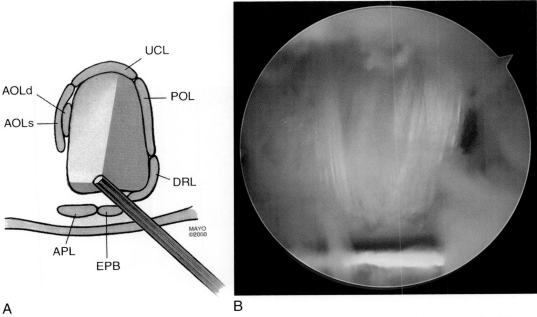

Figure 41–10   Arthroscopic view of the anterior margin of the first carpometacarpal joint through the 1-U portal. A, Drawing showing the superficial anterior oblique ligament (AOLs) and the radial border of the deep anterior oblique ligament (AOLd). B, Arthroscopic view of the structures visible in A. APL, abductor pollicis longus; DRL, dorsoradial ligament; EPB, extensor pollicis brevis; POL, posterior oblique ligament; UCL, ulnar collateral ligament. (A from Bettinger P, Berger R: Functional ligamentous anatomy of the trapezium and trapeziometacarpal joint [gross and arthroscopic]. Hand Clin 17:151-168, 2001.)

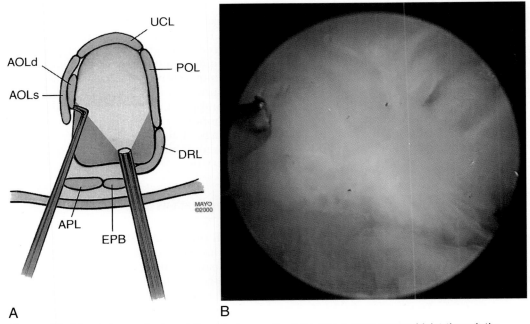

Figure 41–11   Arthroscopic view of the anterior margin of the first carpometacarpal joint through the 1-U portal. A, Drawing showing the ulnar collateral ligament (UCL), superficial anterior oblique ligament (AOLs), and deep anterior oblique ligament (AOLd). B, Arthroscopic view of the structures visible in A. APL, abductor pollicis longus; DRL, dorsoradial ligament; EPB, extensor pollicis brevis; POL, posterior oblique ligament. (A from Bettinger P, Berger R: Functional ligamentous anatomy of the trapezium and trapeziometacarpal joint [gross and arthroscopic]. Hand Clin 17:151-168, 2001.)

4 Wrist and Hand

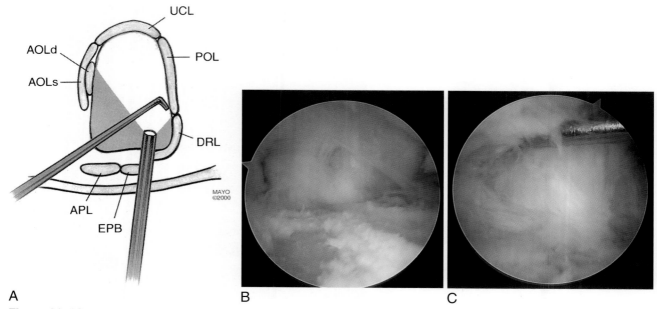

Figure 41-12 Arthroscopic view through the 1-U portal. A, Drawing of an intra-articular view of the first carpometacarpal joint. The 1-U portal is used to visualize the ulnar collateral ligament (UCL), posterior oblique ligament (POL), and dorsoradial ligament (DRL). B and C, Arthroscopic views through the same portal, showing the structures visible in A. AOLd, deep anterior oblique ligament; AOLs, superficial anterior oblique ligament; APL, abductor pollicis longus; EPB, extensor pollicis brevis. (*A* from Bettinger P, Berger R: Functional ligamentous anatomy of the trapezium and trapeziometacarpal joint [gross and arthroscopic]. Hand Clin 17:151-168, 2001.)

remaining portion of the tendon is packed using Adson forceps. The arthroscope is then withdrawn, and the opening of the joint capsule is closed with a single stitch.

At the end of the procedure, traction is relieved, a sterile dressing is applied, the tourniquet is deflated, and a thumb spica splint is applied.

If arthroscopy is being performed for an acute intra-articular fracture, small Kirschner wires (K-wires) are used as joysticks to anatomically reduce fracture fragments under direct visualization before final K-wire fixation.

They recommended a complete arthroscopic trapeziectomy if scaphotrapeziotrapezoid joint arthritis was visualized through a midcarpal portal. Their modified technique included partial or complete resection of the trapezium, pinning of the CMC joint in its anatomic position under fluoroscopic guidance with a 0.045-inch K-wire, and painting of the surrounding joint capsule with a monopolar radiofrequency probe to effect capsular shrinkage. This procedure provided patients with pain relief and stability, with minimal morbidity and a shorter recovery time.

Results

Menon[23] reported 76% complete pain relief in 31 patients (33 hands) who underwent arthroscopic debridement of the first CMC joint, partial resection of the trapezium, and interpositional arthroplasty. The materials he used for interposition were Gore-Tex in 19, palmaris longus in 8, fascia lata (allograft) in 4, and flexor carpi radialis in 2. All patients maintained their preoperative range of motion, were able to touch the base of the little finger with the thumb, had no change in the first web space, and improved their pinch strength from 6 to 11 pounds.

Culp and Rekant[10] reported 88% excellent or good outcomes in 22 patients (24 thumbs) who underwent hemi- or complete trapeziectomy with electrothermal shrinkage for advanced arthritis, followed up to 4 years.

Complications

As with other surgical procedures in the upper extremity, arthroscopy of the first CMC joint is associated with some basic complications. First, the creation or use of arthroscopic portals may cause damage to one or more branches of the superficial radial sensory nerve. This may result in altered sensory function, as well as painful neuroma formation. Second, the radial artery might be inadvertently damaged during the procedure because it courses immediately posterior and ulnar to the arthroscopic field. This may result in loss of perfusion to the thumb or other digits in a hand with radial artery dominance, or in hematoma formation. Third, because the CMC joint is in close proximity to other joints such as the radioscaphoid and scaphotrapezium, inadvertent advancement of the arthroscope into the wrong joint is possible. Other possible complications include a low risk of infection and neurapraxia of any nerve passing under the tourniquet.

These complications can be minimized by a thorough knowledge of the anatomy of the region and an awareness of the location of the branches of the superficial radial nerve and the radial artery. In addition, careful palpation of bony and soft tissue landmarks and the use of blunt dissection are helpful in minimizing complications.

Conclusion

Arthroscopy of the first CMC joint is an appealing alternative to open surgical procedures. It is less invasive, can detect articular damage with excellent visualization long before radiologic changes become evident, the joint capsule is not detached, postoperative pain is significantly less, and patients are discharged the same day. A number of arthroscopic procedures of the first CMC joint have evolved over the past few years, including athroscopic debridement and removal of loose bodies, reduction of intra-articular fracture, capsular shrinkage, and partial or complete trapeziectomy, with good results reported. In other joints of the body, arthroscopy has almost completely replaced open surgical procedures, and the same pattern can be expected for the first CMC joint. However, more studies and published results are needed to validate this technique as a standard procedure for the treatment of the above-mentioned conditions.

References

1. Baratz ME, Klimo GF, Verma RB: The treatment of trapeziometacarpal arthritis with arthrodesis. Hand Clin 17:261-270, 2001.
2. Berger RA: A technique for arthroscopic evaluation of the first carpometacarpal joint. J Hand Surg [Am] 22:1077-1080, 1997.
3. Berger R, Bettinger PC: Functional ligamentous anatomy of the trapeziometacarpal joint (gross and arthroscopic). Hand Clin 17:151-168, 2001.
4. Berger R, Bettinger P, Linscheid R: An anatomic study of the stabilizing ligaments of the trapezium and trapeziometacarpal joint. J Hand Surg [Am] 24:786-798, 1999.
5. Burton RI: Basal joint arthrosis of the thumb. Orthop Clin North Am 4:331-348, 1973.
6. Chamay A, Paget-Morerod F: Arthrodesis of the trapeziometacarpal joint. J Hand Surg [Br] 19:489-497, 1994.
7. Chao EO, Cooney WP: Biomechanical analysis of static forces in the thumb during hand function. J Bone Joint Surg 59:27-36, 1977.
8. Cooney W, Imaeda T: Anatomy of trapeziometacarpal ligaments. J Hand Surg 18:226-231, 1993.
9. Culp RW, Osterman AL: Arthroscopic evaluation and treatment of thumb carpometacarpal joints. Atlas Hand Clin 2:23-28, 1997.
10. Culp RW, Rekant MS:. The role of arthroscopy in evaluating and treating trapeziometacarpal disease. Hand Clin 17:315-319, 2001.
11. Eaton R, Littler J: A study of the basal joint of the thumb: Treatment of its disabilities by fusion. J Bone Joint Surg 55:1655-1666, 1969.
12. Eaton RG, Littler JW: Ligament reconstruction for the painful thumb carpometacarpal joint. J Bone Joint Surg 55:1655-1666, 1973.
13. Glickel SZ: Clinical assessment of the thumb trapeziometacarpal joint. Hand Clin 17:185-195, 2001.
14. Gonzalez MH, Kemmler J, Rinella A, Weinzweig N: Portals for arthroscopy of the trapeziometacarpal joint. Br Soc Surg Hand 22B:574-575, 1997.
15. Haines R:. The mechanism of rotation of the first carpometacarpal joint. J Anat 78:44-46, 1944.
16. Hollenbreg G, Olcott CW, Pelligrini VD Jr: Contact patterns in the trapeziometacarpal joint: The role of the palmar beak ligament. J Hand Surg [Am] 18:238-244, 1993.
17. Jones NF, Maser BM: Treatment of arthritis of the trapeziometacarpal joint with trapeziectomy and hematoma arthroplasty. Hand Clin 17:237-243, 2001.
18. Kaplan E: Functional and Surgical Anatomy of the Hand, 2nd ed. Philadelphia, JB Lippincott, 1965.
19. Katarincic JA: Thumb kinematics and their relevance to function. Hand Clin 17:169-174, 2001.
20. Kuczynski K: Carpometacarpal joint of the human thumb. J Anat 118:119-126, 1974.
21. Kuczynski K, Lamb DW, Pagalidis T: Ligamentous stability of the base of the thumb. Hand 13:29-35, 1981.
22. Linscheid R: The thumb axis joints: A biomechanical model. In Strickland JE (ed): Difficult Problems in Hand Surgery. St. Louis, Mosby, 1982, pp 169-172.
23. Menon J: Arthroscopic management of the trapeziometacarpal joint arthritis of the thumb. Arthroscopy 12:581-587, 1996.
24. Napier J: The form and function of the carpo-metacarpal joint of the thumb. J Anat 89:362-369, 1955.
25. Napier J: Hands. New York, Pantheon Books, 1980, p 71.
26. Pellegrini V: Osteoarthritis of the trapeziometacarpal joint: The pathophysiology of the articular cartilage degeneration. I. Anatomy and pathology of the aging joint. J Hand Surg 16:967-974, 1991.
27. Pellegrini VD Jr: Pathomechanics of the thumb trapeziometacarpal joint. Hand Clin 17:175-183, 2001.
28. Pomerance J: Painful basal joint arthritis of the thumb. Am J Orthop 24:401-408, 1995.
29. Tomaino MM: Treatment of Eaton stage I trapeziometacarpal disease: Ligament reconstruction or thumb metacarpal extension osteotomy. Hand Clin 17:197-205, 2001.
30. Weitbrecht J: Syndesmology. Philadelphia, WB Saunders, 1969, p 1742.
31. Zaidenberg C, Zancolli EA, Zancolli EA Jr: Biomechanics of the trapeziometacarpal joint. Clin Orthop 220:14-26, 1987.

Arthroscopic Management of Triangular Fibrocartilage Complex Tears

JAMES CHOW AND LEONID I. KATOLIK

ARTHROSCOPIC MANAGEMENT OF TRIANGULAR FIBROCARTILAGE COMPLEX TEARS IN A NUTSHELL

History:
Fall onto pronated, extended wrist or traction to ulnar side of wrist; complaints of ulnar-sided wrist pain

Physical Examination:
Ulnar deviation with axial load elicits pain

Imaging:
Plain radiographs, magnetic resonance imaging, arthrogram, wrist arthroscopy

Indications:
Ulnar-sided wrist pain unresponsive to conservative therapy with arthroscopically proven triangular fibrocartilage complex tear

Contraindications:
Prior open surgery, intra-articular fracture, or anatomic abnormalities may preclude arthroscopic repair

Surgical Technique:
Dependent on type of injury—class I (traumatic) or class II (degenerative); treatment ranges from debridement to arthroscopic repair

Postoperative Management:
Debridement: early mobilization and splinting for comfort
Repair: plaster immobilization in 60 degrees of supination for 4 to 6 weeks

Results:
90% or greater good or excellent

Complications:
Irritation of extensor carpi ulnaris or dorsal sensory branch of ulnar nerve by suture knot, nerve entrapment, motion loss, wound complications

Anatomy and Function

The triangular fibrocartilage complex (TFCC) is the major stabilizer of the distal radioulnar joint and supports the ulnar carpus during axial loading. It is located on the ulnar side of the wrist and is divided into two parts: the articular disk and the ulnocarpal ligaments, which are the ulnolunate and ulnotriquetral ligaments.

The TFCC has various functions of load sharing and joint stabilization through flexion-extension, radial

417

deviation, and pronation-supination. The TFCC acts as an extension of the articular surface of the radius, supports the proximal carpal row, and stabilizes the distal radioulnar joint. The volar carpal ligament assists in limiting wrist extension and radial deviation, as well as stabilizing the volar ulnar aspect of the carpus. Individuals with congenital or acquired positive ulnar variance are subject to unusual compressive loads of the central disk of the TFCC between the head of the ulna and the ulnolunate. This unusual compressive load can result in central wear or tear of the TFCC.

Biomechanics

Approximately 20% of the actual load of the forearm is transferred through the ulnar side of the wrist and through the TFCC. The disk portion of the TFCC has thickening of the volar and dorsal margin, known as the volar and dorsal radioulnar ligaments; they help stabilize the distal radioulnar joint. The axial load applied through the triquetrum and ulnar side of the lunate compresses the central disk of the TFCC, tightening the volar and dorsal aspects of the distal radioulnar joint ligaments. Part of the load is transferred back to the radius through these ligaments. In full pronation, the dorsal capsule of the distal radioulnar joint and the volar distal radioulnar joint ligament become tight. Excessive pronation can rupture the volar distal radioulnar joint ligament or the dorsal capsule, allowing the ulna to translate dorsally from the sigmoid notch. In supination, the converse occurs. The volar distal radioulnar joint capsule and the dorsal distal radioulnar joint ligament tighten. Excessive supination can tear these structures and permit volar translation of the ulna from the sigmoid notch.[9]

History

Obtaining the proper history is necessary to determine the mechanism of injury. Patients typically present after a fall onto a pronated, extended wrist or after a traction injury to the ulnar aspect of the wrist. Patients complain of ulnar-sided wrist pain. Acutely, swelling may be noted about the ulnar wrist.

Physical Examination

The physical examination plays an important role in diagnosing a TFCC injury. Provocative testing is recommended to compress the wrist axially, in the position of ulnar deviation, and grind the TFCC between the lunate and ulna, which may reproduce the pain of a TFCC injury. Depending on the type of injury, complete passive pronation-supination may also reproduce the symptoms.

Imaging

Diagnostic tests, including triple-injection arthrography and magnetic resonance imaging (MRI), can help deter-

mine the extent of a TFCC injury; however, it has been proved by numerous authors that wrist arthroscopy is the most sensitive tool for diagnosing injuries of the TFCC.[1,5,6,8]

Diagnostic imaging should begin with routine zero-rotation posteroanterior and lateral views of the wrist to assess ulnar variance, congruence of the distal radioulnar joint, and the presence of nonunited ulnar styloid fractures. Advanced imaging is fraught with diagnostic uncertainty and is highly user dependent. Triple-injection wrist arthrography has a high rate of false-positive results. Investigators have found only 50% agreement between arthroscopy and arthrography, and arthrography has a poor ability to localize tears. More than 50% of asymptomatic individuals older than 50 years have arthrographically evident tears of the articular disk.

Similarly, MRI of the wrist is highly technique and user dependent. Although MRI is useful for identifying central perforations of the TFCC, investigators have found poor interobserver agreement in the interpretation of MRI scans for TFCC pathology, citing low sensitivity and specificity for the presence of tears, as well as poor tear localization. In addition, signal intensity changes on wrist MRI scans have been reported in up to 50% of normal wrists.

Wrist arthroscopy has emerged as the gold standard for the diagnosis and evaluation of TFCC pathology.

Classification

In 1989, Palmer[4] proposed a classification system for TFCC tears. Basically, this system divides TFCC injuries into two categories: class I traumatic injuries (Table 42–1) and class II degenerative injuries (Table 42–2). For class I injuries, there are four subclassifications that describe the location of the injury. For class II injuries, five subclassifications describe the severity of TFCC wear and arthritic changes to the ulnar side of the wrist.

Clinical Presentation and Treatment

Class I: Traumatic Injuries

Class IA

Class IA tears, or perforations, are horizontal tears of the TFCC that are usually 1 to 2 mm wide and located 2 to 3 mm medial to the radial attachment of the sigmoid notch (Fig. 42–1). The patient usually presents with dorsal tenderness of the distal ulna and pain with pronation-supination. A triple arthrogram may demonstrate dye leaking to the distal radioulnar joint. Debridement to remove the unstable flap of the tear is the preferred treatment. Caution is needed to avoid involving the volar and dorsal radioulnar ligaments, which help to stabilize the distal radioulnar joint.

Class IB

Traumatic avulsions of the TFCC from its insertion into the distal ulna, with or without fracture of the ulnar

Table 42–1
Class I Traumatic Injuries

Subclass	Description	Clinical Presentation	Suggested Treatment
IA	Tears or perforations of horizontal portion of TFCC Usually 1-2 mm wide Dorsal palmar slit located 2-3 mm medial to radial attachment of sigmoid notch	Dorsal tenderness of distal ulna Pain with pronation-supination	Debridement to remove unstable flap, taking care to avoid volar and dorsal radioulnar ligament
IB	Traumatic avulsion of TFCC from insertion into distal ulna May be accompanied by fracture of ulnar styloid at its base Usually associated with distal radiocarpal joint instability	Tenderness around site of 6-U portal Pain may be reproduced with ulnar deviation of wrist Triple arthrogram may be negative	Arthroscopic examination, which may show loss of "trampoline sign" Debridement of hypertrophic synovitis to help locate tear Arthroscopic suturing of TFCC and immobilization for 6 wk
IC	Tears of TFCC that result in ulnocarpal instability, such as avulsion of TFCC from distal attachment of lunate or triquetrum	Tenderness of palm over pisiform Locking on ulnar side with firm grip	If no wrist instability, treat conservatively Patients with ulnar carpal instability may need exploration and repair
ID	Traumatic avulsions of TFCC from attachment at distal sigmoid notch	Diffuse tenderness along entire ulnar aspect of wrist Possible hemarthrosis of wrist	Immobilization for ~6 wk or arthroscopic reattachment

TFCC, triangular fibrocartilage complex.

Table 42–2
Class II Degenerative Lesions

Subclass	Description	Clinical Presentation	Suggested Treatment
IIA	Wear of horizontal portion of TFCC distally, proximally, or both, with no perforation Possible ulnar-plus syndrome	Arthritic pain	Arthroscopic debridement
IIB	Wear of horizontal portion of TFCC and chondromalacia of lunate, ulna, or both	Arthritic pain	Ulnar shortening if ulnar-plus syndrome is present
IIC	TFCC perforation and chondromalacia of lunate, ulna, or both	Limitation of movement	Arthroscopic debridement
IID	TFCC perforation and chondromalacia of lunate, ulna, or both Perforation of lunotriquetral ligament	Painful supination-pronation	Wafer procedure if ulnar plus syndrome is present and <4 mm resection is required
IIE	TFCC perforation and chondromalacia of lunate, ulna, or both Perforation of lunotriquetral ligament Ulnocarpal arthritis	Crepitation	If ulnar resection requires >4 mm, ulnar shortening is recommended

TFCC, triangular fibrocartilage complex.

styloid at its base, are class IB injuries (Fig. 42–2A). These are usually associated with distal radiocarpal joint instability. The patient usually has tenderness around the site of the 6-U portal, and the pain may be reproduced with ulnar deviation of the wrist. The triple arthrogram may be negative, and arthroscopic examination usually shows loss of TFCC tension (the "trampoline sign").[4] Hypertrophic synovitis may cover the torn portion of ulnar dorsal TFCC as the body attempts to heal, and debridement of this covering helps locate the tear (Fig. 42–2B). Three arthroscopic suturing techniques have been

described as treatment for class IB injuries: Whipple, Poehling, and Chow.

WHIPPLE TECHNIQUE

For tears that extend dorsally, Whipple,[8] Corso et al.,[1] and Roth and Haddad[6] have described an outside-in technique that involves placing sutures longitudinally to reattach the central cartilage disk to the floor of the fifth and sixth extensor compartment. The arthroscope is normally inserted in the 3-4 portal. After establishment of

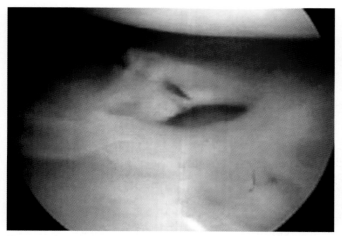

Figure 42–1   Arthroscopic view of a class IA lesion.

the 6-R portal, the central disk and its peripheral attachment are probed for loss of the trampoline sign. Any fibrovascular tissue is debrided, and the dorsal margin of the central disk is freshened with a small motorized shaver. A longitudinal incision, approximately 12 to 15 mm long, is then made, incorporating the 6-R portal. The extensor carpi ulnaris tendon retinaculum is opened, and the tendon is retracted either ulnarly or radially. A curved cannulated needle and suture retriever are introduced through the extensor compartment floor, with the needle at the distal radioulnar joint level and the suture retriever at the radiocarpal level (Fig. 42–3A). The suture is advanced through the needle, brought through the dorsal capsule using the suture retriever's wire loop, and tied over the dorsal capsule (Fig. 42–3B). Normally, only two or three sutures are needed to close the tear. The retinaculum can then

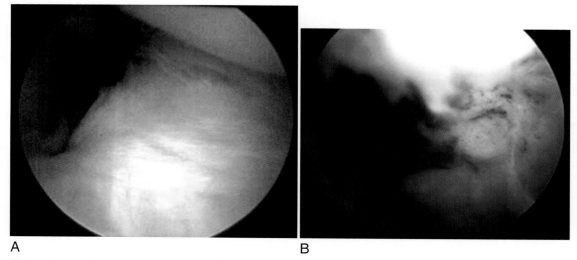

A   B

Figure 42–2   *A,* Arthroscopic view of a class IB lesion. *B,* Hypertrophic synovium covering a IB tear.

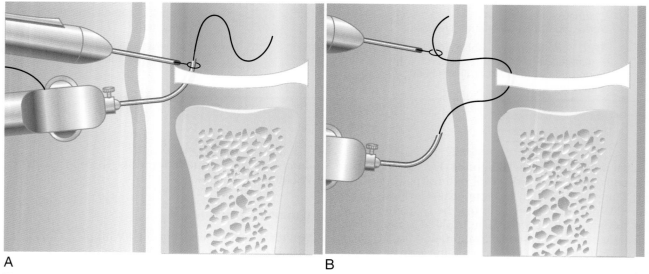

A   B

Figure 42–3   *A,* A curved cannulated needle is introduced through the extensor compartment floor at the distal radioulnar joint level, and a suture retriever is introduced at the radiocarpal level. *B,* The suture is advanced through the dorsal capsule and brought through the dorsal capsule with the use of a suture retriever.

be closed with a single suture, and the skin edges are closed.

It is not necessary to disturb the extensor carpi ulnaris tendon for tears that lie over the ulnar styloid. For these, a 1.5-mm drill hole is made obliquely, under fluoroscopic control, through the base of the ulnar styloid. A straight needle from the Inteq device is used to pass a suture through the drill hole and then distally through the TFCC's ulnar edge. The suture is retrieved through the 6-U portal (made inside the surgical incision) and tied around the volar edge of the styloid process.

The patient is placed in a long arm cast or sugar tong splint in slight supination for 3 weeks, followed by a short arm cast or rigid splint for 3 weeks. The patient should avoid pronation and supination initially.

POEHLING TECHNIQUE

In this technique, the camera is placed in the 4-5 portal, and a 20-gauge Touhy needle is placed in the radiocarpal joint through either the 1-2 or the 3-4 portal. Under direct visualization, it is passed through the torn edge of the TFCC, through the ligamentous tissue above the ulnar styloid, and out through the soft tissue and skin. A 2-0 absorbable suture is threaded through the entire needle and anchored at each end with hemostats (Fig. 42–4A). The needle is then brought back into the joint space and passed through the edge of the tear again, advanced through the ligamentous tissue on the ulnar side of the joint, and out through the soft tissue and skin, with the suture traveling through the soft tissue both inside and outside the needle (Fig. 42–4B and C). The

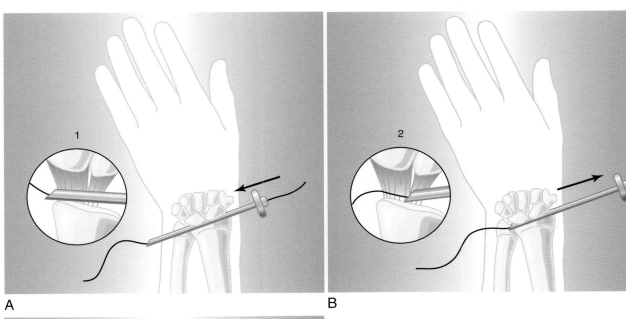

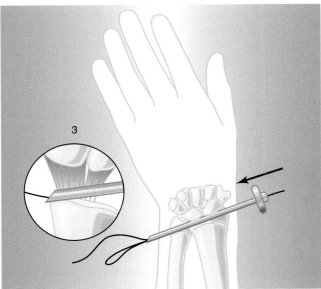

Figure 42–4   *A,* A 2-0 absorbable suture is passed through a 20-gauge Touhy needle placed in the radiocarpal joint, through the torn triangular fibrocartilage complex and ligamentous tissue above the ulnar styloid, and through the soft tissue and skin on the other side. Each end of the suture is anchored with hemostats. *B,* The needle is brought back into the joint space. *C,* It is then passed through the edge of the tear again, advanced through the ligamentous tissue on the ulnar side of the joint, and out the soft tissue and skin again. The suture travels through the soft tissue both inside and outside the needle.

suture is pulled out of the needle on the ulnar side of the wrist. The needle is then withdrawn back into the joint space. Both ends of the suture are anchored in the same manner as before. This is repeated until three sutures are in place, at which point the needle can be removed from the wrist. Blunt subcutaneous dissection is carried out, and under direct visualization from the 4-5 portal, all sutures are pulled back through the skin and out the single incision. They are tied firmly so that the TFCC is pulled against the ulnar side of the wrist. The skin can then be closed over the knots so that they stay subcutaneous. The patient is placed in a splint for 1 month but is allowed to move the fingers and pronate-supinate the forearm.

CHOW TECHNIQUE

The Chow technique uses an InstruMaker meniscus suture set, along with a 25-gauge needle as a guide for suture insertion, to reattach the TFCC to the joint capsule. The arthroscope is normally engaged in the 3-4 portal, using the 6-U portal for assistance (Fig. 42–5). A shaver is introduced to remove the synovium and allow better visualization of the dorsal aspect between the 3-4 and 4-5 portals. The peripheral tear is identified, and the shaver is used to refresh the edges of the torn tissue, preferably to bleeding tissue, but taking care to avoid debriding too much of the joint capsule. Next, a 25-gauge needle, with the head removed to gain access from the outside, is used as a guide for insertion of the repair sutures (Fig. 42–6). The straight needle is then checked to ensure that the wire loop is easy to open and that the sharp-tipped side is pointing down (Fig. 42–7A). The 4-5 and 6-R arthroscopy portals are the most common suturing sites, and if the patient has a large hand, it is recommended that the portals be made at this time to allow easier movement of the needle inside the joint. The wire loop is brought back inside the straight needle, and the needle is inserted on the distal side of the TFCC, following the guide of the 25-gauge needle and being careful that the bevel of the needle is facing up to avoid damage to the articular surface. The second straight needle, containing the suture, is inserted 4 to 5 mm inferior to the first needle, with the bevel inserted facedown and the sharp-tipped edge pointing upward to facilitate puncturing the torn TFCC (Fig. 42–7B). A small bassinet or holder inserted from the 6-U portal is used to assist in

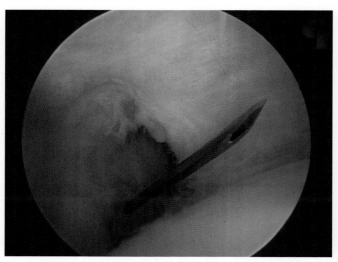

Figure 42–6   A 25-gauge needle is used as a guide for the insertion of repair sutures.

passing the suture by holding the free edge of the tear. Once the needle has passed through the TFCC, the wire loop is advanced from the first needle to loop around the second needle (Fig. 42–7C). Turning the second needle gently, so that the bevel is faceup, engages the wire loop and gently pulls it to further engage the TFCC with the second needle (Fig. 42–7D). The suture is then passed through the second needle and grasped by a grasper inserted through the 6-U portal (Fig. 42–7E). Following this, the second needle is retreated gently through the TFCC to avoid cutting the suture, and the suture is retrieved through the 6-U portal by gently tugging the grasper (Fig. 42–7F). The end of the suture is secured to the second needle with a hemostat, and the wire loop is retracted, pulling the suture back through the 6-U portal and out the dorsal aspect of the wrist, where it is secured. A small incision is made between the sutures, and blunt dissection to the joint capsule is performed with a hemostat under direct visualization, taking care not to trap any tendons or puncture the joint capsule. A probe is inserted into the incision and looped around the suture, above and below, to bring it out the center incision, and hemostats are used to tack down the suture for future tying.

Once the first suture is secured, a second suture can be placed in the same fashion through either the 4-5 or the 6-R portal. If the tear involves the 6-U portal, the flat edge of the TFCC tear should be easily identified. The grasper can be brought in from the portal to hold the TFCC (Fig. 42–8A). A straight needle is passed through the TFCC without difficulty, with the bevel face of the needle pointed down (Fig. 42–8B). Once the needle has gone through the TFCC, the suture is passed through and retrieved by the grasper (Fig. 42–8C). To avoid severing the suture, the needle should be backed out before pulling the suture through (Fig. 42–8D). The suture is then freely tacked onto the TFCC, and the end of the suture is tacked onto the free needle to attach it to the joint capsule (Fig. 42–8E and F). First, the edge of

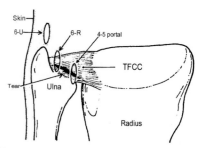

Figure 42–5   The 4-5 and 6-R arthroscopy portals are the most common for suturing. TFCC, triangular fibrocartilage complex.

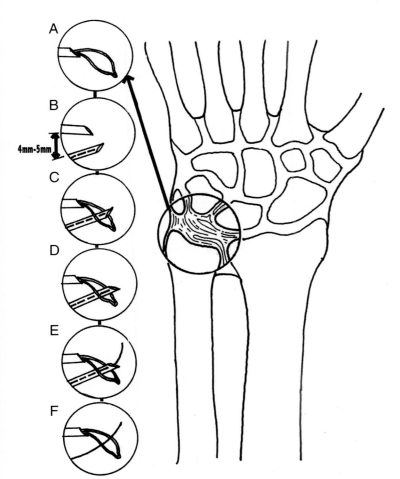

Figure 42–7 *A,* The wire loops should be pointing down to the sharp-tipped side of the needle and should be easy to open. *B,* The bevel of the needle should be faceup to avoid damaging the bone surface–cartilage articular surface. The second straight needle, containing the suture, is inserted 4 to 5 mm inferior to the first needle. *C,* Once the needle has passed through the triangular fibrocartilage complex (TFCC), the wire loop is advanced from the first needle and looped around the second needle. *D,* The wire loop is gently pulled to further engage the TFCC with the second needle. *E,* The suture is then passed through the second needle. *F,* The second needle is retracted gently through the TFCC to avoid cutting the suture with the needle.

the capsule is identified, and the needle is passed through only the joint capsule. A nerve probe is then used just above the joint capsule to loop the suture ends to the center of the incision, allowing the joint capsule to be involved in the tying of only one suture from each side of the portal incisions (Fig. 42–8*G*).

When all the sutures are in place, the tying process begins. The surgeon's knot is preferred for the first knot, followed by insertion of the probe under arthroscopic visualization to ensure that the suture is tight and no tissue or tendons are caught in it. The second suture is then tied. When the suturing is complete, the arthroscope is removed from the joint, and irrigation and closure are performed as usual. The patient's wrist is immobilized in a plaster cast for 4 to 6 weeks. When the cast is removed, active exercise should begin.

Class IC

These are generally peripheral tears of the TFCC, usually involving the distal attachment of the lunate or triquetrum. This type of injury frequently results in ulnar carpal instability, demonstrated by palmar translocation of the ulnar carpus in relation to the radius or ulnar head. The patient usually presents with palmar tenderness over the pisiform bone, with pain and locking on the ulnar side when making a firm grip. Class IC

lesions with no wrist instability are usually treated conservatively. Patients with ulnar carpal instability may need to undergo exploration and repair.

Class ID

Class ID injuries are quite severe and involve traumatic avulsion of the TFCC from the attachment of the distal sigmoid notch, usually associated with a fracture of the sigmoid notch. Patients with this type of injury usually have diffuse tenderness along the entire ulnar aspect of the wrist and may also have hemarthrosis of the wrist joint.

In the past, treatment required cast immobilization for about 6 weeks to allow the body to try to heal the TFCC injury, as the fibrocartilage is intact. More recently, Sagerman and Short[7] suggested arthroscopic reattachment. Following debridement of the bony rim of the sigmoid notch, the radial edge of the horizontal disk is reattached to the bone by drilling two or three holes with small Kirschner wires (K-wires) percutaneously into the joint from the sigmoid notch across the distal radius (Fig. 42–9*A*). Long meniscal repair needles are inserted through the drill holes to place two nonabsorbable sutures into the horizontal disk and out the radial aspect of the wrist (Fig. 42–9*B*). These sutures are tied directly over the radius by means of a small incision. The distal radioulnar joint is then pinned in neutral position

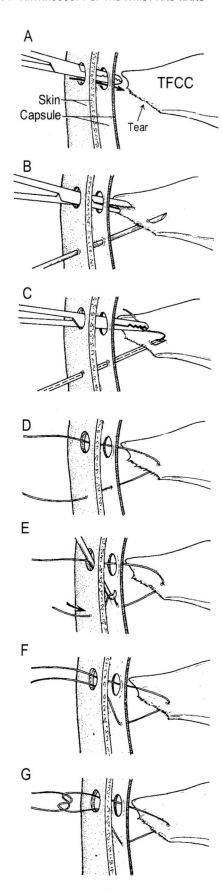

Figure 42–8   *A*, A grasper is brought in from the portal to hold the triangular fibrocartilage complex (TFCC). *B*, A straight needle is passed through the TFCC with the bevel of the needle facedown. *C*, The suture is passed through and retrieved by the grasper. *D*, To avoid severing the suture, the needle should be backed out before pulling the suture through. *E*, The suture is tacked to the TFCC, and the end of the suture is tacked to the free needle to attach it to the joint capsule. *F*, The suture ends are looped to the center of the incision. *G*, The joint capsule is involved in the tying of only one suture from each side of the portal incisions.

using one 0.062-inch K-wire percutaneously (Fig. 42–9*C* and *D*).[2]

Class II: Degenerative Lesions

Classes IIA and IIB

Class IIA lesions consist of wear of the horizontal portion of the TFCC distally, proximally, or both, without perforation. Class IIB lesions consist of the wear of the horizontal portion of the TFCC and chondromalacia of the lunate, ulna, or both, without perforation. Because these lesions involve only wear of the TFCC, with no perforation, simple debridement is recommended to avoid actual perforation of the TFCC.

Classes IIC, IID, and IIE

Class IIC lesions involve TFCC perforation and chondromalacia of the lunate, ulna, or both. Class IID includes all the conditions in class IIC, plus perforation of the lunotriquetral ligament. Class IIE lesions are class IID lesions that have progressed to ulnocarpal arthritis. As in class IIA and IIB lesions, arthroscopic debridement is recommended for classes IIC, IID, and IIE lesions. However, if ulnar plus syndrome is present, a wafer procedure can be performed through the arthroscope.[7]

The wafer procedure involves using a bur to resect 2 to 3 mm of the ulnar head, with visualization gained through the TFCC tear by supinating or pronating the wrist. The most common question regarding the wafer procedure is how much bone needs to be resected. Under normal conditions, less than 4 mm of resection should be sufficient. Precautions should be taken to ensure preservation of the stability of the distal radioulnar joint and the origins of the ulnar carpal ligament. Some surgeons recommend using the laser to resect the ulnar head to the bony section before using the bur.[3,10] However, we do not have enough experience with this technique to comment on its success. If more than 4 mm of ulnar resection is required, ulnar shortening should be considered.

Postoperative Management

After simple debridement of a central tear, patients are splinted for 1 week, followed by the use of a prefabricated wrist splint for comfort for an additional 3 weeks. Gentle range-of-motion exercises begin at 1 week, and strenuous

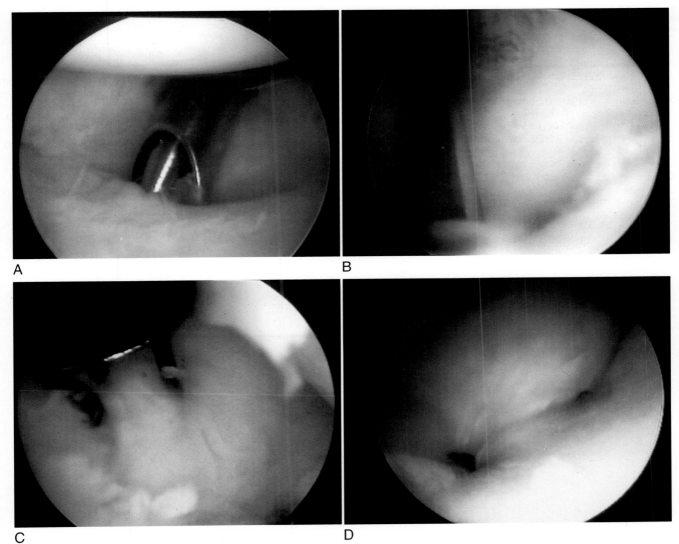

Figure 42–9 *A*, The radial edge of the horizontal disk is reattached to the bone by drilling two or three holes with small K-wires percutaneously into the joint from the sigmoid notch across the distal radius. *B*, Long meniscal repair needles are inserted through the drill holes to place two nonabsorbable sutures into the horizontal disk and out the radial aspect of the wrist. *C*, These sutures are tied directly over the radius by means of a small incision. *D*, The distal radioulnar joint is pinned in the neutral position using one 0.062-inch K-wire percutaneously.

activity with the hand and wrist is avoided for 6 weeks. Formal therapy is rarely needed.

After repair of a peripheral tear, patients are immobilized in a sugar tong splint or long arm cast in 60 degrees of supination for 4 weeks. Range of motion is then initiated to neutral rotation and neutral deviation. Full pronation is not allowed until 5 weeks postoperatively. By 6 weeks, full range of motion can be expected, and rapid grip strengthening can be initiated.

Results

Various authors have reported better than 90% good and excellent results for arthroscopic treatment of TFCC pathology. Factors predicting good outcomes include post-traumatic tears, return of grip strength, and return to work. The timing of repair has not been found to affect results.

Complications

True procedural complications are uncommon but may include irritation of the extensor carpi ulnaris or the dorsal sensory branch of the ulnar nerve by the suture knot, entrapment of the sensory nerve by the repair sutures, loss of full pronation requiring pronation splinting, and local wound complications. Meticulous surgical technique is mandatory. Careful dissection to the ulnar wrist capsule is necessary to avoid injury to the small sensory branches of the ulnar nerve.

4 Wrist and Hand

References

1. Coroso SJ, Savoie FH, Geissler WB, et al: Arthroscopic repair of peripheral avulsions of the triangular fibrocartilage complex of the wrist: A multicenter study. Arthroscopy 13:78-84, 1997.
2. Hermansdorfer JD, Kleinman WB: Management of chronic peripheral tears of the triangular fibrocartilage complex. J Hand Surg [Am] 16:340-346, 1991.
3. Nagle DJ: The use of lasers in wrist arthroscopy. Paper presented at the Fall Meeting of the Arthroscopy Association of North America, Nov 7, 1997, Rosemont, IL.
4. Palmer AK: Triangular fibrocartilage complex lesion: A classification. J Hand Surg [Am] 14:494-606, 1989.
5. Richards RS, Bennet JD, Roth JH, et al: Arthroscopic diagnosis of intra-articular soft tissue injuries associated with distal radius fractures. J Hand Surg [Am] 22:772-776, 1997.
6. Roth JH, Haddad RG: Radiocarpal arthroscopy and arthrography in the diagnosis of ulnar wrist pain. Arthroscopy 2:234-243, 1986.
7. Sagerman SD, Short W: Arthroscopic repair of radial-sided triangular fibrocartilage complex tears. Arthroscopy 12:339-342, 1996.
8. Whipple TL: Arthroscopic Surgery: The Wrist. Philadelphia, JB Lippincott, 1992, pp 103-105.
9. Whipple TL: TFCC injury: Biomechanics, classification and treatment with Whipple technique. In Chow JC (ed): Advanced Arthroscopy. New York, Springer-Verlag (in press).
10. Wnorowki DC, Palmer AK, Werner FW, et al: Anatomical and biomechanical analysis of the arthroscopic wafer procedure. Arthroscopy 8:204-212, 1992.

Arthroscopy of the Hip

Hip: Patient Positioning, Portal Placement, Normal Arthroscopic Anatomy, and Diagnostic Arthroscopy

J. W. THOMAS BYRD

Anesthesia

Hip arthroscopy is commonly performed with the patient under general anesthesia. It can also be performed using epidural anesthesia, but this requires an adequate motor block to ensure optimal distractibility of the joint. A dose of broad-spectrum antibiotic is administered intravenously immediately before beginning the procedure.

Positioning

Most current literature deals with arthroscopy that involves distraction of the joint.[2-4,10,14,15] When the distraction technique is used, the patient can be placed in either the supine or the lateral decubitus position; arthroscopy can be performed with equal effectiveness in either position. There may be minor advantages of one over the other, but this depends largely on the surgeon's preference.

Familiarity with the anatomy and the joint orientation is a possible advantage of both positions. Orthopedic surgeons are familiar with the supine position in association with routine hip fracture management; other surgeons are more comfortable with the lateral position commonly used in total hip arthroplasty procedures. There may be an advantage to the lateral position in severely obese patients, because the excess adipose tissue tends to fall away. The biggest advantage of the supine position is the simplicity and ease of patient positioning. Also, there have been a few case reports of intra-abdominal fluid extravasation as a serious complication of hip arthroscopy.[1,5] Fluid can leak through a fresh acetabular fracture or gain access to the retroperitoneal space along the iliopsoas sheath. These complications have occurred only in the lateral position. It may be that, when placed laterally, the abdominal cavity acts as a sink, collecting fluid. When placed supine, the abdomen is not in such a dependent position.

For the supine position, any standard fracture table can be used. A tensiometer can be incorporated into the footplate, which aids in monitoring the ability to maintain adequate traction intraoperatively. Some fracture tables accommodate the lateral position, and there are also several commercially available distractors that can be used on a regular operating room table.

Regardless of whether the patient is supine or lateral, the same principles of hip positioning are used to achieve safe and effective traction. The perineal post should be oversized and heavily padded, which better distributes the pressure on the perineum. The perineal post is also lateralized against the medial thigh of the operative hip (Fig. 43–1), which distances the point of contact from the pudendal nerve, reducing the risk of compression neurapraxia, and also facilitates achievement of the optimal vector for distraction of the joint (Fig. 43–2). The hip is in approximately 25 degrees of abduction. Excessive abduction is avoided because it may cause the greater trochanter to interfere with optimal access of the portals to the joint.

In the supine position, the hip is maintained in neutral rotation and extension. Rotational position is determined by pointing the patella toward the ceiling. Accounting for anteversion of the femoral neck, this

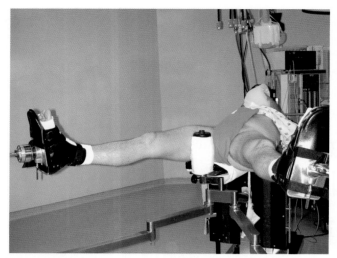

Figure 43–1 The patient is positioned on the fracture table so that the perineal post is placed as far laterally as possible toward the operative hip and resting against the medial thigh.

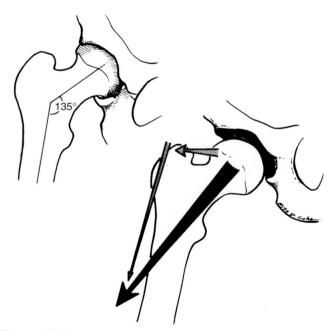

Figure 43–2 The optimal vector for distraction is oblique relative to the axis of the body; this more closely coincides with the axis of the femoral neck than that of the femoral shaft. This oblique vector is partially created by abducting the hip and is partially accentuated by a small transverse component to the vector. (From Byrd JWT: Hip arthroscopy utilizing the supine position. Arthroscopy 10:275-280, 1994. With permission from The Arthroscopy Association of North America.)

maintains a consistent relationship of the joint to the greater trochanter, which is the principal topographic landmark for portal placement.

Some authors believe that slight external rotation may relax the capsule, but this can make the relationship of the trochanter to the joint more variable. Slight hip flexion may also relax the capsule, but excessive flexion

should be avoided because it places traction on the sciatic nerve, making it vulnerable to injury.

Arthroscopy can also be performed without distraction,[8,9,12] allowing visualization of only the peripheral portions of the joint. Access to the posterior aspect is limited, but with hip flexion, an excellent view of the anterior and inferomedial femoral neck can be achieved, as well as the capsule, synovial lining, and peripheral aspect of the acetabular labrum and femoral head. As an isolated procedure, hip arthroscopy without distraction has limited application, but when used in conjunction with distraction of the joint, it is advantageous for select conditions such as synovial disease, loose bodies, and thermal capsulorrhaphy.

Equipment

Specialized arthroscopic instrumentation has been developed for use in the hip, and systems are available from several manufacturers. Two principal features are important. First is extra-length cannulas and instruments for accessing the joint. Second is cannulation of the obturators. Thus, custom spinal needles can be prepositioned in the joint. Once these have been properly placed, a guidewire can be passed through the needle; the arthroscopic cannula, with its accompanying obturator, can then be passed over the guidewire, ensuring reproducible placement within the joint.

Flexible and slotted cannulas allow passage of various hand instruments and curved shaver blades, which are useful for operative arthroscopy within the confines of the hip. Extra-length thermal devices, including laser and radiofrequency, add versatility in selective tissue ablation, especially with the limitations on maneuverability inside the joint.

A high-flow fluid management system markedly enhances the ability to perform various operative procedures. This is important because adequate flow can be maintained for optimal visualization without requiring high fluid pressures, which could cause inordinate fluid extravasation.

Portals

Nomenclature regarding hip portals has not been well standardized. Portals described here as anterolateral and posterolateral may be called paratrochanteric by others.

Although some authors believe that two portals are sufficient for performing hip arthroscopy, it is my opinion that three portals, properly dispersed within the joint, provide optimal visualization and access and minimize the risk of overlooking or incompletely addressing intra-articular pathology.

Portal placement, relationship to the extra-articular structures, and arthroscopic anatomy are the same regardless of whether the procedure is performed with the patient in the supine or the lateral decubitus position. The three standard portals are anterior, anterolateral, and posterolateral (Figs. 43–3 and 43–4). Their

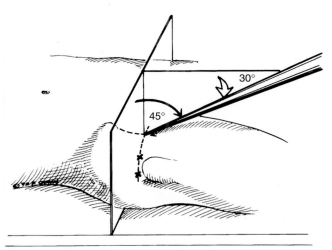

Figure 43–3   The site of the anterior portal coincides with the intersection of a sagittal line drawn distally from the anterior superior iliac spine and a transverse line drawn across the superior margin of the greater trochanter. The direction of this portal courses approximately 45 degrees cephalad and 30 degrees toward the midline. The anterolateral and posterolateral portals are positioned directly over the superior aspect of the trochanter at its anterior and posterior borders. (From Byrd JWT: Hip arthroscopy utilizing the supine position. Arthroscopy 10:275-280, 1994. With permission from The Arthroscopy Association of North America.)

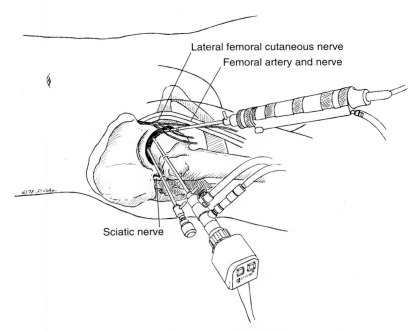

Figure 43–4   Relationship of the major neurovascular structures to the three standard portals. The femoral artery and nerve lie well medial to the anterior portal. The sciatic nerve lies posterior to the posterolateral portal. The lateral femoral cutaneous nerve lies close to the anterior portal. Injury to this structure is avoided by using proper technique in portal placement. The anterolateral portal is established first because it lies most centrally in the safe zone for arthroscopy. (From Byrd JWT: Hip arthroscopy utilizing the supine position. Arthroscopy 10:275-280, 1994. With permission from The Arthroscopy Association of North America.)

5 Hip

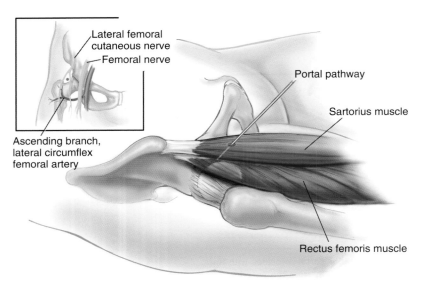

Figure 43–5 Anterior portal pathway and its relationship to the lateral femoral cutaneous nerve, femoral nerve, and lateral circumflex femoral artery. (Courtesy of Smith and Nephew Endoscopy, Andover, MA.)

position and relationship to the extra-articular anatomy have been described elsewhere and are recounted here.[7]

Anterior Portal

The anterior portal (Fig. 43–5) lies an average of 6.3 cm distal to the anterior superior iliac spine. It penetrates the muscle belly of the sartorius and the rectus femoris before entering the anterior capsule.

Typically, the lateral femoral cutaneous nerve is divided into three or more branches at the level of the anterior portal. This portal usually passes within several millimeters of one of these branches (Fig. 43–6). Because of the multiple branches, the nerve is not easily avoided by altering the portal position, but it can

be protected by using meticulous technique in portal placement. Specifically, it is most vulnerable to a skin incision placed too deeply, lacerating one of the branches.

Passing from the skin to the capsule, the anterior portal runs almost tangential to the axis of the femoral nerve and lies only slightly closer at the level of the capsule, with an average minimum distance of 3.2 cm (Fig. 43–7).

Although variable in its relationship, the ascending branch of the lateral circumflex femoral artery is usually approximately 3.6 cm inferior to the anterior portal (Fig. 43–8). In some cadaver specimens, a small terminal branch of this vessel has been identified lying within millimeters of the portal at the level of the capsule. The clinical significance of this is uncertain, and there have been

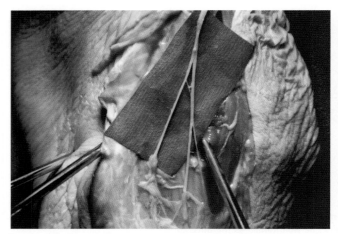

Figure 43–6 Relationship of the anterior portal to the multiple branches of the lateral femoral cutaneous nerve. Multiple branches at the level of the portal are characteristic, and the branches always extend lateral to the portal. (From Byrd JWT, Pappas JN, Pedley MJ: Hip arthroscopy: An anatomic study of portal placement and relationship to the extra-articular structures. Arthroscopy 11:418-423, 1995. With permission from The Arthroscopy Association of North America.)

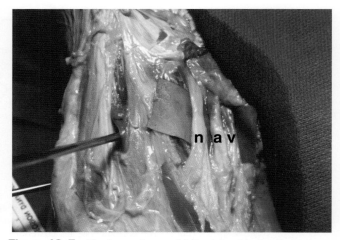

Figure 43–7 The femoral nerve (n) lies lateral to the femoral artery (a) and vein (v). The relationship of the anterior portal as it pierces the sartorius is shown. (From Byrd JWT, Pappas JN, Pedley MJ: Hip arthroscopy: An anatomic study of portal placement and relationship to the extra-articular structures. Arthroscopy 11:418-423, 1995. With permission from The Arthroscopy Association of North America.)

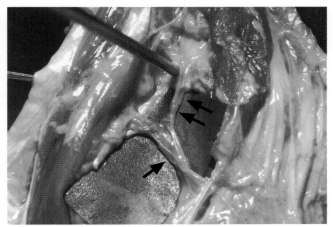

Figure 43–8   The ascending branch of the lateral circumflex femoral artery *(single arrow)* has an oblique course distal to the anterior portal, seen here at the level of the capsule. This specimen demonstrates a terminal branch *(double arrow)* coursing vertically, adjacent to the portal. (From Byrd JWT, Pappas JN, Pedley MJ: Hip arthroscopy: An anatomic study of portal placement and relationship to the extra-articular structures. Arthroscopy 11:418-423, 1995. With permission from The Arthroscopy Association of North America.)

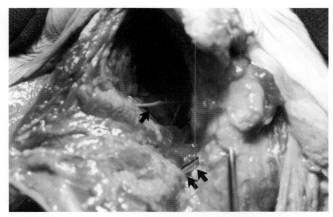

Figure 43–10   The superior gluteal nerve *(single arrow)* courses transversely on the deep surface of the gluteus medius. It passes above the anterolateral portal *(double arrow)*, which is seen between the deep surface of the gluteus medius and the capsule. (From Byrd JWT, Pappas JN, Pedley MJ: Hip arthroscopy: An anatomic study of portal placement and relationship to the extra-articular structures. Arthroscopy 11:418-423, 1995. With permission from The Arthroscopy Association of North America.)

no reported cases of excessive bleeding from the anterior position.

Anterolateral Portal

The anterolateral portal (Fig. 43–9) penetrates the gluteus medius before entering the lateral aspect of the capsule at its anterior margin. The only structure of significance relative to the anterolateral portal is the superior gluteal nerve (Fig. 43–10). After exiting the sciatic notch, it courses transversely, posterior to anterior, across the deep surface of the gluteus medius. Its relationship

to both lateral portals is the same, with an average distance of 4.4 cm.

Posterolateral Portal

The posterolateral portal (Fig. 43–11) penetrates both the gluteus medius and minimus before entering the lateral capsule at its posterior margin. Its course is superior and anterior to the piriformis tendon (Fig. 43–12). It lies closest to the sciatic nerve at the level of the capsule. The distance to the lateral edge of the nerve averages 2.9 cm.

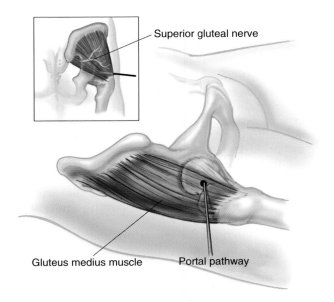

Superior gluteal nerve

Gluteus medius muscle   Portal pathway

Figure 43–9   Anterolateral portal pathway and its relationship to the superior gluteal nerve. (Courtesy of Smith and Nephew Endoscopy, Andover, MA.)

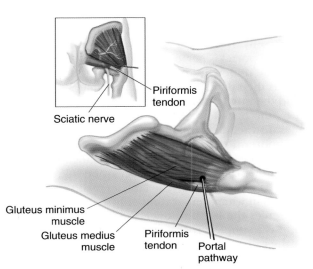

Piriformis tendon

Sciatic nerve

Gluteus minimus muscle
Gluteus medius muscle   Piriformis tendon   Portal pathway

Figure 43–11   Posterolateral portal pathway and its relationship to the sciatic nerve and superior gluteal nerve. (Courtesy of Smith and Nephew Endoscopy, Andover, MA.)

5   Hip

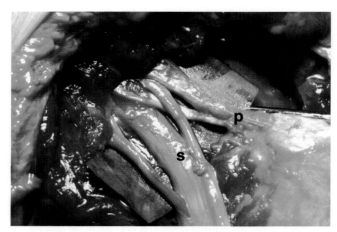

Figure 43–12 Relationship of the posterolateral portal to the piriformis tendon (p) and sciatic nerve (s). Note the anomaly where the sciatic nerve is formed from three divisions distal to the sciatic notch; the lateral-most division passes through a split muscle belly of the piriformis. (From Byrd JWT, Pappas JN, Pedley MJ: Hip arthroscopy: An anatomic study of portal placement and relationship to the extra-articular structures. Arthroscopy 11:418-423, 1995. With permission from The Arthroscopy Association of North America.)

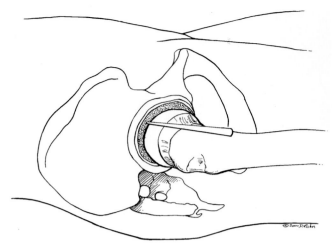

Figure 43–13 With the patient supine, the hip is in neutral rotation, with the patella pointing toward the ceiling. A needle placed at the anterior margin of the greater trochanter (anterolateral position) is maintained in the coronal plane by keeping it parallel to the floor as it enters the joint. Owing to femoral neck anteversion, the entry site will be just anterior to the joint's center. If the entry site is too anterior, it will be crowded with the anterior portal. If it is too posterior, it will be difficult to properly visualize the entry site for the anterior portal. (From Byrd JWT: Avoiding the labrum in hip arthroscopy. Arthroscopy 16:770-773, 2000. With permission from The Arthroscopy Association of North America.)

Portal Placement

The anterolateral portal lies most centrally in the "safe zone" for arthroscopy and is thus the first portal placed.[7] Subsequent portal placements are assisted by direct arthroscopic visualization. This initial portal is placed by fluoroscopic inspection in the anteroposterior plane. However, orientation in the lateral plane is equally important. With the leg in neutral rotation, femoral anteversion leaves the center of the joint just anterior to the center of the greater trochanter. Thus, the entry site for the anterolateral portal at the anterior margin of the greater trochanter corresponds with entry of the joint just anterior to its midportion. This correct entry site is achieved by keeping the instrumentation parallel to the floor during portal placement (Fig. 43–13).

When distracting the hip, a vacuum phenomenon is usually present (Fig. 43–14A). Prepositioning for the anterolateral portal is performed with a 6-inch, 17-gauge spinal needle under fluoroscopic control (Fig. 43–14B). The joint is then distended with approximately 40 mL of fluid, and the intracapsular position of the needle is confirmed by the backflow of fluid. Distention of the joint enhances distraction (Fig. 43–14C).

It is important to note that the needle may inadvertently penetrate the lateral acetabular labrum during initial placement in the joint.[6] This can be felt, because pushing the needle through the labrum results in greater resistance than when penetrating only the capsule. If the needle pierces the labrum, once the joint has been distended, it is a simple process to back the needle up and reenter the capsule below the level of the labrum. Failure to recognize this problem can result in violation of the labrum by the cannula.

A stab wound is made through the skin at the needle site. The guidewire is placed through the needle, and the needle is removed. The cannulated obturator with the 5-mm arthroscopy cannula is passed over the wire into the joint (Fig. 43–14D).

While establishing the portal, the cannula-obturator assembly should pass close to the superior tip of the greater trochanter and then directly above the convex surface of the femoral head. It is important to keep the assembly off the femoral head to avoid inadvertent articular surface scuffing.

Sometimes blood is present within the joint due to the traction force necessary to distract the surfaces. This is difficult to clear until a separate egress has been established. However, venting fluid with the spinal needle from the anterior clears the field of view.

Once the arthroscope has been introduced, the anterior portal is placed. Positioning is now facilitated by visualization from the arthroscope as well as fluoroscopy. The 70-degree scope works best for directly viewing where the instrumentation penetrates the capsule. Prepositioning is again performed with the 17-gauge spinal needle, entering the joint directly underneath the free edge of the anterior labrum. As the cannula-obturator assembly is introduced, it is lifted up to stay off the articular surface of the femoral head while passing underneath the acetabular labrum.

If proper attention is given to the topographic anatomy when positioning the anterior portal, the femoral nerve should lie well medial to the approach.[7] However, the lateral femoral cutaneous nerve lies quite close to this portal. It is best avoided by using proper technique in portal placement. The nerve is most vulnerable to laceration by a skin incision placed too deeply.

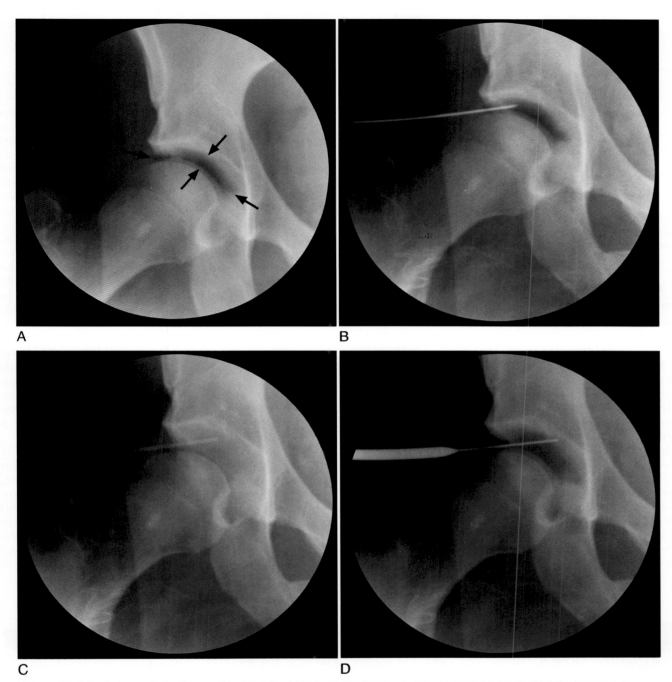

Figure 43–14   Anteroposterior fluoroscopic view of a right hip. *A,* A vacuum effect is apparent due to the negative intracapsular pressure created by distraction of the joint *(arrows). B,* A spinal needle is used in prepositioning for the anterolateral portal. The needle courses above the superior tip of the trochanter and then passes under the lateral lip of the acetabulum entering the hip joint. *C,* Distention of the joint disrupts the vacuum and facilitates adequate distraction. *D,* The cannula-obturator assembly is passed over the nitinol wire that was placed through the spinal needle.

Rarely, access for the anterior portal may be blocked by an overlying osteophyte or simply by the architecture of the patient's acetabular bony anatomy. If necessary, arthroscopy can still be performed using just the lateral two portals.

Last, the posterolateral portal is introduced. The fluoroscopic guidelines are similar to those for the anterolateral portal. Rotating the lens of the arthroscope posteriorly brings the entry site underneath the poste-

rior labrum into view. Placement under arthroscopic control ensures that the instrumentation does not stray posteriorly, potentially placing the sciatic nerve at risk. The hip remains in neutral rotation during placement of the posterolateral portal. External rotation of the hip would move the greater trochanter more posteriorly, and because this is the main topographic landmark, the sciatic nerve might be at greater risk for injury (Fig. 43–15).

5 Hip

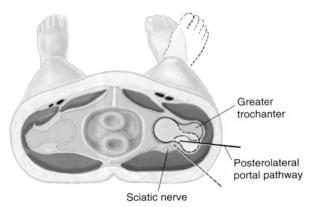

Figure 43–15 Neutral rotation of the operative hip is essential to protect the sciatic nerve during placement of the posterolateral portal. (Courtesy of Smith and Nephew Endoscopy, Andover, MA.)

Portal Placement for Peripheral Joint

After completing arthroscopy of the interior of the hip, the instruments can be removed and traction released for access to the peripheral compartment. The hip is flexed approximately 45 degrees, which relaxes the anterior capsule (Fig. 43–16). From the anterolateral entry site, the spinal needle penetrates the capsule on the anterior neck of the femur under fluoroscopic control (Fig. 43–17A and B). Using the guidewire, the cannula-obturator assembly is then placed (Fig. 43–17C). The 5-mm cannula is preferable, with the inflow attached to the scope.

For instrumentation, an ancillary portal is placed 4 cm distal to the anterolateral portal. Once again, prepositioning is performed with the 17-gauge spinal needle, directly observing through the arthroscope where the needle enters the peripheral compartment (Fig. 43–17D). Many loose bodies reside in this area and can be retrieved. This also provides superior access to the synovial lining and capsule, which is important for

performing a thorough synovectomy and also aids when performing a thermal capsulorrhaphy.

Diagnostic Arthroscopy

When preparing for hip arthroscopy, the surgeon formulates a tentative treatment plan based on the preliminary diagnosis. However, the definitive treatment strategy will be dictated by the findings observed at arthroscopy. With the current limitations of investigative techniques, the arthroscopic findings may differ significantly from those implied by the preoperative studies. Thus, a systematic and thorough initial inspection of the joint is imperative. Once all aspects of the intra-articular pathology have been identified, the surgeon can embark on intervention, making sure to manage the operative time appropriately to address all pathology within the joint. The surgeon should avoid spending considerable time on one obvious aspect of the pathology only to realize that there is other coexistent damage that needs to be addressed as well.

Using the three-portal technique (anterior, anterolateral, and posterolateral), inspection begins from the anterolateral portal (see Fig. 43–4). The 70-degree scope is used initially, as it provides the best view of the outer margins of the joint and allows direct arthroscopic visualization of the location of the other two portals. The anterolateral portal provides the best view of the anterior portion of the joint (Fig. 43–18).

Next, the arthroscope is placed in the anterior portal. Viewing laterally, the relationship of the lateral two portals underneath the lateral labrum is seen (Fig. 43–19). The surgeon should be especially cognizant of the entry site of the anterolateral portal, because this portal is placed with only fluoroscopic guidance, without the benefit of arthroscopic visualization of where the portal enters the joint. Viewing medially from the anterior portal, the surgeon can see the most inferior limit of the anterior labrum (Fig. 43–20).

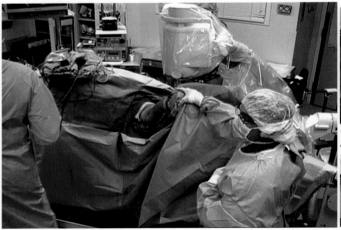

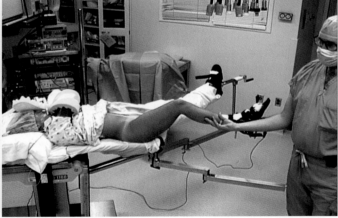

A   B

Figure 43–16 *A,* The operative area remains covered in sterile drapes while the traction is released and the hip is flexed 45 degrees. *B,* Position of the hip without the overlying drape.

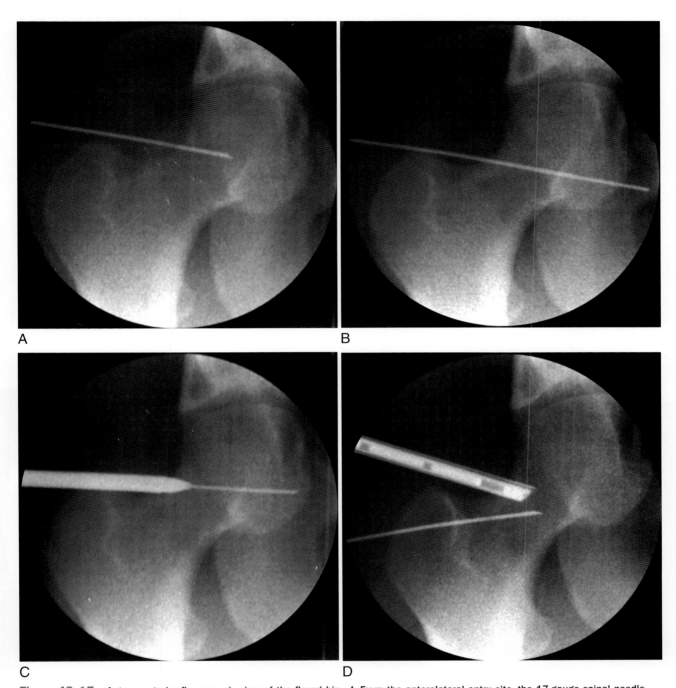

A

B

C

D

Figure 43–17   Anteroposterior fluoroscopic view of the flexed hip. *A,* From the anterolateral entry site, the 17-gauge spinal needle has been repositioned on the anterior neck of the femur. The spinal needle can be felt perforating the capsule before contacting the bone. *B,* The guidewire is placed through the spinal needle. It should pass freely to the medial capsule, as illustrated. *C,* The cannula-obturator assembly is placed over the guidewire. *D,* The position of the 30-degree arthroscope is shown while a spinal needle is being placed for an ancillary portal.

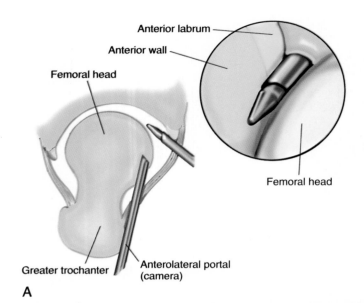

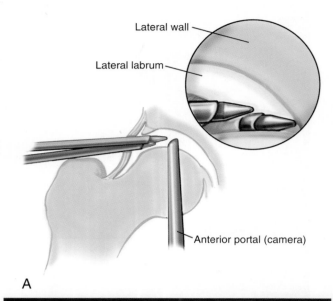

A

A

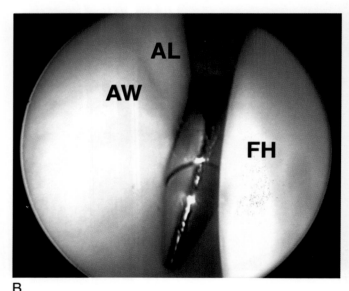

B

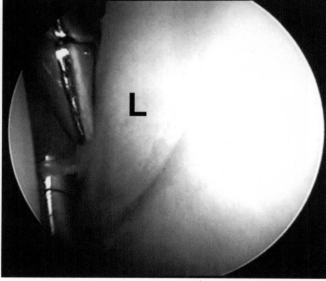

B

Figure 43–18 *A,* Diagram of placement of the anterolateral portal. *B,* Arthroscopic view of a right hip from the anterolateral portal. The anterior acetabular wall (AW) and the anterior labrum (AL) are shown. The anterior cannula is seen entering underneath the labrum, and the femoral head (FH) is on the right. (*A,* Courtesy of Smith and Nephew Endoscopy, Andover, MA. *B,* From Byrd JWT: Hip arthroscopy—the supine position. In McGinty JB, Caspari RB, Jackson RW, Poehling GG [eds]: Operative Arthroscopy. New York, Raven Press, 1996, pp 1091-1099.)

Figure 43–19 *A,* Diagram of placement of the anterior portal. *B,* Arthroscopic view from the anterior portal. The lateral aspect of the labrum (L) and its relationship to the two lateral portals. (*A,* Courtesy of Smith and Nephew Endoscopy, Andover, MA. *B,* From Byrd JWT: Hip arthroscopy—the supine position. In McGinty JB, Caspari RB, Jackson RW, Poehling GG [eds]: Operative Arthroscopy. New York, Raven Press, 1996, pp 1091-1099.)

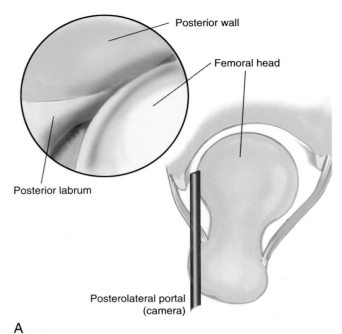

Figure 43–20   View from the anterior portal demonstrates where the inferior aspect of the anterior labrum (L) becomes contiguous with the transverse acetabular ligament (TAL) below the ligamentum teres (LT).

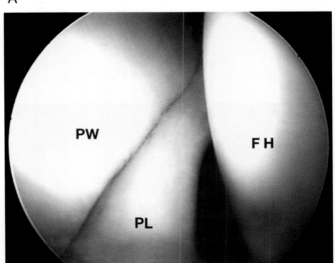

Figure 43–21   *A,* Diagram of placement of the posterolateral portal. *B,* Arthroscopic view from the posterolateral portal. The posterior acetabular wall (PW), posterior labrum (PL), and femoral head (FH) are shown. (*A,* Courtesy of Smith and Nephew Endoscopy, Andover, MA. *B,* From Byrd JWT: Hip arthroscopy—the supine position. In McGinty JB, Caspari RB, Jackson RW, Poehling GG [eds]: Operative Arthroscopy. New York, Raven Press, 1996, pp 1091-1099.)

The arthroscope is then placed in the posterolateral portal, which provides the best view of the posterior regions of the joint, especially the posterior labrum (Fig. 43–21). The posterior labrum is the portion that is least often damaged and that has the most consistent morphologic appearance. Thus, this area is often used as a reference for assessing variations in the anterior or lateral labrum and accompanying pathology.

Each of the three portals provides a different perspective on the acetabular fossa (Fig. 43–22). The 70-degree scope provides a direct view of the ligamentum teres, which resides in the inferior portion of the fossa. The transverse acetabular ligament can also be partially viewed coursing underneath the ligamentum teres. After completing the inspection with the 70-degree scope, the 30-degree scope is used, reversing the sequence of steps among the three portals. The 30-degree scope provides a better view of the central portion of the femoral head and acetabulum and the superior portion of the acetabular fossa.

Once the traction has been released and the hip flexed, the arthroscope is repositioned from the anterolateral portal on the anterior neck of the femur, providing an excellent perspective of the peripheral compartment (Fig. 43–23). This brings into view structures that cannot be seen from inside the joint and also provides a different peripheral perspective on some of the intra-articular structures. The medial synovial fold is consistently visualized adjacent to the anteromedial neck of the femur.

Normal Variants

The lateral and anterior portions of the labrum are the most variable. Sometimes this portion of the labrum is thin, poorly developed, and hypoplastic; at other times it may appear enlarged. In the presence of acetabular dysplasia, the lateral labrum is especially hypertrophic, having more of a stabilizing and weight-bearing role as it substitutes for the absent lateral portion of the bony acetabulum. A labral cleft is sometimes present (Fig. 43–24). This is a normal finding and should not be misinterpreted as a traumatic detachment. The distinguishing features are absence of tissue that looks damaged and absence of any attempted healing response that would be expected in the presence of trauma.

5 Hip

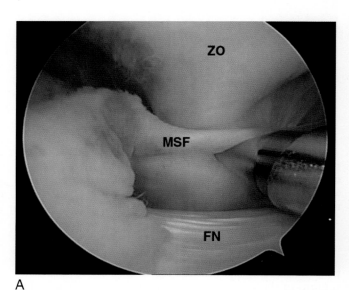

A

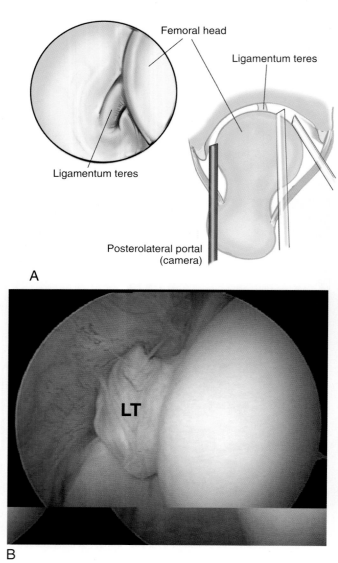

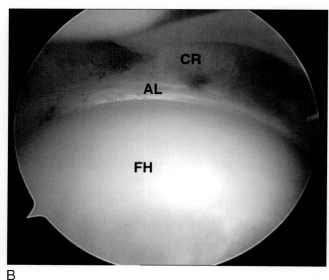

A

B

Figure 43–22 *A*, The acetabular fossa can be inspected from all three portals. *B*, The ligamentum teres (LT), with its accompanying vessels, has a serpentine course from its acetabular attachments. (*A*, Courtesy of Smith and Nephew Endoscopy, Andover, MA.)

Figure 43–23 Arthroscopic image of the peripheral compartment of a right hip. *A*, Viewing medially are the femoral neck (FN), medial synovial fold (MSF), and zona orbicularis (ZO). *B*, Viewing superiorly, the anterior portion of the joint is observed, including the articular surface of the femoral head (FH), anterior labrum (AL), and capsular reflection (CR).

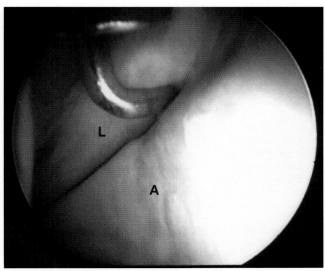

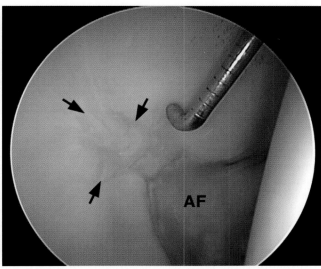

Figure 43–24   The cleft identified by the probe sometimes separates the margin of the acetabular articular surface (A) from the labrum (L). This is a normal variant, without evidence of trauma or an attempted healing response.

Figure 43–26   The stellate crease is frequently found directly superior to the acetabular fossa (AF) and is characterized by a stellate pattern of chondromalacia *(arrows)*. This appears to be a normally occurring process, even in young adults, without clear prognostic significance.

Remnants of the triradiate cartilage may be evident in adulthood as a physeal scar, devoid of overlying articular cartilage, extending in a linear fashion along the medial aspect of the acetabulum anterior or posterior to the fossa (Fig. 43–25). This should not be misinterpreted as an old fracture line.

A commonly encountered observation in adults is a stellate-appearing articular lesion immediately above the acetabular fossa, referred to as the stellate crease (Fig. 43–26). This is unlikely to be of clinical significance as a contributing cause of pain, and its long-term prognostic significance in terms of susceptibility to future degenerative disease is uncertain. Occasionally, this must be dis-

tinguished from traumatic articular lesions, which can occur in the same area, especially from a lateral blow to the hip impacting the femoral head against the superomedial acetabulum.

Complications

The reported complication rate associated with hip arthroscopy is low.[5,11,13] Most of these complications are minor or transient, but a few serious problems have been encountered. The major neurovascular structures are a safe distance from the standard portals.[7] However, careful attention to the topographic anatomy and orientation to the joint and meticulous technique in portal placement are important to ensure safe entry.

An area of particular concern is pressure on the perineum generated by countertraction from the perineal post, which places the pudendal nerve at risk for compression neurapraxia. This problem is best avoided by careful positioning of the perineal post laterally against the medial thigh and heavy padding of the post. Excessive or prolonged traction has also been implicated. With careful attention to these factors, this condition (if it occurs) should be transient, with full recovery anticipated.

There have been a few reports of neurapraxia of the sciatic and femoral nerves. Again, excessive or prolonged traction may be a factor, but extremes of hip position that might place these nerves under greater stretch should be avoided.

The lateral femoral cutaneous nerve arborizes well proximal to the anterior portal.[7] Thus, only small branches exist at this level, but it is possible that one of these branches may be stretched with vigorous instrumentation from the anterior portal, even with careful

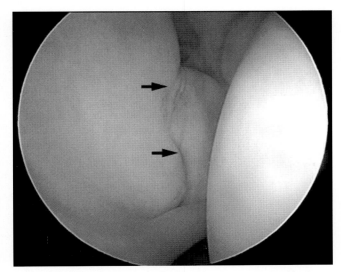

Figure 43–25   The physeal scar *(arrows)* is an area devoid of articular surface that may extend posteriorly from the acetabular fossa (as shown here) or anteriorly, demarcating the area of the old triradiate physis.

attention to initial portal placement. This complication is uncommon, with a less than 1% incidence in my experience. It is usually transient but could result in a small area of reduced sensation in the lateral thigh.

As with any joint, there will be some extravasation of fluid. This is normally readily resorbed, but there have been a few case reports of serious consequences when fluid collected within the abdominal cavity. This has been associated with acute acetabular fractures allowing intrapelvic communication and also with prolonged surgical procedures, when fluid may communicate along the course of the iliopsoas tendon.[1,13] This complication was reported in cases performed in the lateral position. It is unclear whether the problem is unique to that position, but with the patient on his or her side, the abdominal cavity is in a dependent position, creating a sink to collect extravasated fluid.

The most common problem encountered in hip arthroscopy is the potential for iatrogenic intra-articular damage. This risk is inherent in the geometry of the joint. The most likely injury is either perforation of the acetabular labrum or gouging of the femoral articular surface. This emphasizes the importance of meticulous attention to detail and the need to perform this procedure as carefully as possible. This should minimize the risk, but occasionally, some minor scuffing may still be encountered.

It is also important to acknowledge that, perhaps for unclear reasons, the patient may be made worse as a consequence of the procedure. This can be due to the development of complex regional pain syndrome. The surgeon should be especially alert to this possibility when the patient's pain and disability seem to be out of proportion to the objective evidence of pathology.

References

1. Bartlett CS, DiFelice GS, Buly RL, et al: Cardiac arrest as a result of intraabdominal extravasation of fluid during arthroscopic removal of a loose body from the hip joint of a patient with an acetabular fracture. J Orthop Trauma 12:294-299, 1998.

2. Byrd JWT: Hip arthroscopy—the supine position. In McGinty JB, Caspari RB, Jackson RW, Poehling GG (eds): Operative Arthroscopy. New York, Raven Press, 1996, pp 1091-1099.

3. Byrd JWT: Hip arthroscopy utilizing the supine position. Arthroscopy 10:275-280, 1994.

4. Byrd JWT: The supine position. In Byrd JWT (ed): Operative Hip Arthroscopy. New York, Thieme, 1998, pp 123-138.

5. Byrd JWT: Complications associated with hip arthroscopy. In Byrd JWT (ed): Operative Hip Arthroscopy. New York, Thieme, 1998, pp 171-176.

6. Byrd JWT: Avoiding the labrum in hip arthroscopy. Arthroscopy 16:770-773, 2000.

7. Byrd JWT, Pappas JN, Pedley MJ: Hip arthroscopy: An anatomic study of portal placement and relationship to the extra-articular structures. Arthroscopy 11:418-423, 1995.

8. Dienst MRI, Godde S, Seil R, et al: Hip arthroscopy without traction: In vivo anatomy of the peripheral hip joint cavity. Arthroscopy 17:924-931, 2001.

9. Dorfmann H, Boyer T: Arthroscopy of the hip: 12 years of experience. Arthroscopy 15:67-72, 1999.

10. Glick JM: Hip arthroscopy using the lateral approach. Instr Course Lect 37:223-231, 1988.

11. Griffin DR, Villar RN: Complications of arthroscopy of the hip. J Bone Joint Surg Br 81:604-606, 1999.

12. Klapper RC, Dorfmann H, Boyer T: Hip arthroscopy without traction. In Byrd JWT (ed): Operative Hip Arthroscopy. New York, Thieme, 1998, pp 139-152.

13. Sampson TG: Complications of hip arthroscopy. Clin Sports Med 20:831-836, 2001.

14. Sampson TG, Farjo L: Hip arthroscopy by the lateral approach. In Byrd JWT (ed): Operative Hip Arthroscopy. New York, Thieme, 1998, pp 105-122.

15. Sampson TG, Glick JM: Hip arthroscopy by the lateral approach. In McGinty JB (ed): Operative Arthroscopy, 2nd ed. Philadelphia Lippincott-Raven, 1996, pp 1079-1090.

CHAPTER

44

General Techniques for Hip Arthroscopy: Labral Tears, Synovial Disease, Loose Bodies, and Lesions of the Ligamentum Teres

J. W. Thomas Byrd

GENERAL TECHNIQUES FOR HIP ARTHROSCOPY IN A NUTSHELL

History:
Labral Tear
Twisting injury or degenerative process; sharp stabbing pain; reduced performance and twisting ability
Synovial Disease
Gradual onset; groin discomfort; symptoms worse with vigorous activities
Loose Bodies
Due to major trauma or disease; locking, catching, giving-way type of mechanical symptoms
Ruptured Ligamentum Teres
Forceful twisting injury; intermittent pain, catching, and popping
Physical Examination:
Labral Tear
Often normal gait and strength; painful logrolling specific for joint pathology; pain with flexion/internal rotation or abduction/external rotation more severe
Synovial Disease
Often antalgic gait, but strength maintained; discomfort through end ranges of motion
Loose Bodies
Normal gait and strength with intermittent symptoms; pain and catching elicited with forceful rotation maneuvers
Ruptured Ligamentum Teres
Intermittently antalgic gait; painful catching or popping elicited with forceful rotation maneuvers

Continued

Imaging:

Labral Tear

Plain radiographs normal; magnetic resonance imaging may demonstrate labral pathology; magnetic resonance arthrography more sensitive

Synovial Disease

Plain radiographs may show mild osteopenia depending on severity and duration of disease; magnetic resonance imaging shows proliferative synovial disease

Loose Bodies

Radiographs and computed tomography demonstrate bone fragments; arthrographic techniques (arthro-CT or MRA) demonstrate radiolucent loose bodies

Ruptured Ligamentum Teres

Radiographs normal; magnetic resonance imaging rarely demonstrates pathology

Decision-Making Principles:

Labral Tear

Progressive symptoms; failed physical therapy and activity modification; positive physical examination and imaging

Synovial Disease

Progressively destructive process

Loose Bodies

Associated symptoms or incongruent joint

Ruptured Ligamentum Teres

Duration and magnitude of symptoms; positive physical examination findings and index of suspicion

Surgical Technique:

Labral Tear

Resect damaged tissue, creating stable transition zone; chondroplasty of associated articular lesion

Synovial Disease

Synovectomy performed via multiple portals; synovial lining of peripheral capsule resected after traction released

Loose Bodies

Small fragments resected with mechanical shavers; large fragments retrieved with hand instruments, enlarging the portals; monitor for fluid extravasation

Ruptured Ligamentum Teres

Identify tear and resect damaged portion from anterior and posterolateral portals

Postoperative Management:

Functional progression based on pathology and symptoms; crutches for 5 to 7 days; early range of motion, physical therapy, isometric and closed chain rehabilitation

Results:

Labral Tear

20-point improvement in hip score; 70% to 90% successful outcome

Synovial Disease

18-point improvement in hip score

Loose Bodies

28-point improvement in hip score; also important to reduce secondary damage due to third-body wear

Ruptured Ligamentum Teres

43-point improvement in hip score

Labral Tear

Case History

A 20-year-old Division I collegiate hockey player is referred with a 2-year history of progressively worsening sharp, stabbing left hip pain. He is unclear about the exact mechanism of injury, other than his participation in a sport in which high-velocity collisions and forceful twisting mechanisms are common. He has continued to compete, but with greater difficulty and reduced performance. Previous treatment for groin symptoms included activity modification, physical therapy, and various anti-inflammatory medications. Straight plane activities such as jogging are relatively well tolerated, but symptoms are experienced with twisting-type maneuvers.

Physical Examination

On examination, he has a normal gait and full strength. Lying supine, logrolling of the leg back and forth produces symptoms in the anterior groin. He has maintained full range of motion, but maximal flexion combined with internal rotation is painful, again producing groin symptoms. Some discomfort is also experienced with abduction combined with external rotation. These maneuvers reproduce the characteristic symptoms he experiences with activities. There is minimal tenderness to palpation in the groin region and minimal discomfort with resisted hip flexion.

Imaging

Radiographs are unremarkable. Magnetic resonance imaging following gadolinium arthrography reveals evidence of anterior labral pathology (Fig. 44–1).

Decision-Making Principles

Arthroscopy was recommended based on the following factors: severity and duration of symptoms; progressively worsening character, to the point that he could no longer compete effectively; failure of conservative treatment; and physical examination and imaging findings.

Surgical Technique

Arthroscopy was performed on an outpatient basis with the patient under general anesthesia and in the supine position, using a standard three-portal technique. Initial systematic inspection of the hip was performed with the 70- and 30-degree scopes from all three portals. The principal pathology was identified in the anterior portion of the acetabulum. Thus, the inflow was maintained from the posterolateral portal. Operative arthroscopy was achieved by switching the arthroscope and instruments back and forth between the anterolateral and anterior portals.

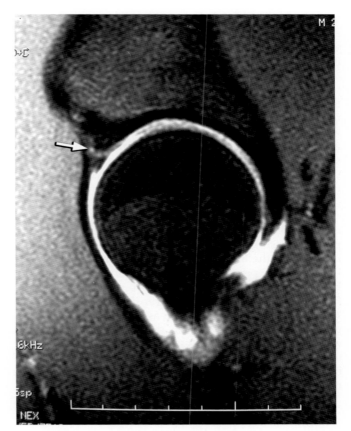

Figure 44–1   Sagittal T2-weighted image of the right hip demonstrates evidence of anterior labral pathology *(arrow)*.

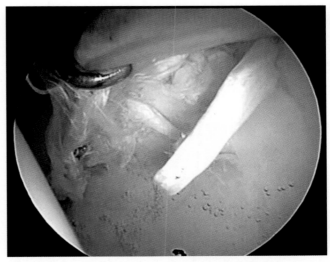

Figure 44–2   Arthroscopic view from the anterolateral portal identifies a radial fibrillated tear of the anterior labrum. The probe was introduced from the anterior portal.

The principal finding was a radial fibrillated tear of the anterior labrum (Fig. 44–2), as seen on preoperative magnetic resonance arthrography. Adjacent to the area of labral pathology was a localized region of deep articular delamination along the anterior rim of the acetabulum. The pathologic tissue was debrided with a full-radius resector (Fig. 44–3), and a stable transition zone with the contiguous healthy labrum was created using a thermal device.

The pattern of labral tears is variable, but the principle of management is the same. The goal is to debride the diseased or damaged labrum while preserving as much healthy, stable tissue as possible. Labral tears uniformly occur at the articular-labral junction. There is usually some element of adjacent articular damage at this site. In fact, the extent of articular pathology may be the determining factor in the response to surgery, as reflected by both the length and the completeness of recovery.

As with other joints, thermal devices should be used in a cautious and conservative fashion. However, they provide great versatility in managing lesions inside the hip, despite the limitations imposed by the constraints of the joint. The principal goal in the management of both labral and articular damage is to remove the unstable fragments and create a stable transition zone while preserving as much healthy tissue as possible. This is sometimes difficult to accomplish using mechanical devices without sacrificing healthy tissue. When properly used, thermal devices can more effectively create this stable transition zone while preserving healthy surrounding tissue.

Results

In my experience, labral debridement results in a median 20-point improvement (based on a 100-point modified Harris hip rating system), with 82% successful outcomes reported in a general population with 5-year follow-up.[5] The results are superior among athletes, with a 31-point improvement and 90% successful results.[4] Farjo et al.[8] reported a 71% success rate in patients without arthritis, and Santori and Villar[17] reported only

67% successful outcomes in a large population. In general, a history of significant trauma is a prognostic indicator that arthroscopy will be successful.[3] An insidious onset of symptoms or a relatively minor precipitating event suggests an underlying predisposition to injury and a less certain prognosis. O'Leary et al.[15] also found that in general, patients with mechanical symptoms such as catching or locking fare better than those who simply experience pain.

Complications

Isolated labral pathology is relatively uncommon. Accompanying articular damage has been reported in 50% to 55% of cases.[5,8] The extent of articular damage is most likely the limiting factor with regard to the success of arthroscopic debridement. Farjo et al.[8] reported a success rate of only 21% for labral debridement in the presence of arthritis.

Synovial Disease

Case History

A 22-year-old woman is referred with a 3-year history of ill-defined left hip pain. There was no history of trauma or precipitating activities; there was simply a gradual onset of groin discomfort. Symptoms were made worse with vigorous activities but remained present even after she accepted a sedentary lifestyle.

Physical Examination

On examination, the patient had a normal gait and good strength on manual testing. There was minimal discomfort with logrolling of the leg back and forth. She maintained full passive range of motion, although she experienced mild groin discomfort at all end ranges.

Imaging

Radiographs were unremarkable except for subtle evidence of regional osteopenia, likely associated with 3 years of altered function from her underlying symptoms (Fig. 44–4). Magnetic resonance imaging revealed evidence of proliferative synovial disease (Fig. 44–5). Serologic testing and review of systems were unrevealing. A previous attempt at aspiration had been unsuccessful at obtaining sufficient fluid for analysis.

Decision-Making Principles

With a diagnosis of an unspecified synovial disorder, arthroscopy was recommended. Although her symptoms were mostly manageable with a sedentary lifestyle, the possibility of a progressively destructive process made intervention prudent, rather than waiting for the symptoms to worsen.

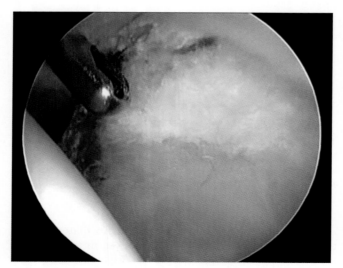

Figure 44–3 The damaged tissue is debrided with a full-radius resector.

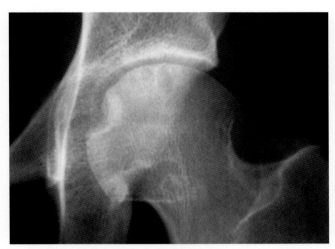

Figure 44–4 Anteroposterior radiograph of a left hip demonstrates joint space preservation with multiple subchondral cysts of the femoral head, suggestive of pigmented villonodular synovitis.

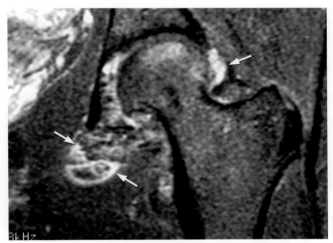

Figure 44–5 Coronal T2-weighted image of the left hip demonstrates evidence of proliferative synovial disease (arrows).

Surgical Technique

Arthroscopy was begun using the standard supine distraction method with three portals. Superficial acetabular chondral changes were identified and debrided, as well as synovial disease from the pulvinar contained within the acetabular fossa (Fig. 44–6). After completing arthroscopy of the intra-articular portion of the joint, the instruments were removed, the traction was released, and the hip was flexed 45 degrees. From the anterolateral portal, the arthroscope was repositioned on the anterior neck of the femur for access to the peripheral compartment. An ancillary portal was established distally for instrumentation. More extensive synovial disease was encountered, and a thorough synovectomy was performed (Fig. 44–7).

The pulvinar appears to be the neural equivalent of the fat pad in the knee. Lesions in this tissue can be quite painful. Synovial disease is sometimes focally localized to this area without involvement of the capsular lining. Reactive hypertrophic fibrotic tissue can also be encountered in this area, with accompanying pain. Sometimes this is the primary lesion causing the patient's symptoms, and sometimes fibrosis of this area occurs as a secondary phenomenon in association with other intra-articular pathology.

For fulminant synovial disease requiring an extensive synovectomy, the region of greatest involvement is the synovial lining of the joint capsule. This is most effectively addressed by arthroscopy of the peripheral compartment with the traction released.

Results

We have reported a median 18-point improvement with synovectomy in patients followed for 5 years.[5] However, this is a heterogeneous group. In many cases, the synovial process is secondary to other intra-articular pathology, most commonly degenerative disease. Synovectomy can improve the symptoms associated with aggressive rheumatoid disorders, and arthroscopy can be quite helpful in both diagnosing and treating various primary synovial disorders, including synovial chondromatosis and pigmented villonodular synovitis. The diagnosis of synovial chondromatosis tends to be more elusive in the hip than in other joints. McCarthy et al.[14] found that less than half of their cases were diagnosed before arthroscopy.

Loose Bodies

Case History

An obese 16-year-old girl sustained a posterior dislocation of the right hip (Fig. 44–8) from a motor vehicle accident. She underwent closed reduction under general anesthesia. A computed tomography scan (Fig. 44–9) and a postreduction radiograph (Fig. 44–10) demonstrated a comminuted femoral head fracture. This included a large, nondisplaced Pipkin I fragment of the inferior femoral head and at least two other entrapped intra-articular fragments, resulting in a nonconcentric reduction. The patient was kept on a strict, protected weight-bearing status and referred for consideration of arthroscopy to remove the intra-articular fragments.

Surgical Technique

Arthroscopy was performed with the standard supine, three-portal technique. An initial systematic inspection was performed to assess all aspects of the pathology as thoroughly as possible. The largest entrapped fragment

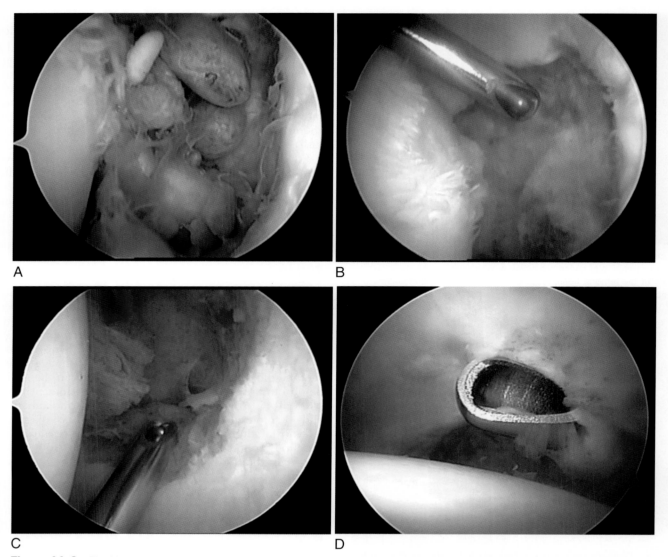

A

B

C

D

Figure 44–6 The hip is viewed from the anterolateral portal. *A,* Synovial disease characteristic of pigmented villonodular synovitis is identified in the acetabular fossa. *B,* Debridement of the fossa is begun with the shaver from the anterior portal. *C,* Debridement of the fossa is completed from the posterolateral portal. *D,* Synovial disease of the posterior capsule extending underneath the posterior labrum is best debrided from the posterolateral portal, as this portion of the capsule is not well accessed from the peripheral compartment.

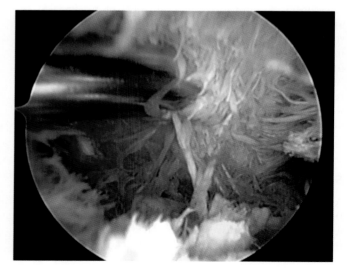

Figure 44–7 With traction released and the hip flexed, the arthroscope has been repositioned from the anterolateral portal into the peripheral compartment. Extensive synovial disease is present, and debridement is performed with the shaver introduced from an ancillary portal. This illustrates the "seaweed" appearance ascribed to pigmented villonodular synovitis.

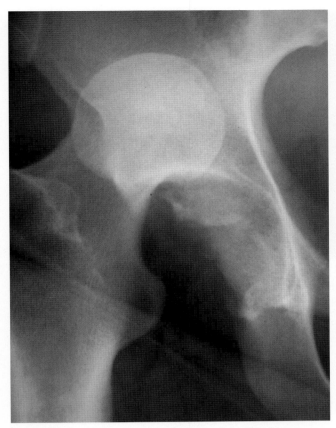

Figure 44–8   Anteroposterior radiograph of the right hip demonstrates a posterior fracture-dislocation.

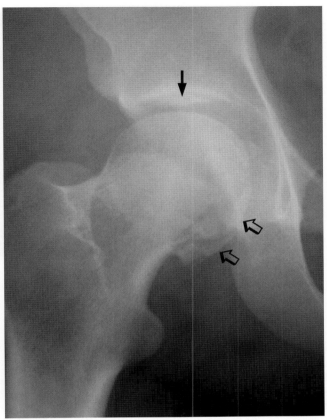

Figure 44–10   Postreduction radiograph reveals a nonconcentric reduction with a bone fragment trapped in the weight-bearing portion of the joint *(arrow)* and a minimally displaced fracture of the inferior femoral head *(open arrows)*.

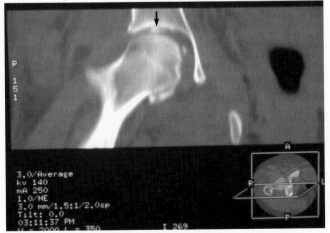

Figure 44–9   Coronal computed tomographic reconstruction illustrates the largest entrapped fragment *(arrow)* within the joint.

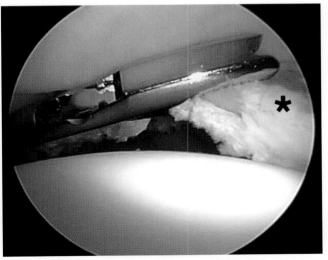

Figure 44–11   Arthroscopic view from the anterolateral portal demonstrates the largest fragment (*), which has been grasped by an instrument brought in from the posterolateral portal.

5 Hip

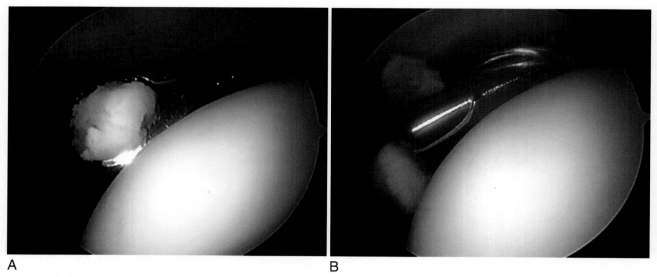

A   B

Figure 44–12   Now viewing from the posterolateral portal, fragments are identified within the acetabular fossa and retrieved from the anterior portal. *A,* One is retrieved with a grasper. *B,* Smaller fragments are debrided with a full-radius resector.

was identified with an attachment of the posterior capsule (Fig. 44–11). Smaller fragments identified in the fossa were retrieved with a grasper and debrided with a shaver (Fig. 44–12). Before the fragments were removed, the skin and capsular incisions were enlarged to ensure passage of the fragments through the soft tissues as they were withdrawn from the joint. It is also important to view the fragments through the arthroscope as they leave the capsule in case they are lost or portions break off and remain undetected in the joint. The postoperative radiograph demonstrates removal of the intra-articular fragments, now with a concentric reduction, and the inferior femoral head fragment remains nondisplaced (Fig. 44–13). Postoperatively, the patient was maintained on antithrombotic prophylaxis because of her obesity, recent trauma, and inactivity.

Removal of free-floating loose bodies can be a challenge. If there is soft tissue attachment, debridement should leave a small tag of tissue attached that tethers the loose body, making it easier to grasp. Manipulating the position of the inflow cannula often flushes pieces up toward the instrument for grasping. Loose bodies associated with disease, such as synovial chondromatosis, may go undetected in the peripheral compartment. Thus, for these conditions, it is important to inspect the periphery of the joint with the traction released.

Loose body removal represents the earliest and clearest indication for arthroscopy.[1,2,16] The importance of loose body removal has been well documented by the work of Epstein.[7] Arthroscopy offers distinct advantages over traditional open techniques, including less morbidity and shortened recovery. Post-traumatic fragments are usually the most obvious; loose bodies associated with synovial chondromatosis may be less evident. Loose bodies are occasionally encountered in association with degenerative disease. In this circumstance, it is important to carefully assess for associated arthritis, as this will be the limiting factor in the procedure's success. With

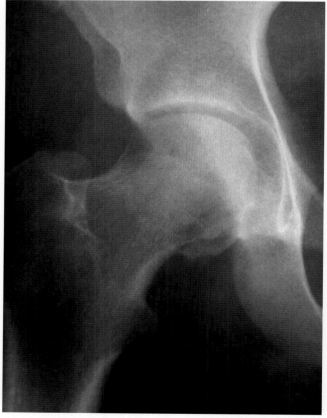

Figure 44–13   Postoperative anteroposterior radiograph demonstrates a concentric reduction; the inferior femoral head fragment remains in place.

advanced degeneration, removing bone fragments may be of no benefit to the patient.

One issue regards the timing of arthroscopy following acute trauma. Fluid extravasation can occur due to loss of the capsular integrity or through acetabular fracture lines. Waiting several weeks may result in sufficient soft tissue healing to create a fluid seal; however, this must be weighed against the consequences of secondary damage incurred from the entrapped fragments. A high-flow fluid management system for arthroscopy is advantageous, as it allows adequate flow for visualization without requiring high pressures, which would accentuate extravasation. However, during this and all arthroscopic hip procedures, it is imperative to be cognizant of the rate of fluid ingress. It is also important that the procedure be completed in a timely and efficient fashion. It is appropriate to abandon the procedure if inordinate fluid extravasation is encountered or if the procedure cannot be completed within a reasonable amount of time.

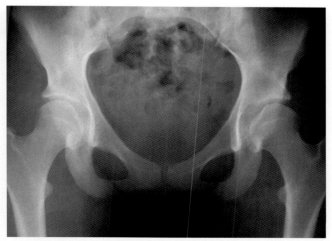

Figure 44–14   Anteroposterior radiograph of the pelvis demonstrates slight widening of the medial joint space of the left hip compared with the right.

Ruptured Ligamentum Teres

Case History

A 16-year-old cheerleader is referred 2 years after a twisting injury to her left hip. Since then, she has had intermittent episodes of pain and catching, necessitating a restriction of activities.

Physical Examination

On examination, she demonstrates a mildly antalgic gait. Logrolling of her hip back and forth is uncomfortable, and maximal flexion combined with internal rotation produces sharp anterior groin pain. Otherwise, she has full range of motion, and there are no other remarkable findings.

Imaging

Radiographs suggest slight widening of the medial joint space of the left hip compared with the right (Fig. 44–14), and magnetic resonance imaging suggests a lesion within the acetabular fossa (Fig. 44–15) suspicious for synovial disease, possibly synovial chondromatosis.

Decision-Making Principles

Given the magnitude and duration of her symptoms, as well as the physical examination findings and the imaging studies suggesting articular pathology, arthroscopy was recommended.

Surgical Technique

Standard three-portal arthroscopy performed with the patient in the supine position revealed a rupture of the ligamentum teres, with the disrupted fibers floating freely in the joint (Fig. 44–16A). Debridement was performed using combinations of straight and curved shaver

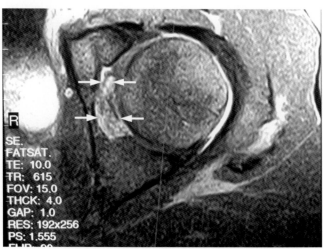

Figure 44–15   Axial T2-weighted image suggests a soft tissue lesion contained within the medial joint and acetabular fossa *(arrows)*.

blades, allowing access to the disrupted ligament around the convex surface of the femoral head. Most of the debridement was performed from the anterior portal, allowing optimal access to the fossa (Fig. 44–16B). External rotation of the hip facilitates delivery of the disrupted ligament anteriorly. However, the acetabular attachment is on the posterior aspect of the fossa, and this portion is often best addressed from the posterior portal (Fig. 44–16C).

Results

Rupture of the ligamentum teres is increasingly recognized as a significant source of persistent mechanical hip pain. Disruption can be expected in association with dislocation of the joint but is more frequently encountered in simple twisting injuries. These lesions are usually not

5 Hip

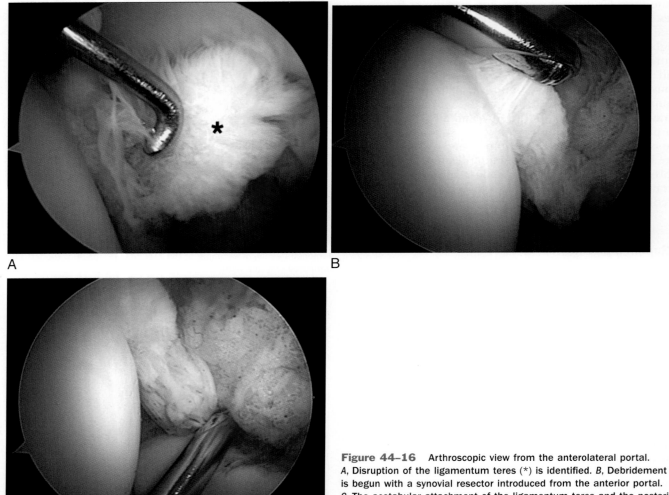

A

B

C

Figure 44–16 Arthroscopic view from the anterolateral portal. *A,* Disruption of the ligamentum teres (*) is identified. *B,* Debridement is begun with a synovial resector introduced from the anterior portal. *C,* The acetabular attachment of the ligamentum teres and the posterior aspect of the fossa are addressed with a shaver from the posterolateral portal.

evident with current imaging methods. They tend to be quite painful and often respond well to arthroscopic debridement.

Indiscriminate debridement of the ligamentum teres should be avoided because of its potential vascular contribution to the femoral head, but selective debridement of the disrupted fibers is indicated. The disrupted portions tend to float freely in the joint and are readily delivered with suction to the shaver blades. Traumatic ruptures can be partial or complete. Degenerative rupture can also occur and is more commonly seen in association with global arthritic disease.

Gray and Villar[9] were the first to recognize arthroscopically the existence of lesions of the ligamentum teres and classified them as partial, complete, and degenerative. We have found disruption of the ligamentum teres to be the third most common disorder encountered in athletes undergoing arthroscopy and demonstrated one of the most successful outcomes.[4] In a separate study of traumatic disruptions, the improvement averaged 43 points, with 96% of patients demonstrating greater than 20-point improvement.[6]

Postoperative Management

Postoperative rehabilitation following hip arthroscopy is similar for most forms of pathology.[10-13] There is a functional progression, with the time frame dictated by the extent of pathology, the patient's residual symptoms, and the ultimate goals of recovery. General exceptions to this protocol include patients with arthritic disease and patients who undergo microfracture.

Crutches are helpful the first few days after surgery, until the patient's gait pattern is normalized. Usually within 5 to 7 days, these can be discontinued. Supervised therapy can begin on the second postoperative day. This may be little more than periodic instruction in the progression of exercises or may be more intense and hands-on, depending on the circumstances. For example, professional athletes can dedicate many hours and resources to their rehabilitation. They tend to be more tolerant of residual discomfort and often have economic incentives to resume competition as quickly as possible, especially given the limited span of their professional careers.

Gentle range-of-motion exercises are begun immediately and are mostly pushed to tolerance. Excessive emphasis on range of motion may only exacerbate symptoms and ultimately prolong recovery. Isometric exercises and closed chain strengthening, such as gentle single leg stance, are also begun right away. Progression to open chain exercises and functional drills is individualized, based on the extent of pathology and the ultimate goals of recovery.

In the presence of arthritic disease, the postoperative recovery is slower and can be expected to be less complete. Typically, crutches may be necessary for the first 2 weeks after surgery to develop a relatively pain-free gait and avoid early setbacks.

Microfracture is sometimes indicated for grade IV lesions with a healthy surrounding articular surface. In these circumstances, the patient is kept on a strict, protected weight-bearing status for 8 to 10 weeks to protect the area of microfracture during the early fibrocartilaginous healing phase. The patient is allowed to bear pressure equivalent to the weight of the leg. This neutralizes the forces across the hip joint and also makes crutch use more tolerable. During this early phase, emphasis is on passive and active assisted range of motion. Some precautions are mandated for the first 3 months after surgery.

References

1. Byrd JWT: Hip arthroscopy for post-traumatic loose fragments in the young active adult: Three case reports. Clin Sports Med 6:129-134, 1996.
2. Byrd JWT: Indications and contraindications. In Byrd JWT (ed): Operative Hip Arthroscopy. New York, Thieme, 1998, pp 7-24.
3. Byrd JWT, Jones KS: Prospective analysis of hip arthroscopy. Arthroscopy 16:578-587, 2000.
4. Byrd JWT, Jones KS: Hip arthroscopy in athletes. Clin Sports Med 20:749-762, 2001.
5. Byrd JWT, Jones KS: Prospective analysis of hip arthroscopy with 5 year follow up. Paper presented at the 69th annual meeting of the American Academy of Orthopaedic Surgeons, Feb 2002, Dallas, TX.
6. Byrd JWT, Jones KS: Traumatic rupture of the ligamentum teres as a source of hip pain. Paper presented at the annual meeting of the Arthroscopy Association of North America, Apr 2002, Washington, DC.
7. Epstein H: Posterior fracture-dislocations of the hip: Comparison of open and closed methods of treatment in certain types. J Bone Joint Surg Am 43:1079-1098, 1961.
8. Farjo LA, Glick JM, Sampson TG: Hip arthroscopy for acetabular labrum tears. Arthroscopy 15:132-137, 1999.
9. Gray AJR, Villar RN: The ligamentum teres of the hip: An arthroscopic classification of its pathology. Arthroscopy 13:575-578, 1997.
10. Griffin KM: Rehabilitation of the hip. Clin Sports Med 20:837-850, 2001.
11. Griffin KM, Henry CO, Byrd JWT: Rehabilitation. In Byrd JWT (ed): Operative Hip Arthroscopy. New York, Thieme, 1998, pp 177-202.
12. Griffin KM, Henry CO, Byrd JWT: Rehabilitation after hip arthroscopy. J Sports Rehab 9:77-88, 2000.
13. Henry C, Middleton K, Byrd JWT: Hip rehabilitation following arthroscopy. Videotape presented at the annual meeting of the American Academy of Orthopaedic Surgeons, Feb 1995, Orlando, FL.
14. McCarthy JC, Bono JV, Wardell S: Is there a treatment for synovial chondromatosis of the hip joint? Arthroscopy 13:409-410, 1997.
15. O'Leary JA, Berend K, Vail TP: The relationship between diagnosis and outcome in arthroscopy of the hip. Arthroscopy 17:181-188, 2001.
16. Sampson TG, Glick JM: Indications and surgical treatment of hip pathology. In McGinty JB (ed): Operative Arthroscopy, 2nd ed. New York, Lippincott-Raven, 1996, pp 1067-1078.
17. Santori N, Villar RN: Acetabular labral tears: Result of arthroscopic partial limbectomy. Arthroscopy 16:11-15, 2001.

5 Hip

Arthroscopic Removal of Post-traumatic Loose Bodies and Penetrating Foreign Bodies from the Hip

David M. Kahler

ARTHROSCOPIC REMOVAL OF POST-TRAUMATIC LOOSE BODIES AND PENETRATING FOREIGN BODIES FROM THE HIP IN A NUTSHELL

History:
Acetabular fracture; low-velocity gunshot wound

Physical Examination:
Mechanical symptoms, pain

Imaging:
Computed tomography (preoperatively); fluoroscopy (intraoperatively)

Indications:
Accessible symptomatic loose body

Surgical Technique:
Examination under anesthesia; distraction; portal placement; arthroscopic shaving; loose body identification and removal

Postoperative Management:
Total hip precautions*; early range of motion; progressive weight bearing

Results:
Good in properly selected patients; if complete removal is not possible, the goal is to ensure that the fragments are extra-articular

---

*Avoid hip flexion past 90 degrees, and avoid adduction or internal rotation past neutral for the first 6 weeks.

Trauma to the hip joint sometimes results in intra-articular loose bodies or foreign bodies. During closed reduction of a traumatic dislocation of the hip, small fragments of the anterior or posterior walls of the acetabulum may inadvertently become entrapped in the joint. These fragments may require removal to eliminate mechanical symptoms and prevent further damage to the articular surface. Occasionally, low-velocity gunshot wounds may also result in intra-articular loose bodies or bullet fragments. Injuries such as these traditionally required formal open exposure and dislocation of the hip joint for the removal of loose bodies. Hip arthroscopy can allow the minimally invasive removal of such fragments, without further jeopardizing the blood supply to the femoral head during surgical dislocation. In the case of retained bullet fragments, thorough inspection, debridement, and lavage of the hip joint space by arthroscopy decrease the risk of the late complication of lead synovitis.[1,4,5]

With the exception of isolated case reports, there has been little literature on the arthroscopic versus open removal of articular fragments and foreign bodies from the hip joint. Nonetheless, hip arthroscopy has been shown to be safe and effective for the removal of labral fragments and loose bodies, with a low complication rate.[2,3] It therefore seems reasonable to consider the use of less invasive techniques to debride the hip joint when trauma results in intra-articular loose bodies.

There are several caveats regarding arthroscopy following hip trauma. The size and location of the fragments should be carefully assessed by computed tomography preoperatively. The surgeon should be aware that small-looking ossific fragments may have relatively large labral or articular cartilage attachments that could hinder removal. Fragments deep in the nonarticular acetabular fossa may be difficult to reach arthroscopically; loose bodies in this location may cause minimal symptoms if they are not mobile and do not impinge on the femoral head, so they can often be ignored (Fig. 45–1). Large loose bodies that resemble a flake of cortical bone are usually attached to a torn labrum and are not amenable to arthroscopic removal (Fig. 45–2). Loose bodies embedded in the femoral head near the anterior and posterior articular margins may be impossible to remove arthroscopically, because joint distraction for arthroscopy only tightens the capsule against these areas. Finally, fragments in the inferior recess of the joint may be visible but inaccessible to the arthroscopist.

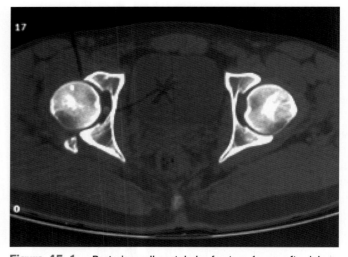

Figure 45–1 Posterior wall acetabular fracture 1 year after injury, demonstrating remodeling of the posterior wall. This fracture was treated nonsurgically and demonstrates a small, asymptomatic retained fragment in the nonarticular fossa.

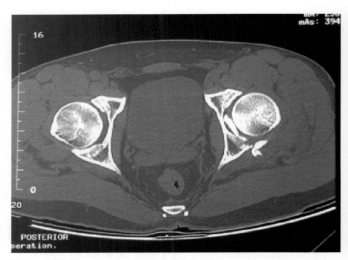

Figure 45–2 This large intra-articular fragment represents a significant portion of the posterior wall and is attached to a torn, infolded acetabular labrum. This case requires a formal open reduction.

Imaging

Penetrating trauma requires additional evaluation before contemplating the removal of loose bodies. Arteriography is advisable whenever there is an entry wound in the vicinity of the femoral triangle. Visceral injury must be ruled out by computed tomography, because peritoneal lavage may be negative when there is retroperitoneal involvement of bowel or vascular structures. The surgeon should also carefully assess the status of the femoral, sciatic, and superior gluteal nerves at the initial evaluation. Because the femoral vessels are relatively tethered beneath the inguinal ligament, the safest course in cases of penetrating trauma may be to explore the contents of the femoral triangle and hip joint through an anterior (Smith-Peterson) approach rather than relying on arthroscopy alone. In cases in which the projectile fragments are clearly intra-articular, novel approaches have been described for their removal.[1,4,5]

Intraoperative C-arm fluoroscopy is probably advisable for all hip arthroscopies, but it is essential in trauma cases. In routine hip arthroscopy, it is usually necessary to vent the hip joint to allow controlled distraction. However, because hip dislocation and penetrating trauma invariably cause some degree of capsular disruption, venting of the joint is usually unnecessary, and it generally requires very little traction to distract the traumatized hip joint adequately on the fracture table. Traction should be applied slowly under fluoroscopic control to avoid excessive distraction and the resultant risk of neurologic injury or vascular compromise to the extremity or femoral head. The standard arthroscopic portals are used for visualizing fragments and inserting tools for removal. The optimal portal for viewing loose bodies is sometimes the optimal portal for fragment removal as well; in these cases, the scope may be replaced by a curved grasper and fragments removed under fluoroscopic (rather than arthroscopic) control.

Case Histories and Surgical Techniques

Case 1

A 37-year-old man was involved in a single-vehicle head-on collision and suffered facial lacerations and a posterior dislocation of the left hip. A small posterior wall acetabular fracture was noted. Sciatic nerve function was normal. Closed reduction of the hip was accomplished under conscious sedation soon after presentation to the emergency department. Postreduction radiographs revealed a slightly widened joint space, and computed tomography confirmed an isolated osteochondral fragment entrapped in the nonarticular fossa of the joint (Fig. 45–3). Although the posterior wall defect appeared innocuous (<30% of the posterior articular arc), the hip was extremely irritable, and the patient was unable to

mobilize with physical therapy. The patient was offered examination under anesthesia and arthroscopic removal of the entrapped fragment. He gave consent for open reduction in the event the hip proved to be unstable under anesthesia.

Following induction of general anesthesia with muscle relaxation, the patient's hip was examined and was found to be stable at the extremes of motion. Significant crepitus was noted during flexion and rotation. The patient was placed in the supine position, as is typical in trauma cases. The hip was then distracted under fluoroscopic control using a standard fracture table. A direct lateral arthroscopic portal was established; despite the capsular disruption resulting from the dislocation, it was necessary to use a banana blade to perform a capsulotomy under fluoroscopic control to facilitate passage of the arthroscopic cannula. Multiple chondral and osteochondral fragments were easily visualized. Under fluoro-

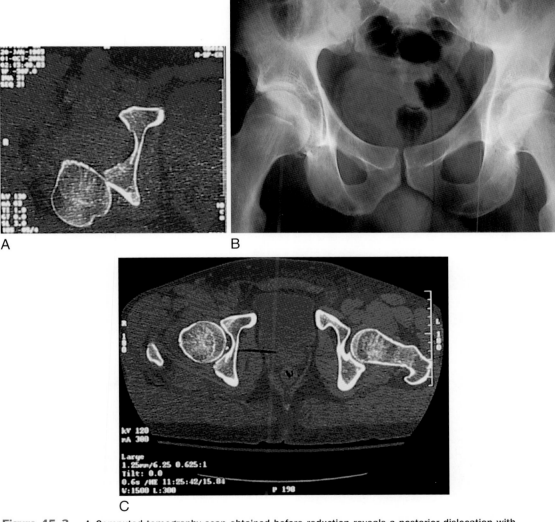

A

B

C

Figure 45–3   *A,* Computed tomography scan obtained before reduction reveals a posterior dislocation with minimal posterior wall defect. *B,* Postreduction film of the pelvis shows very slight widening of the hip joint (note the teardrop distance). *C,* Postreduction computed tomography scan reveals that a small fragment of the posterior wall has been reduced into the hip joint space.

5 Hip

scopic control, a shaver was inserted through the antero-lateral portal, and the smaller cartilaginous fragments were removed during debridement of the posterior wall. A grasper was used to remove the larger osteoarticular fragment (Fig. 45–4). The scope was partially withdrawn to view joint congruity as traction was gradually released, and fluoroscopy confirmed a concentric reduction. The patient was mobilized immediately with total hip precautions (restrictions against excessive hip flexion, adduction, and internal rotation) and a brief period of toe-touch weight bearing. He recovered uneventfully without evidence of instability, arthrosis, or avascular necrosis.

It is often difficult to completely withdraw large fragments through the dense gluteal fascia and musculature, and the goal is simply to ensure that the fragments are extracapsular at the end of the procedure. Viewing of the articular margins during release of traction helps confirm joint congruity and concentric reduction. Following removal of the arthroscope, the hip should be ranged under fluoroscopic visualization to ensure that there is no residual mechanical dysfunction or joint space widening following joint debridement.

Case 2

A 48-year-old marksman accidentally discharged a .22-caliber target pistol into his left groin while exiting his vehicle at a shooting match. He was seen at an outside hospital and underwent emergent exploration of the wound. The bullet had passed through the iliopsoas muscle belly without damaging the femoral nerve or vascular sheath, and the surgeon could not locate the projectile. Computed tomography confirmed that the bullet had lodged at the posterior articular margin of the acetabular fossa (Fig. 45–5). The patient was transferred to our institution, where it was decided to attempt arthroscopic removal of the bullet and several small lead fragments from the hip joint.

Following distraction of the hip joint under fluoroscopic control, the acetabular fossa was visualized with a

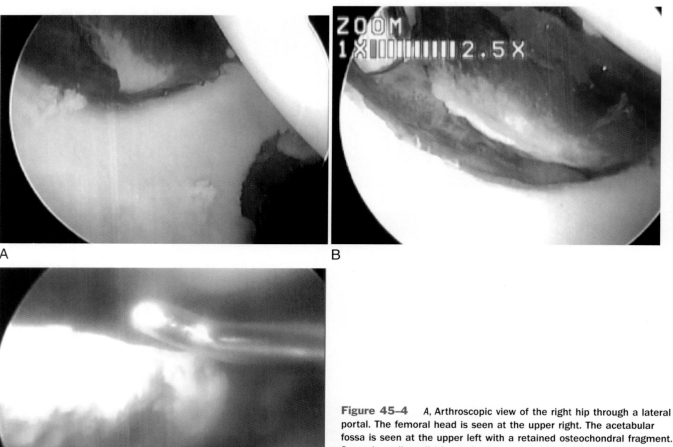

A

B

C

Figure 45–4 *A,* Arthroscopic view of the right hip through a lateral portal. The femoral head is seen at the upper right. The acetabular fossa is seen at the upper left with a retained osteochondral fragment. Several small cartilaginous fragments lie on the posterior articular surface of the acetabulum. The small posterior wall defect is seen at the lower right. *B,* Close-up view of the retained osteochondral fragment. *C,* A probe is used to evaluate chondral flaps adjacent to the posterior wall fracture before debridement with a shaver.

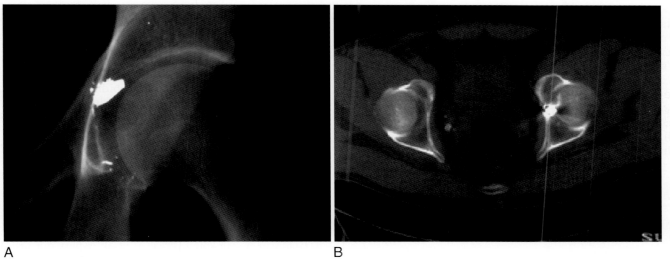

Figure 45–5   *A*, Radiograph reveals a possible intra-articular penetrating foreign body. *B*, Computed tomography scan confirms that the bullet is embedded in the acetabular fossa.

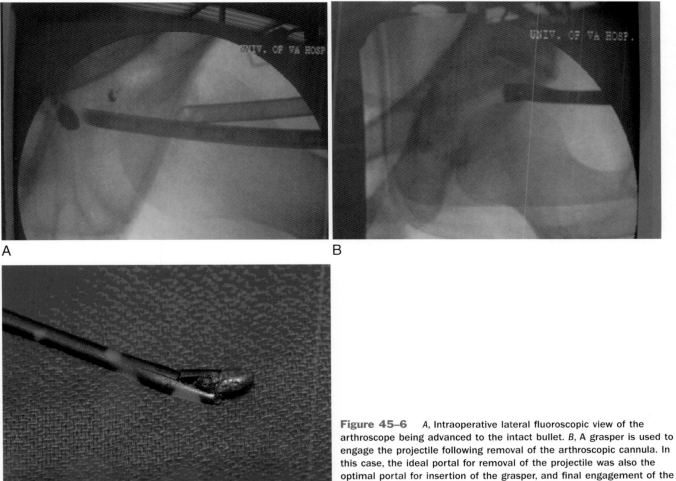

Figure 45–6   *A*, Intraoperative lateral fluoroscopic view of the arthroscope being advanced to the intact bullet. *B*, A grasper is used to engage the projectile following removal of the arthroscopic cannula. In this case, the ideal portal for removal of the projectile was also the optimal portal for insertion of the grasper, and final engagement of the bullet was performed under fluoroscopic control. *C*, The grasper and extracted projectile.

5 Hip

30-degree scope, and a shaver was used to debride the hemorrhagic fatty tissue and several small lead fragments in the acetabular fossa. The bullet was relatively nondeformed and fixed in place and could be well visualized only through the lateral portal. The arthroscopic cannula was removed, and a curved grasper was introduced under fluoroscopic control (Fig. 45–6). The bullet was easily removed, and the scope was reinserted to confirm the removal of all lead fragments. The patient has developed slight nonprogressive narrowing of the hip joint space at 4-year follow-up.

Postoperative Management

Most patients can be mobilized immediately following hip arthroscopy for trauma, with weight bearing as tolerated. A short period of crutch walking usually improves comfort. Most patients with isolated injuries can be managed on an outpatient basis.

Complications

Heterotopic ossification has occasionally been observed following joint distraction for post-traumatic fragment removal. Excessive traction has also been known to cause pudendal nerve palsy. Careful application of traction for joint distraction should minimize these complications. Post-traumatic arthritis may develop as a consequence of any articular injury to the hip joint.

Conclusion

Hip arthroscopy provides a less invasive alternative for the removal of intra-articular loose bodies resulting from trauma. The judicious use of this technology may spare the trauma patient from the morbidity of a traditional open approach. Formal open reduction and joint debridement remain the treatment of choice for posterior wall acetabular fractures that are large enough to cause hip instability and for foreign bodies lodged in the inferior recesses of the joint.

References

1. Goldman A, Minkoff J, Price A, et al: A posterior arthroscopic approach to bullet extraction from the hip. J Trauma 27:1294-1300, 1987.
2. Kashiwagi N, Suzuki S, Seto Y: Arthroscopic treatment for traumatic hip dislocation with avulsion fracture of the ligamentum teres. Arthroscopy 17:67-69, 2001.
3. McCarthy JC, Day B, Busconi B: Hip arthroscopy: Applications and technique. J Am Acad Orthop Surg 3:115-122,1995.
4. Meyer NJ, Thiel B, Ninomiya JT: Retrieval of an intact, intraarticular bullet by hip arthroscopy using the lateral approach. J Orthop Trauma 16:51-53, 2002.
5. Teloken MA, Schmietd I, Tomlinson DP: Hip arthroscopy: A unique inferomedial approach to bullet removal. Arthroscopy 18:E21, 2002.

Arthroscopy of the Knee

Knee: Patient Positioning, Portal Placement, and Normal Arthroscopic Anatomy

Bernard C. Ong, Francis H. Shen, Volker Musahl,

Freddie Fu, and David R. Diduch

General Principles

As arthroscopic equipment, techniques, and surgical skills have improved, the role of arthroscopy in diagnosing and managing various knee pathologies has expanded. It is not the goal of this chapter, nor is it feasible, to describe all the arthroscopic equipment and techniques available. It is more important to understand the general principles and for each surgeon to develop a systematic approach to knee arthroscopy that works for him or her. By evaluating the knee joint in a consistent, reproducible fashion, the surgeon reduces the risk of missing lesions and decreases operative time by minimizing the number of "second passes" necessary. This decreases tourniquet time, operative time, patient morbidity, and complications.

Identification

Before the patient is anesthetized and brought to the surgical suite, it is important that the patient's identity be verified and that the correct operative site be identified by both the patient and the operating surgeon. The American Academy of Orthopaedic Surgeons currently recommends that the patient identify the surgical site and that the operating surgeon sign his or her name or initials on the actual operative site with indelible ink.[1] If the patient is marking the surgical site, use of a checkmark (√) is recommended, because an X may be misconstrued as indicating the incorrect site. This practice decreases the possibility of performing surgery at the wrong site.

Anesthesia

Depending on the procedure, knee arthroscopy can be performed under local, regional, or general anesthesia.[20,30] The choice of anesthetic is affected by the patient's general medical condition, the procedure, and the preference of the patient, surgeon, and anesthesiologist.

Local Anesthesia

The use of local anesthesia with or without intravenous sedation for knee arthroscopy has gained popularity. The decision to use local anesthetic must take into account the procedure performed and the estimated length of time required. Procedures that can be performed in less than 20 minutes and do not require significant joint exposure are best suited for local anesthesia with intravenous sedation.[30] This may include procedures such as diagnostic arthroscopy, removal of loose bodies, and partial meniscectomies. Longer procedures that require significant joint exposure or bone work are not good candidates for local anesthesia.[26] An arthroscopic fluid pump can minimize bleeding because a tourniquet is often poorly tolerated.

At 15 to 30 minutes before the procedure, the planned portal sites are infiltrated with 3 to 5 mL of 1% lidocaine (Xylocaine) as a small skin wheal and infiltrated down to the joint capsule. The knee joint itself is infiltrated with 30 mL of a 1:1 mixture of Xylocaine and bupivacaine to provide both immediate and longer-term analgesia.[5,30] Additional anesthetic can be delivered as needed intraoperatively, staying below the maximum total dose of 300 mg (or 4.5 mg/kg) for Xylocaine[25] and 175 mg for bupivacaine.[24]

Regional Anesthesia

Regional anesthesia, such as a spinal anesthetic, can be considered in patients with significant medical issues for whom general anesthesia may be contraindicated or in those who simply wish to observe the procedure on the monitor. Most arthroscopic knee procedures can be adequately managed with regional anesthesia, if necessary.

General Anesthesia

For the majority of patients, general anesthesia is the preferred method. It allows for adequate joint exposure and complete muscle relaxation, and tourniquet pain is not an issue. Cases requiring bone work or long tourniquet times, such as cruciate ligament reconstruction, are best managed with general anesthesia.[30]

Examination under Anesthesia

Once the patient is anesthetized, an examination under anesthesia should be performed. A systematic physical examination with the patient comfortable or asleep can provide the surgeon with important additional information. The surgeon can correlate the examination with the pathology found arthroscopically, and at teaching insti-tutions, it is the ideal opportunity to practice and improve examination skills.

Patient Positioning

After the examination under anesthesia, if a tourniquet is being used, it is applied to the proximal thigh of the operative extremity. In the absence of a tourniquet, the use of an arthroscopic fluid pump may be desirable to limit bleeding. Position the patient supine on the operating table. The use of either a leg holder or a lateral post allows the surgeon to manipulate the extremity intraoperatively.

A lateral post is advantageous because it leaves the extremity free for intraoperative examination, eliminates the need for leg support when in extension, and makes access to posterior and accessory portals easier (Fig. 46–1). However, it may require that an assistant be available to help manipulate the leg, and use of a post generally makes it more difficult to apply large varus and valgus stresses to the knee.

Alternatively, the use of a proximal leg holder allows the patient's foot to be placed on the surgeon's iliac crest, eliminating the need for an assistant to hold the leg in most cases. It also gives the surgeon the ability to generate greater varus and valgus stresses across the knee, which can be beneficial for visualization of and access to the joint in tight knees, especially postero-

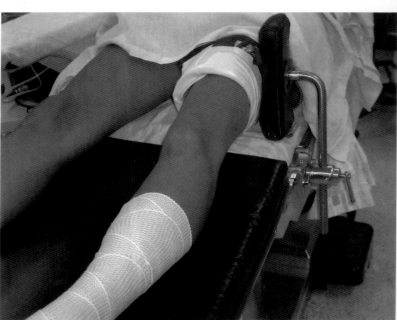
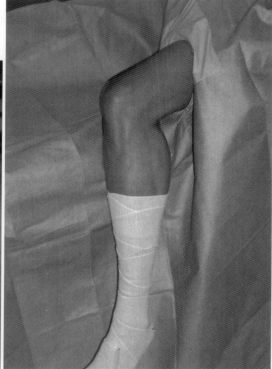

A   B

Figure 46–1   *A* and *B*, Using the lateral post during knee arthroscopy leaves the extremity free for intraoperative examination and eliminates the need for leg support when in extension.

medially. However, a leg holder may be difficult to use, particularly in heavy patients with short thighs. Use of the leg holder is facilitated by positioning the foot of the table with 90 degrees of flexion. The patient must be adequately distal on the operating table to ensure that the knee is beyond the break of the table (Fig. 46–2).

The nonoperative leg should be well padded to prevent potential pressure problems, and consideration can be given to wrapping the nonoperative side to limit venous stasis. The operative extremity is then prepared and draped in the standard surgical fashion with any of the commercially available drapes.

Arthroscopic Equipment

For a surgeon just beginning to learn arthroscopic techniques, the equipment can be confusing. Few of the arthroscopic instruments are the same as those used in open procedures. Although instrumentation has evolved to make complex arthroscopic procedures easier, good fundamental arthroscopic techniques must still be applied. Knowledge of the capabilities and limitations of the arthroscopic equipment is vital to the efficiency, success, and safety of the procedure being performed.

The arthroscopes are named based on the angle between the direction of the viewing lens and the long axis of the arthroscope. The viewing lens of the 0-degree arthroscope is straight ahead, whereas the 70-degree arthroscope "looks off" at 70 degrees from the direction that the arthroscope is pointing.

The most commonly used arthroscope is the 30-degree lens; however, for tight angles, such as when viewing structures in the posteromedial or posterolateral compartments, the 70-degree lens is often helpful.[12,18,27] The 0-degree arthroscope may be helpful when working straight ahead in the intercondylar notch from one of the more anterior portals.[18,27]

Of all the arthroscopic equipment, perhaps the most commonly used and most important diagnostic tool is the arthroscopic probe. When used properly, it is an extension of the surgeon's finger and is essential for the complete evaluation of intra-articular structures.

In general, when working in the medial compartment (in contrast to the lateral compartment), up-going arthroscopic instruments may be easier to use. Because the medial tibial plateau is concave, up-going instruments may conform better to the contours and make certain arthroscopic procedures easier. In contrast, the lateral plateau is convex, and straight instruments are often more effective. Various left- and right-angled instruments are also available to gain access to hard-to-reach areas.

When managing chondral and meniscal lesions, it is important to think "mechanically" rather than "cosmetically." Unstable lesions should be removed or repaired, as appropriate, to minimize mechanical joint wear. Once a stable lesion has been created, contouring should be performed; however, excessive attempts at making chondral or meniscal lesions look perfect increase the likelihood of doing more damage to previously healthy tissue.

When trimming meniscal tears, arthroscopic "biters" and "ducklings" are designed to take wider bites than arthroscopic "punches" do. They are typically used first because they are quicker and cause less trauma to the cartilage. Because the punch is narrower, it leaves a cleaner edge, minimizes debris, and is easier to see around when used in the knee; it is therefore used to trim the corners of flaps or the ends of a bucket handle tear. The suction shaver is generally used to contour the meniscal rim or debride chondral lesions.

Relevant Anatomy

The patella articulates with the anterior aspect of the femur predominantly in the trochlear groove. However, in full extension, the patella is in minimal contact with the articular surface of the femur, riding on the anterior femoral shaft just proximal to the lateral aspect of the trochlear groove.[19]

The articular cartilage on the posterior aspect of the patella is the thickest in the body and reflects the large forces that the patellofemoral joint must sustain.[16] On the femoral side, the V-shaped trochlear groove is about 5 to 6 mm deep and separates the medial and lateral femora. Inferiorly and posteriorly it becomes the intercondylar notch.

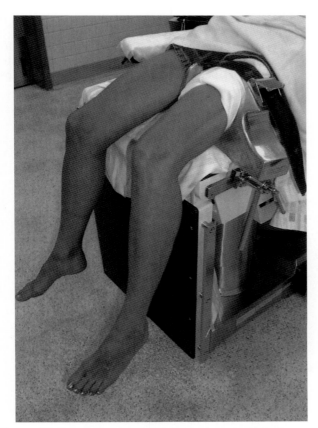

Figure 46–2   When using a thigh holder, have the patient sufficiently distal on the table to allow for adequate intraoperative knee flexion.

A distinct indentation at the midportion of the lateral femoral condyle marks the lateral groove, or sulcus terminalis, which demarcates where the patellofemoral articulation ends and the tibiofemoral articulation begins. This groove can usually be seen on the lateral radiograph and should not be mistaken for an osteochondral defect. Similarly, a smaller medial groove on the medial femoral condyle delineates the most anterior extent of the medial femoral articular surface that contacts the tibia. This medial groove is well forward of the lateral femoral condyle and may be mistaken for a pathologic process caused by a hypertrophic medial plica. It is actually the area where the anterior horn of the medial meniscus abuts the femur when the knee is fully extended.

On the tibial side, the medial tibial plateau is longer in the sagittal plan than is the lateral plateau. Both the medial and lateral plateaus are concave in the coronal plane; in the sagittal plane, however, the lateral plateau is convex, producing a saddle-shaped articulation. Therefore, the articular surfaces of the knee are not congruent. On the medial side, the femur meets the tibia like a wheel on a flat surface; on the lateral side, it is like a wheel on a dome and would produce extremely high stresses if not for the meniscus. By improving joint congruence and increasing contact area, the menisci participate in load sharing.[7,10,14]

The medial meniscus is somewhat more C-shaped than the circular, O-shaped lateral meniscus (Fig. 46–3). The medial meniscus, constituting more than half of the contact surface of the medial plateau, is less mobile than the lateral meniscus, which covers approximately three fourths of the contact surface. Both have firm anterior and posterior attachments to help distribute the protective tensile hoop stresses within the body of the meniscus.[6,14,28] Up to 80% of the total load on an intact joint passes through the menisci,[9,10] and removal of even a portion of the meniscus results in a decreased ability to transmit load across the joint.[2-4]

The anterior and posterior cruciate ligaments cross each other within the notch of the femur and provide anterior and posterior stability. The anterior cruciate ligament, originating from the inner wall of the lateral femoral condyle, has a broad insertion into a nonarticular portion of the tibia between the tibial spines.[8] The posterior cruciate ligament originates from the medial wall of the intercondylar notch and descends posterolaterally, inserting into a groove on the posterior aspect of the tibia 1 to 1.5 cm below the joint line.[22]

Arthroscopy Portals

One of the keys to successful knee arthroscopy is precise placement of the portals of entry. Poorly placed portals translate into poorly positioned arthroscopes and instruments. This can complicate the procedure and lead to articular injury, missed pathology, and instrument damage. Careful palpation of the knee to identify bony and soft tissue landmarks after draping, but before joint distention, can help identify the appropriate entry portals. Surgeons who are new to arthroscopy may benefit from drawing the joint lines, soft tissue, and bony landmarks with a skin marker before making an incision.[31] Flexion and extension of the knee can aid in palpation of the landmarks.

We describe here the most commonly used standard and accessory portals. Although additional entry sites have been described, they are rarely necessary. Most

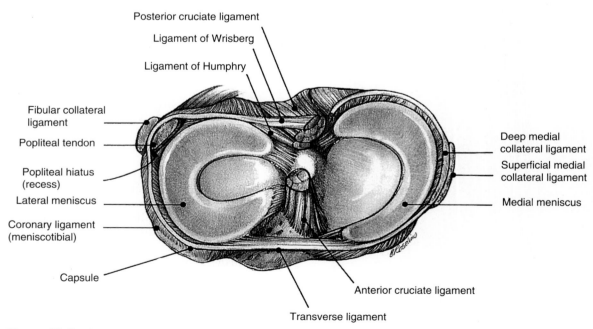

Figure 46–3 Schematic of tibial plateau and associated structures. (From Scott WN [ed]: The Knee. St Louis, Mosby, 1994, p 20.)

arthroscopic knee procedures can be performed through two or three standard portals, although surgeons should be prepared to use additional portals as necessary, depending on the pathology found intraoperatively.

Standard Portals

Anterolateral Portal

The anterolateral portal is the standard viewing portal where the arthroscope is first inserted. It is the most versatile portal and is located in the palpable lateral "soft spot" approximately 1 cm above the lateral joint line and adjacent to the lateral margin of the patellar tendon (Fig. 46–4).[23] The anterolateral site allows visual access to almost all the structures within the knee joint, with the possible exception of the tibial insertion of the posterior cruciate ligament and the undersurface of the anterior horn of the lateral meniscus.

When creating this portal, care should be taken not to make the incision too superiorly or inferiorly. Superior placement restricts access into the patellofemoral joint and suprapatellar pouch. In addition, visualization of the posteromedial structures is difficult owing to the

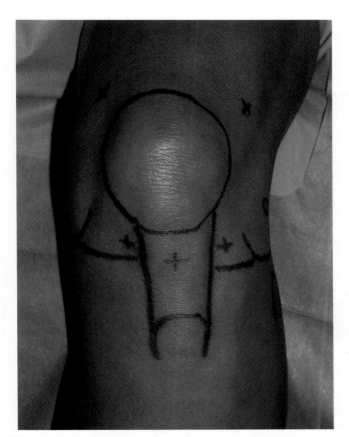

Figure 46–4   Surgeons new to arthroscopy may benefit from drawing the joint line and bony anatomy. This figure demonstrates the anteromedial, anterolateral, superomedial, superolateral, and transpatellar portals (see text).

arthroscope's entering at too steep an angle that is not parallel to the joint space. Inferior placement puts the anterior horn of the meniscus at risk for iatrogenic laceration. The medial tibial spine may block the path of instruments as they are passed across the notch into the lateral compartment. Further, at this level, the arthroscope enters the thickest portion of the infrapatellar fat pad. Excessively medial placement may also result in penetration of the edge of the patellar tendon, restricting maneuverability within the joint.

Anteromedial Portal

The anteromedial portal is the primary working portal. It may be used to introduce arthroscopic instrumentation or as an alternative viewing portal. It is located 1 cm above the medial joint line, 1 cm inferior to the tip of the patella, and adjacent to the medial edge of the patellar tendon in the medial soft spot (see Fig. 46–4).[23] This portal can be made at the same time as the anterolateral portal, or it can be established under arthroscopic visualization after localization with a spinal needle (see Chapter 47).

Superomedial and Superolateral Portals

Either of these portals can be useful for the evaluation of dynamic tracking of the patellofemoral articulation and, if necessary, as a separate portal for an inflow cannula if the scope sheath is not used for irrigation fluid. They are located approximately 2.5 cm superior to the superomedial or superolateral corner of the patella, respectively (see Fig. 46–4).[23] One must make sure that the portal is adjacent to but not through the quadriceps tendon. The superolateral entry site is typically less traumatic to the muscle and therefore less painful for the patient postoperatively. The interval between the vastus lateralis and iliotibial band can be readily defined with manual translation of the patella laterally. Lateral subluxation of the patella tenses the lateral edge of the vastus lateralis and accentuates the interval between the vastus lateralis and the iliotibial band. The cannula is aimed toward the suprapatellar pouch during insertion to avoid inadvertent chondral injury to the patella or femoral trochlea. This portal is useful as an inflow-outflow portal or for assessment of patellofemoral tracking, visualization of the superior chondral surface of the patella and trochlea, and retrieval of loose bodies in the suprapatellar pouch.

Accessory Portals

Posterolateral Portal

This portal is rarely used in routine arthroscopy. It is located behind the lateral collateral ligament anterior to both the biceps tendon and the common peroneal nerve (Fig. 46–5). This portal can be palpated when the joint is fully distended with the knee in a figure-of-four position. It is used primarily for assisting in posterior horn repairs of the lateral meniscus,[21] total synovectomies,[15,29] and occasionally removal of loose bodies.[9,17,30]

6 Knee

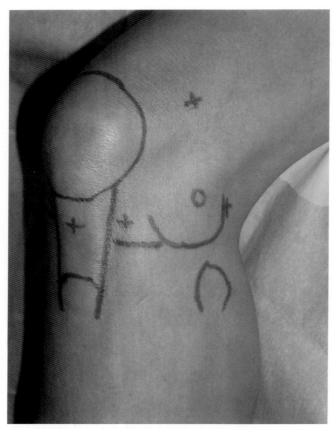

Figure 46–5 Lateral oblique view demonstrating the posterolateral portal. The femoral condyle, fibular head, and joint line have been outlined. The lateral epicondyle is marked with a circle (o).

Posteromedial Portal

Located in a small triangular soft spot formed by the posteromedial edge of the femoral condyle and tibia, this portal offers optimal viewing of and access to the posteromedial compartment structures.[12,13] The location is approximately 2 cm above the posteromedial joint line and 1 to 2 cm posterior to the palpable outline of the femoral epicondyle and the medial collateral ligament origin (Fig. 46–6). Hence, the portal is above and behind the posteromedial compartment, with instruments inserted down and anteriorly to access the joint. This small triangle is often difficult to find, but the landmarks are easier to palpate before joint distention and with the knee flexed to 90 degrees. Transilluminating the skin by passing the arthroscope under the posterior cruciate ligament into the posteromedial compartment also assists in locating this portal while decreasing the risk of saphenous nerve and vein injury by outlining their location. A spinal needle is then introduced, and the location and direction are confirmed intra-articularly under direct vision. For this portal, it is often safest to cut only the skin with the knife blade and then use a straight hemostat to spread bluntly through the soft tissues into the joint to minimize injury to the neurovascular structures.

Transpatellar Portal

First described to facilitate exposure of the intercondylar notch, this portal, as the name implies, is a vertical incision directly through the patellar tendon paralleling its fibers (see Fig. 46–4). Although this portal allows

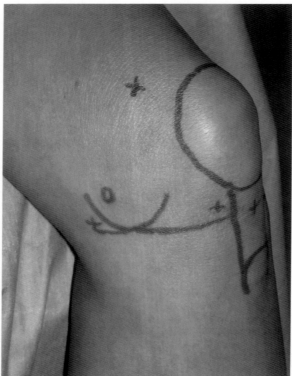

A

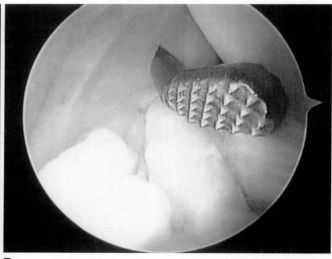

B

Figure 46–6 *A,* Medial oblique view demonstrating the posteromedial portal. The femoral condyle and joint line have been outlined. The medial epicondyle is marked with a circle (o). *B,* A meniscal rasp is placed through the posteromedial portal to access the meniscosynovial junction of the medial meniscus.

excellent visualization of intercondylar notch structures, it can be difficult to manipulate the arthroscope through the patellar tendon.[11] In addition, this portal risks the complications of tendinitis and catastrophic injury to the extensor mechanism. As a result, this portal is seldom used.

Other Accessory Portals

If the surgeon has a clear understanding of the joint anatomy and the location of neurovascular structures that are potentially at risk, accessory portals can be established in almost any area of the knee. The position of these portals is dependent on the location of the pathology and the angle of access required. The same techniques used to establish other portals, such as avoidance of neurovascular structures and localization with a spinal needle under direct vision, are used for establishing these portals.

References

1. American Academy of Orthopaedic Surgeons: "Sign your site" gets strong support from academy members. AAOS Bull 47:35, 1999.
2. Anderson DR, Gershuni DH, Nakhostine M, Danzig LA: The effects of nonweight bearing and limited motion on tensile properties of the meniscus. Arthroscopy 9:440, 1993.
3. Baratz ME, Fu FH, Mengato R: Meniscal tears: The effect of meniscectomy and repair on intra-articular contact areas and stress in the human knee. Am J Sports Med 14:270, 1986.
4. Belzer JP, Cannon WE: Meniscal tears: Treatment in the stable and unstable knee. J Am Acad Orthop Surg 1:41-47, 1993.
5. Boden BP, Fassler S, Cooper S, et al: Analgesic effect of intraarticular morphine, bupivacaine, and morphine/bupivacaine after arthroscopic knee surgery. Arthroscopy 10:104, 1994.
6. Caldwell GL, Allen AA, Fu FH: Functional anatomy and biomechanics of the meniscus. Oper Tech Sports Med 2:152, 1994.
7. Cannon WD, Morgan CD: Meniscal repair. Part II. Arthroscopic repair techniques. J Bone Joint Surg Am 76:294, 1994.
8. Carson WE, Simon PT, Wickiewicz, et al: Revision ACL reconstruction. Am Acad Orthop Surg Instr Course Lect 47:361-368, 1998.
9. Collican MR, Dandy DJ: Arthroscopic management of synovial chondromatosis: Findings and results in 18 cases. J Bone Joint Surg Br 71:498, 1989.
10. DeHaven KE, Arnoczky SP: Meniscal repair. Part I. Basic science, indications for repair and open repair. J Bone Joint Surg Am 76:140-152, 1994.
11. Eriksson E, Sebik A: A comparison between the transpatellar tendon and the lateral approach to the knee joint during arthroscopy: A cadaveric study. Am J Sports Med 8:103, 1980.
12. Gillquist J, Habgerg G, Oretorp N: Arthroscopic visualization of the posteromedial compartment of the knee joint. Orthop Clin North Am 10:545, 1979.
13. Gold DL, Schaner PJ, Sapega AA: The posteromedial portal in knee arthroscopy: An analysis of diagnostic and surgical utility. Arthroscopy 11:139, 1995.
14. Henning CE: Arthroscopic repair of meniscus tears. Orthopedics 6:1130, 1983.
15. Highgenboten CL: Arthroscopic synovectomy. Orthop Clin North Am 13:399, 1982.
16. Hungerford DS, Barry M: Biomechanics of the patellofemoral joint. Clin Orthop 241:203, 1989.
17. Jackson RW: Current concepts review: Arthroscopic surgery. J Bone Joint Surg Am 65:416, 1983.
18. Mariani PP, Gillquist J: The blind spots in arthroscopic approaches. Int Orthop 5:257, 1982.
19. Marquet P: Mechanics and osteoarthritis of the patellofemoral joint. Clin Orthop 144:70, 1979.
20. McGinty JB, Matza RA: Arthroscopy of the knee: Evaluation of an out-patient procedure under local anesthesia. J Bone Joint Surg Am 60:787, 1978.
21. Miller MD: Atlas of meniscal repair. Oper Tech Orthop 5:70 1995.
22. Miller MD, Bergfield JA, Fowler PJ, et al: The posterior cruciate ligament injured knee. Am Acad Orthop Surg Instr Course Lect 48:199-207, 1999.
23. Parisien JS: Normal arthroscopic anatomy portals and techniques. Paper presented at the 62nd annual meeting of the American Academy of Orthopaedic Surgeons, Feb 1995, Orlando, FL.
24. Physicians' Desk Reference, 55th ed. Montvale, NJ, Medical Economic Corporation, 2001, p 599.
25. Physicians' Desk Reference, 55th ed. Montvale, NJ, Medical Economic Corporation, 2001, p 607.
26. Sapega AA, Heppenstall RD, Chance B, et al: Optimizing tourniquet application and release times in extremity surgery: A biomechanical and ultrastructural study. J Bone Joint Surg Am 67:303, 1985.
27. Shahriaree H: O'Connor's Texbook of Arthroscopic Surgery. Philadelphia, JB Lippincott, 1984.
28. Shrive NG, O'Connor JJ, Goodfellow JW: Load-bearing in the knee joint. Clin Orthop 131:279, 1978.
29. Smiley P, Wasilewski SA: Arthroscopic synovectomy. Arthroscopy 6:18, 1990.
30. Yoshiya S, Kurosaka M, Hirohata K, Andrish JT: Knee arthroscopy using local anesthetic. Arthroscopy 4:86, 1988.
31. Zarins B: Knee arthroscopy: Basic technique. Contemp Orthop 6:63, 1983.

47

Knee: Diagnostic Arthroscopy

DAVID R. DIDUCH, FRANCIS H. SHEN, BERNARD C. ONG,

VOLKER MUSAHL, AND FREDDIE FU

Regardless of the planned arthroscopic procedure, the surgeon should perform at least a quick diagnostic arthroscopy. The importance of a systematic approach cannot be overemphasized. In this chapter we describe the major areas of the knee that every arthroscopic examination should include (Table 47–1). The exact sequence is not critical, but performing the examination methodically helps to avoid missed pathology.

Scope Insertion

There are several techniques available for scope insertion. If a separate inflow cannula is used, it is inserted through either a superomedial or a superolateral portal. A small skin incision is made in the direction of Langer's line, and a blunt trocar within its cannula is inserted through the skin and joint capsule and into the suprapatellar pouch by aiming deep to the patella (posteriorly) and toward its superior tip. The posterior path allows for clearance of the patella. Access to the suprapatellar pouch can be confirmed with a side-to-side sweeping motion of the blunt trocar. In general, use of a sharp trocar to enter the knee joint should be avoided to decrease the risk of iatrogenic cartilage injury.

The anterolateral portal is typically established next. However, if the surgeon does not wish to use a separate inflow cannula, the anterolateral portal is established first as the viewing portal, with the inflow attached to the same cannula. The decision whether to use a separate irrigation inflow portal is based on the surgeon's preference. Use of the arthroscopic cannula for inflow eliminates the need for an extra incision and the associated morbidity. Previous concerns about decreased joint distention because of lower volumes through a smaller sheath have been reduced with the availability of high-flow cannulas and optional inflow pumps.

When making the skin incision for the anterolateral portal, a number 11 blade is used, aimed toward the femoral notch. Care is taken to point the blade superiorly and vertically to minimize the risk of cutting the anterior horn of the lateral meniscus. Alternatively, if the anatomic landmarks can be accurately palpated and the surgeon is confident that the incision is above the meniscus, a horizontal incision can be used. Here, the blade is oriented away from the patellar tendon to avoid injury to the fibers. This leaves a more cosmetic scar, but the incision can be difficult to extend if access is limited.

In either case, the blade should be inserted deep enough to penetrate the joint capsule, but not to the point of damaging the femoral condyles. Next, the arthroscopic sheath with a blunt trocar is introduced with a twisting motion toward the intercondylar notch with the knee flexed approximately 60 to 90 degrees. The tip of the trocar is then retracted slightly, and the knee is fully extended slowly to allow the trocar to be passed into the suprapatellar pouch.

If excessive resistance is met, the maneuver should be stopped and the site reassessed. The surgeon should ensure that the trocar is not caught in the intercondylar notch, that the portal is within the patellar tendon, and that the incision is long enough to prevent the scope from binding on the skin or capsule. If the tip of the trocar is caught on the ligamentum mucosum, which comes from the roof of the intercondylar notch to the fat pad, the patella will rotate as the trocar is advanced against resistance. In this case, the trocar should be withdrawn slightly and passed more laterally into the suprapatellar pouch.

Once in the suprapatellar pouch, the trocar is removed and the arthroscope is inserted through the sheath. If the manufacturer's name or logo is facing superiorly toward the head, the scope is oriented correctly so that "up is up." The arthroscopic camera lens generally views an area directed either 30 or 70 degrees away from the side of the light cord attachment (or straight ahead

Table 47-1
Arthroscopic Regions of the Knee

Suprapatellar pouch
Patellofemoral compartment
Lateral gutter
Medial gutter
Medial compartment
Intercondylar notch
Lateral compartment

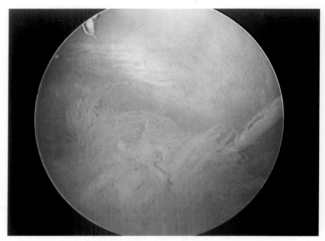

Figure 47-1 Inflamed, thickened synovium with increased vascularity from chronic inflammation.

with the 0-degree scope). In most cases, the 30-degree lens is used. Once the arthroscope is in the suprapatellar pouch, the patella can be used as a visual reference to check the camera orientation.

Suprapatellar Pouch

The suprapatellar pouch is easily visualized and is the starting point for most arthroscopic knee examinations. With the pouch distended and the knee extended, the surgeon should systematically examine the pouch from medial to lateral and superior to inferior to characterize the synovium and look for the presence of adhesions, plicae, or loose bodies. The character of the synovial villi, their vascularity, and the presence of inflammation or crystalline deposits should be noted.[55] Normally, the synovium is a light or pale red in color. When the knee is inflamed from a mechanically impinging meniscal tear or advanced arthrosis, the synovium can be thickened and extremely vascular (Fig. 47-1). Alternatively, the synovium itself can be primarily involved in the disease process, such as rheumatoid arthritis, pigmented villonodular synovitis, and ochronosis.[1,39] If an arthroscopic synovectomy is planned, it may be necessary to use three to five portals to access all knee compartments for a complete synovectomy, including posteromedial and posterolateral portals.[17,55]

Plicae are normal remnants of synovial partitions that remain from embryologic development and are classified according to their anatomic relationship to the patella (Table 47-2). They vary in size, thickness, and clinical significance.[43] Very few plicae are pathologic or contribute to a patient's symptoms.

When present, the suprapatellar plica divides the suprapatellar pouch into two partial or complete compartments. An incidental finding of a centrally placed hole or opening within the suprapatellar plica, called the *porta*, has been described (Fig. 47-2A).[45,46] The significance of the suprapatellar plica lies in the potential for

Table 47-2	
Incidence of Synovial Plicae of the Knee	
Plica	Incidence (%)
Infrapatellar (ligamentum mucosum)	67
Suprapatellar	55
Medial	25
Lateral	<1

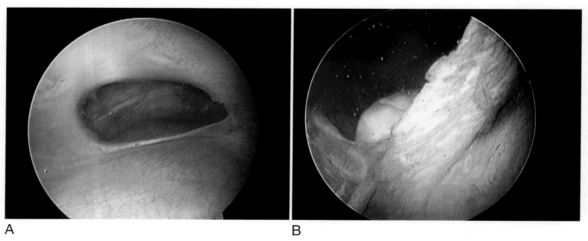

A   B

Figure 47-2 *A,* Porta of the suprapatellar plica. *B,* Loose body hidden behind the porta.

loose bodies to lodge behind the septation, hidden from view (Fig. 47–2*B*).

Patellofemoral Compartment

By withdrawing the scope inferiorly with the lens rotated upward, the undersurface of the patella can be seen. The full width and length of the patella should be examined. Rotating the lens inferiorly allows inspection of the trochlear groove where the patella articulates. Document any changes in the patellar and trochlear articular surfaces.

At this point, the patellar and femoral relationship is assessed (Fig. 47–3*A*). In full extension, normally no more than 20% of the patellar surface overhangs the lateral edge of the femur.[15,20,21] Visualizing the patellofemoral articulation from below as the knee is taken through a limited range of motion demonstrates contact and wear patterns or malalignment and maltracking between the patella and femur.

Normally, the lateral facet aligns at 20 degrees of flexion and the medial facet contacts the trochlear notch at about 50 degrees of flexion.[20,21] Arthroscopic evidence of malalignment is suggested if the patella is not centrally located in the trochlear notch during the first 40 to 50 degrees of flexion (Fig. 47–3*B*).[5,35]

Classification of Chondral and Osteochondral Lesions

If chondral lesions are seen in the patellofemoral joint, or anywhere in the knee, they should be documented carefully both with arthroscopic pictures and in the operative notes. Accurate diagnosis involves visualization as well as palpation with the probe for firmness and surface disruption.[50]

Several classification systems exist to describe chondral injuries. The original Outerbridge[41] classification described both the quality and the size of the chondral damage. Insall et al.[22] subsequently modified this classi-fication system to reflect primarily the depth of cartilage loss (Table 47–3). Because no single classification system is all-inclusive, it is more important for the surgeon to be descriptive and to routinely use one system to document the findings, including the percentage of the surface area involved in each compartment.

Lateral Gutter

The lateral gutter is examined next. If this portion of the arthroscopic examination is not performed early, it is often skipped. This is unfortunate, because the latter gutter is often the site where loose bodies and resected pieces of menisci collect (Fig. 47–4). The lateral gutter is entered with the knee in full extension to relax the soft tissues on the lateral aspect of the knee. When entering from the patellofemoral joint, it is important to lift up on the cannula or retract the arthroscope slightly to

Table 47–3	
Classification of Articular Injury	

Grade	Description
Outerbridge System	
I	Softening and swelling of cartilage
II	Fragmentation and fissuring, <0.5 inch in diameter
III	Fragmentation and fissuring, >0.5 inch in diameter
IV	Erosion of cartilage down to exposed subchondral bone
Insall Modification	
I	Softening and swelling of cartilage
II	Fissuring to subchondral bone
III	Fibrillation of articular surface
IV	Erosion of cartilage down to exposed subchondral bone

6 Knee

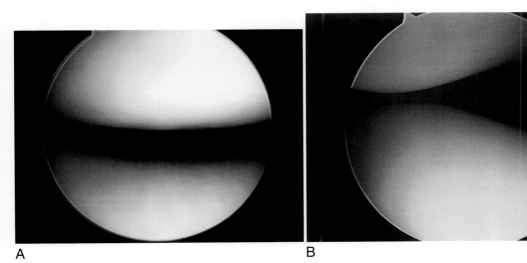

Figure 47–3   *A*, Normal patellofemoral relationship. *B*, Maltracking of the patellofemoral joint.

A   B

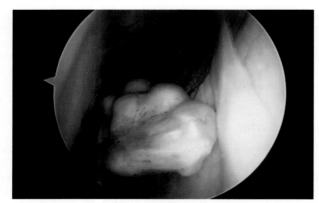

Figure 47–4 Loose body in the lateral gutter.

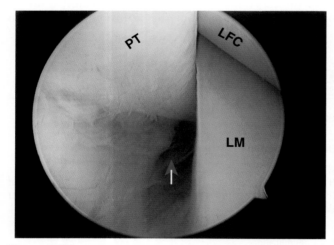

Figure 47–5 Lateral gutter *(arrow)* at the junction of the popliteal tendon (PT), posterior horn of the lateral meniscus (LM), and posterior articular surface of the lateral femoral condyle (LFC).

prevent scuffing the superolateral edge of the lateral femoral condyle. The structures visualized in this position are the posterior horn of the lateral meniscus, the meniscosynovial capsular reflection, the popliteal tendon, the posterior limits of the popliteal hiatus, and the posterior articular surface of the lateral femoral condyle (Fig. 47–5). With the arthroscopic cannula positioned at the hiatus, apply suction through the cannula to help dislodge and remove loose bodies that may have migrated into the popliteal recess. Compressing the back of the knee can also help flush out loose bodies from the inferior portion of the recess. Again being careful not to scuff the superolateral edge of the lateral femoral condyle, return up into the patellofemoral compartment and proceed to the medial side.

Medial Gutter

As the surgeon enters the medial gutter, about 40% of knees have a medial synovial plica running medial and distal to the patella, originating from the medial wall of the suprapatellar pouch and inserting into the fat pad distally (Fig. 47–6).[9] Although this is almost always an incidental finding and asymptomatic, it can occasionally be the cause of anteromedial knee pain and popping, especially with repetitive activities such as cycling.[43] If thickened from trauma or chronic inflammation, it can cause chondromalacial changes due to abrasion on the corner of the medial femoral condyle. By flexing the knee slightly, the area of contact between the plica and the medial femoral condyle can be inspected for damage that suggests the plica as a source of symptoms.[13,53] Occasionally, the arthroscope may need to be partially withdrawn to disengage from a large plica so that the medial compartment can be entered.

Next, advance the arthroscope and look inferiorly over the edge of the medial femoral condyle into the medial gutter. If the scope is entering from the anterolateral portal, as is customary, it will not be possible to "drive" the scope deep into the medial gutter, as was done on the lateral side. Look for loose bodies, synovitis, or traumatic disruptions of the capsule (Fig. 47–7). Palpation of the posteromedial knee joint may help express any hidden loose bodies.

If a leg holder is being used, flex the knee approximately 30 degrees with valgus stress and move the arthroscope into the medial compartment. If a lateral post is being used, 90 degrees of knee flexion over the side of the operating table accomplishes the same result.

Medial Compartment

As the surgeon enters the medial compartment, the medial meniscus helps orient the viewer. Valgus stress with external rotation of the tibia can help open up the medial compartment for the arthroscope. Allow the arthroscope to slip between the medial femoral condyle and the tibial plateau into the space created by the valgus stress on the knee. Forcing the arthroscope can result in gouging and scuffing of the articular surfaces that will never heal, so this should be meticulously avoided. Likewise, withdrawing the arthroscope before releasing the stress on the knee prevents the arthroscope from being

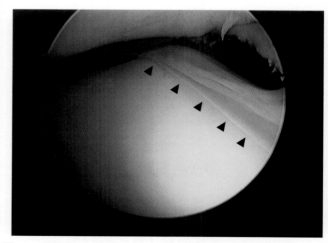

Figure 47–6 Medial synovial plica *(arrowheads)* draped over a corner of the medial femoral condyle.

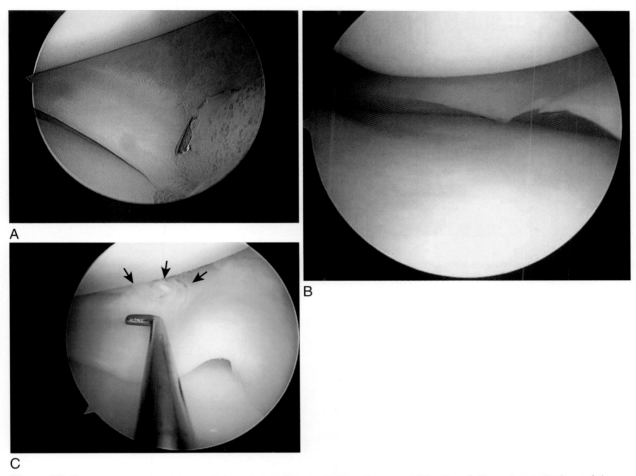

Figure 47–7   *A*, Anterior horn of the medial meniscus with a normal meniscosynovial junction. *B*, Normal posterior horn of the medial meniscus. *C*, Tear *(arrows)* in the posterior horn of the medial meniscus.

caught between the articular surfaces and gouging the cartilage as it is removed.

Creation of the Anteromedial Portal

At this point, if the anteromedial portal has not been created, it can be established under direct vision. With the lens directed medially and anteriorly, an 18-gauge spinal needle is inserted through the planned portal, free of the fat pad and superior to the medial meniscus. The anteromedial portal is adjacent to the patellar tendon, 1 cm above the joint line and in the medial "soft spot" that mirrors the anterolateral portal location.[42] Under direct vision, observe the path of the needle to ensure placement in the appropriate location (Fig. 47–8*A*). A downward and medially directed path improves visualization and allows eventual instrument access to the posterior aspect of the medial compartment.

Remove the needle and make a skin and capsular incision with a number 11 blade directed toward the intercondylar notch (Fig. 47–8*B*). This can be performed under direct vision to prevent damage to the articular cartilage and anterior horn of the medial meniscus. A straight hemostat can be used to help stretch the capsu-

lar opening and improve access for instruments. A probe is then inserted through this portal.

Examination of the Medial Meniscus

For a systematic approach, the meniscus is divided into anterior, middle (or body), and posterior regions. With the lens still directed anteromedially, examine the anterior horn of the meniscus, manipulating the fat pad with a probe or resecting a portion of the fat pad if necessary to obtain a better view. In addition to a visual inspection, a complete meniscal examination should include direct palpation of the upper and undersurfaces of the meniscus with a probe (Fig. 47–9). Simple tears that are not noted on visual inspection can often be demonstrated with probing. Use the probe to lift, depress, and retract the meniscus to help palpate for clefts. This must be done gently, however, because vigorous probing can tear the meniscus, especially if the tip is used.

Follow the meniscus posteriorly to the body of the medial meniscus. Evaluate the meniscosynovial reflection and synovial covering. Probe both the superior and inferior surfaces for stability. Elevate the midportion of the medial meniscus to visualize the deep medial collateral ligament (Fig. 47–10), where the attachment runs

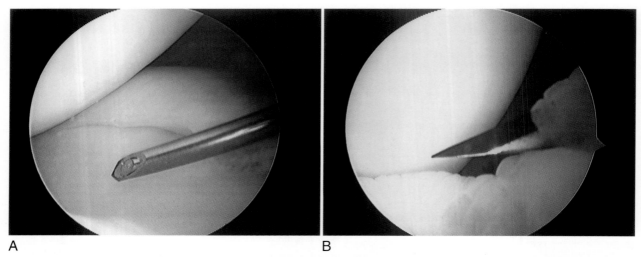

A   B

Figure 47–8 Establish the anteromedial portal under direct vision. *A,* Insert the needle and confirm that the pathology can be reached from this position. *B,* Remove the needle and direct the number 11 blade toward the intercondylar notch.

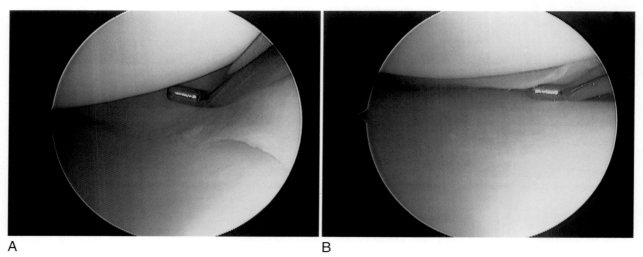

A   B

Figure 47–9 *A* and *B,* A complete examination includes direct palpation of the upper and undersurface of the meniscus.

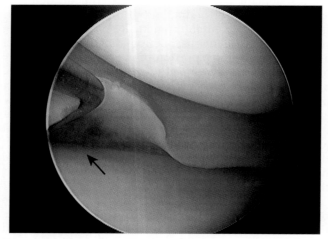

Figure 47–10 Occasionally, acute injuries to the deep medial collateral ligament *(arrow)* can be visualized arthroscopically by elevating the medial meniscus.

from the meniscal rim to the edge of the tibia. If abnormal wrinkling is seen anywhere along the length of the meniscus, a peripheral detachment should be suspected. If a small rim of the medial meniscus is seen instead of a normal-sized one, consideration should be given to either a prior partial medial meniscectomy or a displaced meniscal fragment, possibly lodged posteriorly.

In the case of a bucket handle tear, the loose fragment of the meniscus flips (displaces) into the intercondylar notch, much like the handle of a bucket flips from one side to the other (Fig. 47–11). If the displaced meniscus fills the space between the medial femoral condyle and tibial plateau anteriorly, it can block the arthroscope's access to the medial compartment unless it is manipulated back into its reduced position with a probe. If there is a radial tear associated with the bucket handle tear, the fragment is attached at only one edge and can flip behind the femoral condyle or under the intact portion of the meniscus, where it may be missed.

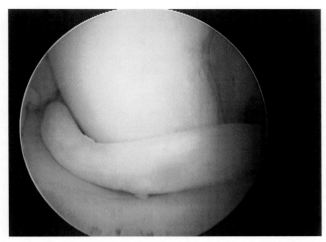

Figure 47–11 Displaced bucket handle tear into the intercondylar notch.

Table 47–4

Considerations for Meniscal Repair			
Parameter	Decreasing Likelihood of Meniscal Repair		
Acuity of tear	Acute	Subacute	Chronic
Location from periphery	Red-red (<3 mm)	Red-white (3–5 mm)	White-white (>5 mm)
Tear pattern	Vertical		Horizontal, radial, complex
Tissue quality	Good		Degenerative, macerated
Tear length	1–4 cm		>4 cm

Now direct the 30-degree arthroscope parallel to the tibia and posteriorly to aid in visualizing the posterior horn, where most medial meniscal tears occur. In tight knees, this region can be difficult to examine; extending the knee and applying a valgus force should help. The peripheral portion of the posterior horn and its attachments may also be visualized by passing the arthroscope under the posterior cruciate ligament in the intercondylar notch (modified Gillquist maneuver) into the posteromedial compartment.[14,37]

Meniscal Tears

If a meniscal tear is discovered, the decision whether to perform a partial meniscectomy versus a meniscal repair is based on several factors. It is beyond the scope of this chapter to fully describe the classification and management of all meniscal tears, but proper management requires that the acuity of the tear, degenerative changes within the tissue, tear pattern, and length and width

of the tear from the periphery be considered (Table 47–4).[3,7,48] Therefore, a complete understanding of the character of the meniscal lesion is essential for proper management. Failure to accurately explore the extent of the tear may result in the needless sacrifice of healthy meniscal tissue.[36] If the location and type of tear make it amenable to repair, this is the preferred treatment.[10,18] If repair is not possible, partial meniscectomy is always preferable to total meniscectomy.[38,44] Leaving an intact, stable, peripheral rim of meniscus provides stability to the joint and protects the articular surface by sharing the load-bearing responsibilities.[3,7] Total meniscectomy decreases the load-bearing protection and reduces joint stability.[3,12,51]

During a partial meniscectomy, the torn, mobile fragment is excised, and the peripheral rim is contoured in an attempt to leave a balanced, stable rim of meniscal tissue (Fig. 47–12).[16] Sharp excision is preferable to morcellation to minimize the debris created in the joint. The blunt short trocar and cannula can be inserted through the instrument portal; the trocar is then removed to "vacuum out" the free-floating meniscal

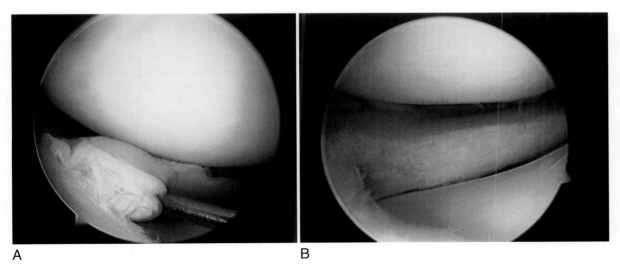

A   B

Figure 47–12 *A*, Probing of the medial meniscus demonstrates a radial tear. *B*, During a partial meniscectomy, contouring of the unstable tear results in a balanced, stable rim of meniscal tissue.

fragments. The suction shaver can complete the process and help contour the meniscal edges. If the shaver is used to remove multiple large meniscal fragments first, it frequently becomes clogged. The remaining peripheral rim must be carefully probed again to ensure that it is balanced and stable and that no additional tears are present.

Examination of the Femoral and Tibial Condyles

The articular surfaces of the femoral and tibial condyles should be systematically examined through a range of motion. It is important to note that early articular wear on the medial femoral condyle is typically located slightly posteriorly, making contact with the tibia when the knee is flexed 30 to 50 degrees (Fig. 47–13). These arthroscopic findings correlate with standing flexion (Rosenberg) radiographs.[47]

Systematic palpation with the probe is important to demonstrate softening of the cartilage (chondromalacia),[50] collapse of the underlying subchondral bone (avascular necrosis, osteonecrosis),[28] osteochondritis dissecans,[2,31,56,60] or unstable chondral flaps (Fig. 47–14).[19] The tip of the probe can be used as an "arthroscopic ruler" to measure the dimensions of the lesion. With the lens directed superolaterally, the medial femoral condyle can be followed into the intercondylar notch.

Intercondylar Notch

The structures to examine in the intercondylar notch include the infrapatellar fat pad, ligamentum mucosum, medial and lateral tibial spines, attachments of both menisci, anterior and posterior cruciate ligaments, ligaments of Humphry and Wrisberg (meniscofemoral ligaments), and intermeniscal ligament.

Ligamentum Mucosum

The ligamentum mucosum, or infrapatellar plica, is the most commonly encountered plica in the knee and rarely produces any symptoms.[43] It runs from the superior intercondylar notch down to the fat pad and, in some cases, can be confused with the anterior cruciate ligament. The distinction is easily made by visualizing the attachment of the ligamentum mucosum to the anterior roof of the intercondylar notch; the anterior cruciate ligament attaches much more posteriorly in the back of the notch.

The ligamentum mucosum may be a thin, narrow band of synovium or a complete septum dividing the medial and lateral compartments.[43] An enlarged ligamentum mucosum (Fig. 47–15) or a complete septum can make passing the arthroscope from the medial to lateral compartments difficult and obscure the view of the intercondylar notch. Although this structure has no clinical significance, it should be debrided only when necessary because it is well vascularized and bleeding may occur.

Anterior Cruciate Ligament

The ligaments within the intercondylar notch are best viewed with the knee flexed 60 to 90 degrees. Because 80% of anterior cruciate ligament tears are from its femoral attachment, it is important to visualize the origin clearly. This can be performed with the scope through the anterolateral portal by rotating the lens until the medial aspect of the lateral femoral condyle is visualized (approximately 10 o'clock on right knees and 2 o'clock on left knees). Alternatively, the knee can be placed in the figure-of-four position to tension the anterior cruciate ligament and view it from the lateral compartment by looking toward the notch. Check the integrity of the anterior cruciate ligament by probing along its length and, most importantly, its femoral origin (Fig. 47–16). Occasionally, inspection of the anterior cruciate ligament is best performed with the arthroscope through an anteromedial portal.

The appearance of the anterior cruciate ligament varies from patient to patient. Normally, a thin synovial lining covers the ligament. If significant synovitis exists and an injury is suspected, this tissue may need to be removed to adequately visualize the underlying ligament. In recent anterior cruciate ligament ruptures, considerable hemorrhage can be seen within the synovial tissues, and the torn bundles of the cruciate can be seen as white "rope end" structures. The tibial stump of the injured anterior cruciate ligament can also hypertrophy until a rounded mass termed a Cyclops lesion exists (Fig. 47–17).[34,40] This can impinge in the intercondylar notch, blocking extension.[34]

An anterior drawer test performed when the torn anterior cruciate ligament is directly viewed demonstrates that the ligament does not tense appropriately (Fig. 47–18A), or it may be completely avulsed from its femoral origin—the empty lateral wall sign (Fig. 47–18B). Often, at first glance, the ligament may appear to be intact.[6,30,33] However, careful probing of the origin reveals that the ligament is lax or that it is scarred down to the posterior cruciate ligament, giving the appearance

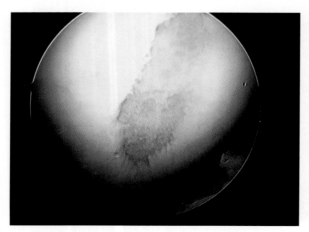

Figure 47–13 Early medial femoral condyle arthritis is typically located more posteriorly and often is not visualized until the knee is flexed 30 to 50 degrees.

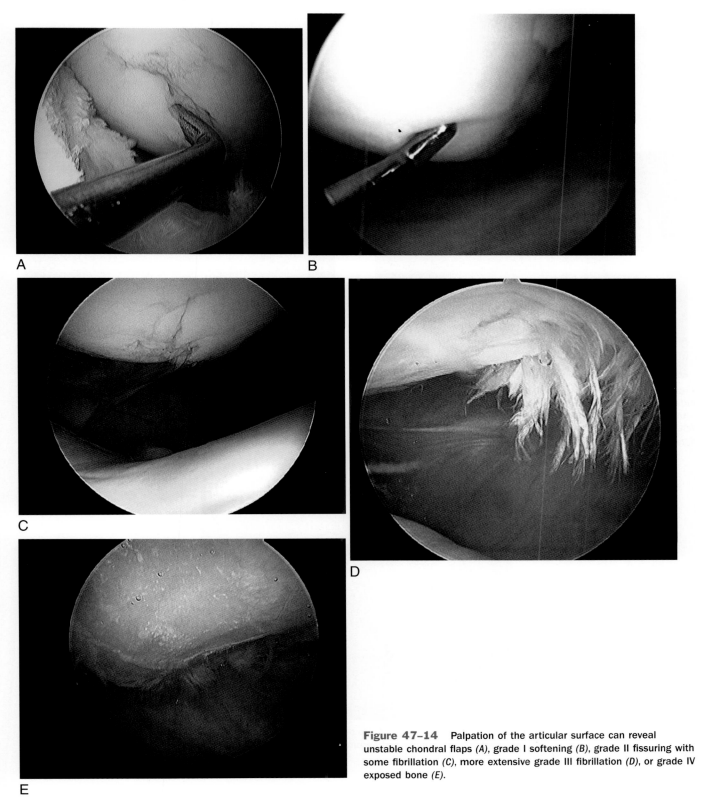

Figure 47–14   Palpation of the articular surface can reveal unstable chondral flaps *(A)*, grade I softening *(B)*, grade II fissuring with some fibrillation *(C)*, more extensive grade III fibrillation *(D)*, or grade IV exposed bone *(E)*.

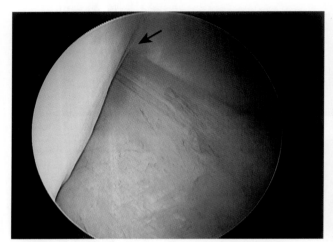

Figure 47-15 Note that the ligamentum mucosum can be differentiated from the anterior cruciate ligament (ACL) by its attachment to the anterior roof of the intercondylar notch (*arrow*). The ACL, which in this patient is completely obscured by an enlarged ligamentum mucosum, attaches more posteriorly in the notch.

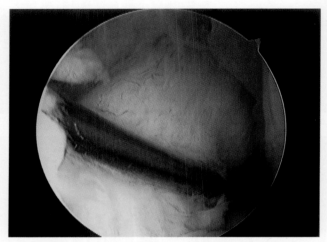

Figure 47-16 An intact anterior cruciate ligament tensions normally when the anterior drawer test is performed with the arthroscopic probe.

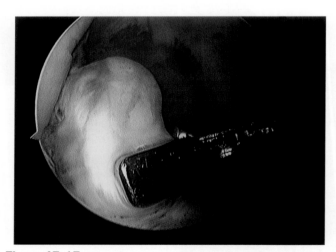

Figure 47-17 The tibial stump of an injured anterior cruciate ligament can hypertrophy and become a Cyclops lesion.

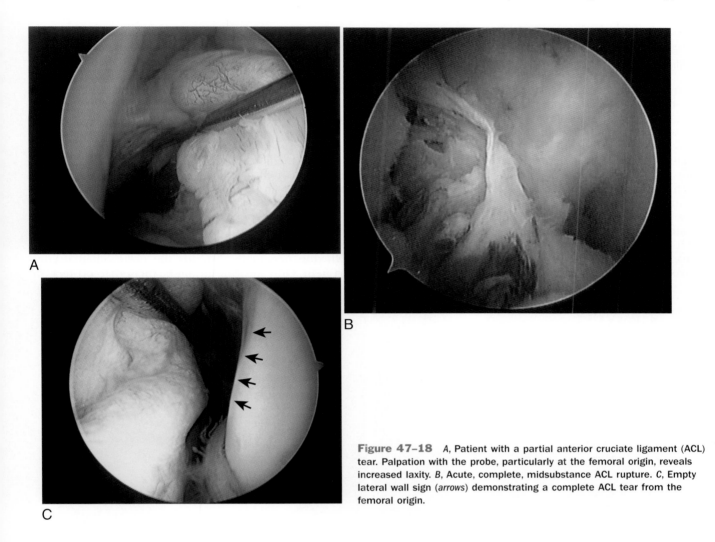

A

B

C

Figure 47–18   *A*, Patient with a partial anterior cruciate ligament (ACL) tear. Palpation with the probe, particularly at the femoral origin, reveals increased laxity. *B*, Acute, complete, midsubstance ACL rupture. *C*, Empty lateral wall sign (*arrows*) demonstrating a complete ACL tear from the femoral origin.

of an intact ligament but not providing any functional stability.

Posterior Cruciate Ligament

Next, the femoral insertion of the posterior cruciate ligament, which is also covered by synovial tissue, is inspected. It arises from the lateral aspect of the medial femoral condyle and runs in a more vertical direction, just over the back of the tibia to insert approximately 1 cm below the articular surface. Palpation of the posterior cruciate ligament is performed by probing the undersurface of the femoral attachments and pulling anteriorly (Fig. 47–19).[32]

Meniscofemoral Ligaments

The two meniscofemoral ligaments are the ligament of Humphry and the ligament of Wrisberg. Either or both of these meniscofemoral ligaments can be seen originating adjacent to the posterior cruciate ligament and attaching to the posterior horn of the lateral meniscus in up to 83% of patients.[29,59] The ligament of Humphry

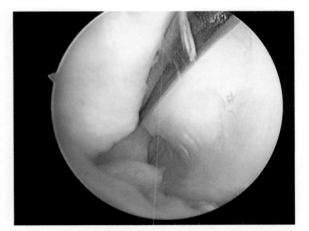

Figure 47–19   Palpate the posterior cruciate ligament by probing the undersurface of the femoral attachment and pulling anteriorly.

runs anterior to the ligament of Wrisberg, which is easily remembered by the fact that alphabetically Humphry precedes Wrisberg. Their function is to help stabilize the posterior horn attachment of the lateral meniscus.[4,29,59]

6 Knee

Examination of the Posteromedial Compartment through the Intercondylar Notch— Modified Gillquist Maneuver

Whenever loose bodies are suspected, or to better visualize the posteromedial meniscal attachment, the posteromedial compartment can be viewed by passing the arthroscope through the intercondylar notch from the anterolateral portal (modified Gillquist maneuver).[37] Visualization may be aided by the use of a 70-degree scope.[14,52] Structures to examine include the peripheral attachment of the posterior horn of the medial meniscus, the distal half of the posterior cruciate ligament, the posterior femoral condyle, and the posteromedial joint capsule. Free loose bodies and meniscal fragments also gravitate to this region.

To perform the modified Gillquist maneuver, the arthroscope is passed between the posterior cruciate ligament and medial femoral condyle (Fig. 47–20).[14,52] Ninety degrees of knee flexion with valgus stress may help pass the arthroscope. To avoid damage to the joint surface or the arthroscope, "drive" the arthroscope into the notch under the origin of the posterior cruciate ligament and rest it gently against the medial femoral condyle. While holding the cannula in this position, replace the arthroscope with the blunt trocar. With gentle pressure and a twisting motion, advance the trocar along the medial femoral condyle, under the posterior cruciate ligament, and into the posteromedial compartment. Once in, remove the trocar and reinsert the arthroscope.

An accessory posteromedial instrument portal can then be established under direct vision, using a spinal needle to locate the optimal portal site. Placing the knee in flexion maximally distends the posteromedial compartment. Only the skin should be incised, to protect the

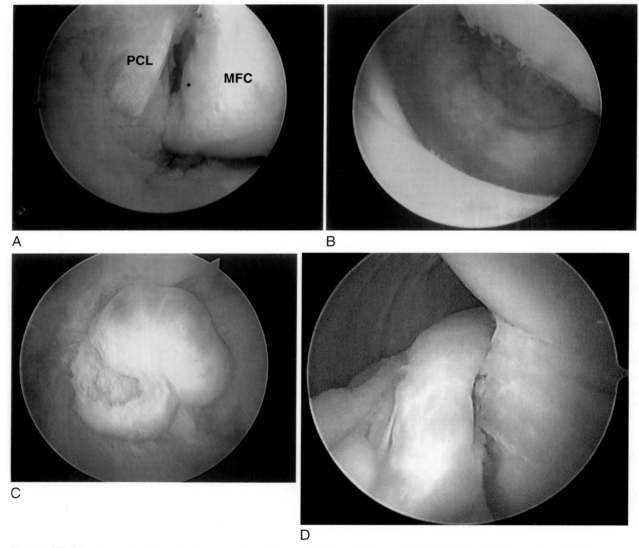

Figure 47–20 Access to the posterior compartment is possible through the modified Gillquist portal. The posteromedial compartment *(A)* can be entered by passing the arthroscope between the posterior cruciate ligament (PCL) and the medial femoral condyle (MFC). The star locates the position where the arthroscope should rest on the medial femoral condyle. Once the posterior compartment *(B)* is entered, loose bodies *(C)* or a peripheral meniscal tear *(D)* may be seen.

nearby saphenous nerve and vein. A blunt hemostat is passed through the skin and subcutaneous tissue along the posterior aspect of the medial femoral condyle. Be careful to glance off the condyle posteriorly rather than directing the instrument too deeply into the posterior soft tissues. Penetrate the capsule with the tip of the hemostat under direct vision, and then replace the hemostat with the arthroscopic cannula using the blunt trocar.

The arthroscopic camera can be inserted through the cannula directly into the posteromedial portal. The posterior aspect of the medial femoral condyle helps orient the surgeon. Turn the lens inferiorly to visualize the meniscocapsular junction of the posterior horn of the medial meniscus. Farther down, the tibial insertion of the posterior cruciate ligament can also be seen. Palpate the posterior horn of the meniscus and the posterior cruciate ligament by passing a probe from the anterolateral portal through the intercondylar notch between the posterior cruciate ligament and the medial femoral condyle into the posteromedial compartment.

By rotating the lens posteriorly, occasionally the opening of a popliteal (Baker's) cyst can be visualized as a fold of synovium. If the cyst is oriented appropriately, passage of the arthroscope into the popliteal cyst may be possible.

Examination of the Posterolateral Compartment through the Intercondylar Notch

If the specific pathology warrants, such as loose bodies, the posterolateral compartment can be accessed from either the anterolateral or the anteromedial portal using a maneuver similar to the one used to enter the posteromedial compartment.[37] Direct the arthroscope back into the notch, but this time between the anterior cruciate ligament and the lateral femoral condyle. Again, if difficulty is encountered, a cannula and blunt trocar can be used to slide along the edge of the lateral femoral condyle. Exchange the trocar for the arthroscope and rotate the lens to view the meniscus posterolaterally.

Lateral Compartment

The lateral compartment can be viewed with the arthroscope through either the anteromedial or, more commonly, the anterolateral portal. When using a lateral post, this compartment is best visualized by placing the leg in the figure-of-four position with flexion and abduction of the hip and flexion of the knee (Fig. 47–21). If additional varus stress is required, have the assistant push down on the thigh just above the knee, resulting in varus and internal rotational opening of the lateral compartment. When using a leg holder, varus stress on a slightly flexed knee with internal rotation of the tibia provides the same lateral opening.

With the arthroscope in the anterolateral portal, sweep the scope laterally from the intercondylar notch into the lateral compartment. Examine and palpate the meniscus with the probe coming from the anteromedial

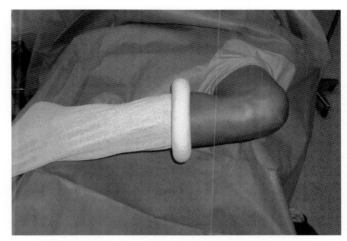

Figure 47–21   Figure-of-four position creates a varus stress, opening the lateral compartment.

portal. If a hypertrophic, edematous fat pad blocks the view of the anterior horn of the lateral meniscus, partial resection of the fat pad may be necessary. Excessive shaving in this area can result in inadvertent destabilization of the rim attachment of the anterior horn of the lateral meniscus and should be minimized.

Occasionally, a prominent intercondylar eminence forces the probe superiorly, making palpation of the posterior third of the lateral meniscus difficult. Also, because the lateral meniscus is more circular than the medial meniscus,[7] the anterior horn attachment is more posterior in the intercondylar notch, forcing arthroscopic instruments to come more superiorly over the anterior horn before entering the lateral compartment. In this instance, the portals for the probe and the arthroscope can be switched.

Examination of the Lateral Meniscus and Popliteal Tendon

Rotate the lens posteriorly and examine the lateral meniscus systematically from posterior to anterior. Note that the mobile lateral meniscus tends to ride up off the lateral tibial condylar surface. Probe both the inferior and superior surfaces of the meniscus to check for tears and assess the integrity of the meniscosynovial attachment. Note that the intercondylar attachment of the posterior horn of the lateral meniscus is located more anteriorly than on the medial side.

In the posterolateral corner of the lateral compartment, the obliquely coursing popliteal tendon within the popliteal hiatus can be easily seen (Fig. 47–22). Lifting up on the meniscus can enhance visualization of the tendon as it heads inferiorly toward its muscular origin on the back of the tibia. In this region, the increased mobility of the meniscus to probing is normal, and the gap in the coronary ligament attachment between the meniscal edge and capsule should not be confused with a peripheral meniscal tear.[3,27] The anterior and posterior horn should remain attached with a smooth synovial reflection, and the body of the meniscus should not translate beyond the apex of the convex lateral femoral

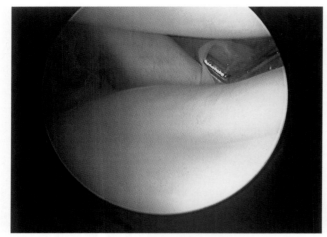

Figure 47–22 Obliquely coursing popliteal tendon within the popliteal hiatus.

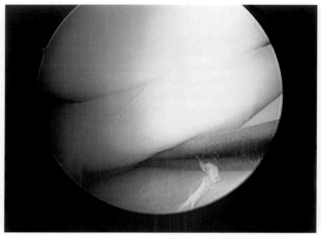

Figure 47–23 Normal translation of the lateral meniscus with palpation.

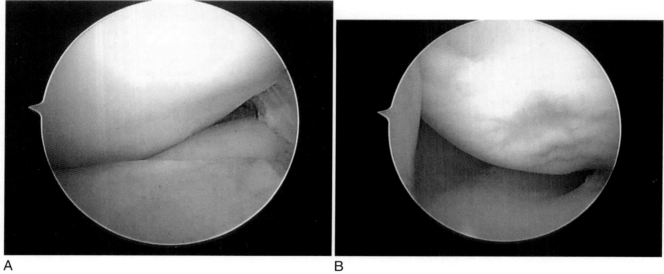

A   B

Figure 47–24 The normal sulcus terminalis (A) indentation is not the same as the traumatic chondral injury (B) commonly seen in the same location and associated with anterior cruciate ligament tears.

condyle (Fig. 47–23).[7,27] After examination of the meniscus, the articular surfaces of the femoral and tibial condyles should be examined and probed with the same technique used for the medial compartment. The sulcus terminalis is a normal indentation demarcating the junction between the patellofemoral and femorotibial articulations (Fig. 47–24A). This should be distinguished from a traumatic chondral injury that might be seen with the bone bruises commonly associated with anterior cruciate ligament tears (Fig. 47–24B).

Documentation of the Arthroscopic Examination

Clear documentation of the arthroscopic findings and surgical intervention is imperative. This should include both arthroscopic images and concise operative notes.

Arthroscopic pictures of all pathology should be obtained before and after the surgical intervention. In the case of a meniscal tear, for example, arthroscopic pictures should demonstrate the unstable tear before and after repair or partial meniscectomy. These images can be reviewed with the patient and family postoperatively; this often improves their understanding of the knee pathology and what was done to treat it.

Operative notes should be concise but descriptive. Preoperative and postoperative diagnoses and procedures performed should be accurately listed at the beginning of the operative dictation. A separate section listing the operative findings can also be included at the beginning of the notes before the full description of the procedure. This is often helpful for the surgeon because it allows a quick review of the pertinent findings of the arthroscopic examination without having to dissect the body of the operative notes. In this section, the locations and types of chondral lesions can be described, based on the modified Outerbridge classification,[22,41] along with the size of the lesions in terms of the percentage of the articular surface involved. Descriptions of meniscal tears should include the percentage of stable meniscal rim remaining if a partial meniscectomy was performed.

Complications

Complications associated with knee arthroscopy are uncommon. In a series of more than 8000 arthroscopic knee procedures, the overall complication rate was 1.68% (Table 47–5).[54] Infection, loss of range of motion,[58] and iatrogenic articular cartilage injuries are the most common complications.[6,8,23,26]

Iatrogenic cartilage injuries can be minimized with proper portal placement, careful technique, and adequate visualization.[8] Careless and forceful movements and inappropriate use of arthroscopic tools should be avoided. Surgeons should pay attention to the "feel" of the arthroscope and arthroscopic tools. Remember that the arthroscope and cannula together create a long lever arm capable of generating large forces at the tip. With increased proficiency, "surgeonmalacia" and "divotoses" can be minimized.

Infection, which occurs in less than 1% of all knee arthroscopies, can be a devastating complication.[54,63] Surgeons should not be cavalier about arthroscopic knee surgery, and care should be taken to use strict sterile technique. Although the routine use of preoperative prophylactic antibiotics is not recommended by the American Academy of Orthopaedic Surgeons, it is a common practice.[60-62]

Staphylococcus epidermidis and *Staphylococcus aureus* are frequently the offending pathogens and can be difficult to diagnose in the immediate postoperative period.[25,54,55] Aspirations should be performed and the fluid sent for Gram stain, culture, sensitivity, and cell count. White blood cell count greater than $25,000/mm^3$ with a polymorphonuclear predominance in the aspirate is typical. Sedimentation rates and C-reactive protein levels are usually elevated, but this is a nonspecific finding.

Treatment should include early arthroscopic debridement and lavage and intravenous antibiotics to help erad-

icate the infection.[24] Arthroscopic treatment of septic arthrosis offers the advantage of high-volume fluid lavage and debridement of fibrinoid material and infected debris. It may reduce morbidity and shorten hospitalization. Smith[57] studied 30 patients treated with arthroscopic debridement and lavage combined with parenteral and oral antibiotics. Twenty-eight patients had excellent results, and two had good results; no cases of osteomyelitis were reported.

Standard arthroscopy equipment, setup, and portals are used to treat infections. Do not exsanguinate the extremity. Repeat aspirates can be sent at the beginning of the case. Use a large-bore cannula or an arthroscopic pump for irrigation. Complete debridement of necrotic and infected tissue and thorough lavage with 9 L of fluid may enhance the chances of a good outcome. All compartments, including the medial and lateral gutters, should be addressed. Following the procedure, place suction drain tubes through the arthroscopic cannula, and close the incisions loosely. Debridement and lavage can be repeated, if necessary, at 24 to 72 hours. Early rehabilitation may help decrease permanent knee stiffness.

The use of a tourniquet for longer than 50 minutes has been found to increase the incidence of deep vein thrombosis.[11,47,49] Pulmonary embolism may occur in up to a quarter of these cases, especially in older patients.[26] A high index of suspicion should be maintained. Postoperative calf tightness, pain, and swelling may be the only signs. In rare cases, warfarin (Coumadin) prophylaxis may have an acceptable role in extremely high risk patients.

Table 47–5
Complications of Arthroscopic Knee Surgery

Postoperative hemarthrosis
Infection
Arthrofibrosis
Deep vein thrombosis
Anesthetic complications
Instrument failure
Complex regional pain syndrome (reflex sympathetic dystrophy)
Iatrogenic ligament injury
Iatrogenic fracture
Neurologic injury

References

1. Bronstein RD, Sebastianelli WJ, DeHaven KE: Case report: Localized pigmented villonodular synovitis presenting as a loose body in the knee. Arthroscopy 9:596, 1993.
2. Cahill BR: Osteochondritis dissecans of the knee: Treatment of juvenile and adult forms. J Am Acad Orthop Surg 3:237, 1995.
3. Cannon WD, Morgan CD: Meniscal repair. Part II. Arthroscopic repair techniques. J Bone Joint Surg Am 76:294, 1994.
4. Carpenter WA: Meniscofemoral ligament stimulating tear of the lateral meniscus: MR features. J Comput Assist Tomogr 14:1033-1034, 1990.
5. Casscells SW: The arthroscope in the diagnosis of disorders of the patellofemoral joint. Clin Orthop 144:45, 1979.
6. Coward DB: Principles of arthroscopy of the knee. In Chapman MW (ed): Chapman's Orthopaedic Surgery, 3rd ed. Philadelphia, Lippincott Williams & Wilkins, 2001, pp 2269-2298.
7. DeHaven KE, Arnoczky SP: Meniscal repair. Part I. Basic science, indications for repair and open repair. J Bone Joint Surg Am 76:140-152, 1994.
8. DeLee JC: Complications of arthroscopy and arthroscopic surgery: Results of a national survey. Arthroscopy 1:214, 1985.
9. Dupont JY: Synovial plica of the knee: Controversies and review. Clin Sports Med 16:87, 1997.
10. Eggli S, Wegmuller H, Kosina J, et al: Long-term results of open meniscal repair. Am J Sports Med 23:715, 1995.

11. Fahmy NR, Patel DG: Hemostatic changes and postoperative deep vein thrombosis associated with use of a pneumatic tourniquet. J Bone Joint Surg Am 63:461, 1981.

12. Fairbank TJ: Knee joint changes after meniscectomy. J Bone Joint Surg Br 30:664, 1948.

13. Flanagan JP, Trakru S, Meyer M: Arthroscopic excision of symptomatic medial plica: A study of 118 knees with 1–4 year follow-up. Acta Orthop Scand 65:408, 1994.

14. Gillquist J, Habgerg G, Oretorp N: Arthroscopic visualization of the posteromedial compartment of the knee joint. Orthop Clin North Am 10:545, 1979.

15. Grood ES, Suntag WJ, Noyes FR, Butler DL: Biomechanics of the knee-extension exercise. J Bone Joint Surg Am 66:725, 1984.

16. Guhl JF: Excision of flap tears. Orthop Clin North Am 13:387, 1982.

17. Highgenboten CL: Arthroscopic synovectomy. Orthop Clin North Am 13:399, 1982.

18. Horibe SH, Shino K, Maeda A, et al: Results of isolated meniscal repair evaluated by second-look arthroscopy. Arthroscopy 12:150, 1996.

19. Hubbard MJ: Arthroscopic surgery for chondral flaps in the knee. J Bone Joint Surg Br 69:794-796, 1987.

20. Huberti HH, Hayes WC: Patellofemoral contact pressures: The influence of Q-angle and tendofemoral contact. J Bone Joint Surg Am 66:715, 1984.

21. Hungerford DS, Barry M: Biomechanics of the patellofemoral joint. Clin Orthop 241:203, 1989.

22. Insall J, Falvo KA, Wise DW: Chondromalacia patellae: A prospective study. J Bone Joint Surg Am 58:1, 1976.

23. Irrang JJ, Harner CD: Loss of motion following knee ligament reconstruction. Sports Med 19:150, 1995.

24. Jackson RW: Current concepts review: Arthroscopic surgery. J Bone Joint Surg Am 65:416, 1983.

25. Jackson RW: The septic knee, arthroscopic treatment. Arthroscopy 1:194, 1985.

26. Kieser C: A review of the complications of arthroscopic knee surgery. Arthroscopy 8:79, 1992.

27. Kimura M, Shirakura K, Hasegawa A, et al: Anatomy and pathophysiology of the popliteal tendon area in the lateral meniscus: Arthroscopic and anatomical investigation. Arthroscopy 8:419, 1992.

28. Koshino T, Okamoto R, Takamura K, Tsuchiya K: Arthroscopy in spontaneous osteonecrosis of the knee. Orthop Clin North Am 10:609, 1979.

29. Lee BY, Jee WH, Kim JM, et al: Incidence and significance of demonstrating the meniscofemoral ligament on MRI. Br J Radiol 73:271-274, 2000.

30. Lerat JL, Moyen BL, Cladiere F, et al: Knee instability after injury to the anterior cruciate ligament: Quantification of the Lachman test. J Bone Joint Surg Br 82:42-47, 2000.

31. Linden B: Osteochondritis dissecans of the knee. J Bone Joint Surg Br 53:448, 1971.

32. Lysholm J, Gillquist J: Arthroscopic examination of the posterior cruciate ligament. J Bone Joint Surg Am 63:363, 1981.

33. McGuire DA, Wolchok JC: Arthroscopic Lachman test: A new technique using anatomic references. Arthroscopy 14:641-642, 1998.

34. McMahon PJ, Dettling JR, Yocum LA, Glousman RE: The Cyclops lesion: A cause of diminished knee extension after rupture of the anterior cruciate ligament. Arthroscopy 15:757-761, 1999.

35. Metcalf RW: An arthroscopic method of lateral release of the subluxating or dislocating patella. Clin Orthop 167:9, 1983.

36. Miller MD: Meniscal surgery and treatment. Oper Tech Orthop 10:161-244, 2000.

37. Morin WD, Steadman JR: Arthroscopic assessment of the posterior compartments of the knee via the intercondylar notch: The arthroscopist's field of view. Arthroscopy 9:284, 1993.

38. Newman AP, Anderson DR, Daniels AU, et al: Mechanics of the healed meniscus in a canine model. Am J Sports Med 17:164, 1989.

39. Ogilvie-Harris DJ, Basinski A: Arthroscopic synovectomy of the knee for rheumatoid arthritis. Arthroscopy 7:91, 1991.

40. Olson PN, Rud P, Griffiths HJ: Cyclops lesion. Orthopedics 18:1041, 1044-1045, 1995.

41. Outerbridge RE: The etiology of chondromalacia patellae. J Bone Joint Surg Br 43:752, 1961.

42. Parisien JS: Normal arthroscopic anatomy portals and techniques. Paper presented at the 62nd annual meeting of the American Academy of Orthopaedic Surgeons, Feb 1995, Orlando, FL.

43. Patel D: Arthroscopy of the plicae-synovial folds and their significance. Am J Sports Med 6:217, 1978.

44. Perdue PS, Hummer CD, Offosimo AJ, et al: Meniscal repair: Outcomes and clinical follow-up. Arthroscopy 12:694, 1996.

45. Pianka G, Combs J: Arthroscopic diagnosis and treatment of symptomatic plicae. In Scott WN (ed): Arthroscopy of the Knee: Diagnosis and Treatment. Philadelphia, WB Saunders, 1990, p 83.

46. Rand JA: Arthroscopic diagnosis and management of articular cartilage pathology. In Scott WN (ed): Arthroscopy of the Knee: Diagnosis and Treatment. Philadelphia, WB Saunders, 1990, p 113.

47. Rosenberg TD, Paulos LE, Parker RD, et al: The 45-degree flexion weight bearing radiograph of the knee. J Bone Joint Surg Am 70:1479, 1988.

48. Rosenberg TD, Scott SM, Coward DB, et al: Arthroscopic meniscal repair evaluated with repeat arthroscopy. Arthroscopy 2:13, 1986.

49. Sapega AA, Heppenstall RD, Chance B, et al: Optimizing tourniquet application and release times in extremity surgery: A biomechanical and ultrastructural study. J Bone Joint Surg Am 67:303, 1985.

50. Schonholtz GJ, Ling B: Arthroscopic chondroplasty of the patella. Arthroscopy 1:92, 1985.

51. Seehom BB, Hargreaves DJ: Transmission of the load in the knee joint with special reference to the role of the menisci. Eng Med 8:220, 1979.

52. Shahriaree H: O'Connor's Texbook of Arthroscopic Surgery. Philadelphia, JB Lippincott, 1984.

53. Sherman RMP, Jackson RW: The pathological medial plica: Criteria for diagnosis and prognosis. J Bone Joint Surg Br 71:351, 1989.

54. Small NC: Complications of arthroscopic surgery performed by experienced arthroscopists. Arthroscopy 4:215, 1988.

55. Smiley P, Wasilewski SA: Arthroscopic synovectomy. Arthroscopy 6:18, 1990.

56. Smillie I: Treatment of osteochondritis dissecans. J Bone Joint Surg Br 39:248, 1957.

57. Smith M: Arthroscopic treatment of the septic knee. Arthroscopy 2:30, 1986.

58. Sprague NF III, O'Connor RL, Fox JM: Arthroscopic treatment of postoperative knee fibroarthrosis. Clin Orthop 166:165, 1982.

59. Vahey TN, Bennet HT, Arrington LE, et al: MR imaging of the knee: Pseudotear of the lateral meniscus caused by the meniscofemoral ligament. AJR Am J Roentgenol 154:1237-1239, 1990.

60. Vince KG: Osteochondritis dissecans of the knee. In Scott WN (ed): Arthroscopy of the Knee: Diagnosis and Treatment. Philadelphia, WB Saunders, 1990, p 175.

61. Wertheim SB, Gillespie S, Klaus R: Role of prophylactic antibiotics in arthroscopic knee surgery. Orthop Trans 4:1101, 1993.
62. Wieck JA, Jackson JK, O'Brien TJ, et al: A prospective, randomized, double-blinded evaluation of the efficacy of antibiotics in arthroscopic surgery. Paper presented at the annual meeting of the American Academy of Orthopaedic Surgeons, 1995.
63. Williams RJ III, Laurencin CT, Warren RF, et al: Septic arthritis after arthroscopic anterior cruciate ligament reconstruction: Diagnosis and management. Am J Sports Med 25:261-267, 1997.

6 Knee

Arthroscopic Synovectomy in the Knee

ROBERT SELLARDS, RODNEY STANLEY, AND CHARLES A. BUSH-JOSEPH

ARTHROSCOPIC SYNOVECTOMY IN THE KNEE IN A NUTSHELL

History:
Pain, stiffness, swelling, warmth, mechanical symptoms

Physical Examination:
Localized or diffuse synovial thickening, with or without loss of joint motion

Imaging:
Plain radiographs may show typical findings of inflammatory disease, including osteopenia, erosions, and symmetrical joint space narrowing; magnetic resonance imaging is often diagnostic for synovial thickening

Indications and Contraindications:
Surgery is indicated for chronic synovitis refractory to medical management in patients with inflammatory conditions; patients with significant joint space narrowing on plain radiographs are generally poor candidates for synovectomy

Surgical Technique:
Synovectomy requires multiple portals and advanced arthroscopic skills to ensure adequate synovial resection and avoid complications

Postoperative Management:
Control of postoperative swelling with the use of drains and joint aspiration is critical to avoid motion loss; early restoration of active and passive range of motion is critical to avoid permanent motion loss

Results:
Variable, depending on the cause of synovitis: synovectomy for localized conditions such as pigmented villonodular synovitis may be effective in up to 88% of cases; in generalized conditions, including rheumatoid arthritis, synovectomy may be effective in 80% of cases

Synovium is specialized mesenchymal tissue that is essential to proper joint function. Synovial disorders comprise various conditions that can affect multiple joints (Table 48–1). These vary from the massive, total joint involvement of rheumatoid arthritis to the isolated lesion of plica syndrome. Elements that are important for diagnosis include the history, clinical findings, and radiographic analysis. Orthopedic management of synovial disorders begins after medical management has been exhausted. The same basic surgical techniques are employed for most conditions and vary only in the amount of synovium debrided.

History

A thorough medical history is important in evaluating patients with synovial disorders. It is important to determine the duration of pain, exacerbating factors,

Table 48–1
Synovial Disorders

Rheumatoid arthritis
Pigmented villonodular synovitis
Plicae
Synovial hemangioma
Synovial osteochondromatosis
Intra-articular adhesions
Fibrotic fat pad
Fibrotic ligamentum mucosum
Post-traumatic synovitis
Hemophilic synovitis

interference with daily activities, and any other affected joints. Patients with rheumatoid arthritis often have an insidious onset of morning stiffness and polyarthritis, initially involving the hands and feet.

Pigmented villonodular synovitis (PVNS) is usually a monoarticular process affecting adults in the third or fourth decade of life.[7] The knee joint is most commonly involved, and symptoms may be similar to those associated with mechanical causes, including meniscal tears.[20] Clinical symptoms include an insidious onset of localized warmth, swelling, and stiffness. The patient may complain of occasional locking with a palpable mass. The presentation of localized PVNS is more episodic than that of its diffuse counterpart.

Physical Examination

A comprehensive physical examination is important in evaluating patients with rheumatic disorders. Typical findings in patients with inflammatory conditions include multiple joint involvement, joint warmth and swelling, and muscle atrophy. Patients often have an effusion coupled with synovial thickening. The loss of terminal flexion and extension is a common finding in chronic cases. Patients with bony malalignment or collateral ligament insufficiency often have more severe articular loss and are generally poor candidates for synovectomy. Subcutaneous nodules are seen in up to 20% of rheumatoid patients in their lifetime. Laboratory findings include an elevated erythrocyte sedimentation rate, elevated C-reactive protein level, and positive rheumatoid factor titer in most patients. Joint fluid analysis can reveal rheumatoid factor, decreased complement levels, and increased inflammatory cells.

Physical examination of a knee affected with PVNS is often nonspecific. There may be a palpable mass, depending on the amount of joint involvement. An effusion is often associated with diffuse involvement. Ligamentous instability is uncommon. Palpation of the joint can reveal warmth and tenderness. Aspiration of joint fluid in patients with PVNS reveals a dark brownish fluid consistent with recurrent bleeding into the joint.

Imaging

Adequate radiographic evaluation of the knee is necessary to understand the extent of joint involvement. Radiographic characteristics of rheumatoid arthritis include symmetrical periarticular erosions and osteopenia. Preoperative flexion and extension films of the cervical spine are necessary to rule out any cervical instability in the rheumatoid population. Significant joint space narrowing or malalignment on standing radiographs would lead to a more guarded prognosis with arthroscopic synovectomy.

Imaging of the joint affected with PVNS involves both radiographs and magnetic resonance imaging. Plain radiographs can reveal erosive, cystic, and sclerotic lesions of the articular surface.[9] Often there are no changes on plain radiographs, and joint spaces are maintained. Soft tissue masses of increased density can be visualized on radiographs owing to the hemosiderin-laden synovium. Magnetic resonance imaging is useful for preoperative assessment of joint involvement. Characteristic findings include nodular intra-articular masses of low signal intensity on T1- and T2-weighted images (Fig. 48–1). The low signal is attributed to the deposition of hemosiderin.[2,15]

Indications and Contraindications

Surgery can provide definitive treatment of synovial disorders or alleviate many of the symptoms interfering with joint function. In the case of disorders associated with localized pathology, such as synovial plica or localized PVNS, arthroscopic treatment allows the surgeon to remove the lesion in its entirety.[3,11,12,17]

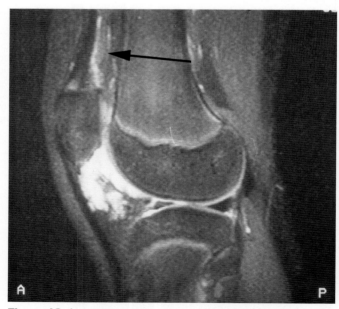

Figure 48–1   Magnetic resonance imaging scan of a 15-year-old boy with diffuse pigmented villonodular synovitis. Note the synovial thickening in the suprapatellar pouch *(arrow)*.

With diffuse conditions, synovectomy can be expected to reduce the severity of symptoms experienced by the patient. An example of an indication for synovectomy is a patient with rheumatoid arthritis and *minimal* degenerative changes on radiographs. Significant joint space narrowing or mechanical malalignment is a relative contraindication to synovectomy for inflammatory synovial diseases of the knee. Hemophilic synovitis, also associated with aggressive joint destruction, has responded well symptomatically to arthroscopic synovectomy.[5,10,21] Unlike most forms of the disorder, hemophilic synovitis usually requires a short period of hospitalization for arthroscopic treatment. The procedure has been effective in reducing recurrent hemarthrosis and maintaining range of motion. However, joint deterioration continues to occur, although probably at a slower rate.

Surgical Technique

Arthroscopic synovectomy requires the use of multiple portals to allow visualization and working access to all areas of the knee joint (Table 48–2). The surgical setup is critical to allow unimpeded access to both the anterior and posterior compartments of the knee.

Positioning

The patient is placed in the supine position to allow full access to the anterior and posterior compartments of the knee with the foot of the operating table dropped (Fig. 48–2). An arthroscopic leg holder is not used because it may prohibit use of the superomedial and superolateral portals.

A well-padded thigh tourniquet is placed high on the operative leg. If the tourniquet is placed too low on the thigh, work in the superomedial and superolateral portals may be difficult, possibly affecting the quality of the synovectomy. The contralateral leg is placed in a leg

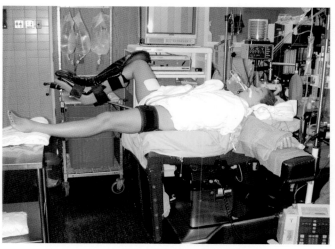

Figure 48–2 Arthroscopic setup and patient positioning.

holder. Compressive wrapping or sequential compression stockings should be used on the contralateral leg, owing to the length of the procedure. The foot of the bed is dropped, and the leg is allowed to hang free.

If the patient is in the supine position with the foot of the bed in extension, an arthroscopic lateral post must be positioned midthigh on the side of the operative bed. A tourniquet is positioned high on the thigh. The patient is maneuvered to the edge of the bed, ensuring that the leg can be easily hung over the side. Advantages of the lateral post include ease of establishing superomedial and superolateral portals and unlimited knee flexion, for there is no restraining leg holder on the thigh.

Examination under Anesthesia

The knee is first evaluated without a tourniquet on the extremity. Range of motion, ligamentous stability, patellar mobility, patellar tracking, and presence of effusion are determined. An evaluation of the contralateral leg is also performed for comparison.

Specific Surgical Steps

1. The extremity is exsanguinated, and the tourniquet is inflated to 250 to 300 mm Hg.
2. A number of arthroscopic portals are used for access to various areas of the knee. The procedure begins with the outflow cannula in the superomedial portal, because this portal is rarely needed for viewing (Fig. 48–3).
3. The initial diagnostic arthroscopy is performed (Fig. 48–4).
4. The synovectomy begins with the arthroscope in the inferolateral portal and the shaver in the superolateral portal. The synovium is resected from the suprapatellar pouch and lateral gutter. The shaver is then moved to the inferomedial portal. The synovium is removed from the medial gutter and medial aspect of the suprapatellar pouch.

Table 48–2		
Surgical Technique: Complete Synovectomy		
Camera Portal	Working Portal	Compartments
Inferolateral	Superolateral	Suprapatellar pouch, lateral gutter
Inferolateral	Inferomedial	Suprapatellar pouch, medial gutter, intercondylar notch
Inferolateral	Superomedial	Suprapatellar pouch, medial gutter
Superolateral	Inferolateral	Retropatellar pouch, inferolateral gutter
Superolateral	Inferomedial	Retropatellar pouch, inferomedial gutter
Inferolateral	Posteromedial	Posteromedial
Inferomedial	Posterolateral	Posterolateral

6 Knee

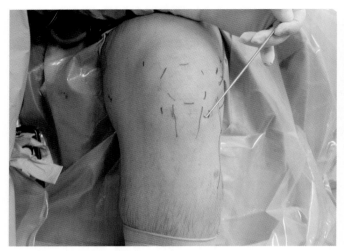

Figure 48–3 Typical arthroscopic portals used for synovectomy.

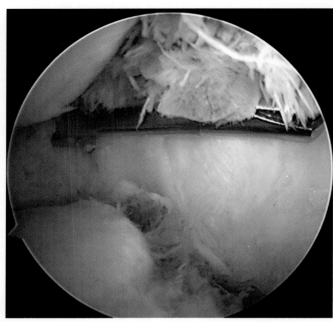

Figure 48–5 Arthroscopic view from the superolateral portal with the shaver inferomedial.

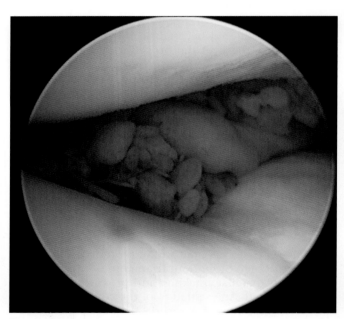

Figure 48–4 Initial scope appearance, with brownish synovium.

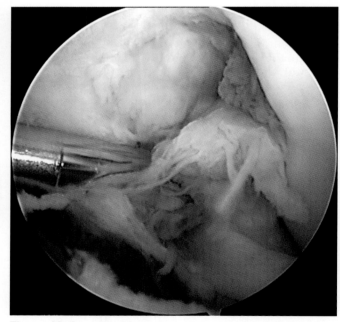

Figure 48–6 Arthroscopic view from the inferolateral portal with the shaver in the intercondylar notch.

5. The shaver is positioned in the superomedial portal to complete resection of the synovium in the medial gutter and medial aspect of the suprapatellar pouch.
6. For the next phase, the arthroscope is placed in the superolateral portal and the shaver in the inferolateral portal. This allows synovial resection from the retropatellar space and inferolateral gutter.
7. The shaver is placed in the inferomedial portal to complete the synovectomy of the retropatellar space and inferomedial gutter (Fig. 48–5).
8. The arthroscope is returned to the inferolateral portal, and the shaver is maintained in the inferomedial portal. Synovium is resected in the intercondylar notch and around the cruciate ligaments (Fig. 48–6). Care must be taken to distinguish synovium from ligament.

9. Once the synovium has been removed from the anterior portion of the knee, attention is turned to the posterior compartments. Proper posterior portal placement is critical to allow full access. The resection begins in the posteromedial compartment. A blunt-tipped trocar is placed in the arthroscopic sheath and inserted into the inferolateral portal. The medial femoral condyle is palpated with the instrument tip, and the trocar is pushed posteriorly

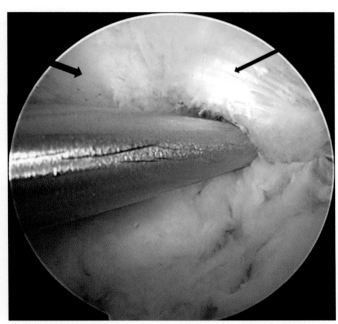

Figure 48–7   Blunt-tipped trocar used to enter the posterior compartment. The thin arrow indicates the posterior cruciate ligament, and the thick arrow depicts the medial femoral condyle.

through the interval between the medial femoral condyle and the posterior cruciate ligament (Fig. 48–7). The hand is raised to remain parallel with the posterior tibial plateau slope. The trocar should push into the posteromedial compartment without too much force. If excessive force is required, a central patellar tendon portal may allow easier access

to the posterior compartment. The trocar is removed, and the arthroscope is inserted. From this position, the surgeon should see the posterior aspect of the medial femoral condyle and the posterior horn of the medial meniscus.

10. While looking medially, a posteromedial working portal is created. A spinal needle is inserted into the posteromedial compartment under direct visualization. The needle is inserted anterior to the medial head of the gastrocnemius to avoid the neurovascular structures. Once the portal site is selected, a small longitudinal incision is made through the skin. Using a hemostat, the soft tissue is spread until the capsule is reached. The hemostat or scalpel can then be pushed through the capsule into the joint. The hemostat is replaced with a blunt-tipped trocar and arthroscopic cannula to establish a working portal. The shaver is inserted through this cannula, and the posteromedial compartment synovium is resected (Fig. 48–8).

11. A blunt-tipped trocar in the arthroscopic cannula is placed in the inferomedial portal, in the notch between the lateral femoral condyle and the anterior cruciate ligament. Again, the hand is raised to accommodate the posterior slope of the tibial plateau. One should feel the trocar give way, indicating passage into the posterolateral compartment. If resistance is encountered, one should not push hard, for fear of piercing the posterior capsule and damaging the neurovascular structures. Instead, one should simply try again until the trocar is inserted into the posterolateral compartment. The arthroscope is placed into the cannula, and the posterior aspect of the lateral femoral condyle, as well as the

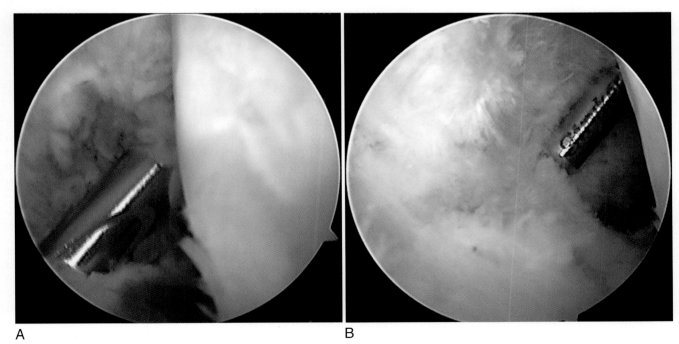

A   B

Figure 48–8   Arthroscopic view of the posteromedial compartment before *(A)* and after *(B)* synovial resection.

posterior horn of the lateral meniscus, should be seen.

12. To establish a posterolateral portal, insert a spinal needle into the compartment under direct visualization. The soft spot anterior to the biceps femoris muscle and posterior to the iliotibial tract protects the peroneal nerve. The needle should be inserted posterior to the fibular collateral ligament and anterior to the lateral head of the gastrocnemius. In a manner similar to establishing the posteromedial portal, the skin is incised with a scalpel, and a hemostat is used to dissect to the posterior capsule. One may puncture the capsule with the instrument under direct visualization. Maintaining the same angle, the hemostat is replaced with a blunt trocar in an operative cannula. The shaver is inserted, and the posterolateral compartment is debrided.

13. Be sure to obtain enough tissue for pathologic evaluation (Fig. 48–9).

14. After completion of the synovectomy, the tourniquet is released, and hemostasis is achieved with electrocautery. A suction drain is typically used for 24 hours postoperatively to minimize hemarthrosis. Light compressive dressing and cryotherapy are used to minimize swelling and encourage early joint motion.

Pearls and Pitfalls

Performing an arthroscopic synovectomy requires a well-planned procedure using multiple arthroscopic portals and a variety of instruments, including shavers and electrocautery. The surgeon must be prepared to view the knee and its pathology from multiple angles.

Depending on the extent of synovium involved, the procedure can be lengthy. General anesthesia rather than local anesthesia is recommended. An epidural can also be used when medically indicated, and it may aid in postoperative pain relief. A Foley catheter may be used in anticipation of prolonged anesthesia.

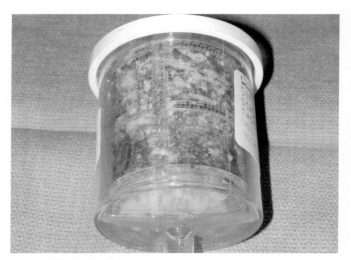

Figure 48–9 Typical volume of synovium collected with total synovectomy.

Correct portal placement is crucial to successful resection of the synovium. Before each portal is created, an 18-gauge spinal needle should be used to find the correct portal site. Each portal should be dilated with a straight hemostat to ensure atraumatic entry of the cannula into the joint.

Failure to obtain hemostasis at the end of the procedure will result in a large hemarthrosis and necessitate a repeat procedure. Excessive bleeding is prevented by not resecting the overlying soft tissue.

Most important, the surgeon must have a preoperative plan for approaching the lesion. This includes the appropriate instrumentation and a well-thought-out sequence of steps to excise the synovium in its entirety. Excellent results are possible with arthroscopic synovectomy if the surgeon employs good technique.

Postoperative Management

After the procedure, the patient may bear weight as tolerated on the extremity. For complete synovectomy, continuous passive range of motion is initiated in the hospital for 1 to 3 days, advancing the arc of motion as pain and swelling allow. In ambulatory patients, physical therapy is started on postoperative day 1 after removal of the drain. The emphasis in physical therapy is on closed chain exercises. Regaining and maintaining full knee extension and quadriceps function is also critical in the early phase of rehabilitation. Other modalities include the stationary bicycle, patellar mobilization, and nonimpact aerobic exercises. Flexion is also desirable but is not as important for ambulation.

Ideally, therapy should be initiated under the guidance of a physical therapist. In this setting, proper techniques can be learned by the patient and continued at home. Additional modalities can be employed by the therapist to complement the range-of-motion and strengthening exercises, including muscle stretching, electrical stimulation, and muscle massage.

Results

Arthroscopic synovectomy has proved to be effective in patients with rheumatoid arthritis, reducing both pain and swelling. It is a relatively safe procedure that can usually be performed on an outpatient basis. When combined with current rheumatoid medications, it can reduce inflammation and preserve range of motion.[6] Success rates, based on the relief of pain and swelling, have been as high as 80% in the treatment of rheumatoid arthritis.[19]

Arthroscopic synovectomy has also enjoyed success in the treatment of PVNS. Open synovectomy is associated with complications, including stiffness and incisional pain. Recurrence rates after arthroscopic synovectomy of diffuse PVNS have been as low as 11%, with improved range of motion.[1,8,18]

Localized PVNS has responded best to arthroscopic treatment. Multiple series have reported no recurrences at follow-up after excision of the lesion.[4,14,16,18,22] The procedure allows improved visualization of lesions and facilitates the discovery of small, localized forms of PVNS.

Complications

Complications following arthroscopic synovectomy include recurrent hemarthrosis requiring aspiration or arthroscopic irrigation and debridement. Usually the blood can be aspirated with a large-bore needle. If the blood has coagulated and aspiration is unsuccessful, repeat arthroscopy is occasionally indicated.

Joint stiffness and loss of extension can be problematic after arthroscopic synovectomy.[7,13,22] The use of extension boards and dynamic bracing may be helpful in this situation. Joint sepsis and neurovascular injury have been reported anecdotally. These complications can be prevented by judicious use of the tourniquet, adequate padding of the operative and nonoperative extremities, and meticulous posterior portal placement.

References

1. Beguin J, Locker B, Vielpeau C, Souquieres G: Pigmented villonodular synovitis of the knee: Results from 13 cases. Arthroscopy 5:62-64, 1989.
2. Bessette PR, Cooley PA, Johnson RP, Czarnecki DJ: Gadolinium-enhanced MRI of pigmented villonodular synovitis of the knee. J Comput Assist Tomogr 16:992-994, 1992.
3. Comin JA, Rodriguez-Merchan EC: Arthroscopic synovectomy in the management of painful localized posttraumatic synovitis of the knee joint. Arthroscopy 13:606-608, 1997.
4. Delcogliano A, Galli M, Menghi A, Belli P: Localized pigmented villonodular synovitis of the knee: Report of two cases of fat pad involvement. Arthroscopy 14:527-531, 1998.
5. Eickhoff HH, Koch W, Radershadt G, Brackmann HH: Arthroscopy for chronic hemophilic synovitis of the knee. Clin Orthop 343:58-62, 1997.
6. Fiacco U, Cozzi L, Rigon C, et al: Arthroscopic synovectomy in rheumatoid and psoriatic knee joint synovitis: Long-term outcome. Br J Rheumatol 35:463-470, 1996.
7. Flandry F, Hughston JC: Current concepts review: Pigmented villonodular synovitis. J Bone Joint Surg Am 69:942-949, 1987.
8. Flandry FC, Hughston JC, Jacobson KE, et al: Surgical treatment of diffuse pigmented villonodular synovitis of the knee. Clin Orthop 300:183-192, 1994.
9. Flandry F, McCann SB, Hughston JC, Kurtz DM: Roentgenographic findings in pigmented villonodular synovitis of the knee. Clin Orthop 247:208-219, 1989.
10. Gilbert MS, Radomisli TE: Therapeutic options in the management of hemophilic synovitis. Clin Orthop 343:88-92, 1997.
11. Highgenboten CL: Arthroscopic synovectomy. Arthroscopy 1:190, 1985.
12. Klein W, Jensen KU: Arthroscopic synovectomy of the knee joint: Indication, technique and follow-up results. Arthroscopy 4:63, 1988.
13. Klug S, Wittmann G, Weseloh G: Arthroscopic synovectomy of the knee joint in early cases of rheumatoid arthritis: Follow-up results of a multicenter study. Arthroscopy 16:262-267, 2000.
14. Lee BI, Yoo JE, Lee SH, Min KD: Localized pigmented villonodular synovitis of the knee: Arthroscopic treatment. Arthroscopy 14:764-768, 1998.
15. Lin J, Jacobson JA, Jamadar DA, et al: Pigmented villonodular synovitis and related lesions: The spectrum of imaging findings. AJR Am J Roentgenol 172:191-197, 1999.
16. Mancini GB, Lazzeri S, Bruno G, Pucci G: Localized pigmented villonodular synovitis of the knee. Arthroscopy 14:532-536, 1998.
17. McEwen C: Multicenter evaluation of synovectomy in the treatment of rheumatoid arthritis: A report of results at the end of five years. J Rheumatol 15:764, 1988.
18. Ogilvie-Harris DJ, McLean J, Zarnett ME: Pigmented villonodular synovitis of the knee. J Bone Joint Surg Am 74:119-123, 1992.
19. Ogilvie-Harris DJ, Weisleder L: Arthroscopic synovectomy of the knee: Is it helpful? Arthroscopy 11:91-95, 1995.
20. Van Meter CD, Rowdon GA: Localized pigmented villonodular synovitis presenting as a locked lateral meniscal bucket handle tear: 2 cases and a review of the literature. Arthroscopy 10:309-312, 1994.
21. Wiedel JD: Arthroscopic synovectomy of the knee in hemophilia: 10 to 15 year follow-up. Clin Orthop 328:46-53, 1996.
22. Zvijac JE, Lau AC, Hechtman KS, et al: Arthroscopic treatment of pigmented villonodular synovitis of the knee. Arthroscopy 15:613-617, 1999.

6 Knee

CHAPTER

49

Meniscus: Diagnosis and Decision Making

Marc R. Safran and Gabriel Soto

Our understanding of the meniscus and its function has grown from thinking that it is an embryologic or useless remnant of leg muscle to knowing that it is an important structure critical to the function and health of the knee.[4] Injury to the meniscus commonly occurs as a result of athletic activities and activities of daily living. Injury to the meniscus may occur in isolation or in combination with other knee injuries, particularly ligament injuries. Arthroscopic meniscal surgery is one of the most commonly performed surgeries in the United States.

Anatomy and Biomechanics

The meniscus is a semicircular fibrocartilaginous structure with bony attachments at its anterior and posterior aspects to the tibial plateau (Fig. 49–1). The medial meniscus is C-shaped. In addition to its bony attachments, the medial meniscus has a capsular attachment, known as the coronary ligament. A thickening of the capsular attachment at its midportion from the tibia to the femur is known as the deep medial collateral ligament. The lateral meniscus is more semicircular and covers a larger portion of the tibial plateau compared with its medial counterpart. The meniscus is thick at its periphery and thin centrally. Discoid variants of the lateral meniscus occur in up to 5% of cases and cover much of the lateral tibial plateau (Fig. 49–2).[38] The popliteal tendon runs posterolateral to the posterior insertion of the lateral meniscus, in an area called the popliteal hiatus. In addition to its bony attachments, the lateral meniscus is attached to the capsule except at the area of the popliteal hiatus.[34] Its capsular attachments are less well developed compared with the medial side, allowing for more motion of the meniscus with knee flexion-extension (Fig. 49–3).[37]

The menisci are composed of coarse collagen bundles that run mainly circumferentially, with binding fibers that run radially (Fig. 49–4).[3] This allows the meniscus to disperse compressive loads (hoop stresses). Sixty percent to 70% of the meniscus is composed of collagen, primarily type I collagen. At birth, the entire meniscus is vascular; however, by 10 years of age, only the peripheral 10% to 25% of the lateral meniscus and 10% to 30% of the medial meniscus has a blood supply, which is how it remains through adulthood (Fig. 49–5).[19] The blood supply comes from the geniculates through a perimeniscal capillary plexus.[1] Owing to its lack of capsular attachment, the lateral meniscus at the popliteal hiatus is relatively avascular. Nutrition of the inner 66% of the meniscus is through diffusion or mechanical pumping; the outer meniscus receives nutrition through its blood supply.[23] Neural elements are present in the outer portion of the meniscus, at the capsular junction and the insertional horns.

The menisci are important in many aspects of knee function, including load sharing, shock absorption, reduction of joint contact stresses, increase in joint congruity and contact area, articular cartilage nutrition, passive or secondary stabilization, limitation of extreme flexion and extension, and possibly proprioception.[2,13,18,23,28,33]

Historical Aspects

The meniscus was once thought to be a functionless remnant of intra-articular knee muscle and was routinely removed. Although Fairbank[12] published a paper in 1948 suggesting that the meniscus was important based on postmeniscectomy radiographs, it was not until the mid-1970s that retention of the meniscus began to be discussed. The annual incidence of meniscal tears is 60 to 70 per 100,000 general population.[14,26] Meniscal tears are more common in males (2.5 to 4:1), with a peak incidence between 21 and 30 years of age in males and 11

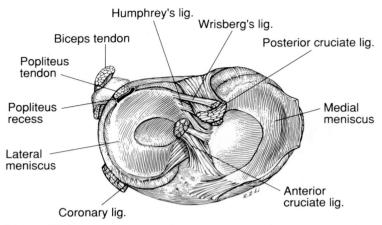

Figure 49–1 View of the tibial plateau from above. Note the degree of coverage of the medial and lateral tibial plateau due to the different shapes of the medial and lateral menisci. (From Tria AJ Jr, Klein KS: An Illustrated Guide to the Knee. New York, Churchill Livingstone, 1992.)

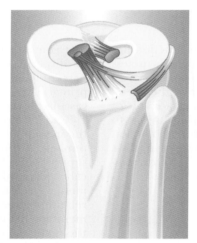

Figure 49–2 Schematic representation of a discoid lateral meniscus, covering most of the lateral tibial plateau. (From Fu F, Harner C: Knee Surgery. Philadelphia, Lippincott, Williams & Wilkins, 1994.)

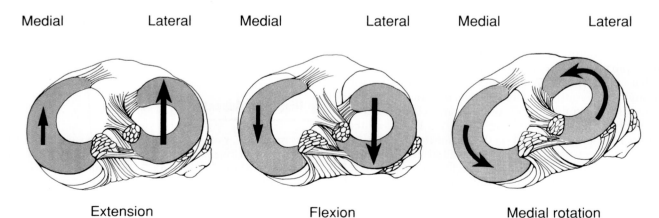

Medial   Lateral   Medial   Lateral   Medial   Lateral

Extension   Flexion   Medial rotation

Figure 49–3 Kinematics of the different menisci with knee flexion, extension, and rotation. Note that even though the lateral meniscus and lateral tibial plateau have a smaller anteroposterior width, the lateral meniscus moves more than the medial meniscus through each range of motion. (From Tria AJ Jr, Klein KS: An Illustrated Guide to the Knee. New York, Churchill Livingstone, 1992.)

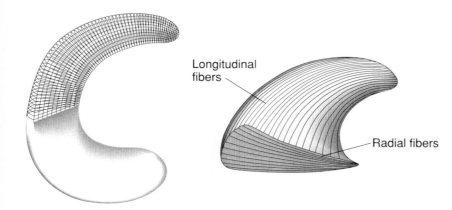

Figure 49–4   Drawing of the meniscus showing most of the collagen fibers aligned longitudinally, with some fibers radially oriented to hold the longitudinal fibers together. These longitudinally oriented fibers allow for dissipation of compressive forces via hoop stresses. (From Tria AJ Jr, Klein KS: An Illustrated Guide to the Knee. New York, Churchill Livingstone, 1992.)

Longitudinal fibers

Radial fibers

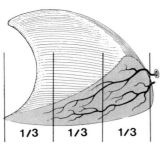

Figure 49–5   **Blood supply within the meniscus.** (From Tria AJ Jr, Klein KS: An Illustrated Guide to the Knee. New York, Churchill Livingstone, 1992.)

and 20 years in females.[27] Degenerative meniscal tears commonly occur after the third decade in men.

Mechanism of Injury

In older patients, tears may occur with activities of daily living, including squatting and deep knee flexion. Younger patients usually sustain a twisting, cutting, or hyperflexion injury, or they suffer a meniscal injury in conjunction with an anterior cruciate ligament (ACL) tear or tibial plateau fracture.

Clinical Evaluation

The diagnosis of meniscal tear can be made from a careful history, physical examination, and appropriate diagnostic tests.

History

The onset of symptoms and mechanism of injury are often clues to the diagnosis. With an injury mechanism as described earlier, there may be an acute onset of pain and swelling. Complaints of locking or catching may be present, but these may be due to other pathology. Loss of motion with mechanical block to extension may be due to a displaced bucket handle tear. Degenerative tears

tend to occur in patients older than 40 years, frequently with an atraumatic, chronic history of mild joint swelling, joint line pain, and mechanical symptoms.

Physical Examination

Inspection should be performed to assess for effusion (present in 51% to 74% of cases; positive predictive value, 50%), quadriceps muscle atrophy, and any joint line swelling that may occur with a meniscal cyst. Range of motion must be assessed to determine whether there is a mechanical block to extension. A complete ligamentous examination and patellofemoral evaluation are important to rule out concomitant pathology or other sources of knee pain. Numerous tests have been described to evaluate the meniscus for tears, including joint line tenderness (sensitivity, 61% to 86%; specificity, 29%)[41]; pain on forced flexion (sensitivity, 50%; specificity, 68%); McMurray test (sensitivity, 16% to 59%; specificity, 93 to 98%; positive predictive value, 83%), which is enhanced when seen with loss of extension (sensitivity, 85%; specificity, 95%); Apley grind test; and others (Fig. 49–6).[7,11,20]

It has been shown that no single predictive test can make the diagnosis of meniscal tear. It has also been shown that concurrent ACL injury negatively impacts the accuracy of physical findings for meniscal pathology.[32] Most investigators have found that a composite of physical examination findings is more accurate at predicting meniscal pathology than any single test is.[35,36]

Imaging

Although plain radiographs do not show meniscal tears, they are important in any knee evaluation to assess for bony pathology and to look for joint space narrowing. A radiographic series consists of a flexion weight-bearing posteroanterior (Rosenberg) view (which is most sensitive for evaluating joint space narrowing, as this occurs in 30 to 45 degrees of flexion), a true lateral view, and a tangential patellofemoral radiograph.[30] Fairbank's changes—flattening of the medial femoral condyle, joint space narrowing, and osteophyte formation—are

6 Knee

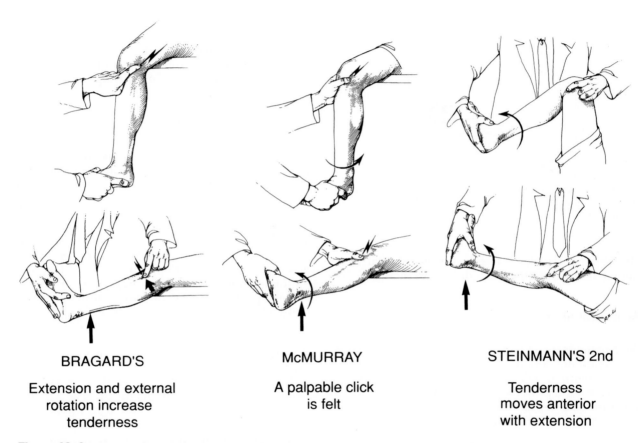

BRAGARD'S	McMURRAY	STEINMANN'S 2nd
Extension and external rotation increase tenderness	A palpable click is felt	Tenderness moves anterior with extension

Figure 49–6 Various physical examination tests to evaluate the meniscus. (From Tria AJ Jr, Klein KS: An Illustrated Guide to the Knee. New York, Churchill Livingstone, 1992.)

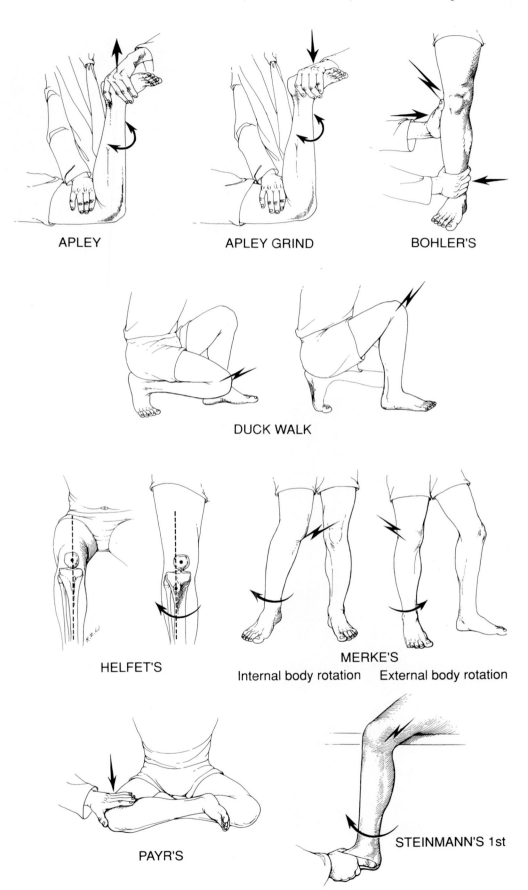

APLEY

APLEY GRIND

BOHLER'S

DUCK WALK

HELFET'S

MERKE'S

Internal body rotation   External body rotation

PAYR'S

STEINMANN'S 1st

Figure 49–6, cont'd

6 Knee

indicative of degenerative changes seen with chronic untreated meniscal tears or after meniscectomy (Fig. 49–7).

Many studies suggest that magnetic resonance imaging (MRI) is very sensitive (95%) for the detection of meniscal tears (Fig. 49–8).[24] However, several investigators found that the overall accuracy of clinical examination (81% to 95%) was as good as or better than that of MRI (74% to 96%) for diagnosing torn menisci.[16,22,29] In a comparison between clinical examination and MRI, the positive predictive value was similar (92% versus 97%), the negative predictive value was better for clinical examination (99% versus 92%), the sensitivity was similar (97% versus 98%), and the specificity was virtually the same (87% versus 86%).[24] In a prospective study, Miller[22] concluded that preoperative MRI did not prevent unnecessary surgery in any case. In fact, many authors have reported that MRI has a high false-positive rate (5% to 36%) for torn menisci.[5,17] The finding of age-dependent degeneration of the meniscus manifesting as increased MRI signal in asymptomatic adults has been well documented. Similarly, among a group of asymptomatic athletes, 50% demonstrated "significant baseline

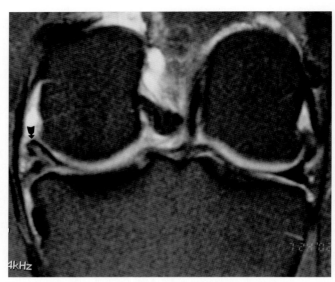

Figure 49–8 Magnetic resonance imaging scan of a typical meniscal tear. The arrow points to the medial meniscus with a complex tear pattern.

MRI abnormalities." Studies in children have also failed to show an enhanced diagnostic utility of MRI over clinical examination. In fact, clinical examination was significantly more sensitive than MRI for detecting lateral discoid menisci (88.9% versus 38.9%). Further, Rose and Gold[29] found that clinical examination had an accuracy of 79% for meniscal lesions, compared with 72% accuracy for MRI. All these studies emphasize the need for clinicians to match clinical signs and symptoms with MRI findings before embarking on surgical treatment.

Classification

Meniscal tears can be classified in many ways, although the most common is based on the pattern of tear seen at arthroscopy. Commonly described patterns include vertical longitudinal (including bucket handle tears), oblique (also known as flap or parrot beak tears), radial (transverse), horizontal, and complex (a combination of tears, including degenerative tears) (Fig. 49–9).

MRI classification of meniscal changes is as follows: grade 0, normal with homogeneous signal intensity; grades I and II, high signal intensity within the meniscus that does not go to the surface; and grade III, high signal intensity that goes to the surface of the meniscus and is indicative of a tear (Fig. 49–10). The repairability of menisci cannot be inferred from MRI findings.

Associated Injuries

Meniscal tears may occur in isolation, although approximately one third of them are associated with ACL tears—lateral meniscal tears with acute ACL injuries, and medial meniscal tears with chronic ACL deficiency.[10,27] Meniscal tears also frequently occur with tibial plateau fractures.[39]

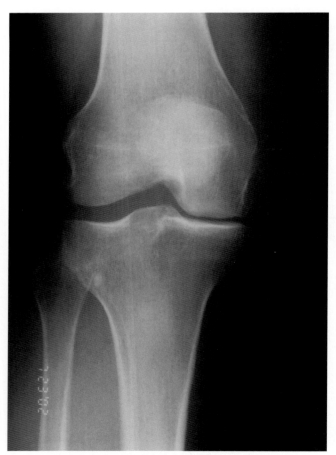

Figure 49–7 Radiographs of a 40-year-old woman seen 28 years after an anterior cruciate ligament–medial meniscus injury that was treated nonoperatively. Note the narrowing of the medial compartment joint space, sclerosis, flattening of the medial femoral condyle, and marginal osteophytes.

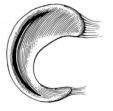
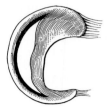
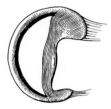

Complete longitudinal   Bucket handle   Displaced bucket handle

Figure 49–9   *A*, **Schematic representation of types of meniscal tears.** *B*, **Meniscal cyst.** (*A*, From Tria AJ Jr, Klein KS: An Illustrated Guide to the Knee. New York, Churchill Livingstone. 1992. *B*, From Safran M, Stone DA, Zachezewski J: Instructions to Sports Medicine Patients. Philadelphia, WB Saunders, 2002.)

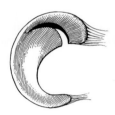
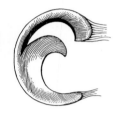
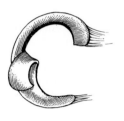

Parrot beak   Flap   Displaced flap

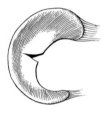
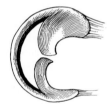
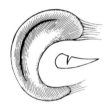

Radial   Double flap   Incomplete longitudinal

A

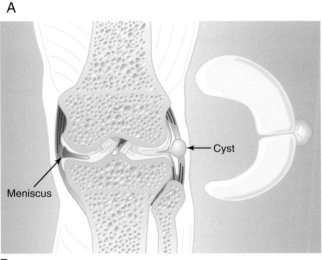

Cyst

Meniscus

B

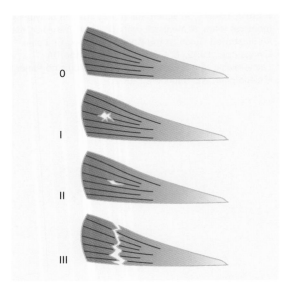

Figure 49–10 Magnetic resonance imaging classification of meniscal tears. (From Fu F, Harner C: Knee Surgery. Philadelphia, Lippincott, Williams & Wilkins, 1994.)

Treatment Options: Indications and Contraindications

Nonoperative

Many meniscal tears are asymptomatic, especially in older patients. Further, some symptomatic tears may become asymptomatic with conservative management consisting of activity modification, anti-inflammatory medications (including a cortisone injection), and a rehabilitation program. Thus, nonoperative management for 3 months should be the initial treatment if the patient has full range of motion, especially in older patients. Although chronic tears with a superimposed acute injury usually do not heal with nonsurgical treatment, they may become asymptomatic with conservative therapy alone. The chance of spontaneous healing of an acute injury is inversely proportional to the size of the tear and the amount of displacement and is impaired by concurrent ACL injury. It has been shown that more than 90% of athletes with symptomatic meniscal tears are unable to return to sports; thus, nonoperative management is usually not recommended.

Operative

Indications for surgery include (1) daily symptoms of meniscal injury that affect sports or activities of daily living or work, such as frequent locking and repeated or chronic effusions; (2) physical findings consistent with a meniscal tear; (3) failure of nonoperative management; and (4) absence of other causes of knee pain based on a complete evaluation.[21] Loss of motion due to a displaced meniscal tear should be addressed urgently with surgery. Every attempt should be made to preserve as much meniscus as possible, and the meniscus should be repaired if feasible (in conjunction with ACL reconstruction if there is concomitant ACL deficiency). Currently, only vertical longitudinal tears involving the outer 25% to 30% of the meniscus (within 3 to 5 mm of the meniscocapsular junction, where there is a blood supply), with no degeneration and a stable knee, have the potential to heal and should be repaired. Almost all other tears should be managed with meniscectomy, with the following exceptions: short, stable, vertical longitudinal tears (<10 mm); stable partial-thickness tears (<50% of meniscal thickness); and small radial tears (<3 mm).[15]

Meniscal reconstruction is a controversial topic, including the indications. The senior author's indications for meniscus transplantation are patients who have undergone complete or subtotal meniscectomy with symptoms of joint pain in the ipsilateral compartment, recurrent effusions, or failed ACL reconstruction thought to be due to loss of the medial meniscus.

Rehabilitation

After Nonoperative Treatment

The goals of nonoperative management are to decrease inflammation and effusion, attain or maintain range of motion, and increase quadriceps strength before performing sports-specific activities to allow a return to competition. These goals are achieved through a phased program, including icing and electrical stimulation, stretching, and closed chain strengthening exercises, in addition to straight leg raises and isometric quadriceps strengthening.

After Operative Treatment

The goals after surgery are to decrease inflammation, restore motion, increase strength, and facilitate a safe return to competition. This is usually achieved through a phased program with set goals, although it is important to emphasize measures to prevent reinjury. Following meniscectomy, there is usually no need for bracing or range-of-motion restrictions. Measures include immediate full weight bearing, ice to reduce effusion, anti-inflammatory drugs as needed if there are no contraindications, and quadriceps exercises.[42] The patient can return to sports when full range of motion is achieved, there is no effusion, and strength is 80% of the uninjured side (usually 4 to 6 weeks).

A meniscal repair needs to be protected in the early phases. For meniscal suturing, this usually means weight bearing with the knee locked in full extension for 4 to 6 weeks and no weight bearing with the knee flexed greater than 90 degrees for 4 to 6 months. For meniscal implants, weight bearing should be additionally restricted for the first few weeks. Return to sports usually occurs after 6 months, as long as quadriceps strength is within 80% of the contralateral extremity. The rehabilitation for meniscal reconstruction still lacks a scientific basis and is empirical at this time; however, this procedure is not performed in those expecting to return to sports.

Results

Arthroscopy has had a tremendous impact on the ability to treat meniscal injuries while reducing morbidity (Fig. 49–11). Although open total meniscectomy was once the standard of care for meniscal injuries, several long-term follow-up studies found that these patients have poor outcomes and are significantly more likely to develop arthritic changes in the operated knee.[25] Several authors compared open total meniscectomy with arthroscopic partial meniscectomy and found that leaving some of the meniscus behind led to significantly better results and reduced the rate of degenerative arthritis.[25,31]

Meniscal repair has been shown to be successful in healing the tear and retaining the meniscus. Open repair has the longest follow-up, with excellent results and retention of the healed meniscus.[9] Arthroscopic repair has comparable results in the short and medium terms.[6,8,40]

Meniscal reconstruction can be helpful in reducing symptoms associated with total meniscectomy, such as pain and effusion. However, many factors have been shown to adversely affect outcome, including extremity malalignment, irradiated grafts, lyophilized grafts, and advanced degenerative articular changes. Meniscus transplantation has not been shown to prevent arthritis or joint degeneration.

Complications

Early reports of the initial experience with arthroscopic fluid pumps found complication rates as high as 1.4%. Improved instrumentation and techniques, however, have made these complications incredibly rare. As with other surgeries, potential complications include infection, bleeding, arteriovenous fistula, and nerve injury (particularly the saphenous, as well as the peroneal and popliteal neurovasculature). Other complications of arthroscopic meniscal surgery that have been reported and should be discussed with the patient preoperatively include deep vein thrombosis and pulmonary embolism, recurrent effusions, incomplete tear removal, synovial cutaneous fistula, iatrogenic arthroscopic joint lesions, osteonecrosis (usually in the elderly), popliteal pseudo-aneurysm, inability to repair the meniscus, nonhealing of meniscal repair, nonhealing of meniscal reconstruction, arthritis, complications from implants (including articular cartilage injury), and the need for further surgery.

Future Directions

The last 20 years have led to an explosion in knowledge about the meniscus and its treatment. However, there is still much to be learned about meniscal injury and healing. Further understanding of meniscal injury, such as the difference between isolated tears and traumatic tears; the ability to repair tears other than vertical longitudinal tears at the periphery; and the determination of the long-term success of meniscal repair in preventing arthritis are but a few areas to be studied. An understanding of meniscus transplantation, including the ability to properly size a meniscus preoperatively and to place it simply and reproducibly, and scientific study of the appropriate rehabilitation are critical before we can determine whether meniscal reconstruction prevents arthritis. Last, the ability to heal meniscal tears of any type or of any vascularity with gene therapy, making arthroscopy unnecessary, would be an ideal goal for the future.

References

1. Arnoczky SP, Warren RF: Microvasculature of the human meniscus. Am J Sports Med 10:90-95, 1982.
2. Baratz ME, Fu FH, Mengato R: Meniscal tears: The effect of meniscectomy and of repair on intraarticular contact areas and stress in the human knee. A preliminary report. Am J Sports Med 14:270-275, 1986.
3. Beaupre A, Choukroun R, Guidouin P, et al: Knee menisci: Correlation between microstructure and biomechanics. Clin Orthop 208:72-75, 1986.
4. Bland-Sutton J (ed): Ligaments: Their Nature and Morphology, 2nd ed. London, JK Lewis, 1897.
5. Boden SD, Davis DO, Dina TS, et al: A prospective and blinded investigation of magnetic resonance imaging of the knee: Abnormal findings in asymptomatic subjects. Clin Orthop 282:177-185, 1992.
6. Cannon WD Jr: Arthroscopic meniscal repair: Inside-out technique and results. Am J Knee Surg 9:137-143, 1996.
7. Corea JR, Mousa M, Othman A: McMurray's test tested. Knee Surg Sports Traumatol Arthrosc 2:70-72, 1994.

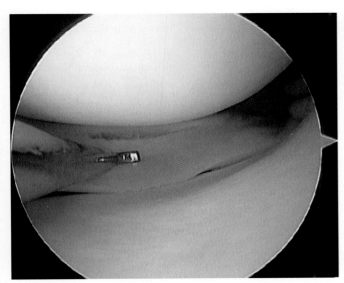

Figure 49–11 Arthroscopic picture of a longitudinally torn meniscus.

8. DeHaven KE: Meniscus repair. Am J Sports Med 27:242-250, 1999.

9. DeHaven KE, Lohrer WA, Lovelock JE: Long-term results of open meniscal repair. Am J Sports Med 23:524-530, 1995.

10. Duncan JB, Hunter R, Purness M, Freeman J: Meniscal injuries associated with acute anterior cruciate ligament tears in alpine skiers. Am J Sports Med 23:170-172, 1995.

11. Evans PJ, Bell GD, Frank C: Prospective evaluation of the McMurray test. Am J Sports Med 21:604-608, 1993.

12. Fairbank TJ: Knee joint changes after meniscectomy. J Bone Joint Surg Br 30:664-670, 1948.

13. Fukubayashi T, Kurosawa H: The contact area and pressure distribution pattern of the knee: A study of normal and osteoarthritic knee joints. Acta Orthop Scand 51:871-879, 1980.

14. Hede A, Jensen DB, Blyme P, Sonne-Holm S: Epidemiology of meniscal lesions of the knee: 1215 open operations in Copenhagen 1982–1984. Acta Orthop Scand 61:435-437, 1990.

15. Henning CE, Clark JR, Lynch MA, et al: Arthroscopic meniscus repair with a posterior incision. Instr Course Lect 37:209-221, 1988.

16. Kocher MS, DiCanzio J, Zurakowski D, Micheli LJ: Diagnostic performance of clinical examination and selective magnetic resonance imaging in the evaluation of intraarticular knee disorders in children and adolescents. Am J Sports Med 29:292-296, 2001.

17. LaPrade RF, Burnett QM II, Veenstra MA, Hodgman CG: The prevalence of abnormal magnetic resonance findings in asymptomatic knees: With correlation of magnetic resonance imaging to arthroscopic findings in symptomatic knees. Am J Sports Med 22:739-745, 1994.

18. Levy IM, Torzilli PA, Warren RF: The effect of medial meniscectomy on anterior-posterior motion of the knee. J Bone Joint Surg Am 64:883-888, 1982.

19. McDevitt CA, Webber RJ: The ultrastructure and biochemistry of meniscal cartilage. Clin Orthop 252:8-18, 1990.

20. Medlar RC, Mandiberg JJ, Lyne ED: Meniscectomies in children: Report of long-term results (mean 8.3 years) of 26 children. Am J Sports Med 8:87-92, 1980.

21. Metcalf RW, Burks RT, Metcalf MS, McGinty JB: Arthroscopic meniscectomy. In McGinty JB, Caspari RB, Jackson RW, Poehling GC (eds): Operative Arthroscopy, 2nd ed. Philadelphia, Lippincott-Raven, 1996, pp 263-297.

22. Miller GK: A prospective study comparing the accuracy of the clinical diagnosis of meniscus tear with magnetic resonance imaging and its effect on clinical outcome. Arthroscopy 12:406-413, 1996.

23. Mow VC, Fithian DC, Kelly MA: Fundamentals of articular cartilage and meniscus biomechanics. In Ewing JW (ed): Articular Cartilage and Knee Joint Function: Basic Science and Arthroscopy. New York, Raven Press, 1990, pp 1-18.

24. Muellner T, Weinstabl R, Schabus R, et al: The diagnosis of meniscal tears in athletes: A comparison of clinical and magnetic resonance imaging investigations. Am J Sports Med 25:7-12, 1997.

25. Neyret P, Donell ST, Dejour H: Results of partial meniscectomy related to the state of the anterior cruciate ligament: Review at 20 to 35 years. J Bone Joint Surg Br 75:36-40, 1993.

26. Nielsen AB, Yde J: Epidemiology of acute knee injuries: A prospective hospital investigation. J Trauma 31:1644-1648, 1991.

27. Poehling GG, Ruch DS, Chabon SJ: The landscape of meniscal injuries. Clin Sports Med 9:539-549, 1990.

28. Radin EL, de Lamotte F, Maquet P: Role of the menisci in the distribution of stress in the knee. Clin Orthop 185:290-294, 1984.

29. Rose NE, Gold SM: A comparison of accuracy between clinical examination and magnetic resonance imaging in the diagnosis of meniscal and anterior cruciate tears. J Arthrosc Rel Surg 12:398-405, 1996.

30. Rosenberg TD, Paulos LE, Parker RD, et al: The forty-five-degree posteroanterior flexion weight-bearing radiograph of the knee. J Bone Joint Surg Am 70:1479-1483, 1988.

31. Schimmer RC, Brulhart KB, Duff C, Glinz W: Arthroscopic partial meniscectomy: A 12-year follow-up and two-step evaluation of the long-term course. Arthroscopy 14:136-142, 1998.

32. Shelbourne KD, Martini DJ, McCarroll JR, Van Meter CD: Correlation of joint line tenderness and meniscal lesions in patients with acute anterior cruciate ligament tears. Am J Sports Med 23:166-169, 1995.

33. Shoemaker SC, Markolf KL: The role of the meniscus in the anterior-posterior stability of the loaded anterior cruciate deficient knee: Effects of partial versus total excision. J Bone Joint Surg Am 68:71-79, 1986.

34. Simonian PT, Sussman PS, van Trommel M, et al: Popliteomeniscal fasciculi and lateral meniscal stability. Am J Sports Med 25:849-853, 1997.

35. Solomon DH, Simel DL, Bates DW, et al: The rational clinical examination: Does this patient have a torn meniscus or ligament of the knee? Value of the physical examination. JAMA 286:1610-1620, 2001.

36. Terry GC, Tagert BE, Young MJ: Reliability of the clinical assessment in predicting the cause of internal derangements of the knee. Arthroscopy 11:568-576, 1995.

37. Thompson WO, Thaete FL, Fu FH, Dye SF: Tibial meniscal dynamics using three-dimensional reconstruction of magnetic resonance images. Am J Sports Med 19:210-216, 1991.

38. Vandermeer RD, Cunningham FK: Arthroscopic treatment of the discoid lateral meniscus: Results of long-term follow-up. Arthroscopy 5:101-109, 1989.

39. Vangsness CT Jr, Ghaderi B, Hohl M, Moore TM: Arthroscopy of meniscal injuries with tibial plateau fractures. J Bone Joint Surg Br 76:488-490, 1994.

40. Venkatachalam S, Godsiff SP, Harding ML: Review of the clinical results of arthroscopic meniscal repair. Knee 8:129-133, 2001.

41. Weinstabl R, Muellner T, Vecsei V, et al: Economic considerations for the diagnosis and therapy of meniscal lesions: Can magnetic resonance imaging help reduce the expense? World J Surg 21:363-368, 1997.

42. Wheatley WB, Krome J, Martin DF: Rehabilitation programmes following arthroscopic meniscectomy in athletes. Sports Med 21:447-456, 1996.

CHAPTER

50

Arthroscopic Meniscectomy

GABRIEL SOTO AND MARC R. SAFRAN

ARTHROSCOPIC MENISCECTOMY IN A NUTSHELL

History:
Twisting hyperflexion injury

Physical Examination:
Joint line tenderness; McMurray maneuver; stable ligamentous examination

Imaging:
Plain radiographs normal; magnetic resonance imaging shows a tear

Indications:
Failed physical therapy and anti-inflammatory medications

Surgical Technique:
Perform diagnostic arthroscopy; assess repairability; remove loose pieces, flaps, mobile segments; use biters first, then shaver; use different portals and biters
Bucket handle: bite posterior then anterior; grab and remove
Discoid: saucerize if torn
Cyst: partial meniscectomy, cyst decompression, biter and shaver

Postoperative Management:
Weight bearing as tolerated; ice, other modalities; range of motion; return to sports ~1 month

Results:
Lateral: 54% to 92% good to excellent
Medial: 79 to 100% good to excellent

Case History

MM is a 15-year-old high school track long jumper and basketball and football player. He injured his left knee while performing a long jump 6 weeks before evaluation in the senior author's office. The pain and swelling started 2 days after a twisting hyperflexion injury upon landing from the jump. He presented to a physician, who prescribed nonsteroidal anti-inflammatory medications, referred the athlete to physical therapy, and obtained a magnetic resonance imaging (MRI) scan for a suspected meniscal tear. He was referred to the senior author 1 month later with lateral joint line pain but no complaints of locking or buckling. His pain is along the lateral joint line. He has been unable to return to sports due to the lateral knee pain.

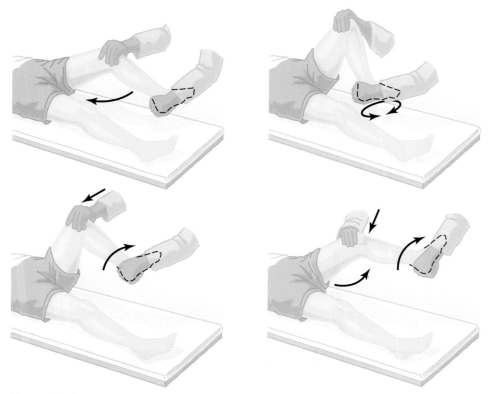

Figure 50–1   McMurray maneuver. The knee is flexed maximally while one hand is on the heel and the thumb of the other hand is on the lateral joint line and the fingers are across the medial joint line. Valgus stress is applied with the hand on the knee while the other hand applies an external rotation force to the heel and the knee is extended. A palpable clunk on the lateral side of the knee is consistent with a lateral meniscal tear. Similarly, a varus stress with an internal rotation force while extending the knee loads the medial meniscus, and a clunk is consistent with a medial meniscus tear. (From Fu FH, Harner CD: Knee Surgery. Philadelphia, Williams & Wilkins, 1994.)

Physical Examination

On physical examination, MM was 6 feet tall and weighed 155 pounds. His feet were normal and ambulated with a nonantalgic gait. He had full range of motion (0 to 135) and mild atrophy of his quadriceps muscles on the left side. He had no patellofemoral tenderness or crepitation, with a symmetrical patellar glide measuring 1 quadrant medially and laterally. He had no ligamentous laxity or signs of ligamentous instability in the varus-valgus plane or the anteroposterior plane. He had lateral joint line tenderness and a positive McMurray test (Fig. 50–1).

Imaging

This patient's radiographs revealed a widened lateral joint space (Fig. 50–2) with closed growth plates. There were no loose bodies or evidence of osteochondritis dissecans. MRI revealed a discoid lateral meniscus, as

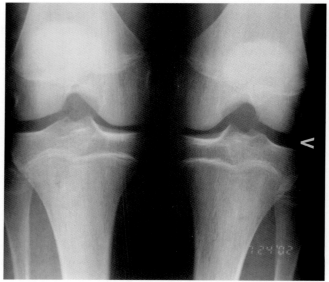

Figure 50–2   Radiograph showing a widened lateral joint space (*arrowhead*), consistent with a discoid lateral meniscus.

evidenced by the multiple cuts where the meniscus was in continuity. There also was evidence of a grade III radial signal at the junction of the anterior and middle portions of the lateral meniscus on MRI, consistent with a radial tear (Fig. 50–3). The medial meniscus was normal, and there were no other signs of pathology.

Decision-Making Principles

This patient had had 1 month of physical therapy and anti-inflammatory medications with no resolution of symptoms. Owing to his young age and activity level, the traumatic onset, and evidence of a discoid lateral meniscus with a radial tear involving the avascular central region, it was thought that this tear could best be managed by surgical intervention. The surgery considered was excision of the radial tear and saucerization of the torn discoid meniscus.

Surgical Technique

Positioning, Anesthesia, and Diagnostic Arthroscopy

Positioning and diagnostic arthroscopy are discussed in detail elsewhere in this book; however, a few points need to be addressed. First, the patient is positioned supine with the nonoperative leg in a leg holder that brings the extremity into flexion at the hip and knee. This allows access to the posteromedial portal without obstruction for meniscal repair and to address posteromedial loose bodies or other pathology (Fig. 50–4). The choice of anesthesia is at the discretion of the surgeon, patient, and anesthesiologist. Local anesthesia can be used for meniscectomy.[30] Examination under anesthesia may be performed to rule out ligamentous pathology, and it may be easier to perform a McMurray maneuver when the patient is asleep.

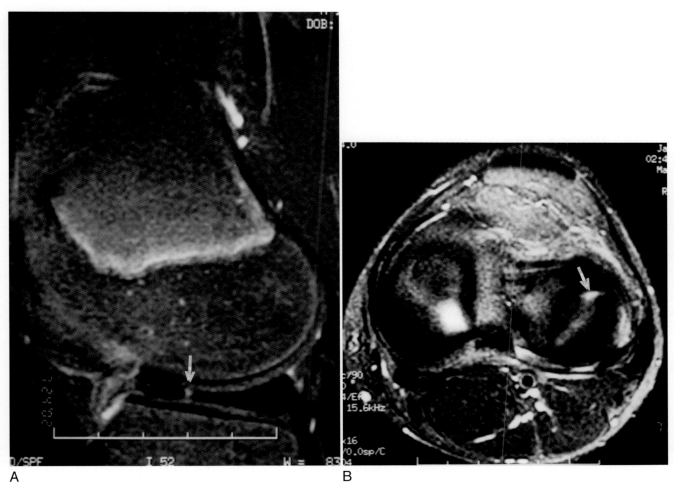

Figure 50–3   Magnetic resonance imaging scan showing a radial tear of a discoid lateral meniscus. *A,* Sagittal section. The arrow is pointing to the tear. *B,* Cross-sectional view of the same knee showing the meniscus covering a large portion of the lateral tibial plateau. The arrow is pointing to the anterolateral radial tear. (Anterior is at the top of the figure.)

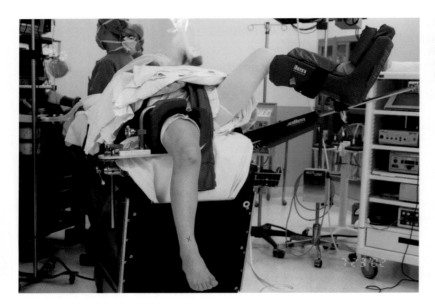

Figure 50–4 Intraoperative photograph of patient positioning for meniscal surgery. The well leg is positioned in a leg holder in flexion and abduction to allow easy access if a posteromedial portal is needed or a medial meniscal repair is necessary.

After the diagnostic arthroscopy is completed for the whole knee, including palpating the articular surfaces and both surfaces of the meniscal cartilage, the meniscal tear is addressed. The meniscus is inspected to assess tear type and repairability. When the meniscus is inspected, a waviness (meniscal flounce) may be observed; if so, close inspection is needed, because there is likely a tear. For tears that are not repairable, all mobile fragments that can be pulled past the inner margin of the meniscus into the center of the joint should be removed. The remaining meniscus should be contoured to reduce the risk of leaving a tear that may propagate to become a larger tear. The meniscal rim does not need to be perfectly smooth. Removing the whole tear and contouring are weighed against the risk of removing too much meniscus, because the risk of degeneration is directly proportional to the amount of meniscus removed. During and after the partial meniscectomy, it is important to palpate the remaining meniscus repeatedly to assess the mobility and texture of what remains and to ensure that the whole tear has been removed. It is important to protect the meniscocapsular junction and peripheral meniscal rim to maintain the function of the remaining meniscus. In general, the key is to remove the tear entirely while removing as little meniscus as possible and preserving as much meniscal function as possible.

Specific Surgical Steps

Conventional Tears

For conventional tears, the goal is to amputate the mobile segment at its base and then contour the remaining meniscus, leaving as wide and functioning a rim as possible (Fig. 50–5). Any tags or pieces that may catch in the joint or can be displaced into the center of the joint are resected. Usually the tear is removed with meniscal biters (basket forceps); these are precise instruments that cause minimal collateral damage. Full-radius resectors

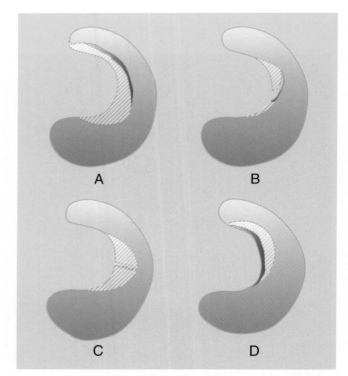

Figure 50–5 Principles of partial meniscectomy. Shaded areas show the different types of meniscal tears: vertical longitudinal (A), oblique (B), radial (C), and horizontal (D). The surgeon must remove the tear and leave as much normal meniscus as possible. The meniscus is also contoured for a smooth edge. (Adapted from Newman AP, Daniels AU, Burks RT: Principles and decision making in meniscal surgery. Arthroscopy 9:33-53, 1993.)

and motorized suction shavers can also remove damaged cartilage, smooth the repair, and remove loose pieces of cartilage generated by the meniscal biters. Controversy exists over the management of horizontal cleavage tears: some resect the superior and inferior leaves back to a stable rim, and some resect one leaf—the upper or lower leaf—leaving the other to function. There are no good studies to resolve this controversy.

Bucket Handle Tears

For bucket handle tears, it is easier to remove the posterior attachment first with a meniscal biter. The anterior horn is removed last to prevent the tear from displacing into the posterior compartment of the knee, which can increase the difficulty of the procedure (Fig. 50–6). There is a new meniscal back-biting cutter that allows for easier visualization while cutting the posterior horn of the bucket handle tear. Alternatively, a third working portal can be made to allow grasping and application of tension on the cut anterior horn to keep the meniscus from displacing posteriorly when a bucket handle tear is first cut from the anterior portion.

Further, when removing a torn meniscus, flap tear, or bucket handle tear, it may be easiest to remove all but a few strands of meniscal tissue with the meniscal biter. Then a grasping device can be introduced, and the remaining meniscus with its few strands of tissue attached can be avulsed or twisted and removed. This helps prevent the meniscus from becoming a loose body that the surgeon must then locate, grasp, and remove.

Meniscectomy with Cyst Decompression

Meniscal cysts are usually associated with degenerative meniscal tears, particularly horizontal cleavage tears. The irritation from the tear produces fluid that pushes the capsule; at an area of capsular weakness, an outpouching occurs, which is the cyst. It is thought that a one-way valve exists, which is why the cyst can get bigger but does not spontaneously get smaller. The senior author's approach is to perform an arthroscopic partial meniscectomy to remove the irritating source (the meniscus) and the valve. This often requires removing almost all the meniscus to the meniscocapsular rim. With free and open communication with the joint, the cyst decompresses on its own. Manual compression of the cyst at the time of surgery hastens the disappearance of the cyst from the patient's perspective. Some surgeons may enter the cyst from within by probing or inserting a shaver into it to ensure decompression.

Saucerization of Discoid Meniscus

If a discoid meniscus is identified incidentally at the time of arthroscopy and there is no tear, we recommend doing nothing to the meniscus. Saucerization of the discoid meniscus can help eliminate symptoms caused by a tear (Figs. 50–7, 50–8, and 50–9). Removal of the central

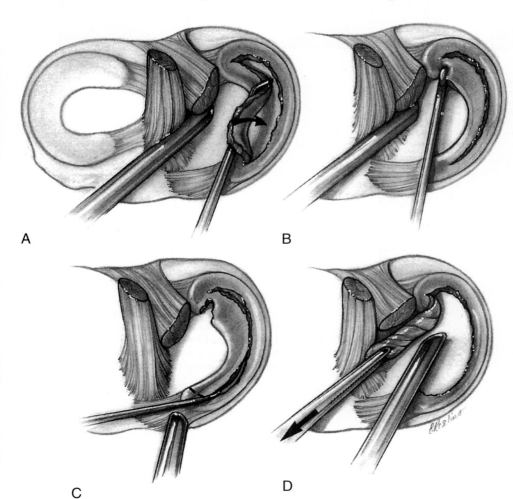

Figure 50–6 Principles of meniscectomy for bucket handle tear. The displaced fragment is reduced into its normal position with a probe. The posterior attachment is nearly transected under direct vision using a meniscal biter. The anterior attachment is transected using meniscal biters or knife. The fragment is grasped in line with the bulk of the meniscus, avulsed (rotating the meniscus may help) from its remaining posterior attachment, and removed. (From Scott N: The Knee. St. Louis, Mosby Year Book, 1994.)

A

B

C

D

6 Knee

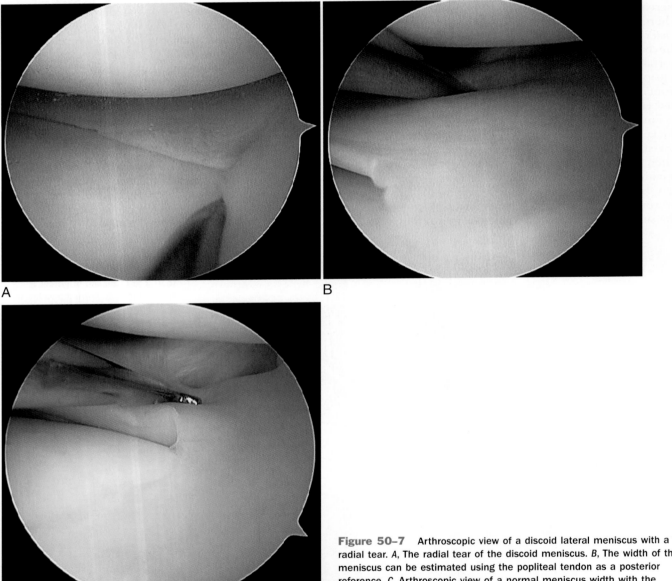

A

B

C

Figure 50–7   Arthroscopic view of a discoid lateral meniscus with a radial tear. *A*, The radial tear of the discoid meniscus. *B*, The width of the meniscus can be estimated using the popliteal tendon as a posterior reference. *C*, Arthroscopic view of a normal meniscus width with the popliteal tendon posteriorly for comparison with *B*.

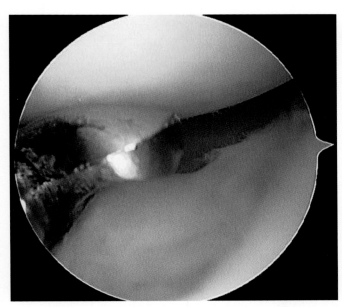

Figure 50–8 Arthroscopic partial meniscectomy of a discoid lateral meniscus using meniscal biters.

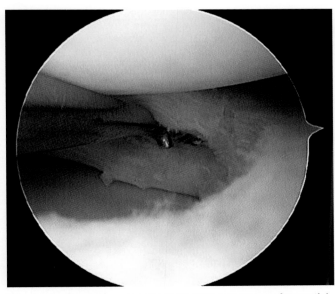

Figure 50–9 Appearance of discoid lateral meniscus after partial meniscectomy. A horizontal tear was seen after removal of the radial tear. This was debrided to a stable edge.

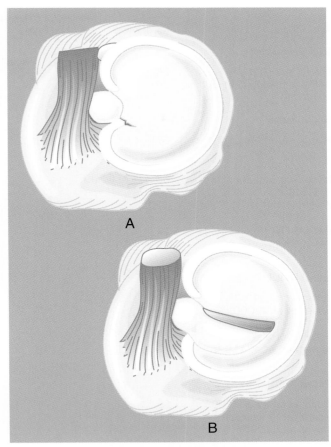

Figure 50–10 Schematic representation of the approach to the discoid meniscus. *A*, The tear, usually a radial tear, is continued radially until it is approximately 1 cm from the peripheral margin. *B*, The meniscus is cut anteriorly, contouring a more normal-sized meniscus. The meniscus is trimmed posteriorly to normal size. (From Scott N: The Knee. St. Louis, Mosby Year Book, 1994.)

The Role of Lasers

The role of lasers in arthroscopic meniscectomy is still controversial. Although some authors have found lasers to be beneficial in the treatment of chondromalacia and synovitis, no one has demonstrated a significant difference in global clinical results between laser and conventional debridement.[32,36] In addition, a number of recent published reports have implicated the use of lasers in the occurrence of postoperative chondrolysis and osteonecrosis.[21] These findings, in concert with the high cost of laser instrumentation, is why the senior author does not use the laser for routine arthroscopic meniscectomy.

Postoperative Management

The goal is to decrease inflammation, restore motion, increase strength, and facilitate a safe return to competition.[35] This begins with a phased program with set goals, with an emphasis on preventing reinjury.

portion of the meniscus with meniscal biters of varying angles can be difficult to perform initially due to visualization problems. The removal is most easily performed in a piecemeal fashion. The key is to leave a rim about the width of a normal meniscus (Fig. 50–10). This remaining rim has a thick edge that transforms over time to a more normal appearance (see Figs. 50–7 through 50–9). Care should be taken, as there may be more than one tear in a discoid meniscus.

6 Knee

Table 50–1
Results of Meniscectomy

Author (Date)	No. of Knees	Average Age (yr)	Follow-up (yr)	Results	Radiographic Changes	Comment
Total Meniscectomy						
Dai et al. (1995)[11]	60		10-30	58.3% g-e	87.5%	All totals
Andersson-Molina et al. (2002)[2]	36		14	70% normal	33% partial; 70% total	
Medial Partial						
Higuchi et al. (2000)[14]	67		12.2	79% satisfied	48%	Increased OA with medial and large resection
Matsusue and Thomas (1996)[22]	68	49.7	7.8	87% excellent (no OA)		Medial
Kruger-Franke et al. (1999)[18,19]	100		7	96% g-e	33%	Medial; increased OA in women
Biedert (1993)[5]	11	30.4	2.2	100% normal		Medial; randomized (75% normal in control)
Lateral Partial						
Yocum et al. (1979)[37]	26			54% satisfied		
Hoser et al. (2000)[15]	31		10.3	58% g-e	97%	Lateral; 29% reoperation
Scheller et al. (2001)[28]	75		12.3	77% g-e	84%	Lateral
Jaureguito et al. (1995)[17]	27		8	92% g-e	No change	Lateral; 48% at preinjury level
Discoid Partial						
Washington et al. (1995)[34]	15	10.5	17	87% g-e	0%	
Aglietti et al. (1991)[1]	17	13.6	10	94% g-e	65%	
Atay et al. (1997)[3]	14	12.8	2.7	100% g-e		
ACL Deficient						
Kwiatkowski (1995)[20]	107		3	62% g-e		ACL deficient
Neyret et al. (1993)[23]	195		20	92%/74% satisfied		6%/38% reoperation; ACL intact/deficient
Umar (1997)[33]	139/49			93%/75% g-e		ACL intact/deficient
Hazel et al. (1993)[13]	63		4.5	84% improved	65%	ACL deficient
OA as a Factor						
Crevoisier et al. (2001)[10]	95	74	4	81% satisfied (no OA) 55% satisfied (OA)		
Barrett et al. (1998)[4]	36	64.9	3	94% improved (no OA) 80% improved (OA)		
Results Decline						
Schimmer et al. (1998)[29]	119		4/12	91.7%/78.1% g-e		
Medial-Lateral Mixed						
Rangger et al. (1995)[27]	284		4.6		38% medial, 24% lateral	
Burks et al. (1997)[8]	146		14.7	88% g-e		Mixed—no difference; increased OA in females
Bonamo et al. (1992)[7]	118	57	3.3	83% satisfied		
Chatain et al. (2001)[9]	317	38 ± 11	11.5	91% normal	40.3%	
Desai and Ackroyd (2000)[12]	43		6	50% satisfied		
Hulet et al. (2001)[16]	74 (in 54 patients)	36	12	95% satisfied	22.4%	
Osti et al. (1994)[25]	41	26	3	85% g-e		98% returned to sports in 55 days; worse with OCD
Raber et al. (1998)[26]	17		19.8	76% normal	59%	

ACL, anterior cruciate ligament; g-e, good to excellent; OA, osteoarthritis; OCD, osteochondritis dissecans.

- No brace or range-of-motion restrictions.
- Immediate full weight bearing with crutches as needed to prevent low back pain and compensatory injuries associated with limping.
- Icing of the knee for 20 minutes every 2 to 3 hours while awake.
- Begin a nonsteroidal anti-inflammatory drug at 2 weeks if no contraindications.
- Active, passive, and active assisted range of motion immediately postoperatively.
- Straight leg raise exercises immediately.
- Return to sports when full range of motion, no effusion, and strength at 80% of uninjured side (usually 4 to 6 weeks).

Results

Although open total meniscectomy was once the standard of care for meniscal injuries, several long-term follow-up studies have shown that these patients have poor outcomes and are significantly more likely to develop arthritic changes in the operated knee. Northmore-Ball et al.[24] compared open total meniscectomy with arthroscopic partial meniscectomy and found that leaving some of the meniscus behind led to significantly improved results (90% versus 68% good to excellent results). Andersson-Molina et al.[2] went further and compared arthroscopic total and partial meniscectomy and demonstrated improved outcomes with partial excision.

Most researchers investigating meniscectomy have looked at both functional outcomes and radiographic findings of osteoarthritis to evaluate the effect of meniscectomy on patients. Although many authors have shown that even partial meniscectomy can lead to an increased incidence of arthritis, these findings have generally not correlated with clinical outcomes.

Clinical outcomes after lateral partial meniscectomy (54% to 92% good to excellent results) have generally been worse than those for medial partial meniscectomy (79% to 100% good to excellent results). Rangger et al.[27] found an increased incidence of osteoarthritis following medial partial meniscectomy compared with lateral; however, this did not correlate with clinical outcomes. Several other authors have also found increased degenerative changes following medial meniscectomy compared with lateral.[14,18,19]

Partial meniscectomy for discoid meniscus in children has generally been successful, with 87% to 100% good to excellent results. There have been varying reports of degenerative changes in these patients. Washington et al.[34] found no evidence of degeneration at 17 years, whereas Aglietti et al.[1] found a 65% incidence of some radiographic changes at 10 years' follow-up.

Schimmer et al.[29] reported a decline in patient outcomes over time, with good to excellent results dropping from 91.7% at 4 years to 78.1% at 12 years. These findings are supported by the work of other authors who have followed their patients beyond 10 years.[1-3,8,9,14-16,28,34] There have been some reports, however, of continued high rates of good to excellent results with follow-up as long as 20 years.[11,23] Two factors that predict a worse result following partial meniscectomy are preexisting osteoarthritis (55% to 80% good to excellent) and ACL deficiency (62% to 84% good to excellent).

Published results are summarized in Table 50-1.

Complications

Early studies of the initial experience with arthroscopic fluid pumps reported complication rates as high as 1.4% from fluid extravasation during knee arthroscopy.[6] Fortunately, with improved instrumentation and techniques, these types of complications are rare. Other complications that have been reported and should be discussed with the patient preoperatively include deep vein thrombosis with or without pulmonary embolism, recurrent effusions, incomplete removal of tear, synovial-cutaneous fistula, iatrogenic arthroscopic joint lesions, osteonecrosis in the elderly, arteriovenous fistula, and popliteal pseudoaneurysm.[31]

References

1. Aglietti P, Bertini FA, Buzzi R, Beraldi R: Arthroscopic meniscectomy for discoid lateral meniscus in children and adolescents: 10-year follow-up. Am J Knee Surg 12:83-87, 1999.
2. Andersson-Molina H, Karlsson H, Rockborn P: Arthroscopic partial and total meniscectomy: A long-term follow-up study with matched controls. Arthroscopy 18:183-189, 2002.
3. Atay OA, Doral MN, Aksoy MC, et al: Arthroscopic partial resection of the discoid meniscus in children. Turk J Pediatr 39:505-510, 1997.
4. Barrett GR, Treacy SH, Ruff CG: The effect of partial lateral meniscectomy in patients >60 years. Orthopedics 21:251-257, 1998.
5. Biedert RM: Intrasubstance meniscal tears: Clinical aspects and the role of MRI. Arch Orthop Trauma Surg 112:142-147, 1993.
6. Bomberg BC, Hurley PE, Clark CA, McLaughlin CS: Complications associated with the use of an infusion pump during knee arthroscopy. Arthroscopy 8:224-228, 1992.
7. Bonamo JJ, Kessler KJ, Noah J: Arthroscopic meniscectomy in patients over the age of 40. Am J Sports Med 20:422-429, 1992.
8. Burks RT, Metcalf MH, Metcalf RW: Fifteen-year follow-up of arthroscopic partial meniscectomy. Arthroscopy 13:673-679, 1997.
9. Chatain F, Robinson AH, Adeleine P, et al: The natural history of the knee following arthroscopic medial meniscectomy. Knee Surg Sports Traumatol Arthrosc 9:15-18, 2001.
10. Crevoisier X, Munzinger U, Drobny T: Arthroscopic partial meniscectomy in patients over 70 years of age. Arthroscopy 17:732-736, 2001.
11. Dai L, Zhang W, Zhou Z, Xu Y: Long-term results after meniscectomy in 60 patients. Chin Med J (Engl) 108:591-594, 1995.
12. Desai VV, Ackroyd CE: Resection of degenerate menisci—is it useful? Knee 7:179-182, 2000.

13. Hazel WA Jr, Rand JA, Morrey BF: Results of meniscectomy in the knee with anterior cruciate ligament deficiency. Clin Orthop 292:232-238, 1993.

14. Higuchi H, Kimura M, Shirakura K, et al: Factors affecting long-term results after arthroscopic partial meniscectomy. Clin Orthop 377:161-168, 2000.

15. Hoser C, Fink C, Brown C, et al: Long-term results of arthroscopic partial lateral meniscectomy in knees without associated damage. J Bone Joint Surg Br 83:513-516, 2001.

16. Hulet CH, Locker BG, Schiltz D, et al: Arthroscopic medial meniscectomy on stable knees. J Bone Joint Surg Br 83:29-32, 2001.

17. Jaureguito JW, Elliot JS, Lietner T, et al: The effects of arthroscopic partial lateral meniscectomy in an otherwise normal knee: A retrospective review of functional, clinical, and radiographic results. Arthroscopy 11:29-36, 1995.

18. Kruger-Franke M, Kugler A, Trouillier HH, et al: Clinical and radiological results after arthroscopic partial medial meniscectomy: Are there risk factors? Unfallchirurg 102:434-438, 1999.

19. Kruger-Franke M, Siebert CH, Kugler A, et al: Late results after arthroscopic partial medial meniscectomy. Knee Surg Sports Traumatol Arthrosc 7:81-84, 1999.

20. Kwiatkowski K: Arthroscopic meniscectomy in anterior cruciate ligament deficient knees. Chir Narzadow Ruchu Ortop Pol 60:205-209, 1995.

21. Lubbers C, Siebert WE: Holmium:YAG-laser-assisted arthroscopy versus conventional methods for treatment of the knee: Two-year results of a prospective study. Knee Surg Sports Traumatol Arthrosc 5:168-175, 1997

22. Matsusue Y, Thomson NL: Arthroscopic partial medial meniscectomy in patients over 40 years old: A 5- to 11-year follow-up study. Arthroscopy 12:39-44, 1996.

23. Neyret P, Donell ST, Dejour H: Results of partial meniscectomy related to the state of the anterior cruciate ligament: Review at 20 to 35 years, J Bone Joint Surg Br 75:36-40, 1993.

24. Northmore-Ball MD, Dandy DJ, Jackson RW: Arthroscopic, open partial, and total meniscectomy: A comparative study. J Bone Joint Surg Br 65:400-404, 1983.

25. Osti L, Liu SH, Raskin A, et al: Partial lateral meniscectomy in athletes. Arthroscopy 10:424-430, 1994.

26. Raber DA, Friederich NF, Hefti F: Discoid lateral meniscus in children: Long-term follow-up after total meniscectomy. J Bone Joint Surg Am 80:1579-1586, 1998.

27. Rangger C, Klestil T, Gloetzer W, et al: Osteoarthritis after arthroscopic partial meniscectomy. Am J Sports Med 23:240-244, 1995.

28. Scheller G, Sobau C, Bulow JU: Arthroscopic partial lateral meniscectomy in an otherwise normal knee: Clinical, functional, and radiographic results of a long-term follow-up study. Arthroscopy 17:946-952, 2001.

29. Schimmer RC, Brulhart KB, Duff C, Glinz W: Arthroscopic partial meniscectomy: A 12-year follow-up and two-step evaluation of the long-term course. Arthroscopy 14:136-142, 1998.

30. Shapiro MS, Safran MR, Crockett HR, Finerman GAM: Local anesthesia for knee arthroscopy: Efficacy and cost containment. Am J Sports Med 23:50-53, 1995.

31. Small NC: Complications in arthroscopic surgery of the knee and shoulder. Orthopaedics 16:985-988, 1993.

32. Thal R, Danziger MB, Kelly A: Delayed articular cartilage slough: Two cases resulting from holmium:YAG laser damage to normal articular cartilage and a review of the literature. Arthroscopy 12:92-94, 1996.

33. Umar M: Ambulatory arthroscopy knee surgery results of partial meniscectomy. J Pak Med Assoc 47:210-213, 1997.

34. Washington ER 3rd, Root L, Liener UC: Discoid lateral meniscus in children: Long-term follow-up after excision. J Bone Joint Surg Am 77:1357-1361, 1995.

35. Wheatley WB, Krome J, Martin DF: Rehabilitation programmes following arthroscopic meniscectomy in athletes. Sports Med 21:447-456, 1996.

36. Yakin DE, Rogers VP: Conventional instrument vs laser-assisted arthroscopic meniscectomy. Lasers Surg Med 25:435-437, 1999.

37. Yocum LA, Kerlan RK, Jobe FW, et al: Isolated lateral meniscectomy: A study of twenty-six patients with isolated tears. J Bone Joint Surg Am 61:338-342, 1979.

51

Arthroscopic Meniscus Repair

Akbar Nawab, Peter W. Hester,
and David N. M. Caborn

ARTHROSCOPIC MENISCUS REPAIR IN A NUTSHELL

History:
Twisting injury, pain, ± associated anterior cruciate ligament tear

Physical Examination:
Joint line tenderness; McMurray test; rule out locked knee

Imaging:
Radiographs normal; magnetic resonance imaging shows peripheral meniscal tear

Indications:
Symptomatic tear ± concurrent anterior cruciate ligament tear

Surgical Technique:
Device specific
Reduce tear; assess repairability; rasp tear and periphery; pass suture, cannula, and device; repeat at 3- to 5-mm intervals; tension and secure fixation

Postoperative Management:
Flexion limited to less than 90 degrees for 3 to 6 weeks; partial weight bearing for 3 to 6 weeks; no running for 3 months

Results:
Suture: 75% to 90% good to excellent results
T-Fix: 88% success
Arrow: 85% good to excellent results

The essential and complex biomechanical functions of the meniscus make this small structure an integral component of the knee. Based on the substantial literature stressing its preservation, especially for articular cartilage integrity, it is best to attempt meniscal repair rather than debridement, whenever possible. The optimal repair technique affords adequate stability; is performed relatively easily; allows anatomic reapproximation; is non-traumatic to the meniscus, cartilage, and neurovascular structures; is easily removable; and uses low-profile or absorbable materials.

This chapter reviews arthroscopic repair methods, including the Meniscal Arrow (Bionx Implants Inc., Bluebell, PA), inside-out suture repair, outside-in suture repair, meniscal repair enhancement, and all-inside repair.

Meniscal Arrow

Case History

A 25-year-old man sustained a twisting injury to his right knee. He reported joint line tenderness and giving way when pivoting.

Physical Examination

On physical examination, effusion was present. Range of motion was 0 to 110 degrees. The McMurray test was positive. Medial joint line tenderness was noted, and the ligaments were stable.

Imaging

Radiographs were normal. Grade III signal change in the posterior horn of the medial meniscus was demonstrated on gadolinium-enhanced magnetic resonance imaging (MRI).

Indications

The Meniscal Arrow is indicated for vertical, longitudinal, and bucket handle tears in the vascular zone of the meniscus. In a young, active patient with a large meniscal tear, the approach should emphasize repair of the medial meniscus.

Surgical Technique

Positioning

The operative extremity is placed in the arthroscopic leg holder with a padded tourniquet around the proximal thigh and the nonoperative leg in the well-leg holder.

Examination under Anesthesia

In this patient, the examination under anesthesia did not demonstrate any ligamentous compromise.

Diagnostic Arthroscopy

Diagnostic arthroscopy demonstrated a 15-mm longitudinal, full-thickness, unstable posterior horn medial meniscal tear located in the peripheral third.

Device and Instrumentation

The Meniscal Arrow is available in 10 mm for the middle third of the medial meniscus, 13 mm for the posterior horn of the medial meniscus and the middle third of the lateral meniscus, and 16 mm for the posterior horn of the lateral meniscus. The Arrows are made of a self-reinforced copolymer (96% poly-L-, 4% poly-D-lactic acid) that provides an ultra-high-strength microstructure. The instrument set consists of six zone-specific cannulas, obturator, needle, perforator, pusher, and hammer.[15]

Specific Surgical Steps

With the meniscal tear well visualized, the zone-specific cannula is aligned perpendicular to the meniscal surface, reducing the tear. The obturator is removed, and the perforator is placed through the cannula across the reduced meniscus. The perforator is removed, and the implant is loaded into the cannula. The inflow should be turned off before insertion of the implant to avoid ejecting the Arrow out the back end of the cannula. The deployment rod is fully depressed, passing the Arrow across the tear site. Complete seating of the device head is imperative (Fig. 51–1). Implants should be spaced 3 to 4 mm apart.

Pearls and Pitfalls

Reducing a tear can be accomplished using the cannula or a probe introduced simultaneously through the same portal.

Selecting the appropriate implant length is critical. Palpating the meniscal perforator under the skin and measuring how far it has advanced may allow one to downsize the implant length before insertion. The 16-mm implant should be used with caution, as vital structures are at risk, especially with posterior horn repairs.

A hybrid repair may be the best indication for Arrow use. The Arrow can be utilized to hold an unstable tear reduced, to allow arthroscopic suture repair.

Some of the cannulas have a dual barrel for the implant and for a guidewire, which can be inserted across the meniscus to prevent cannula migration. It is best to leave the perforator or guidewire across the meniscus until the implant is ready to be deployed. Holding the cannula firmly when removing the perforator and advancing the implant prevents the implant from missing the meniscotomy and slipping over the surface of the meniscus, resulting in the implant being either lost or driven into the capsule.

Results

Hurel et al.[10] reported the 1-year follow-up results for 26 repairs using the Biofix Meniscal Arrow. Eight of these patients also had concomitant anterior cruciate ligament (ACL) reconstruction. Of the 26 patients, 22 achieved excellent or good outcomes based on the Modified Marshall Knee Score.

Complications

Femoral condyle articular cartilage damage in the form of "troughing" has been reported.[1,25] To prevent this problem, the head of the device must be buried in the substance of the meniscus. Coloring the head of the implant with a marker can help one visualize the seated

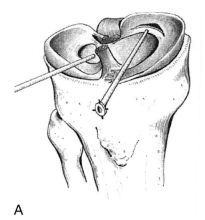

A

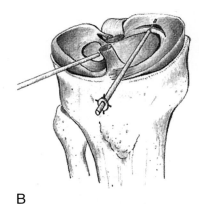

B

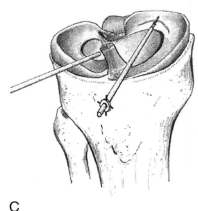

C

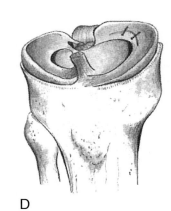

D

Figure 51–1   *A*, Cannula delivery. *B*, Perforator placed across tear. *C*, Arrow delivery across tear with pusher or obturator. *D*, Reduced tear. (Illustration by Robin Nyland.)

6 Knee

position. This complication can be avoided with lower-profile implants such as the Arthrex Dart.

Menche et al.[14] first described a local reactive synovitis, a histiocytic and giant cell inflammatory response, to degradation of the crystalline poly-L-lactic acid 6 months after implantation. At follow-up arthroscopy, the meniscal tear was not healed.

The Arrow has been found as a subcutaneous foreign body, with fracture at the shaft-barb juncture, between 1 and 10 months postoperatively.[21,25] If the Arrow is placed too centrally, a difference in implant absorption is created between the vascular and avascular zone, which may result in implant fracture.[15]

Up to 30% of patients report pain for 4 to 6 months after repair. In Whitman and Diduch's[32] patients, the pain abated by 6 months, corresponding to anticipated partial resorption. They believed that the tip of the Arrow may stretch or penetrate the joint capsule, irritating posterior structures.

Kurzweil and Friedman[12] described a complication rate of 50% due to implant fracture from early weight bearing and aggressive rehabilitation. This rate decreased to 16% when patients were kept non–weight bearing for 4 weeks. They also found this implant more difficult to work with than those that were driven over a guidewire, such as the lower-profile BioStinger

(Linvatec, Largo, FL), which also has a better pullout strength.

Inside-Out Suture

Case History

While playing basketball, a 12-year-old boy twisted his knee when landing after a jump. He had an immediate large effusion and was unable to extend his knee.

Physical Examination

On physical examination, a 3+ effusion was present. Range of motion was 30 to 70 degrees. There was medial joint line tenderness. Both the McMurray test and ligament examination were guarded.

Imaging

Radiographs of the right knee were negative. MRI with gadolinium revealed a bucket handle tear displaced into the intercondylar notch.

Indications

Large bucket handle tears, long vertical and longitudinal tears, are well suited for inside-out repair. The patient was taken to the operating room expeditiously to avoid extension or amputation of the tear.

Surgical Technique

Positioning

The operative extremity is placed in the arthroscopic leg holder with a padded tourniquet around the proximal thigh and the nonoperative leg in the well-leg holder.

Examination under Anesthesia

The knee is examined gently, avoiding testing maneuvers that might injure the displaced bucket handle component. In this patient, range of motion still demonstrated an extension block at 20 degrees.

Diagnostic Arthroscopy

The displaced bucket handle is reduced by levering a blunt trocar on the displaced fragment as the knee is brought from flexion into extension with simultaneous valgus loading and external rotation.

Device and Instrumentation

Inside-out repair requires a double-loaded 2-0 PDS or Ticron suture on long Keith needles. Zone-specific cannulas are necessary to accommodate the posterior, middle, and anterior portions of the medial and lateral menisci. The surgeon, controlling the cannula, manually advances the needle with a needle driver. The Sharp-shooter (Linvatec, Largo, FL) has a single-hand dual function, allowing the surgeon to position the zone-specific cannula and advance the needle with a ratcheting trigger. A long retractor is necessary to allow visualization posteriorly, safeguarding against neurovascular injury from stray needle passage.

Specific Surgical Steps

Inside-out repair requires an incision to allow for needle capture, knot tying, and neurovascular structure identification and protection.

MEDIAL EXPOSURE

A longitudinal incision is made in the interval of the tibial collateral ligament and posterior oblique ligament. The sartorius fascia is identified, along with the infrapatellar branches of the saphenous nerve (Fig. 51–2). An incision is made in the sartorius fascia. A spoon, pediatric speculum, or other retracting device is placed posteriorly, deep to the sartorius fascia (Figs. 51–3 and 51–4).

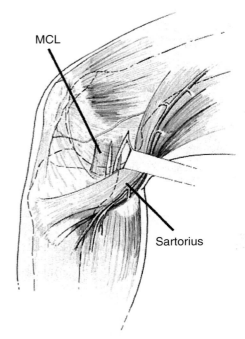

Figure 51–2   Medial incision. MCL, medial collateral ligament.

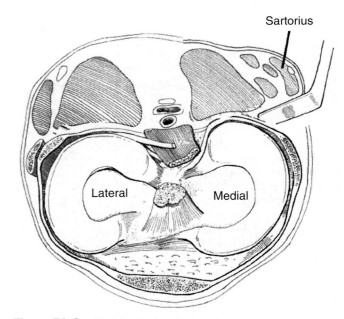

Figure 51–3   Medial retractor placement.

LATERAL EXPOSURE

A longitudinal incision is made anterior to the fibular collateral ligament (Fig. 51–5). The interval between the iliotibial band and biceps tendon is developed. Deep to this interval is the collateral ligament and the lateral inferior geniculate artery passing deep and medial to the ligament. Retraction of the biceps exposes the lateral head of the gastrocnemius (Fig. 51–6). Gastrocnemius retraction provides access to the posterolateral capsule

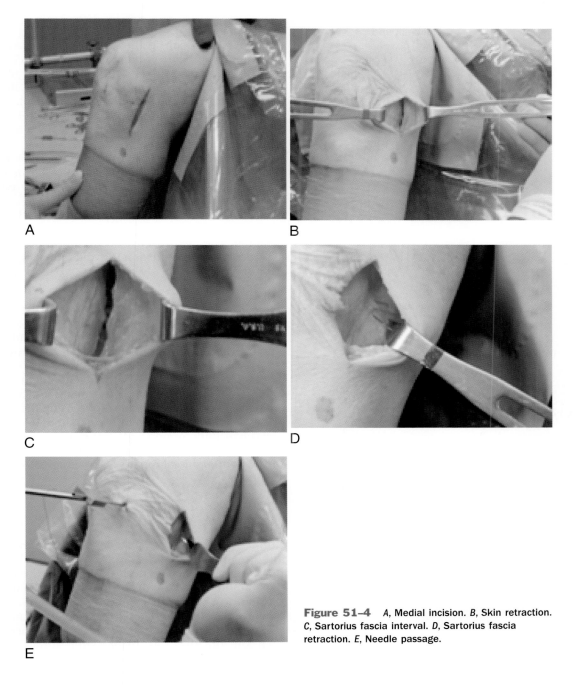

Figure 51–4   *A*, Medial incision. *B*, Skin retraction.
C, Sartorius fascia interval. *D*, Sartorius fascia
retraction. *E*, Needle passage.

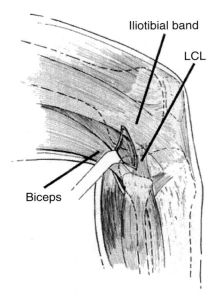

Figure 51–5   Lateral incision. LCL, lateral collateral ligament.

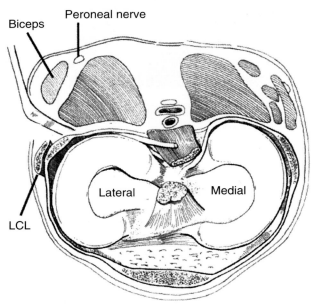

Figure 51–6   Lateral retractor placement. LCL, lateral collateral ligament.

and safeguards the peroneal nerve against injury (Fig. 51–7).

The smaller, single-barrel cannulas are preferred over the double-barrel ones for easier maneuvering. The cannulas are usually best introduced through the contralateral portal but may be passed through the ipsilateral one if this provides better orientation to the tear. The double-armed long meniscal repair needles are advanced within 5 mm of one another (Fig. 51–8). During needle advancement, attention to the position of the knee is important to avoid neurovascular injury. When working laterally, flexion to 90 degrees allows the peroneal nerve to move posteriorly.

Pearls and Pitfalls

Adequate exposure is the key to inside-out repair. Take the time to provide good visualization posteriorly.

Sutures can be passed on the femoral or tibial side of the meniscus. Once the needle has passed through the capsule, its course may be difficult to control, particularly in posterior third repairs. One must reevaluate the course of the needle if the tip is not seen after advancing 15 mm.

Laterally, one must be particularly wary of the peroneal nerve, popliteus, and lateral inferior geniculate artery. Knee flexion of 90 degrees helps move these structures posteriorly.

Medially, one must identify the infrapatellar branch of the saphenous nerve to avoid injury and neuroma formation. The medial side is secured with the knee held in 20 to 30 degrees of flexion to avoid tethering the capsule, limiting extension.

Results

Rosenberg et al.[24] repaired 29 menisci and examined them arthroscopically 3 months later. Twenty-four had healed fully. Four of the five partially healed tears occurred in unstable ACL-deficient knees. They were able to access all areas of the meniscus. Stone et al.[26] reported good to excellent results, using the Hospital for Special Surgery knee rating system, in 81% of 31 patients who had undergone inside-out repair an average of 4.1 years earlier. Miller[16] showed a 91% success rate in 96 inside-out meniscal repairs followed up an average of 39 months.

Complications

Injury to the infrapatellar branch of the saphenous nerve and the peroneal nerve has been reported.[4] Inadvertent passing of the needle posteriorly places the neurovascular bundle at risk. With flexion, the meniscus translates posteriorly, and with extension, the meniscus resumes its anterior station. Therefore, tying the knot down in flexion greater than 90 degrees may place excessive tension on the soft tissues and subsequently limit extension.

Outside-In Suture

Case History

A 23-year-old volleyball player twisted her knee upon landing from a jump.

Physical Examination

On physical examination, a 2+ effusion was present. Range of motion was 5 to 110 degrees. The McMurray test was positive. There was medial joint line tenderness, and the ligaments were stable.

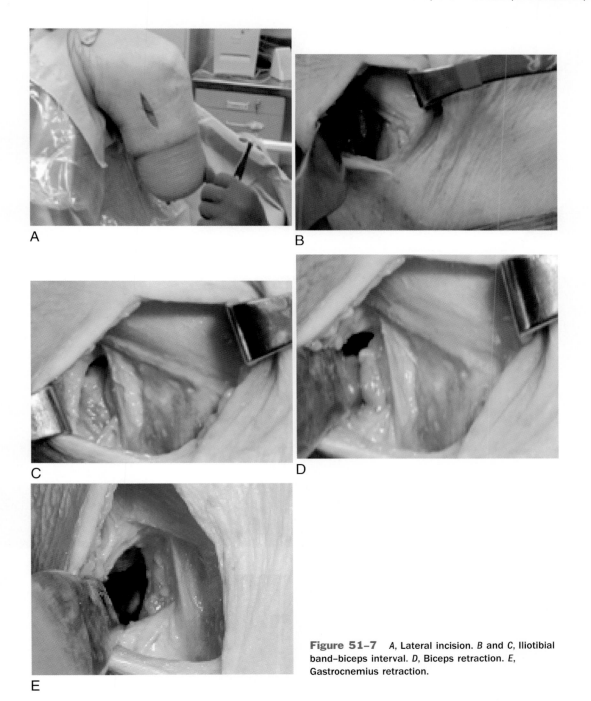

Figure 51–7   *A*, Lateral incision. *B* and *C*, Iliotibial band–biceps interval. *D*, Biceps retraction. *E*, Gastrocnemius retraction.

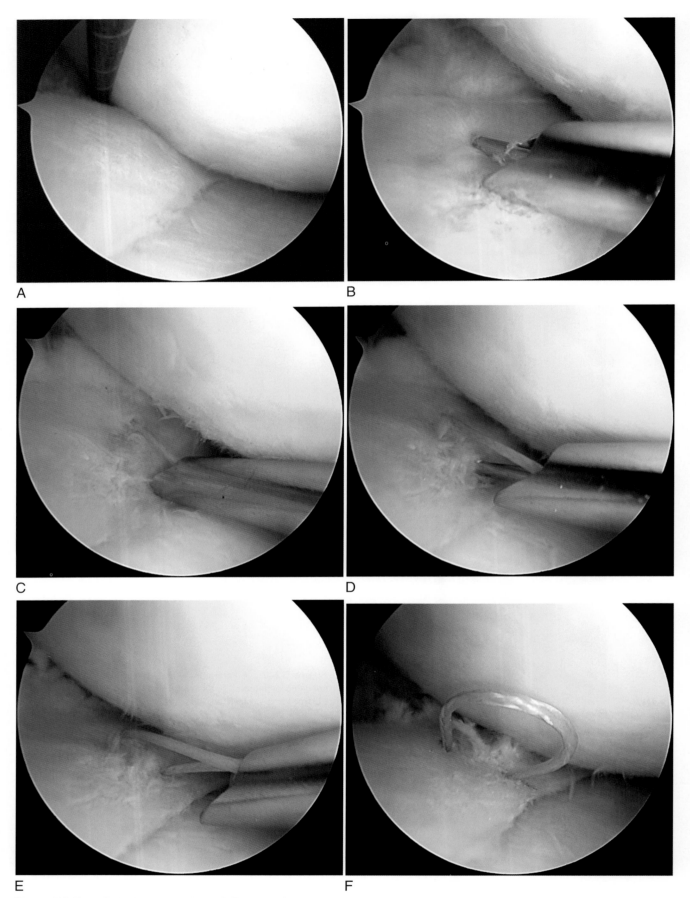

Figure 51–8   *A*, Probe in peripheral tear. *B*, Zone-specific cannula reducing tear, with first needle penetrating meniscus. *C*, Cannula in position for second needle. *D*, Needle delivery. *E* and *F*, Suture passage.

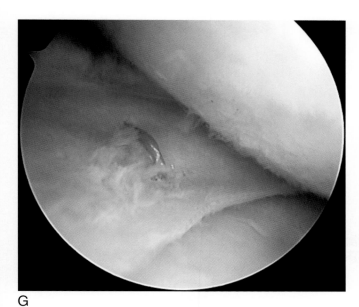

G

Figure 51–8, cont'd. *G*, Knot tied with proper tension, and reduced tear.

Imaging

Plain films of the right knee were negative. MRI with gadolinium demonstrated a grade III signal of the central third of the medial meniscus.

Indications

An isolated full-thickness, longitudinal, nondisplaced tear in an active 23-year-old demands an attempt at repair. The outside-in technique is recommended for tears of the anterior third and middle third of the meniscus and for radial tears.

Surgical Technique

Positioning

The operative extremity is placed in the arthroscopic leg holder with a padded tourniquet about the proximal thigh and the nonoperative leg in the well-leg holder.

Examination under Anesthesia

The examination under anesthesia demonstrated a mild effusion, with near full range of motion.

Diagnostic Arthroscopy

The nondisplaced medial meniscal tear was in the central third, approximately 20 mm long, and unstable with probing.

Device and Instrumentation

This technique requires basic instrumentation consisting of three 18-gauge, 1.5-inch spinal needles; 2-0 PDS suture

or a wire loop; and an arthroscopic grasper or small hemostat.

Specific Surgical Steps

Placing a vertical or horizontal outside-in suture requires two cannulas (spinal needles). Cannula 1, threaded with a 2-0 PDS suture (suture 1), is passed through the skin, across the meniscal tear, and into the medial or lateral compartment (Fig. 51–9). A horizontal 3- to 4-mm skin incision is made adjacent to the cannula and spread down to the capsule using a hemostat. The skin incision should be made before withdrawing the needle to avoid cutting the suture. Through this same incision and anterior to cannula 1, cannula 2, threaded with a looped 2-0 PDS suture (suture 2), is passed across the meniscal tear in an appropriate orientation and location relative to cannula 1 (see Fig. 51–9).

A grasping device is advanced through the ipsilateral anterior portal, passes through the loop of suture 2, and grasps the free end of suture 1. After cannula 1 is pulled back, the forceps pulls the free end of suture 1 out the anterior portal. It is important to retrieve cannula 1 before pulling suture 1 to avoid cutting the suture. The suture 2 loop and cannula 2 are then pulled back out, bringing with them the free end of suture 1 (Figs. 51–9 and 51–10). Knot tying advances from posterior to anterior.

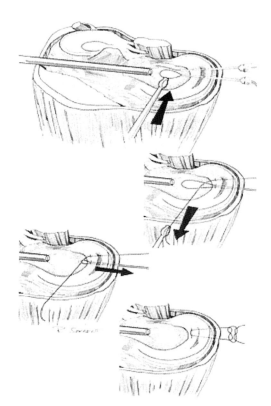

Figure 51–9 Diagram of outside-in technique. (Illustrations by Rick Sergeant.)

6 Knee

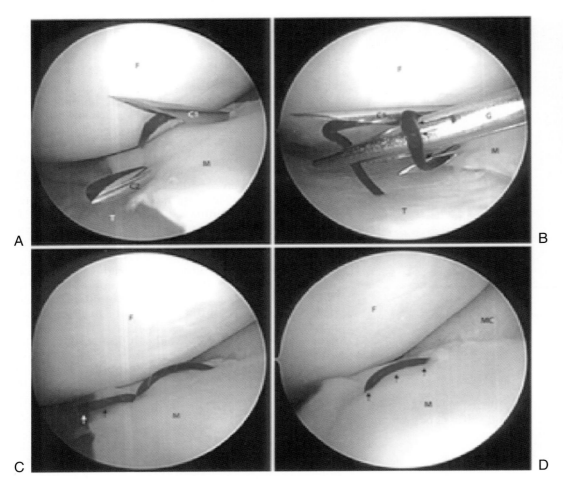

Figure 51-10
Arthroscopic view of outside-in technique.
A, **Passage of needles.**
B, **Retrieval of suture.**
C and *D,* **Reduced tear and knot tied.** (From Strobel MJ: Meniscus treatment. In Strobel MJ [ed]: Manual of Arthroscopic Surgery. Strabing, Germany, Springer-Verlag, 2001, p. 139.)

Pearls and Pitfalls

Load the needle with both ends of the suture through the sharp end of the needle, creating a loop through which a grasper can fit. Preparing the needle by passing the suture from the sharp end is easier than passing it through the cap end.

Palpation and transillumination provide adequate localization for the needle entry site. Place the looped suture needle (cannula 2) *anterior* to the cannula 1 meniscal repair suture to allow for easier suture capture, rather than having to backtrack through a posteriorly positioned loop. Counterpressure on the meniscus with a probe or a blunt trocar through the anteromedial portal may assist with needle advancement.

Tears located far posteriorly may make suture placement perpendicular to the tear difficult. This often yields obliquely oriented sutures that provide less coaptation force across the tear. Alternating sutures between the femoral and tibial surfaces more evenly coapts the meniscus to the capsule.[19,29]

Medially, the saphenous nerve and infrapatellar branch pass anterior to the semitendinosus when the knee is extended. Use the light source to transilluminate these structures, extend the knee, and start the needle entry point posterior to the semitendinosus tendon. Posterior sutures are secured in extension, which reduces the posterior horn to the capsule and prevents flexion contractures by avoiding entrapment of the posterior capsule.

Avoiding peroneal nerve injury is the primary focus of lateral meniscal repair with this or any other technique. Flexing the knee to 90 degrees allows the nerve to translate posteriorly. Keeping the needles anterior to the biceps further ensures safe needle passage. The lateral inferior geniculate artery is also vulnerable as it courses along the joint line and between the popliteus and fibular collateral ligament.

Anterior horn tears are best approached with the knee in 50 to 60 degrees of flexion and the needle placed anterior to the pes tendons and saphenous branches. A cannula should be used to avoid the sutures becoming tangled in soft tissue.

Results

Morgan et al.,[17] by way of second-look arthroscopy in 74 repairs, reported 84% healing, with 65% complete and 19% partial. Eleven of the 12 failures were of medial posterior horn tears. Mariani et al.[13] reported good clinical results in 17 of 22 repairs performed along with ACL reconstruction. Among Warren's[31] 90 patients, 87% had good outcomes. Of the 38 knees undergoing concomitant ACL reconstruction, only two meniscal repairs failed. Eleven of 72 medial repairs failed, compared with only 1 of 18 lateral repairs.

Complications

One must watch the needle as it presents just below the meniscal surface in an effort to avoid multiple perforations and risk further injury to both the meniscus and the articular cartilage.

The incision for this procedure, being only 4 to 6 mm, does not allow good visualization; however, one needs to clear the capsule of all soft tissue interposed, especially any branches of the saphenous nerve to avoid neuroma formation. Proper knee position and needle placement are critical for avoiding neurovascular injury.

Van Trommel et al.[29] used second-look arthroscopy, arthrography, MRI, or a combination of these techniques to follow 51 patients who underwent outside-in meniscal repair. Of the patients with partial or no healing, 62% had meniscal injuries located in the middle to posterior third of the medial meniscus. These results emphasize the difficulty of achieving suture placement perpendicular to the meniscal tear and with maximal coaptive force in the posterior horn of the medial meniscus.

Enhancement Techniques

Case History

Ten months after ACL allograft reconstruction and partial medial meniscectomy, a 41-year-old man noted a pop and instability while doing rotatory exercises in therapy.

Physical Examination

On physical examination, a 2+ effusion was present. Range of motion was 0 to 120 degrees. There was medial and lateral joint line tenderness. Both McMurray and Lachman tests were positive.

Imaging

Gadolinium MRI showed a signal change in the femoral insertion of the ACL and postoperative changes in the medial meniscus.

Indications

With a recent history of trauma and an examination consistent with ACL disruption, the treatment plan called for repeat arthroscopy and possible reconstruction.

Surgical Technique

Positioning

The operative extremity is placed in the arthroscopic leg holder with a tourniquet about the proximal thigh and the nonoperative leg in the well-leg holder.

Examination under Anesthesia

The examination under anesthesia demonstrated straight anterior instability with a mild effusion.

Diagnostic Arthroscopy

Inspection of the notch confirmed a torn allograft on the femoral side. The lateral compartment demonstrated a partial posterior horn tear of the lateral meniscus.

Specific Surgical Steps

DEBRIDEMENT AND RASPING

This technique is used mostly for freshening a partial- or full-thickness tear. The meniscal tear is identified. A rasp or shaver is taken over the femoral and tibial surfaces, lightly abrading both sides of the tear (Fig. 51–11).

TREPHINATION AND VASCULAR ACCESS CHANNEL

Arnoczky[2] first described avascular meniscal tear healing by placing a spinal needle in radial orientation from the peripheral toward the inner rim (Fig. 51–12). This technique develops small vascular access channels across the otherwise avascular inner third of the meniscus. As the needle nears the surface, a small bulge should be appreciated in the substance of the meniscus. Avoid piercing the meniscal surfaces.

FIBRIN CLOT

This technique requires 40 mL of the patient's blood obtained by venipuncture. The blood is stirred in a sterile glass dish with a glass rod for 3 to 5 minutes, until the clot adheres to the rod. The 1- to 2-cm clot is rinsed and blotted. Repair sutures are placed loosely across the tear site before clot introduction. The clot is secured to one of the repair sutures and advanced arthroscopically into the tibial side of the tear. Sutures are tied, trapping the fibrin clot.[3,9,23]

Pearls and Pitfalls

Rasping is good for partial tears, but care must be taken to abrade the meniscus without causing further damage. It is also important to address both tibial and femoral surfaces if possible.

For trephination, use the light source to transilluminate and locate the entry point for the needle. The needle should bulge, not pierce, the meniscal surface. A small-bore needle is recommended to avoid excessive injury to the meniscus.

Be sure the fibrin clot is fully formed before manipulation. Turn off the pump to avoid dislodging the clot from the suture. Placement on the tibial side of the

6 Knee

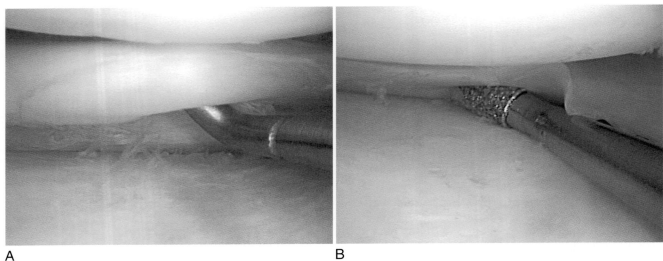

A

B

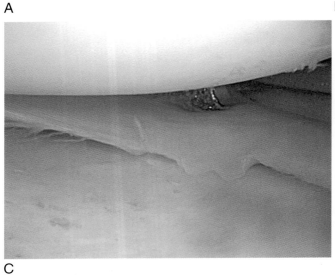

C

Figure 51–11 *A,* Probe in a partial posterior horn meniscal tear. *B,* Tibial rasping. *C,* Femoral rasping.

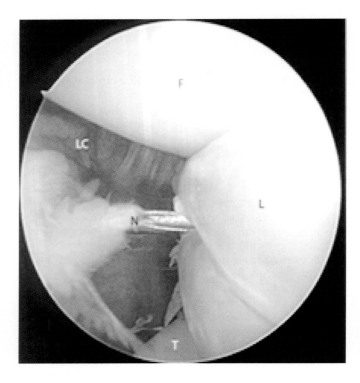

Figure 51–12 Arthroscopic view of meniscal trephination. **F,** femur; **L,** lateral meniscus; **LC,** lateral condyle; **N,** Needle; **T,** tibia. (From Strobel MJ: Meniscus treatment. In Strobel MJ [ed]: Manual of Arthroscopic Surgery. Strabing, Germany, Springer-Verlag, 2001, p. 105.)

meniscus helps capture the clot against the plateau. It is best inserted through a large cannula without a stopper.

Results

Talley and Grana[27] reported on 44 partial, stable meniscal tears treated with limited synovial abrasion at the time of ACL reconstruction. At a median of 12 months, 4 of 19 (21%) medial meniscal tears and 1 of 25 (4%) lateral meniscal tears had failed to heal and required debridement. Okuda et al.[20] treated full-thickness longitudinal tears in the avascular zones of rabbit medial menisci with synovial abrasion. At 2 to 4 weeks, the experimental menisci demonstrated hypertrophic synovium, with near complete healing by 8 to 16 weeks. The contralateral, nontreated control meniscal tears remained unhealed. Significant differences were noted between the rasped group and the control group in tensile strength and stiffness. Nakhostine et al.[18] evaluated the effect of abrasion on a longitudinal full-thickness tear in the avascular inner rim of sheep lateral menisci. They noted that the distance from the defect to the peripheral vasculature supply did not allow for sufficient cellular ingrowth.

In 1988, Arnoczky et al.[3] reported the introduction of autologous fibrin clot to the meniscal tear site to assist with healing. The clot acted as a chemotactic and mitogenic stimulus for reparative cells, as well as a scaffolding for fibrous connective tissue proliferation, with subsequent conversion to fibrocartilaginous tissue. This method is best used in the case of an isolated tear. Van Trommel et al.[29] reported on three patients treated with the fibrin clot technique for radial split tears in the avascular zone of the lateral meniscus, anterior to the popliteus. MRI demonstrated complete healing at an average of 71 months' follow-up.

Complications

A full-thickness trephination channel is required, but this disrupts the peripheral circumferential collagen fibers, which are necessary for meniscal biomechanical function. The main complication of these techniques, used mostly for red-white or white-white tears, is incomplete healing. Although preliminary evidence suggests that lesions in the avascular region of the menisci can be repaired directly or with a concurrent fibrin clot, complex meniscal tears still necessitate removal in some instances. Understanding which tears can be addressed by enhancement techniques and which require debridement is a cornerstone of successful results.

All-Inside Repair

Case History

Two years after ACL reconstruction, a 24-year-old man reinjures his knee with a twisting mechanism while playing basketball.

Physical Examination

On physical examination, effusion was noted. Range of motion was 10 to 110 degrees, and there was medial joint line tenderness. The McMurray test was positive, and the Lachman test was +1.

Imaging

Gadolinium MRI demonstrated a bucket handle meniscal tear.

Indications

In this young, active patient, meniscal repair would be more beneficial than debridement to avoid further stress and increase the longevity of the ACL reconstruction. The all-inside arthroscopic repair is appropriate for posterior horn tears.

Surgical Technique

Positioning

The operative extremity is placed in the arthroscopic leg holder with a tourniquet about the proximal thigh and the nonoperative leg in the well-leg holder.

Examination under Anesthesia

The examination under anesthesia demonstrates that the mechanical block to full extension is still present, with a slight increased anterior translation.

Diagnostic Arthroscopy

The intercondylar notch is notable for frayed fibers of the ACL graft and a displaced, complex medial meniscal bucket handle tear.

Device and Instrumentation

The FasT-Fix implant consists of two 5-mm polymer suture bars and a pretied, sliding number 0 USP braided polyester suture with a self-locking knot. The anchors are inserted via a curved or straight delivery needle (17 gauge). The split cannula allows introduction of the delivery needles to avoid the inadvertent grasping of soft tissue. A depth penetration limiter and a safety sleeve provide the surgeon with a means of restricting the depth of needle insertion. The FasT-Fix system has biomechanical properties comparable to those of the vertical suture technique.

The RapidLoc implant consists of a PDS or poly-lactic acid backstop with an eyelet through which a 2-0 or 0 Panacryl or Ethibond suture is threaded. A sliding TopHat is attached to the suture such that it can slide against the backstop. Three different delivery needles are available for ease of implantation: 0-, 12-, and 27-degree curved. The delivery device has a gun handle that affords less kickback. This can be used with or without a working cannula. Silicone tubing is attached 13 mm proximal to the tip of the delivery needle to assist with meniscal reduction. A clear cannula or malleable graft retractor is available for the working portal, although these are not essential.

Specific Surgical Steps

FasT-Fix

The depth penetration limiter (the dark blue plastic sleeve) allows the introduction of the delivery needle to a preset depth of 25 mm, which extends 17 mm from the back of the implant. For a second depth measurement, the white safety sleeve can be used. The meniscal width across which the implant must pass to penetrate the meniscocapsular junction is measured with a probe; then, 4 mm is added to accommodate soft tissue clearance. The white safety sleeve, marked at 2-mm intervals, is trimmed and placed over the depth penetration limiter.

The FasT-Fix[7] delivery needle and split cannula sheath are inserted through a portal with or without an arthroscopic cannula. Once the needle is visualized, the split cannula sheath can be removed. The inner fragment is penetrated first, rotating the delivery needle 90 degrees. Once it is through the meniscus and extracapsular, as indicated by a tactilely sensed "pop," the delivery needle is oscillated 5 to 10 degrees to release the first implant (Figs. 51–13 and 51–14).

To load the second implant, fully advance the gold trigger on the delivery needle handle. Without passing

through the loose suture loops, maneuver the delivery needle to its next insertion site, optimally 4 to 5 mm from the first implant site. Insert the delivery needle, appreciate the "pop," and pull the delivery needle back out the portal (Fig. 51–15).

The single free end of the suture should extend from the portal. Pulling on the suture tightens the knot. To further secure the knot, one can pull the suture through the FasT-Fix knot pusher and suture cutter, which also serves to countersink the knot. To cut the suture, rest the tip against the knot and slide the gold trigger, leaving a 2- to 3-mm tail. A standard knot pusher and arthroscopic scissors may be used instead (Fig. 51–16).

RapidLoc

The meniscal tear is prepared with a shaver or rasp. The delivery needle is inserted and placed along the inner fragment. The tear can be reduced with the silicone sleeve and needle, or a probe can be used through the ipsilateral portal. As with the FasT-Fix, the needle is passed through the meniscus into the capsule, indicated by a tactilely sensed "pop." While maintaining forward pressure, the trigger is depressed, releasing the backstop. The delivery needle is removed. Using the arthroscopic knot pusher, the TopHat is gently slid down to the meniscus. Similar to the tying of arthroscopic knots, alternating push and pull advancement on the suture allows seating of the TopHat, while keeping the meniscus reduced. Dimpling the meniscus with the TopHat ensures proper tension. The suture is cut with any type of arthroscopic cutter, leaving at least 2 mm of suture (Fig. 51–17).

Pearls and Pitfalls

The FasT-Fix needle should be kept in the blue sheath until it is visualized in the compartment, to avoid tissue laceration or soft tissue entrapment of the implant. Compared with the straight delivery system, the curved needle allows for easier manipulation and delivery of both implants. Although the RapidLoc silicone tubing allows 13 mm of needle length, it will collapse to allow extracapsular backstop delivery.

Perpendicular suture placement is essential and makes for easier knot sliding. Anterior horn fixation may require a far medial or lateral portal. Body tears are approached from the contralateral portal. For posterior tears, the ipsilateral portal is used for implant introduction.

The FasT-Fix can be placed through either the tibial or femoral surface of the meniscus to assume a vertical, horizontal, or oblique orientation. Oblique placement of the suture construct, working from posterior-superior forward to anterior-inferior, may allow for easier cinching of the knot, as well as more peripheral knot placement. In a vertical repair, the superior implant should be placed first.

The RapidLoc should be placed on the femoral surface. Dimpling the meniscus helps prevent any possibility of chondral abrasion. Care should be taken to avoid overzealous reduction or risk meniscal perforation with the TopHat.

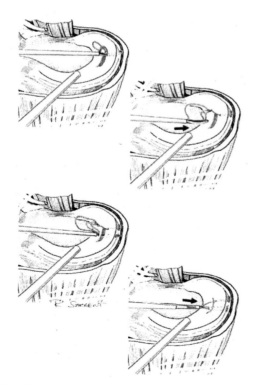

Figure 51–13 Diagram of FasT-Fix technique. (Illustrations by Rick Sergeant.)

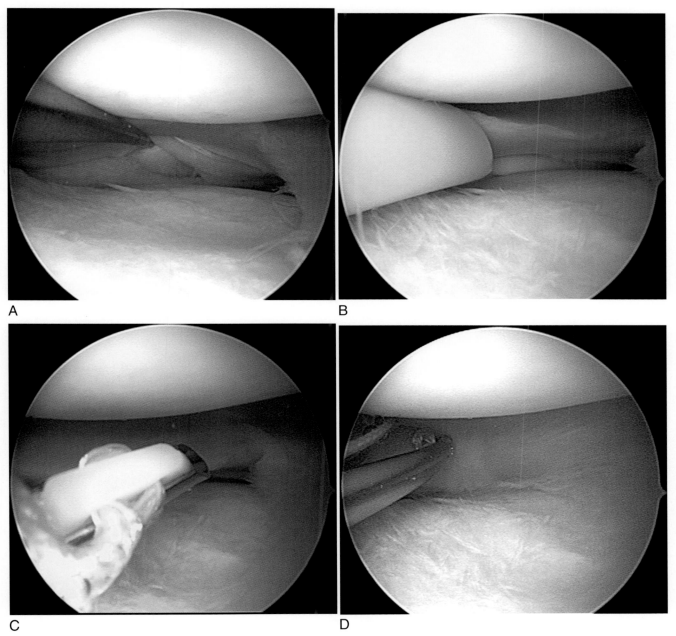

Figure 51–14   *A,* Probe in posterior horn tear of medial meniscus. *B,* FasT-Fix with sheath. *C,* Sheath removed. *D,* First anchor delivered through tear.

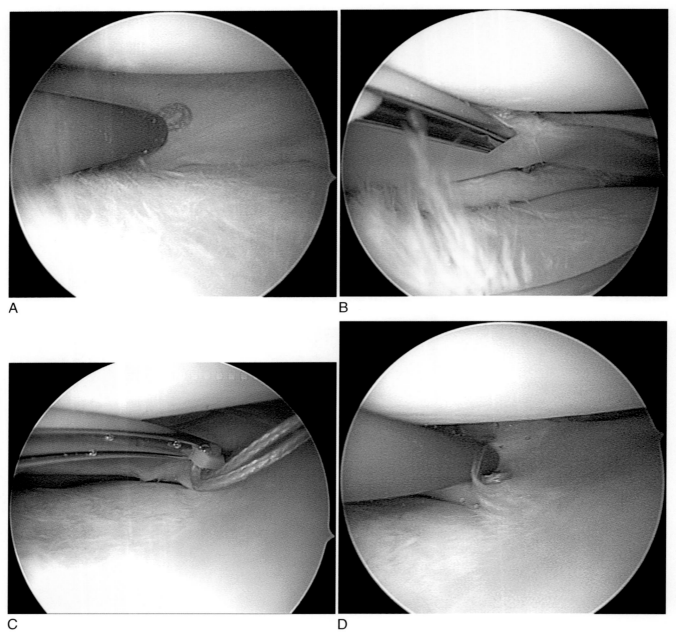

Figure 51–15   *A,* First anchor fully seated. *B,* Visualization of anchor penetrating tear. *C,* Second anchor loaded. *D,* Second anchor fully seated.

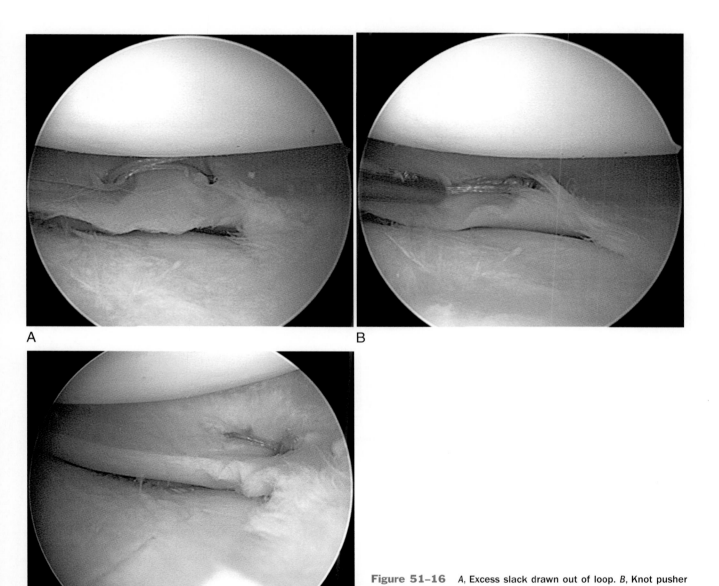

A

B

C

Figure 51–16   *A*, Excess slack drawn out of loop. *B*, Knot pusher tightening slipknot. *C*, Suture cut with properly tensioned knot, and reduced tear.

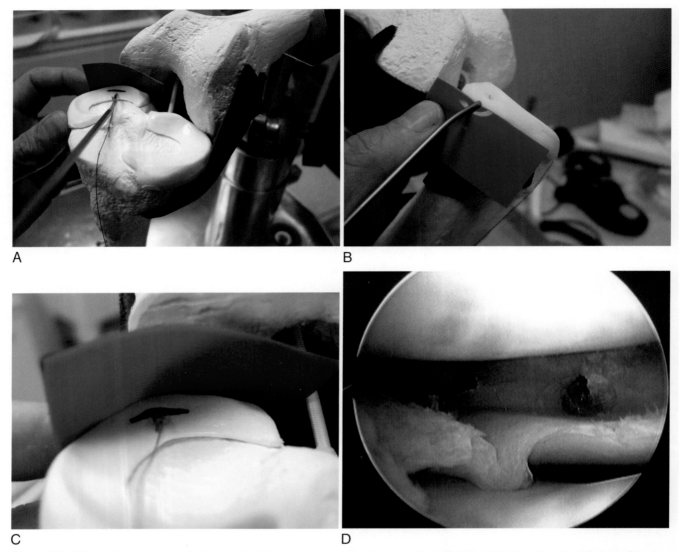

A

B

C

D

Figure 51–17 *A*, Meniscus reduced with needle. *B*, Backstop delivered extracapsularly. *C*, TopHat seated to reduced meniscal surface. *D*, Repaired meniscus with TopHats properly spaced and tensioned. (Courtesy of Mark Miller.)

The sutures should be oriented perpendicular to the meniscus to ensure proper knot sliding. Use the knot pusher to avoid premature knot tightening. This also helps countersink the knot for the FasT-Fix.

The arthroscopic knot pusher must be used with the RapidLoc to properly seat the TopHat.

Results

The T-Fix device was developed as the next generation of all-inside implants but requires intra-articular knot tying. Borden et al.[6] reported an 88% success rate in 55 meniscal repairs. Five of the seven failures were in acute injuries.[6]

Because these second-generation implants are new to the arthroscopy community, there are almost no mid- or long-term data on them. Caborn's unpublished series with the FasT-Fix has reported only 2 failures among 72 treated menisci. One of the failures was due to a ramp lesion that was not captured in the initial repair. The second failure was in an active wrestler with a large bucket handle tear. Caborn noted that there is an initial learning curve, but the implant is easy to use, with all areas of the meniscus accessible. Cyclic loading has found the FasT-Fix to be comparable to vertical mattress sutures. There are no reports in the literature on cyclic loading results for the RapidLoc device.

The Johnson and Johnson Company performed pullout studies with the RapidLoc device that demonstrated 39% higher strength than its predecessor meniscal repair device. The RapidLoc caused less chondral injury compared with the Bionix Arrow in sheep 12 weeks after meniscal repair.

Complications

Once these devices have been inserted, they cannot be retrieved from an extracapsular position. The FasT-Fix implants and sutures are nonabsorbable. If the surgeon is unable to secure the knot completely, the sutures are either left in their loose state or must be cut out. To combat this difficulty, use the knot pusher or cutter before tightening.

Although no reports have been published, a prominent TopHat could provide a mechanism for chondral abrasion.

Avoid driving the FasT-Fix blue depth penetration limiter into the substance of the meniscus, as this may compound the injury.

Coen et al.[8] showed in a cadaveric study that T-Fix placement within the posterior meniscal horns created a 15-mm "buffer zone" from the popliteal neurovascular bundle. Care must be taken with both implants when working posterolaterally to avoid penetrating the popliteus.

Principles of Meniscal Repair

Biomechanical work has been done in human, cow, pig, goat, and rabbit menisci, comparing the effects on load to failure of the various suture orientations, meniscal implants, and suture thicknesses.

Kohn and Siebert[11] detailed the superior qualities of vertical sutures in meniscal repair and explained that such an orientation captures a greater number of the predominant circumferential meniscal fibers. Several studies have documented the failure of vertical repairs by suture breakage and horizontal repairs by suture pullout or tissue failure.

Post et al.[22] showed that suture material is most important for vertical repair and of less importance for horizontal mattress repair. Barrett et al.[5] reported fewer clinical symptoms and a lower failure rate using nonabsorbable sutures for meniscal repair.

The knee is positioned in 10 to 20 degrees of flexion for medial meniscal repair. A valgus load serves to open the medial compartment as well as approximate the meniscus to the capsule. Sutures should be positioned 4 to 5 mm apart.

Lateral meniscal tears have superior healing rates compared with medial ones. For this reason, there are broader indications to attempt lateral meniscal repair.

The highest rates of healing of meniscal pathology have been found with concomitant ACL reconstruction, exceeding the success rates of repairs done in knees with stable cruciate ligaments. Repairing meniscal tears before ligament reconstruction avoids stressing the repair, as one may have to position or rotate the knee in the extreme to adequately access a tear. When repairing a meniscus with a concomitant ACL tear, one should place the meniscal sutures, then perform and secure the ACL reconstruction, then tie down the meniscal repair sutures.

Bucket Handle Repair Technique

Starting in flexion, a blunt trocar is inserted through the ipsilateral portal, and an attempt is made to lever the bucket handle back into the reduced position as the knee is brought into extension with a valgus force applied to open the medial joint line. At least three sutures are required for bucket handle repair. It is best to start with an all-inside repair of the posterior horn if possible. Horizontal sutures are easier to place than vertical ones, but they frequently cause puckering. To avoid puckering, one should consider alternating adjacent suture placement between the superior and inferior surfaces. Vertical suturing not only is stronger but also allows for broader coaptation and avoids buckling of the meniscus. For large bucket handle tears, placing the first suture in the center of the tear facilitates the reduction.

Ramp Lesion Repair Technique

These tears occur at the peripheral attachment of the posterior horn of the medial meniscus. They are frequently associated with ACL insufficiency. The ramp lesion site is best seen by flexing the knee to 90 degrees and passing the scope through the contralateral portal, across the intercondylar area, and into the posteromedial recess. Repair should always be considered, because resection of this lesion will most likely require a near-total meniscectomy. The FasT-Fix is a good option for these tears.

Radial Tear Repair Technique

After freshening of the tear with debridement, rasping, and trephination, an outside-in technique may be used to reapproximate the anterior and posterior segments. The FasT-Fix also works well. Radial tears located in the posterior horn have better healing potential than those in the middle third owing to better vascularity. Compressive loading is converted to axial loads, keeping the tear reduced (Fig. 51–18).

Postoperative Management

Flexion is limited to 90 degrees for the first 3 weeks for standard, nondisplaced meniscal repairs and for as long as 6 weeks following complex procedures such as bucket handle repairs and meniscal reconstruction. Thompson[28] has shown that with flexion, the meniscus translates posteriorly. At less than 60 degrees of flexion, this posterior translation is minimal and easily justifies permitting at least this amount of motion immediately after repair.

Patients are kept weight bearing as tolerated with an assistive device. Discontinuing the crutches depends on quadriceps control, gait mechanics, and range of motion.

6 Knee

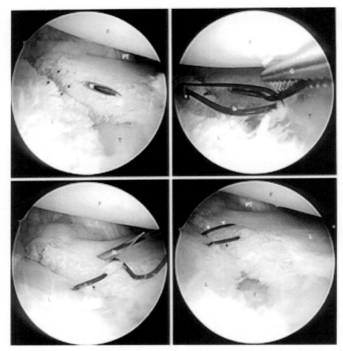

Figure 51–18 Radial tear repair via outside-in technique. (From Strobel MJ: Meniscus treatment. In Strobel MJ [ed]: Manual of Arthroscopic Surgery. Strabing, Germany, Springer-Verlag, 2001, p. 163.)

A long-leg hinged knee brace locked in extension is used for the first 3 weeks in unstable cases. Discontinuing the brace depends on quadriceps control, appropriate gait mechanics, and concomitant ligament reconstruction. A functional brace may be provided at that time.

Core strengthening and quadriceps exercises are started immediately. Bicycling is permitted as range of motion returns after the time restrictions for flexion. In-line running may begin at 12 weeks, and running with subtle change of direction begins at 16 weeks. Cutting with sharp stop-and-go exercises is anticipated shortly thereafter. These guidelines are dependent on satisfactory functional performance evaluation.

Results

Tables 51–1 to 51–5 list the load-to-failure strengths of the various meniscal repair techniques.

Table 51–1 Load to Failure of Meniscal Repair Techniques[4]

Technique	Maximum Pullout Strength Load to Failure (N)
Arrow	33.4 (hand)/33.6 (crossbow)
T-Fix	50.4
Horizontal suture	55.9
BioStinger	56.6
Dart	61.6
Vertical suture (single)	81.6
Vertical suture (double)	113.3

Table 51–2 Load to Failure of Meniscal Sutures[22]

Technique	Suture Type	Mean Load to Failure (N)
Vertical mattress	2-0 Ethibond	89.3 ± 23.8
	0 PDS	115.9 ± 28.5
	1 PDS	146.3 ± 17.1
Horizontal mattress	2-0 Ethibond	59.7 ± 20.4
	0 PDS	66.1 ± 28.7
	1 PDS	73.81 ± 31.3
Mulberry knot	0 PDS	68.6 ± 13.7
	1 PDS	69.3 ± 11.4

Table 51–3 Load to Failure of Meniscal Sutures[11]

Technique	Suture Type	Mean Load to Failure (N)
Vertical mattress	2-0 Vicryl	105 ± 4
Horizontal mattress		
Surface	2-0 Vicryl	89 ± 4
Buried open	2-0 Vicryl	44 ± 18
Mulberry knot	0 PDS	24 ± 9

Table 51–4 Load to Failure of Meniscal Sutures[30]

Technique	Suture Type	Mean Load to Failure (N)
Arrow		44.3
Horizontal suture	3 metric Ethibond	63.2
Vertical suture (single)	3 metric Ethibond	73.9

Table 51–5 Load to Failure of Meniscal Fixation Devices[6]

Device	Load to Failure (N)	Stiffness (N/mm)
FasT-Fix	104	7.69
Vertical mattress	102	7.74
Meniscal Arrow	49	6.07

References

1. Anderson K, Marx RG, Hannafin J, Warren RF: Chondral injury following meniscal repair with a biodegradable implant. Arthroscopy 16:749-753, 2000.
2. Arnoczky SP, Warren RF: The microvasculature of the meniscus and its response to injury. An experimental study in the dog. Am J Sports Med 11:131-141, 1983.
3. Arnoczky SP, Warren RF, Spivak JM: Meniscal repair using an exogenous fibrin clot: An experimental study in dogs. J Bone Joint Surg 70:1209-1217, 1988.

4. Barber A: Arthroscopic Meniscal Repair. Orlando, FL, ICL, 2000.
5. Barrett GR, Richardson K, Ruff CG, Jones A: The effect of suture type on meniscus repair: A clinical analysis. Am J Knee Surg 10:2-9, 1997.
6. Borden P, Nyland J, Caborn DNM, Pienkowski D: Biomechanical comparison of the FasT-Fix meniscal repair suture system to vertical mattress sutures and meniscus arrows. Am J Sports Med 31(3):374–378, 2003.
7. Caborn D: Meniscal Repair with the FasT-Fix Suture System Technique. Andover, MA, Smith and Nephew, 2002.
8. Coen MJ, Caborn DNM, Urban W, et al: An anatomic evaluation of T-Fix suture device placement for arthroscopic all-inside meniscal repair. Arthroscopy 15:275-280, 1999.
9. Henning CE, Lynch MA, Yearout KM, et al: Arthroscopic meniscal repair using an exogenous fibrin clot. Clin Orthop 22:64-72, 1990.
10. Hurel C, Mertens F, Verdonk R: Biofix resorbable meniscus arrow for meniscal ruptures: Results of a 1-year follow-up. Knee Surg Sports Traumatol Arthrosc 8:46-52, 2000.
11. Kohn D, Siebert W: Meniscus suture techniques: A comparative biomechanical cadaver study. Arthroscopy 5:324-327, 1989.
12. Kurzweil PR, Friedman MJ: Meniscus: Resection, repair and replacement. Arthroscopy 18:33-39, 2002.
13. Mariani PP, Santori N, Adriani E, Mastantuono M: Accelerated rehabilitation after arthroscopic meniscal repair: A clinical and magnetic resonance imaging evaluation. Arthroscopy 12:680-686, 1996.
14. Menche DS, Phillips GI, Pitman MI, Steiner GC: Inflammatory foreign body reaction to an arthroscopic bioabsorbable meniscal arrow repair. Arthroscopy 15:770-772, 1999.
15. Meniscus Arrow: Surgical Technique. Bluebell, PA, Bionx Implants, 1998.
16. Miller DB Jr: Arthroscopic meniscus repair. Am J Sports Med 16:315-320, 1988.
17. Morgan CD, Wojtys EM, Casscells CD, Casscells SW: Arthroscopic meniscal repair evaluated by second look arthroscopy. Am J Sports Med 19:632-637, 1991.
18. Nakhostine M, Gershuni DH, Anderson R: Effects of abrasion therapy on tears in the avascular region of sheep menisci. Arthroscopy 6:280-287, 1990.
19. Nicholas SJ, Rodeo SA, Ghelman B, et al: Arthroscopic meniscal repair using the outside-in technique. Paper presented at the AAOS, AOSSM Specialty Day, 1991, Anaheim, CA.
20. Okuda K, Ochi M, Shu N, Uchio Y: Meniscal rasping for repair of meniscal tears in the avascular zone. Arthroscopy 15:281-286, 1999.
21. Oliverson TJ, Lintner DM: Biofix arrow appearing as a subcutaneous foreign body. Arthroscopy 16:652-655, 2000.
22. Post WR, Akers SR, Kish V: Load to failure of common meniscal repair techniques: Effects of suture technique and suture material. Arthroscopy 13:731-736, 1997.
23. Rodeo SA: Arthroscopic meniscal repair with use of the outside-in technique. Instr Course Lect 49:192-206, 2000.
24. Rosenberg TD, Scott SM, Coward DB, et al: Arthroscopic meniscal repair evaluated with repeat arthroscopy. Arthroscopy 2:14-20, 1986.
25. Ross G, Grabill J, McDevitt E: Chondral injury after meniscal repair with bioabsorbable arrows. Arthroscopy 16:754-756, 2000.
26. Stone RG, Frewin PR, Gonzales S: Long-term assessment of arthroscopic meniscus repair: A two- to six-year follow-up study. Arthroscopy 6:73-78, 1990.
27. Talley MC, Grana WA: Treatment of partial meniscal tears identified during anterior cruciate ligament reconstruction with limited synovial abrasion. Arthroscopy 16:6-10, 2000.
28. Thompson WO, Thaete FL, Fu FH, Dye SF: Tibial meniscal dynamics using three-dimensional reconstruction of magnetic resonance images. Am J Sports Med 19:210-215, 1991.
29. Van Trommel MF, Simonian PT, Potter HG, Wickiewicz TL: Arthroscopic meniscal repair with fibrin clot of complete radial tears of the lateral meniscus in the avascular zone. Arthroscopy 14:360-365, 1998.
30. Walsh SP, Evans SL, O'Doherty DM, Barlow IW: Failure strengths of suture versus biodegradable arrow and staple for meniscal repair: An in vitro study. Knee 8:151-156, 2001.
31. Warren RF: Arthroscopic meniscus repair. Arthroscopy 1:170-172, 1985.
32. Whitman TL, Diduch DR: Transient posterior knee pain with the meniscal arrow. Arthroscopy 14:762-763, 1998.

6 Knee

52

Arthroscopic Meniscus Transplantation: Plug and Slot Technique

E. Marlowe Goble

ARTHROSCOPIC MENISCUS TRANSPLANTATION: PLUG AND SLOT TECHNIQUE IN A NUTSHELL

History:
Prior meniscectomy; pain and swelling, activity restriction; twisting hyperflexion injury

Physical Examination:
Not obese; range of motion within 5 degrees of normal; joint line tenderness with or without effusion; alignment

Imaging:
Weight-bearing films (degenerative joint disease); long leg cassette (alignment); lateral (sizing); magnetic resonance imaging (tear)

Indications:
Failed physical therapy and anti-inflammatory medications; skeletally mature; stable ligament; normal alignment; prior total meniscectomy with current symptoms; grade III or lower chondrosis; realistic expectations

Surgical Technique:
Lateral: prepare graft (block); prepare meniscal rim; prepare trough; drill holes for suture passage; pass sutures (trough and posterolateral capsule); pass graft (varus stress); secure block; suture meniscus
Medial: prepare graft (plugs); prepare meniscal rim; prepare tunnel (anterior cruciate ligament guide); pass sutures (tunnels and posteromedial capsule); pass graft (varus stress); secure plugs; suture meniscus

Postoperative Management:
No weight bearing for 8 weeks; ice and other modalities; physical therapy; range of motion; return to play ~1 month; sports at 4 months

Results:
Lateral: 54% to 92% good to excellent
Medial: 79% to 100% good to excellent

Partial or total meniscectomy increases the incidence of knee joint degeneration. Therefore, significant effort should be made to prevent meniscal injury and to repair meniscal tissue appropriately when injury occurs.[1-4] Nevertheless, meniscectomy, or even total removal of the meniscus, is sometimes indicated when a patient presents with pain and swelling of the knee.

If a meniscus is discovered to be nonfunctional, the surgeon must determine the cause of the meniscal disease before he or she can recommend appropriate treatment. If meniscal allograft transplantation (MAT) is considered, the source of the meniscal damage must be mechanical, not degenerative,[5] and it cannot be caused by synovial disease, because the transplant would suffer the same fate as the original meniscus.

The lateral meniscus carries most of the load in the lateral compartment. The medial meniscus shares more of the medial compartment load with the articular cartilage.[6] Therefore, lateral meniscectomy accelerates degeneration in its compartment relative to medial meniscectomy.

Meniscectomy eventually leads to joint space narrowing, flattening of the femoral condyle, and spurring. These changes, described by Fairbank,[7] cause mechanical malalignment that must be corrected before MAT can be successful.

Immunologically, MAT elicits both B- and T-cell responses. Samuelson showed that the host immune response is rarely strong enough to destroy an osteochondral transplant.

History

On average, a typical MAT candidate is 33 years old (range, 19 to 44 years). Males predominate over females 2:1. Typically, the patient is active athletically and is concerned about the immediate future with regard to participating in his or her children's athletic activities, meeting the physical demands of his or her occupation, and achieving personal athletic goals. The patient has probably consulted an average of four physicians and is generally more self-educated than the average person with a knee disorder. This patient will consider a short-term good result to be a success. A history of injury, subsequent meniscectomy, a period of good knee function (2 to 15 years), followed by complaints of (single compartment) pain and swelling with activity is the usual presentation.

Physical Examination

A proper physical examination includes an assessment of the following:

1. Height and weight: Obesity is a contraindication to MAT.
2. Hip function: Examination of the hip should reveal adequate range of motion and full extension and flexion without pain.
3. Quadriceps strength: Usually atrophy and decreased muscle tension are present because of chronic pain and swelling of the knee. The circumferential measurement should be recorded. Extension lag should be corrected before MAT.
4. Knee range of motion: Extension should be within 5 degrees of normal, and flexion should exceed 125 degrees. Any restriction in preoperative range of motion is likely to increase postoperatively.
5. Ligament stability: A complete examination that records varus or valgus stability, rotational stability, and translational stability (Lachman test, anterior and posterior drawer test, pivot shift) is required. In 40% of MAT candidates, an anterior cruciate ligament (ACL) deficiency exists. Anterior and posterior cruciate ligament deficiencies must be corrected before or at the same time as MAT.
6. Mechanical femoral-tibial alignment: Deviation of greater than 2 degrees from the normal contralat-

eral varus-valgus alignment requires osteotomy for correction.
7. Pain: Joint line tenderness is present in the affected compartment. Sometimes, physical exertion is required to produce pain symptoms. Have the patient jump, squat, or run to test for compartment intolerance of activity.
8. Effusion: The presence of joint fluid without activity suggests a grade III (or greater) state of compartment degeneration.
9. Patellofemoral alignment and function: Patellofemoral pain should be minimal; otherwise, symptoms will increase after MAT. Any chondromalacia or malalignment problem should be treated before MAT.
10. Meniscal dysfunction (McMurray test): Not valid when considering MAT.

Imaging

Weight-bearing anteroposterior and lateral radiographs of both knees are required to evaluate the degenerative state of the knee. Additional anteroposterior and lateral radiographs, including a calibration device, are required when sizing for MAT. The instructions from the allograft processor must be followed to properly size for the allograft.

Magnetic resonance imaging is desirable to document the condition of any remaining meniscus and any articular cartilage defects. Subchondral bone sizing can also be performed using magnetic resonance imaging.

Indications and Contraindications

Table 52–1 lists the indications for MAT, and Table 52–2 the contraindications.

Table 52–1
Indications for Meniscus Transplantation

Skeletal maturity
Stable ligaments
Normal femorotibial alignment
Mechanical meniscal disorder (i.e., meniscal injury resulting from trauma, not synovial or metabolic disease)
Absence of an intact meniscal rim
No greater than grade III chondral wear (preferably, grade I or II)
At least one recent opinion from a knee specialist
Realistic expectations (i.e., the patient understands that the benefits are relatively short term)
No obesity
Intact immune system
Pain

Table 52-2	Contraindications for Meniscus Transplantation

Skeletal immaturity
Unstable knee
Varus or valgus malalignment
Synovial disease
Intact meniscal rim extending to the "red-white" zone
Grade IV chondral wear
No second opinion
Obesity
Immune deficient
Painless, meniscus-deficient compartment without
   radiographic changes (debatable)

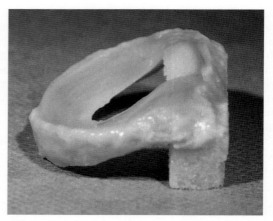

Figure 52–1 The thawed lateral meniscal allograft is prepared on the back table simultaneously with preparation of the lateral tibial plateau of the recipient. (From Goble EM, Kane SM: Meniscal allograft transplantation. In Insall JN, Scott WN [eds]: Surgery of the Knee, 3rd ed. New York, Churchill Livingstone, 2001.)

Surgical Technique

Lateral MAT is most commonly performed as an arthroscopic or arthroscopically assisted procedure. Medial MAT is currently an arthroscopically assisted or open surgical technique.

Lateral Meniscal Transplantation

The frozen allograft is carefully thawed, with consideration of the method of freezing. Lyophilized (freeze-dried) tissue requires sufficient time for rehydration—about 40 minutes in a room-temperature sterile saline solution. Too little hydration of lyophilized meniscal allograft may result in central substance fibrocartilaginous fracture, even though the surface architecture appears ductile.

Deep-frozen allograft tissue, although not in need of hydration, must be thoroughly thawed to eliminate all crystalline water content. Mechanical microtrauma can result from manipulation of the space-occupying ice crystal within the tissue.

Cryopreserved meniscal allograft tissue does not contain water in the crystalline state, and the tissue is not dehydrated. However, slow thawing in appropriate solvents is mandatory to preserve cellular viability. The surgeon must carefully follow the step-by-step directions (supplied by the manufacturer, Cryolife, Kennesaw, GA) to prepare the tissue mechanically and histologically for implantation.

The lateral meniscal allograft is prepared immediately before or during the surgical procedure. The lateral meniscus is prepared with a single rectangular bone block rigidly joining the anterior and posterior horns in an anatomic relationship. All nonmeniscal soft tissue is sharply removed from the specimen (Fig. 52–1).

A variable number of sutures are preinserted into the meniscal edge to facilitate spreading of the meniscus around the margins of the host compartment after insertion of the graft through the expanded lateral arthroscopic portal. Critical meniscal suture placement sites include (1) the posterolateral corner; (2) the edge of the anterior horn, 15 mm lateral to its insertion into the

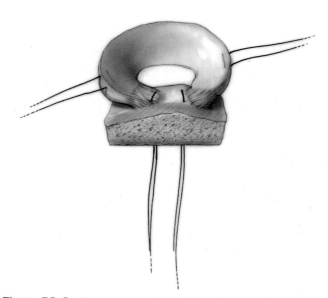

Figure 52–2 Sutures are preinserted into the posterolateral edge of the meniscus, into the anterior horn of the meniscus, and into the bone block. (From Goble EM, Kane SM: Meniscal allograft transplantation. In Insall JN, Scott WN [eds]: Surgery of the Knee, 3rd ed. New York, Churchill Livingstone, 2001.)

bone; and (3) two sutures, 10 cm apart, through the common bone block (Fig. 52–2).

The bone block is precisely debrided of excess bone until it fits within the appropriate slot on the sizing block. Usually, the diameter of the bone block chosen is 8, 9, or 10 mm. A silicone template, originally measuring 40 mm long and 10 mm in diameter, is trimmed until it exactly matches the finished bone block (Fig. 52–3).

Medial and lateral arthroscopic portals are prepared immediately adjacent to the patellar tendon. The medial portal is placed in the "soft spot" just below the lower

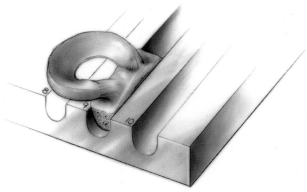

Figure 52–3   Bone blocks are sized within the "bone block sizer." (From Goble EM, Kane SM: Meniscal allograft transplantation. In Insall JN, Scott WN [eds]: Surgery of the Knee, 3rd ed. New York, Churchill Livingstone, 2001.)

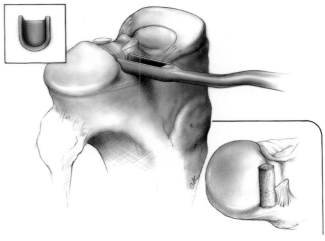

Figure 52–4   Large-gouge cutting trough. (From Goble EM, Kane SM: Meniscal allograft transplantation. In Insall JN, Scott WN [eds]: Surgery of the Knee, 3rd ed. New York, Churchill Livingstone, 2001.)

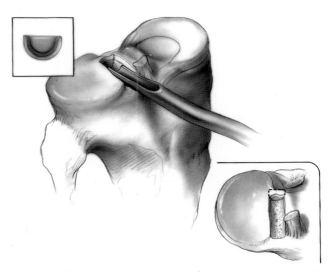

Figure 52–5   Quarter-round gauge removing the posterior trough. (From Goble EM, Kane SM: Meniscal allograft transplantation. In Insall JN, Scott WN [eds]: Surgery of the Knee, 3rd ed. New York, Churchill Livingstone, 2001.)

border of the patella. The lateral portal is placed 1 cm distal to the patella–patellar tendon junction, because there is no need to elevate the scope over the anterior portion of the meniscus.

The original meniscal remnants are debrided, except for the most peripheral border of the meniscus, where it attaches to the capsule; 1 to 2 mm of peripheral meniscal edge is left intact to "receive" the MAT. It is vital that the meniscocapsular junction be exposed and bleeding. Do not waste time removing the meniscal insertions into bone (anterior and posterior), because these insertion sites will be easily accessible after preparing the bony trough.

Enlarge the lateral portal by inserting a number 15 blade into the arthroscopic portal and incising distally until reaching the tibial plateau. This enlarges the portal sufficiently to allow insertion of an index finger when the knee is flexed greater than 45 degrees. Surprisingly, this enlarged portal does not allow excessive loss of pressurized fluid from the joint, because the vertical borders of the portal are drawn tightly together when the knee is flexed beyond 60 degrees.

Place the 30-degree arthroscope into the medial portal, and visualize the lateral footprint of the ACL and the lateral tibial eminence. Insert the meniscal gouge (8-, 9-, or 10-mm diameter) into the lateral portal, and select the proper handle angle, usually 20 degrees. Remove bone from anterior to posterior while remaining in close proximity to the lateral border of the ACL (Fig. 52–4). It may be necessary to remove some lateral fibers of the ACL. Begin the trough 1 cm posterior to the anterior edge of the lateral tibial plateau. Remove short, bony segments while progressing posteriorly, deepening the channel to the upper margins of the meniscal trough gouge. Be careful not to exit the bone posteriorly, because the popliteal neurovascular structures lie on the posterior border of the joint capsule (Fig. 52–5).

Using a power bur, hand gouge (Fig. 52–6), and meniscal trough rasp, prepare the trough to receive the silicone trough template, which should exactly match the prepared graft bone block (Fig. 52–7).

Make a 2-cm longitudinal incision medial to the tibial tuberosity. Using an ACL tibial guide, place two transosseous holes, 10 mm apart, in the middle of the trough, exiting the tibia adjacent to the tibial tuberosity (Fig. 52–8).

Pull each of the sutures inserted in the graft bone block through the lateral portal and into their respective transosseous holes in the bottom of the bone trough. Each suture should exit the tibia medial to the tibial tuberosity (Fig. 52–9).

Place a 16-gauge spinal needle, from outside in, at the posterolateral corner of the knee. Insert a monofilament suture through the needle into the joint. Pull that suture across the joint and out the lateral portal. Attach this suture to the suture that was preinserted into the

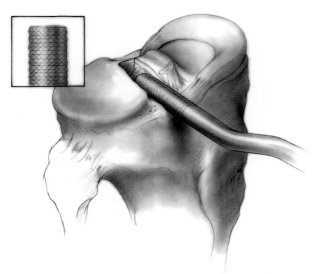

Figure 52–6 **Rasping trough.** (From Goble EM, Kane SM: Meniscal allograft transplantation. In Insall JN, Scott WN [eds]: Surgery of the Knee, 3rd ed. New York, Churchill Livingstone, 2001.)

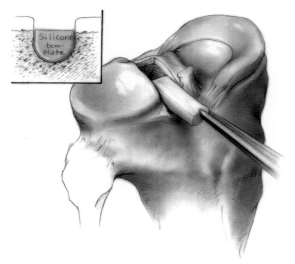

Figure 52–7 **Template within the trough, with articular cartilage above the template.** (From Goble EM, Kane SM: Meniscal allograft transplantation. In Insall JN, Scott WN [eds]: Surgery of the Knee, 3rd ed. New York, Churchill Livingstone, 2001.)

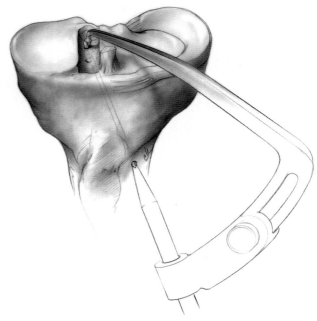

Figure 52–8 **The receiving trough lies adjacent to the anterior cruciate ligament (ACL). Two transosseous suture holes are prepared using a tibial ACL guide.** (From Goble EM, Kane SM: Meniscal allograft transplantation. In Insall JN, Scott WN [eds]: Surgery of the Knee, 3rd ed. New York, Churchill Livingstone, 2001.)

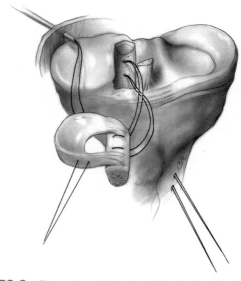

Figure 52–9 **The preinserted posterolateral suture is pulled through the posterolateral capsule.** (From Goble EM, Kane SM: Meniscal allograft transplantation. In Insall JN, Scott WN [eds]: Surgery of the Knee, 3rd ed. New York, Churchill Livingstone, 2001.)

posterolateral edge of the meniscal graft. Pull this suture assembly through the joint and out the posterolateral corner of the knee (the knot will pass through this hole) (see Fig. 52–9).

The meniscal allograft is now ready for insertion. While gently pulling on each of the guide sutures (posterolateral knee and medial tibial tuberosity), urge the graft through the lateral portal and into the bony trough. Place a varus stress on the knee while flexing the knee 30 degrees. The varus stress should open the lateral compartment sufficiently for the posterolateral guide suture to expand the folded meniscus into the peripheral compartment.

Pull on the sutures attached to the bone block to guide it securely into the trough. Range the knee joint 10 times from 0 to 100 degrees, and the lateral meniscal graft should seat itself anatomically within the lateral compartment. Match the coincidental slopes of the host-donor lateral tibial eminences. Expose the peroneal nerve at the level of the posterolateral joint line to avoid suture needle trauma. Tie the two bone trough sutures together at the medial edge of the tibial tuberosity while visualizing the position of the donor bone block within the trough. Suture the periphery of the meniscal graft at the capsule from the popliteal tendon, posteriorly, to the anterior horn. Use the preinserted anterior horn suture in the meniscus to close the lateral portal at the end of the procedure (Fig. 52–10).

Medial Meniscal Transplantation

The medial MAT is preferably performed with bony anchors at its anterior and posterior horns. This surgical implantation is accomplished by using either separated bone plugs or a single cylindric bone island joining the two horns, similar to the technique employed for lateral meniscal transplantation.

Separate Bone Plugs

Two separate bone plugs of the desired diameter and length (I prefer 9-mm diameter and 10-mm length) are sculptured or "hole-saw" drilled from the thawed en bloc allograft. All the soft tissue attachments to bone can be preserved with 9-mm-diameter plugs. Nonabsorbable number 2 braided polyethylene sutures are attached to each bone plug through 1.5-mm drill holes located at the center of each plug. Each of these sutures will eventually be pulled, via the medial portal, through individual transosseous tunnels located in the bottom of each recipient anterior and posterior bone hole (Fig. 52–11).

The arthroscope is placed laterally, and the medial arthroscopic portal is expanded in a manner analogous to the lateral meniscal technique.

An ACL tibial guide directs a ³⁄₃₂-inch guidewire from just lateral of the tibial tuberosity to the anatomic center of each horn (anterior and posterior). The guidewires are overdrilled with a 6-mm cannulated drill. The proximal "mouth" of each 6-mm hole is then expanded intra-articularly with a curet to a 10-mm diameter. A posteromedial portal is best used to locate the anatomic position of the posterior horn and then expand the diameter of the hole to 10 mm. The location of the anterior horn attachment is anterior to the footprint of the ACL at the anterior margin of the tibial plateau (Fig. 52–12).

After elongating the medial portal distally to bone, the posteromedial suture that was preinserted in the posteromedial body of the meniscus is passed, via the medial portal, through the medial compartment, exiting through the posteromedial portal. The anterior and posterior horn bone plug sutures are passed through each transosseous hole, exiting adjacent to the tibial tuberosity in the anterolateral tibia (Fig. 52–13).

While maintaining tension on each guide suture, the meniscal graft is urged through the medial portal and into the joint. Valgus stress should open the medial compartment sufficiently to allow the meniscus to "unfold" and "spread out" by pulling on the posteromedial guide suture (Fig. 52–14).

The posterior bone block is manipulated into its hole. Sometimes it may be necessary to remove the top of the medial tibial eminence in order to pass the posterior bone block (Fig. 52–15).

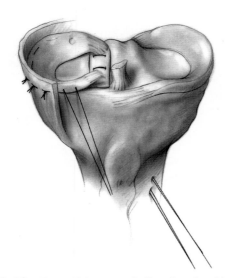

Figure 52–10 The graft is anatomically reduced and held in this position with the critical guide sutures. Note the reestablishment of the slope of the lateral tibial eminence. A meniscal screw secures the posterior horn to the capsule. (From Goble EM, Kane SM: Meniscal allograft transplantation. In Insall JN, Scott WN [eds]: Surgery of the Knee, 3rd ed. New York, Churchill Livingstone, 2001.)

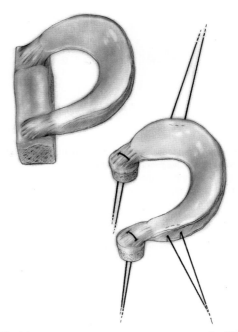

Figure 52–11 Nonabsorbable sutures are centered within each bone block. Guide sutures (which help spread out the meniscus within the medial compartment) are preinserted into the posteromedial and anterior portions of the allograft. (From Goble EM, Kane SM: Meniscal allograft transplantation. In Insall JN, Scott WN [eds]: Surgery of the Knee, 3rd ed. New York, Churchill Livingstone, 2001.)

6 Knee

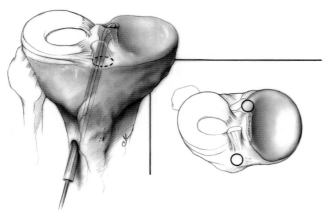

Figure 52–12 The anterior horn attachment is at the anterior margin of the tibial plateau. The posterior horn attachment is on the posterior slope of the medial intercondylar eminence. The "top" of the medial tibial eminence is removed. (From Goble EM, Kane SM: Meniscal allograft transplantation. In Insall JN, Scott WN [eds]: Surgery of the Knee, 3rd ed. New York, Churchill Livingstone, 2001.)

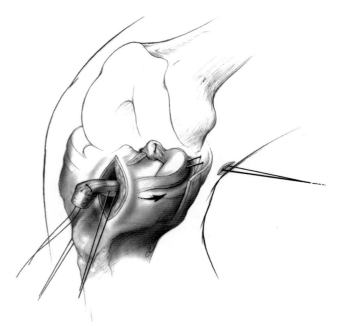

Figure 52–14 The allograft is gently urged through the expanded medial portal. The posteromedial suture and the anterior suture are tensioned to spread out the meniscus within the compartment. (From Goble EM, Kane SM: Meniscal allograft transplantation. In Insall JN, Scott WN [eds]: Surgery of the Knee, 3rd ed. New York, Churchill Livingstone, 2001.)

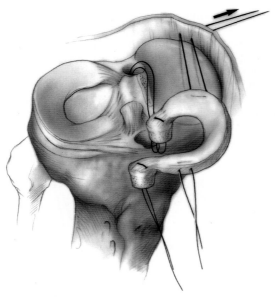

Figure 52–13 The posteromedial preinserted suture is passed into the joint through the medial portal and out of the joint through a hole in the posteromedial capsule. (From Goble EM, Kane SM: Meniscal allograft transplantation. In Insall JN, Scott WN [eds]: Surgery of the Knee, 3rd ed. New York, Churchill Livingstone, 2001.)

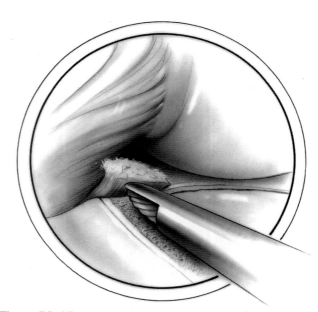

Figure 52–15 Removing the top of the tibial eminence. (From Goble EM, Kane SM: Meniscal allograft transplantation. In Insall JN, Scott WN [eds]: Surgery of the Knee, 3rd ed. New York, Churchill Livingstone, 2001.)

The anterior bone block is guided into its recipient hole. Arthroscopic visualization of this step may be difficult, and it can best be confirmed by digital palpation through the medial portal.

The knee joint is taken through several range-of-motion cycles. This motion should seat the meniscus properly.

The periphery is sewn with horizontal mattress sutures from posterior to anterior, closing the medial portal with the preinserted anterior horn suture (Fig. 52–16). The bone plug sutures are then tied over bone in the anterolateral tibia while the proper reduction of each bone plug within its hole is visualized (Fig. 52–17).

Single Bone Plug

The insertion sites of the horns of the medial meniscus are much wider apart than those of the lateral meniscus. Therefore, insertion of a long, cylindric bone plug

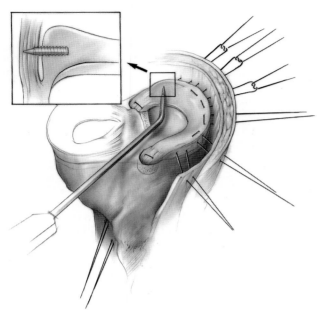

Figure 52–16   Zone-specific inside-out reabsorbable sutures are placed around the graft periphery. A meniscal screw (Clearfix) is inserted posteriorly. The preinserted anterior suture closes the medial (capsular) portal. (From Goble EM, Kane SM: Meniscal allograft transplantation. In Insall JN, Scott WN [eds]: Surgery of the Knee, 3rd ed. New York, Churchill Livingstone, 2001.)

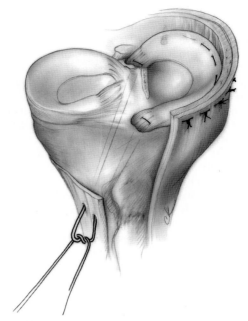

Figure 52–17   Each of the peripheral sutures is tied over fascia before tying the transosseous bone plug sutures together. (From Goble EM, Kane SM: Meniscal allograft transplantation. In Insall JN, Scott WN [eds]: Surgery of the Knee, 3rd ed. New York, Churchill Livingstone, 2001.)

joining the anterior horn to the posterior horn is more difficult than in the lateral meniscal technique.

The technique for a single bone plug installation is the same as that employed for the lateral procedure, with the following exceptions: Develop the medial trough beginning at the anterior margin of the tibial plateau below the fat pad. Remove bone from anterior to posterior in line with the axis of the medial tibial eminence. Extend the trough to the posterior tibial margin but not beyond. I prefer a graft diameter of 8 mm for this technique. It is often necessary to reinforce this plug by inserting a $\frac{1}{16}$-inch threaded guidewire through the middle of the bony graft. This reinforcing wire is left within the bone block.

Open Medial Meniscal Transplantation

If arthroscopic installation is not possible, or if a more secure peripheral suturing and bony fixation technique is preferred, an open surgical procedure should be performed.

The knee is flexed to 80 degrees and supported in a proximal thigh leg-holder device. A medial curvilinear incision is made beginning medial to the patellar tendon at the joint line and extending proximally and posterior to a point just proximal and posterior to the medial femoral epicondyle. The interval is developed along the patellar tendon from the anteromedial joint line to a level proximal to the patella. The synovium is incised deep to this interval and retracted posteriorly, placing a long Army-Navy retractor cephalad and caudad to the soft tissues originating from the medial epicondyle.

One should then be able to visualize the medial gutter, including the medial articular border of the medial femoral condyle. The superior, inferior, and anterior margins of the medial epicondyle and its soft tissue attachments are well exposed when visualized from the distal incision. A curved 1-inch osteotome is inserted, and the medial epicondyle is removed from distal to proximal and anterior to posterior. The bone is carefully scored distal and posterior to the medial epicondyle to prevent extension of this osteotomy to the margin of the femoral articular border. The medial epicondyle is elevated from anterior to posterior, and the posterior capsular attachment is sharply dissected from the posteromedial femur with the curved osteotome. Valgus stress now completely exposes the contents of the medial compartment.

The peripheral attachments of any remaining medial meniscus should be sharply excised with a number 15 blade. Two 10-mm holes can now be directly approached and prepared at the anatomic site of each horn's insertion into bone.

A 4-mm cancellous screw, 20 mm long, is preinserted into the middle of each graft bone plug. Each plug can therefore be compressed within its appropriate recipient hole using a lag screw technique rather than a transosseous suture fixation. Alternatively, a reabsorbable 7-mm-diameter interference screw can be inserted alongside the bone block.

If one desires to use a single anterior to posterior bone plug, the trough is prepared under direct visualization, as opposed to arthroscopically, and the bone graft is fixated with two cancellous screws.

6 Knee

An advantage of this open technique is the ability to preinsert all peripheral sutures within the meniscal graft. It is more accurate and less traumatic to the surface of the graft to sew into the edge of the meniscus rather than to introduce sutures through the meniscal face, which is in contact with femoral hyaline articular cartilage. Each preinserted suture can be mounted on a small, free needle and sewn directly into the adjacent capsule, beginning from the posterior horn and extending to the anterior horn.

Finally, the medial epicondyle is reattached to the femur through screw and washer or staple technique, and a standard closure is completed.

It is my opinion that the open technique is more precise and stable than the arthroscopic technique. Patients undergoing the open procedure are discharged as outpatients on the same day and require no more analgesics than do arthroscopic patients. All muscle groups function immediately, and rehabilitation is no different from that following arthroscopic meniscal insertion, except for the need to protect the medial collateral ligament during the early postoperative period. Aside from the larger scar, no other differences have been noted in early outcome studies.

Postoperative Management

Postoperative rehabilitation is similar to the standard ACL protocol:

- A device for injecting bupivacaine (Marcaine) over 48 hours is inserted into the knee (e.g., Pain Care 3000, Breg, Vista, CA).
- The catheter is removed by the physical therapist at 48 hours.

- The knee is braced (long leg with adjustable hinge) at 30 degrees of flexion.
- Physical therapy visits begin 4 to 5 days after surgery.
- Crutches, allowing partial weight bearing, are used for 3 weeks, followed by use of a cane and full weight bearing.
- Bicycling, with increasing resistance as tolerated, is begun at 10 days.
- Unrestricted sports activity is possible at 4 months postoperatively.

References

1. Johnson RJ, Kettlekamp DB, Clark W, Weaverton O: Factors affecting late results after meniscectomy. J Bone Joint Surg Am 56:719-729, 1974.
2. Lynch MA, Henning CE: Osteoarthritis in the ACL deficient knee. In Feagin JA Jr (ed): The Cruciate Ligaments, 1st ed. New York, Churchill Livingstone, 1988, pp 385-391.
3. Lynch MA, Henning CE, Glick KR: Knee joint surface changes: Long-term follow-up meniscus tear treatment and stable anterior cruciate ligament reconstruction. Clin Orthop 172:148-153, 1983.
4. O'Brien WR: Degenerative arthritis of the knee following anterior cruciate ligament injury: Role of the meniscus. Sports Med Arthrosc Rev 1:114-118, 1993.
5. Ward H, Lie SH, Yang R: Destruction of a cryopreserved meniscal allograft: A case for acute rejection, case report, arthroscopy. J Arthrosc Rel Surg 13:517-521, 1997.
6. Veltri DM, Warren RF, Wickiewicz TL, O'Brien SJ: Current status of allograft meniscal transplantation. Clin Orthop 303:44-55, 1994.
7. Fairbank TJ: Knee joint changes after meniscectomy. J Bone Joint Surg Br 30:664-670, 1984.

53

Arthroscopic Meniscus Transplantation: Bridge in Slot Technique

KEVIN B. FREEDMAN, BRIAN J. COLE, AND JACK FARR

ARTHROSCOPIC MENISCUS TRANSPLANTATION: BRIDGE IN SLOT TECHNIQUE IN A NUTSHELL

History:
Previous meniscectomy, ipsilateral joint line pain, activity-related swelling

Physical Examination:
Joint line pain; evaluate for malalignment or ligament insufficiency

Imaging:
Standing radiographs, including 45-degree posteroanterior and mechanical axis views; magnetic resonance imaging and bone scan usually unnecessary

Indications:
Prior meniscectomy, normal alignment, stable knee, intact articular cartilage (less than grade III)

Contraindications:
Significant articular disease (grade III or IV), inflammatory arthritis, uncorrected comorbidities (malalignment, cartilage defects, ligament insufficiency)

Preoperative Planning:
Meniscus sizing: anteroposterior (meniscus width) and lateral (meniscus length [×0.8 for medial, ×0.7 for lateral meniscus]) radiographs, corrected for magnification
Meniscus preservation: fresh-frozen or cryopreserved

Surgical Technique:
Arthroscopic preparation: debride remaining meniscus to 1- to 2-mm rim; limited notchplasty; meniscus repair exposure on ipsilateral side
Exposure: mini-arthrotomy on ipsilateral side of patellar tendon
Slot preparation: in line with anterior and posterior horns; slot created with 4-mm bur; drill guide used for guide pin insertion; ream over guide pin; do not penetrate posterior cortex; box cutter and rasp
Meniscal allograft preparation: debride meniscus to attachment sites; bone bridge 7 mm wide and 1 cm high; remove bone beyond posterior horn; leave bone beyond anterior horn; number 0 PDS vertical mattress traction suture at posterior one-third junction
Meniscus insertion: nitinol pin to pass traction suture through repair incision; meniscus inserted through arthrotomy and reduced
Meniscus fixation: allograft bone screw for fixation of bone bridge in slot; inside-out vertical mattress sutures in meniscus
Closure: standard arthrotomy closure

Postoperative Management:
Hinged knee brace; range of motion 0 to 90 degrees first 4 weeks, then full motion; partial to full weight bearing over first 4 weeks, then weight bearing as tolerated; return to sports at 4 to 6 months

Contemporary understanding of the natural history and biomechanical consequences of the meniscectomized knee has led to a commitment to preserve the meniscus. However, there is an existing population of patients who have already undergone subtotal meniscectomy, in addition to cases in which meniscal preservation is not possible. In these cases, the knee suffers from the loss of meniscus function, including load sharing, shock absorption, joint stability, joint nutrition, and protection of the articular cartilage. In an effort to restore normal knee anatomy and biomechanics, meniscal allografts are used to replace the native meniscus in select symptomatic individuals. Excellent pain relief and improved function can be achieved with rigid adherence to surgical indications.

History

Patients typically report a history of one or more previous meniscectomies, performed arthroscopically or open. Usually, there is a near immediate and complete resolution of symptoms following open or arthroscopic meniscectomy. Over time, however, there is an increase in ipsilateral joint line pain, activity-related swelling, and generalized achiness affected by changes in the ambient barometric pressure. Occasionally, there are complaints of giving way and crepitus. A thorough history should elicit the mechanism of injury, associated injuries, and previous treatments, such as ligament reconstruction or management of articular cartilage lesions.

Physical Examination

Typically, patients experience tenderness along the ipsilateral joint line and may have palpable bony changes along the edges of the femoral or tibial condyle. The location of previous incisions should be noted and may provide evidence of prior meniscectomy. It is essential to evaluate for concomitant pathology that would modify treatment recommendations, such as malalignment or ligament deficiency. Because only minor degrees of arthritic change are considered acceptable in candidates for meniscus transplantation, motion is generally preserved.

Imaging

Diagnostic imaging should begin with a standard weight-bearing anteroposterior (AP) radiograph of both knees in full extension, a non–weight-bearing 45-degree-flexion lateral view, and an axial view of the patellofemoral joint. Additionally, a 45-degree-flexion weight-bearing posteroanterior radiograph is recommended to help identify subtle joint space narrowing that traditional extension views may fail to identify. Special studies such as a long-cassette mechanical axis view or magnetic resonance imaging should be ordered if there is any degree of clinical malalignment or

suspicion of chondral injury, respectively. Generally, magnetic resonance imaging should be reserved for difficult cases in which the diagnosis remains unknown, especially in the setting of completely normal radiographs. Techniques include two-dimensional fast spin echo and three-dimensional fat suppression with and without intra-articular gadolinium. When questions remain about the source of a patient's symptoms, a three-phase technetium bone scan is potentially useful. Both magnetic resonance imaging and bone scan may demonstrate increased signals in the affected compartment related to stress overload due to the meniscal deficiency.

Indications and Contraindications

Indications for meniscus transplantation are prior meniscectomy with persistent pain in the involved compartment, intact articular cartilage (less than grade III), normal alignment, and a stable joint. Simultaneous or staged ligament reconstruction or realignment procedures can be performed in patients who otherwise have appropriate indications for the procedure. In addition, patients with recurrent failure of anterior cruciate ligament (ACL) reconstruction who have medial meniscal deficiency may be candidates for combined ACL reconstruction and medial meniscus transplantation to increase knee stability. Contraindications are most commonly significant articular disease (grade III or IV) or radiographic osteoarthritic changes. Localized chondral defects can be treated concomitantly with cartilage restoration techniques. Additional contraindications are inflammatory arthritis, obesity, and previous infection.

Preoperative Planning

Concomitant Procedures

In cases of significant limb malalignment and ligament insufficiency, these deformities should be corrected either before or concomitant with meniscus transplantation. Technical considerations regarding the simultaneous performance of these procedures are discussed later.

Meniscus Sizing

Meniscal allografts are size and compartment specific. Precise preoperative measurements are obtained from AP and lateral radiographs with magnification markers placed on the skin at the level of the joint line. The meniscus width is determined on the AP radiograph (from the edge of the ipsilateral tibial spine to the edge of the tibial plateau), and the meniscus length is determined on the lateral radiograph (AP dimension of the ipsilateral tibial plateau). Following correction for magnification, this number is multiplied by 0.8 for the medial and 0.7 for the lateral meniscus (Fig. 53–1).

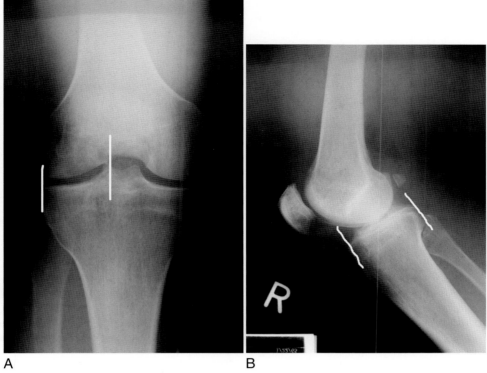

A   B

Figure 53–1   Meniscus sizing is performed by first correcting for magnification. *A*, Meniscus width (coronal plan) is calculated on the anteroposterior radiograph by measuring the distance from the peak of the tibial eminence (medial or lateral) to the tibial metaphyseal margin, ignoring marginal osteophytes. *B*, Meniscus length (sagittal plane) is determined on the lateral radiograph. The medial meniscal length is 80%, and the lateral mensical length is 70%, of the sagittal tibial plateau distance measured at the joint line between a line parallel to the anterior tibia and one tangential to the posterior plateau margin perpendicular to the joint line.

Meniscal Graft Processing and Preservation

Meniscal allografts are harvested using sterile surgical technique within 24 hours of death. Following the harvest, the tissue is preserved by one of four methods: fresh, cryopreservation, fresh-frozen, or lyophilization. Unlike in fresh osteochondral allografts, cell viability in meniscal allografts does not seem to improve the morphologic or biochemical characteristics of the grafts; thus, the most commonly implanted grafts are either fresh-frozen or cryopreserved. The risk of disease transmission is minimized through rigid donor screening, graft culturing, and polymerase chain reaction testing for human immunodeficiency virus (HIV).

Surgical Technique

Positioning

Depending on surgeon preference, the limb can be placed in a standard leg holder or maintained in the unsupported supine position. The posteromedial or posterolateral corner of the joint must be freely accessible to perform an inside-out meniscus suturing technique.

Examination under Anesthesia

An examination under anesthesia should be performed to confirm full range of motion and the absence of concomitant ligamentous laxity.

Diagnostic Arthroscopy

In most cases, diagnostic arthroscopy has been performed before surgery to confirm meniscal deficiency. However, at the time of surgery, meniscal deficiency and the integrity of the articular surface should be confirmed. In general, if chondral changes greater than grade III are present on the femoral condyle or tibial plateau, meniscus transplantation is not indicated, because the results will be compromised.

Specific Surgical Steps

Arthroscopic Preparation

The initial steps for medial and lateral meniscus transplantation are similar and are performed in the ipsilateral compartment only. The remaining meniscus is

6 Knee

arthroscopically debrided to a 1- to 2-mm peripheral rim until punctate bleeding occurs (Fig. 53–2). The remnant of the anterior and posterior meniscal horns can be maintained to provide a footprint for subsequent allograft placement. In addition, performing a limited notchplasty along the most inferior and posterior aspects of the femoral condyle adjacent to the cruciate ligaments is helpful to visualize the posterior horn and to pass the meniscus into the recipient slot. A standard meniscus repair exposure on the posteromedial or posterolateral joint line is performed and is situated one third above the joint line and two thirds below it to protect the neurovascular structures during an inside-out meniscus repair.

Exposure

It is necessary to perform a mini-arthrotomy in line with the anterior and posterior horns of the involved meniscus to permit accurate, "in-line" guide placement during slot formation and introduction of the meniscus. Depending on the surgeon's preference, the mini-arthrotomy may be immediately adjacent to the patellar tendon or in a portion of the patellar tendon in line with its fibers.

Slot Preparation

A slot is created based on the normal anatomy of the meniscus attachment sites. Using electrocautery, a line is marked to connect the centers of the anterior and posterior horn attachment sites. With this line as a guide, a 4-mm bur is used to create a superficial reference slot equal to the height of the bur and parallel to the sagittal slope of the tibial plateau (Fig. 53–3). A level slot

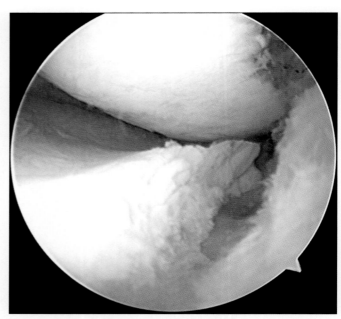

Figure 53–3   Arthroscopic view of the reference slot created in line with the anterior and posterior horns of the medial meniscus using a 4-mm arthroscopic bur to create a flat subchondral surface. This is facilitated by making a satellite portal through the patellar tendon at the level of the joint line in line with the horn insertion sites.

should be confirmed by placing a depth gauge in the reference slot; the depth gauge should also be used to determine the AP length of the tibial plateau. Using a drill guide, an insertion pin is placed under fluoroscopic guidance in a parallel fashion (Fig. 53–4). Care should be taken to ensure that the pin does not overpenetrate the posterior cortex. A reamer is then used to drill over the guide pin with a 7- or 8-mm cannulated drill bit (Fig. 53–5). The posterior cortex of the tibia should be maintained. A 7- or 8-mm box cutter is then used to create a slot 7 or 8 mm wide by 10 mm deep. A 7- or 8-mm rasp is used to smooth the final slot. This ensures that the bone bridge will slide smoothly into the slot (Fig. 53–6).

Meniscal Allograft Preparation

This technique creates a slotted meniscus within a 1-mm-undersized bone bridge. The undersized bridge prevents inadvertent bridge fracture during insertion. The attachment sites of the meniscus are identified on the bone block, and the accessory attachments to the meniscus are debrided. Only the true attachment sites should remain, usually 5 to 6 mm wide. The bone bridge is then cut to a width of 7 mm and a height of 1 cm. Any bone that extends beyond the posterior horn attachment should be removed. However, bone extending beyond the anterior horn attachment is left intact, because this provides graft integrity during insertion. A temporary vertical mattress traction suture is placed at the junction of the posterior middle third of the meniscus using a number 0 PDS suture (Fig. 53–7). The anterior horn of the medial meniscus usually extends to the anteriormost extent of the tibial plateau for its attachment. In addition, the

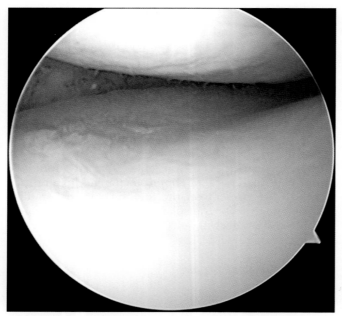

Figure 53–2   Arthroscopic view demonstrating the periphery of the host medial meniscus debrided to within 1 to 2 mm of the capsule to promote punctate bleeding.

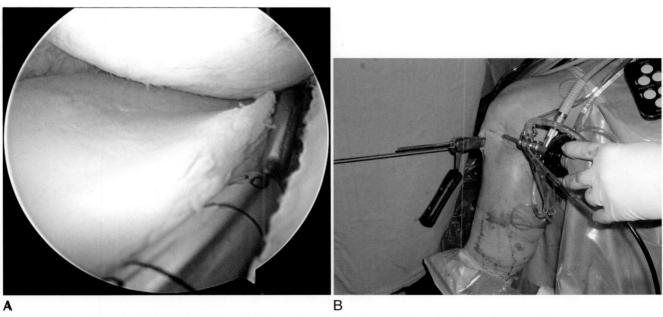

A   **B**

Figure 53–4   *A,* The reference arm (depth gauge) is placed through the top hole of the drill guide and rests within the reference slot. *B,* An insertion pin is placed in a parallel fashion through the inferior hole. To ensure that the pin does not overpenetrate the posterior cortex, it should be placed under fluoroscopic guidance.

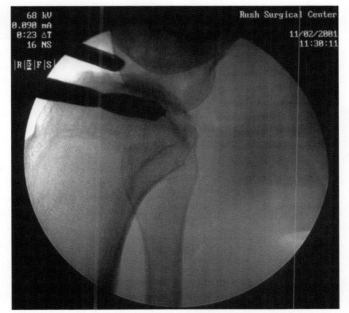

Figure 53–5   Fluoroscopic view of a 7-mm reamer passing over the guide pin, taking care to avoid penetrating the posterior cortex.

6 Knee

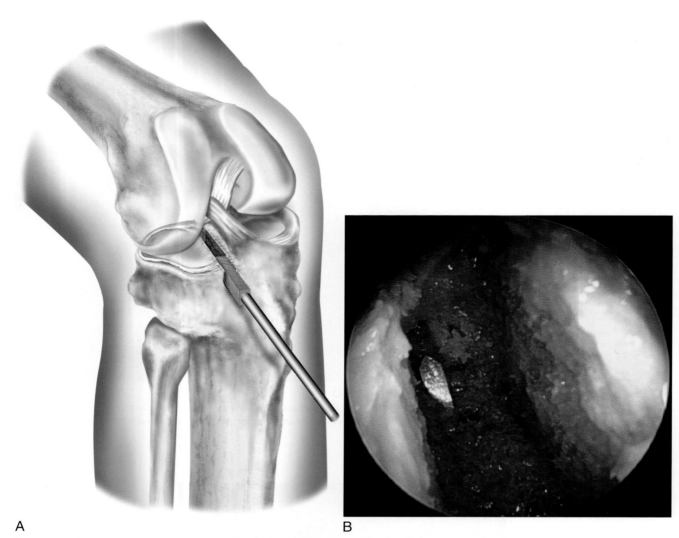

A   B

Figure 53–6 *A,* A 7- or 8-mm three-sided rasp is used to create the rectangular recipient slot. *B,* The recipient slot is uniform in nature from anterior to posterior, as seen arthroscopically. (Courtesy of Regeneration Technologies, Inc., Alachua, FL.)

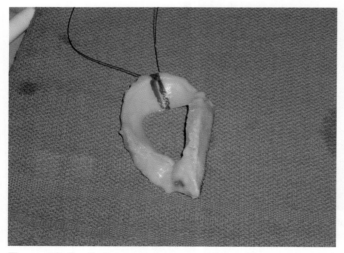

Figure 53–7 Medial meniscus prepared by creating a rectangular slot 7 mm wide and 1 cm deep, measured at the insertion of the anterior and posterior horns. A traction suture is placed at the junction of the posterior and middle third of the body of the meniscus to facilitate introduction into the knee.

anterior horn attachment can be 7 to 9 mm wide. If the anterior horn width is greater than 7 mm, the attachment should be left intact, and the width of the bone bridge should be increased appropriately in the area underneath the anterior horn only. The remainder of the bone bridge should be trimmed to 7 mm as planned. Before insertion, the most anterior aspect of the recipient slot should be widened to fit the enlarged bone bridge.

Meniscus Insertion and Fixation

A single-barrel zone-specific cannula for inside-out suture technique is placed in the contralateral portal and is used to advance a long nitinol suture-passing pin through the knee capsule at the attachment site of the posterior middle third of the meniscus. This should exit the accessory posteromedial or posterolateral incision. The proximal end of the nitinol pin is then withdrawn from the arthrotomy site to facilitate passage of the meniscus into the knee. The traction sutures are passed through the loop of the nitinol pin, and the sutures are withdrawn through the accessory incision.

The meniscus is inserted through the arthrotomy, taking care to align it with the recipient slot while gently pulling on the traction suture. The meniscus should be appropriately reduced. The proper size and position of the meniscus are confirmed by cycling the knee through its range of motion. An allograft cortical bone interference screw is used to achieve final fixation of the bone bridge in the slot (Fig. 53–8). The meniscus is then fixed with standard vertical mattress sutures using an inside-out technique (Fig. 53–9).

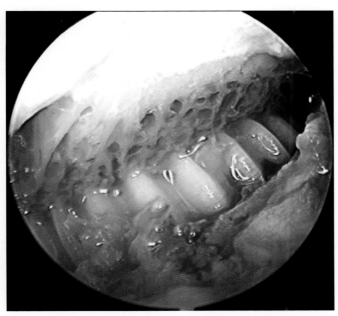

Figure 53–8 A fully threaded interference cortical bone screw is placed adjacent to the meniscus, achieving rigid fixation.

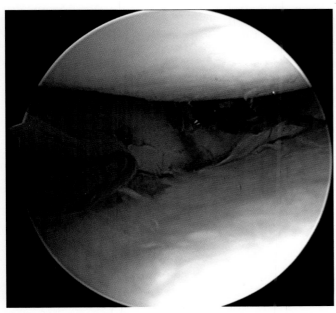

Figure 53–9 Medial meniscus is reduced and sutured to the periphery using 2-0 nonabsorbable vertically placed mattress sutures.

Closure

Standard closure of the arthrotomy and accessory incisions is performed.

Postoperative Management

There is progression from partial to full weight bearing with crutches over the first 4 postoperative weeks. The patient is placed in a hinged knee immobilizer and is allowed immediate motion from 0 to 90 degrees. Flexion with weight bearing is limited beyond 90 degrees for the first 4 weeks to protect the meniscus repair. At 4 weeks, full range of motion is allowed, and gentle strengthening is performed. In-line running is permitted at 12 weeks, and return to full activity is allowed at 4 to 6 months, provided lower extremity strength is at least 80% to 85% that of the nonoperated leg.

Results

Following meniscal allograft transplantation, good to excellent results are achieved in nearly 85% of cases, and patients demonstrate a measurable decrease in pain and increase in activity level (Table 53–1). The risk of graft failure seems to be greatest with irradiated grafts and in patients with grade III to IV osteoarthritic changes.[6]

Table 53–1	Clinical Results of Meniscal Allograft Transplantation	
Author (Date)	**Follow-up**	**Outcome**
Milachowski et al. (1989)[5]	14 mo mean	19 of 22 (86%) successful
Garrett (1993)[3]	2-7 yr	35 of 43 (81%) successful
Noyes et al. (1995)[6]	30 mo mean (range, 22-58 mo)	56 of 96 (58%) failed
van Arkel and de Boer (1995)[9]	2-5 yr	20 of 23 (87%) successful
Cameron and Saha (1997)[1]	31 mo mean (range, 12-66 mo)	58 of 63 (92%) successful
Goble et al. (1996)[4]	2 yr minimum	17 of 18 (94%) successful
Carter (1999)[2]	48 mo mean	45 of 51 (88%) successful
Rodeo (2001)[8]	2 yr minimum	22 of 33 (67%) successful 14 of 16 (88%) bone fixation 8 of 17 (47%) no bone fixation
Rath et al. (2001)[7]	5.4 yr mean (range, 2-8 yr)	14 of 22 (64%) successful

Complications

Complications are rare and are similar to those following meniscus repair. These include incomplete healing of the meniscus repair, infection, arthrofibrosis, and neurovascular injury related to the repair technique. Persistent symptoms despite meniscal allograft are most frequently related to improper patient selection. Traumatic tears of the meniscus occur occasionally following meniscus transplantation and can be treated with standard arthroscopic meniscal repair techniques or partial meniscectomy when necessary.

Technical Considerations for Concomitant Procedures

High Tibial Osteotomy

Patients with a history of meniscectomy who develop secondary varus or valgus deformity should be treated with concomitant high tibial or distal femoral osteotomy, respectively. If performed as separate procedures, the limb realignment should be done first. When performed simultaneously, the meniscus transplant is completed first. Otherwise, the varus and valgus stress during the transplantation procedure could create excessive stress at the osteotomy site. Extreme caution must be used to avoid creating a fracture through the slot to the osteotomy site.

Anterior Cruciate Ligament Reconstruction

Any concomitant ligamentous laxity must be addressed at the time of meniscus transplantation. When the surgeon is performing an ACL reconstruction and meniscus transplantation, all the soft tissue portions of the transplant technique should be performed first; then the ACL tibial and femoral tunnels should be reamed before meniscus slot placement. Placing the tibial ACL tunnel as close to the midline as possible decreases the interference between the tunnel and the meniscus slot. In addition, the meniscus bone bridge is trimmed at the site of the intersection with the ACL tunnel. When using a patellar tendon graft, the bone bridge of the meniscal allograft is temporarily elevated to allow passage of the bone and is then reduced, as the tendon portion occupies a much smaller volume of the tunnel.

Autologous Chondrocyte Implantation or Osteochondral Allografting

If an isolated chondral defect exists, it should be treated at the time of meniscus transplantation. It is typically easier and safer for the chondral procedure to be performed after all the steps of the meniscus transplant have been completed. This avoids any inadvertent damage to the articular cartilage graft during instrumentation or suture placement.

References

1. Cameron JC, Saha S: Meniscal allograft transplantation for unicompartmental arthritis of the knee. Clin Orthop 337:164-171, 1997.
2. Carter TR: Meniscal allograft transplantation. Sports Med Arthrosc Rev 7:51-62, 1999.
3. Garrett JC: Meniscal transplantation: A review of 43 cases with two to seven year follow-up. Sports Med Arthrosc Rev 1:164-167, 1993.
4. Goble EM, Kane SM, Wilcox TR, Doucette SA: Meniscal allografts. In McGinty JB, Caspari RB, Jackson RW, Poehling GG (eds): Operative Arthroscopy. Philadelphia, Lippincott-Raven, 1996, pp 317-331.
5. Milachowski KA, Weismeir K, Wirth CJ: Homologous meniscus transplantation: Experimental and clinical results. Int Orthop 13:1-11, 1989.
6. Noyes FR, Barber-Westin SD: Irradiated meniscus allografts in the human knee: A two to five year follow-up. Orthop Trans 19:417, 1995.
7. Rath E, Richmond J, Yassir W, et al: Meniscal allograft transplantation: Two to eight year results. Am J Sports Med 29:410-414, 2001.
8. Rodeo SA: Current concepts: Meniscus allografts—where do we stand? Am J Sports Med 29:246-261, 2001.
9. van Arkel ERA, de Boer HH: Human meniscal transplantation: Preliminary results at 2- to 5-year follow-up. J Bone Joint Surg Br 77:589-595, 1995.

54

Knee Cartilage: Diagnosis and Decision Making

KEVIN B. FREEDMAN, JEFF A. FOX, AND BRIAN J. COLE

Articular cartilage is vulnerable to irreversible traumatic injury and degenerative disease. Damaged articular cartilage has a limited ability to heal without intervention owing to two primary factors: lack of a vascular response, and relative absence of an undifferentiated cell population to respond to injury. The rationale for early surgical intervention for articular cartilage injuries is based on the symptomatic nature of focal chondral lesions and the potential for these lesions to progress.

The surgical management of articular cartilage defects is based on several underlying principles, including the reduction of symptoms, improvement in joint congruence and force distribution, and prevention of additional cartilage damage. This chapter reviews the anatomy and biomechanics of articular cartilage, discusses the clinical evaluation of these injuries, and provides a practical approach to the treatment of symptomatic articular cartilage injuries.

Anatomy and Biomechanics

The function of articular cartilage is to provide for smooth, pain-free gliding of the joints during skeletal motion. The architecture of articular cartilage is such that it provides a low coefficient of friction to allow smooth motion throughout a lifetime. However, normal function requires maintenance of the structural properties and the metabolic function of cartilage.

Articular cartilage is composed of a large extracellular matrix including type II collagen and proteoglycan aggregates. Collagen fibers give cartilage its form and tensile strength, and water constitutes 75% to 80% of the extracellular matrix, functioning largely in compression. In addition, chondrocytes synthesize and degrade proteoglycans and are responsible for cartilage homeostasis.

The structure of articular cartilage can be divided into three zones—superficial, transitional, and deep—each of which imparts mechanical properties contributing to the ultimate function of the articular surface. The superficial zone is composed primarily of collagen fibers oriented parallel to the joint surface, and it primarily resists shear forces. The middle, or transitional, zone is composed of obliquely oriented collagen fibers and primarily resists compressive forces. The fibers in the deep zone are oriented perpendicular to the subchondral plate, and this zone resists both compressive and shear forces. Injury to any one of these layers, the chondrocytes, or the subchondral bone can disrupt the normal biomechanical properties of articular cartilage, leading to further degeneration.

Historical Aspects

Both partial- and full-thickness lesions have limited capacity for repair. The avascular nature of articular cartilage and the limited stem cell population limit the healing response following injury. In addition, the constant load of articular cartilage, particularly in the knee, creates a challenging mechanical environment for an appropriate healing response.

The natural history of asymptomatic focal chondral defects is not well documented. It is thought that chondral injuries lead to the development of degenerative arthritis, although this has not been proved. Recent studies of unipolar, unicompartmental, full-thickness articular cartilage lesions following debridement have shown progression to radiographic joint space narrowing.[22] Symptomatic lesions, however, are unlikely to become quiescent without significant activity restriction or some form of surgical intervention.

Clinical Evaluation

History

Patients with chondral or osteochondral injuries typically report either a twisting, shearing-type injury combined with an axial load or significant blunt trauma causing an impaction injury. In addition, these lesions are commonly associated with other soft tissue injuries about the knee, including condylar lesions from ligament rupture (anterior cruciate ligament tears), or patellar or trochlear lesions following patellar dislocation. Full-thickness chondral injuries can account for 5% to 10% of the pathology following acute hemarthrosis and must be suspected in sports- or work-related injuries.[26]

Symptomatic chondral lesions typically present as knee pain localized to the affected compartment: the medial or lateral hemijoint for medial or lateral condyle injuries, and the patellofemoral joint for patellar or trochlear lesions. Weight-bearing activities typically aggravate symptoms from lesions on the medial or lateral femoral condyle. Activities such as sitting, stair climbing, and squatting aggravate patellofemoral lesions. In addition, recurrent effusions, catching, and locking can occur with symptomatic chondral lesions. Patients with documented lesions who have atypical symptoms should be critically evaluated to prevent inadvertent treatment of coexisting incidental lesions.

Physical Examination

Patients are typically tender along the ipsilateral joint line or condyle. Patients with patellar or trochlear lesions typically have patellar crepitation and a positive patellar grind and inhibition test. An effusion may be present as well. It is essential to evaluate for concomitant pathology that would modify treatment recommendations, such as malalignment or ligament deficiency. For medial or lateral condyle injuries, careful attention must be paid to any varus or valgus limb alignment. For patellar or trochlear lesions, maltracking of the patella, including a tight lateral retinaculum or high Q angle, must be evaluated. In addition, signs of meniscal pathology must be evaluated, because coexisting disease is frequently present. Finally, any ligamentous injury must be noted; failure to address these injuries can lead to early failure of any articular cartilage repair technique.

Imaging

Standard diagnostic imaging should include a standard weight-bearing anteroposterior radiograph of both knees in full extension, a non–weight-bearing 45-degree-flexion lateral view, and an axial view of the patellofemoral joint. In addition, a 45-degree-flexion weight-bearing posteroanterior radiograph is recommended to identify subtle joint space narrowing that traditional extension views may miss. If there is any degree of clinical malalignment, a long-cassette mechanical axis view should be ordered to evaluate the mechanical axis of the limb.

Magnetic resonance imaging can be helpful in delineating the extent of articular cartilage lesions, especially in the setting of completely normal radiographs. It can define the location, size, and depth of chondral injuries and can evaluate any subchondral fractures, bone bruises, or osteochondritis dissecans lesions. Magnetic resonance imaging can also assess the stability of an osteochondral lesion: fluid behind the lesion indicates an unstable lesion that may be amenable to surgical stabilization. Evolving techniques, including two-dimensional fat suppression, three-dimensional fast spin-echo sequences, and gadolinium enhancement, provide accurate information on the presence and size of articular cartilage lesions and may assist in the evaluation of patients after cartilage restoration procedures.

Classification

Focal chondral defects of the femur are a specific subset of articular cartilage injuries. The Modified International Cartilage Repair Society Chondral Injury Classification System classifies chondral injuries based on the amount and depth of the cartilage lesion. Most commonly, these lesions are classified using the modified Outerbridge system (Table 54–1).[27] Other important factors that affect the ability of cartilage lesions to heal with operative treatment include the location and size of the lesion, the depth and condition of the subchondral bone, the condition of the surrounding normal cartilage, and coexisting knee pathology. In addition, it is important to recognize any bony deficiency that may alter the treatment plan for the repair of chondral injuries

In addition to classifying lesions by depth and size, it is important to consider other factors when determining the appropriate treatment. These include whether the defect is acute or chronic, the defect's location, associated ligamentous instability, integrity of the meniscus, and tibiofemoral or patellofemoral malalignment. Many patient factors must also be considered, including age, activity level, occupation, expectations, body weight, presence of systemic disease, and results of previous treatment attempts.

Associated Injuries

The most common associated injuries are ligament and meniscus tears. The meniscus functions in both load

Table 54–1 Modified Outerbridge Classification of Cartilage Lesions

Grade	Description
I	Softening of articular cartilage
II	Fibrillation or superficial fissures of cartilage
III	Deep fissuring of cartilage without exposed bone
IV	Exposed subchondral bone

From Outerbridge R: The etiology of chondromalacia patellae. J Bone Joint Surg Br 43:752-757, 1961.

distribution and shock absorption. The detrimental effects of meniscal deficiency, leading to excessive articular cartilage load and the development of osteoarthritis, have been well documented.[17,33,34] Although meniscal and chondral injuries can occur concomitantly, it is likely that many chondral injuries occur secondary to meniscal deficiency. Alternatively, a highly irregular articular surface may predispose a patient to a meniscus tear. Every attempt should be made to preserve and repair the meniscus, especially in the presence of a chondral defect. If a chondral defect is present in a meniscus-deficient knee, it is essential that the meniscal deficiency be addressed (e.g., with meniscal allograft transplantation) when treating the articular cartilage lesion. In addition, any ligamentous instability must be addressed before or at the time of articular cartilage repair. Knee instability will lead to excessive shear forces and early failure of articular cartilage repair.

If varus malalignment exists in the presence of medial condyle disease, a valgus-producing high tibial osteotomy should be performed to improve the predictability of the repair. Similarly, valgus malalignment should be treated with distal femoral osteotomy. When treating patellar or trochlear chondral lesions, there is an increasing trend toward distal realignment with anteriorization or anteromedialization of the tibial tubercle, even in the face of normal patellar tracking. This is performed primarily to unload the patellofemoral compartment and protect the cartilage repair site.

Treatment Options

Nonoperative

Nonoperative treatment for chondral injuries is generally reserved for asymptomatic lesions. Small, incidental chondral lesions can be treated with benign neglect in the absence of clinical symptoms, although defect progression is possible. Nonoperative treatment of symptomatic lesions is unlikely to be successful but includes a regimen similar to that for osteoarthritis. This includes nonsteroidal anti-inflammatory medications, physical therapy, intra-articular corticosteroid or hyaluronic acid injections, and nutritional supplementation with chondroitin and glucosamine sulfate. Unfortunately, in higher-demand patients with symptoms attributable to the defect, nonoperative treatment is rarely successful. If symptoms persist despite nonsurgical treatment, surgical intervention is warranted. Although there are no definitive guidelines for the length of nonsurgical treatment, it is generally believed that symptomatic chondral lesions should be treated aggressively, because progression and further cartilage deterioration may limit the benefits of cartilage restoration.

Operative

The principal goals in the surgical management of symptomatic chondral defects are to reduce symptoms, improve joint congruence, and prevent additional cartilage deterioration. Primary repair should be attempted for all traumatic lesions and symptomatic unstable osteochondritis dissecans lesions with a viable osteoarticular fragment of at least $1\,cm^2$ and an adequate bony bed for fixation.

For those lesions that cannot be primarily repaired, the treatment options can be characterized as palliative, reparative, or restorative. Palliative procedures, such as debridement and lavage, are used for incidentally discovered lesions or symptomatic lesions in low-demand patients with a preponderance of mechanical symptoms or signs of meniscal pathology. In these instances, there is no attempt to repair or replace the damaged articular cartilage. Reparative procedures, such as marrow-stimulating techniques (drilling, abrasion arthroplasty, or microfracture), promote a fibrocartilage healing response in the area of the defect. Restorative techniques replace the damaged cartilage with new articular cartilage; these include autologous chondrocyte implantation, osteochondral autografting, and fresh osteochondral allografting. Taking into account the factors previously discussed, a treatment algorithm has been developed to guide the implementation of these options (Fig. 54–1).

Primary Repair

For acute osteochondral lesions or in situ and unstable osteochondritis dissecans, primary repair should be attempted. The size and location of the lesion are the primary determinants of whether the fragment needs to be removed or can be stabilized. Every attempt should be made to fix large fragments ($>1\,cm^2$) from the weight-bearing portion of the femoral condyles. Some lesions are amenable to arthroscopic fixation, but an arthrotomy may be necessary for adequate reduction and fixation of the fragment. Fixation is usually performed provisionally with K-wires and then with bioabsorbable pins or metal screws (Fig. 54–2). Typically, patients are kept non–weight bearing following repair, and the screws are removed 8 to 10 weeks postoperatively. Continuous passive motion may be used, or patients are asked to perform 600 to 800 cycles/day without the use of a formal machine. If headless screws are used and are sufficiently recessed in the subchondral bone, there may be no need for removal.

Debridement and Lavage

Palliative procedures such as debridement and lavage are reserved for lower-demand patients with incidentally discovered chondral lesions or those with small lesions (<2 to $3\,cm^2$) and limited symptoms. Debridement can be particularly helpful for patients with mechanical symptoms from a loose chondral flap. However, relief from debridement and lavage may be incomplete and temporary. Postoperative rehabilitation is relatively straightforward and should include weight bearing and resumption of activities as tolerated.

Thermal debridement of partial-thickness articular cartilage injuries is currently being investigated. Proponents of thermal debridement advocate this treatment

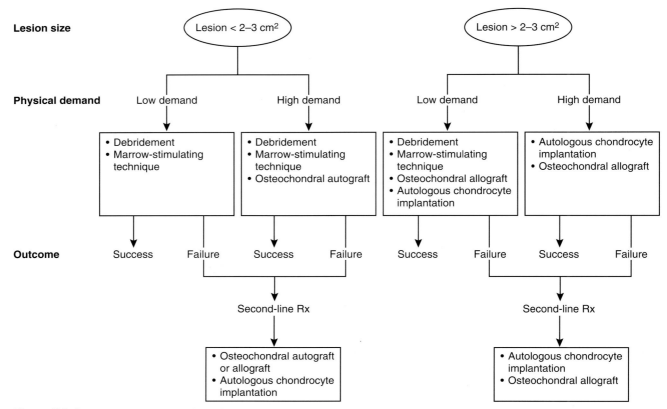

Figure 54–1 Treatment algorithm for articular cartilage lesions.

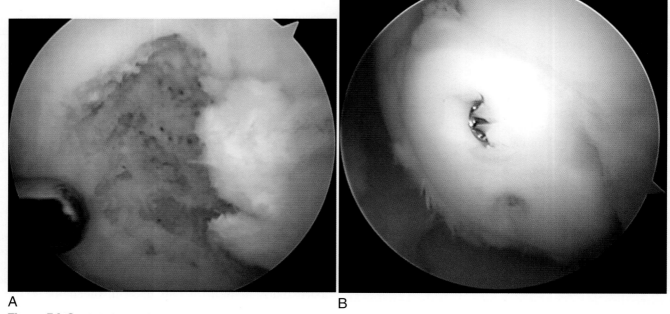

Figure 54–2 *A*, Arthroscopic example of an unstable osteochondritis dissecans lesion of the medial femoral condyle considered amenable to repair. *B*, Arthroscopic picture of the lesion repaired with two variably pitched headless screws.

for the smoothing of articular cartilage and the containment of articular cartilage lesions (preventing propagation). However, if improperly used, thermal treatment can cause injury to the underlying or surrounding normal cartilage and potentially affect the subchondral bone.[7,21] Therefore, thermal treatment of articular cartilage injuries must be approached with caution.

Marrow-Stimulating Techniques

For patients with small to moderate-sized lesions (1 to 5 cm^2) and moderate demands, marrow-stimulating techniques such as drilling, abrasion arthroplasty, and microfracture can be used. All these techniques are used to stimulate fibrocartilage ingrowth into the chondral defect. Abrasion arthroplasty was initially developed by Pridie[31] as an open technique in 1959,[18] and it was later modified for arthroscopic use by Johnson.[19] Abrasion arthroplasty has been used mostly for osteoarthritic knees rather than focal chondral defects. At this time, microfracture is the most commonly accepted technique for marrow stimulation (Fig. 54–3). It involves providing fibrocartilage repair tissue to the focal chondral defect by debriding the lesion through the calcified layer and penetrating the subchondral plate with specialized awls in an effort to expose the damaged area to progenitor cells present within the subchondral bone. In many cases, microfracture is used as a first-line treatment for focal chondral defects in the hope that larger cartilage restoration procedures can be avoided. Optimal results following microfracture come from rigid adherence to the postoperative protocol, so the procedure should not be performed casually. Postoperative management requires a prolonged period of non–weight bearing (4 to

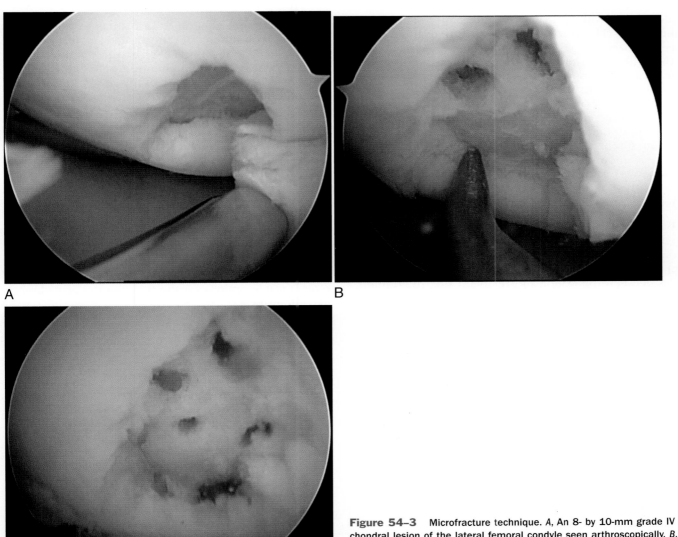

Figure 54–3 Microfracture technique. *A*, An 8- by 10-mm grade IV chondral lesion of the lateral femoral condyle seen arthroscopically. *B*, Microfracture awls are used to penetrate the subchondral bone to allow the marrow elements to enter the lesion. *C*, The final prepared lesion.

6 weeks) with continuous passive motion, or patients are asked to perform 600 to 800 cycles/day without the use of a formal machine.

Cartilage Restoration Techniques

AUTOLOGOUS CHONDROCYTE IMPLANTATION

Autologous chondrocyte implantation (ACI; Fig. 54–4) is indicated for intermediate- to high-demand patients with symptomatic articular cartilage lesions who have failed at least an attempt at arthroscopic debridement. This technique is used primarily for larger (2 to $10\,cm^2$) symptomatic lesions of the knee, principally of the femoral condyles. Recent literature supports its use for trochlear and patellar lesions, especially when combined with distal realignment procedures.[29] ACI is a two-stage technique in which 200 to 300 mg of autologous chondrocytes are biopsied arthroscopically in the first stage and implanted through an arthrotomy in the second stage. Coverage is obtained by a periosteal patch sewn with 6-0 Vicryl suture and sealed with fibrin glue. The repair tissue from this technique has been shown to be durable, mechanically firm, and hyaline-like in histology.[29] Lesions of osteochondritis dissecans are also appropriate candidates for ACI, provided that the depth of bone loss is less than 6 to 8 mm. The postoperative course is demanding, with a prolonged period of protected weight bearing and range of motion with continuous passive motion for 4 to 6 weeks. Symptom relief is generally predictable, but it may take 12 to 18 months for some lesions (e.g., patellofemoral lesions).

OSTEOCHONDRAL AUTOGRAFT TRANSPLANTATION

Osteochondral autograft transplantation (Fig. 54–5) is generally used for chondral lesions of the femoral condyle. These grafts are not generally recommended for the patella, owing to a mismatch of cartilage thickness between the donor and recipient site. In addition, care must be taken to match the curvature of the trochlea when such grafts are used for these lesions. They are generally used for small to medium-sized lesions (0.5 to $3\,cm^2$), owing to limited donor site availability. Donor grafts can be harvested arthroscopically or through a small incision from the intercondylar notch or the lateral femoral trochlea. For larger lesions, the "mosaicplasty" technique of multiple plugs can be used. The advantages of osteochondral autografts are that they are autogenous tissue and have immediate normal hyaline architecture. There are several disadvantages of osteochondral autografts, however, including donor site morbidity, technical difficulty in achieving proper graft orientation and placement, residual gaps between the cartilage plugs, and the potential for cartilage or subchondral bone breakdown resulting from graft handling or improper placement.

OSTEOCHONDRAL ALLOGRAFT TRANSPLANTATION

Fresh osteochondral allograft transplantation (Fig. 54–6) involves the implantation of a composite cadaveric graft that includes the subchondral bone and overlying hyaline cartilage in the site of the chondral defect. Osteochondral allograft transplants are used for medium to large articular cartilage lesions in relatively high-demand patients who tend to be somewhat older and often have associated bone loss (>6 to 8 mm) or for larger articular cartilage lesions ($3\,cm^2$ up to an entire hemicondyle) in both low- and high-demand patients. These grafts are most commonly used on the femoral condyles but can also be used for the patella, trochlea, and medial and lateral tibial plateau along with the donor meniscus. Another relative consideration is patient age, with patients older than 40 years possibly being better candidates for allografting than for ACI because of biologic considerations and perhaps the patient's unwillingness to engage in the prolonged recovery process associated with ACI. Additionally, young patients with superficial chondral injury only may best be treated with ACI rather than osteochondral allografting simply because the subchondral bone is left undisturbed with the former procedure.

Osteochondral allograft transplantation depends on anatomic restitution of the articular surface with size-matched donor tissue. Fresh osteochondral tissue demonstrates good donor chondrocyte viability (60% or greater) at biopsy.[11] A major advantage of osteochondral allografts is the ability to replace large osteochondral defects with a single-stage procedure; disadvantages include availability, technical difficulty, cost, and possible disease transmission. Postoperatively, patients are kept non–weight bearing for 6 to 8 weeks and use continuous passive motion.

ARTHROPLASTY

Although the focus of this chapter is on other alternatives for the repair or restoration of articular cartilage defects, prosthetic arthroplasty techniques, including unicondylar, patellofemoral, and total knee arthroplasty, remain viable options for the treatment of articular cartilage injuries.

Rehabilitation Principles

The specific rehabilitation regimens for each procedure for cartilage repair or restoration are outlined in the chapters on specific techniques. However, several general principles apply. Rehabilitation following palliative procedures allows a rapid return to activities with no restrictions on weight bearing or range of motion. Reparative procedures require strict protection of the lesion from loading to allow healing of the defect, while encouraging full range of motion for cartilage nutrition. Similarly, restorative procedures require protection of the healing articular surface from weight bearing, while encouraging range of motion. After 6 weeks of protection, weight bearing is usually advanced. The return to full activity depends on the procedure performed and can take from 4 to 18 months.

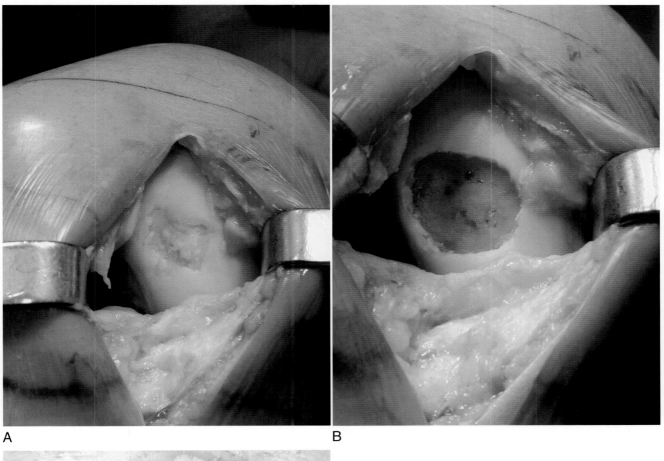

A

B

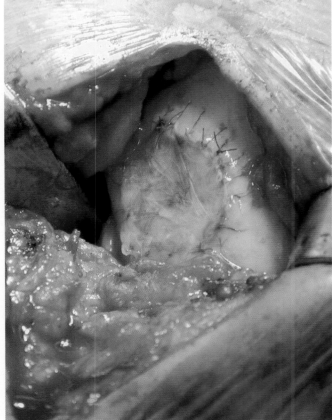

C

Figure 54–4   Autologous chondrocyte implantation. *A*, A 20- by 15-mm grade IV chondral lesion of the medial femoral condyle seen via a mini-arthrotomy before preparation for transplantation. *B*, The lesion is prepared for transplantation. *C*, The periosteal patch is sewn in place and sealed with fibrin glue, and the cells are injected.

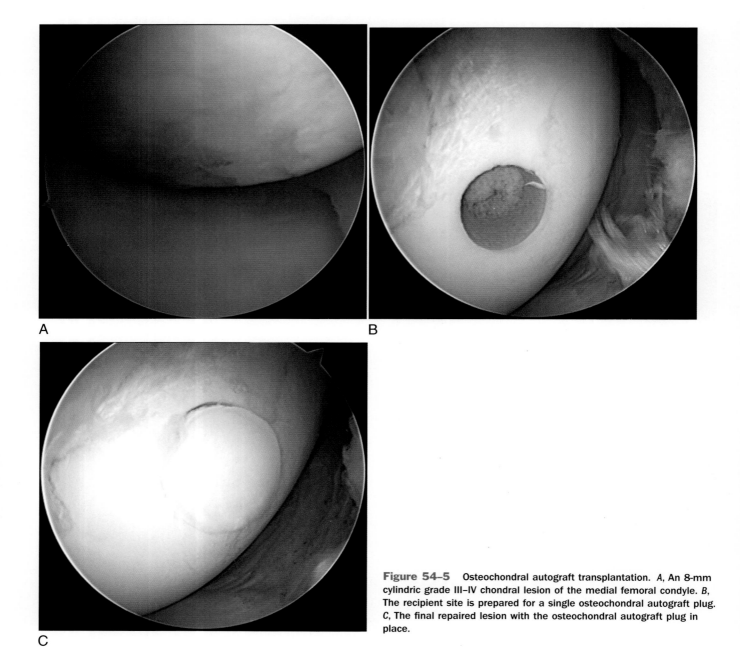

A

B

C

Figure 54–5 Osteochondral autograft transplantation. *A,* An 8-mm cylindric grade III–IV chondral lesion of the medial femoral condyle. *B,* The recipient site is prepared for a single osteochondral autograft plug. *C,* The final repaired lesion with the osteochondral autograft plug in place.

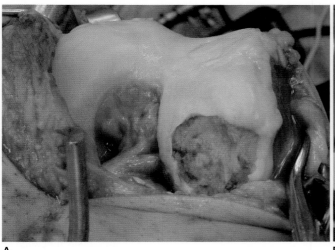

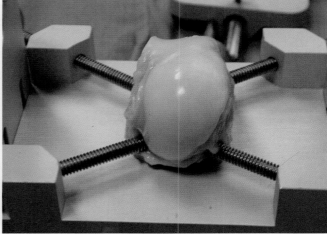

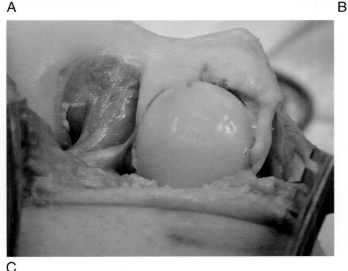

Figure 54-6 Osteochondral allograft transplantation. *A,* A 24- by 28-mm irregular grade IV lesion of the lateral femoral condyle. *B,* The allograft hemicondyle is placed in the cutting jig for preparation of the donor allograft plug. *C,* The osteochondral allograft plug fills the large chondral defect.

Results

There are many published reports on the results on each type of treatment for articular cartilage injuries; however, there are very few trials comparing treatment options. In addition, given the varying indications for each procedure, it is important to recognize the difficulty in comparing the results of treatment options for articular cartilage lesions. Population differences among trials, including patient age, lesion size, lesion location, and concomitant pathology, all affect the ability to make comparisons. In addition, it is important to recognize that good results can be achieved with each treatment technique in the appropriate patient population.

The results for articular cartilage debridement are limited to predominantly older studies in arthritic knees. Federico and Reider[8] performed simple mechanical debridement for traumatic and atraumatic chondromalacia patellae and achieved 58% good or excellent results in traumatic patients and 41% good or excellent results in atraumatic patients. Another study found that

superior clinical outcomes were obtained with patellar debridement using bipolar frequency versus a mechanical shaver for isolated patellar chondral lesions.[28] Simple debridement, with removal of loose cartilaginous flaps, can be performed for incidentally discovered asymptomatic lesions or small symptomatic lesions in low-demand patients.

The results for marrow-stimulating techniques, including abrasion arthroplasty and microfracture, are listed in Table 54-2. Overall, the results of abrasion arthroplasty have been unpredictable, and recurrent symptoms often develop within 2 to 3 years. Microfracture has shown promising results as first-line treatment in smaller chondral lesions, but there are few published clinical studies documenting the success rate of the procedure.

The results for cartilage restoration techniques (osteochondral autografts, osteochondral allografts, and autologous chondrocyte transplantation) are shown in Table 54-3. Success has been achieved in a high proportion of patients using each of these procedures, indicating that they are acceptable options for patients with articular cartilage lesions. However, the different patient populations

Table 54–2

Clinical Results of Marrow-Stimulation Techniques

Author (Date)	Technique	No. of Patients	Indications	Mean Follow-up	Outcome
Rand (1991)[32]	Abrasion arthroplasty	28	Degenerative arthritis	3.8 yr	39% good/excellent 29% unchanged/fair 32% worse/poor
Bert and Maschka (1989)[2]	Abrasion arthroplasty	59	Degenerative arthritis	60 mo	51% good/excellent 16% unchanged/fair 33% worse/poor
Friedman et al. (1984)[9]	Abrasion arthroplasty	73	Degenerative arthritis	>6 mo	60% good/excellent 34% unchanged/fair 6% worse/poor
Gill and MacGillivray (2001)[12]	Microfracture	100	Focal chondral defect	6 yr	Significant reduction in pain and swelling and improved function
Gill and MacGillivray (2001)[12]	Microfracture	19	Focal chondral defect	3 yr	74% minimal or no pain 63% good/excellent
Steadman et al. (2002)[35]	Microfracture	71	Focal chondral defect	11 yr	Lysholm improved Tegner improved (3.1–5.8, mean)

Table 54–3

Clinical Results of Cartilage Restoration Techniques

Author (Date)	Technique	Type/Location	No. of Patients	Mean Follow-up	Outcome
Hangody et al. (2001)[15]	OC autograft	Femur	461	>1 yr	92% good/excellent
		Patella, trochlea	93		81% good/excellent
		Tibia	24		88% good/excellent
Kish et al. (1999)[20]	OC autograft	Femur	52	>12 mo	100% good/excellent
Bradley (1999)[3]	OC autograft	—	145	18 mo	43% good/excellent 43% satisfactory 12% poor
Hangody et al. (1998)[16]	OC autograft	Femur, patella	57	48 mo	91% good/excellent
Aubin et al. (2001)[1]	OC allograft	Femur	60	10 yr	66% good/excellent 20% failure
Bugbee et al. (2000)[5]	OC allograft	Femur	122	5 yr	91% successful 5% failure
Chu et al. (1999)[6]	OC allograft	Femur, tibia, patella	55	6.3 yr	76% good/excellent 16% failure
Gross (1997)[14]	OC allograft	Femur, tibia, patella	123	7.5 yr	85% successful
Garrett (1994)[10]	OC allograft	Femur	17	3.5 yr	94% successful
Meyers et al. (1989)[23]	OC allograft	Femur, tibia, patella	39	3.6 yr	78% successful 22% failure
Peterson et al. (2002)[29]	ACI	Femur	18	>5 yr	89% good/excellent
		OCD	14	>5 yr	86% good/excellent
		Patella	17	>5 yr	65% good/excellent
		Femur, ACL	11	>5 yr	91% good/excellent
Minas (2001)[25]	ACI	Femur, tibia, patella, trochlea	169	>1 yr	85% significant improvement
Micheli et al. (2001)[24]	ACI	Femur, patella, trochlea	50	>3 yr	84% significant improvement
Peterson et al. (2000)[30]	ACI	Femur	25	>2 yr	92% good/excellent
		Patella	19	>2 yr	65% good/excellent
		Femur, ACL	16	>2 yr	75% good/excellent
		Multiple	16	>2 yr	67% good/excellent
Gillogly et al. (1998)[13]	ACI	Femur, patella, tibia	25	>1 yr	88% good/excellent
Brittberg et al. (1994)[4]	ACI	Femur, patella	16	39 m	88% good/excellent
		Patella	7	36 m	29% good/excellent

ACI, autologous chondrocyte implantation; ACL, anterior cruciate ligament; OC, osteochondral; OCD, osteochondritis dissecans.

and the nonstandardized reporting of results make it difficult to recommend one procedure over another on a scientific basis.

Complications

Complications following the treatment of articular cartilage injuries are rare and mimic those seen following arthroscopy. The most common complication is incomplete resolution of symptoms or recurrence of pain. In such situations, one would typically advance from a first-line to a second-line treatment. Other major complications include postoperative stiffness, especially with combined procedures (e.g., meniscal allograft transplantation) or those performed on patellar or trochlear lesions. Reparative techniques are unlikely to cause complications other than recurrence of symptoms. Subchondral drilling, however, can cause thermal injury to bone, which is why microfracture is the preferred technique for marrow stimulation.

Restorative techniques have complications unique to each procedure. Some complications associated with ACI, including hypertrophy and detachment, are related to the periosteum. These may be amenable to arthroscopic debridement. In addition, osteochondral grafts can be complicated by dislodgment of the graft from the transplant site, which is rare with the press-fit technique. Additionally, graft collapse can occur through biomechanical overload or biologic failure of the chondral or subchondral components.

Treatment Algorithm

Rigid adherence to the technical and postoperative requirements of each procedure is critical to the success of any treatment option; however, appropriate patient selection for a specific treatment is paramount to successfully reducing symptoms and improving function. In addition, there is substantial overlap between treatment options, and multiple factors must be considered, adding to the complexity of the treatment decision. Primary factors that must be considered include defect-specific factors such as size, depth, location, and degree of containment. Patient-specific factors include the results of prior treatment, comorbidities (e.g., ligament insufficiency, meniscal deficiency), patient age, current and desired activity level, patient expectations, and surgeon comfort and experience.

When considering the three major factors in the treatment decision—lesion size, patient demand, and whether this is primary or secondary treatment—an algorithm can be formulated to help guide the decision (see Fig. 54–1). Our preferred treatment for each arm of the algorithm is highlighted. However, these treatment recommendations are commonly modified based on additional patient factors, as mentioned previously.

In general, we prefer simple debridement only in small to medium-sized lesions (<2 to $5\,cm^2$) in low-demand patients. For small lesions in higher-demand patients, we initially attempt microfracture as a marrow-stimulating technique. If this fails to resolve symptoms, we progress osteochondral autografting. For medium-sized lesions in this population, ACI is frequently used. Lesions with significant bone loss (>6 to $8\,mm$) may be treated best with fresh osteochondral allografting.

For larger lesions, our primary treatment is debridement or microfracture for older, lower-demand patients. Although we may also microfracture these defects in higher-demand or younger patients, we often consider performing a biopsy for ACI, given the more guarded prognosis that microfracture has in this population. If there is a significant bony defect or the defect is particularly large, consideration is given to osteochondral allografting as a secondary treatment. Secondary treatment of patients who fail ACI may include osteochondral allografting as well. Although several factors can modify the treatment decision, including coexisting pathology that needs to be addressed concomitantly, having a general approach to these lesions helps determine the optimal treatment (Table 54–4 summarizes the decision-making process).

Future Directions

Undoubtedly, cartilage restoration techniques will evolve over the next several decades. It is likely that gene therapy techniques will increase the capacity for natural healing of articular cartilage lesions. Alternative tissue techniques will be available to replace damaged articular cartilage, or modifications of existing technology will lead to better results or fewer complications. In addition, continued advances in arthroscopic techniques will allow procedures that are commonly performed through an open arthrotomy to be performed arthroscopically.

Table 54–4	
Summary of Decision Making in Articular Cartilage Injuries	

Clinical Evaluation

History	Pain in ipsilateral compartment; recurrent effusions
Physical examination	Pain in ipsilateral compartment; rule out coexisting pathology
Imaging	Standing radiographs, including 45-degree posteroanterior, and mechanical axis views; magnetic resonance imaging commonly shows articular cartilage lesion
Classification	Outerbridge classification (see Table 54–1)
Associated injuries	Evaluate for knee instability, meniscal deficiency, malalignment

Treatment Options

Nonoperative	Low-demand patients, small lesions ($<1\,cm^2$)
Operative	
Primary repair	Osteochondral lesions
Debridement and lavage	Low-demand patients
	Small to medium lesions ($0.5\text{-}3\,cm^2$)
Marrow stimulation (microfracture)	Moderate-sized lesions ($1\text{-}3\,cm^2$)
	Low- or high-demand patients
	Fibrocartilage repair tissue
Osteochondral autograft	Small to medium lesions ($1\text{-}3\,cm^2$)
	Autogenous tissue with normal hyaline architecture
	Consider donor site morbidity and availability
Autologous chondrocyte implantation	Medium to large lesions ($2\text{-}10\,cm^2$)
	Hyaline-like tissue
	Durable
Osteochondral allograft	Medium to large lesions (up to hemicondyle)
	Allograft tissue
	Good for lesions with bony defects
Postoperative rehabilitation	Protect repair tissue from weight bearing for 6 wk
	Immediate range of motion
	Gradual return to weight bearing and activities based on technique

References

1. Aubin PP, Cheah HK, Davis AM, Gross AE: Long-term follow-up of fresh femoral osteochondral allografts for posttraumatic knee defects. Clin Orthop 391(suppl):S318-S327, 2001.
2. Bert J, Maschka K: The arthroscopic treatment of unicompartmental gonarthrosis: A five-year follow-up study of abrasion arthroplasty plus arthroscopic debridement and arthroscopic debridement alone. Arthroscopy 5:25-32, 1989.
3. Bradley JP: Osteochondral autograft transplantation clinical outcome study. Paper presented at Metcalf Memorial Meeting, 1999, Sun Valley, ID.
4. Brittberg M, Lindahl A, Nilsson A, et al: Treatment of deep cartilage defects in the knee with autologous chnodrocyte implantation. N Engl J Med 331:889-895, 1994.
5. Bugbee WD: Fresh osteochondral allografting. Oper Tech Sports Med 8:158-162, 2000.
6. Chu C, Covery F, Akeson W, Meyers M: Articular cartilage transplantation. Clin Orthop 360:159-168, 1999.
7. Edwards RB, Lu Y, Nho S, et al: Thermal chondroplasty of chondromalacic human cartilage: An ex vivo comparison of bipolar and monopolar radiofrequency devices. Am J Sports Med 30:90-97, 2002.
8. Federico D, Reider B: Results of isolated patellar debridement for patellofemoral pain in patients with normal patellar alignment. Am J Sports Med 25:663-669, 1997.
9. Friedman M, Berasi D, Fox J: Preliminary results with abrasion arthroplasty in the osteoarthritic knee. Clin Orthop 182:200-205, 1984.
10. Garrett JC: Fresh osteochondral allografts for treatment of articular defects in osteochondritis dissecans of the lateral femoral condyle in adults. Clin Orthop 303:33-37, 1994.
11. Ghazavi M, Pritzker K, Davis A, Gross A: Fresh osteochondral allografts for posttraumatic defects of the knee. J Bone Joint Surg Br 79:1008-1013, 1997.
12. Gill TJ, MacGillivray JD: The technique of microfracture for the treatment of articular cartilage defects in the knee. Oper Tech Orthop 11:105-107, 2001.
13. Gillogly S, Voight M, Blackburn T: Treatment of articular cartilage defects of the knee with autologous chondrocyte implantation. J Orthop Sports Phys Ther 28:241-251, 1998.
14. Gross AE: Fresh osteochondral allografts for post-traumatic knee defects: Surgical technique. Oper Tech Orthop 7:334-339, 1997.
15. Hangody L, Feczko P, Bartha L, et al: Mosaicplasty for the treatment of articular cartilage defects of the knee and ankle. Clin Orthop 391(suppl):S328-S336, 2001.
16. Hangody L, Kish G, Karpati Z: Arthroscopic autogenous osteochondral mosaicplasty: A multicenter, comparative, prospective study. Index Traumat Sport 5:3-9, 1998.
17. Higuchi H, Kimura M, Shirakura K, et al: Factors affecting long-term results after arthroscopic partial meniscectomy. Clin Orthop 377:161-168, 2000.
18. Insall J: The Pridie debridement operation for osteoarthritis of the knee. Clin Orthop 101:61-67, 1974.

19. Johnson LJ: Arthroscopic abrasion arthroplasty historical and pathologic perspective: Present status. Arthroscopy 2:54-69, 1986.

20. Kish G, Modis L, Hangoody L: Osteochondral mosaicplasty for the treatment of focal chondral and osteochondral lesions of the knee and talus in the athlete: Rationale, indications, technique, and results. Clin Sports Med 18:45-66, 1999.

21. Lu Y, Edwards RB, Kalscheur VL, et al: Effect of bipolar radiofrequency energy on human articular cartilage: Comparison of confocal laser microscopy and light microscopy. Arthroscopy 17:117-123, 2001.

22. Messner K, Maletius W: The long-term prognosis for severe damage to weight-bearing cartilage in the knee. Acta Orthop Scand 67:165-168, 1996.

23. Meyers M, Akeson W, Convery F: Resurfacing of the knee with fresh osteochondral allograft. J Bone Joint Surg Am 71:704-713, 1989.

24. Micheli L, Browne JE, Erggelet C, et al: Autologous chondrocyte implantation of the knee: Multicenter experience and minimum 3 year follow-up. Clin J Sports Med 11:223-228, 2001.

25. Minas T: Autologous chondrocyte implantation for focal chondral defects of the knee. Clin Orthop 391(suppl):S349-S361, 2001.

26. Noyes FR, Bassett RW, Grood ES, Butler DL: Arthroscopy in acute traumatic hemarthrosis of the knee. J Bone Joint Surg Am 62:687-695, 1980.

27. Outerbridge R: The etiology of chondromalacia patellae. J Bone Joint Surg Br 43:752-757, 1961.

28. Owens BD, Stickles BJ, Balikian P, Busconi BD: Prospective analysis of radiofrequency versus mechanical debridement of isolated patellar chondral lesions. Arthroscopy 18:151-155, 2002.

29. Peterson L, Brittberg M, Kiviranta I, et al: Autologous chondrocyte transplantation: Biomechanics and long-term durability. Am J Sports Med 30:2-12, 2002.

30. Peterson L, Minas T, Brittberg M, et al: Two- to 9-year outcome after autologous chondrocyte transplantation of the knee. Clin Orthop 374:212-234, 2000.

31. Pridie KW: A method of resurfacing osteoarthritic knee joints. J Bone Joint Surg Br 41:618-619, 1959.

32. Rand J: Role of arthroscopy in osteoarthritis of the knee. Arthroscopy 7:358-361, 1991.

33. Rangger C, Klestil T, Gloetzer W, et al: Osteoarthritis after arthroscopic partial meniscectomy. Am J Sports Med 23:240-244, 1995.

34. Schimmer RC, Brulhart KB, Duff C, Glinz W: Arthroscopic partial meniscectomy: A 12-year follow-up and two-step evaluation of the long-term course. Arthroscopy 14:220-228, 1998.

35. Steadman JR, Kocher MS, Briggs KK, et al: Outcomes of patients treated arthroscopically by microfracture for traumatic chondral defects of the knee: Average 11-year follow-up. Paper presented at the annual meeting of the Arthroscopy Association of North America, 2002, Washington, DC.

6 Knee

CHAPTER

55

Debridement of Articular Cartilage in the Knee

MARK A. KWARTOWITZ AND BRUCE REIDER

DEBRIDEMENT OF ARTICULAR CARTILAGE IN THE KNEE IN A NUTSHELL

History:
Knee pain when ambulating stairs, rising from a low chair, and squatting or kneeling

Physical Examination:
Crepitus with full active range of motion of the knee; palpable effusion with compression of the suprapatellar pouch; tenderness with palpation of the patellar facets

Imaging:
Standard and weight-bearing radiographs

Indications:
Continued pain that affects activities of daily living after failed conservative treatment

Surgical Technique:
Initial diagnostic arthroscopy to inspect the entire articular surface of the knee, probing and looking for damaged articular cartilage; the extent of chondral damage and whether it involves the weight-bearing surface should be noted

Arthrotome blade and basket forceps allow a controlled debridement without putting normal cartilage at risk

An accessory portal can be established to help reach difficult areas of damaged cartilage

After debridement, the lesion's size is measured with a calibrated probe, and the location is noted

Postoperative Management:
Range-of-motion exercises are begun immediately after surgery; a noncrepitant strengthening program is started, followed by a progressive return to activities

Results:
Encouraging; surgery had a beneficial effect in 32 of 36 patients after a 59-month follow-up

Patients with traumatic chondrosis had a higher percentage of good or excellent results after surgery compared with atraumatic cases

No significant correlation between the grade of chondral damage and improvement with surgery

Arthroscopic debridement of the knee may improve function and decrease pain but is not a curative procedure

---

Debridement of damaged articular cartilage is a common arthroscopic procedure performed most often for chondrosis of the patellofemoral joint. Its use is not without controversy, because the biologic or biomechanical basis for its effectiveness has never been fully elucidated.[3-10,16,21,22,27,28] Debridement does not restore the articular surface to its normal, pristine state.[17,18,20] It is thus not surprising that the expected result is amelioration, not elimination, of symptoms. Nevertheless, its relatively low morbidity makes it a popular treatment for joint symptoms that have not responded to conservative measures. In our experience, key factors in the successful use of chondral debridement are great care in patient selection and proper patient education regarding realistic postoperative expectations.

Case History

A 30-year-old woman was carrying a laundry basket downstairs when she missed a step and fell, landing directly on her right knee. She had immediate pain in the knee and a gradual onset of swelling over the next 12 hours. The patient presented to the office 6 months later complaining of anterior knee pain and intermittent swelling. Climbing or descending stairs, rising from a low chair, and squatting or kneeling exacerbated the pain. Prolonged sitting sometimes elicited pain as well. She denied any mechanical symptoms such as catching or locking but did note frequent crepitus. There was no history of any symptoms before the fall, and no pain in any other joints.

Physical Examination

The patient walked without a limp. The overall knee alignment appeared normal: her Q angle measured about 14 degrees (Fig. 55–1), and her tubercle-sulcus angle was about 5 degrees. Mild quadriceps atrophy was

visualized on the injured extremity, with a circumferential measurement difference of 1 cm.

Seated on the examining table, the patient was able to fully extend her knee against gravity, although retropatellar crepitus could be felt during this maneuver. Aside from the crepitus, the patella seemed to track smoothly, with a small lateral deviation near full extension. Active flexion was to 130 degrees.

Compression of the suprapatellar pouch produced a small visible fluid wave (Fig. 55–2). Patellar glide was about 1 cm both medially and laterally. The patellar apprehension test was negative. Both the medial and lateral facets seemed tender (Fig. 55–3). There was no tenderness of the patellar tendon or the tibiofemoral joint lines. The Lachman test, varus and valgus stress

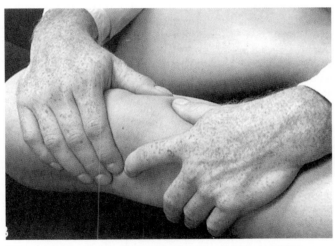

Figure 55–2   Demonstration of a palpable fluid wave. (From Reider B: The Orthopaedic Physical Examination. Philadelphia, WB Saunders, 1999, p 227.)

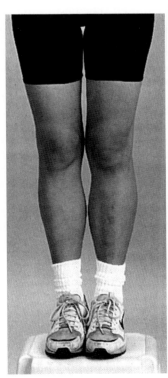

Figure 55–1   Position for examining knee alignment. (From Reider B: The Orthopaedic Physical Examination. Philadelphia, WB Saunders, 1999, p 211.)

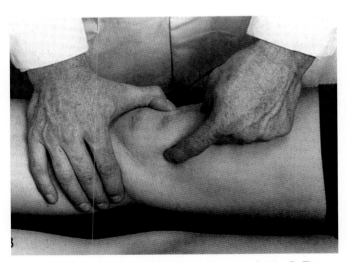

Figure 55–3   Palpation of patellar facets. (From Reider B: The Orthopaedic Physical Examination. Philadelphia, WB Saunders, 1999, p 219.)

6 Knee

tests, posterior drawer test, and McMurray test were normal.

Imaging

Standard radiographs were obtained, including a standing anteroposterior view of both knees, standing posteroanterior view in flexion ("skier's view"), lateral view, and skyline view taken in 30 degrees of flexion. In this case, the radiographs were all normal. Weight-bearing radiographs allow assessment of joint space narrowing and other signs of tibiofemoral osteoarthritis. Occasionally, osteochondral fragments can be seen on anteroposterior and lateral radiographs. The axial radiograph is helpful in evaluating patellar alignment, if it is done in a standardized manner (Fig. 55–4), and for detecting patellar avulsion fragments and ectopic calcifications that may be associated with patellar instability. Patellar osteophytes can be appreciated on the lateral or axial projections. We do not routinely perform magnetic resonance imaging in cases of apparent patellofemoral pain, as it rarely adds to the evaluation. It is most helpful when the diagnosis is uncertain and another entity such as a meniscus tear is a possibility.

Indications and Contraindications

Surgery is not the primary treatment of patellofemoral pain. In most instances, the patient is given a simple home exercise program emphasizing light knee extension exercises in the nonpainful or noncrepitant arc of motion. In most cases, crepitus is felt near terminal extension, so exercise is recommended in a flexed arc, such as 105 to 40 degrees. Patients who are more severely disabled or who have failed a home exercise program are referred for supervised physical therapy. The goal is to devise a nonpainful strengthening program appropriate

for each patient. Patellar taping may be used as an adjunct to exercise if it is effective in reducing the patient's pain. Biofeedback techniques can also be helpful if quadriceps muscle inhibition is present.

Nonsteroidal anti-inflammatory drugs are not routinely used but are prescribed for a specified course if an effusion or other signs of inflammation are present. Glucosamine may be beneficial, although its efficacy is still being evaluated. Some patients find that patellar knee sleeves are helpful when worn during activities. If the patient shows evidence of a flattened longitudinal arch and in-facing (squinting) patellas, a simple semirigid orthosis should be tried.

Finally, activity modification is recommended. Usually this consists of reduction or modification of athletic or daily living activities that exacerbate the patient's symptoms. These changes may be temporary, although some patients may need to permanently avoid squatting or kneeling.

In this case, the patient underwent a structured physical therapy program for 4 months consisting of quadriceps strengthening, patellar taping, and lower extremity flexibility training. She was given an oral nonsteroidal anti-inflammatory medicine to resolve her effusion. The patient had improved muscle tone in the knee but still complained of severe pain affecting her activities of daily living.

The primary indication for surgery in cases of patellofemoral pain is debilitating pain that is intractable to nonsurgical treatment. Patients whose pain is treatable by a reasonable level of activity modification should probably not be offered surgery. Once a decision has been made that surgery is indicated, the best procedure must be identified. The best candidates for patellar chondroplasty have (1) normal patellofemoral alignment,[12,14,15,26] (2) normal patellar mobility, (3) history of a direct injury to the patella, (4) normal radiographs, and (5) a discrete lesion of the articular surface surrounded by normal articular cartilage. Obviously, this last requirement can be definitively determined only at the time of the arthroscopic procedure.

Patients should have realistic expectations about the results of surgery. Specifically, we tell them that (1) the goal of surgery is to improve function and reduce pain; (2) most, but not all, patients will experience improvement, but the amount of improvement is unpredictable in any given patient; (3) it is unlikely that the knee will feel perfectly normal after surgery; and (4) certain activities, especially kneeling directly on the patella and deep squatting, will probably not be possible even after the surgery.

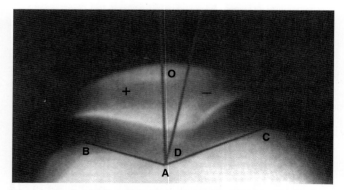

Figure 55–4 Skyline view. BAC represents the angle of the trochlear sulcus. AO is the bisector of this angle. AD is the line between the apex of the trochlear sulcus and the apex of the patella. The angle OAD is one measurement of patellar alignment. As the patella shifts laterally, this angle becomes positive.[19] (From Reider B: The Orthopaedic Physical Examination. Philadelphia, WB Saunders, 1999, p 371.)

Surgical Technique

Positioning

The patient is positioned supine on the operating table. A tourniquet is applied to the proximal thigh, and a lateral post is situated to help visualize the medial compartment of the knee. The tourniquet is not normally used for the procedure but is put in place as a precaution.

Diagnostic Arthroscopy

A superolateral portal is made for placement of the outflow cannula. We prefer the superolateral portal to the superomedial portal to avoid possible inhibition of the vastus medialis obliquus postoperatively. Standard anteromedial and anterolateral portals are used for insertion of the surgical instruments and the arthroscope. A diagnostic arthroscopy is begun, starting in the suprapatellar pouch and the medial and lateral gutters to look for any loose chondral fragments. When evaluating the patella, it is important to make sure that the entire articular surface is systematically inspected. A flexion contracture of the knee or a large, tethered fat pad can obstruct visualization of the patella from the joint line portals. If difficulty is experienced while attempting to visualize the patella, the arthroscope should be shifted to the superolateral portal.

Specific Surgical Steps

The patella is probed, looking for softening and determining the extent of fibrillations and fissuring. We do not recommend debriding areas that are softened but have a normal, intact surface. In this case, the inferomedial portion of the patella showed grade III chondral damage with fibrillation measuring 1 by 1.5 cm. In addition to the patella, the femoral trochlea should be examined from the proximal border distally to the roof of the intercondylar notch (Figs. 55–5 and 55–6). Lesions of the femoral trochlea carry a worse prognosis than do lesions of the patella.

After the patellofemoral joint has been inspected, the knee is gradually flexed while assessing the medial and

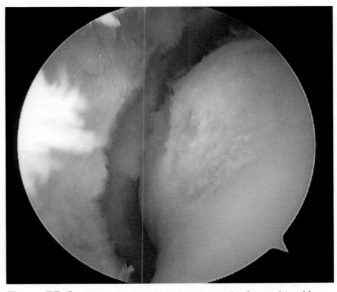

Figure 55–6   Grade III chondral changes to the femoral trochlea.

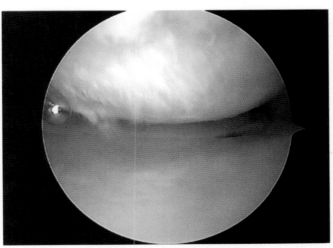

Figure 55–7   Grade III chondral changes to the medial femoral condyle.

lateral femoral condyles. The size and location of chondral lesions should be noted. Especially important to note are whether the principal weight-bearing surface is involved and at what degree of flexion a condylar lesion makes contact with the tibia. Obviously, a large lesion that involves the weight-bearing surface and makes contact near extension is more of a problem than a small lesion to the side of the weight-bearing surface that makes contact in 90 degrees of flexion. In this case, the medial femoral condyle had grade III changes measuring 1.5 by 2 cm on the weight-bearing surface with the knee in full extension (Figs. 55–7 and 55–8). Completion of the diagnostic arthroscopy includes visualizing and probing the cruciate ligaments and menisci for tears and assessing the medial and lateral gutters for loose bodies.

Our general guideline for debridement of the knee is to be conservatively aggressive. This means selecting

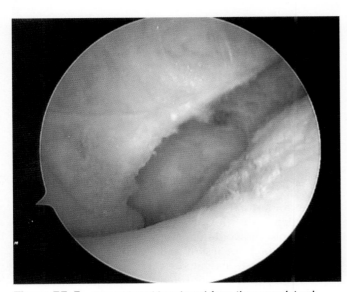

Figure 55–5   Femoral trochlea viewed from the superolateral portal.

6 Knee

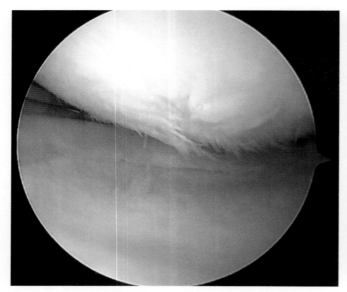

Figure 55–8 Medial femoral condyle with knee in full extension.

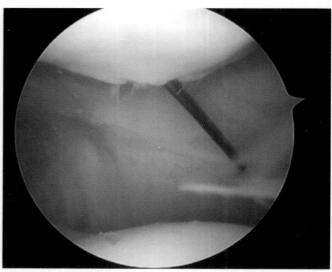

Figure 55–9 Establishing a superomedial accessory portal with an 18-gauge needle.

patients who have truly failed conservative treatment and choosing instrumentation that is capable of debriding degenerated cartilage without putting normal cartilage at risk. The arthroscopic instruments used most often for debridement and chondroplasty of the knee are basket forceps and a gently scalloped arthrotome blade. The arthrotome blade is first used to remove fibrillated, degenerated cartilage. Little pressure on the arthrotome and a moderate amount of suction are required for this portion of the procedure. The basket forceps are then used to resect firmer, undermined flaps of cartilage that may lie along the edges of the lesion. The lesion is carefully probed to identify which areas are still significantly soft and fibrillated and require further resection. The mouth of the blade should always face the degenerated cartilage to avoid injury to normal, healthy cartilage. If necessary, an accessory portal should be created to approach inaccessible lesions without damaging normal articular cartilage. The medial facet of the patella can often be a difficult area to adequately debride from either the anterior or superolateral portal. An 18-gauge needle is helpful to localize the best placement of an accessory portal for debridement of the medial patella (Fig. 55–9).

As a chondral lesion is debrided, greater pressure is often required to resect the more sessile fragments (Fig. 55–10). The goal is to create smooth contours with stable surrounding borders (Fig. 55–11). When debridement appears to be complete, the area of resection is carefully examined and probed to verify that no further debridement is required and that all edges are stable. The arthroscope should be moved from the anterior portal to the superolateral portal to view any resection performed to the patellofemoral joint. This allows a different vantage point and often reveals residual areas of fibrillation. If subchondral bone is exposed during debridement, it is lightly curetted to encourage the ingrowth of fibrocartilage. Using a calibrated probe, the length and breadth

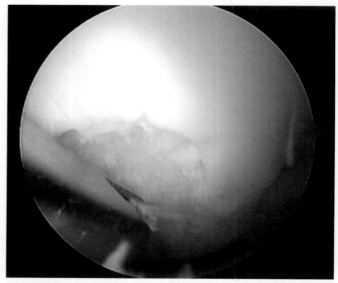

Figure 55–10 Arthrotome blade debridement of sessile fragments.

of the lesion, as well as its location and depth, are recorded. The location of patellofemoral lesions can be helpful in customizing the postoperative exercise regimen. Distal patellar lesions and proximal trochlear lesions make contact near extension, whereas proximal patellar and distal trochlear lesions make contact in greater degrees of flexion. We usually instruct the physical therapist to avoid quadriceps exercises in the arc of motion in which the lesion is likely to make contact. The knee is copiously irrigated to remove any remaining loose fragments from debridement. The portal sites are closed with single nylon sutures, and the knee is sterilely dressed and bandaged with a compressive wrap.

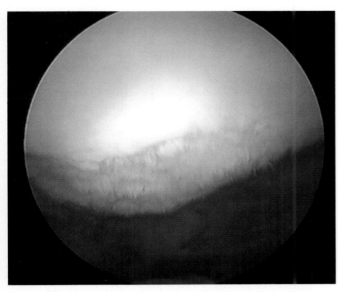

Figure 55–11   Patella after debridement with stable borders.

Postoperative Management

Range-of-motion exercises are initiated immediately after surgery. Progression to full weight bearing as tolerated is usually possible within the first couple of postoperative days. The patient is encouraged to ice and elevate the surgical extremity to decrease swelling. A rehabilitation program is started after the first follow-up office visit. The patient is instructed on noncrepitant range-of-motion strengthening exercises for chondral lesions involving the patellofemoral joint. Closed chain quadriceps exercises are initiated, followed by a progressive return to sporting activities as tolerated. The need for activity modification, particularly the avoidance of kneeling and squatting, is stressed to the patient.

Results

We reviewed 36 patients who underwent arthroscopic patellar debridement for patellofemoral pain with isolated chondromalacia patellae noted during arthroscopy.[24,25] Nineteen patients had traumatic events to the patellofemoral joint that initiated their symptoms. The patients had continued pain after a minimum of 4 months of physical therapy (noncrepitant arc quadriceps muscle strengthening, stretching, electrical stimulation, and ultrasound). No patient had a history of patellar instability or malalignment. All patients had Outerbridge grade II[1] or worse chondromalacia at the time of debridement; 61% had grade III lesions (53% traumatic, 47% atraumatic). The lesions were debrided according to the guidelines described earlier. Follow-up and evaluation consisted of the Fulkerson-Shea patellofemoral joint evaluation score, subjective outcome rating, activity level, questionnaire, and independent physical examination. Average follow-up was 59 months. All but four patients subjectively reported that surgery had had a beneficial effect. There was significant improvement in the patellofemoral joint evaluation score from the preoperative level to the maximal and final postoperative level. Patients with traumatic chondrosis had a higher percentage of good or excellent results compared with atraumatic cases (57.9% vs. 41.1%). Patients with milder grades of chondral damage had higher patellofemoral joint evaluation scores. Patients with traumatic chondrosis had a significantly greater improvement in their pain scores than did those without a history of trauma. All but one patient in the traumatic group had an average improvement of 14.2 points on a 35-point patellofemoral pain scale. There was no significant correlation between the grade of chondral damage and the improvement after surgery in the two groups. Fifty-three percent of the traumatic group and 59% of the atraumatic group had improved stair-climbing ability. Surgery decreased symptoms of crepitation in 58% of the traumatic group and 53% of the atraumatic group. Twenty-seven of 29 patients were active in sports at final follow-up; 14 of these patients were at a lower activity level, however. There was a direct correlation between the patients' final symptoms and the amount of articular tenderness present on physical examination. Overall, patients had an 89% rate of subjective improvement with patellar debridement.

Friedman et al.[11] reviewed arthroscopic debridement of 110 patients with grade IV articular changes. Patients who had the most improvement from debridement were younger than 40 years and had treatment isolated to the patellofemoral joint. Baumgaertner et al.[2] reviewed arthroscopic debridement of 49 knees with a 33-month follow-up. Patients with a longer duration of symptoms, advanced arthritis on preoperative radiographs, and malalignment had poorer results. Debridement of the knee had a beneficial effect on the patients' function with regard to walking endurance and the need for assistive walking devices. Symptoms of swelling and giving way improved postoperatively. Rand[23] reported that normal preoperative radiographs did not correlate with arthroscopic findings of grade III and IV changes. All patients who were worse at final follow-up had radiographic evidence of osteoarthritis. Harwin[13] retrospectively reviewed 204 knees that underwent arthroscopic debridement. Standing radiographs were taken to evaluate limb alignment. Harwin concluded from statistical analysis that patients with less deviated axes did better than those with greater knee malalignment. Bert and Maschka[5] reported a 5-year follow-up comparing arthroscopic debridement alone and debridement with abrasion arthroplasty. Results showed that 66% of patients had good or excellent results with debridement alone, compared with 51% of those also undergoing abrasion arthroplasty. Half the patients who had abrasion arthroplasty showed joint space widening, but there was no correlation with symptomatic improvement. They concluded that arthroscopic joint debridement should be considered in selected patients when conservative measures have failed.

6 Knee

Complications

There were no postoperative complications in our series, although patients who undergo arthroscopic chondroplasty are presumably at risk for the usual complications associated with arthroscopy of the knee, such as infection, thromboembolic disease, hematoma, and arthrofibrosis.

Conclusion

Arthroscopic chondroplasty of the patellofemoral joint can improve pain and function in a properly selected group of patients. Patients must understand that the procedure does not restore a normal articular surface and rarely leads to complete resolution of all symptoms. The duration of improvement has yet to be determined with long-term prospective studies.

References

1. Bauer M, Jackson RW: Chondral lesions of the femoral condyles: A system of arthroscopic classification. Arthroscopy 4:97-102, 1988.
2. Baumgaertner MR, Cannon WD, Vittori JM, et al: Arthroscopic debridement of the arthritic knee. Clin Orthop 253:197-202, 1990.
3. Bentley G: The surgical treatment of chondromalacia patellae. J Bone and Joint Surg Br 60:74-81, 1978.
4. Bentley G, Dowd G: Current concepts of etiology and treatment of chondromalacia patellae. Clin Orthop 189:209-228, 1984.
5. Bert JM, Maschka K: The arthroscopic treatment of unicompartmental gonarthrosis: A five-year follow-up study of abrasion arthroplasty plus arthroscopic debridement and arthroscopic debridement alone. Arthroscopy 5:25-32, 1989.
6. Buckwalter JA, Lohmander S: Current concepts review: Operative treatment of osteoarthrosis. J Bone Joint Surg Am 76:1405-1418, 1994.
7. Buckwalter JA, Mankin HJ: Articular cartilage: Tissue design and chondrocyte-matrix interactions. J Bone Joint Surg Am 79:600-611, 1997.
8. Burks RT: Arthroscopy and degenerative arthritis of the knee: A review of the literature. Arthroscopy 6:43-47, 1990.
9. Casscells SW: Editorial: What, if any, are the indications for arthroscopic debridement of the osteoarthritic knee? Arthroscopy 6:169-170, 1990.
10. Dandy DJ: Editorial: Arthroscopic debridement of the knee for osteoarthrtitis. J Bone Joint Surg Br 73:877-878, 1991.
11. Friedman MJ, Berasi CC, Fox JM, et al: Preliminary results with abrasion arthroplasty in the osteoarthritic knee. Clin Orthop 182:200-205, 1984.
12. Grana WA, Hinkley B, Hollingsworth S: Arthroscopic evaluation and treatment of patellar malalignment. Clin Orthop 186:122-128, 1984.
13. Harwin SF: Arthroscopic debridement for osteoarthritis of the knee: Predictors of patient satisfaction. Arthroscopy 15:142-146, 1999.
14. Hvid I, Andersen L, Schmidt H: Chondromalacia patellae: The relationship to abnormal patellofemoral joint mechanics. Acta Orthop Scand 52:661-666, 1981.
15. Insall JN, Aglietti P, Tria AJ: Patellar pain and incongruence. II. Clinical application. Clin Orthop 176:225-232, 1983.
16. Kaplan L, Uribe JW, Sasken H, et al: The acute effects of radiofrequency energy in articular cartilage: An in vitro study. Arthroscopy 16:2-5, 2000.
17. Kim HK, Moran ME, Salter RB: The potential for regeneration of articular cartilage in defects created by chondral shaving and subchondral abrasion: An experimental investigation in rabbits. J Bone Joint Surg Am 73:1301-1315, 1991.
18. Mankin HJ: The response of articular cartilage to mechanical injury. J Bone Joint Surg Am 64:460-466, 1982.
19. Merchant AC, Mercu RL, Jacobsen RH, et al: Roentgenographic analysis of patellofemoral congruence. J Bone Joint Surg Am 56:1391-1396, 1974.
20. Milgram JW: Injury to articular cartilage joint surfaces. I. Chondral injury produced by patellar shaving: A histopathologic study of human tissue specimens. Clin Orthop 192:168-173, 1985.
21. Moseley JB, Wray NP, Kuykendall D, et al: Arthroscopic treatment of osteoarthritis of the knee: A prospective, randomized, placebo-contolled trial. Results of a pilot study. Am J Sports Med 24:28-34, 1996.
22. Ogilvie-Harris DJ, Jackson RW: The arthroscopic treatment of chondromalacia patellae. J Bone Joint Surg Br 66:660-665, 1984.
23. Rand JA: Role of arthroscopy in osteoarthritis of the knee. Arthroscopy 7:358-363, 1991.
24. Reider B, Federico DJ: Arthroscopic patellar debridement. Oper Tech Sports Med 2:285-290, 1994.
25. Reider B, Federico DJ: Results of isolated patellar debridement for patellofemoral pain in patients with normal alignment. Am J Sports Med 25:663-669, 1997.
26. Sojbjerg AO, Lauritzen J, Boe S: Arthroscopic determination of patellofemoral malalignment. Clin Orthop 215:243-247, 1987.
27. Sprague NF: Arthroscopic debridement for degenerative knee joint disease. Clin Orthop 160:118-123, 1981.
28. Yang SS, Nisonson B: Arthroscopic surgery of the knee in the geriatric patient. Clin Orthop 316:50-58, 1995.

Microfracture Technique in the Knee

KEVIN B. FREEDMAN AND BRIAN J. COLE

MICROFRACTURE TECHNIQUE IN THE KNEE IN A NUTSHELL

History:
    Pain in ipsilateral compartment; recurrent effusions

Physical Examination:
    Pain in ipsilateral compartment; rule out coexisting pathology

Imaging:
    Standing radiographs, including 45-degree posteroanterior and mechanical axis views; magnetic resonance imaging commonly shows articular cartilage lesion

Indications:
    Grade III or IV lesions, 2 to 3 cm^2

Contraindications:
    Larger lesions (>3 cm^2 in high-demand patients); diffuse degenerative lesions

Surgical Technique:
    Diagnostic arthroscopy: position to allow full flexion of knee for evaluation of all surfaces; evaluate lesion for size and depth; evaluate and treat concomitant pathology
    Arthroscopic debridement: use shaver or curet to debride unstable flaps
    Use curet to create vertical walls for adherence of clot
    Use curet to remove calcified layer from base of lesion; this provides a better surface for adherence of clot and improved chondral nutrition
    Microfracture defect: use an awl to place holes 3 to 4 mm apart; progress peripheral to central; do not allow holes to become confluent
    Confirm adequate penetration: stop arthroscopic pump to confirm marrow elements flowing from area of microfracture

Postoperative Management:
    Femoral condyle: continuous passive motion 6 to 8 hours for 4 to 6 weeks; touch-down weight bearing for 6 to 8 weeks
    Patella/trochlea: continuous passive motion 6 to 8 hours for 4 to 6 weeks; weight bearing as tolerated in hinged brace with 30-degree-flexion stop for 8 weeks

Without intervention, articular cartilage injuries have a limited ability to heal. Two main factors contribute to this limited intrinsic repair capacity: the avascular nature of the tissue, and the relative absence of an undifferentiated cell population that can respond to injury. Many of the surgical techniques used to treat full-thickness lesions of articular cartilage are designed to stimulate a local influx of undifferentiated mesenchymal cells from the subchondral marrow.

The technique of microfracture was popularized by Steadman.[7,10] The premise of this technique is to repair a focal chondral defect with fibrocartilage. Fibrocartilage repair occurs through surgical penetration of the subchondral plate, which exposes the damaged area to progenitor cells that reside within the subchondral bone. Microfracture is theoretically favored over subchondral drilling and abrasion arthroplasty for several reasons: (1) it is less destructive to the subchondral bone because it creates less thermal injury than drilling does, (2) it allows better access to difficult areas of the articular surface, (3) it provides controlled depth penetration, and (4) use of a correctly angled awl permits the microfracture holes to be made perpendicular to the surface of the subchondral plate.[9,10]

History

Patients with symptomatic chondral lesions typically complain of knee pain localized to the particular compartment affected by the lesion. Weight-bearing activities typically aggravate symptoms from lesions on the medial or lateral femoral condyle. Patellofemoral lesions are aggravated by sitting, stair climbing, and squatting. Recurrent effusions can occur with symptomatic chondral lesions.

Physical Examination

Typically, patients are tender along the ipsilateral joint line. A positive patellar grind test can indicate a patellar or trochlear lesion. An effusion may be present. It is essential to evaluate for concomitant pathology that would modify treatment recommendations, such as malalignment or ligament deficiency.

Imaging

Diagnostic imaging should begin with a standard weight-bearing anteroposterior radiograph of both knees in full extension, a non–weight-bearing 45-degree-flexion lateral view, and an axial view of the patellofemoral joint. Additionally, a 45-degree-flexion weight-bearing posteroanterior radiograph is recommended to identify subtle joint space narrowing that traditional extension views may fail to show. Special studies such as a long-cassette mechanical axis view should be ordered if there is any degree of clinical malalignment. Magnetic resonance imaging can help delineate the extent of articular cartilage lesions, especially in the setting of completely normal radiographs. Techniques include two-dimensional fast spin echo and three-dimensional fat suppression with or without intra-articular gadolinium. Evolving magnetic resonance imaging techniques provide accurate information about the presence and size of articular cartilage lesions, which can aid in diagnosis and preoperative planning.

Indications and Contraindications

The microfracture technique can be used to treat patients with moderate symptoms and midsized lesions, grade III or IV, by the modified Outerbridge classification (Fig. 56–1).[6] Specifically, microfracture is recommended for active patients with small lesions (<2 to 3 cm^2) and no more than moderate symptoms, or for lower-demand patients with larger lesions (>2 to 3 cm^2) and mild symptoms.[1] Results in higher-demand patients with larger lesions are generally less favorable and shorter lived. In general, microfracture should not be used for defects more than 10 mm deep.[2]

Preoperative Planning

It is important to address any concomitant pathology at the time of microfracture. In addition, it is essential to discuss postoperative restrictions with the patient before performing the microfracture technique, because success depends on strict adherence to the postoperative treatment regimen, including 6 to 8 weeks of partial weight bearing.

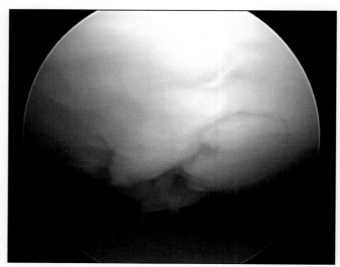

Figure 56–1 Symptomatic grade IV chondral lesion of the medial femoral condyle before preparation for microfracture.

Surgical Technique

Examination under Anesthesia

An examination under anesthesia should be performed to confirm full range of motion and that there is no concomitant ligamentous laxity.

Positioning

Depending on surgeon preference, the limb can be placed in a standard leg holder or maintained in the unsupported supine position. However, a leg holder, with the end of the table flexed, may provide better access to the extreme flexion surface of the femoral condyle.

Diagnostic Arthroscopy

A routine, 10-point diagnostic arthroscopy is performed, with careful examination of the posterior aspects of the medial and lateral femoral condyles. A probe is used to assess the quality of the cartilage surface, and any changes on the articular cartilage surface are noted. If global chondral changes are found, microfracture is not performed. However, multiple isolated chondral lesions in separate compartments of the knee can be treated concomitantly.

Arthroscopic Preparation of the Lesion

The initial step for arthroscopic preparation is debridement of the focal chondral defect. An arthroscopic shaver or curet can be used to sharply debride any unstable cartilage flaps (see Fig. 56–1). A curet is then used to create vertical walls around the cartilage defect (Fig. 56–2). In addition, debridement of the calcified cartilage

layer from the base of the lesion is necessary. Both these steps—creating vertical walls and removing the calcified cartilage layer—are crucial. The vertical walls provide an area for the clot of progenitor cells to form and adhere, as well as a discrete load-bearing transition zone. Removal of the calcified cartilage layer provides a better surface for adherence of the clot and improved chondral nutrition through subchondral diffusion, which can increase the percentage of the defect that is filled.

Microfracture

Any associated intra-articular disease should be addressed before microfracture is performed. A surgical awl (Linvatec, Largo, FL) is used to create multiple small holes in the exposed bone of the chondral defect (Fig. 56–3). The microfracture holes are first made in the periphery and then brought toward the center of the lesion. The holes should be placed 3 to 4 mm apart (three to four holes per cm^2) (Fig. 56–4). The holes should not connect or become confluent in order to protect the integrity of the subchondral plate. To aid healing of the repair tissue to the surrounding normal articular cartilage, the most peripheral aspects of the lesion at the transition zone should be microfractured.

After completion of the procedure, the arthroscopic pump is stopped, and blood and fat droplets should be seen flowing from the area of the microfracture (Fig. 56–5). Intra-articular drains should not be placed, to allow adherence and stabilization of the blood clot to the lesion.

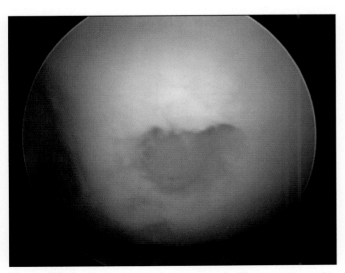

Figure 56–2   The lesion has been prepared with a curet to create stable vertical walls and debride the calcified cartilage layer.

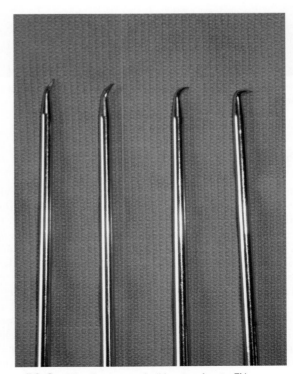

Figure 56–3   Microfracture awls (Linvatec, Largo, FL).

6 Knee

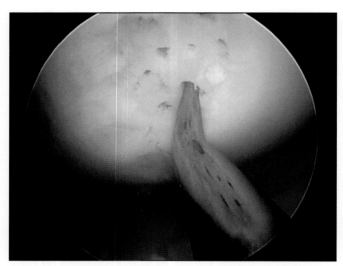

Figure 56–4 The microfracture awl is used to penetrate the subchondral plate, with holes spaced 3 to 4 mm apart.

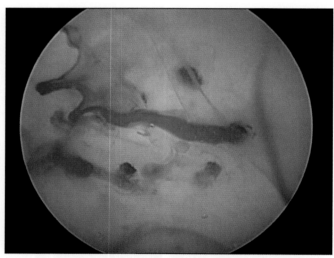

Figure 56–5 The arthroscopic pump is stopped, and bleeding is confirmed from the microfracture site.

Postoperative Management

Postoperative rehabilitation plays a vital role in achieving the best results from microfracture.[5,7,9] All patients should use a continuous passive motion machine on the day of surgery and continue it at home for 4 to 6 weeks, 6 to 8 hours a day. Full knee passive range of motion can be performed without a machine—500 repetitions, three times a day.[7,9]

The anatomic location and size of the defect dictate the amount of postoperative weight bearing. If the microfractured area is in the medial or lateral compartment, the patient is kept on strictly touch-down weight bearing (15% weight bearing) for 6 to 8 weeks. If the lesion is in a non–weight-bearing region of the compartment, weight bearing may begin earlier, depending on

the size of the affected area. Patients with patellar and trochlear groove lesions should be placed in a hinged brace with a 30- to 45-degree-flexion stop for at least 8 weeks. However, patients with these lesions may be allowed weight bearing as tolerated with these motion restrictions.[9] The brace protects the lesion because the median ridge of the patella does not engage the trochlear groove until after 30 degrees of flexion.

After the period of protected weight bearing, patients begin active range-of-motion exercises and progress to full weight bearing. No cutting, twisting, or jumping sports are allowed until at least 4 to 6 months postoperatively.[9,10]

Results

The clinical results of microfracture treatment for focal chondral defects are limited (Table 56–1). Steadman et al.[9] reported that the microfracture procedure has been performed in more than 1800 patients. The first study of the long-term results of microfracture was presented at the first annual meeting of the International Cartilage Repair Society.[4] A summary of these results was provided by Gill and MacGillivray.[3] The results of microfracture were reviewed in more than 100 patients with full-thickness chondral defects, with an average follow-up of 6 years. Microfracture resulted in statistically significant reduction in pain, swelling, and all functional parameters studied.[3] The ability to walk 2 miles, descend stairs, perform activities of daily living, and do strenuous work showed significant improvement. Maximal functional improvement was achieved 2 to 3 years after the microfracture procedure.[3,4]

Gill and MacGillivray reviewed the results of microfracture for isolated chondral defects (mean size, $3.2 \, cm^2$) of the medial femoral condyle at the Hospital for Special Surgery.[3] The study included 19 patients at a mean follow-up time of 3 years. The calcified cartilage layer was not routinely debrided, and patients did not routinely use continuous passive motion or limited weight bearing for 6 weeks. Seventy-four percent of these patients reported minimal or no pain, and 63% rated

Table 56–1

Clinical Results of Microfracture

Author (Date)	Mean Follow-up (yr)	No. of Patients	Outcome
Gill and MacGillivray (2001)[3]	6	100	Significant reduction in pain and swelling and improved function
Gill and MacGillivray (2001)[3]	3	19	74% minimal or no pain; 63% good or excellent
Steadman et al. (2002)[8]	11	71	Lysholm score improved (55.8 to 88.9); Tegner score improved (3.1 to 5.8)

their overall condition as good or excellent. In addition, magnetic resonance imaging was performed on all patients postoperatively. Despite the good subjective results, only 42% of the patients had 67% to 100% fill of the defect, 21% had 31% to 66% fill, and the remaining 37% had 0 % to 30% fill.[3]

The results of microfracture for the treatment of traumatic, full-thickness chondral defects were recently presented.[8] Seventy-one knees were treated, with a follow-up of 7 to 17 years. There was significant improvement in both the Lysholm and the Tegner scores from preoperative to postoperative status in these patients. The authors concluded that microfracture leads to statistically significant improvement in pain and function in patients with traumatic chondral defects.

Complications

Complications of microfracture are rare and mimic those seen following arthroscopic debridement and lavage. Occasionally, if a steep perpendicular rim is made in the trochlear groove during preparation of the cartilage defect, patients may experience catching or locking as the apex of the patella rides over this lesion.[9] These symptoms generally dissipate within 3 months. In addition, a recurrent painless effusion can persist following microfracture and can be treated conservatively.[9] Progressive cartilage degeneration and recurrent symptoms are the most common complications, and close postoperative monitoring of patients is required.

References

1. Cole BJ, Cohen B: Chondral injuries of the knee, a contemporary view of cartilage restoration. Orthopaedics (Special Edition) 6:71-76, 2000.
2. Gill TJ: Technique in the treatment of full-thickness chondral injuries. Oper Tech Sports Med 8:138-140, 2000.
3. Gill TJ, MacGillivray JD: The technique of microfracture for the treatment of articular cartilage defects in the knee. Oper Tech Orthop 11:105-107, 2001.
4. Gill TJ, Steadman JR, Rodrigo JJ: Indications and long-term clinical results of microfracture. Paper presented at the Second Symposium of the International Cartilage Repair Society, 1998, Boston.
5. Hagerman GR, Atkins JA, Dillman CJ: Rehabilitation of chondral injuries and chronic degenerative arthritis of the knee in the athlete. Oper Tech Sports Med 3:127-135, 1995.
6. Outerbridge RE: The etiology of chondromalacia patellae. J Bone Joint Surg Br 43:752-767, 1961.
7. Rodrigo JJ, Steadman JR, Silliman JF, Fulstone HA: Improvement of full-thickness chondral defect healing in the human knee after debridement and microfracture using continuous passive motion. Am J Knee Surg 7:109-116, 1994.
8. Steadman JR, Kocher MS, Briggs KK, et al: Outcomes of patients treated arthroscopically by microfracture for traumatic chondral defects of the knee: Average 11-year follow-up. Paper presented at the annual meeting of the Arthroscopy Association of North America, 2002, Washington, DC.
9. Steadman JR, Rodkey WG, Rodrigo JJ: Microfracture: Surgical technique and rehabilitation to treat chondral defects. Clin Orthop S391: S362-S369, 2001.
10. Steadman JR, Rodkey WG, Singleton SB, Briggs KK: Microfracture technique for full thickness chondral defects: Technique and clinical results. Oper Tech Orthop 7:300-304, 1997.

6 Knee

Primary Repair of Osteochondritis Dissecans in the Knee

BERNARD C. ONG, JON K. SEKIYA, AND CHRISTOPHER D. HARNER

PRIMARY REPAIR OF OSTEOCHONDRITIS DISSECANS IN THE KNEE IN A NUTSHELL

History:
Occult trauma; pain, swelling, catching

Physical Examination:
Localized tenderness, effusion

Imaging:
Plain films (flexion weight-bearing views); magnetic resonance imaging (size, depth, location, and stability)

Indications:
Symptomatic juvenile OCD that fails conservative management; most adult OCD

Surgical Technique:
In situ: pinning
In situ detached: hinge open, debride bed, with or without bone graft, internal fixation
Detached: debride bed, tailor fragment, bone graft, internal fixation or salvage (microfracture, mosaicplasty, autologous chondrocyte implantation, allograft)

Postoperative Management:
Extension bracing for 1 to 2 weeks; continuous passive motion for 4 to 6 weeks; partial weight bearing for 4 to 6 weeks; hardware removal 4 to 6 months postoperatively

Results:
Good

Osteochondritis dissecans (OCD) is a relatively rare disorder that has been estimated to occur in 15 to 21 cases per 100,000 knees.[4] OCD is a condition in which a fragment of subchondral bone and its overlying articular cartilage become separated from the underlying bone. Multiple causes for OCD have been proposed in the literature, including spontaneous necrosis, macro- or microtrauma, an ischemic event, epiphyseal abnormality, endocrine imbalance, and familial predisposition.[7,8,11] Approximately 40% to 60% of patients with OCD have a history of prior knee trauma to a mild or moderate degree[3]; however, the exact cause of OCD remains unknown.

OCD lesions can occur in multiple areas of the knee. Aichroth[1] described the location of typical lesions, including the classic lesion in the lateral portion of the medial femoral condyle, which was present in 69% of his cases. The medial femoral condyle is involved in 85% of cases, the lateral femoral condyle in 13%, the trochlea in 2%, and the patella in less than 1%.[1,2]

Plain radiographs can usually detect the presence of an OCD lesion. A standard series should include anteroposterior, lateral, Merchant, and flexion weight-bearing posteroanterior views of the knees. The flexion weight-bearing view is best for identifying the typical lesion located at the lateral aspect of the medial femoral condyle.[6]

Magnetic resonance imaging is a useful tool in the diagnosis of OCD. It can help determine the size, depth, location, and stability of the lesion, depending on the various imaging criteria. The presence of fluid or granulation tissue at the interface between the fragment and its bed, best seen on T2-weighted images, indicates an unstable lesion. Magnetic resonance imaging staging, which is similar to arthroscopic staging, is as follows[5,9]:

Stage 0: normal

Stage I: signal changes consistent with articular cartilage injury, without disruption, and with normal subchondral bone

Stage II: high signal intensity; breach of the articular cartilage with a stable subchondral fragment

Stage III: partial chondral detachment with a thin high-signal rim (on T2-weighted images) behind the osteochondral fragment, representing synovial fluid

Stage IV: loose body in the center of the osteochondral bed or free in the joint space

Management of OCD is determined by several factors, including the age of the patient, the level of skeletal maturity, and the location and size of the lesion. Two forms of OCD have been described: juvenile and adult. In juvenile OCD, the presence of open physes is the most important determinant of treatment. Conservative management of juvenile OCD has had good results, with a reported healing potential between 50% and 91%.[2,3] In juvenile OCD patients in whom conservative management fails and in patients with symptomatic adult OCD, operative treatment is often necessary.

We use the following approach when treating OCD at the University of Pittsburgh (Fig. 57–1). OCD lesions are subdivided according to the integrity of the overlying cartilage. There are three types of lesions: in situ, in situ detached, and detached. In situ lesions have an intact articular cartilage surface and are best treated with in situ pinning. The goals are to stabilize the lesion, promote healing, and halt the progression of the disease process. In situ detached lesions have a partially disrupted articular cartilage surface. The bed of the lesion communicates with the joint and synovial fluid via the break in the overlying hyaline cartilage surface. The bed is often coated with a fibrous tissue that prevents healing of the fragment. Treatment consists of hinging the fragment open, debriding the fibrous base to bleeding bone, bone grafting (if necessary), and internal fixation. Finally, detached lesions (i.e., osteochondral loose bodies) require debridement of the bed, tailoring of the fragment, bone grafting (if necessary), and internal fixation if possible.[10]

Several fixation methods have been described in the literature, including Kirschner wires, headless variable-pitch compression screws, cannulated screws, bone pegs, and bioabsorbable pins and screws.[3] Despite the

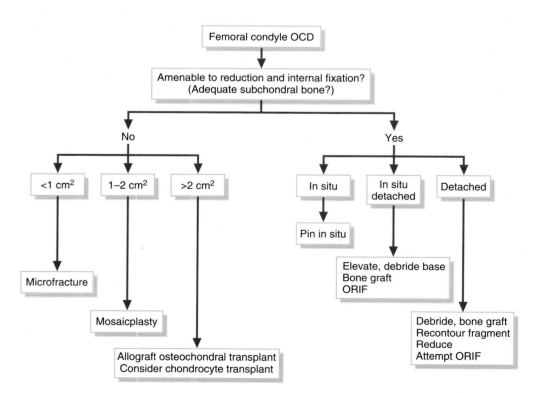

Figure 57–1 Treatment algorithm for osteochondral lesions of the knee. OCD, osteochondritis dissecans; ORIF, open reduction and internal fixation.

variations in fixation methods, the ultimate goal is to attain stability and compression to promote healing of the fragment.

Case History 1: Fixation and Bone Grafting of Unstable in Situ Detached OCD of the Medial Femoral Condyle

History

RA is a 36-year-old truck driver who complains of pain and "catching" in his right knee. The first episode of pain began 2 months ago while he was walking to work. At that time, he felt a "pop" and sharp pain in the center of his knee. There was no history of trauma. Since then, he has had several episodes of "catching, swelling, and giving way" with ambulation. The pain is intermittent and is localized to the anteromedial aspect of the knee. He has significant discomfort with running, kneeling, and squatting.

His past medical history and past surgical history are noncontributory. He takes no medications.

Physical Examination

RA is 5 feet 10 inches tall and weighs 190 pounds. He ambulates with a bent knee, antalgic gait. His standing alignment is 2 degrees of valgus bilaterally. Range of motion is 3 to 135 degrees on the right and 0 to 140 degrees on the left. The involved knee demonstrates approximately 10% quadriceps atrophy and a small effusion.

Examination of the patellofemoral joint reveals symmetry with a 0-degree patellar tilt, two quadrants of medial and lateral patella glide, no facet tenderness, no crepitation, and no apprehension. His knee is stable, with a normal and symmetrical ligament examination. There is tenderness along the anteromedial femoral condyle at 90 degrees of knee flexion, but no significant joint line tenderness. There is a positive Wilson test, with pain elicited on internal rotation of the tibia at approximately 45 degrees of knee flexion and relieved with external rotation.

Imaging

Radiographs of the right knee were obtained, including posteroanterior flexion weight-bearing, lateral, and Merchant views (Fig. 57–2). These images reveal a large OCD lesion of the lateral aspect of the medial femoral condyle.

Magnetic resonance imaging is performed and reveals an unstable in situ detached lesion, with disruption of the overlying chondral surface. T2-weighted images reveal joint fluid between the osteochondral fragment and its base (Fig. 57–3).

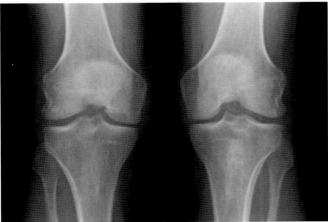

A

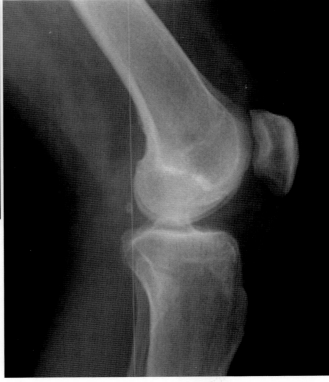

B

Figure 57–2 Flexion weight-bearing posteroanterior (A) and lateral (B) views of the right knee. Note the radiolucent area of the osteochondritis dissecans lesion at the classic site—the lateral aspect of the medial femoral condyle.

6 Knee

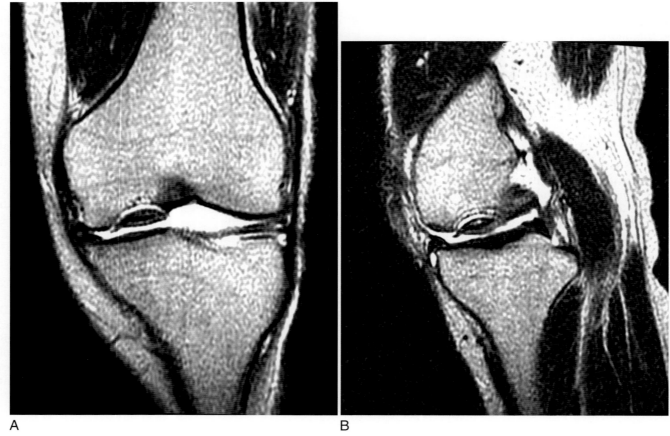

A   B

Figure 57–3   Coronal *(A)* and sagittal *(B)* T2-weighted images. Note the increased signal between the osteochondritis dissecans fragment and its bed. This is an in situ detached lesion.

Surgical Technique

Positioning and Preparation

The patient is placed in the supine position. All bony prominences are well padded to avoid pressure necrosis of the skin. A sandbag is secured to the foot of the table to support the heel at 90 degrees of knee flexion. A side post is positioned at the level of the tourniquet, which is inflated only as needed. The knee is prepared and draped to the proximal thigh to allow full knee access and unrestricted motion of the knee.

Examination under Anesthesia

During the examination under anesthesia, RA is found to have a moderate effusion. There is a symmetrical range of motion from 0 to 140 degrees with a palpable "click" at the anteromedial joint line. Ligament examination reveals a 1+ Lachman test with a firm endpoint, a normal tibial step-off, and no varus-valgus or posterolateral rotatory instability.

Diagnostic Arthroscopy

Standard superolateral, anteromedial, and anterolateral portals are used. The arthroscope is introduced through the anterolateral portal, and a systematic evaluation is performed. Examination of the patellofemoral joint and lateral compartment demonstrates no evidence of chondral or meniscal pathology. Examination of the medial compartment reveals an in situ detached OCD lesion with an intact medial border. The lesion measures approximately 2.5 by 3 cm. A probe is used to palpate the lesion, with care taken not to disrupt the medial chondral hinge (Fig. 57–4). The bed is examined and reveals fibrous tissue interposition (Fig. 57–5). A mini–medial parapatellar arthrotomy is performed for improved access to the lesion.

Specific Surgical Steps

MINI–MEDIAL PARAPATELLAR ARTHROTOMY

The knee is positioned at 90 degrees of flexion, and the anteromedial portal is extended in a superior and inferior direction for a total of 4 cm. The subcutaneous layer is carefully dissected to the capsule, and sensory branches of the infrapatellar saphenous nerve are protected (Fig. 57–6). These branches cross the inferior portion of the incision. The anteromedial portal site is defined, and the capsulotomy is enlarged. Inferior extension is performed with great care to avoid injury to the anterior horn of the medial meniscus (see Fig. 57–6). A

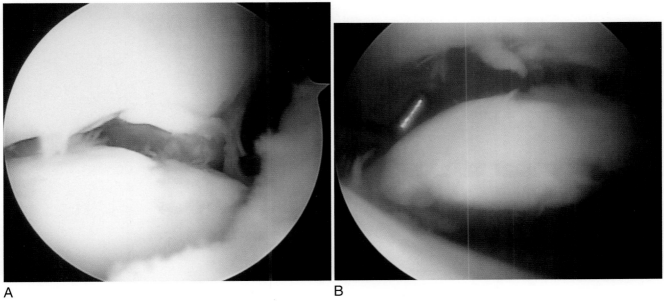

Figure 57–4   *A,* The chondral surface is disrupted at the anterior, posterior, and lateral aspects of the osteochondritis dissecans lesion. *B,* The lesion is hinged on the intact medial chondral surface to evaluate the bed.

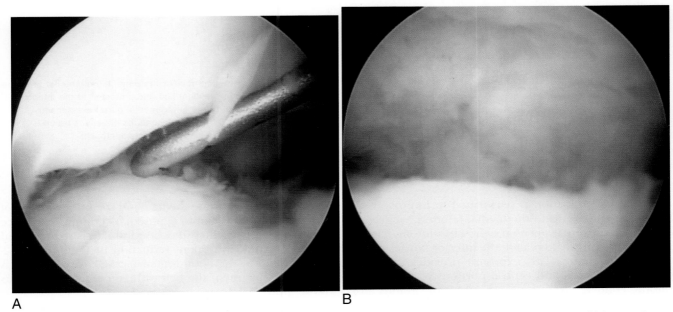

Figure 57–5   The undersurface *(A)* and bed *(B)* of the osteochondritis dissecans lesion are covered with fibrous tissue, which prevents healing of the fragment.

6 Knee

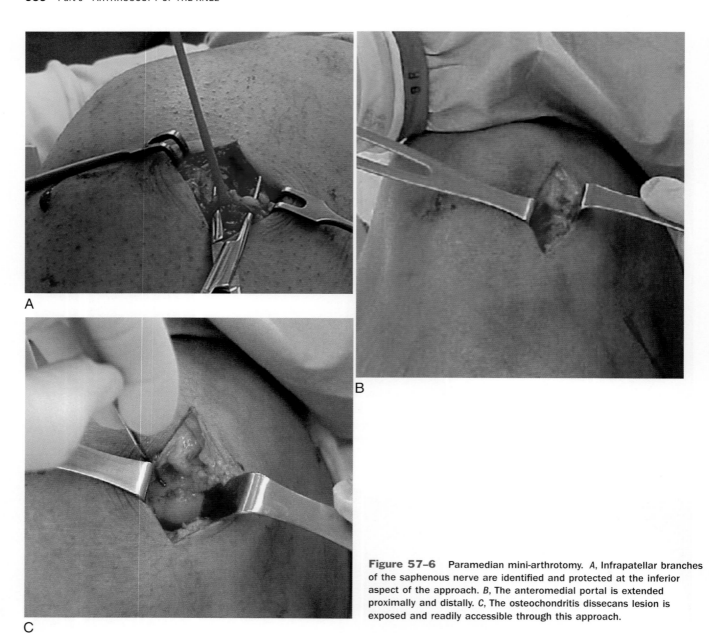

Figure 57–6   Paramedian mini-arthrotomy. *A,* Infrapatellar branches of the saphenous nerve are identified and protected at the inferior aspect of the approach. *B,* The anteromedial portal is extended proximally and distally. *C,* The osteochondritis dissecans lesion is exposed and readily accessible through this approach.

limited fat pad resection is performed to improve visualization of and access to the medial femoral condyle. If additional exposure is necessary, the capsulotomy can be extended proximally to release the inferior border of the medial retinaculum. This exposure provides excellent access to the lateral and central portions of the medial femoral condyle. Anterior and posterior lesions are easily visualized with extension or flexion of the knee, respectively.

ASSESSMENT AND FIXATION

The OCD lesion is identified at the lateral aspect of the medial femoral condyle at 90 degrees of knee flexion. The area of chondral separation is hinged on the intact medial border of the lesion to reveal the fibrous bed. A

curet is used to debride the bed and the undersurface of the osteochondral flap to exposed, bleeding bone. Once this is performed, the osteochondral flap is reduced and assessed. A noncongruent reduction is noted, with a 2-mm step-off at the chondral surface. At this point, it is decided to augment the bed with autologous cancellous bone graft.

Cancellous autograft is harvested from the ipsilateral limb at Gerdy's tubercle. A 2-cm longitudinal incision is made over Gerdy's tubercle, and the subcutaneous tissue is dissected down to the periosteum. The periosteum is incised and reflected. A 1-cm cortical window is created to gain access to the metaphyseal bone of the proximal lateral tibia. A curet is used to harvest the cancellous bone. The cortical window is replaced, the periosteum is repaired, and the incision is closed.

The bone graft is placed into the bed and successively impacted. Reduction is repeated, and the chondral surface is reassessed. Once adequate bone graft has been applied and the reduction is congruent, the lesion is held in place with 1.6-mm Kirschner wires. These wires are carefully spaced to avoid crowding of areas where the final fixation will be placed.

Fixation is achieved with a 4-mm partially threaded cancellous screw. The screw is placed at the center of the lesion and perpendicular to the chondral surface. The screw head is countersunk below the chondral surface to avoid injury to the articular surface of the tibia. Over-tightening of the screw is avoided, because aggressive compression can fracture the osteochondral fragment. The periphery of the lesion is secured with two 1.5- by 20-mm SmartNails (Bionix, Blue Bell, PA) placed perpendicular to the chondral surface. Final assessment demonstrates a congruent reduction with secure fixation (Fig. 57–7). Postoperative radiographs are obtained to ensure proper positioning and length of the screw (Fig. 57–8).

The wounds are irrigated with copious amounts of antibiotic solution. The arthrotomy is closed with number 2 braided, nonabsorbable suture. The subcutaneous layer and skin are closed in a standard fashion.

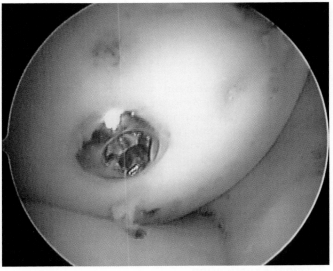

Figure 57–7 The bed is bone grafted, and the osteochondritis dissecans lesion is reduced and secured with a 4-mm partially threaded cancellous screw and two bioabsorbable SmartNails (Bionix, Blue Bell, PA).

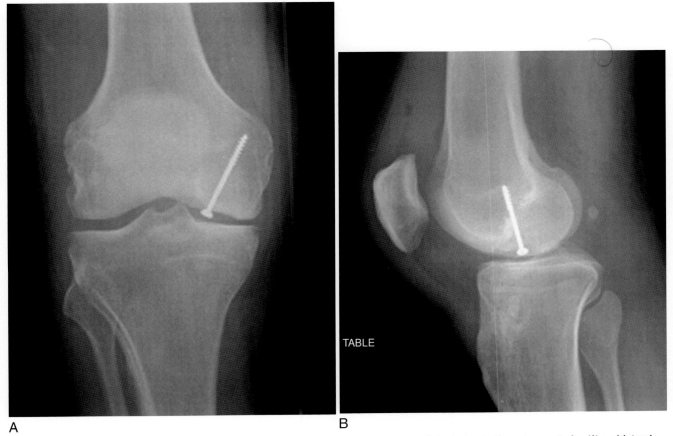

A

B

Figure 57–8 Postoperative radiographs. Note that the screw is placed in the center of the lesion in the anteroposterior *(A)* and lateral *(B)* planes.

6 Knee

Case History 2. Arthroscopic Retrograde Fixation of in Situ Detached OCD of the Patella

History

The patient is a 15-year-old male cross-country runner who presents with a 3-month history of right anterior knee pain. He has been unable to run because of peripatellar knee discomfort. His pain is exacerbated by running downhill. Treatment to date has included an intra-articular steroid injection and nonsteroidal anti-inflammatory medications, but his symptoms have persisted. He is referred by his local orthopedic surgeon. The patient is otherwise healthy, his only medication is the prescribed nonsteroid anti-inflammatory medicine, and he is a nonsmoker.

Physical Examination

The patient is 5 feet 11 inches tall and weighs 170 pounds. He stands with 2 degrees of valgus alignment bilaterally. There is an antalgic gait, and squat is limited to 90 degrees with pain anteriorly. There is approximately 5% quadriceps atrophy and a small effusion. Range of motion is symmetrical and 0 to 130 degrees. The ligament examination is normal. The patellofemoral examination reveals a 0-degree patellar tilt, negative lateral patellar apprehension, and two quadrants of medial and lateral patellar glides with mild, fine crepitation. There is tenderness at the medial and lateral patellar facets. There is no joint line tenderness.

Imaging

Flexion weight-bearing, lateral, and Merchant views are obtained (Fig. 57–9). An OCD lesion is noted on the lateral facet of the patella and is best seen with the Merchant view. Magnetic resonance imaging is performed and demonstrates an intact chondral surface (Fig. 57–10). The lesion appears to be an in situ lesion.

Surgical Technique

Positioning

The patient is placed in a supine position on a radiolucent table. An image intensifier (C-arm fluoroscope) is positioned on the contralateral side of the operating table and is set to obtain lateral and Merchant views of the patella (Fig. 57–11). The optimal position of the limb and C-arm is determined before prepping and draping.

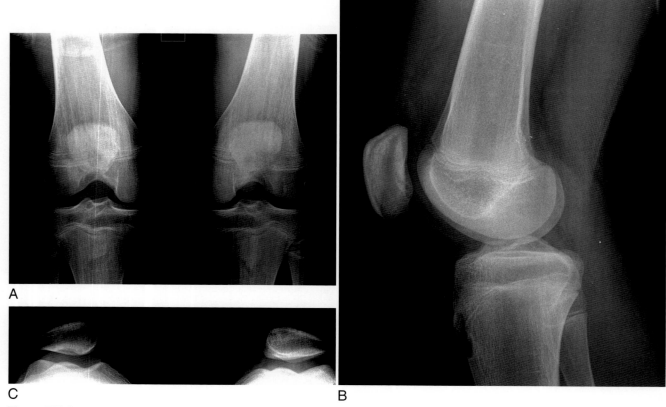

Figure 57–9 Flexion weight-bearing posteroanterior (A), lateral (B), and Merchant (C) views. Note the radiolucent area on the lateral facet of the patella, best seen on the Merchant view.

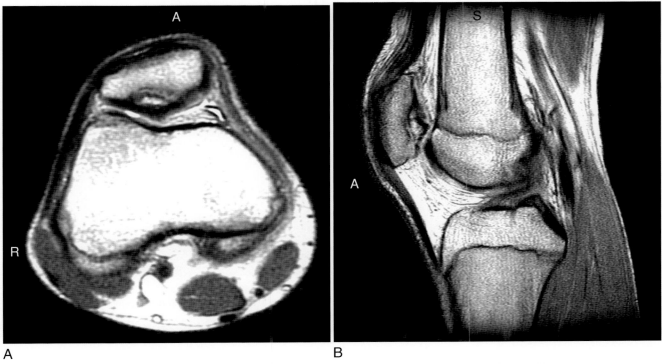

Figure 57–10   Magnetic resonance imaging scans of the involved knee. Axial *(A)* and sagittal *(B)* images demonstrate an in situ lesion. The chondral surface appears to be intact.

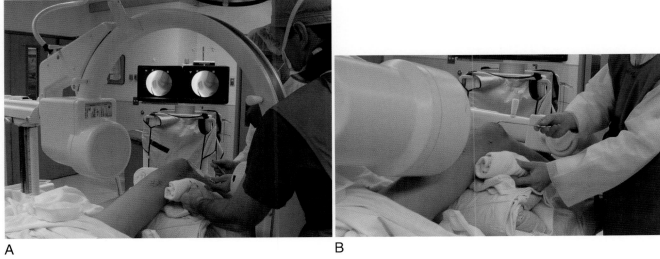

Figure 57–11   Optimal positions of the leg and fluoroscope are determined before preparation and draping of the patient. The location of the osteochondritis dissecans lesion is identified in both the lateral *(A)* and the Merchant *(B)* views.

The knee is prepared and draped to the proximal thigh to allow full access of the knee and unrestricted motion of the knee. A tourniquet is used as needed.

Examination under Anesthesia

During the examination under anesthesia, there is symmetrical range of motion from 0 to 130 degrees bilaterally. The ligament examination is normal. The patella examination reveals two quadrants of medial and lateral

patellar glide and a 0-degree patellar tilt. Patellofemoral "clicking" and crepitation are noted on patellar grind testing.

Diagnostic Arthroscopy

Standard superolateral, anteromedial, and anterolateral portals are used. The OCD lesion is identified and viewed with a 70-degree arthroscope in the superolateral portal and with a 30-degree arthroscope in the anterolateral

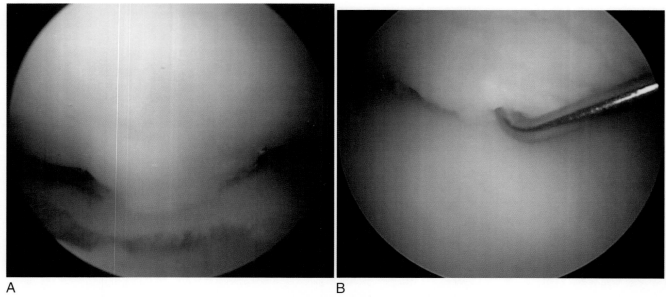

A   B

Figure 57–12   The osteochondritis dissecans lesion is evaluated thoroughly, with a 70-degree scope in the superolateral portal *(A)* and a 30-degree scope in the anterolateral portal. The chondral surface is soft but intact *(B)*.

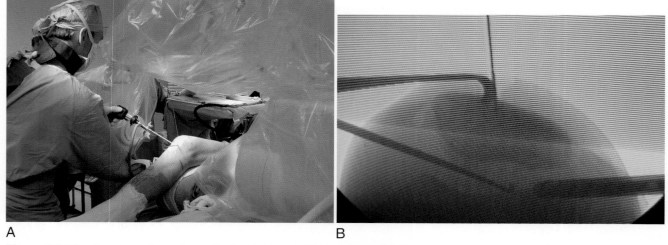

A   B

Figure 57–13   Fluoroscopy is used to guide the placement of fixation in the lateral *(A)* and Merchant *(B)* views. The guidewire is centered on the lesion and perpendicular to its bed. Counterpressure is applied with a probe on the chondral surface. Chondral penetration is avoided by the use of fluoroscopy and direct visualization of the surface with the arthroscope.

portal. A probe is used to assess the extent of the lesion. The chondral surface is soft and has areas of fissuring; however, it is intact. There is slight motion of the lesion on palpation, indicating that the underlying fragment is detached, despite an intact chondral surface. The size of the lesion is 1.5 by 2 cm (Fig. 57–12).

Specific Surgical Steps

FIXATION

Fluoroscopy is used to identify the level of the lesion in the lateral and Merchant views. The skin is marked, and a 2-cm longitudinal incision is made over the patella.

The guidewire is aimed to enter the center of the OCD lesion, perpendicular to its base. Fluoroscopy is used to position the guide pin (Fig. 57–13). The pin is advanced through the subchondral bone without penetration of the chondral surface. The arthroscope views the chondral surface as the guide pin is advanced. A cannulated depth gauge is placed over the guide pin to measure screw length. One cannulated Acutrak screw (Acumed, Beaverton, OR) is placed over the guide pin and used to secure the fragment. The differential pitch on this screw provides compression across the defect. Final screw placement is visualized in perpendicular planes using fluoroscopy and plain radiographs to ensure proper orientation and length (Fig. 57–14). The OCD lesion is

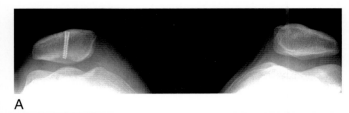

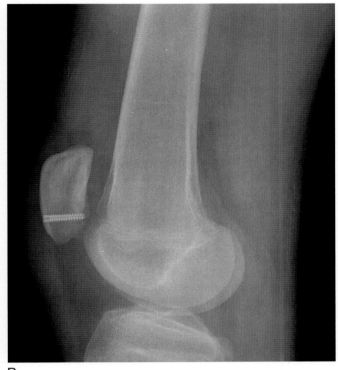

Figure 57–14   Postoperative radiographs showing the central placement of the variable-pitch Acutrak screw (Acumed, Beaverton, OR) on the Merchant *(A)* and lateral *(B)* views.

now stable to probing. The chondral surface remains intact. The incisions are irrigated and closed in a standard fashion.

Postoperative Management

The knee is held in extension in a hinged knee brace for 1 to 2 weeks. The brace is locked at all times except for self-guided exercises. A continuous passive motion machine is used for 4 to 6 weeks. Quadriceps sets, heel slides, straight leg raises, and calf pumps are started immediately. Touch-down weight bearing is permitted during the first 4 to 6 weeks, followed by progressive weight bearing. Radiographs are obtained on the first postoperative visit 1 week after surgery and on successive follow-up visits every 4 weeks. Physical therapy is focused on range-of-motion exercises for the first 2 weeks, after which gentle, progressive strengthening is initiated. Once adequate radiographic healing is confirmed, approximately 4 to 6 months after surgery, the screw is removed percutaneously. At that time, the status of the

hyaline chondral surface is assessed arthroscopically, as is the stability and healing of the OCD lesion.

Summary

Femoral condyle OCD lesions may be approached arthroscopically and through mini-open techniques. The anatomy of the knee can make a pure arthroscopic approach very difficult, if not impossible in certain cases. We routinely perform a mini–medial or lateral parapatellar arthrotomy, which in most cases allows direct access and visualization of the lesion. Internal fixation can be placed perpendicular to the fragment, which maximizes the stability and compression obtained. Lesions involving the patella can be especially challenging, given the orientation of the articular surface. The medial or lateral patellar facet can be approached through a small arthrotomy, although some degree of patellar eversion is necessary to place the fixation perpendicular to the chondral surface. We prefer retrograde fixation of patellar OCD lesions, using fluoroscopic guidance and arthroscopic assistance; this allows the fixation to be placed perpendicular to the lesion, and the chondral surface is not violated.

Primary repair of OCD lesions of the knee should be attempted whenever possible. Reduction, bone grafting (if necessary), and internal fixation can stabilize the fragment and maximize healing potential. Further, restoration of joint congruity should be a priority and can help retard the progression of degenerative joint disease.

References

1. Aichroth P: Osteochondritis dissecans of the knee: A clinical survey. J Bone Joint Surg Br 53:440, 1971.
2. Cahill BR, Phillips MR, Navarro R: The results of conservative management of juvenile osteochondritis dissecans using joint scintigraphy: A prospective study. Am J Sports Med 17:601, 1989.
3. Cain EL, Clancy WG: Treatment algorithm for ostechondral injuries of the knee. Clin Sports Med 20:321-342, 2001.
4. Linden B: The incidence of osteochondritis dissecans in the condyles of the femur. Acta Orthop Scand 47:664, 1976.
5. Loredo R, Sanders TG: Imaging of osteochondral injuries. Clin Sports Med 20:249-278, 2001.
6. Milgram JW: Radiological and pathological manifestations of osteochondritis dissecans of the distal femur. Diagn Radiol 126:305, 1978.
7. Mubarack SJ, Carroll NC: Familial osteochondritis dissecans of the knee. Clin Orthop 140:131, 1979.
8. Mubarak SJ, Carroll NC: Juvenile osteochondritis dissecans of the knee: Etiology. Clin Orthop 157: 200, 1981.
9. Nelson DW, DiPaola J, Colville M, et al: Osteochondritis dissecans of the talus and knee: Prospective comparison of MR and arthroscopic classifications. J Comput Assist Tomogr 14:804-808, 1990.
10. Petrie RS, Klimkiewicz JJ, Harner CD: Surgical management of chondral and osteochondral lesion of the knee. In Harner CD, Vince KG, Fu FH (eds): Techniques in Knee Surgery. Philadelphia, Lippincott Williams & Wilkins, 2001, pp 140-158.
11. Schenck RC, Goodnight JM: Osteochondritis dissecans. J Bone Joint Surg Am 78:439, 1996.

6 Knee

Avascular Necrosis Drilling in the Knee

DAVID R. DIDUCH AND BRETT J. HAMPTON

AVASCULAR NECROSIS DRILLING IN THE KNEE IN A NUTSHELL

History:
  Multiple sclerosis, high-dose oral steroids, progressively worsening knee pain

Physical Examination:
  Trace effusion and lateral joint line tenderness; stable to ligamentous examination and full range of motion; McMurray test negative for click or pain

Imaging:
  Plain radiographs unremarkable, without evidence of arthrosis, collapse, altered density, or malalignment; magnetic resonance imaging reveals serpiginous foci of subchondral high-signal abnormality on T2-weighted images within the femoral condyles and lateral tibial plateau

Indications:
  Immediate core decompression indicated for stage I, II, or III symptomatic knees with avascular necrosis

Surgical Technique:
  See Table 58–1 for antegrade and retrograde (distal femur) and retrograde (proximal tibia) techniques

Postoperative Management:
  50% weight bearing for 2 weeks until radiographs rule out collapse, then advance as tolerated; physical therapy three times a week for 4 weeks for quadriceps strengthening and active and passive range-of-motion exercises

Results:
  Core decompression for stage I, II, and III symptomatic knees provides symptomatic relief, with 79% of patients having good or excellent results at 7 years; a repeat core decompression with arthroscopic debridement may be of some benefit for those failing initial core decompression

---

Avascular necrosis (AVN), or atraumatic osteonecrosis of the knee, involves a loss of blood supply to a segment of bone, which can lead to bone death and subchondral fracture with collapse of the joint surface. The knee is the second most common location for osteonecrosis and is affected approximately 10% as often as the hip.[8-10] The disease may affect the distal femur, proximal tibia, or both. Atraumatic osteonecrosis usually occurs in patients younger than 55 years, involves multiple condyles, and is bilateral in more than 80% of cases. These patients are predominantly women, have osteonecrosis of other large

joints in 60% to 90% of cases, and frequently have a history of systemic lupus erythematosus, sickle-cell disease, alcoholism, or systemic corticosteroid use. The pathologic lesion may be located in the diaphysis, metaphysis, or epiphysis.[8]

AVN is different from spontaneous osteonecrosis of the knee (SONK). SONK usually occurs in patients older than 55 years, involves only one condyle (medial femoral condyle most commonly), and is unilateral in 99% of cases.[8] It rarely involves other joints and is three times more common in women.[2] The pathologic lesion in

Table 58–1

Avascular Necrosis Drilling Techniques

Retrograde Technique (Distal Femur)

Fluoroscopy required
2-mm guidewire used to pierce skin down to bone
Fluoroscopy used to identify starting location for guidewire in AP and lateral views
Advance guidewire in AP view to within a few millimeters of articular surface
Confirm position in lateral view by placing probe against target condyle's distal articular surface
Advance guidewire using arthroscopic visualization to just barely pierce articular surface
Use 4.5-mm cannulated drill bit to perform drilling decompression, advancing bit by hand for better control as it approaches articular surface; drill bit should stop 2 mm short of articular surface
Two to three passes with guidewire and cannulated drill bit required for each lesion

Retrograde Technique (Proximal Tibia)

No fluoroscopy required
ACL guide used to target lesion
Place 2-mm guidewire through ACL guide and allow it to just pierce articular surface
Use 4.5-mm cannulated drill bit to perform drilling decompression, stopping drill bit just beneath articular surface

Antegrade Technique (Distal Femur)

No fluoroscopy required
Make multiple drill holes in lesion with smooth, 1- to 2-mm guidewire of sufficient depth to penetrate lesion
After drilling, motorized shaver with suction can be used to aspirate drilled tract for bleeding

ACL, anterior cruciate ligament; AP, anteroposterior.

SONK is located in the subchondral bone and extends to the articular surface. Collapse of the weakened subchondral bone results in joint incongruity and pain. In contrast, AVN characteristically involves a larger area of subchondral bone, with extension well into the epiphysis and even the metaphysis.

Treatment options for symptomatic AVN of the knee include nonoperative therapy (e.g., restricted weight bearing and administration of analgesics) and observation.[1,9,10] Surgical treatment can include arthroscopic debridement,[7,8] core decompression,[4,8,10] high tibial osteotomy,[8] vascularized bone grafting,[12] and resurfacing with osteoarticular allografts.[3,6] Unicompartmental arthroplasty[5] and total knee arthroplasty[9] are additional treatment options for patients with condylar collapse and secondary arthrosis.

Magnetic resonance imaging (MRI) is the diagnostic imaging modality of choice, although bone scanning may be used in patients unable to tolerate the special demands of MRI. It should be noted, however, that one recent study found that technetium-99m bone scanning missed lesions in 16 of 56 knees (29%) with AVN, reflecting its lack of sensitivity.[8]

This chapter focuses on the arthroscopic treatment of AVN, specifically core decompression and debridement, and emphasizes the special techniques and equipment required.

Case History

A 30-year-old white woman with multiple sclerosis presents with a 3-month history of progressively worsening bilateral knee pain, left greater than right. The patient has received multiple high-dose oral steroid preparations for treatment of her condition and for optic neuritis. The knee pain has begun to interfere with her activities of daily living and caused her to miss work as a critical care nurse. Her pain is described as deep within the knee, sharp and stabbing in quality, and not dependent on weight bearing or position. She denies hip pain bilaterally and complains of only occasional bilateral ankle pain.

Physical Examination

On physical examination, the left knee has a trace effusion and lateral joint line tenderness. The right knee has no effusion and no tenderness to palpation. Both knees are stable to ligamentous examination and have full range of motion. The McMurray test is negative for click or pain.

Imaging

Plain radiographs of both knees are unremarkable, without evidence of arthrosis, collapse, altered density, or malalignment, as are screening radiographs of her pelvis and ankles. The left knee MRI reveals serpiginous foci of high-signal abnormality on T2-weighted images within the femoral condyles and lateral tibial plateau. These areas have the characteristic appearance of AVN and are primarily subchondral in location (Fig. 58–1). The right knee MRI reveals multiple serpentine high-signal areas on T2-weighted images within the medial and lateral femoral condyles, medial and lateral tibial plateaus, and superior pole of the patella. Screening MRI studies are also performed of the pelvis and both ankles. The pelvic MRI demonstrates bilateral femoral head AVN without collapse. The bilateral ankle studies are unremarkable. It is decided that this patient will undergo arthroscopic treatment first for her more symptomatic left knee.

Surgical Technique

Positioning and Diagnostic Arthroscopy

The patient is placed supine at the distal end of the operating table to facilitate fluoroscopy access, and a tourniquet is placed on her left thigh. A lateral post is used to

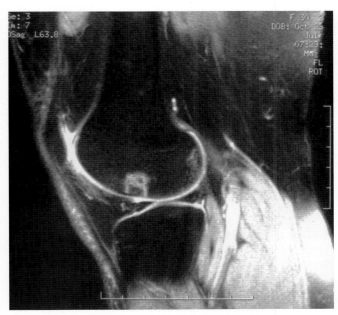

Figure 58–1   Magnetic resonance imaging scan revealing an avascular necrosis lesion.

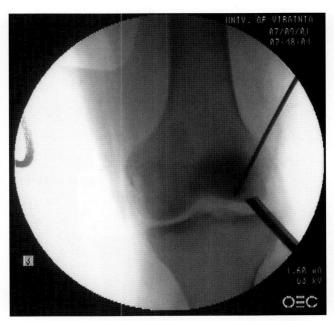

Figure 58–2   Fluoroscopic image of the guidewire advanced to the articular surface and the arthroscope using the retrograde technique.

stabilize the extremity for valgus stress, while also facilitating hip rotation into a figure-of-four position for lateral knee access and fluoroscopic imaging. The left lower extremity is prepared and draped, and the tourniquet is inflated. The arthroscope is introduced into the knee through a standard inferolateral portal, and a systematic arthroscopic evaluation of the knee is performed. The inferomedial portal is established under direct vision. In the lateral compartment, there is softening of an area on the distal femur that corresponds to the MRI localization of the AVN lesion.

Specific Surgical Steps

Retrograde drilling of the lateral condyle lesion is performed. The retrograde technique permits a larger-diameter channel for decompression than could safely be achieved by drilling antegrade through the cartilage surface. Slightly anterior and proximal to the palpable lateral epicondyle, a 2-mm smooth guidewire is used to pierce the skin and subcutaneous tissue down to bone. Fluoroscopy is used to assist in identifying the starting location for the guidewire in the anteroposterior and lateral projections. By rotating the leg into a figure-of-four position, the fluoroscopy C-arm can be left in place with only minor rotational changes. The guidewire is then carefully advanced in the anteroposterior view to within a few millimeters of the articular surface (Fig. 58–2). The position of the guidewire is confirmed in the lateral projection. Identification of the target condyle and its articular surface is facilitated by an arthroscopic probe placed against the distal articular surface of the condyle (Fig. 58–3). The articular surfaces form overlapping shadows, and this technique eliminates confusion on the lateral radiographic projection by identifying

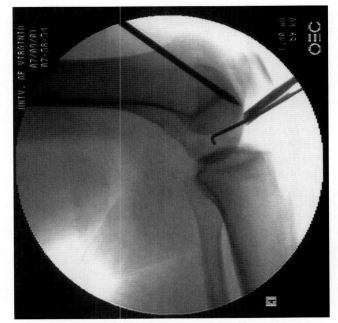

Figure 58–3   Fluoroscopic image of the target condyle identified in the lateral projection using the arthroscopic probe placed against the distal articular surface of the condyle.

which profile represents the target condyle. The guidewire is then advanced and viewed through the arthroscope as the tip is allowed to just barely pierce the articular surface of the condyle. A 4.5-mm cannulated drill bit from the Endobutton set (Smith and Nephew Endoscopy, Andover, MA) is passed over the guidewire to perform the drilling decompression (Fig.

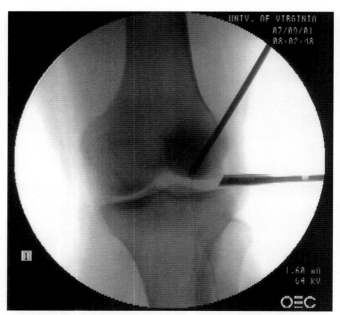

Figure 58-4 Fluoroscopic image of the cannulated drill bit over the guidewire using the retrograde technique.

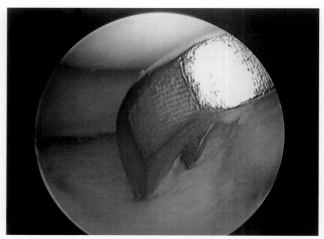

Figure 58-5 Anterior cruciate ligament guide used to target a tibial avascular necrosis lesion using the retrograde technique.

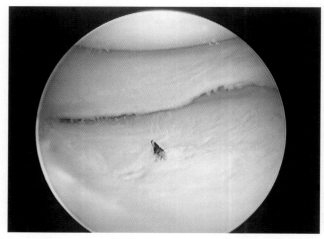

Figure 58-6 Guidewire piercing the tibial articular surface using the retrograde technique.

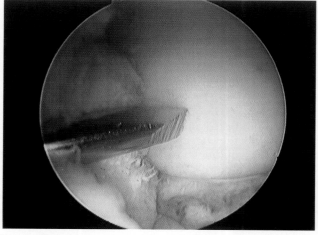

Figure 58-7 Perforating the distal femur articular surface with a smooth guidewire using the antegrade technique.

58–4). The bit is advanced by hand for better control as it approaches the articular surface, stopping 2 mm short of the surface using fluoroscopic visualization. Generally, two or three passes with the guidewire and cannulated drill bit are performed for each lesion on the condyle. Similarly, soft areas in the medial distal femur, which also correspond to the MRI identification of the AVN lesions, are treated with arthroscopic retrograde drilling as described earlier.

For lesions in the proximal tibia, retrograde drilling of the lesion with the use of an anterior cruciate ligament (ACL) guide for targeting is another valuable technique. In this situation, the lesion is identified by intra-articular inspection and correlated with MRI findings, as described earlier. The ACL guide is then used to target the lesion as the guidewire is placed through the ACL guide and allowed to just pierce the articular surface (Figs. 58–5 and 58–6). This guided retrograde technique does not require fluoroscopy. Overdrilling with the 4.5-mm cannulated drill bit is then performed, stopping just as the edge of the drill bit begins to be visible beneath the articular cartilage.

An alternative technique involves antegrade drilling from the articular surface into the lesion. In this technique, the articular surface softening is correlated with the MRI scan to localize the lesion. Multiple drill holes are then made directly into the lesion using a smooth, 1- to 2-mm guidewire to sufficient depth to penetrate through the lesion into healthy bone (Fig. 58–7). After completion of the drilling, a motorized shaver with suction can be used to aspirate the drilled tract for bleeding (Fig. 58–8). This would indicate decompression and evidence of drilling completely through the subchondral dead bone.

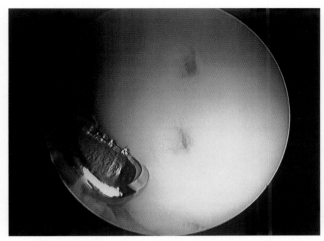

Figure 58-8   Motorized shaver with suction aspirates the drilled tract for bleeding using the antegrade technique.

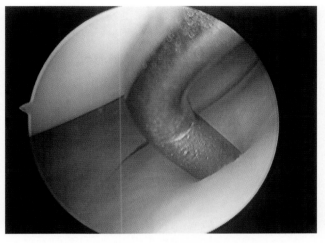

Figure 58-9   Lateral tibial plateau demonstrating softening.

Postoperative Management

Postoperative management consists of 50% weight bearing for 2 weeks until radiographs are performed in the office to rule out collapse. Then weight bearing is advanced as tolerated. At that point, patients may benefit from physical therapy three times a week for 4 weeks for quadriceps strengthening and active and passive range-of-motion exercises. This patient had arthroscopy and drilling of her right knee approximately 1 month later in a similar manner.

Results

AVN of the knee is classified using the system of Ficat and Arlet as modified for the knee.[8] In this radiographic staging system, stage I knees have a normal appearance. Stage II knees have cystic or osteosclerotic lesions or both, with a normal contour of the bone without subchondral collapse or flattening of the articular surface. Stage III knees have a crescent sign or subchondral collapse. Stage IV knees have narrowing of the joint space with secondary degenerative changes on the opposing joint surface, such as cysts, marginal osteophytes, and destruction of cartilage. If untreated, AVN can progress from articular surface softening (Fig. 58-9) to fragmentation (Figs. 58-10 and 58-11) and finally collapse (Figs. 58-12 and 58-13). Treatment of symptomatic AVN with nonoperative methods such as restricted weight bearing, analgesics, and observation has a greater than 80% rate of clinical failure.[11] An immediate core decompression of symptomatic knees is now recommended, with observation for asymptomatic knees. Core decompression for stage I, II, or III symptomatic knees has been demonstrated to provide symptomatic relief, with 79% of patients having good or excellent Knee Society scores at a mean of 7 years.[8] For those who fail an initial core decompression, a repeat core decompression with

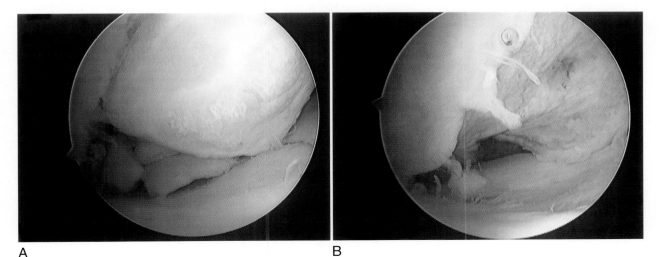

A   B

Figure 58-10   *A*, Fragmentation of the distal femoral condyle. *B*, After debridement.

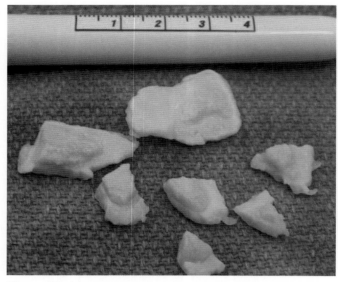

Figure 58–11 Fragments removed arthroscopically.

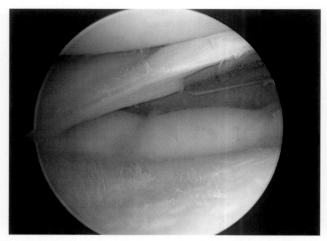

Figure 58–12 Collapse of the medial tibial articular surface.

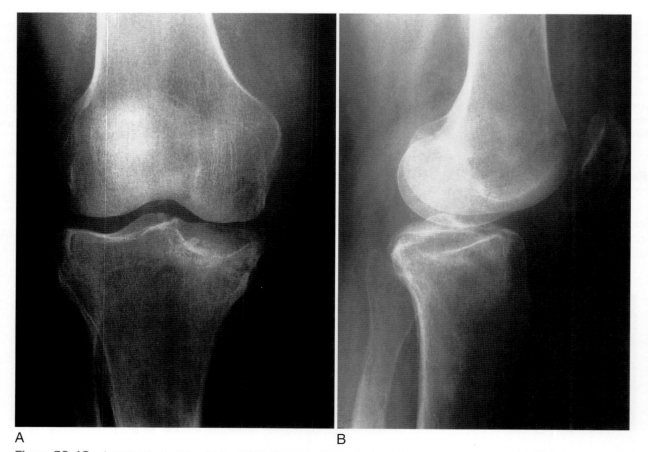

A

B

Figure 58–13 Anteroposterior *(A)* and lateral *(B)* radiographs demonstrating collapse of the tibial articular surface.

arthroscopic debridement may provide some benefit, with results almost as good as those for initial attempts.[8] Arthroscopic drilling and debridement are valuable tools in the treatment of AVN of the knee, with the ability to provide lasting pain relief, delay radiographic progression, identify and treat associated intra-articular pathology, effect healing of the lesion, and delay or obviate the need for joint arthroplasty.

Complications

Complications of AVN drilling are generally limited and include inability to localize the lesion, penetration of the articular surface with the drill bit, soft tissue irritation or burn if a number 11 blade is not used to open a skin incision, and other risks inherent to knee arthroscopy, including infection and deep venous thrombosis.

References

1. Ahlback S, Bauer GC, Bohne W, et al: Spontaneous osteonecrosis of the knee. Arthritis Rheum 11:705-733, 1968.
2. Ecker ML, Lotke PA: Spontaneous osteonecrosis of the knee. J Am Acad Orthop Surg 2:173-178, 1994.
3. Flynn JM, Springfield DS, Mankin HJ, et al: Osteoarticular allografts to treat distal femoral osteonecrosis. Clin Orthop 303:38-43, 1994.
4. Jacobs MA, Loeb PE, Hungerford DS, et al: Core decompression of the distal femur for avascular necrosis of the knee. J Bone Joint Surg Br 71:583-587, 1989.
5. Marmor L: Unicompartmental arthroplasty for osteonecrosis of the knee joint. Clin Orthop 294:247-253, 1993.
6. Meyers MH, Akeson W, Convery FR, et al: Resurfacing of the knee with fresh osteochondral allograft. J Bone Joint Surg Am 71:704-713, 1989.
7. Miller GK, Maylahn DJ, Drennan DB, et al: The treatment of idiopathic osteonecrosis of the medial femoral condyle with arthroscopic debridement. Arthroscopy 2:21-29, 1986.
8. Mont MA, Baumgarten KM, Rifai A, et al: Atraumatic osteonecrosis of the knee. J Bone Joint Surg Am 82:1279-1290, 2000.
9. Mont MA, Rifai A, Baumgarten KM, et al: Total knee arthroplasty for osteonecrosis. J Bone Joint Surg Am 84:599-603, 2002.
10. Mont MA, Tomek IM, Hungerford DS: Core decompression for avascular necrosis of the distal femur. Clin Orthop 334:124-130, 1997.
11. Motohashi M, Morii T, Koshino T, et al: Clinical course and roentgenographic changes of osteonecrosis in the femoral condyle under conservative treatment. Clin Orthop 266:156-161, 1991.
12. Ochi M, Kimori K, Sumen Y, et al: A case of steroid induced osteonecrosis of femoral condyle treated surgically. Clin Orthop 312:226-231, 1995.

59

Osteochondral Autologous Plug Transfer in the Knee

KORNELIS A. POELSTRA, ERIC S. NEFF, AND MARK D. MILLER

OSTEOCHONDRAL AUTOLOGOUS PLUG TRANSFER IN THE KNEE IN A NUTSHELL

History: Trauma, recurrent swelling, ± mechanical symptoms
Physical Examination: Effusion ± joint line tenderness
Imaging: Plain radiographs often normal; magnetic resonance imaging is becoming more sensitive
Indications: Recurrent effusion ± positive magnetic resonance imaging scan; failure of nonoperative management
Surgical Technique: Diagnostic arthroscopy; geographic planning; perpendicular harvest (mini-arthrotomy); perpendicular delivery
Postoperative Management: Protective weight bearing for 6 weeks; continuous passive motion
Results: Good incorporation of plugs at 6 weeks with good midterm results

---

"If we consult the standard Chirurgical Writers from *Hippocrates* down to the present Age, we shall find, that an ulcerated Cartilage is universally allowed to be a very troublesome Disease; that it admits of a Cure with more Difficulty than a carious bone; and that, when destroyed, it is never recovered."[10] More than 250 years after this observation, we have come a long way, but we have not yet discovered a "cure" for cartilage injuries. We must resist the temptation to promote ourselves rather than ensure the welfare of our patients. We also need to remain objective as equipment companies develop newer and "better" instruments and techniques that are aggressively promoted.

Although physical examination is the mainstay of diagnostic testing in orthopedics, osteochondral injuries are hard to appreciate on physical examination alone, and there are no disease-specific findings. We should

consider articular cartilage injuries in patients with chronic effusions, especially when other causes are not obvious. Unfortunately, articular cartilage lesions are most often discovered during arthroscopy, when neither the surgeon nor the patient is prepared for the consequences.

Case History

A healthy 16-year-old female athlete presents with intermittent right knee pain and a moderate effusion. Her soccer coach and physical therapist managed her complaints with rest, ice, and nonsteroidal anti-inflammatory drugs, but pain and incidental locking persisted. She does not remember a specific trauma.

Physical Examination and Imaging

Her examination showed a 1+ effusion with some medial joint line tenderness, negative Lachman test, stable varus-valgus testing, and negative posterior drawer test. The McMurray test was negative but exhibited some crepitus and pain medially; pivot shift was negative. The patient appeared to be neurovascularly intact and experienced only some popping in the knee when jumping off the table, with moderate pain. Her radiographic evaluation did not show a bony injury, but magnetic resonance imaging (Fig. 59–1) revealed a focal chondral defect on the medial condyle with some degenerative changes.

Surgical Technique

Multiple reports have shown that attempts at replantation of cartilage flaps or loose bodies that have no bone attached do not succeed, nor does replantation of articular cartilage attached to dead bone. For articular cartilage transplants to remain viable, a healthy and supportive subchondral bone is necessary.[22] Recently, techniques have been developed to harvest cylindric plugs from a normal, nonarticulating joint surface and transplant them into chondral and osteochondral defects, as diagnosed in this case.

Diagnostic Arthroscopy

Diagnostic arthroscopy revealed no patellofemoral pathology or loose bodies in the medial or lateral gutter. The anterior and posterior cruciate ligaments were intact

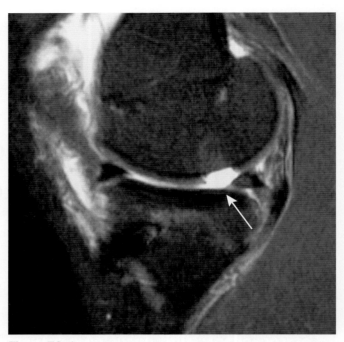

Figure 59–1 Sagittal magnetic resonance imaging scan showing the focal chondral defect on the medial condyle of the right femur (arrow).

on examination of the notch, and the superiorly unstable cartilaginous fragment was encountered on the medial femoral condyle, flapping in and out of a defect (Fig. 59–2).

This area was partly debrided using a straight basket and motorized shaver, improving exposure of the subchondral bone. The scope was placed under the

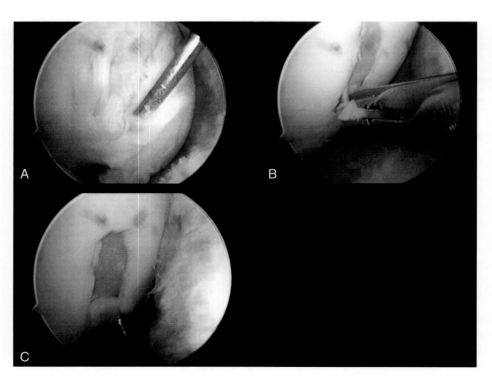

Figure 59–2 Arthroscopic views identifying the focal chondral defect (A) and subsequent debridement of the loose, nonviable cartilaginous flap (B). C, A 6- by 9-mm area of bare subchondral bone was exposed.

posterior cruciate ligament and advanced into the posterior recess of the knee, where a small loose body was removed. It must be emphasized that all compartments of the knee need to be thoroughly examined for loose bodies when encountering an osteochondral defect. Suction and lavage techniques should be used to mobilize hidden flakes from under the menisci, and the back of the knee must be visualized. Also, allow for hyperflexion of the knee as needed to examine the entire femoral condyles for defects.

The optimal angle of the drill to reach the defect properly was from the inferomedial portal, to obtain perpendicularity. A spinal needle should be placed to determine the most perpendicular access, and additional portals (including a transpatellar tendon portal) may be used. The knee had to be held in 110 degrees of flexion as well, and in this case, the fat pad had to be shaved to improve access.

Specific Surgical Steps

Harvest Procedure

A 2.5-cm full-thickness incision is made (in extension), lateral to the patella. Easy access is obtained through the capsule to the articular cartilage of the trochlear ridge (Fig. 59–3). Note that the arthrotomy must allow

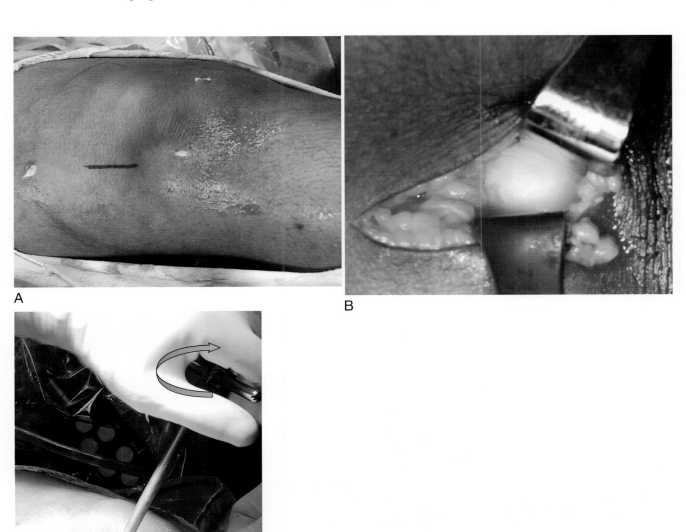

A

B

C

Figure 59–3   Superolateral incision *(A)* and exposure of the lateral trochlear ridge *(B)* with easy access and ability to perform a perpendicular harvest. *C,* The T-handle needs to be rotated 360 degrees to cut the plug at its base. For a more detailed view of the cutting tip, see Figure 59–4C.

excellent access to the site of harvest to permit perpendicularity of the harvest instruments. It is better to sacrifice another centimeter of incision for visualization and positioning than to struggle and obtain inferior grafts.

We use the Mitek/COR variable-depth harvester and confirm the location by slight indentation of the cartilage surface before harvesting. A 12-mm-deep by 6-mm-diameter plug is harvested from the superolateral trochlear ridge without difficulty. This is transferred to the clear insertion tube, to prepare for delivery (Fig. 59–4).

In addition to harvesting plugs from the lateral trochlear ridge of the femur, plugs can be harvested from the medial trochlear ridge and the femoral condyles in the notch.[3,5,11,13,21,23,26,27]

After plug harvesting, the variable-depth drill is used to drill the subchondral bone of the focal lesion. In this case, the transfer of one 6-mm-diameter plug, 12 mm long, was planned to fill the defect; however, the use of multiple plugs in a mosaic pattern is sometimes indicated for larger defects. Depending on the company supplying the equipment, different plug diameters can be used. Typical plugs sizes are 6, 8, and 10 mm in diameter, and they are prepared using color-coded instruments.

While drilling the hole, it is important to keep the drill perpendicular to the surface and not allow the drill to stray into softer bone or an adjacent drill hole if a mosaicplasty is planned (Fig. 59–5).

After drilling to the desired depth (usually 12 to 15 mm), it is wise to manipulate the scope so that the defect is visualized all the way to the bottom and under direct sight, cleared from debris with the motorized shaver (Fig. 59–6). Loose chondral flakes need to be removed from the edges to achieve a smooth chondral surface all around.

The next step is to introduce the plug into the defect (again perpendicularly) and tamp the inserter while keeping the clear tube steady with the other hand. It is important to almost sink the plug completely before removing the clear inserter tube. Failure to do so can result in shearing off of the cartilage surface from the subchondral bone when the transplant positioning is

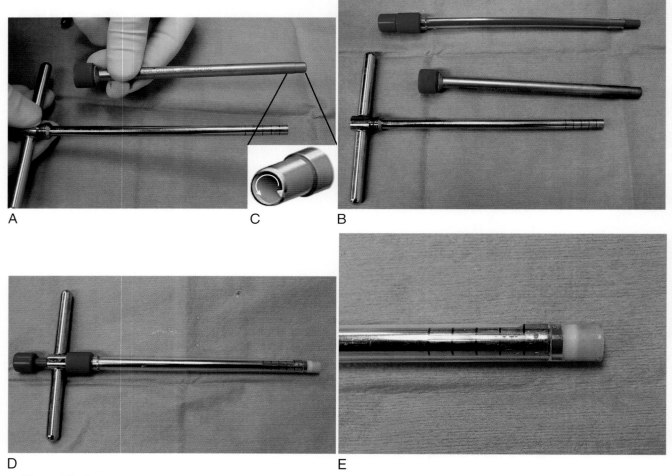

A   C   B

D   E

Figure 59–4 *A* and *B*, Mitek osteochondral plug harvest tool for 6-mm plugs. The T-handle is used for harvesting, after which the plug is transferred to the clear plastic cannula by pushing it out of the T-handle with the blue plunger. *C*, Tip of the T-handle with a triangular cutter that allows the harvested plug to be cut at its base and retrieved when the T-handle is rotated 360 degrees. *D* and *E*, The harvested 6-mm osteochondral plug is in the clear plastic inserter tube, ready for placement. The perpendicularity of the cartilage surface can be seen clearly at the bottom right.

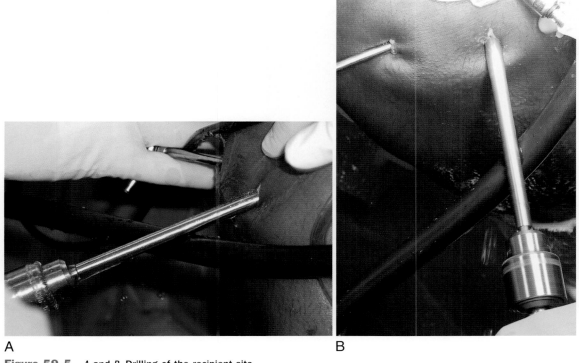

Figure 59–5   *A* and *B*, Drilling of the recipient site.

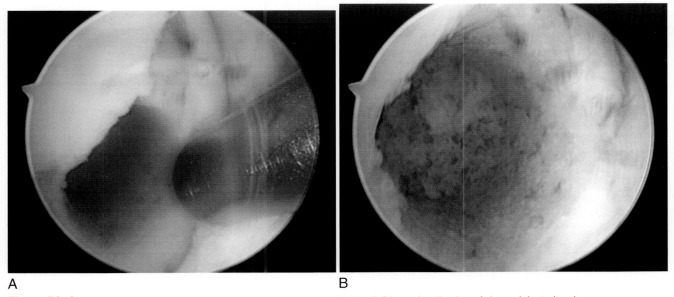

Figure 59–6   *A*, Clearing the edges and inside of the drilled recipient site. *B*, Direct visualization of the recipient site shows no remaining debris that could prevent the plug from being placed flush with the surrounding cartilage surface.

finalized using the shallow tamp to make the surface flush with the surrounding cartilage (Fig. 59–7). Note that placement 1 mm too prominent will cause severely increased contact pressure (and shear), whereas ideal, 0.25-mm placement below the surrounding surface will result in 50% reduction of joint pressure.[27]

After perfect positioning of the plug is achieved by following the preceding steps, the knee is ranged and again examined for the presence of loose bodies. The scope is withdrawn, excess arthroscopy fluid is expressed from the joint, and portals are closed with 3-0 nylon sutures. The arthrotomy is lavaged with saline and bacitracin via a bulb syringe and closed with interrupted 2-0 Vicryl deep and superficial sutures and also with 3-0 nylon. A sterile Xeroform dressing, 4×4s, and soft roll are applied, covered with an elastic wrap.

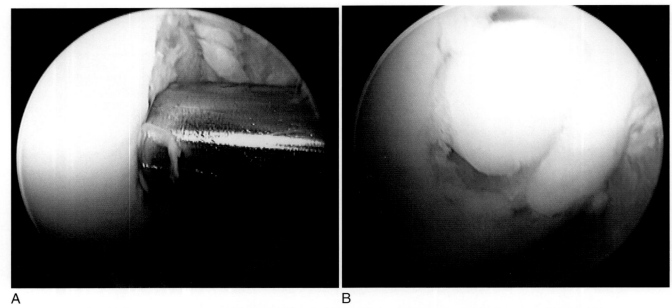

A   B

Figure 59–7 *A* and *B*, Finalizing plug insertion with the shallow tamp. Note the flush surface with the surrounding cartilage.

If no instability is expected, use of an expensive brace can be avoided. Postoperative administration of oral antibiotic prophylaxis is at the discretion of the surgeon; however, toe-touch weight-bearing (~20 pounds) precautions need to be observed rigorously for 6 weeks to allow ingrowth of the transplanted plug.

Large Defects

In cases in which large osteochondral fragments are encountered, it is possible to use multiple plugs (Fig. 59–8).[18] Extra care must be taken not to allow the drill to stray into an adjacent hole, because each plug needs

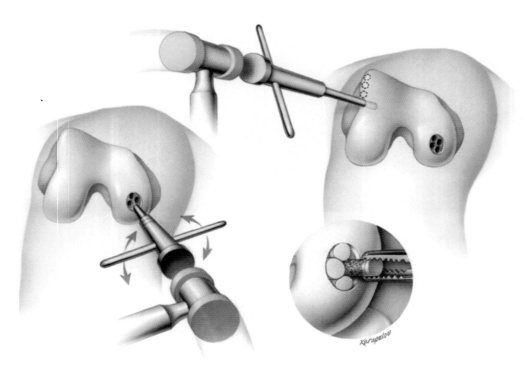

Figure 59–8   Mosaicplasty of the medial femoral condyle using four plugs from the lateral trochlear ridge. (From Miller MD, Cole BJ: Atlas of chondral injury treatment. Oper Tech Orthop 11:145-150, 2001.)

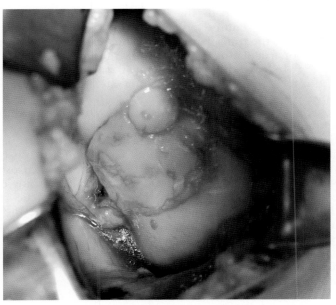

Figure 59–9 In certain cases, use of a mosaicplasty can be avoided if an osteochondral fragment can be "pinned in situ" using an osteochondral plug. Minimal debridement was performed in this patient. The fragment was stable inferiorly and was secured with a single plug superiorly; several bioabsorbable pins were placed in the body of the lesion. This does not work for chondral flaps, because viability is significantly compromised.

to have circumferential cancellous bony contact to maintain its position when loaded.

If multiple (more than six) plugs are placed to cover a large defect, restoration of the convexity of the recipient surface sometimes requires nonperpendicular graft harvest. In the center of the defect, the cartilage cap needs to be placed perpendicularly and thus must be harvested in the same orientation. Toward the periphery, an obliquity of 10 to 15 degrees is sometimes required, which is hard to achieve arthroscopically. When seating the graft, we sometimes prefer to insert the plug only 20% to 25% and manipulate the inserter tube so that the oblique cartilage cap corresponds to the convexity of the surface. This can conveniently be done under direct vision with the clear plastic inserter tube in place.

In cases in which an osteochondral (*not* chondral) flap is pedunculated but still appears to be viable and firmly attached on one side, it can potentially be rescued. We have learned that securing a partly separated osteochondral flap (Fig. 59–9) using a similar-type plug as described earlier allows for acceptable fixation and good clinical results.

Postoperative Management

We perform most osteochondral plug transfers and mosaicplasties as outpatient procedures. Patients do not receive braces when no ligamentous instability was encountered before the procedure and no ligamentous procedures were performed. Stitches are removed after

10 to 14 days, and minimal weight-bearing precautions are rigorously observed for 6 weeks. Passive range of motion is begun immediately to prevent stiffness of the joint (via continuous passive motion machine, as needed). Unless a large defect was repaired, full weight bearing is encouraged after 6 to 8 weeks.

Our study using gadolinium-enhanced magnetic resonance imaging scans of transferred osteochondral plug showed that vascular bridging occurs only after 6 weeks postoperatively. Full weight bearing before this time could significantly compromise graft viability[24] or lead to subsidence.[14] Heavy labor and athletic exercise are delayed until 12 weeks postoperatively.

Our experience is that patients have significantly improved joint motion when they are encouraged to seek the assistance of a physical therapist during the immediate postoperative period. Knee stiffness is much more common in patients who did not receive early assistance from either a therapist or continuous passive motion. This can significantly compromise outcome.

Results

Hyaline cartilage is remarkably durable and unique in tolerating the repetitive impacts and shear loads applied to it. Injury often results in progressive degeneration and accompanying symptoms. The treatment of osteochondral defects in the weight-bearing regions of the knee presents a therapeutic challenge, particularly in young patients who wish to remain active.

6 Knee

Improved techniques have been developed for autogenous cartilage transplant. Open procedures[15,16,19] have become arthroscopic and allow for the transplantation of cylindric plugs from a nonarticulating joint surface area to another.[2,3,6,8,14,17,20,25] In cases in which large defects are encountered, this technique allows for the transplantation of multiple plugs (mosaicplasty) close to each other, leading to a "cobblestone" appearance (see Fig. 59–8). This technique was developed in 1991 by Hangody and Karpati of Hungary and resulted in hyaline cartilage plugs with fibrocartilage "grout."[7] Five-year follow-up of 155 mosaicplasties was encouraging, with histologic evidence of incorporation.[7] In a more recent study in which seven patients consented to second-look arthroscopy and biopsy analysis of their grafted sites, all showed maintenance and integrity of the grafts, with living chondrocytes and osteocytes.[1] The donor sites were not grafted, but they had all filled in and were covered with fibrocartilaginous scar tissue. The contour was normal, and no discontinuity with adjacent cartilage was observed.

We agree that there is no need to graft the harvest site. Only 7 months after the initial procedure, typical fibrocartilage had filled the defect in our patient in Figure 59–10, and no donor site morbidity from this part of the knee has been observed in any of our cases.

When up to 12 plugs measuring 6 to 7 mm were taken, surface irregularities have been reported, leading to donor site morbidity.[12] For the long term, the importance of this effect is unknown, and it may lead to the development of biomaterials to fill the donor holes. The scarcity of grafting material, however, prevents the potential problem of additional loose bodies inside the knee.

The reasons for the effectiveness of osteochondral plug transfer in relieving joint pain remain uncertain, but it may be partly attributable to the removal of an innervated segment of subchondral bone and its replacement with a graft that lacks innervation. Decrease in the local intraosseous pressure has also been suggested as playing a role.[4]

This procedure is particularly useful in patients with osteochondritis dissecans.[28] This disease is usually responsible for a clear osteochondral defect at a classic location: the lateral side of the medial femoral condyle (Fig. 59–11). Magnetic resonance imaging is typically needed to determine the extent of the injury; there is usually joint effusion with a focal cartilage defect and subchondral edema.

To reduce morbidity, arthroscopic technique should be applied when possible. Despite encouraging results with arthroscopy, however, both large and posterior osteochondral defects usually require an arthrotomy. Also, although short-term success has been achieved using this technique, no long-term results have been reported.[3,7,9,17]

A number of systems for autologous osteochondral transplantation are commercially available (e.g., Acufex Mosaicplasty, Smith and Nephew, Andover, MA; Osteochondral Autograft Transfer System [OATS], Arthrex, Naples, FL; Mitek/COR Systems, Innovasive Devices, Marlborough, MA), and all perform well clinically. Most important is that meticulous technique and correct postoperative management be rigorously observed.

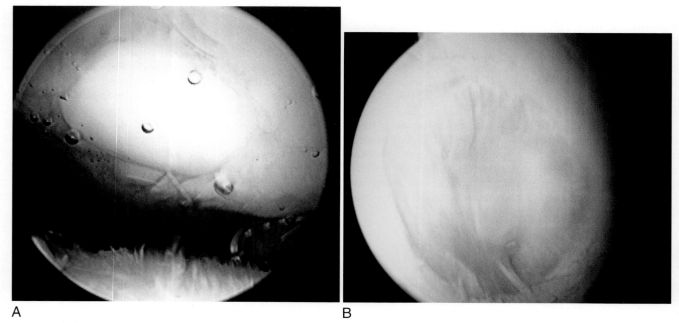

A   B

Figure 59–10 Second-look arthroscopy 7 months after osteochondral plug transfer. *A,* Recipient site with excellent incorporation of the graft. *B,* Donor site showing fibrocartilaginous filling of the defect. The patient did not have any donor site morbidity.

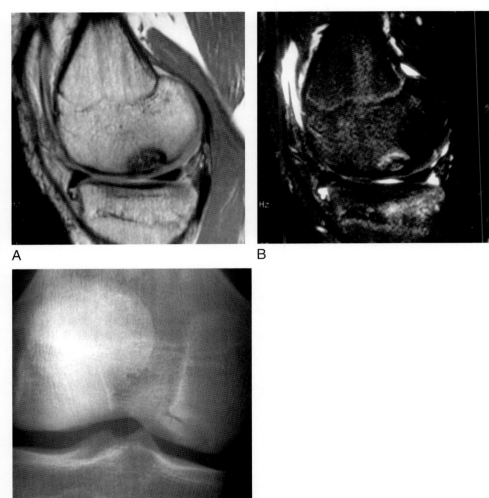

Figure 59-11 *A*, Sagittal, proton density-weighted, fast spin-echo magnetic resonance imaging scan showing the osteochondral defect on the mid–weight-bearing surface of the medial femoral condyle. *B*, T2-weighted fat-suppressed fast spin-echo image. *C*, Anteroposterior view of the right knee showing characteristic lateral osteochondritis dissecans of the medial femoral condyle without other bony injury. (From Berlet GC, Mascia A, Miniaci A: Treatment of unstable osteochondritis dissecans lesions of the knee using autogenous osteochondral grafts [mosaicplasty] Arthroscopy 15:312-316, 1999.)

6 Knee

References

1. Barber FA, Chow JCY: Arthroscopic osteochondral transplantation: Histologic results. Arthroscopy 17:832-835, 2001.
2. Berlet GC, Mascia A, Miniaci A: Treatment of unstable osteochondritis dissecans lesions of the knee using autogenous osteochondral grafts (mosaicplasty). Arthroscopy 9:312-316, 1999.
3. Bobic V: Arthroscopic osteochondral autograft transplantation in anterior cruciate ligament reconstruction: A preliminary clinical study. Knee Surg Sports Traumatol Arthrosc 3:262-264, 1996.
4. Buckwalter JA: Articular cartilage injuries. Clin Orthop 402:21-37, 2002.
5. Campanacci M, Cervellati C, Donati U: Autogenous patella as replacement for a resected femoral or tibial condyle: A report of 19 cases. J Bone Joint Surg Br 67:557-563, 1985.
6. Czitrom AA, Keating S, Gross AE: The viability of articular cartilage in fresh osteochondral allografts after clinical transplantation. J Bone Joint Surg Am 72:574-581, 1990.
7. Hangody L, Kish G, Karpati Z, Eberhardt R: Osteochondral plugs: Autogenous osteochondral mosaicplasty for the treatment of focal chondral and osteochondral articular defects. Oper Tech Orthop 7:312-322, 1997.
8. Hangody L, Kish G, Karpati Z, et al: Arthroscopic autogenous osteochondral mosaicplasty for the treatment of femoral condylar articular defects: A preliminary report. Knee Surg Sports Traumatol Arthrosc 5:262-267, 1997.
9. Hangody L, Kish G, Karpati Z, et al: Treatment of osteochondritis dissecans of the talus: Use of the mosaicplasty

technique: A preliminary report. Foot Ankle Int 18:628-634, 1997.

10. Hunter W. Of the structure and disease of articular cartilages. Philos Trans R Soc Lond B Biol Sci 42:514-521, 1743.

11. Jacobs JE: Follow-up notes on articles previously published in the journal: Patellar graft for severely depressed comminuted fractures of the lateral tibial condyle. J Bone Joint Surg Am 47:842-847, 1965.

12. Jackob RP, Franz T, Gautier E, Mainil-Varlet P: Autologous osteochondral grafting in the knee: Indication, results and reflections. Clin Orthop 401:170-184, 2002.

13. Karpinski MR, Blotting TD: Patellar graft for late disability following tibial plateau fractures. Injury 15:197-202, 1983.

14. Kish G, Modis L, Hangody L: Osteochondral mosaicplasty for the treatment of focal chondral and osteochondral lesions of the knee and talus in the athlete: Rationale, indications, techniques, and results. Clin Sports Med 18:45-66, 1999.

15. Maletius W, Lundberg M: Refixation of large chondral fragments on the weight-bearing area of the knee joint: A report of two cases. Arthroscopy 10:630-633, 1994.

16. Marcacci M, Kon E, Zaffagninni S, Visani A: Use of autologous grafts for reconstruction of osteochondral defects of the knee. Orthopedics 22:595-600, 1999.

17. Matsusue Y, Yamamuro T, Hama H: Arthroscopic multiple osteochondral transplantation to the chondral defect in the knee associated with anterior cruciate ligament disruption. Arthroscopy 9:318-321, 1993.

18. Miller MD, Cole BJ: Atlas of chondral injury treatment. Oper Tech Orthop 11:145-150, 2001.

19. Muller W: Osteochondritis dissecans. Prog Orthop Surg 3:135, 1978.

20. Ohlendorf C, Thomford WW, Mankin HJ: Chondrocyte survival in cryopreserved osteochondral articular cartilage. J Orthop Res 14:413-416, 1996.

21. Outerbridge HK, Outerbridge AR, Outerbridge RE: The use of lateral patellar autologous graft for the repair of a large osteochondral defect in the knee. J Bone Joint Surg Am 77:65-77, 1995.

22. Radin EL, Rose RM: Role of subchondral bone in the initiation and progression of cartilage damage. Clin Orthop 213:34-40, 1986.

23. Roffman M: Autogenous grafting for an osteochondral fracture of the femoral condyle: A case report. Acta Orthop Scand 66:571-572, 1995.

24. Sanders TG, Mentzer KD, Miller MD, et al: Autologous osteochondral "plug" transfer for the treatment of focal chondral defects: Postoperative MR appearance with clinical correlation. Skeletal Radiol 30:570-578, 2001.

25. Schachar N, McAllister D, Stevenson M, et al: Metabolic and biochemical status of articular cartilage following cryopreservation and transplantation: A rabbit model. J Orthop Res 10:603-609, 1992.

26. Wilson WJ, Jacobs JE: Patellar graft for severely depressed comminuted fracture of the lateral tibial condyle. J Bone Joint Surg Am 34:436-442, 1952.

27. Wu JZ, Herzog W, Hasler EM: Inadequate placement of osteochondral plugs may induce abnormal stress-strain distributions in articular cartilage—finite element simulations. Med Eng Phys 24:85-97, 2002.

28. Yamashita F, Sakakida K, Suzu F, Takai S: The transplantation of an autologenic osteochondral fragment for osteochondritis dissecans of the knee. Clin Orthop 201:43-50, 1985.

Osteochondral Allografting in the Knee

KEVIN F. BONNER AND WILLIAM D. BUGBEE

OSTEOCHONDRAL ALLOGRAFTING IN THE KNEE IN A NUTSHELL

History:
Pain and mechanical symptoms of traumatic or insidious onset; previous cartilage procedures

Physical Examination:
Check for focal tenderness or effusion and for malalignment

Imaging:
Radiographs: weight-bearing anteroposterior, 45-degree-flexed posteroanterior, lateral, Merchant, long-alignment views
Magnetic resonance imaging: size assessment of defect, bone involvement, other pathology, accurate graft sizing

Decision-Making Principles:
Malalignment, ligamentous instability, and meniscal insufficiency must be addressed before or at the time of the resurfacing procedure
Generally considered a salvage operation for younger patients who have failed other procedures and in whom arthroplasty is not desirable
Primary treatment considered for large lesions or when bone loss is greater than 6 to 10 mm deep

Surgical Technique:
Press-fit technique
Shell allograft technique

Postoperative Management:
Toe-touch weight bearing for 6 to 12 weeks; continuous passive motion for 6 weeks, light sports at 4 to 6 months, depending on several factors

Results:
Overall, approximately 85% of unipolar grafts rated successful at 6.5- to 10-year follow-up; radiographic degenerative arthritis common with longer follow-up

Complications:
Deep infection: graft removal, debridement, antibiotics
Subsidence: expect 1 to 3 mm of subsidence; 28% get 4 to 5 mm of subsidence
Fragmentation or collapse: consider salvage with repeat osteochondral graft or reconstructive procedure
Progressive degenerative joint disease: treat symptomatically; eventually requires reconstructive procedure

The use of fresh osteochondral allografts in the reconstruction of lesions of the femoral condyle has a long clinical history, extending over 2 decades.[2,4,6-11,14-19,21-23] Fresh allograft transplantation has gained widespread popularity, owing to the increased availability of fresh tissue as well as the interest among both the orthopedic community and the general public in the biologic resurfacing and restoration of diseased or damaged cartilage. Fresh allografts are most useful in treating large osteochondral lesions such as those seen with osteochondritis dissecans or osteonecrosis, in the reconstruction of osteochondral fractures, and in selected cases of degenerative arthrosis. Allografts have also become increasingly important in the salvage of knees that have failed other cartilage resurfacing procedures such as microfracture, autologous chondrocyte implantation, and osteochondral autologous transfer.

History

Typically, the patient has a history of osteochondritis dissecans diagnosed in adolescence. However, we often encounter adults in the fourth or even fifth decade of life with no previous diagnosis who present for the first time with knee pain and are found to have a displaced osteochondral fragment consistent with osteochondritis dissecans. Patients may present with a history of trauma or an insidious onset of knee dysfunction. Pain is generally present but is often a minor symptom, particularly in younger individuals; in these patients, mechanical symptoms such as catching, locking, or giving way may be more pronounced. Some individuals present with a longtime history of the knee's "not working as well as the other side" but without a specific incident or diagnosis. It is important to evaluate both knees, as this condition can occur bilaterally in up to 50% of individuals.

Physical Examination

Patients may or may not present with effusion. Generally, range of motion is maintained, but occasionally, individuals are unable to fully extend, particularly in the case of large medial femoral condyle lesions. Atrophy of the quadriceps is also a common finding, suggesting a prolonged period of knee dysfunction. Patients may present with classic signs of loose body or with profound catching or crepitation in the involved compartment. Meniscal injury is common, particularly with larger lesions, and at times, visible or audible catching or locking can be noted. Often, these lesions are tender to palpation, and a key component of the physical examination is deep palpation of the affected condyle with the knee in a flexed position, which often elicits focal tenderness over the lesion. All patients should be examined carefully for subtle or obvious instability, and most importantly, the angular alignment of the limb should be evaluated. A medial femoral condyle lesion with associated varus is not uncommon, and this mechanical situation profoundly affects the pathology and treatment of the osteochondritis lesion. Consideration should be given to unloading osteotomy in conjunction with allografting.

Imaging

Lesions of osteochondritis dissecans are commonly visible on plain radiographs. The standard radiographic images include a standing anteroposterior, a notch or tunnel view, a lateral view with the knee in 90 degrees of flexion, and a patellar view. Medial femoral condyle lesions are commonly seen just medial to the notch in the standing anteroposterior and lateral views. Lateral femoral condyle lesions will be missed in the standing anteroposterior view but often become evident with the knee in 30 to 60 degrees of flexion. Frequently, the lateral view most clearly demonstrates the extent and depth of the osseous lesion. Long-alignment films are also indicated when there is a question of angular malalignment.

Magnetic resonance imaging is the modality of choice for evaluating osteochondral lesions. With proper sequences, the images show the osseous component as well as the chondral component. One can determine whether the articular cartilage is intact or depressed over the lesion. It is important to evaluate whether there is a layer of fluid or edema around the lesion, suggesting an unstable fragment or a so-called empty nest. Imaging studies can also evaluate other pathology, such as meniscal lesions, and can help determine the extent and depth of osseous involvement. Care should be taken not to misinterpret the magnetic resonance imaging scan, as it is very sensitive to subchondral edema, which does not always translate into significant osseous pathology.

Indications and Contraindication

The most commonly encountered clinical situation in which an allograft might be considered is osteochondritis dissecans of the medial or lateral femoral condyle. These lesions are typically large (≥ 2 cm) and include both an osseous and a chondral component. The classic lesions of osteochondritis dissecans are located in the lateral aspect of the medial femoral condyle or the central portion of the lateral femoral condyle. Generally, an allograft is considered in stage III or IV lesions or when the individual has failed other treatments, including drilling, stabilization, or bone grafting, or when there is an empty defect that cannot be reconstructed with the patient's own tissue. Fresh osteochondral allografts are well suited for these types of lesions because they can restore both the osseous and the chondral components and provide an anatomically precise graft that restores articular anatomy.

Patients for whom fresh osteochondral allografts are indicated include a select group of young individuals in whom arthroplasty is not desirable.[18] Generally, osteochondral allografting is considered a salvage procedure for patients who have failed prior cartilage procedures.

Primary treatment can be considered for large lesions for which other procedures may be inadequate or when there is bone involvement greater than 6 to 10 mm deep.[6,12,25] Patients with localized, unipolar, traumatic, nondegenerative chondral lesions; osteochondritis dissecans; or osteonecrosis are thought to be optimal candidates for fresh osteochondral allografting.[3,6,18]

Associated kissing lesions of the tibiofemoral or patellofemoral articulation are generally considered contraindications. Malalignment, ligamentous instabilities, and meniscal insufficiency must be addressed either before or at the time of the resurfacing procedure.[18]

Case History

History

A 16-year-old girl was referred for progressive lateral-sided knee pain that had been unresponsive to treatment. She had first been diagnosed with osteochondritis dissecans at age 11. She had a history of three prior surgeries to address the lesion, as well as a near-complete lateral meniscectomy. She complained of increasing knee pain, without any significant relief from the prior procedures. She has been unable to participate in gym class and currently has pain walking short distances. She is planning on going to college next year, and her goal is to be able to walk across campus without the severe pain she is currently experiencing.

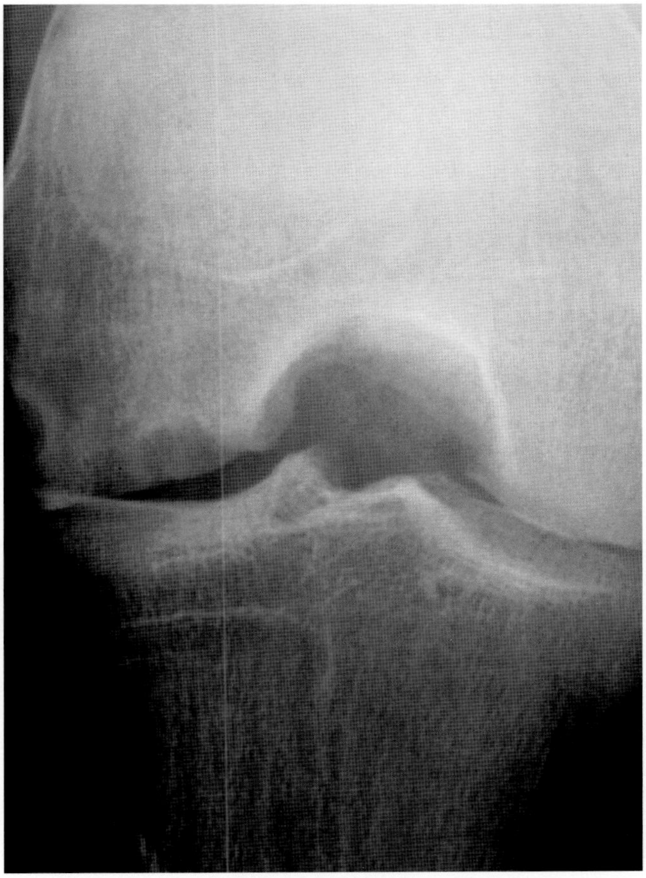

Physical Examination

The patient walked with an antalgic gait. She had normal alignment with no medial thrust. Her knee had a mild effusion, with moderate tenderness over the lateral joint line and lateral femoral condyle. Her active and passive range of motion was from full extension to 130 degrees of flexion, associated with mild to moderate lateral-sided pain. She lacked 10 degrees of flexion compared with the contralateral side, which may have been due to the effusion. The ligamentous and patellofemoral examinations were normal.

Imaging

Plain radiographs included weight-bearing anteroposterior in extension, weight-bearing posteroanterior in 45 degrees of flexion, lateral, Merchant, and long-alignment views. Radiographs were significant for a large osteochondral defect involving the lateral femoral condyle (Fig. 60–1). There was mild joint space narrowing, with no associated degenerative changes. The patient's mechanical axis fell within normal limits.

Magnetic resonance imaging was performed to evaluate the extent of the osteochondral lesion involving the lateral femoral condyle (Figs. 60–2 and 60–3). The cartilage defect measured 22 by 25 mm and associated with up to 8 mm of bone loss.

Figure 60–1   Anteroposterior radiograph revealing an osteochondral lesion of the lateral femoral condyle in a 16-year-old girl.

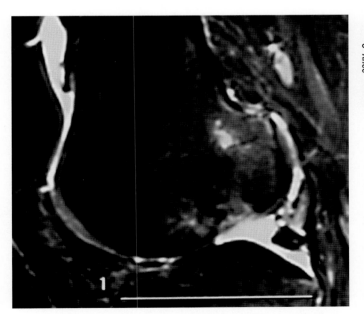

Figure 60–2   Magnetic resonance imaging scan showing cartilage and bone involvement of an old osteochondritic lesion in the lateral femoral condyle.

6 Knee

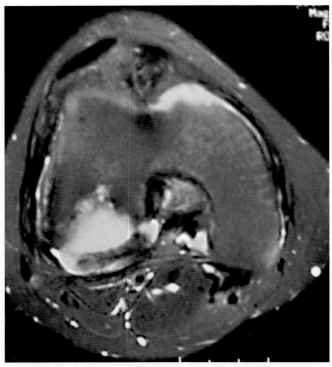

Figure 60–3 Magnetic resonance imaging scan showing cartilage and bone involvement of an old osteochondritic lesion in the lateral femoral condyle.

Decision-Making Principles

Several algorithms have been proposed for the treatment of chondral lesions of the knee (Fig. 60–4).[5,13,20,24] There are many factors to consider when deciding on the best treatment option, and they can be divided into patient factors and lesion factors (Table 60–1).

In this case, the teenaged patient had a large osteochondral defect that had failed several prior procedures. She had moderate bone loss from the fragmented osteochondral lesion. Her alignment was normal, and she had no ligamentous instability. She did have some flattening of the lateral femoral condyle, but the remainder of the cartilage in the compartment was reasonably well preserved, based on magnetic resonance imaging scans and a review of pictures from her last arthroscopy.

The patient had a large cartilage lesion (>4 cm²) associated with a moderate osseous defect; thus a marrow stimulating technique was not appropriate. The bone loss of up to 8 mm was considered both too large and too deep for autologous osteochondral transfer. Viable options for this patient included primary versus staged autologous chondrocyte implantation and fresh osteochondral allograft transplant. The choice of a fresh osteochondral allograft was based on its ability to immediately restore subchondral bone stock while providing viable hyaline cartilage to the defect.[6,18] In preparation for obtaining a size-matched fresh osteochondral allograft, the magnetic resonance imaging scan was sent to a proprietary tissue bank to await an appropriate graft. The patient was scheduled to undergo a lateral meniscus

Table 60–1	Factors in the Evaluation of Patients with Chondral Lesions
Patient-Related Factors	**Defect-Related Factors**
Age	Size
Activity level	Location
Alignment	Containment
Ligament instability	Cause
Expectations	Bone involvement
Time availability	Prior surgical treatment and response
	Associated degenerative changes

transplant during the same procedure owing to her prior complete lateral meniscectomy.

Surgical Technique

Positioning

The patient is positioned supine with a proximal thigh tourniquet. A leg holder is valuable in this procedure to position the leg in 70 to 100 degrees of flexion and permit access to the lesion. Alternatively, a sandbag can be taped on the table to help keep the knee flexed in an optimal position. The technique of fresh osteochondral allografting generally relies on an open procedure, including an arthrotomy of variable size (depending on the position and extent of the lesion). For most femoral condyle lesions, eversion of the patella is not necessary.

Diagnostic Arthroscopy

In most situations, a diagnostic arthroscopy has been performed recently and is not a necessary component of the allografting procedure; however, if there are any unanswered questions regarding the status of the meniscus or other compartments, a diagnostic arthroscopy can be performed before the allografting procedure.

Specific Surgical Steps

The fresh graft, which has been placed in chilled saline on the back table, is inspected to confirm the size match and the tissue quality before opening the knee joint.

A standard midline incision is made from the center of the patella to the tip of the tibial tubercle. This incision is elevated subcutaneously, either medially or laterally, to the patellar tendon, depending on the location of the lesion (medial or lateral). A retinacular incision is then made from the superior aspect of the patella inferiorly. Great care is taken to enter the joint and incise the fat pad without disrupting the anterior horn of the meniscus. In some cases in which the lesion is posterior or very large, the meniscus must be taken down; generally, this can be done safely, leaving a small cuff of tissue adjacent to the anterior attachment of the meniscus.

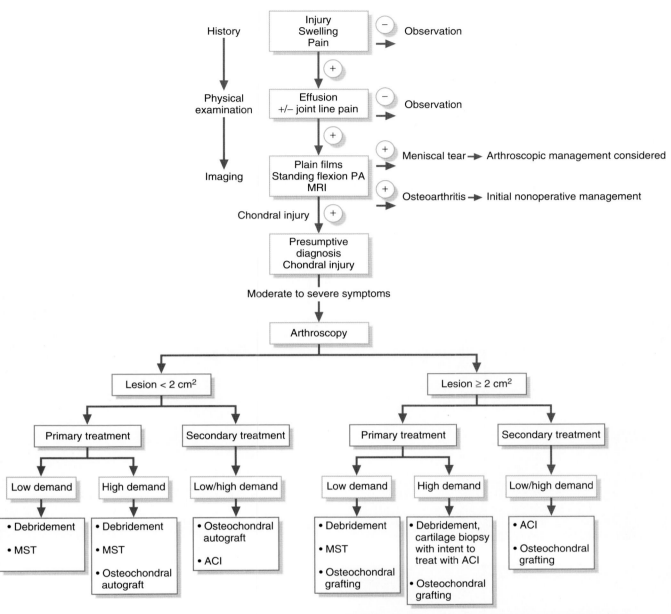

Figure 60–4 Treatment algorithm for the management of chondral injuries. ACI, autologous chondrocyte implantation; MRI, magnetic resonance imaging; MST, marrow stimulating technique; PA, posteroanterior. (From Miller M, Cole B: Atlas of chondral injury treatment. Oper Tech Orthop 11:145-150, 2001.)

Once the joint capsule and synovium have been incised and the joint has been entered, retractors are placed medially and laterally. Care is taken when positioning the retractor within the notch to protect the cruciate ligaments and articular cartilage. The knee is then flexed or extended to find the proper degree of flexion that presents the lesion in the arthrotomy site. Excessive degrees of flexion limit the ability to mobilize the patella. The lesion is then inspected and palpated with a probe to determine the extent, margins, and maximum size.

The two commonly used techniques for the preparation and implantation of osteochondral allografts are the press-fit plug technique and the shell graft technique.

Each technique has advantages and disadvantages. The press-fit plug technique is similar in principle to autologous osteochondral transfer systems. This technique is optimal for contained condylar lesions between 15 and 35 mm in diameter. Fixation is generally not required owing to the stability achieved with the press fit. Disadvantages include the fact that many lesions are not amenable to the use of a circular coring system; this includes tibial, patellar, and trochlear lesions. Additionally, the more ovoid a lesion is, the greater the amount of normal cartilage that must be sacrificed at the recipient site to accommodate the circular donor plug. Shell grafts are technically more difficult to perform and typically require fixation. However, depending on the technique used, less normal cartilage may be sacrificed. Also, tibial, patellar, and many trochlear lesions are more amenable to shell allografts because of their location.

Press-Fit Allograft

Several proprietary instrumentation systems are currently available for the preparation and implantation of press-fit plug allografts up to 35 mm in diameter. Only one of the instrumentation systems is discussed here; however, most systems are similar (Fig. 60–5).

Following exposure of the lesion, all abnormal cartilage is identified (Fig. 60–6). Of paramount importance is to correctly reconstruct the normal geometry of the condyle with an orthotopic donor graft. Precise orientation of the axis of the recipient hole will be matched with the orientation of the axis of the donor plug. This is achieved by initially placing a cylindric sizing guide over the defect. A circumferential mark is placed around the guide, and a mark is placed in the twelve o'clock position of the recipient cartilage. A drill guide pin is inserted into the defect to a depth of 2 to 3 cm (Figs. 60–7 and 60–8). A cartilage scoring device is placed over the guide pin, and the peripheral cartilage is scored to the underlying subchondral bone by hand (Fig. 60–9). An appropriate-sized counterbore is drilled to create the defect into the subchondral bone to a minimum depth of 8 to 10 mm or until a bleeding bone surface is achieved (Fig. 60–10). Precise measurements of the depth of the cylindric defects are recorded in four quadrants. These measurements will be referenced in the final preparation of the articular cartilage allograft.

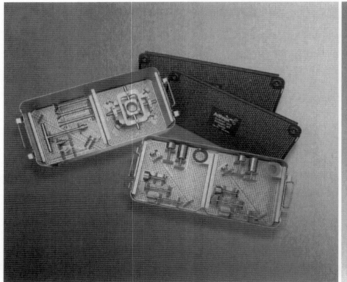

A

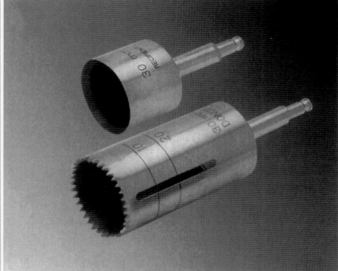

B

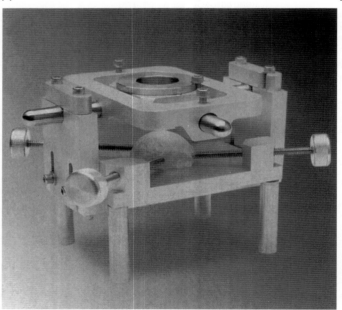

C

Figure 60–5 Allograft Osteoarticular Transfer System (OATS, Arthrex, Inc., Naples, FL). *A,* Allograft instrumentation cases. *B,* Allograft instrumentation harvester. *C,* Allograft instrumentation workstation. (From Garrett J, Wyman J: The operative technique of fresh osteochondral allografting of the knee. Oper Tech Orthop 11:132-137, 2001.)

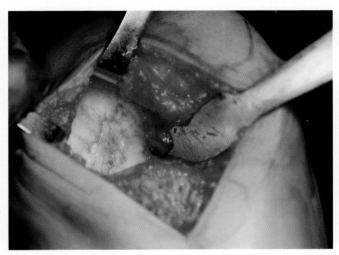

Figure 60–6   Through a lateral parapatellar arthrotomy, the chondral defect is identified.

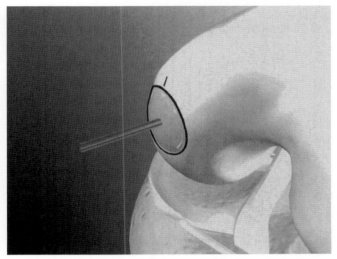

Figure 60–8   A reference mark is made at the 12 o'clock position outside the recipient site to align the orientation of the graft. (From Miller M, Cole B: Atlas of chondral injury treatment. Oper Tech Orthop 11:145-150, 2001.)

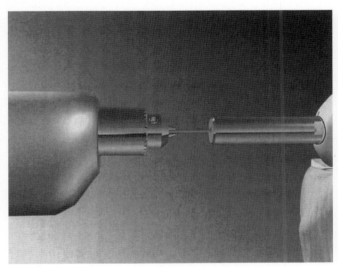

Figure 60–7   The optimal plug diameter is determined and marked before placement of a centering pin, which is inserted to a depth of 2 to 3 cm. (From Garrett J, Wyman J: The operative technique of fresh osteochondral allografting of the knee. Oper Tech Orthop 11:132-137, 2001.)

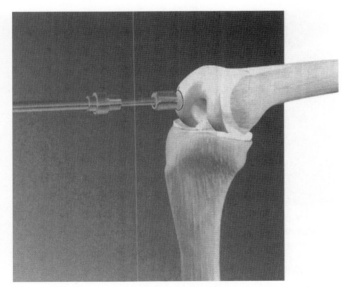

Figure 60–9   The peripheral hyaline cartilage edge is scored before preparation of the recipient socket with a counterbore. (From Garrett J, Wyman J: The operative technique of fresh osteochondral allografting of the knee. Oper Tech Orthop 11:132-137, 2001.)

6 Knee

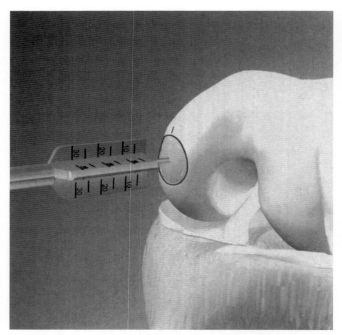

Figure 60–10 The socket is drilled to a depth of 10 to 12 mm, or until bleeding bone is established. (From Garrett J, Wyman J: The operative technique of fresh osteochondral allografting of the knee. Oper Tech Orthop 11:132-137, 2001.)

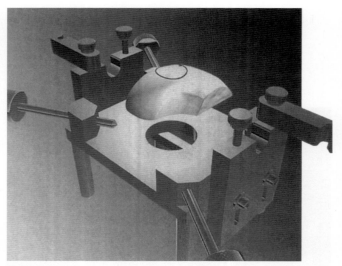

Figure 60–12 The cancellous base of the graft is trimmed to properly align the graft plug in the workstation. (From Garrett J, Wyman J: The operative technique of fresh osteochondral allografting of the knee. Oper Tech Orthop 11:132-137, 2001.)

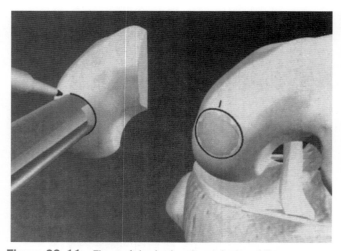

Figure 60–11 The graft is sized and matched, and the corresponding donor site is marked to fit the exact geometric contour of the articular surface to be re-created. (From Garrett J, Wyman J: The operative technique of fresh osteochondral allografting of the knee. Oper Tech Orthop 11:132-137, 2001.)

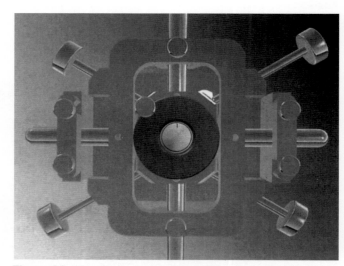

Figure 60–13 The bushing that matches the intended graft diameter is seated into the workstation and aligned with the marked allograft. (From Garrett J, Wyman J: The operative technique of fresh osteochondral allografting of the knee. Oper Tech Orthop 11:132-137, 2001.)

Preparation is begun on the previously size-matched fresh medial or lateral femoral condyle. The donor condyle is secured in the allograft workstation after the appropriate donor site has been determined and outlined (Figs. 60–11 and 60–12). The bushing of the corresponding size is placed into the top housing over the graft and set to the exact angle necessary to match the recipient's condylar contour (Fig. 60–13). Once the housing is securely fastened, a donor harvester is passed into the proximal graft housing and rested on the graft's surface. The graft is drilled through its entire depth (Fig. 60–14). The graft is extracted from the donor harvester, with care taken not to damage the articular surface (Fig. 60–15). The depth measurement guide is used to mark the graft equal to the recipient depth in four quadrants (Fig. 60–16). The allograft is secured in the allograft-holding forceps and trimmed by a saw to achieve precise height-matching of the recipient socket depth (Fig. 60–17).

A calibrated dilator is inserted into the recipient's socket site to achieve an additional 0.5 mm of dilation. The corners of the allograft may be slightly beveled to

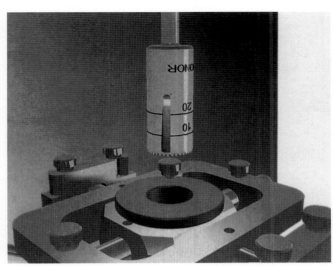

Figure 60–14 A donor harvester is passed through the graft station housing, and the donor plug is created. (From Garrett J, Wyman J: The operative technique of fresh osteochondral allografting of the knee. Oper Tech Orthop 11:132-137, 2001.)

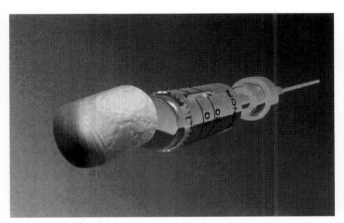

Figure 60–15 The graft is removed from the donor harvester, taking care not to damage the articular surface. (From Garrett J, Wyman J: The operative technique of fresh osteochondral allografting of the knee. Oper Tech Orthop 11:132-137, 2001.)

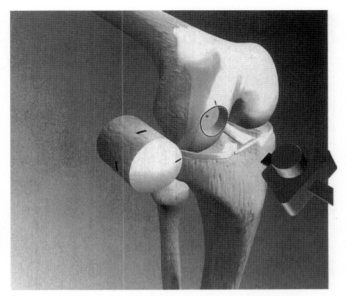

Figure 60–16 Depth measurements of the recipient socket are matched to the graft in four quadrants. (From Garrett J, Wyman J: The operative technique of fresh osteochondral allografting of the knee. Oper Tech Orthop 11:132-137, 2001.)

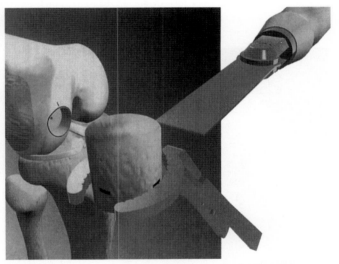

Figure 60–17 The donor allograft is trimmed to the exact depth of the recipient. (From Garrett J, Wyman J: The operative technique of fresh osteochondral allografting of the knee. Oper Tech Orthop 11:132-137, 2001.)

enhance insertion. The graft is press-fit while the appropriate marking is referenced with relation to depth into the recipient bed (Fig. 60–18). Press-fitting the graft by hand avoids injury to the articular surfaces. An oversized tamp may also be used to ensure that the articular surface of the graft is flush with the surrounding cartilage rim (Fig. 60–19).

Once the graft is seated, a determination is made whether additional fixation is required. Typically, absorbable polydioxanone pins are used, particularly if the graft is large or has an exposed edge within the notch. Often the graft needs to be trimmed in the notch region to prevent impingement. The knee is then brought through a complete range of motion to confirm that the graft is stable and there is no catching or soft tissue obstruction. At this point, the wound is irrigated copiously, and routine closure is performed.

In the case of the 16-year-old patient presented earlier, this technique was used to resurface the large osteochondral lesion on the lateral femoral condyle (Fig. 60–20). A lateral meniscal transplant from the same donor was performed following placement of the osteochondral transplant.

Shell Allograft

In the shell allograft technique (Fig. 60–21), the defect is identified through the previously described arthrotomy. The circumference of the lesion is marked with a

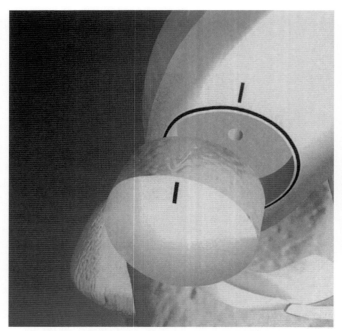

Figure 60–18 The orientation marks are aligned to ensure that geometric curvature of the articular surface is reestablished. (From Garrett J, Wyman J: The operative technique of fresh osteochondral allografting of the knee. Oper Tech Orthop 11:132-137, 2001.)

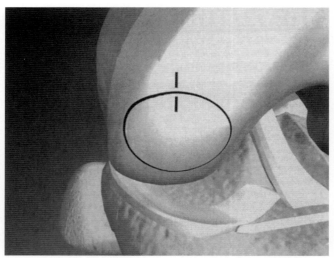

Figure 60–19 It is recommended that the graft be inserted by hand. An oversized tamp is used to ensure that the graft is seated flush with the adjacent condyle. (From Garrett J, Wyman J: The operative technique of fresh osteochondral allografting of the knee. Oper Tech Orthop 11:132-137, 2001.)

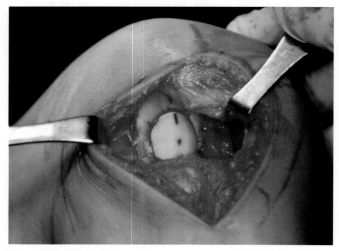

Figure 60–20 Sixteen-year-old patient with the osteochondral plug press-fit into the lateral femoral condyle.

surgical pen. An attempt is made to create a geometric shape that is amenable to hand crafting a shell graft; however, the sacrifice of normal cartilage should be kept to a minimum. A number 15 blade is used to cut around the lesion. Sharp ring curets are used to remove all tissue inside this tidemark. Using both a motorized 4-mm bur and sharp curets, the defect is debrided down to a depth of 4 to 5 mm.

One of the authors (KFB) has found a foil template useful to achieve a precisely sized graft. The large piece of foil from the suture packs can be used. The foil is manually molded over the involved femoral condyle, trochlea, or the like to create a template for the unprepared allograft. The foil is pressed into the defect around the entire lesion while maintaining the foil mold of the surrounding bone. The defect is cut out on the foil, and the foil mold is placed back over the lesion to ensure a precise match. The molded foil is placed over the matched allograft, and the future orthotopic graft area is marked with a surgical pen. This demarcated cartilage can be used as a guide to meticulously prepare a shell graft with 4 to 5 mm of remaining subchondral bone. Initially, the graft should be slightly oversized; bone and cartilage can be carefully removed as necessary through multiple trial fittings. If there is deeper bone loss in the defect, more bone can be left on the graft, and the defect can be grafted with cancellous bone before graft insertion. The graft is placed flush with the articular surface. The need for fixation is based on the degree of inherent stability. Bioabsorbable pins are typically used when fixation is required, but compression screws can be used as an alternative.

Postoperative Management

Postoperative management is based on the size, location, stability, and containment of the graft. General rehabilitation guidelines are outlined in Table 60–2.

Early postoperative management includes the use of continuous passive motion while the patient is in the hospital. Extended continuous passive motion is desirable but optional. Patients are generally allowed full range of motion unless other reconstructive procedures (e.g., meniscal repair, anterior cruciate ligament reconstruction, osteotomy) have been performed that would alter the rehabilitation plan. Patients are begun on early

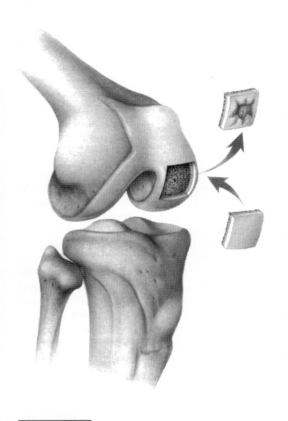

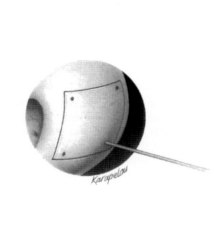

Figure 60–21 **Shell allografting procedure.** (From Garrett J, Wyman J: The operative technique of fresh osteochondral allografting of the knee. Oper Tech Orthop 11:132-137, 2001.)

Table 60–2	**Rehabilitation Protocol Following Osteochondral Allograft Implantation**
Modality	**Time Frame**
Brace	6-12 wk (patellofemoral grafts)
Continuous passive motion machine	6-8 wk (optional)
Weight-bearing status	
Press-fit graft	Toe-touch or non–weight bearing 6-12 wk (based on size of graft)
Shell graft	Toe-touch or non–weight bearing 10-12 wk; progressive weight bearing thereafter
Activity	
Closed chain exercises	Only activity for first 12 wk
Straight leg raises	Immediately postoperatively
Stationary bicycling	Started at 4-8 wk
Light recreational sports	Considered at 4-6 mo*
High-impact sports	Not recommended for larger lesions; considered at 6 mo for smaller lesions

*Use extreme caution with larger lesions when considering specific sporting activities.

range-of-motion exercises and quadriceps strengthening and are maintained in a toe-touch-only weight-bearing status for at least 8 weeks and often as long as 12 weeks, depending on the size of the graft and radiographic evidence of incorporation.

At 4 weeks, patients are allowed closed chain exercises such as cycling. Progressive weight bearing as tolerated is usually allowed at 3 months, and if functional rehabilitation is complete, the patient is allowed to return to recreation and sports at approximately 6 months. Patients are generally cautioned about excessive impact loading of the allograft, particularly in the first year.

Typically, braces are not used unless the graft involves the patellofemoral joint, in which case flexion is limited to less than 45 degrees for the first 4 to 6 weeks. If bipolar tibial femoral grafts were used, an unloader or range-of-motion brace is worn to prevent excessive stress on the grafted surfaces.

Results

One of the authors (WDB) treated 66 patients (69 knees) with osteochondritis dissecans of the femoral condyle using fresh osteochondral allografts. All allografts were implanted within 5 days of procurement. Patients were prospectively evaluated using an 18-point modified D'Aubigne and Postel scale, and subjective assessment was performed with a patient questionnaire. In this group there were 49 males and 17 females, with a mean age of 28 years (range, 15 to 54 years). Forty lesions involved the medial femoral condyle, and 29 the lateral femoral condyle. An average of 1.6 surgeries had been performed on each knee before the allograft procedure. Allograft size was highly variable, ranging from 1 to 13 cm^2; the average allograft size was 7.4 cm^2. Two knees were lost to follow-up, and mean follow-up in the remaining 67 knees was 5.2 years (range, 1 to 14 years). Overall, 50 of 67 knees (75%) were rated good or excellent, scoring 15 or higher on the 18-point scale; 12 of 67 knees (18%) were rated fair; and 5 of 67 knees (7%) were rated poor after an average of 72.4 months' follow-up. The average clinical score improved from 13.0 preoperatively to 15.8 postoperatively ($P < .01$). Six patients had reoperations on the allograft: one was converted to total knee arthroplasty, and five underwent revision allografting at 1, 2, 5, 7, and 8 years after the initial allograft. Thirty-six of 66 patients completed questionnaires: 95% reported satisfaction with their treatment, and 86% felt they were significantly improved. Subjective knee function improved from a mean of 3.2 to 7.8 on a 10-point scale.

Chu et al.[11] reported on 55 consecutive knees undergoing osteochondral allografting. This group included patients with diagnoses such as traumatic chondral injury, avascular necrosis, osteochondritis dissecans, and patellofemoral disease. The mean age of this group was 35.6 years, with follow-up averaging 75 months (range, 11 to 147 months). Of the 55 knees, 43 were unipolar replacements and 12 were bipolar resurfacing replacements. On an 18-point scale, 42 of 55 knees (76%) were rated good to excellent, and 3 of 55 (5%) were rated fair, for an overall success rate of nearly 82%. It is important to note that 84% of the knees that underwent unipolar femoral grafts were rated good to excellent, and only 50% of the knees with bipolar grafts achieved good or excellent status. No realignment osteotomies were reported in this series. Many of the patients who underwent unipolar replacement were allowed to return to recreational and competitive sports.

McDermott et al.[22] reported on the Toronto experience with fresh osteochondral grafts implanted within 24 hours of harvest. Patients with a unifocal traumatic defect of the tibial plateau or femoral condyle had a 75% success rate after an average follow-up of 3.8 years. Patients with osteoarthritis and osteonecrosis fared much worse, with failure rates of 58% and 79%, respectively. Ghazavi et al.[19] reported on 126 knees in 123 patients with an average follow-up of 7.5 years. In 85% of the patients, the procedure was rated successful. Eighteen patients had failed procedures. Factors related to failure included age older than 50 years, bipolar defects, malalignment, and workers' compensation cases. Aubin et al.[2] reported on the long-term results of fresh femoral grafts implanted for post-traumatic lesions in patients who were part of the cohort reported earlier. Kaplan-Meier survivorship analysis showed 85% graft survival at 10 years and 74% survival at 15 years. Sixty-eight percent of patients underwent simultaneous realignment osteotomy, and 17% had concomitant meniscal transplantation. Radiographic analysis revealed that 52% of knees had moderate to severe arthritis at latest follow-up.

Garrett and Garrett and Wyman[18] reported on their experience using fresh osteochondral allografts as both a press-fit plug and a large shell graft in the treatment of osteochondritis dissecans. Among 113 patients with follow-up ranging from 1 to 18 years, 103 (91%) reported that they were free of pain, stiffness, and swelling.[17] Six of 113 patients underwent concomitant correctional osteotomy for angular malalignment of 5 degrees or greater. Patients were counseled to refrain from running and jumping sports. All 10 failures were due to frag-

mentation of the graft. Garrett[17] also reported successful results in 14 of 15 patients with unipolar defects of the patellofemoral joint.

Complications

Infection following the implantation of a fresh osteochondral allograft is rare, but its consequences can be devastating. Generally, all grafts are harvested and tested in accordance with American Association of Tissue Banks standards.[1] However, allograft-associated bacterial infections have been reported. Death in the immediate postoperative period has occurred as a result of implantation of a contaminated fresh osteochondral graft.[27] As with most procedures, infection may become apparent days to weeks after surgery. Deep infection needs to be distinguished from superficial infection by means of physical examination findings and joint aspiration. In our opinion, deep infection needs to be addressed immediately by removing the allograft, because there is a possibility that the fresh tissue is the source of the infection. The graft may also serve as a nidus for infection. Patients need to be informed of this risk preoperatively and counseled to look for signs of infection before and after discharge from the hospital.

Transmission of viral disease is another important issue. Although fresh allograft donors undergo rigorous screening and serologic testing, there is a risk of viral transmission through the allograft. This risk is estimated to be similar to that associated with blood transfusion.

Although the issues of disease transmission associated with fresh allografts are unique, the relative risk is quite small. In one of the author's (W.D.B.) series from the University of California at San Diego including more than 400 knee and ankle grafts, to date, there has been no documented bacterial or viral infection related to the allograft material. Surgeons who choose to use fresh allografts have a responsibility to understand these risks and should have a working knowledge of tissue banking procedures.

Graft fragmentation or collapse is a complication that may take months to years to occur.[17] Fragmentation and collapse typically occur in areas of unvascularized allograft bone. Patients typically present with new-onset pain or mechanical symptoms. Radiographs may show joint space narrowing, cysts, or sclerotic regions. Magnetic resonance imaging shows areas of graft collapse, but care must be taken in interpreting these images, because even normal, well-functioning allografts demonstrate signal abnormalities. If fragmentation produces loose bodies within the joint, they can typically be removed arthroscopically. Graft failure is treated on an individual basis. Ultimately, a decision is made by the physician and patient whether to attempt to salvage the joint with a repeat fresh allografting procedure. Revision allografting is the most common approach to salvaging a failed allograft procedure and is usually successful in the absence of marked degenerative changes. Progressive degenerative arthritic changes are treated symptomatically, similar to other causes of degenerative joint disease. It is not uncommon to turn to reconstructive procedures, including unicompartmental and total knee arthroplasty, following failure of a grafting procedure if salvage is not an option.

An immune response to fresh osteochondral allografts has been observed.[28] Approximately 50% of individuals develop anti-HLA antibodies, but the clinical consequences of this finding are unclear. Histologic evaluation of failed fresh allografts has not demonstrated significant evidence of cell-mediated immune rejection.[26] Presently, no tissue or blood matching is performed between donor and recipient, but this is an area of active research.

Other complications that may occur but are relatively uncommon include nonunion, stiffness, reflex sympathetic dystrophy, and wound complications.[21] Large grafts such as hemicondyle or tibial plateau grafts may subside 1 to 3 mm. Approximately 30% may subside up to 4 to 5 mm.[21] It is unusual for smaller femoral condyle grafts to demonstrate any measurable subsidence on serial radiographs. As long as there is not frank collapse, most of these patients can be observed, because they tend to be relatively asymptomatic.

Summary

Fresh osteochondral allografts are useful for a wide range of articular pathology, particularly conditions that include both an osseous and a chondral defect. Many clinical and basic scientific studies support the theoretical foundation and efficacy of small fragment allografting.

The surgical technique for femoral condyle lesions is straightforward but demands precision. Further understanding of graft procurement and storage, as well as advances in surgical technique, should continue to improve clinical outcomes.

References

1. American Association of Tissue Banks: Standards for Tissue Banking. Arlington, VA, American Association of Tissue Banks, 1987.
2. Aubin PP, Cheah HK, Davis AM, Gross AE: Long-term follow-up of fresh femoral osteochondral allografts for posttraumatic knee defects. Clin Orthop 391:S318-S327, 2001.
3. Ball ST, Chen AC, Tontz WL Jr, et al: Preservation of fresh human osteochondral allografts: Effects of storage conditions on biological, biochemical, and biomechanical properties. Trans Orthop Res Soc 27:441, 2002.
4. Beaver RJ, Mahomed M, Backstein D, et al: Fresh osteochondral allografts for post traumatic defects in the knee: A survivorship analysis. J Bone Joint Surg Br 74:105-110, 1992.
5. Browne JE, Branch TP: Surgical alternatives for treatment of articular cartilage lesions. J Am Acad Orthop Surg 8:180-189, 2000.
6. Bugbee WD: Fresh osteochondral allografting. Oper Tech Sports Med 8:158-162, 2000.
7. Bugbee WD: Fresh osteochondral allografts. Semin Arthroplasty 11:1-7, 2000.
8. Bugbee WD, Convery FR: Osteochondral allograft transplantation. Clin Sports Med 18:67-75, 1999.
9. Bugbee WD, Emmerson B: Fresh osteochondral allografting in the treatment of osteochondritis dissecans of the femoral dondyle. Poster no. 135. Presented at the annual meeting of the International Cartilage Repair Society, June 2002, Toronto, Canada.
10. Bugbee WD, Jamali A, Rabbani R: Fresh osteochondral allografting in the treatment of tibiofemoral arthrosis. Paper presented at the 69th annual meeting of the American Academy of Orthopaedic Surgeons, 2002, Dallas, TX.
11. Chu CR, Convery FR, Akeson WH, et al: Articular cartilage transplantation—clinical results in the knee. Clin Orthop 360:159-168, 1999.
12. Cole BJ, D'Amato M: Autologous chondrocyte implantation. Oper Tech Orthop 11:115-131, 2001.
13. Cole BJ, Farr J: Putting it all together. Oper Tech Orthop 11:151-154, 2001.
14. Convery FR, Akeson WH, Myers MH: The operative technique of fresh osteochondral allografting of the knee. Oper Tech Orthop 47:340-344, 1997.
15. Convery FR, Meyers MH, Akeson WH: Fresh osteochondral allografting of the femoral condyle. Clin Orthop 273:139-145, 1991.
16. Czitrom AA, Keating S, Gross AE: The viability of articular cartilage in fresh osteochondral allografts after clinical transplantation. J Bone Joint Surg Am 72:574-581, 1990.
17. Garrett J: Fresh osteochondral allografts for treatment of articular defects in osteochondritis dissecans of the lateral femoral condyle in adults. Clin Orthop 303:33-37, 1994.
18. Garrett J, Wyman J: The operative technique of fresh osteochondral allografting of the knee. Oper Tech Orthop 11:132-137, 2001.
19. Ghazavi MT, Pritzker KP, Davis AM, et al: Fresh osteochondral allografts for post-traumatic osteochondral defects of the knee. J Bone Joint Surg Br 79:1008-1013, 1997.
20. Mandelbaum BR, Browne JE, Fu F, et al: Current concepts: Articular cartilage lesions of the knee. Am J Sports Med 26:853-861, 1998.
21. Marwin SE, Gross AE: Fresh osteochondral allografts in knee reconstruction. In Fu FH, Vince KG, Harner CD (eds): Knee Surgery. Baltimore, Williams & Wilkins, 1994, pp 1223-1234.
22. McDermott AG, Langer F, Pritzker PH, Gross AE: Fresh small-fragment osteochondral allografts: Long-term follow-up study on first one hundred cases. Clin Orthop 197:96-102, 1985.
23. Meyers MH, Akeson W, Convery R: Resurfacing of the knee with fresh osteochondral allograft. J Bone Joint Surg Am 71:704-713, 1989.
24. Minas T: A practical algorithm for cartilage repair. Oper Tech Sports Med 8:141-143, 2000.
25. Minas T, Peterson L: Autologous chondrocyte transplantation. Oper Tech Sports Med 8:144-157, 2000.
26. Oakeshott RD, Farine I, Pritzker KP, et al: A clinical and histologic analysis of failed fresh osteochondral allografts. Clin Orthop 233:283-294, 1988.
27. Public Health Dispatch. Update: Unexplained deaths following knee surgery—Minnesota, 2001. MMWR Morb Mortal Wkly Rep 50:1080, 2001.
28. Sirlin CB, Brossman J, Boutin RD, et al: Shell osteochondral allografts of the knee: Comparison of MR imaging findings and immunological responses. Radiology 219:35-43, 2001.

Autologous Chondrocyte Implantation in the Knee

KEVIN B. FREEDMAN AND BRIAN J. COLE

AUTOLOGOUS CHONDROCYTE IMPLANTATION IN THE KNEE IN A NUTSHELL

History:
Pain in ipsilateral compartment; recurrent effusions; prior cartilage treatment common

Physical Examination:
Pain in ipsilateral compartment of lesion; rule out coexisting pathology

Imaging:
Standing radiographs, including 45-degree posteroanterior and mechanical axis views; magnetic resonance imaging commonly shows articular cartilage lesion

Indications:
Grade III or IV lesions, 2 to 10 cm^2

Contraindications:
Diffuse degenerative lesions; bipolar lesions

Surgical Technique:
Diagnostic arthroscopy: evaluate lesion for size and depth; evaluate and treat concomitant pathology
Articular cartilage biopsy: full-thickness biopsy from superomedial trochlea, superolateral trochlea, or intercondylar notch; can be stored up to 18 months
Implantation: surgical exposure; parapatellar arthrotomy; can use mini-arthrotomy for condyle lesions
Defect preparation: debride to subchondral bone; vertically oriented walls; hemostasis; size defect
Periosteum harvest: 3-cm medial incision, 5 fingerbreadths below joint line; #15 blade to incise periosteum; oversize 2-mm sharp periosteal elevator, smooth forceps
Securing of the patch: 6-0 Vicryl sutures, 3 to 4 mm apart; leave small opening
Watertightness testing: saline-filled tuberculin syringe; look for leakage around periphery; seal with fibrin glue and retest; aspirate saline from defect
Chondrocyte injection: sterile aspiration and resuspension; slowly inject through opening, filling entire defect; sew defect in patch and seal with fibrin glue

Postoperative Management:
Continuous passive motion beginning after 6 to 8 hours; touch-down weight bearing for 4 to 6 weeks, then advance; return to activities at 8 to 12 months

Symptomatic chondral lesions are likely to lead to diminished knee function and progressive deterioration over time. Owing to the inability of cartilage lesions to heal, several technologies have emerged for the replacement of articular cartilage defects. Many techniques to treat articular cartilage injuries are palliative or reparative and therefore have a limited capacity to restore hyaline or hyaline-like tissue to the defect. Autologous chondrocyte implantation attempts to replace the articular cartilage defect with hyaline-like cartilage tissue. This process involves taking a biopsy of healthy articular cartilage, which then undergoes enzymatic degradation to proliferate chondrocytes. The chondrocytes are subsequently reimplanted into the knee under a periosteal patch, with the goal of restoring normal articular cartilage to the defect. Autologous chondrocyte implantation can lead to good or excellent results in appropriate candidates provided there is strict adherence to the surgical technique and rehabilitation protocol.

History

Patients with symptomatic chondral lesions typically complain of pain localized to the compartment affected by the lesion. Patients may also complain of swelling after activities, locking, catching, and crepitation. For lesions in the medial and lateral femoral condyles, weight-bearing activities typically aggravate the symptoms. Lesions in the patella or trochlea are aggravated by sitting, stair climbing, and squatting activities. In patients who are candidates for autologous chondrocyte implantation, it is important to review previous operative notes and arthroscopic pictures, because many patients have undergone prior surgical treatment.

Physical Examination

Patients with symptomatic chrondral lesions are typically tender on the ipsilateral joint line or over the affected portion of the condyle. They may also have an effusion. Particular attention should be paid to lower limb malalignment for medial or lateral femoral condyle injuries. For patella or trochlea lesions, the patellar grind test may be positive. In addition, the patient should be evaluated for lateral retinacular tightness, patellar apprehension, and abnormal Q angle. A thorough ligament examination should also be performed to rule out any ligamentous laxity.

Imaging

Diagnostic imaging should include a standard weight-bearing anteroposterior radiograph of both knees in full extension, a 45-degree-flexion posteroanterior weight-bearing radiograph, and non–weight-bearing lateral and Merchant or skyline views. The evaluation should be performed to rule out global osteoarthritis and any bony involvement of the lesion (e.g., osteochondritis disse-

cans) and to evaluate alignment. If malalignment is a concern, a full-length mechanical axis view should be obtained. Magnetic resonance imaging can be helpful for delineating the extent of articular cartilage lesions, assessing subchondral bone, and detecting any associated ligament or meniscal injures.

Indications and Contraindications

The indications for autologous chondrocyte implantation are symptomatic, unipolar, full-thickness (Outerbridge[6] grade III or IV) articular cartilage lesions. Lesions of the medial or lateral femoral condyles are most common, but patellar and trochlear lesions are also amenable to autologous chondrocyte implantation. Commonly, patients have failed previous treatments, including debridement, marrow stimulation, and osteochondral autograft techniques. Osteochondritis dissecans is not a contraindication for autologous chondrocyte implantation, provided the bone loss is less than 6 to 8mm. If the bone loss is greater than 8mm, advanced techniques for autologous chondrocyte implantation with single- or two-stage bone grafting can be performed. Bipolar lesions (greater than grade II chondral lesion on the opposing surface) are considered a contraindication to the procedure. Malalignment and ligament instability are not contraindications, but they must be addressed concomitantly with bony realignment or ligament reconstruction.[2] In addition, meniscal deficiency in the affected compartment must be addressed with allograft meniscal transplantation. Patellofemoral lesions are commonly treated with simultaneously performed anteromedialization of the tibial tubercle.

Surgical Technique

Arthroscopic Assessment and Biopsy

Positioning

Depending on the surgeon's preference, the limb may be placed in a standard leg holder or maintained in the unsupported supine position.

Examination under Anesthesia

An examination under anesthesia should be performed to confirm full range of motion and the absence of concomitant ligamentous laxity or malalignment.

Diagnostic Arthroscopy

A careful and systematic assessment of the entire joint must be performed. Once the chondral defect is identified, a probe is used to assess the quality of the articular surface. Surrounding areas of softening and fissuring must be noted as well. The defect assessment includes measuring its dimensions (both anterior and posterior and medial and lateral) as well as noting the lesion location, depth, quality of surrounding tissue, and condition of the opposing surface. All these factors determine whether the lesion is amenable to autologous chondrocyte implantation (Fig. 61–1).

Articular Cartilage Biopsy

When there is an intention to treat a cartilage lesion with autologous chondrocyte implantation, an articular cartilage biopsy is performed with either a gouge or a sharp ring curet. The preferred technique of the senior author is to perform the biopsy in the lateral intercondylar notch (Fig. 61–2). This is the region where anterior

cruciate ligament notchplasty is regularly performed. Alternative sites include the lateral, medial, or proximal aspects of the trochlea. The biopsy specimen should be a full-thickness area of articular cartilage measuring approximately 5 by 10 mm. This biopsy represents 200 to 300 mg in total weight, containing between 200,000 and 300,000 cells. The specimen should cover the bottom of the biopsy specimen container (Fig. 61–3). The specimen is placed via sterile technique into the vial containing the culture medium and sent for next-day delivery at 4°C to Genzyme Biosurgery Corporation (Cambridge, MA) for processing. The cellular expansion process takes 3 to 5 weeks. The specimen can be stored for up to 18 months before expiration. Once processed, the suspension of autologous chondrocytes contains 12 million cells per 0.4 mL of culture medium. For larger or multiple lesions, two or more vials of chondrocytes can be requested.

Implantation of Autologous Chondrocyte Cells

Positioning

The patient is positioned supine on a standard operating table. Access to the entire lower extremity is necessary. A tourniquet should be placed on the thigh. A lower extremity positioning device can be helpful as well.

Specific Surgical Steps

SURGICAL EXPOSURE

A standard midline incision with a medial parapatellar arthrotomy can provide access to medial and lateral femoral condyle lesions, as well as patella and trochlea lesions. Smaller incisions are often possible with certain

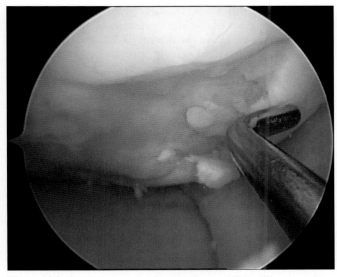

Figure 61–1 Arthroscopic photograph of a 20- by 25-mm grade IV symptomatic chondral lesion of the medial femoral condyle as measured with an arthroscopic probe.

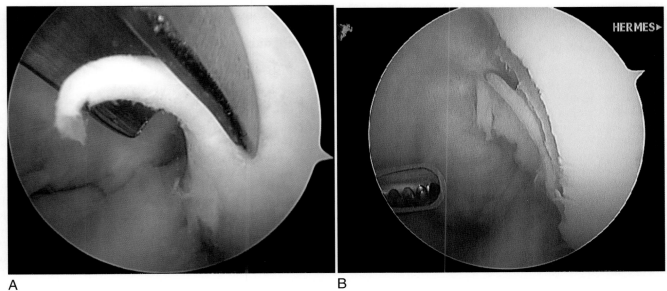

A

B

Figure 61–2 *A*, Arthroscopic photograph showing the lateral intercondylar notch during arthroscopic biopsy using a gouge. Care is taken to avoid the weight-bearing area of the lateral femoral condyle. *B*, Arthroscopic photograph of the intercondylar notch following biopsy.

6 Knee

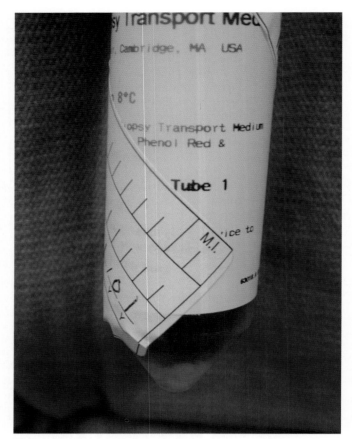

Figure 61–3 The cartilage biopsy specimen fills the bottom of the specimen container.

defect locations. Laterally based lesions are often approached through a lateral retinacular release only. Medially based lesions are often approached through a mini-arthrotomy. The patella can then be subluxated using a Z-type retractor in the intercondylar notch.

DEFECT PREPARATION

Once the defect has been identified, it must be prepared. Defect preparation requires that the surrounding cartilage walls be healthy, full thickness, and firmly attached (Fig. 61–4). Using a fresh number 15 scalpel blade, the defect is outlined, and a sharp ring curet is used to excise the cartilage down to the level of the subchondral bone. Care is taken not to penetrate the subchondral bone to prevent bleeding into the defect. The walls of the remaining cartilage are prepared so that they are vertically oriented. It is important to keep the lesion contained so that there is a rim for the periosteum to be sewn. Once the defect is prepared, adequate hemostasis must be achieved. Neuropatties soaked with a dilute 1:1000 epinephrine and saline solution can be applied using thumb pressure. If bleeding is difficult to control, hemostasis can be obtained with a needle-tip electrocautery device; this should be used with caution, however. Bleeding may be especially problematic in patients who have previously undergone a marrow stimulating technique.

Once the defect is prepared, it must be accurately sized using a sterile ruler. A piece of paper from the sterile surgical glove wrapping can be used to trace the outline of the defect and create a template for the appropriate periosteal patch configuration.

PERIOSTEAL PATCH HARVEST

A 3-cm incision is made on the medial border of the proximal tibia, approximately 5 fingerbreadths distal to the joint line, 2 cm distal to the pes anserinus tendon attachments. Blunt dissection is used to develop the plane between the periosteum and the overlying subcutaneous fat and fascia. Electrocautery should not be used on the periosteum. Using the defect template and a fresh number 15 scalpel blade, the periosteum is incised down to the underlying bone on the medial, lateral, and distal borders. The proximal border can be left intact until the harvest is nearly complete. A sharp, curve-tipped periosteal elevator is used to perform the subperiosteal dissection from distal to proximal (Fig. 61–5). Smooth forceps are used to provide gentle traction on the periosteal edges. Once an adequate piece of periosteum is obtained, it is amputated at its proximal portion. Owing to the tendency for the periosteum to shrink slightly after harvest, the patch should be oversized by 2 mm in each dimension. If the periosteum tears during harvest, it can be repaired during suturing, although this is not ideal. The periosteum should be kept moist at all times. In addition, the outer surface of the periosteum should be marked to distinguish it from the inner cambium layer, which will face the implanted cells. If a tourniquet was used up to this point, it should be deflated, and hemostasis should be obtained at the site of the periosteal harvest as well as at the area of defect preparation.

SECURING OF THE PERIOSTEAL PATCH

At this point, the periosteum is laid over the defect and trimmed to the appropriate size. The periosteum is secured with a 6-0 absorbable Vicryl suture on a P-1 cutting needle (Fig. 61–6). Sterile mineral oil or glycerin should be used to lubricate the suture for smooth passage. The periosteum is secured so that there is no overlap of the overlying cartilage. In addition, the periosteum is tented over the defect to allow adequate filling with the injected cells. Particular attention must be paid to contouring trochlear defects, ensuring that the periosteum is not tented beyond the normal contour of the articular surface. It is usually most efficient to start by placing the sutures at the four corners of the defect. The suturing technique involves passing the needle through the periosteum from outside to inside approximately 2 mm from the tissue edge. The needle then enters the cartilage perpendicular to the inside wall of the defect 2 mm below the articular surface and exits the articular surface a minimum of 3 mm from the edge of the defect. The sutures are then tied, with the knot placed over the periosteal patch at the junction of the patch and the articular cartilage. The sutures are placed approximately 3 to 4 mm apart to provide a watertight seal. A small

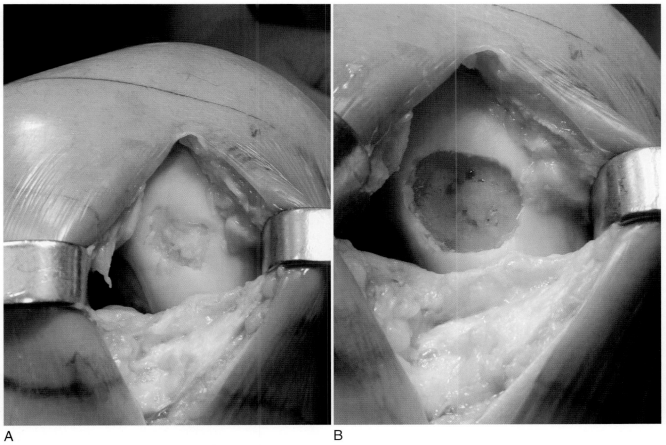

A   B

Figure 61–4   *A,* Lesion of the medial femoral condyle exposed through a mini-arthrotomy before preparation. *B,* The same lesion after defect preparation, with vertical walls at the transition zone.

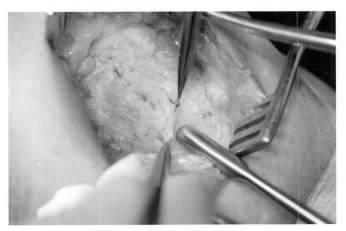

Figure 61–5   Periosteum is harvested from a small incision on the medial aspect of the tibia below the pes anserinus tendons. Smooth forceps are used to provide gentle traction on the periosteum while a periosteal elevator is used to lift the flap.

6 Knee

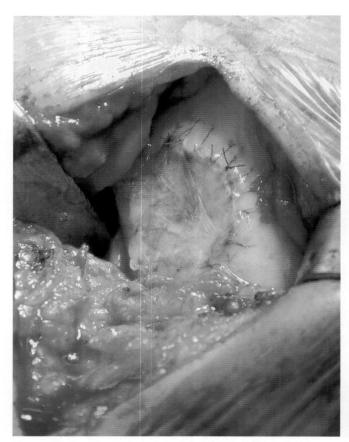

Figure 61–6 The periosteal patch is sewn into place over the defect using 6-0 Vicryl interrupted sutures.

opening approximately 5 mm wide is left at the proximal end of the defect to allow insertion of the cells. If the defect is uncontained, one may need to suture to the surrounding synovium or through small drill holes made with a Kirschner wire. Alternatively, mini bone anchors can be placed, preloaded with the suture material.

Watertightness testing is performed with a saline-filled tuberculin syringe and an 18-gauge catheter. The catheter is placed in the opening in the patch, and the saline is injected. Any leakage seen around the periphery of the defect should be sealed with additional sutures. After the test, the saline should be aspirated from the defect to prevent cellular dilution. Once the defect is deemed watertight, the periosteal patch is sealed with fibrin glue. Commercially available fibrin glue (Tisseel, Baxter Health Care, Glendale, CA) is preferred by the senior author. The fibrin glue is applied along the edges of the defect, and a second watertightness test is performed.

CHONDROCYTE HANDLING AND INJECTION

The autologous chondrocyte cells are delivered in a small vial. The exterior of the vial is not sterile, and careful handling is required to ensure that the cells remain sterile during resuspension, aspiration, and implantation. The vial should be held in the vertical position with the plastic cap removed. The top of the vial is wiped with

alcohol, and a sterile 18-gauge catheter with the metal needle in place is inserted into the vial and advanced until the tip is just above the fluid level. The metal needle is withdrawn, and a sterile tuberculin syringe is attached to the plastic catheter, which remains in the vial. The fluid is then aspirated in the syringe, leaving the cells behind. The fluid is gently ejected back into the vial to resuspend the cells. This is performed approximately three times to achieve a uniform suspension. The catheter with the cells is then carefully withdrawn from the vial.

The catheter with the cells is placed at the opening at the top of the prepared defect (Fig. 61–7). It is advanced to the distal end of the lesion, and the cells are slowly injected into the bed with a side-to-side motion. The catheter is slowly withdrawn, and the opening at the proximal end of the defect is closed with additional sutures and sealed with fibrin glue.

WOUND CLOSURE

Once the defect is sealed, the knee is extended, and no further motion of the knee is allowed for the next 6 to 8 hours. This permits the cells to adhere before the initia-

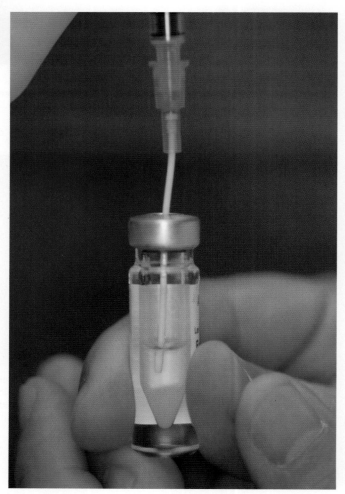

Figure 61–7 The nonsterile vial containing the cells following cellular expansion. The cells are aspirated using a tuberculin syringe.

tion of continuous passive motion. Standard wound closure is performed in layers by closing the arthrotomy, subcutaneous tissue, and skin. A soft sterile dressing is applied to the knee, and the use of drains is avoided to prevent damage to the periosteal patch.

Postoperative Management

Early Phase (0 to 6 Weeks)

Continuous passive motion is initiated 8 hours after surgery, once cell adherence has occurred. This is performed 6 to 8 hours a day at 1 cycle/minute for 2-hour increments. We begin continuous passive motion at 0 to 45 degrees of flexion and increase it as tolerated. Currently, we allow only touch-down weight-bearing for the first 4 weeks to protect the implantation site. However, clinical results suggest that earlier weight bearing may be tolerated, depending on lesion containment. Therapy focuses primarily on quadriceps reactivation with isometric contraction and modalities to limit pain and effusions. Patellofemoral lesions are limited to about 45 degrees of flexion when using continuous passive motion, but patients are permitted to flex to 90 degrees several times a day to prevent motion loss.

Transition Phase (6 to 12 Weeks)

At this stage, full motion should be achieved, and weight bearing is progressed as tolerated to full. Strengthening and exercises can include closed chain activities and functional training.

Maturation and Final Phase (3 to 18 Months)

After 3 months, full motion should be maintained, and strengthening and functional training can start to progress. Resumption of full activities should be delayed at least 8 months to protect the lesion while it continues to mature. It may take up to 18 months for the lesion to mature to a level at which full activities can be tolerated.

Results

The results of autologous chondrocyte implantation were initially reported from Sweden in 1994 (Table 61–1).[1] The first 23 patients treated consisted of 16 with femoral condyle lesions and 7 with patella lesions, with an average follow-up of 39 months. Fourteen of the 16 patients with femoral condyle lesions had good or excellent results, whereas only 2 of the 7 with patella defects achieved good or excellent results.[1] The poor results in the latter group were explained by the failure to address patellar malalignment at the time of implantation.

Two studies with longer follow-up were subsequently published on the Swedish experience with autologous chondroctye implantation.[7,8] Peterson et al.[8] published the results in 94 patients with a 2- to 9-year follow-up.[8] Ninety-two percent of patients with isolated femoral condyle lesions had good or excellent results. Again, the results for patella lesions were not as good, with only 65% achieving good or excellent results. Histologic analysis of biopsy specimens from 37 knees showed a correlation between hyaline-like tissue in the defect and good to excellent clinical results. Another follow-up study by Peterson et al.[7] demonstrated the durability of the results at a mean of 7.4 years. Of 50 patients who had achieved good or excellent result at 2 years, all continued to have good or excellent results at 5 to 11 years after implantation.

The senior author's experience includes 103 chondral defects treated in 83 patients between September 1997 and September 2002. Thirty patients had a minimum follow-up period of 24 months (mean, 33.9 months; range, 24 to 60 months). Significant improvements were seen in all patients using the Modified Cincinnati, International Knee Documentation Committee (IKDC),

Table 61–1

Results of Autologous Chondrocyte Implantation

Author (Date)	Lesion Location	No. of Patients	Mean Follow-up	Significant Improvement (%)	Good or Excellent Results (%)
Peterson et al. (2002)[7]	F	18	>5 yr		89
	OCD	14	>5 yr		86
	P	17	>5 yr		65
	F, ACL	11	>5 yr		91
Minas (2001)[5]	F, Tr, P, T	169	>1 yr	85	
Micheli et al. (2001)[4]	F, Tr, P	50	>3 yr	84	
Peterson et al. (2000)[8]	F	25	>2 yr		92
	P	19	>2 yr		65
	F, ACL	16	>2 yr		75
	Multiple	16	>2 yr		67
Gillogly et al. (1998)[3]	F, P, T	25	>1 yr	88	88
Brittberg et al. (1994)[1]	F, P	16	39 mo		88
	P	7	36 mo		29

ACL, anterior cruciate ligament; F, femur; OCD, osteochondritis dissecans; P, patella; T, tibia; Tr, trochlea.

Tegner, Lysholm, Knee Injury and Osteoarthritis Outcome Score (KOOS), and Short Form-12 (SF-12) scoring systems. Despite the inclusion of patellofemoral lesions and complex pathology (e.g., multiple defects, combined meniscus transplantation and autologous chondrocyte implantation), improvements were 40% to 80% above baseline, depending on the group analyzed and the scoring systems used. Additional series have also been reported from the United States, with patients achieving an 85% success rate at short to medium follow-up.[3-5]

Complications

The most common complications following autologous chondrocyte implantation are periosteal graft hypertrophy and arthrofibrosis. Graft hypertrophy typically occurs between 3 and 7 months postoperatively. This may be related to abrasion of the periosteal patch with motion, especially with patch overlap at the host cartilage edge. This can be treated with careful arthroscopic debridement of the hypertrophic tissue. Arthrofibrosis following autologous chondrocyte implantation is possible, especially with patella and trochlea lesions and when combined with distal realignment. For this reason, range of motion must be initiated early in physical therapy.

Graft failure with delamination or degeneration of the repaired tissue is another possible complication. The patient may be a candidate for repeat autologous chondrocyte implantation or may require an alternative procedure such as osteochondral allograft transplantation.

References

1. Brittberg M, Lindahl A, Nilsson A, et al: Treatment of deep cartilage defects in the knee with autologous chondrocyte implantation. N Engl J Med 331:889-895, 1994.
2. Cole BJ, D'Amato M: Autologous chondrocyte implantation. Oper Tech Orthop 11:115-131, 2001.
3. Gillogly S, Voight M, Blackburn T: Treatment of articular cartilage defects of the knee with autologous chondrocyte implantation. J Orthop Sports Phys Ther 28:241-251, 1998.
4. Micheli L, Browne JE, Erggelet C, et al: Autologous chondrocyte implantation of the knee: Multicenter experience and minimum 3 year follow-up. Clin J Sports Med 11:223-228, 2001.
5. Minas T: Autologous chondrocyte implantation for focal chondral defects of the knee. Clin Orthop 391:S349-S361, 2001.
6. Outerbridge R: The etiology of chondromalacia patellae. J Bone Joint Surg Br 43:752-757, 1961.
7. Peterson L, Brittberg M, Kiviranta I, et al: Autologous chondrocyte transplantation: Biomechanics and long-term durability. Am J Sports Med 30:2-12, 2002.
8. Peterson L, Minas T, Brittberg M, et al: Two- to 9-year outcome after autologous chondrocyte transplantation of the knee. Clin Orthop 374:212-234, 2000.

Anterior Cruciate Ligament: Diagnosis and Decision Making

BERNARD R. BACH, JR., AND SHANE J. NHO

Injury to the anterior cruciate ligament (ACL) can be devastating. It generally occurs in younger patients, and misdiagnosis, delayed diagnosis, recurrent injury, and improper surgical technique may leave a teenage athlete with a knee that is destined to develop premature arthritis. Fortunately, perspectives on the management of ACL-injured knees are changing.[11,33,35] Our ability to diagnose an ACL injury is markedly improved,[2,5-8] and surgical results are much more predictable, with less morbidity.[2-4,6,7,9,10,12,38,39,41,53] ACL reconstruction can be performed on an outpatient basis.[40] Meniscal preservation, characterized by limited partial meniscectomy, nontreatment of stable partial-thickness tears, and meniscal repair, has evolved concurrently with our improved understanding of ACL injuries. It is well recognized that there is a clear disability associated with an ACL-deficient knee, and patients must be willing to modify athletic activities if treated conservatively.[22,42]

Many of our continuing education courses deal with the surgical controversies surrounding ACL management. Graft tissue selection, graft placement, methods of graft fixation, variations in the rehabilitation protocol, postreconstruction functional bracing, and criteria for return to sports remain controversial issues. A particularly critical question is who needs ACL reconstructive surgery—which patients can be treated nonoperatively, and which patients should have surgical reconstruction?

Anatomy and Biomechanics

There are several concepts with regard to overall ACL management. Acute combined ACL–medial collateral ligament (MCL) injuries do not require emergent surgical treatment.[49] In addition, reconstructive surgery is not required on all ACL-injured knees. Although some middle-aged patients are willing to modify their activities and may do well with conservative treatment, many active

middle-aged patients are pursuing surgical options.[13] Disability associated with ACL deficiency is higher than previously recognized.[29] Gait analysis data demonstrate that patients acquire an adaptive gait pattern with an ACL-deficient knee that is time dependent and also affects the opposite knee.[10,12] The significance of this rebalancing between the quadriceps and hamstrings is unknown.

Natural History

The natural history of ACL injuries is not completely understood, and long-term studies are currently unavailable. Existing studies have multiple variables, making comparison difficult.[38] Differences in patient populations (acute, chronic, previous surgical procedures, skill level, age, gender biases), pathology (multiple ligament injury, meniscal surgery, chondral pathology, patellofemoral pathology), treatment protocols, and rehabilitation protocols, as well as potential inherent bias by the treating surgeon, affect the ability to compare studies. There are few prospective studies available.

Before considering the factors that influence the recommendation for surgical or nonsurgical treatment, it is critical to understand the mechanism of injury and the important aspects of the clinical evaluation leading to an accurate diagnosis of an ACL-deficient knee.

Mechanism of Injury

ACL injuries can have contact or, more frequently, noncontact mechanisms of injury. They may occur with internal or external rotation maneuvers (Figs. 62–1 and 62–2). Noncontact injuries generally involve a deceleration, change-of-direction maneuver. Patients usually recollect a sensation of the knee buckling and collapsing to the ground. They may describe this with the "two fist"

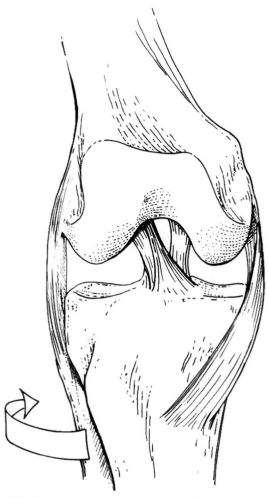

Figure 62–1 External rotation may result in "unwinding" of the anterior cruciate ligament, making it more parallel with the posterior cruciate ligament.

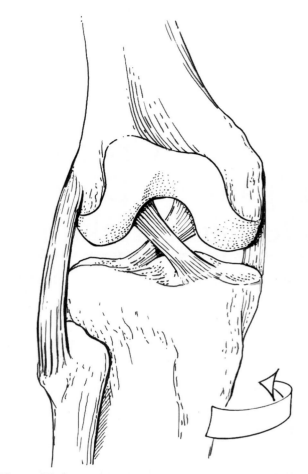

Figure 62–2 Tibial internal rotation mechanism that can result in anterior cruciate ligament injury.

sign in an attempt to characterize the joint instability (Fig. 62–3). An audible pop or tearing sensation is heard in 80% of acute ACL injuries. Almost universally, the athlete is unable to continue participation owing to significant pain. The knee frequently develops a hemarthrosis within 3 hours, but in some patients there may be a gradual onset of swelling over 24 hours. In an acutely injured knee, meniscal tears occur more frequently laterally than medially[9] (Fig. 62–4). In the chronic setting, medial meniscal tears occur more frequently. Displaced bucket handle tears occur nearly four times more frequently medially than laterally (Fig. 62–5). Occasionally, a patient's initial presenting symptoms in the office may be a locked, displaced bucket handle tear superimposed on a chronic ACL-deficient knee. In an acute or subacute setting, patients may lack extension due to incarceration of the ACL stump, which lies in the anterolateral joint space. The frequency of osteochondral fractures associ-

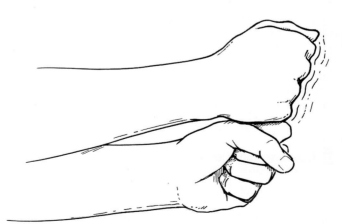

Figure 62–3 The "two fist" sign may be used by some patients when they attempt to describe the sensation of the knee "shifting" or "coming apart."

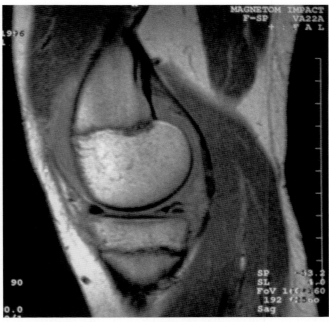

Figure 62–4   Sagittal magnetic resonance imaging scan demonstrates a posterior horn medial meniscal tear in a skeletally immature patient with an anterior cruciate ligament–deficient knee.

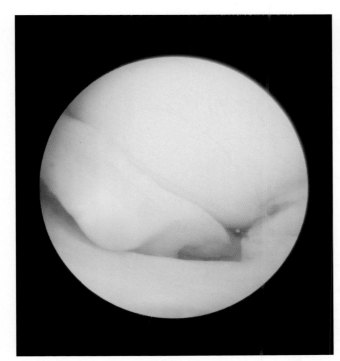

Figure 62–5   Arthroscopic photograph demonstrates a displaced bucket handle medial meniscal tear.

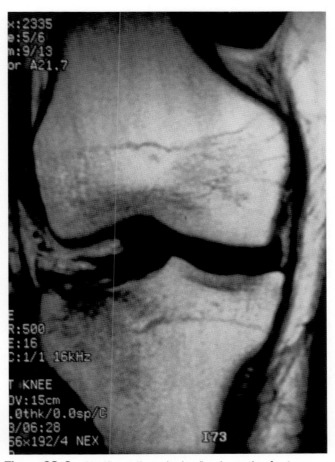

Figure 62–6   Significant "bone bruises" or impaction fractures may be noted on magnetic resonance imaging. Most frequently, they are observed on the lateral femoral and tibial condyles.

Clinical Evaluation

Physical Examination

The three major clinical tests used to establish the diagnosis of an ACL-deficient knee are the Lachman, anterior drawer, and pivot shift tests. The Lachman test is the most sensitive test in the office setting, whereas the pivot shift test is pathognomonic of an ACL-deficient knee. The anterior drawer test has poor sensitivity.

The Lachman test is performed with the knee flexed at 15 to 20 degrees (Fig. 62–7). The thigh is stabilized with one of the examiner's hands, and the other hand grasps the proximal lower leg. An anterior translation is placed on the tibia in an attempt to assess the translation of the tibia, and the presence or absence of an endpoint is determined. The Lachman test is graded as 1 (1 to 5 mm of translation compared with the opposite knee), 2 (6 to 10 mm), or 3 (>10 mm).

The anterior drawer test is performed with the knee flexed at 90 degrees and is graded similarly. The examiner generally sits on the patient's foot to stabilize the lower leg and applies an anterior translation similar to the Lachman test with the knee in further flexion. This

ated with acute injuries is unknown; however, bone contusions are almost universally noted with acute ACL-deficient knees and are most frequently noted on the lateral, femoral, and tibial condyles (Fig. 62–6).

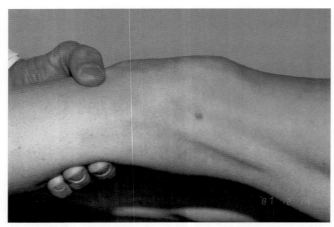

Figure 62–7 The Lachman test is most sensitive for diagnosing an anterior cruciate ligament–deficient knee. It assesses the amount of translation (grade 1, 2, or 3) and the presence or absence of an endpoint.

test is poorly sensitive but may provide a better sense of whether there is a concomitant posterior cruciate ligament (PCL) injury. For example, if the anterior translation of the anterior drawer test is greater than that of the Lachman test, the examiner should suspect a PCL injury.

The pivot shift test demonstrates a relative subluxation reduction phenomenon of the ACL-deficient knee (Fig. 62–8). The test is performed with an axial load and valgus force applied to the knee.[8] With an ACL-deficient knee in extension, the tibia subluxes anteriorly. As the knee is flexed with applied valgus and axial loads, the knee reduces between 15 and 20 degrees of flexion. The magnitude of the pivot shift phenomenon is classified as grade 1 (slip or spin), grade 2 (jump), or grade 3 (transient lock). The pivot shift test must be differentiated from the reverse pivot shift test, which may be noted with a posterolateral corner injury. In the latter situation, the tibia is subluxed in flexion and reduces in extension.

Along with the standard ACL tests, one should perform a PCL examination that includes the posterior drawer and posterior sag tests. Varus-valgus testing at 0 and 30 degrees is performed to exclude the presence of a medial or lateral collateral ligament injury. Assessments of posterolateral spin and thigh-foot angles are performed at 90 and 30 degrees to detect PCL and posterolateral corner pathology (Figs. 62–9 and 62–10). Tenderness along the joint line and discomfort with rotational maneuvers may be highly suggestive of associated meniscal pathology.

If the patient presents acutely to the office, aspiration of the knee frequently demonstrates a hemarthrosis. An injured ACL is the most common cause of a hemarthro-

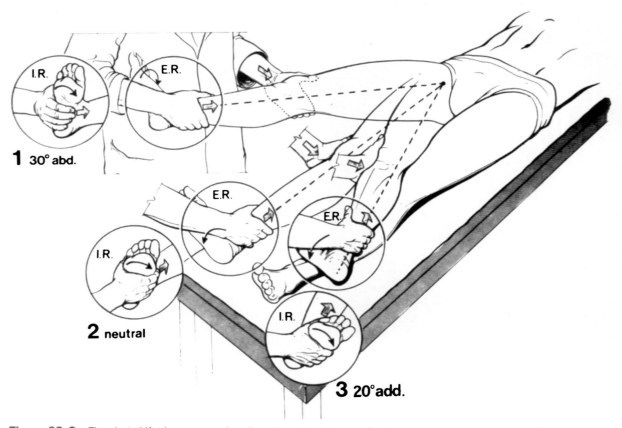

Figure 62–8   The pivot shift phenomenon describes the subluxation-reduction sensation of anterior cruciate ligament deficiency. The magnitude of this test is affected by thigh position, hip flexion, tibial rotation, axial load and valgus force applied, and injured secondary restraints. (From Bach BR Jr, Warren RF, Wickiewicz TL: The pivot shift phenomenon: Results and description of a modified clinical test for anterior cruciate ligament insufficiency. Am J Sports Med 16:571-576, 1988.)

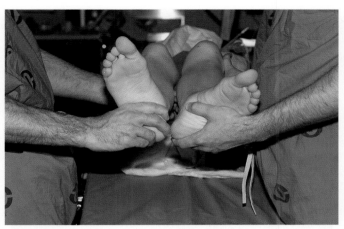

Figure 62–9   Examination under anesthesia demonstrates an increased external rotation of the foot at 30 degrees, indicative of a posterolateral corner injury. This injury may occur in conjunction with an anterior cruciate ligament injury.

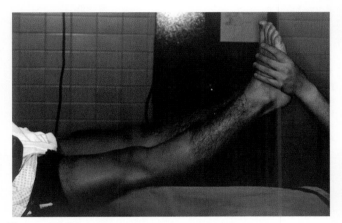

Figure 62–10   Photograph demonstrates the marked asymmetrical recurvation occurring from a severe hyperextension mechanism.

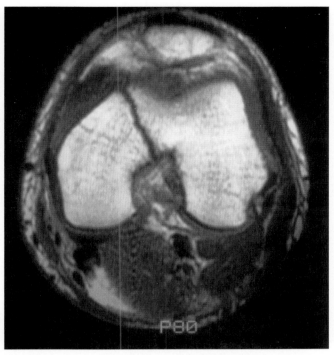

Figure 62–11   Axial magnetic resonance imaging scan shows a nondisplaced Salter III medial femoral condyle fracture in a 15-year-old football player. The rapid onset of a hemarthrosis suggested an anterior cruciate ligament injury, but aspiration yielded fat globules, indicative of an intra-articular fracture.

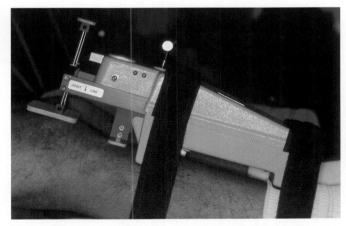

Figure 62–12   KT-1000 arthrometer, an instrumented laxity-testing device used in our practice since 1986.

sis, but other diagnoses must be kept in mind, including osteochondral fracture, peripheral meniscal tear, patellar instability, PCL injury, and avulsion of the popliteal tendon. If fat globules are noted in the hemarthrosis, the patient has an osteochondral fracture (Fig. 62–11).

The KT-1000 arthrometer is an instrumented laxity-testing device that we have had extensive experience with since the mid-1980s[3,4,16,18] (Fig. 62–12). This device is used for preoperative assessment as well for following patients after reconstruction. Anterior and posterior forces are applied to the device to obtain 15-pound, 20-pound, and maximum manual translation results. Several criteria are helpful in assessing the ACL-injured knee arthrometrically. Normal knees generally do not exceed 10 mm of anterior translation. The compliance index measurement, representing the difference between 20- and 15-pound readings, is generally 2 mm or less in a normal knee. The side-to-side difference on maximum manual translation is less than 3 mm in normal knees. For example, if the patient's uninjured knee has readings of 4, 5, and 7 mm at 15 pounds, 20 pounds, and maximum manual testing, respectively, and the injured knee is 7, 9, and 15 mm, we know that the ACL is injured. In this example, the compliance index of the injured knee is 2 versus 1 mm, and the maximum manual side-to-side difference is 8 mm. Preoperatively, approximately 20% of patients with ACL injuries have side-to-side differences of less than 3 mm, whereas after reconstruction, 80% of our patients have side-to-side differences of 3 mm or less.

6 Knee

Imaging

Standard radiographs should be obtained, including anteroposterior, lateral, tunnel, and skyline views. The major reason to obtain radiographs is to exclude a concomitant fracture. Avulsion fractures of the ACL's tibial insertion site occur infrequently but may be seen in young adolescents or in patients in their 30s or 40s who have early diminished bone density (Fig. 62–13). Periarticular spurring, blunting of the intercondylar eminence, and intercondylar notch osteophytes may be suggestive of a chronic ACL-deficient knee (Fig. 62–14). The Segond fracture (lateral capsular avulsion fracture) may be visualized as a small avulsion fracture slightly distal to the articular surface in the anterior aspect of the tibia (Fig. 62–15). This is generally thought to be pathognomonic of an associated ACL injury. In chronic ACL-deficient knees, a recurrent injury may result in accentuation of the sulcus terminalis; this finding has been reported as the "lateral notch" sign[51] (Fig. 62–16). Infrequently, this sign may also be noted in acute ACL injuries. The area is also abnormal on magnetic resonance imaging (MRI).

MRI is frequently used in cases of suspected ACL injury and is helpful in assessing for meniscal pathology, bone contusion, tibial eminence fracture, intra-articular fracture, and associated ligamentous injury (see Figs.

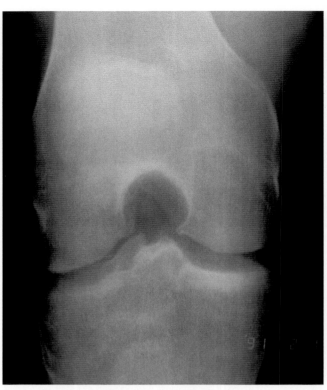

Figure 62–14 This 31-year-old recreational athlete has a chronic anterior cruciate ligament (ACL)–deficient knee and has never had surgical treatment. Radiographs reveal intercondylar notch spurring and blunting of the intercondylar eminence, suggestive of a chronic ACL-deficient knee.

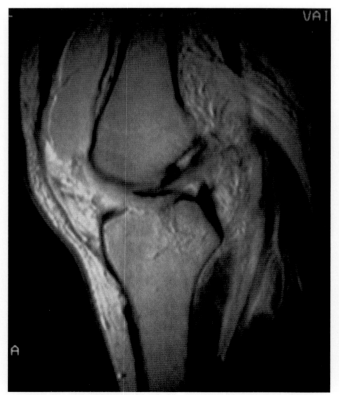

Figure 62–13 This 45-year-old skier sustained a displaced tibial eminence avulsion fracture that required surgical fixation. Without radiographs or magnetic resonance imaging, the physical examination would suggest an anterior cruciate ligament injury.

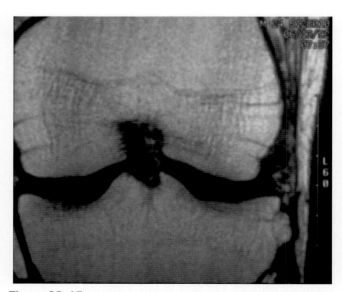

Figure 62–15 Sagittal magnetic resonance imaging scan reveals a Segond, or lateral capsular avulsion, fracture from the lateral tibial plateau. It is almost always associated with an anterior cruciate ligament injury. It is also noted radiographically on the anteroposterior view.

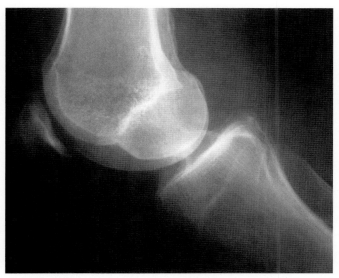

Figure 62-16   Lateral radiograph depicts an exaggerated indentation of the sulcus terminalis. This is generally noted in chronic anterior cruciate ligament–deficient knees. The area of impaction is frequently noted to have a "bone bruise" on sagittal magnetic resonance imaging views.

62–1, 62–4, 62–6, 62–11 to 62–13, and 62–15; Fig. 62–17). We rarely use MRI to establish the diagnosis of an ACL injury, which is done by means of the history and physical examination. Further, MRI is not used to differentiate between partial and complete ACL injuries. Nevertheless, MRI is an important adjunct in the evaluation of ACL-injured knees.

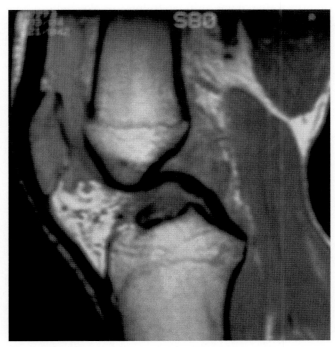

Figure 62-17   Magnetic resonance imaging scan shows a torn anterior cruciate ligament.

Classification

There is some controversy over the diagnosis and prevalence of partial versus complete ACL injuries. Partial ACL injuries are extremely uncommon. We define a partial injury as an asymmetrical Lachman test with a negative pivot shift examination performed under anesthesia. Additionally, arthroscopic documentation of some degree of injury is noted. In general, the KT-1000 side-to-side differences are lower, usually in the 3- to 4-mm range. Using these criteria, we have confirmed the diagnosis of partial ACL injuries in only 65 patients, whereas the senior author has performed more than 1000 ACL reconstructions. It is our opinion that an asymmetrical pivot shift test of any degree is consistent with an ACL-deficient knee.

Treatment Options

Once the diagnosis of an ACL injury has been established, one must consider the multiple variables that affect the decision-making process for nonsurgical or surgical treatment. The most critical factor is the sports activity level, as described by Daniel et al.[17] Sports that require hard cutting, pivoting, and jumping maneuvers such as basketball, football, and soccer are considered level 1 sports. Sports such as baseball, racquet sports, and skiing, which require lateral motion but less jumping or hard cutting, are defined as level 2 sports. Level 3 sports are generally linear sports, including jogging and running. It is thought that patients who participate in level 1 sports are clear candidates for ACL reconstructive surgery and that most patients involved in level 2 sports should consider reconstruction. Daniel et al. also addressed occupational levels, with level 1 occupations being comparable to level 1 sports. Level 2 occupations included heavy manual work, climbing, and working on uneven surfaces, and level 3 included occupational activity levels consistent with activities of daily living. Clearly, patients in occupational levels 1 and 2 should consider ACL reconstructive surgery.

Age may be a consideration in recommending surgical treatment. Ciccotti et al.[13] reviewed ACL management in adults between 40 and 60 years of age. They reported satisfactory outcomes of nonsurgical treatment in more than 80% of their patient but indicated that activity modification was mandatory and that patients should be placed in guided rehabilitation programs. Nevertheless, some of these patients may require surgery. We have found that an increasing number of patients, particularly those in the fifth decade of life, are extremely active in recreational sports and are unwilling to modify their activity levels. These individuals frequently play tennis three to four times a week, ski several weeks per season at the advanced level, and are unwilling to use ACL orthoses. Based on the nature of our referral practice, 8% to 10% of our patients undergoing ACL reconstruction annually are older than 35 years. We previously published a clinical follow-up study of this patient subpopulation, and the results were similar to those of other subgroups with regard to stability, patient satisfaction, and complications.[41]

At the other end of the spectrum are skeletally immature patients. Increasing numbers of ACL injuries are being diagnosed in adolescents. The previously accepted pediatric orthopedic concept that skeletally immature patients do not sustain ligament injuries but instead sustain growth plate fractures has been refuted. The literature has demonstrated that ACL deficiency has similar effects in both skeletally immature patients and adults.[19,24,31,34,36,43] Mizuta et al.[36] retrospectively reviewed 18 patients at a mean age of 12.8 years who were followed a minimum of 36 months after arthroscopic documentation of ACL deficiency. At index arthroscopy, 72% of the patients demonstrated meniscal tears. Six patients (33%) subsequently required reconstruction, 60% demonstrated radiographic evidence of degenerative joint disease at follow-up, and 100% had symptoms. Six percent of the athletes returned to their preinjury sports, and 33% developed secondary meniscal tears. The Lysholm rating was 64 in this patient population. The conclusions of this study were that ACL injuries in this age group do poorly with nonoperative treatment.

The majority of adolescent, skeletally immature ACL patients we see are 13 to 14 years old. An important guideline for determining skeletal maturity in girls is whether menses have commenced. Generally, girls grow for an additional 2 years after the onset of menses. This is more difficult to predict in male patients. Skeletal age is determined and correlated with chronologic age with a posteroanterior view of the left hand compared with the Greunlich-Pyle radiographic classification. Major concerns with regard to surgical intervention in adolescents include premature growth arrest and the development of angular deformities, along with concerns about future growth. Because 60% of lower extremity growth occurs at the knee joint (55% distal femur, 45% proximal tibia), this is an obvious concern. We have observed that most adolescent patients are noncompliant with ACL orthosis use, and few significantly modify their activity levels to reduce the likelihood of reinjury with conservative treatment. The general principles of operative treatment in adolescents include the use of centrally placed tibial tunnels and hamstring or soft tissue grafts, which obviate the need to place a bone plug across the growth plate. We generally place soft tissue grafts "over the top" rather than through a femoral socket. Care must be taken to avoid the placement of hardware or violation of the periosteum about the lateral femoral condylar region. In a patient who has a skeletal age of 14.5 years or greater, we generally use our primary graft construct, a patellar tendon autograft.

In a study by Daniel et al.,[17] risk of reinjury was assessed prospectively. The patients were divided into four groups: (1) early stable, (2) early unstable "copers," (3) early reconstructed, and (4) later reconstructed. The authors concluded that the KT-1000 maximum manual side-to-side difference and sports activity level correlated with reinjury. Using the KT-1000 side-to-side difference and sports hours per year for level 1 and 2 sports (as defined earlier), Daniel et al. were able to prognosticate

the level of reinjury. We have used a side-to-side difference of 3 mm or greater as consistent with ACL injury. Daniel's group defined the 3- to 5-mm range as "copers" and those with 5 mm or greater differences as "noncopers." If the maximum manual difference was less than 5 mm and the athlete was involved in less than 4 hours of sports per week, there was a low likelihood of reinjury, whereas an athlete participating for more than 4 hours per week placed the knee at moderate risk. If the side-to-side difference was between 5 and 7 mm, more than 1 hour of sports per week placed the knee at moderate risk, and more than 4 hour of sports per week placed the knee at high risk. If the maximum manual difference was greater than 7 mm, 1 to 4 hours of sports per week placed the knee at high risk. These observations serve as valuable guidelines when discussing treatment options with patients. We recommend ACL surgery for athletes involved in level 1 sports with a KT-1000 maximum manual difference greater than 5 mm who are participating in sports several hours per week. This clearly includes virtually any high school or college athlete participating in level 1 or 2 sports.

Daniel's study also concluded that arthrosis demonstrated radiographically or by technetium bone scan was greatest in patients who underwent meniscal surgery in both ACL-deficient and ACL-reconstructed patients and that the "copers" had less joint pathology by bone scan than the ACL-reconstructed patients with intact menisci.[17] There are several criticisms with regard to these conclusions. The study included multiple surgeons using multiple surgical techniques. The reconstructed patients had a higher incidence of chondral injuries, and reconstructions were generally based on instability and symptoms (i.e., the worse cases were removed from the "natural history"). Thirty-six percent and 52% of the early and late reconstructed patients, respectively, had a demonstrable pivot shift at follow-up. We believe that these radiographic and bone scan conclusions are reflective of failed ACL surgery rather than ACL surgery in general.

Skill level is another consideration when recommending nonsurgical versus surgical treatment. We consider whether athletes are recreational, interscholastic, intercollegiate, or professional. The recreational athlete may be approached in a nonsurgical fashion, using an ACL orthosis, activity modification, and rehabilitation. Nevertheless, as stated earlier, the majority of these individuals who wish to continue participating in recreational sports are opting for ACL surgical treatment.

There are sport-specific considerations as well. In many interscholastic athletes who play more than one sport per season, the timing of reconstruction may be based on optimizing the rehabilitation interval to prepare for the next season. We generally tell patients that we prefer at least a 4-month interval before the return to athletics, but in appropriately rehabilitated patients who have the potential for an athletic scholarship, we have occasionally returned athletes to play at 3 months postreconstruction.

The frequency of recurrent instability in the ACL-deficient knee has not been well addressed in the literature with regard to recommending surgical treatment. We attempt to differentiate between major and minor episodes. A major episode is defined as an event in which the athlete collapses to the ground. Grana, in a 1995 American Academy of Orthopaedic Surgeons course, recommended that if an athlete is having two major episodes of instability a year, reconstruction is warranted (personal communication).

Associated ligament pathology may play a role, along with a displaced bucket handle meniscal tear. In the acutely ACL-MCL–injured knee, we generally defer surgical treatment of the MCL and initially brace and rehabilitate the patient until motion is recovered, along with documentation of "tightening" of the MCL examination.[49] In appropriate patients, ACL reconstruction is then performed in a semielective fashion. However, in an acute ACL posterolateral injury, we are more likely to intervene acutely, with an emphasis on repair with or without augmentation of the posterolateral corner injury. In the acute ACL-PCL ("bicruciate")–injured knee, we generally do not perform acute reconstruction and have observed that the PCL examination may tighten over the course of approximately 6 to 8 weeks postinjury. In these situations, we frequently perform isolated ACL reconstruction. In an increasing variety of injuries, such as ACL-PCL-MCL injury or knee dislocation, ACL reconstruction is recommended and performed earlier, along with reconstruction of the other injured ligaments.

Patient compliance and motivation are critical. Frequently, we see a patient several times in an effort to get a sense of his or her level of motivation and dedication to rehabilitation. Dr. Jack Hughston has frequently been quoted as stating, "There is nothing that can't be made worse by surgery." This takes into consideration the effects of bracing and failure of nonoperative treatment. Noyes et al.[42] popularized the "rule of thirds"—that one third of patients will do well with a brace, one third will modify their sports activity level but be able to participate, and one third will continue to have major episodes of giving way, necessitating surgery.

Displaced meniscal tears present additional considerations. Lateral meniscal tears are more frequent in the acutely injured ACL, whereas medial meniscal tears are more frequent in the chronic ACL-deficient knee.[9] Bucket handle tears occur three to four times more frequently medially than laterally. With an acute displaced bucket handle tear, a decision must be made whether to perform single or staged repair and reconstruction. In our opinion, this is more germane in the acutely ACL-injured knee than in the chronic ACL-deficient knee that presents with a displaced bucket handle tear.

Motion considerations play a role in the setting of meniscal tears, as well as in ACL injuries in general.[14,15,23,25,26,28,30,32,37,44-48,50,52] The current concept is to defer acute surgical reconstruction until motion has been achieved. Particular attention must be paid to regaining full extension or hyperextension comparable to that of the opposite knee. In a patient with a displaced meniscal tear, we will accept a few degrees of loss of extension and intervene earlier. Many patients who present with an acute displaced bucket handle tear, if given a week to 10 days to "quiet down," rapidly recover the majority of their extension and lack only 3 to 5 degrees compared with the opposite knee. Flexion issues may be a concern with an associated MCL injury. Robins et al.[46] observed that the proximally injured MCL is more likely to result in delayed motion recovery. Therefore, in an acutely injured ACL-MCL patient who has proximal tenderness, we defer any surgical treatment until flexion has been recovered.

Loss of motion may occur due to secondary hamstring spasm; ACL tissue "pseudolocking," resulting in incarceration of the acutely torn ACL fragment in the anterolateral joint line; bucket handle meniscal tears; or associated MCL sprains. Overall, the principles of surgical intervention include delaying acute surgery and allowing the inflammatory response to subside. We want patients to have near-normal motion, demonstrate quadriceps control, and have resolution of effusion.

Social issues have been understated in the literature but are a major factor in the recommending of surgery and the timing of surgical intervention. There may be anticipation of a job or career change, or a change in the health care delivery system. Some patients recognize that because of an imminent change in their health insurance, they face the issue of a "preexisting" condition. Other patients may be on the verge of becoming ineligible under their parents' health care plan and face uncertainty regarding future insurance coverage. Numerous patients have presented desiring ACL surgery based on the timing of family planning. Women are concerned about how their ACL-deficient knees will function during pregnancy and with the associated weight gain. Other patients wish to have maximally stabilized knees so that they can "play sports" with their kids. As previously noted, the timing of reconstruction relative to athletic seasons is effectively a social issue, and timing relative to school vacations is an understated but important consideration. We generally try to time surgery based on summer and other extended vacations to minimize time lost from school. One study of college students demonstrated that ACL reconstruction during the course of a semester resulted in a high likelihood of dropping classes and a significant reduction in academic performance during the recovery period.

Summary

The last decade has resulted in changing perspectives on ACL treatment and indications for surgery (Table 62–1).[1,20,21,27] Improved diagnosis and surgical techniques, accelerated rehabilitation programs, reduced morbidity, and enhanced patient expectations have impacted decision making regarding ACL surgery. Simply stated, surgical recommendations in the acutely injured ACL are based on an active lifestyle, and in the chronic ACL-deficient knee, on recurrent instability. Reinjury, sports participation level, patient age, and KT-1000 maximum manual differences play a major role in our decisions regarding surgical recommendations.

6 Knee

Table 62–1	Anterior Cruciate Ligament Evaluation and Indications for Surgery

History

Deceleration mechanism, pain, pop, hemarthrosis, inability to continue sports participation
Chronic—recurrent instability, meniscal tear, loss of confidence in knee

Physical Examination

ACL tests—Lachman, anterior drawer, pivot shift
Rule out associated patholaxities (e.g., posterolateral corner)

Surgical Considerations and Indications

Active lifestyle, age
Hard-cutting, decelerating sports (e.g., level 1) >5 hr sports/wk
KT-1000 maximum manual difference >6 mm
Associated repairable meniscal tear
Skeletal age in adolescents
Caveat: acute reconstruction
Caveat: associated MCL injury
Motion must be achieved before reconstruction
Recurrent instability
Skill level
Social considerations

ACL, anterior cruciate ligament; MCL, medial collateral ligament.

References

1. Bach BR Jr: Arthroscopy assisted patellar tendon substitution for anterior cruciate ligament insufficiency: Surgical technique. Am J Knee Surg 2:3-20, 1989.
2. Bach BR Jr: ACL surgical techniques. In Wojtys E (ed): The ACL Deficient Knee. AAOS Monograph Series. Rosemont, IL, American Academy of Orthopaedic Surgeons, 1994, pp 46-63.
3. Bach BR Jr, Flynn W, Wickiewicz TL, Warren RF: Arthrometric evaluation of knees that have a torn anterior cruciate ligament. J Bone Joint Surg Am 72:1299-1307, 1990.
4. Bach BR Jr, Jones GT, Hager CA, Sweet F: Arthrometric aspects of arthroscopic assisted ACL reconstruction using patellar tendon substitution. Am J Sports Med 23:179-185, 1995.
5. Bach BR Jr, Jones GT, Sweet F, Hager CA: Arthroscopic assisted ACL reconstruction using patellar tendon substitution: Two year follow up study . Am J Sports Med 22:758-767, 1994.
6. Bach BR Jr, Levy ME, Bojchuk J, et al: Single-incision endoscopic anterior cruciate ligament reconstruction using patellar tendon autograft: Minimum two year follow-up evaluation. Am J Sports Med 26:30-40, 1998.
7. Bach BR Jr, Tradonsky S, Bojchuk J, et al: Arthroscopically assisted anterior cruciate ligament reconstruction using patellar tendon autograft: Five to nine tear follow-up evaluation. Am J Sports Med 26:20-29, 1998.
8. Bach BR Jr, Warren RF, Wickiewicz TL: Observations on the effects of the hip and foot position on the pivot shift phenomenon: Results and description of a modified clinical test for ACL insufficiency. Am J Sports Med 16:571-576, 1988.
9. Bellabarba C, Bush-Joseph CA, Bach BR Jr: Patterns of meniscal tears in ACL deficient knee: A review of the literature. Orthopaedics 26:18-23, 1997.
10. Berchuck M, Andriacchi TP, Bach BR Jr: Gait adaptations by patients who have a deficient anterior cruciate ligament. J Bone Joint Surg Am 72:871-877, 1990.
11. Bonomo J, Fay C, Firestone T: The conservative treatment of the ACL knee. Am J Sports Med 18:618-623, 1990.
12. Bush-Joseph CA, Hurwitz DE, Patel RR, et al: Dynamic function during walking, stair walking and jogging activities following ACL reconstruction with autologous patella tendon. Am J Sports Med 29:36-41, 2001.
13. Ciccotti MG, Lombardo SJ, Nonweiler B, Pink W: Nonoperative treatment of ruptures of the anterior cruciate ligament in middle aged patients. J Bone Joint Surg Am 76:1315-1321, 1994.
14. Cosgarea AJ, DeHaven KE, Lovelock JE: The surgical treatment of arthrofibrosis of the knee. Am J Sports Med 22:184-191, 1994.
15. Cosgarea AJ, Sebastianelli WJ, DeHaven KE: Prevention of arthrofibrosis after anterior cruciate ligament reconstruction using the central third patellar tendon autograft. Am J Sports Med 23:87-92, 1995.
16. Daniel DM, Malcom LL, Losse G, et al: Instrumented measurement of anterior laxity of the knee. J Bone Joint Surg Am 67:720-726, 1985.
17. Daniel DM, Stone ML, Dobson BE, et al: Fate of the ACL-injured patient: A prospective outcome study. Am J Sports Med 22:632-644, 1994.
18. Daniel DM, Stone ML, Sachs R, Malcom L: Instrumented measurement of anterior knee laxity in patients with acute anterior cruciate ligament disruption. Am J Sports Med 13:401-407, 1985.
19. DeLee JC, Curtis R: Anterior cruciate insufficiency in children. Clin Orthop 172:112-118, 1983.
20. Ferrari JD, Bush-Joseph CA, Bach BR Jr: Double incision arthroscopically assisted ACL reconstruction using patellar tendon substitution. Tech Orthop 13:242-252, 314-317, 1998.
21. Ferrari JD, Bush-Joseph CA, Bach BR Jr: Arthroscopically assisted ACL reconstruction using patellar tendon substitution via endoscopic technique. Tech Orthop 13:262-274, 1998.
22. Fetto JF, Marshall JL: The natural history and diagnosis of anterior cruciate ligament insufficiency. Clin Orthop 147:29-42, 1980.
23. Fisher SE, Shelbourne KD: Arthroscopic treatment of symptomatic extension block complicating anterior cruciate ligament reconstruction. Am J Sports Med 21:558-564, 1993.
24. Graf BK, Lange RH, Fujisaki CK, et al: Anterior cruciate tears in skeletally immature patients: Meniscal pathology at presentation and after attempted conservative treatment. Arthroscopy 8:229-233, 1992.
25. Graf BK, Ott JW, Lange RH, Keene JS: Risk factors for restricted motion after anterior cruciate reconstruction. Orthopedics 17:909-912, 1994.
26. Hardin GT, Bach BR Jr, Bush-Joseph C: Extension loss following arthroscopic ACL reconstruction. Orthop Int 1:405-410, 1993.
27. Hardin GT, Bach BR Jr, Bush-Joseph C, Farr J: Endoscopic single incision ACL reconstruction using patellar tendon autograft: Surgical technique. Am J Knee Surg 5:144-155, 1992.
28. Harner CD, Irrgang JJ, Paul J, et al: Loss of motion after anterior cruciate ligament reconstruction. Am J Sports Med 20:499-506, 1992.

29. Hawkins RJ, Misamore GW, Merritt TR: Followup of the acute nonoperated isolated anterior cruciate ligament tear. Am J Sports Med 14:205-210, 1986.

30. Hunter RE, Mastrangelo J, Freeman JR, Purnell ML: The impact of surgical timing on post-operative motion and stability following anterior cruciate ligament reconstruction. Paper presented to the Arthroscopy Association of North America, Apr 1994, Orlando, FL.

31. Lipscomb AB, Anderson AF: Tears of the anterior cruciate ligament in adolescents. J Bone Joint Surg Am 68:19-28, 1986.

32. Marzo JM, Bowen MK, Warren RF, et al: Intraarticular fibrous nodule as a cause of loss of extension following anterior cruciate ligament reconstruction. Arthroscopy 8:10-18, 1992.

33. Marzo JM, Warren RF: Results of treatment of anterior cruciate ligament injury: Changing perspectives. Adv Orthop Surg 15:59-69, 1991.

34. McCarroll JR, Rettig AC, Shelbourne KD: Anterior cruciate ligament injuries in the young athlete with open physes. Am J Sports Med 16:44-47, 1988.

35. McDaniel WJ Jr, Dameron TB Jr: Untreated ruptures of the anterior cruciate ligament: A follow up study. J Bone Joint Surg Am 62:696-705, 1980.

36. Mizuta H, Kubota K, Shiraishi M, et al: The conservative treatment of complete tears of the anterior cruciate ligament in skeletally immature patients. J Bone Joint Surg Br 77:890-894, 1995.

37. Mohtadi NGH, Webster-Bogaert S, Fowler PJ: Limitation of motion following anterior cruciate ligament reconstruction. Am J Sports Med 19:620-624, 1991.

38. Nedeff D, Bach BR Jr: Arthroscopy assisted ACL reconstruction using patellar tendon autograft: A comprehensive review of contemporary literature. Am J Knee Surg 14:243-258, 2001.

39. Nogalski MP, Bach BR Jr: A review of early anterior cruciate ligament surgical repair or reconstruction: Results and caveats. Orthop Rev 22:1213-1223, 1993.

40. Novak PJ, Bach BR Jr, Bush-Joseph CA, Badrinath S: Cost containment: A charge comparison of anterior cruciate ligament reconstruction. Arthroscopy 12:160-164, 1996.

41. Novak PJ, Bach BR Jr, Hager CA: Clinical and functional outcome of anterior cruciate ligament reconstruction in the recreational athlete over the age of 35. Am J Knee Surg 9:111-116, 1996.

42. Noyes FR, Mooar PA, Matthews DS, Butler DL: The symptomatic anterior cruciate deficient knee. Part I. The long term functional disability in athletically active individuals. J Bone Joint Surg Am 65:154-162, 1983.

43. Parker AW, Drez D Jr, Cooper JL: Anterior cruciate ligament injuries in patients with open physes. Am J Sports Med 22:44-47, 1994.

44. Patel DV, Shelbourne DK, Martini DJ: Classification and management of arthrofibrosis of the knee following anterior cruciate ligament reconstruction. Paper presented at the annual meeting of the American Academy of Orthopaedic Surgeons, Feb 22, 1996, Atlanta, GA.

45. Paulos LE, Rosenberg TD, Drawbert J, et al:. Infrapatellar contracture syndrome: An unrecognized cause of knee stiffness with patellar entrapment and patella infera. Am J Sports Med 15:331-341, 1987.

46. Robins AJ, Newman AP, Burks RT: Postoperative return of motion in anterior cruciate ligament and medial collateral ligament injuries: The effect of medial collateral ligament rupture location. Am J Sports Med 21:20-25, 1993.

47. Sachs RA, Daniel DM, Stone ML, et al: Patellofemoral problems after anterior cruciate ligament reconstruction. Am J Sports Med 17:760, 1989.

48. Shelbourne KD, Johnson GE: Outpatient surgical management of arthrofibrosis after anterior cruciate ligament surgery. Am J Sports Med 22:192-197, 1994.

49. Shelbourne KD, Porter DA: ACL-MCL injury: Nonoperative management of the MCL tears with ACL reconstruction. Am J Sports Med 20:283-286, 1992.

50. Shelbourne KD, Wilckens JH, Mollabashy A, DeCarlo M: Arthrofibrosis in acute anterior cruciate ligament reconstruction: The effect of timing of reconstruction and rehabilitation. Am J Sports Med 19:332-336, 1991.

51. Warren RF, Kaplan N, Bach BR Jr: The lateral notch sign of anterior cruciate ligament insufficiency. Am J Knee Surg 1:119-124, 1988.

52. Wasilewski SA, Covall DJ, Cohen S: Effect of surgical timing on recovery and associated injuries after anterior cruciate ligament reconstruction. Am J Sports Med 21:338-342, 1993.

53. Wexler G, Bach BR Jr, Bush-Joseph CA, et al: Outcomes of ACL reconstruction in patients with workmans' compensation claims. Arthroscopy 16:49-58, 2000.

6 Knee

Patellar Tendon Autograft for ACL Reconstruction

BERNARD R. BACH, JR.

PATELLAR TENDON AUTOGRAFT FOR ACL RECONSTRUCTION IN A NUTSHELL

History:
Contact or noncontact injury, "pop" (80%); rapid effusion within 3 hours (80%), pain, sense of knee shifting

Two-fist sign describes instability, determines whether acute or major reinjury; concurrent meniscal tears common, displaced bucket handle meniscal tears (ACL) injury until proven otherwise

Physical Examination:
Varus-valgus test; Lachman test; anterior drawer test, pivot shift phenomenon

Imaging:
Radiographs; magnetic resonance imaging

Decision-Making Principles:
Level of sports activity; frequency of instability; presence of meniscal pathology; KT-1000 maximum manual side-to-side difference; sport level of intensity; hours of activity per week; willingness to modify activities

Surgical Technique:
Expose patellar tendon, tibial tubercle, and distal patella; use oscillating saw to cut bone plugs; do not lever with osteotomes

Size graft for 10-mm sizing tubes

Arthroscopically remove remnant of anterior cruciate ligament tissue

Perform notchplasty as needed and define "over-the-top" position

Determine placement of tibial aimer; assess medial-lateral orientation; use variable-angle aimer and generally a 55-degree angle; remember "N + 10" rule

After drilling $\frac{3}{32}$-inch pin, assess position in knee extension

Overream tibial pin with 11-mm reamer and collect bone reamings for grafting patellar defect

At 80 degrees of knee flexion, place 7-mm offset femoral aimer retrograde and "key off" the over-the-top position at 11 o'clock (right knee) or 1 o'clock (left knee); drill 1.5-inch depth

Overream with 10-mm Acorn cannulated reamer; create endoscopic footprint; assess posterior rim (1 to 2 mm) and complete to 35-mm depth

Collect bone reamings for patellar and tibial tubercle grafting; pass arthroscope retrograde into femoral socket to confirm integrity

Pass graft retrograde using "push-in" technique; grasp graft with hemostat, and guide into femoral socket with cortex oriented posteriorly

Place hyperflex wire and advance with knee in hyperflexion; insert 7- by 25-mm cannulated screw at 100 to 110 degrees of knee flexion

Cycle graft and assess "gross isometry"; place tibial screw (9 by 20 mm) on anterior and cortical surface with knee extended; inspect graft

Continued

PATELLAR TENDON AUTOGRAFT FOR ACL RECONSTRUCTION IN A NUTSHELL—cont'd

If construct mismatch, consider graft rotation (e.g., 540 degrees), "free bone block" modification, staples, screw and post, or femoral graft advancement

Assess stability on table

Graft patellar and tibial tubercle defects; close patellar tendon defect loosely with knee flexed 70 degrees

Postoperative Management:
Early weight-bearing program; physical therapy 1 week postoperatively

Results:
Restores stability (90% of cases)

Case History

An 18-year-old three-sport interscholastic athlete sustained a left knee injury during what was described as a cutting deceleration move. He recollected hearing a pop and experiencing a sensation of his knee shifting. He collapsed to the ground and was unable to continue playing. After being transported off the field, he was seen at a local emergency room, where radiographs were taken and interpreted as normal. According to the patient, no specific diagnosis was made in the emergency room. Within approximately 2 weeks, the patient's swelling had completely resolved. He believed that his knee had recovered and attempted to resume athletics. At his first practice, the knee gave way again, causing him to collapse to the ground. He was subsequently seen in the office for consultation purposes. Before the index injury, he recollected no specific injury to his knee.

Physical Examination

Physical examination in the office revealed a soft effusion. The extensor mechanism was intact, and the patient was able to perform a straight leg raise. Varus-valgus testing at 0 and 30 degrees was normal. The Lachman test was grade II with a soft endpoint. The anterior drawer test was grade I. A demonstrable grade I pivot shift was detected. There was no evidence of posterolateral corner injury, and the posterior cruciate ligament examination, consisting of the posterior drawer and posterior sag tests, was normal. At this point, the patient demonstrated complete symmetrical extension with flexion to 130 degrees. There was no joint line tenderness and no meniscal rotation signs.

Imaging

Radiographs of the left knee were obtained, including anteroposterior, lateral, tunnel, and skyline views. The anteroposterior view revealed a Segond fracture consistent with a lateral capsular avulsion, pathognomonic of an anterior cruciate ligament (ACL) injury.[7] Magnetic resonance imaging revealed signal changes consistent with an ACL injury and a bone contusion of the lateral femoral and tibial condyle. No evidence of a meniscal tear was noted.

Decision-Making Principles

The basic factors considered in patients with ACL-deficient knees include the level of sports activity, frequency of instability, presence of meniscal pathology, KT-1000 maximum manual side-to-side difference, force level intensity, hours of sports activity per week, and willingness or unwillingness to modify activities.[1] In this patient, who was involved in three sports—soccer, basketball (both category I sports), and baseball (category II)—the KT-1000 maximum manual difference was 8 mm, and he participated in sports more than 12 hours a week. Radiographs revealed that he was skeletally mature. Based on these considerations, ACL reconstruction was discussed with this patient.

Graft Selection and Rationale

I consider a middle-third patellar tendon autograft the primary "workhorse" for ACL surgery. Surveys at my institution (with 2- to 4-year and 5- to 9-year follow-up) have demonstrated that this technique has a predictable outcome, a low incidence of patellar pain, and an extremely high patient satisfaction level.[2-4,10,14,15,19] In preoperative discussions, patients are told that the procedure has a less than 1% major complication rate for infection, deep vein thrombosis, pulmonary embolus, extensor mechanism rupture, or patellar fracture. The reoperation rate for symptomatic knee flexion contractures has varied between 1% and 2% annually since 1994. Clinical stability rates approach 90%, and 95% of patients are mostly or completely satisfied. Additionally, when queried whether they would opt to have the contralateral ACL reconstructed if that knee were injured, 95% of patients respond yes.[2-4]

Surgical Technique

The following surgical technique has been used since 1991 with minor refinements and modifications. Descriptions of the technique have been published previously.[11-13]

Positioning

The patient is positioned supine. The waist of the table is flexed slightly to take the lumbar spine out of extension. The contralateral leg is positioned with the hip and knee flexed in a well-padded gynecologic leg holder to protect the common peroneal and femoral nerves. The surgical leg is placed in an arthroscopic leg holder after a meticulous examination under anesthesia is performed. A padded thigh tourniquet is placed but is generally not used. The knee should be able to be flexed to 110 degrees in the leg holder. The leg is prepared with Duraprep ×2, and preoperative first-generation cephalosporin antibiotics are used.

Examination under Anesthesia

As noted, examination under anesthesia is documented before securing the leg in the leg holder. The Lachman, anterior drawer, and pivot shift tests are graded and compared with the opposite knee. Careful assessment is made for any varus-valgus laxity or posterolateral corner injury.

Diagnostic Arthroscopy

Germane to the ACL-injured knee are several points pertaining to arthroscopic evaluation. Condylar injuries are frequently noted. In clinical follow-up studies, approximately 25% of patients have demonstrable chondromalacia patellae at the time of the index reconstruction.[2-4] Approximately 50% of patients have had arthroscopic surgery before the ACL reconstruction.[2-4] Meniscal tears are extremely common. In acute or subacute ACL injuries, the lateral meniscus is more frequently torn, whereas in chronic ACL-deficient knees, the medial meniscus is more frequently torn.[6] With regard to bucket handle tears, the medial meniscus is affected more often, with a 4:1 prevalence. Partial tears should be assessed for stability; if they are less than 1 cm and peripheral, they may be treated conservatively. In chronic ACL-deficient knees, a chondral lateral notch sign consistent with recurrent injuries, resulting in indentation of the normal sulcus terminalis region, should be documented.[18] Additionally, intercondylar notch osteophytes may be detected in chronic ACL injuries. The intercondylar notch should be assessed for an abnormal configuration or narrowness. It is critical to carefully assess the ACL, because frequently it is torn proximally and may scar to the adjacent posterior cruciate ligament; this results in a more vertical orientation, which has been termed the vertical strut sign.[5] In this situation, an empty space may be noted between the normal orientation of the ACL and the lateral wall ("empty wall" sign).

Specific Surgical Steps

If the patient has a demonstrable pivot shift and normal radiographs, I generally harvest the patellar tendon graft first. An 8-cm longitudinal incision is made, paralleling the medial edge of the patellar tendon from the distal pole to slightly below the tibial tubercle (Fig. 63–1). The skin is scored and infiltrated with 0.25% bupivacaine (Marcaine) with epinephrine, and dissection is carried through the subcutaneous tissues down to Marshall's layer 1. This layer is incised, and Metzenbaum scissors are used to incise the fascia proximally and distally; it is then retracted medially and laterally with Senn retractors. An Army-Navy retractor is positioned proximally.

The patellar tendon is visualized proximally and distally, and its width is measured distally and documented

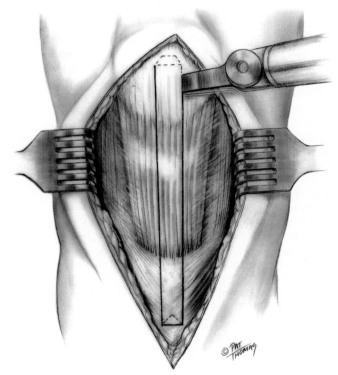

Figure 63–1 A free central-third graft is harvested using an 8- to 9-cm incision. The deep fascia is incised and extended proximally and distally, exposing the patella, patellar tendon, and tibial tubercle region. The patellar tendon width should be measured and documented in the operative report. A number 238 oscillating saw blade is used to create the bone plug cuts. Note that a graft with a triangular profile is harvested on the tibial tubercle, and a graft with a trapezoidal profile is harvested on the patella. Saw cuts should proceed from the tendo-osseous junctions distally and proximally on the tibial tubercle and patellar sides, respectively. The graft width is generally 10 mm. The patellar cut is 6 to 8 mm deep. (From Bach BR: Arthroscopy-assisted patellar tendon substitution for anterior cruciate ligament insufficiency: Surgical technique. Am J Knee Surg 2:3-20, 1989.)

in the operative notes. The central distal patellar pole and central midline portion of the patellar tendon distally are marked with a sterile marking pen. A curved ⅜-inch osteotome, which is effectively 10 mm wide, is used as the cutting template to outline the middle-third patellar tendon bone-tendon-bone graft. One should begin on the patella, extending into the patellar tendon, and maintain visualization of the distal orientation of the tendon incision. The Army-Navy retractor is positioned distally to protect the skin, and once the tendo-osseous junction is defined distally, the tendon incision is extended another 2 to 2.5 cm. This is then repeated, thus creating a 10-mm-wide graft.

A number 238 oscillating saw blade is used to create bone cuts. One should begin on the tibial tubercle side, as this is technically easier and prevents blood from dripping down into the surgical wound region if the patella bone plug is created initially. Senn retractors are positioned distally, and the orientation of the saw blade is such that a graft with an equilateral triangular profile is harvested. A cut on the right side of the bone plug is made with the right hand, and on the left side it is made with the saw held in the left hand. In this way, one's view is not blocked. Then one moves proximally and makes the cuts for the patellar plug. The saw is placed initially at the tendo-osseous junction. The cortex is outlined with the saw, and one works from distal to proximal, effectively moving the saw much like a cast saw, feeling a sense of give as it enters the cancellous bone. The depth of the saw should not exceed 6 to 8 mm. This is repeated on the left side of the bone plug, and the orientation is such that one is trying to create a rhomboid on profile. The transverse cut is then made with the saw angled to reduce the likelihood of creating a stress riser. A ⅜-inch and a ¼-inch curved osteotome are used to carefully remove the bone plugs from their osseous bed. One begins distally, and once the tibial tubercle plug has been removed, it is left attached to the underlying fat pad. Then one moves proximally to remove the bone plug from the patellar bed. Once this has been performed, the tibial tubercle plug is wrapped and held with a laparotomy sponge, and Metzenbaum scissors are used to carefully dissect the fat pad from the undersurface of the patellar tendon. Once the graft is obtained, it is transported by the surgeon to the back table for preparation. The graft should not be handed off; this reduces the likelihood of the graft being dropped on the floor.

At the back table, the graft is prepared by the first assistant. It is sized for 10-mm sizing tubes (Fig. 63–2). A spherical bur or rongeur may be used to fine-tune the shape of the graft to fit the sizing tubes. A "push-in" technique is used; therefore, two drill holes are made with a smooth 0.062 K-wire drill parallel to the cortex of the bone plug, which will reside within the tibia. A number 5 Ticron suture is placed through each of these holes. The tendo-osseous junctions are marked with a sterile marking pen. The cortical edge of the plug, which will be placed on the tibial side, is identified with a marking pen. The graft is placed in a moist sponge and set aside in a kidney basin. All personnel are informed of its location so that it is not inadvertently passed off the operating table in the sponge.

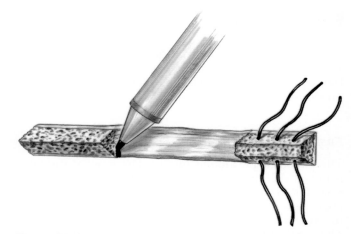

Figure 63–2 The graft is measured and sized for 10-mm sizing tubes. Bone plug lengths and soft tissue construct lengths should be measured. The soft tissue length influences the angle selected for tibial tunnel creation. Because a "push-in" technique is used, two or three drill holes are made with a 0.062 K-wire drill parallel and adjacent to the cortex, and number 5 Ticron sutures are placed through these holes. The tendo-osseous junction is then marked with a sterile marking pen. This transition zone can be visualized arthroscopically.

While the graft is being prepared, a periosteal flap is created in the medial metaphyseal region of the tibia, taking care not to violate the superficial medial collateral ligament, the pes anserinus, or remaining third of the medial patellar tendon. A medial-based ¾- by ¾-inch periosteal flap is elevated with a Cobb elevator after outlining it with electrocautery. This represents the general site for the tibial tunnel entrance.

Through retracted skin edges, the arthroscope is inserted through a standard inferolateral portal placed immediately lateral to the patellar tendon at the level of the distal pole of the patella. A working portal is established inferomedially at the same level, and a superomedial portal is used for pump outflow or inflow purposes. Diagnostic arthroscopy is performed in the standard fashion, with careful attention to articular surfaces and meniscal pathology. Attention is then directed toward intercondylar notch preparation and notchplasty if warranted. Residual ACL tissue is removed with a combination of arthroscopic scissors, arthroscopic osteotome, arthroscopic electrocautery, and motorized shaver (Fig. 63–3). One begins at the tibial insertion and defines the interval between the remnant ACL and the posterior cruciate ligament. The elevator is used to reflect tissue off the lateral intercondylar wall as well. Once it is debrided and hemostasis is achieved with electrocautery, attention is directed toward intercondylar notchplasty. This may be performed with a ¼-inch curved osteotome, mallet, and grasper and fine-tuned with a motorized spherical bur. A spherical bur is preferred to a barrel-shaped bur because it is unlikely to create troughs and channels. Notchplasty is performed from anterior to posterior, working along the lateral wall toward the over-the-top position (Fig. 63–4). One must be certain to perform debridement beyond the "resident's ridge." The over-the-top position

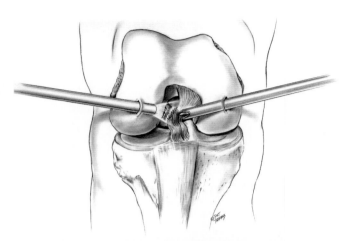

Figure 63–3 Remnant anterior cruciate ligament tissue is debrided with a combination of arthroscopic shaver, scissors, osteotome, and electrocautery. I prefer debridement of the tibial insertion directly down to bone to identify this anatomic footprint. (From Bach BR: Arthroscopy-assisted patellar tendon substitution for anterior cruciate ligament insufficiency: Surgical technique. Am J Knee Surg 2:3-20, 1989.)

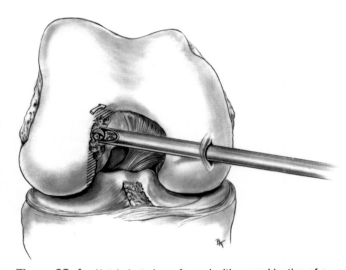

Figure 63–4 Notchplasty is performed with a combination of a ¼-inch curved osteotome, mallet, and grasper or with a spherical motorized bur. Some patients may require minimal or no notchplasty. The goal is to have enough space for graft placement and visualization purposes. Notchplasty should not extend cephalad to the intercondylar apex. Generally, a 3- to 5-mm notchplasty is performed, depending on the width of the intercondylar notch. (From Bach BR: Arthroscopy-assisted patellar tendon substitution for anterior cruciate ligament insufficiency: Surgical technique. Am J Knee Surg 2:3-20, 1989. OR Hardin GT, Bach BR Jr, Bush-Joseph CA, Farr J: Endoscopic single-incision ACL reconstruction using patellar tendon autograft: Surgical technique. Am J Knee Surg 5:144-155, 1992.)

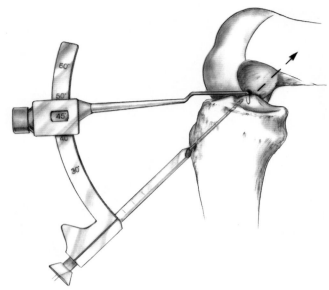

Figure 63–5 Tibial pin placement is generally performed at an angle 10 degrees greater than the length of the graft soft tissue construct. For example, a 45-mm soft tissue construct is generally drilled at 55 degrees. This schematic demonstrates that if a steeper angle is selected, it may be more difficult to place the femoral tunnel anatomically. Additionally, if the tibial tunnel is drilled too horizontally, it may create a femoral tunnel that "blows out" the "over-the-top" position. Tibial pin placement is centered within the middle third of the former anterior cruciate ligament insertion region. I prefer the pin to exit at a point in the coronal plane tangent with the posterior edge of the anterior horn lateral meniscus. Once the pin has been drilled, the knee is brought out to complete extension to make certain that the pin clears the intercondylar apex by 3 to 4 mm. It is particularly important to avoid placing the pin in a sagittal plane. There should be an appropriate mediolateral orientation that directs the pin at an 11 o'clock (right knee) or 1 o'clock (left knee) orientation.

ent on the length of the soft tissue component of the graft construct (e.g., 45 mm soft tissue = 55-degree angle [N + 10]). A "point-to-point" or "point-to-elbow" aimer may be used (Fig. 63–6). A general reference point is the posterior edge of the anterior horn of the lateral meniscus. I generally use a point-to-elbow aimer, and the stylet of the aimer is placed 3 to 4 mm posterior to the posterior edge of the anterior horn of the lateral meniscus within the former ACL insertion region. Attention must be paid to the medial-to-lateral orientation so that one can achieve an 11 o'clock orientation on a right knee or a 1 o'clock orientation on a left knee. Accurate femoral tunnel preparation is contingent on orientation of the tibial tunnel. Provisional pin placement is performed with a ³⁄₃₂-inch smooth Steinmann pin. The aiming device is removed, and the knee is brought out into complete extension. The site should be between 3 and 4 mm posterior to the intercondylar notch in extension or hyperextension. Because of the oblique orientation and placement of this pin, the farther it is drilled intraarticularly, the more lateral it appears to have been placed. After appropriate placement of this tibial pin, it is overreamed with a cannulated reamer. An 11-mm reamer is generally used, although I size for a 10-mm graft. This is done for ease of graft passage. Before

should be hooked with a probe. I prefer to have 10 mm of space between the lateral edge of the posterior cruciate ligament and the lateral intercondylar wall.

After notchplasty is performed, attention is directed toward tibial tunnel placement (Fig. 63–5). A variable-angle tibial aimer is used. The angle selected is depend-

6 Knee

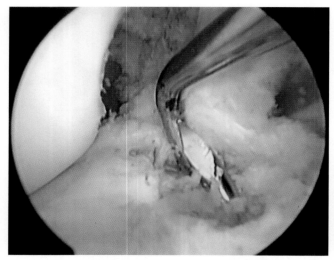

Figure 63–6 Arthroscopic photograph demonstrating the intra-articular entrance of a tibial pin with a "point-to-elbow" tibial aimer.

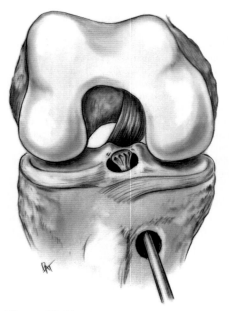

Figure 63–7 Once the tibial pin has been overreamed with a 10- or 11-mm cannulated reamer, the posterior edge is smoothed with a chamfer reamer and hand rasp. This facilitates placement of the femoral aimer in the "over-the-top" position without having to extend the knee. (From Hardin GT, Bach BR Jr, Bush-Joseph CA, Farr J: Endoscopic single-incision ACL reconstruction using patellar tendon autograft: Surgical technique. Am J Knee Surg 5:144-155, 1992.)

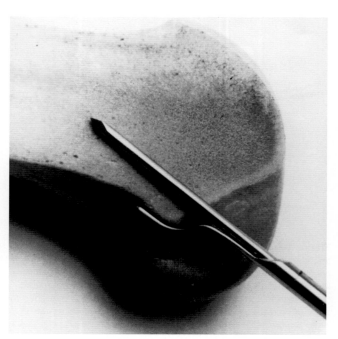

Figure 63–8 Photograph depicting a 7-mm retrograde femoral offset aimer. Using a 10-mm-diameter reamer creates a 2-mm posterior cortical rim.

reaming, the pin is tapped into the roof of the intercondylar notch. This helps stabilize the pin and reduces the amount of posterior tibial wall smoothing that would otherwise be necessary. Before entering intra-articularly, the inflow is turned off. A cannulated bone chip collector is placed over the tibial reamer to collect cancellous bone reamings, which can be used to graft the distal patella and tibial tubercle defects. Once the tibial tunnel has been reamed, a chamfer reamer and hand rasp are used to smooth the posterior tibial tunnel wall intra-articularly (Fig. 63–7). Intra-articular fragments can be removed with an arthroscopic grasper.

The knee is reirrigated and suctioned dry, and the femoral socket is created. A 7-mm femoral offset aimer is used (Fig. 63–8). This is placed retrograde by the tibial tunnel with the knee flexed at approximately 80 degrees. The aimer is "walked" off the intercondylar roof to the over-the-top position and oriented toward the 11 o'clock position (Fig. 63–9). Once it is confirmed that this is secured in the over-the-top position, the aimer can be slightly rotated to fine-tune the position of the femoral pin. It should be done with the knee flexed at approximately 80 degrees. If extension of the knee is necessary to place the femoral aimer, this implies that the tibial tunnel is too far anterior. O'Donnell[17] popularized placement of the femoral aimer through an accessory inferomedial portal with the knee hyperflexed 110 to 120 degrees (Fig. 63–10). Femoral socket creation should be easily performed between 75 and 90 degrees of knee flexion. A $\frac{3}{32}$-inch Steinmann pin is drilled to a depth of 1.5 inches. The aiming device is removed, and the pin is overreamed with a cannulated 10-mm endoscopic Acorn reamer (Fig. 63–11). An endoscopic footprint is created. The reamer is drilled to a depth of approximately 6 to 8 mm, backed out, and inspected for preservation of the posterior cortex. A thin 1- to 2-mm cortical edge should be maintained (Fig. 63–12). Once this is established, the reaming is completed, generally to a depth of 35 mm. The pin and reamer are then removed. Once again, bone reamings can be flushed from the knee and collected on an Owens gauze for grafting of the distal patella and tibial tubercle defects.

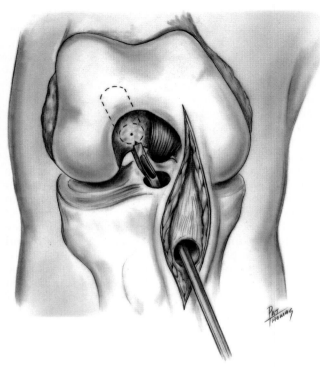

Figure 63–9 Retrograde placement of a 7-mm femoral offset aimer through the tibial tunnel. The knee should be flexed 75 to 90 degrees. (From Hardin GT, Bach BR Jr, Bush-Joseph CA, Farr J: Endoscopic single-incision ACL reconstruction using patellar tendon autograft: Surgical technique. Am J Knee Surg 5:144-155, 1992.)

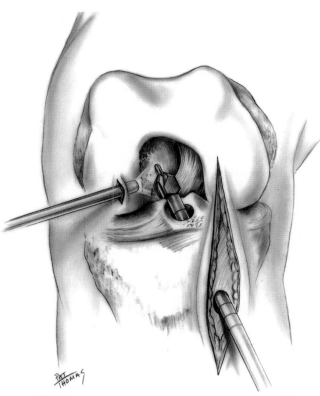

Figure 63–11 The pin is overreamed with a cannulated 10-mm endoscopic reamer, creating an endoscopic footprint. This is done to ensure that the posterior cortex is appropriately preserved and the tunnel is correctly oriented. Once this is confirmed, reaming is completed, generally to a depth of 35 mm. (From Hardin GT, Bach BR Jr, Bush-Joseph CA, Farr J: Endoscopic single-incision ACL reconstruction using patellar tendon autograft: Surgical technique. Am J Knee Surg 5:144-155, 1992.)

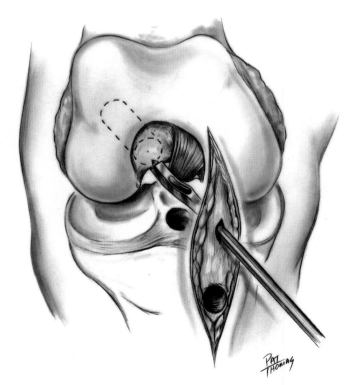

Figure 63–10 Alternatively, an accessory inferomedial portal can be used to position the aimer. The knee should be flexed at least 110 degrees. (From Hardin GT, Bach BR Jr, Bush-Joseph CA, Farr J: Endoscopic single-incision ACL reconstruction using patellar tendon autograft: Surgical technique. Am J Knee Surg 5:144-155, 1992.)

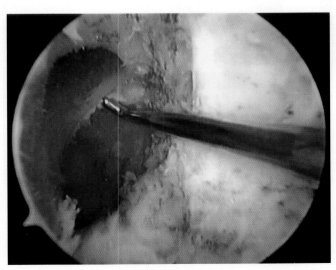

Figure 63–12 Photograph demonstrating the orientation of the femoral socket. A thin 1- to 2-mm cortical edge is palpated with an arthroscopic probe.

The next step is phase II notchplasty. If the reamer has skived along the lateral wall, this suggests that additional expansion of the lateral wall may be necessary. A shaver is used to elevate the anterior edge of the femoral tunnel, which facilitates passage of the graft and insertion of the nitinol hyperflex wire used for screw placement. The arthroscope is removed from the knee retrograde past the tibial tunnel up into the femoral socket. The tunnel is irrigated and inspected to confirm that the femoral socket is intact and that a 1- to 2-mm posterior cortical rim has been maintained (see Fig. 63–12). The arthroscope is reinserted through the inferolateral portal, the knee is reirrigated, and attention is directed toward graft passage. As noted, the graft is positioned using a "push-in" rather than a "pull-through" technique (Fig. 63–13). A curved hemostat is inserted through the inferomedial portal and positioned with the curved tips facing cephalad over the tibial tunnel. A barbed pusher is then used to push the bone plug that will reside in the femur up through the tibial tunnel. When this has entered the intra-articular region at approximately half its length, it is grasped with a hemostat. The graft should be oriented with the cortex in the coronal plane and posteriorly. It is then grasped and guided up into the femoral socket. If difficulty is encountered pushing the graft up into the femoral socket, it may be because the tibial bone plug has not been introduced into the tibial tunnel. Before completely positioning the femoral bone plug, it is left slightly prominent, thus acting as a skid. A hemostat is used to create a slight pilot hole at approximately the 11:30 position, and a 14-inch nitinol hyperflex wire is placed in the inferomedial portal at the 11:30 position.

The knee is then hyperflexed to approximately 100 to 110 degrees, and the pin is slid up in the gap space interface until this "bottoms out" within the recess of the femoral socket (Fig. 63–14). The knee is brought back to the resting position of approximately 80 degrees of flexion, and a variety of devices can be used to push the bone plug flush to the articular margin. At this point, it is held in position, and one inspects distally to determine whether there is any construct mismatch. If there is no mismatch, femoral bone plug fixation is begun.

A 7- by 25-mm cannulated metal interference screw is used for fixation purposes. This is inserted through the inferomedial portal and, in some situations, through an accessory inferomedial portal. It is pushed directly up to the bone-tendon interface; then the knee is hyperflexed to 110 degrees, and under direct vision, with the knee generally dry, the screw is inserted (Figs. 63–15 and 63–16). Once it has been inserted approximately half its distance, the cannulated wire is removed. During the course of screw insertion, one is inspecting to ensure that rotation of the soft tissue component of the graft does not occur. If it does, one must be concerned that the screw may be wrapping around the graft and could lacerate it. Once the femoral bone plug is secured, manual tension is placed on the graft to assess for fixation, and

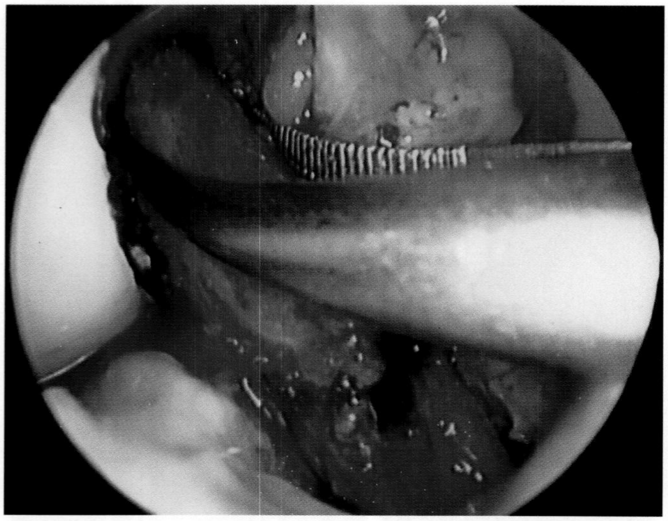

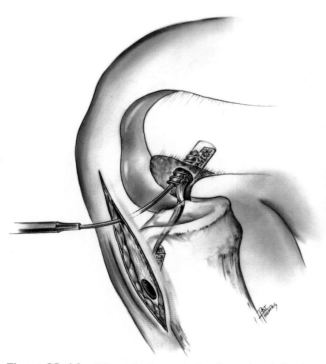

Figure 63–13 A "push-in" technique is used to advance the graft intra-articularly. It is grasped with a hemostat and guided up into the femoral socket. The graft is initially left slightly prominent, for placement of a 14-inch hyperflexed nitinol pin through an inferomedial or accessory inferomedial portal. The knee is then further flexed, and the pin is advanced until it bottoms out within the femoral tunnel. At this point, an arthroscopic "push-in" device is used to place the bone plug flush to the articular margin. Graft construct mismatch is assessed before placement of an interference screw.

Figure 63–14 Schematic demonstrating femoral graft fixation using a metal interference screw, generally 7 by 25 mm long. This is placed over a flexible 14-inch nitinol wire that has been positioned through an inferomedial or accessory inferomedial portal. The knee should be hyperflexed at this point, generally between 100 and 110 degrees. This reduces the likelihood of graft soft tissue injury during placement of the interference screw. (From Hardin GT, Bach BR Jr, Bush-Joseph CA, Farr J: Endoscopic single-incision ACL reconstruction using patellar tendon autograft: Surgical technique. Am J Knee Surg 5:144-155, 1992.)

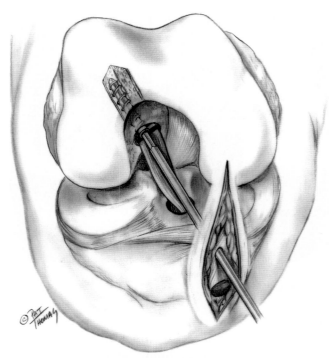

Figure 63–16 Anteroposterior view showing placement of the femoral screw against the cancellous portion of the femoral plug. Note that the soft tissue is not rotating or twisting as the screw is inserted. (From Hardin GT, Bach BR Jr, Bush-Joseph CA, Farr J: Endoscopic single-incision ACL reconstruction using patellar tendon autograft: Surgical technique. Am J Knee Surg 5:144-155, 1992.)

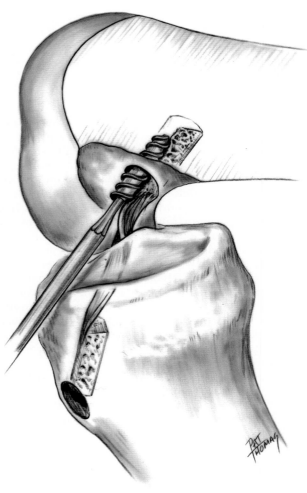

Figure 63–15 Lateral schematic depicting placement of the femoral interference screw. Note that hyperflexion is necessary to reduce the likelihood of screw divergence. (From Hardin GT, Bach BR Jr, Bush-Joseph CA, Farr J: Endoscopic single-incision ACL reconstruction using patellar tendon autograft: Surgical technique. Am J Knee Surg 5:144-155, 1992.)

the "rock" test is performed. Enough tension is placed on the graft to oscillate the patient on the table. Gross isometry is assessed by holding the distal sutures in the bone plug, placing the thumb at the tibial tunnel aperture, and extending the knee from 90 degrees to complete extension. Generally 1 to 2 mm of graft shortening occurs in the terminal 20 degrees of extension. After multiply cycling the knee, attention is directed toward tibial bone plug fixation.

Tibial bone plug fixation is performed with the knee in extension and axially loaded. Many surgeons prefer to do this at 20 to 30 degrees of knee flexion, but I prefer to do it in extension to ensure that the fixation has not "captured" the knee. The tibial bone plug is rotated with a hemostat such that the cortex is facing anteriorly and in the coronal plane. Thus, I routinely rotate the graft 180 degrees. In general, this is secured with a cannulated 9- by 20-mm interference screw. If there is a component of construct mismatch, several options are available. In

general, I prefer not to use staple fixation. Many surgeons prefer proximal recession of the graft. However, the farther the bone plug resides within the femoral socket, the more likely it is that the graft will be lacerated with femoral screw fixation. For this reason, I generally resort to one of two options. The graft can be rotated up to 540 degrees, which may shorten the graft 7 to 8 mm. This gives the graft more of a cable-type appearance when assessed arthroscopically. Alternatively, with a more significant construct mismatch, the distal bone plug can be sharply removed from the tendon, and a Krackow suture can be run up the tendon, thus creating a "pseudo–quadriceps tendon" graft.[16] The graft is secured on the femoral side. The bone plug, which has two sutures in it to prevent it from being pushed into the joint, is placed on the anterior surface of the soft tissue, and an interference screw is used for fixation purposes. Both these technique modifications have been assessed biomechanically, and I have approximately 8 years' experience with them. Once the tibial bone plug has been secured, Lachman, anterior drawer, and pivot shift tests are performed on the table, and the graft is inspected (Fig. 63–17).

Attention is then directed toward closure. Bone reamings are packed in the distal patella and tibial tubercle defects.[8,9] The patellar tendon rent is closed with an absorbable suture while the knee is flexed at approximately 70 degrees. Subcutaneous tissue in the periosteal flap overlying the tibial tunnel is also closed with an

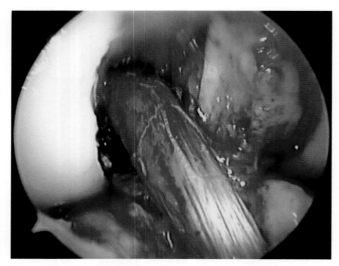

Figure 63–17 Arthroscopic photograph of the graft after femoral and tibial fixation.

absorbable suture. The skin is closed with a running subcuticular Prolene closure. Bupivacaine is injected into the knee joint and within the deep surgical wound region. Owens gauze, unclipped sponges, Kerlix, a motorized cryotherapy device, and a hinged knee brace are placed on the knee with the knee locked in extension.

Postoperative Management

This procedure has been performed exclusively on an outpatient basis since April 1994, and I have completed nearly 800 outpatient arthroscopic ACL reconstructions. Patients are started on an early weight-bearing program with the knee locked in extension.[20] A drop-lock brace is used for the first 6 weeks to protect the donor site. The patient is encouraged to sleep with the brace locked in extension, but the brace can be removed for flexion exercises. Patients begin supervised physical therapy at 1 week postoperatively. General guidelines include progression to a stationary bicycle by a week to 10 days, a stair-stepper at 4 to 6 weeks, running at 3 months, and return to sports at 4 months if motion and strength goals have been achieved. Early on, the focus is on patellar immobilization and recovery of quadriceps activation, and closed chain quadriceps extension exercises are emphasized. Open chain quadriceps extension exercises are not used in the postoperative regimen, nor is isokinetic strength training or testing. Patients are sent for supervised physical therapy, which can be expected to last for approximately 4 months.

Patients are seen at 10 days for suture removal. If they have met their motion goal of complete extension to 90 degrees, they are seen again at 6 weeks postoperatively. If they have not met their motion goal, they are seen on a weekly basis until motion recovery is acceptable. Patients are then seen at 6-week intervals until 6 months postoperatively, and then again at 9 months and 1 year.

KT-1000 testing is performed at 6-week intervals.[1] Functional testing is used as a guideline for strength recovery and return to sports.

Results

Clinical results have been reported in several articles.[2-4,10,14,15,19] My colleagues and I have evaluated the endoscopic and two-incision patellar tendon autograft procedure at 2- to 4-year intervals and our two-incision technique at 5- to 9-year intervals. With the endoscopic technique, the infection rate is less than 1%. There have been no patellar tendon ruptures or patella fractures. The reoperation rate for motion problems has been 1% to 2% since 1994. The stability rate is 90%, demonstrated by clinical evaluation and negative pivot shift testing and KT-1000 testing. Approximately 4% of our patients have a KT-1000 maximum manual side-to-side difference of 5 mm or greater. On average, functional testing generally demonstrates side-to-side differences of less than 5% on single-leg jump, vertical jump, and timed single-leg jump over 20 feet. In 40% of our patients, functional testing scores are actually higher on the surgical side. In a recent study, 12% of our patients had minimal to mild pain associated with stair climbing. Subjective satisfaction levels are extremely high, with 95% of patients completely or mostly satisfied, and 95% indicating that they would repeat the procedure if they tore the contralateral ACL.

Conclusion

Endoscopic ACL reconstruction with patellar tendon autograft is a predictable surgical procedure for stabilizing the ACL-deficient knee. This is an extremely detail-oriented technique, and meticulous attention must be paid during each step of the procedure. At every phase—graft harvest and preparation, tunnel creation, graft placement and fixation—multiple pitfalls exist that can affect the outcome.

References

1. Bach BR Jr, Jones GT, Hager CA, Sweet F: Arthrometric aspects of arthroscopic assisted ACL reconstruction using patellar tendon substitution. Am J Sports Med 23:179-185, 1995.
2. Bach BR Jr, Jones GT, Sweet F, Hager CA: Arthroscopic assisted ACL reconstruction using patellar tendon substitution: Two year follow up study. Am J Sports Med 22:758-767, 1994.
3. Bach BR Jr, Levy ME, Bojchuk J, et al: Single-incision endoscopic anterior cruciate ligament reconstruction using patellar tendon autograft: Minimum two year follow-up evaluation. Am J Sports Med 26:30-40, 1998.
4. Bach BR Jr, Tradonsky S, Bojchuk J, et al: Arthroscopically assisted anterior cruciate ligament reconstruction using patellar tendon autograft: Five to nine year follow-up evaluation. Am J Sports Med 26:20-29, 1998.

5. Bach BR Jr, Warren RF: "Empty wall" and "vertical strut" signs of ACL insufficiency. Arthroscopy 5:137-140, 1989.
6. Bellabarba C, Bush-Joseph CA, Bach BR Jr: Patterns of meniscal tears in ACL deficient knee: A review of the literature. Orthopedics 26:18-23, 1997.
7. Bush-Joseph C, Franco M, Bach BR Jr: The lateral capsular sign associated with posterior cruciate ligament tear: A case report. Am J Knee Surg 5:210-212, 1992.
8. Daluga D, Johnson JC, Bach BR Jr: Primary bone grafting following graft procurement for ACL insufficiency. Arthroscopy 6:205-208, 1990.
9. Ferrari JD, Bach BR Jr: Bone graft procurement for patellar defect grafting in anterior cruciate ligament reconstruction. Arthroscopy 14:543-545, 1998.
10. Ferrari J, Bach BR Jr, Bush-Joseph CA, et al: ACL reconstruction in men and women: An outcome analysis comparing gender. Arthroscopy 17:588-596, 2001.
11. Ferrari JD, Bush-Joseph CA, Bach BR Jr: Arthroscopically assisted ACL reconstruction using patellar tendon substitution via endoscopic technique. Tech Orthop 13:262-274, 1998.
12. Ferrari JD, Bush-Joseph CA, Bach BR Jr: Anterior cruciate ligament reconstruction using bone patellar tendon bone grafts: Autograft and allograft endoscopic techniques and two incision autograft technique. Oper Tech Sports Med 7:155-171, 1999.
13. Hardin GT, Bach BR Jr, Bush-Joseph CA, Farr J: Endoscopic single incision ACL reconstruction using patellar tendon autograft: Surgical technique. Am J Knee Surg 5:144-155, 1992.
14. Nedeff D, Bach BR Jr: Arthroscopy assisted ACL reconstruction using patellar tendon autograft: A comprehensive review of contemporary literature. Am J Knee Surg 14:243-258, 2001.
15. Novak PJ, Bach BR Jr, Hager CA: Clinical and functional outcome of anterior cruciate ligament reconstruction in the recreational athlete over the age of 35. Am J Knee Surg 9:111-116, 1996.
16. Novak PJ, Williams JS, Wexler G, et al: Comparison of screw post fixation and free bone block interference fixation for anterior cruciate ligament soft tissue grafts: Biomechanical considerations. Arthroscopy 12:470-473, 1996.
17. O'Donnell JB, Scerpella TA: Endoscopic anterior cruciate ligament reconstruction: modified technique and radiographic review. Arthroscopy 11:577-584, 1995.
18. Warren RF, Kaplan N, Bach BR Jr: The lateral notch sign of anterior cruciate ligament insufficiency. Am J Knee Surg 1:119-124, 1988.
19. Wexler G, Bach BR Jr, Bush-Joseph CA, et al: Outcomes of ACL reconstruction in patients with Workers' Compensation claims. Arthroscopy 16:49-58, 2000.
20. Williams JS Jr, Bach BR Jr: Rehabilitation of the ACL deficient and reconstructed knee. Sports Med Arthrosc Rev 3:69-82, 1996.

6 Knee

Hamstring Tendons for ACL Reconstruction

KEITH W. LAWHORN AND STEPHEN M. HOWELL

HAMSTRING TENDONS FOR ACL RECONSTRUCTION IN A NUTSHELL

History:
Noncontact pivot injury, immediate swelling, ± pop, giving way; acute versus chronic

Physical Examination:
Acute: pain, effusion, positive Lachman test, guarding
Chronic: painless, positive Lachman test, pivot shift

Imaging:
Radiographs: anteroposterior, lateral, sunrise, and notch views
Magnetic resonance imaging: supportive, identifies associated injuries; not necessary

Initial Management:
Control edema, restore range of motion

Treatment:
Nonoperative: sedentary lifestyle, no instability
Operative: repairable meniscus, instability, multiple ligaments

Advantages:
Less morbidity than patellar tendon graft; strongest and stiffest autogenous graft; quick harvest; easy preparation

Indications:
Professional and low-demand athletes; females and males; skeletally mature and immature

Contraindications:
None; in the skeletally immature, do not put fixation devices across open physis

Surgical Technique:
Graft harvest: leave tendons attached to tibia; remove all branches from semitendinosus and gracilis; use blunt, open-ended tendon stripper
Graft preparation: sew a whipstitch to each tendon; double-loop tendons to form graft; measure diameter using sizing sleeve; use diameter that slides freely to ream tunnels
Portal placement: medial portal touches medial border of patellar tendon; transpatellar portal in lateral one third of tendon
Tibial tunnel: guide pin aligned at 65 degrees in coronal plane, drilled 4 to 5 mm posterior to intercondylar roof in extended knee; avoids posterior cruciate ligament and roof impingement
WasherLoc counterbore: aim counterbore guide toward fibular head; ream posterior and parallel to tibial tunnel toward fibula; ream until flush with posterior wall of tunnel
Femoral tunnel: insert size-specific femoral aimer through tibial tunnel; hook aimer over top and rotate laterally away from posterior cruciate ligament; leaves thin, 1-mm back wall

Continued

The views expressed in this chapter are those of the authors and do not necessarily represent the views of the United States Air Force or the United States Government.

HAMSTRING TENDONS FOR ACL RECONSTRUCTION IN A NUTSHELL—cont'd

Bone Mulch Screw (BMS) tunnel: center guide pin in femoral tunnel using U-guide; ream 7-mm tunnel in soft bone and 8-mm tunnel in hard bone; do not ream medial wall

BMS insertion: expand BMS tunnel 2 mm anterior and posterior; screw BMS two thirds across femoral tunnel; loop suture around BMS with passer; seat BMS in medial wall

Graft passage: remove suture loop passer without twisting; tie posterior suture to graft; pull graft into knee over post

Graft tension: tie sutures attached to each tendon together to form closed loop; put metal rod in suture loop; tension graft and cycle knee

WasherLoc insertion: extend knee; pull on metal rod to equally tension strands of graft; impact WasherLoc toward fibula; insert WasherLoc screw

Postoperative Management:
Brace-free, aggressive; safe return to unrestricted activities at 4 months; no late loss of stability or graft stretch-out

Results:
90% of knees rated normal or nearly normal in terms of function, stability, and overall outcome at 2 years using International Knee Documentation Committee scoring system

Complications:
Rare; avoid difficulty passing graft by correctly performing four steps: (1) sew graft, (2) size graft, (3) center BMS guidewire, (4) expand BMS tunnel

---

A tear of the anterior cruciate ligament (ACL) is devastating to athletes and workers because an unstable knee may prevent them from performing their sports or jobs. Obtaining a careful history, performing the physical examination, and organizing an effective treatment plan can minimize the disability from an ACL tear. This chapter discusses the evaluation and treatment of a patient with a torn ACL.

Case History

A 21-year-old college basketball player presented to the orthopedic clinic 7 days after sustaining a noncontact pivot injury to her left knee. She had been dribbling the basketball and cutting down the lane when she felt her knee buckle and give way. She felt a "pop" and was unable to continue playing. She noted a softball-sized swelling of the knee within hours of the injury. A primary care physician evaluated the injury and instructed her to ice and elevate the knee and to use crutches. The physician referred the patient to an orthopedic surgeon.

The goal of obtaining a history from a patient with an injured knee is to develop an impression of how likely it is that the ACL was torn. To develop this impression, it is important to determine how the injury occurred, what movements or positions reproduce the instability symptoms, and the timing of the injury (i.e., acute or chronic). In this case, the patient described the classic mechanism of a noncontact, change-of-direction, pivot injury associated with a "pop" followed by pain and immediate swelling. The injury was severe enough to halt play. A knee with an acute tear of the ACL typically swells significantly within 12 hours and remains swollen and stiff for several weeks.

Other mechanisms of injury can tear the ACL. Hyperextension can injure the ACL, and this mechanism can also tear the posterior cruciate ligament (PCL).[4,19] A

contact mechanism can disrupt the ACL; this typically involves a force to the lateral knee with a resultant valgus load while the foot is planted. Contact injuries may increase the likelihood of damage to the collateral ligaments, PCL, or extensor mechanism.

Physical Examination

At the initial evaluation, the patient had a moderate effusion and a limited active range of motion of 5 to 95 degrees in the injured left knee. She had passive full extension and passive flexion to 110 degrees. The patient had full active range of motion of the contralateral normal knee. Lachman testing revealed increased translation and a soft endpoint of the left knee compared with the contralateral normal side. KT-1000 arthrometry measurements were not performed, given the patient's pain and a moderate-sized knee effusion. Large effusions have been shown to decrease the reliability of KT testing.[38] Pivot shift testing was attempted but was unreliable, given the patient's discomfort and guarding. The remaining examination revealed no increase in external rotation of the knee at 30 or 90 degrees of flexion, negative posterior drawer testing, and negative varus and valgus laxity. There was no joint line tenderness to suggest a meniscal tear and no retinacular pain to suggest a patellar dislocation. Straight leg raise testing revealed only a very mild extension lag.

When evaluating a patient with a suspected acute rupture of the ACL, it is important to perform a comprehensive knee examination to avoid missing any associated injuries (Table 64–1). It is easy to miss even the ACL injury in the acute setting, because the examination may be limited by the patient's pain, swelling, and guarding. Often, the examination is more revealing several weeks to months later, after the resolution of pain and swelling (Table 64–2).

Table 64–1
Provocative Examination Tests

Examination	Purpose
Lachman, pivot shift tests	ACL injury
Straight leg raise	Extensor mechanism injury
Patella apprehension	Patella instability
Medial retinacular pain	Patella instability
Varus-valgus laxity at 30 degrees	Collateral ligament injury
Tibial external rotation at 30 degrees	Posterolateral corner injury
Tibial external rotation at 90 degrees	PCL injury
Posterior drawer at 90 degrees	PCL injury
Quadriceps active test	PCL injury
Joint line tenderness	Meniscal tear, chondral injury, capsular avulsion
Tibial plateau tenderness	Bone bruise, fracture

ACL, anterior cruciate ligament; PCL, posterior cruciate ligament.

Table 64–2 Examination Findings in Acute versus Chronic Anterior Cruciate Ligament (ACL)–Deficient Knees

Acute ACL Injury	Chronic ACL Injury
Swelling, hemarthrosis	Minimal or no swelling
Painful	Typically painless
Decreased range of motion	Normal to near-normal range of motion
Lachman test—positive	Lachman test—positive
Pivot shift limited by pain	Pivot shift—positive
Consider knee aspiration	Pain—suspect meniscal tear, bone bruise

▎Imaging

Radiographs

Standing anteroposterior, lateral, notch, and sunrise views are required to rule out associated lesions such as fractures, degenerative arthritis, Osgood-Schlatter disease, or patella baja, which may affect the choice of graft material, or a Segond fracture and any other capsular avulsions that may indicate damage to the ACL. Avulsion fractures of the fibular head signify a posterolateral corner injury, and patella alta may suggest a patellar ligament rupture.

Magnetic Resonance Imaging

Surgeons should not rely solely on magnetic resonance imaging (MRI) to diagnose a torn ACL. MRI scans can be misinterpreted, particularly if the slice angle of the study is incorrect. The integrity of the ACL cannot be

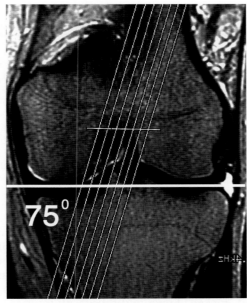

Figure 64–1 Imaging an anterior cruciate ligament (ACL) from origin to insertion requires the correct slice angle and slice thickness. An ACL graft should be imaged with the slice angled at 75 degrees in the coronal plane with respect to the medial joint line, which captures the ACL from origin to insertion on one slice. The slice should be 3 mm thick.

correctly determined unless the image plane is oriented obliquely in the sagittal plane.[11] The coronal angle of the slice should be angled at 75 degrees with the medial tibial joint line, which is the normal orientation of the ACL (Fig. 64–1).[17] The thickness of the slice should be no greater than 3 mm so that at least one slice captures the ACL from origin to insertion. MRI can demonstrate associated pathology, including meniscal tears, collateral ligament injuries, chondral injuries, and bone marrow edema patterns. MRI is not needed for patients who are planning on having ACL reconstruction.

▎Initial Management

Initially, the patient was continued on icing and was instructed to progress to weight bearing as tolerated. She continued range-of-motion exercises to restore her full range of motion and worked on strengthening as well. Once the swelling had diminished and the patient had full range of motion of her injured knee, she underwent operative reconstruction of the torn ACL using her medial hamstring tendons.

The initial management of an ACL injury should consist of counseling the patient about the nature of the injury and the treatment alternatives. The patient must understand the need to regain motion and decrease swelling following the injury, and that rehabilitation of the injured knee requires several weeks. Both nonoperative and operative treatments exist (Table 64–3). Bracing the ACL-deficient knee does not restore anteroposterior laxity to normal, does not decrease internal

Table 64–3
Factors Influencing Treatment Decisions

Nonoperative Treatment	Operative Treatment
Sedentary patient	Athlete, high-demand patient
Arthritis	Repairable meniscus
Willing to alter lifestyle	Unwilling to or cannot alter lifestyle
No symptomatic instability	Symptomatic instability
Willing to accept increased rate of meniscal injury rates	Instability with activities of daily living
	Multiple ligament injuries

rotatory instability, does not restore external rotatory laxity to normal, and does not prevent instability.[18] In patients requiring operative repair, surgery should be deferred until normal knee range of motion has been achieved.[30] However, patients with displaced meniscal tears and "locked" knees and those with injuries to their primary restraints require acute surgical intervention.

Decision-Making Principles

The decisions that need to be made when planning endoscopic reconstruction of the torn ACL include the choice of graft tissue (e.g., autografts or allografts), the technique for positioning the tibial and femoral tunnels, the fixation methods, the use of a postoperative brace, and the use of aggressive rehabilitation. Each of these decisions can affect motion, stability, and the clinical outcome.

The Bone Mulch Screw and WasherLoc technique is effective in patients undergoing reconstruction of ACL-deficient knees using a variety of soft tissue grafts. Our preference is to use an autogenous double-looped semitendinosus gracilis (DLSTG) graft, but this technique is also effective with a single-loop anterior or posterior tibialis allograft. The DLSTG graft is the strongest and stiffest autogenous graft tissue available for ACL reconstruction.[7,9,35] Use of the hamstring tendons avoids the morbidity and complications of patellar tendon graft harvest.[1,2,5,26,28] The strength, stiffness, and slippage of the fixation achieved with a DLSTG graft can be better than that of a bone–patellar tendon–bone graft at implantation, depending on the method of fixation,[15,22,35] so aggressive rehabilitation can be safely performed.[15,16]

The Bone Mulch Screw and WasherLoc devices can be used in skeletally immature patients if care is taken to place the Bone Mulch Screw at least 30 mm into the femoral tunnel and to direct the WasherLoc slightly more posteriorly, to avoid injury to the tibial tubercle physis. Radiographic assessment during hardware placement can also minimize the risk of injury to the physis, which may lead to focal growth arrest and angular deformity. It is a contraindication to place the Bone Mulch Screw and WasherLoc devices (or any other fixation device) into the open physis of the lateral epicondyle and the tibial tubercle of a skeletally immature patient.

Surgical Technique

Fixation Methods

Bone Mulch Screw

The Bone Mulch Screw (Arthrotek, Inc., Warsaw, IN) is an endoscopic femoral fixation method for the DLSTG graft whose structural properties (1126 N, 225 N/mm) in human bone exceed the performance criteria for aggressive rehabilitation.[35] The implant is countersunk within the lateral femoral condyle, and a post is positioned 23 mm inside a 30-mm-long closed-end femoral socket. The entire graft is fixed by pulling both tendons around the post under direct view; in contrast, impaction-type cross-pins spear or capture only a portion of each tendon, which may weaken or cut the graft. Compaction of bone through the hollow body of the Bone Mulch Screw fills the voids between the tendon and the femoral tunnel wall; increases stiffness 41 N/mm; improves the formation of the biologic interface; and produces reciprocal tensile behavior of the anterior and posterior tendon bundles, similar to the increase in load sharing in the anteromedial bundle with flexion and in the posterolateral bundle with extension in the normal ACL.[35,37]

WasherLoc

The WasherLoc (Arthrotek) is a tibial fixation device designed for the DLSTG graft whose structural properties (905 N, 248 N/mm) in human bone exceed the performance criteria for aggressive rehabilitation.[22] The WasherLoc—with 4 peripheral, 11-mm-long spikes and 13 central, 6-mm-long spikes—is compressed into the graft and the bone using a 4.5-mm-diameter cortical or 6-mm-diameter cancellous lag screw. The screw and washer are countersunk inside the distal end of the tibial tunnel to avoid irritation, which is common with other cortical devices placed subcutaneously on the tibia. The slippage of a DLSTG graft under cyclic load is less than that obtained with interference screw fixation of a bone–patellar tendon–bone graft.[21,22] Studies demonstrate that the healing of soft tissue grafts to bone takes longer than bone-to-bone healing does.[27,33,36] Unlike interference screw fixation of soft tissue grafts, the WasherLoc, using cortical bone to secure the graft at the distal end of the tunnel, maintained fixation strength over time, increased complex stiffness, and resulted in excellent biologic bonding properties of the graft to the bone tunnel wall 4 weeks after implantation in an animal model.[33]

Authors' Preferred Surgical Technique

Setup

Position the patient supine on the table, with the lower extremity free and flexed at the knee. Perform an examination under anesthesia. Place a tourniquet around the proximal thigh. Use a padded leg holder to secure the operative extremity. Place the well leg in a leg holder in a comfortable position, and pad all bony prominences. We prefer to use a tourniquet because it provides a bloodless field for improved visualization and ease of tendon harvest. Prepare and drape the extremity in the usual fashion.

Tendon Harvest

We begin with the tendon harvest because, in most cases, we are certain of the existence of an ACL injury based on the history, clinical examination, and intraoperative evaluation. Harvesting the tendon first prevents suturing of the tendon, which can occur if a repair of the medial meniscus is required. Center a 3- to 4-cm vertical or transverse incision approximately three finger-breadths distal to the medial joint line on the antero-medial crest. The transverse incision minimizes injury and numbness to the saphenous nerve. The vertical incision is used if the patient has a large leg. Place the vertical incision slightly posterior to allow for identification of any posteroinferior fascial slips on the hamstring tendons. Expose the sartorius fascia. Palpate the gracilis tendon and split the sartorius fascia along the inferior border of the gracilis tendon. Flex the knee and pass the index finger posteromedially. With the tip of the finger pointed toward the medial soft tissue, flex the index finger toward the tibia to loop the gracilis tendon. Isolate the tendon with a Penrose drain. Cut any fascial slips to the sartorius or medial gastrocnemius. Free the gracilis tendon and then locate the semitendinosus deep and inferior to the gracilis. Isolate the tendon with a Penrose drain, and release the fascial slips. Up to five fascial slips to the medial gastrocnemius or sartorius fascia can exist. Strip the freed tendons using an open-ended tendon stripper, leaving the tendons attached distally on the tibia (Fig. 64–2). Alternatively, release the grafts from the tibia and remove them from the patient for preparation by an assistant.

Graft Preparation

Remove the muscle at the proximal portion of each tendon by stripping it off the tendinous portion with curved Mayo scissors or a periosteal elevator. Using number 1 Vicryl, whipstitch 36-inch sutures of different colors in the ends of each tendon. The different-colored sutures allow for intra-articular identification of each tendon during passage over the post of the Bone Mulch Screw. The whipstitch is a running stitch encircling approximately four fifths of the tendon diameter for 1 to 2 cm proximally, beginning at the end of the tendon (Fig. 64–3). Once this distance is reached, reverse direction, moving distally along the tendon but continuing to encircle the tendon in the same direction. Once the end of the tendon is reached, remove the needle, and tension the sutures to ensure a "Chinese finger trap" effect—that is, tapering of the end of the tendon with increasing tension on the sutures. After the tendons have been prepared, double-loop the tendons over Mersiline tape to form the graft. Size the graft by passing sizing sleeves of

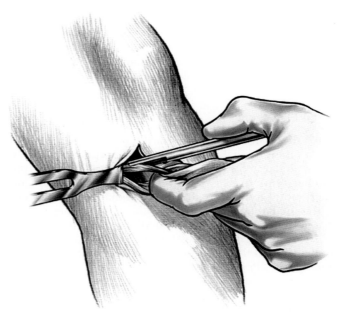

Figure 64–2 The tendon is removed by placing an open-ended tendon stripper around it and pushing (not rotating) the stripper proximally while applying countertraction on the tendon using a finger.

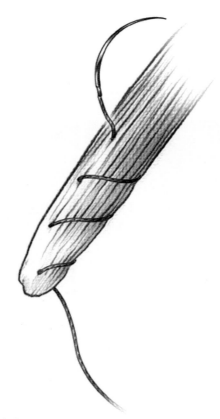

Figure 64–3 Using a running whipstitch, 4 cm of the end of each tendon is sutured. The whipstitch is performed by encircling four fifths of the body of the tendon with each throw of the suture.

6 Knee

varying diameters over the graft and noting the smallest-diameter sleeve that passes freely over the prepared graft to determine the diameter of the tibial and femoral tunnels. If the tendons were left attached to the tibia, coil them around two fingers and store them deep to the sartorius fascia.

Portal Placement

Once the graft has been prepared, establish the portals. Use a superomedial portal for outflow, and place a lateral transpatellar tendon portal in the lateral third of the patellar tendon. This portal allows for visualization up the femoral tunnel. Establish the medial portal adjacent to the medial border of the patellar tendon (Fig. 64–4). It is important to place the medial portal immediately adjacent to the medial border of the tendon to prevent a tibial tunnel that is too medial when using the Howell tibial guide. Perform a full diagnostic arthroscopy and meniscal stabilization before reconstruction, if necessary.

Tibial Tunnel Placement

The tibial tunnel is the key to the transtibial endoscopic ACL reconstruction technique, because the femoral tunnel is drilled through the tibial tunnel. The transtibial endoscopic technique requires distinct guidelines for drilling the tibial tunnel, not only to prevent intercondylar roof and PCL impingement but also because free placement of the femoral tunnel is not possible when the femoral tunnel is drilled through the tibial tunnel.[13] Positioning the tibial tunnel anatomically in both planes ensures that the femoral tunnel is placed in the correct location using a transtibial tunnel femoral aimer.[13,17] In flexion, the graft tension is normal when the femoral tunnel is drilled through a 60-degree tibial

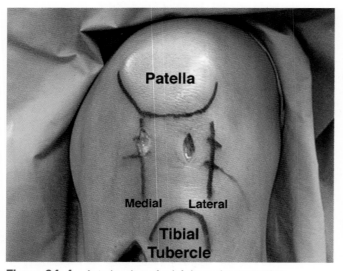

Figure 64–4 Anterior view of a left knee demonstrating landmarks for placing the medial portal and the transpatellar tendon portal. Both portals begin 1 cm distal to the inferior pole of the patella. The medial portal grazes the medial edge of the patellar tendon. The transpatellar tendon portal is made two thirds the width of the patellar tendon lateral to the tendon's medial edge.

tunnel in the coronal plane. The graft tension increases abnormally when the femoral tunnel is drilled through a 70- or 80-degree tibial tunnel because the graft impinges on or tightens around the posterior cruciate ligament in flexion.[32] A knee loses flexion and has more anterior laxity with a graft in a 75-degree or greater tibial tunnel.[14]

Once the stump of the native ACL is removed, place the 65-degree Howell guide (Arthrotek) in the medial portal, and place the tip into the intercondylar notch. If necessary, use an angled osteotome to perform a wallplasty (i.e., remove bone from the medial wall of the lateral femoral condyle) until the tip of the guide passes freely between the posterior cruciate ligament and the lateral femoral condyle. Extend the knee fully and place the heel on a Mayo stand. With the heel of the palm putting gentle downward pressure on the anterior patella while lifting the tibial guide anteriorly with the same hand, the guide will come to rest along the intercondylar roof and customize the sagittal plane angle of the tibial tunnel based on the patient's intercondylar roof angle.[10] The intercondylar roof is the key landmark for judging the position of the tibial guidewire to prevent roof impingement; in addition, the intercondylar roof determines the sagittal position of the native ACL, because the native ligament lies against the intercondylar roof in the extended knee.[12,34] Place the alignment rod through the most proximal alignment hole in the 65-degree Howell guide when viewing the guide from the lateral side. Rotate the guide in the coronal plane until the alignment rod is parallel to the joint line and perpendicular to the long axis of the tibia. Positioning the alignment rod in this orientation places the tibial guidewire at 65 degrees with respect to the medial joint line of the tibia and minimizes impingement of the graft on the PCL (Fig. 64–5).[14,32] Once the rod is positioned, drill a guide pin into the tibia with the knee in full extension. Use of the 65-degree Howell guide with the coronal alignment guide consistently positions the graft anatomically, without roof or PCL impingement, eliminating the need for an intraoperative radiograph.[14]

Tap the guide pin into the joint and assess its position arthroscopically. Proper placement is indicated when the tibial pin bisects the tibial spines, enters the notch lateral to the PCL, and forms a triangle between the pin and the superior border of the PCL (Fig. 64–6). Drill the tibial tunnel using the appropriate-diameter drill bit, based on graft sizing. Extend the knee and pass an impingement rod that matches the diameter of the tibial tunnel into the intercondylar notch. If insertion is blocked, perform a roofplasty (i.e., remove bone from the intercondylar roof). Free passage of the rod into the notch with the knee in maximum extension confirms that the graft is positioned without roof impingement.

Femoral Tunnel Placement

The key step in placing the femoral aimer is removing the ACL origin from the over-the-top position on the femur; this is done with a 70-degree angled curet. Removal of the ACL origin allows the tip of the femoral aimer to rest directly on bone, which prevents blowout

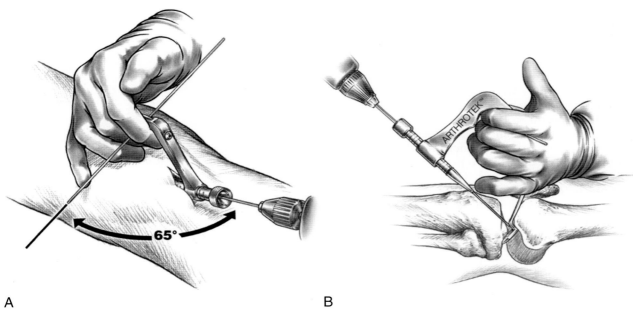

A   B

Figure 64–5 Proper positioning of the 65-degree Howell tibial guide in the coronal plane *(A)* and sagittal plane *(B)*. In the coronal plane, the guide is rotated so that the alignment rod forms a 65-degree angle with respect to the medial joint line of the tibia, which avoids impingement of the posterior cruciate ligament. In the sagittal plane, the guide is inserted into the notch, and the knee is maximally extended. Lifting the guide places the guide pin 4 to 5 mm posterior and parallel to the intercondylar roof, which avoids roof impingement.

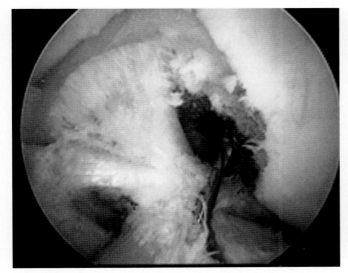

Figure 64–6 Arthroscopic view of a left knee showing the guide pin placed lateral to the proximal two thirds of the posterior cruciate ligament and crossing the notch at a 65-degree angle with respect to the medial joint line of the tibia.

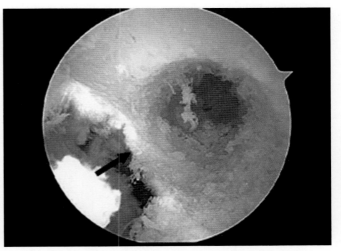

Figure 64–7 Arthroscopic view of a left knee showing the 1-mm-thick posterior wall of the femoral tunnel *(arrow)*.

of the posterior wall of the femoral tunnel. Place the femoral aimer (Arthrotek), which is selected based on the diameter of the tunnel, through the tibial tunnel, and lock it in the over-the-top position. Rotate the femoral aimer laterally, minimizing impingement of the graft against the PCL during knee flexion. The femoral aimer allows for preparation of a femoral tunnel with a

1-mm-thick posterior wall (Fig. 64–7). Flex the knee until the femoral aimer locks itself into place and drill a guidewire into the femur to the far cortex. Using the same-diameter acorn reamer as for the tibial tunnel, drill the femoral tunnel over the guidewire to a depth of 30 mm. Once the femoral tunnel has been drilled, remove the drill and guide pin. This endoscopic technique for placing the femoral tunnel produces an in vivo tension pattern in the DLSTG graft similar to that of the intact ACL, provided the tibial tunnel is properly placed in the sagittal and coronal planes.[17,32,37]

6 Knee

Preparation of the Tibia for the WasherLoc

Remove a thumbnail-sized area of soft tissue surrounding the distal end of the tibial tunnel entrance. Place the counterbore guide in the tibial tunnel and advance it as far proximally as possible. Aim the guide toward the fibular head so that the WasherLoc screw exits the tibia anterior to the posterior cortex and avoids injury to the neurovascular structures. Insert the awl into the guide and the posterolateral wall of the tibial tunnel (Fig. 64–8). Seat the counterbore reamer into the pilot hole created by the awl, taking care to position the reamer in the same direction as the awl. Gently ream until the counterbore is flush with the wall of the tibial tunnel (Fig. 64–9). Save the bone from the flutes of the reamer for bone mulch.

Placement of the Tunnel for the Bone Mulch Screw

Pass the U-shaped guide through the tibial tunnel, across the joint, and seat it completely into the femoral tunnel. Make a small stab incision anterior to the lateral epicondyle and posterior to the lateral border of the patella. Dissect the soft tissues down to bone. Seat the bullet-tip guide on the bone, and measure the length of the Bone Mulch Screw using the markings on the guide. If the length of the screw is between etched markings, select the smaller screw. Drill a guide pin across the lateral condyle until it strikes the U-shaped guide. Remove the guide and tap the guide pin across the femoral tunnel into its medial wall. Advance an 8-mm-diameter cannulated drill over the guidewire until it enters the femoral

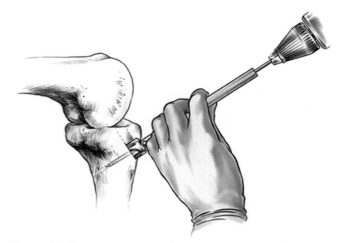

Figure 64–9 A counterbore is created in the distal end of the tibial tunnel to recess the WasherLoc inside the tibia, which avoids symptoms from prominent hardware. The counterbore is created by inserting the reamer in the pilot hole made by the awl, directing the tip of the reamer toward the fibula, and orienting the flat cutting surface of the reamer parallel to the wall of the tibial tunnel. The counterbore is complete when the reamer is flush with the wall of the tibial tunnel.

tunnel. Advance the drill while simultaneously viewing the femoral tunnel using a 30-degree arthroscope placed in the transpatellar lateral portal. Take care not to advance the drill into the medial wall. Remove the drill, and save the bone from the flutes for later use as bone mulch. Use the router or ring curet to remove an additional 1 to 2 mm of bone from the anterior and posterior tunnel walls. Screw the appropriate-size Bone Mulch Screw under arthroscopic guidance until the tip of the screw has crossed the center of the tunnel. Insert a suture loop passer through the tibial tunnel and into the femoral tunnel, and loop the suture around the post of the Bone Mulch Screw (Fig. 64–10). Advance the post of the Bone Mulch Screw until the step-off of the post is buried in the medial wall to ensure that the screw is countersunk in the lateral femoral condyle to avoid hardware symptoms. Withdraw the suture loop passer without rotating to avoid twisting the suture.

Graft Passage and Fixation

Tie the posterior limb of the suture to the graft sutures. Pass the graft in a posterior to anterior direction over the post of the Bone Mulch Screw (Fig. 64–11). Pull the graft over the post until all strands of the graft are taut. Place tension on the graft, and cycle the knee 20 to 30 times. When the knee is flexed from 0 to 30 degrees, the graft may exit the tibial tunnel 1 to 2 mm and then remain isometric during the remainder of flexion.[23] After cycling the knee, position the knee in full extension on a Mayo stand. Tie the graft sutures together. Instruct an assistant to put traction on the graft using an impingement rod to equally tension all four strands (Fig. 64–12). Select an 18-mm WasherLoc for a graft 9 mm or greater in diameter, and use a 16-mm WasherLoc for a graft 8 mm or smaller in diameter. Assemble the WasherLoc washer on

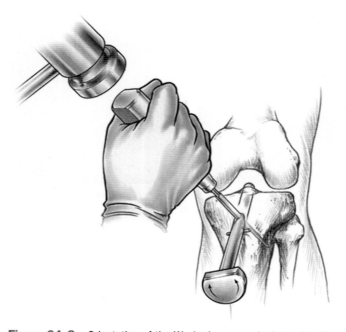

Figure 64–8 Orientation of the WasherLoc screw is determined by creating a pilot hole in the tibia with an awl. The awl is inserted into the counterbore guide, and the tip is rotated toward the fibula. Creating the pilot hole while aiming at the head of the fibula prevents the WasherLoc screw from penetrating the posterior cortex of the tibia and damaging the neurovascular structures.

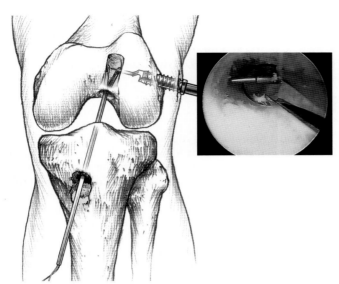

Figure 64–10 A monofilament suture is threaded through the fork and down the stem of the suture loop passer. The suture loop passer is inserted through the tibial tunnel and into the femoral tunnel. The fork is rotated so that the suture is looped over the tip of the Bone Mulch Screw *(inset)*. The Bone Mulch Screw is screwed into the medial wall of the femoral tunnel, which prevents the suture loop from slipping off the tip.

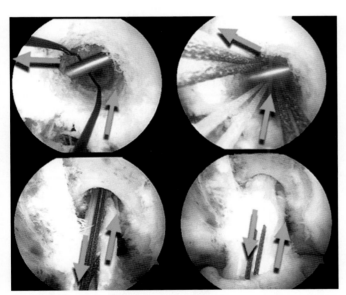

Figure 64–11 Arthroscopic view of the passage of sutures and tendons over the post of the Bone Mulch Screw inside the femoral tunnel. The suture loop *(upper left)* pulls the sutures attached to each tendon from posterior to anterior *(arrows)* around the post of the Bone Mulch Screw *(upper right)*. Pulling the blue suture passes the semitendinosus tendon, and pulling the white suture passes the gracilis tendon *(lower left and right)*.

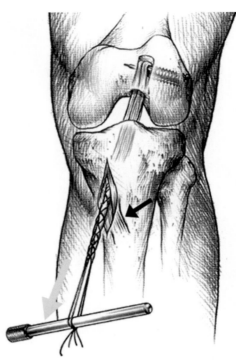

Figure 64–12 Pulling on an impingement rod *(yellow arrow)* inserted through a closed loop places equal tension on the four strands of the double-looped semitendinosus gracilis graft. The closed loop is formed by leaving the semitendinosus and gracilis tendons attached to the tibia *(black arrow)*, looping the tendons over the Bone Mulch Screw inside the femoral tunnel, and tying together the sutures attached to the two tendons distal to the tibial tunnel.

washer into the graft and the tibia using a mallet. Remove the awl, place a 3.2-mm drill through the drill guide, and drill a hole through the far cortex. Remove the drill and drill guide, and determine the screw length using the depth gauge.

Screw in the appropriate-length 6-mm cancellous screw (Fig. 64–13). At this time, perform a Lachman test to determine stability. Compact bone mulch through the Bone Mulch Screw using the sleeve that seats into the head of the screw, an impaction rod, and a mallet to fill any voids in the femoral tunnel. Continue to add bone until the desired knee stability is obtained. Impact additional bone graft into the tibial tunnel if desired, and remove the excess tendons. Close the wounds in layers. Obtain anteroposterior and lateral radiographs of the knee in full extension in the recovery room to confirm satisfactory placement of the tibial and femoral tunnels and hardware (Fig. 64–14).

Postoperative Management

Postoperatively, the patient begins a brace-free, aggressive rehabilitation program. This protocol is safe to use with this reconstruction technique,[16] but aggressive rehabilitation should be used only with fixation methods that provide high strength and stiffness.[15] Multiple studies have shown that there are no detectable benefits to

the drill guide and the awl. Place the tip of the awl in the previous pilot hole in the tibial tunnel, aiming toward the fibula, and position all four bundles of the graft inside the four large washer spikes. With tension maintained on the graft and the knee in full extension, impact the

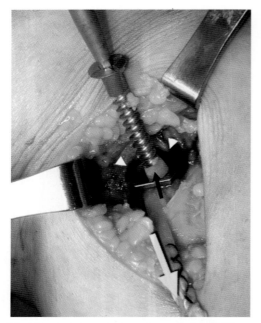

Figure 64–13   Technique for inserting cancellous screw between the four strands of the double-looped semitendinosus gracilis graft to compress the WasherLoc at the distal end of the tibial tunnel. Bone wax *(black arrow)* is applied over the first three threads of the cancellous screw, which prevents the threads from damaging the tendons. Tension is applied to the tendons *(yellow arrow)*, and the screw is inserted.

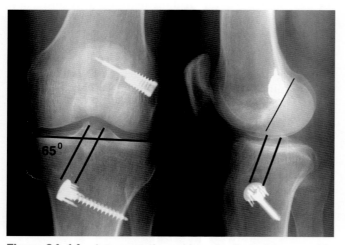

Figure 64–14   Anteroposterior and lateral radiographs are used to check the placement of the tibial tunnel and hardware. In the anteroposterior view *(left)*, the tibial tunnel should enter the notch between the tibial spines and at a 65-degree angle with respect to the medial joint line, the Bone Mulch Screw should be countersunk under the lateral femoral cortex, and the WasherLoc screw should course toward the fibula and penetrate the lateral cortex of the tibia. In the lateral view *(right)*, the tibial tunnel should be posterior and parallel to the intercondylar roof, the Bone Mulch Screw should not exit the posterior femoral cortex, and the WasherLoc screw should not exit the posterior cortex of the tibia.

postoperative bracing.[6,8,20,24] Patients with DLSTG grafts using high-strength and high-stiffness fixation can safely return to sports at 4 months, with no deterioration in stability 2 years after the reconstruction[13,16,29] (Table 64–4).

Results

The importance of using high-strength and high-stiffness fixation devices, such as the Bone Mulch Screw and WasherLoc combination with hamstring grafts, is supported by clinical studies. These types of devices stabilized nearly all knees, whereas low-strength, low-stiffness fixation methods stabilized a smaller percentage of knees. For example, the incidence of a stable knee was best (91%) with the Bone Mulch Screw and either tandem staples[13] or the WasherLoc,[14] somewhat less (70%) with the Endobutton and suture bridge,[31] 55% with the Endobutton and bone staples,[25] and worst (35%) with interference screw fixation (Fig. 64–15).[3]

Table 64–4

Postoperative Rehabilitation

Time	Activity
0-2 wk	WBAT, no brace, crutches, AROM, PROM exercises
2-8 wk	Stationary bike, continue SAQs, hamstring curls, leg press
8-12 wk	Jogging, open/closed chain exercises with light weights
12-16 wk	Continue weights, add agility exercises
>16 wk	Return to sport if SLH > 85% of normal leg

AROM, active range of motion; PROM, passive range of motion; SAQs, short arc quad sets; SLH, single-legged hop; WBAT, weight bearing as tolerated.

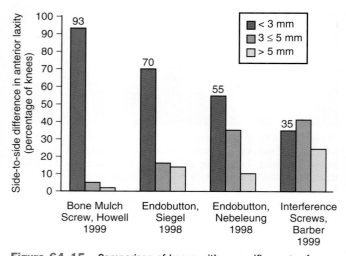

Figure 64–15   Comparison of knees with a specific range of stability for different fixation methods. Stability was measured as the side-to-side difference between the reconstructed and normal knees using an arthrometer. Knees with a less than 3-mm side-to-side difference had the best stability. Knees reconstructed with the Bone Mulch Screw were most stable.

The most likely explanation for this variability in stability is the difference in structural properties (i.e., strength, stiffness, slippage) among fixation methods.[15]

Complications

The most common but easily avoided complication of the Bone Mulch Screw–WasherLoc technique is the inability to pass the graft over the post of the screw. This problem can arise as a result of incorrect suturing of the tendons, undersizing of the tunnels, not centering the post of the Bone Mulch Screw in the femoral tunnel, and not expanding the femoral tunnel. The tendon must be tapered to a point, and tension on the whipstitch should also taper the tendon. The post of the Bone Mulch Screw should be centered in the femoral tunnel as precisely as possible, and the double-looped graft should pass freely through the desired sizing sleeve.

Last, it is important to direct the WasherLoc toward the fibular head to minimize the risk of injury to the popliteal vessels. Injury to the popliteal vessels is prevented when the WasherLoc screw exits the lateral cortex (see Fig. 64–14).

Summary

The disability caused by a torn ACL can be minimized for active athletes and workers by careful evaluation and treatment of the injury. The history and physical examination remain the mainstays of the diagnostic evaluation. Imaging can identify associated pathology such as meniscal tears, ligament injuries, and bone bruises; however, it is not required to make the diagnosis of ACL injury. Nonoperative treatment plays only a limited role in active patients with ACL injuries; surgical reconstruction is the treatment of choice. When possible, knee range of motion should be restored before reconstructing the ACL. The key to a successful ACL reconstruction is proper placement of the tibial and femoral tunnels. The use of hamstring tendons secured with the Bone Mulch Screw and WasherLoc provides a fixation construct with biomechanical properties superior to those of interference screw fixation using both hamstring and patellar tendon bone grafts. This unique reconstruction technique allows the safe use of a brace-free, aggressive rehabilitation protocol, affording the patient the opportunity for an early return to work or sports. Careful attention to the details of the surgical technique will provide a more consistent and satisfying outcome for patients with torn ACLs.

References

1. Aglietti P, Buzzi R, D'Andria S, Zaccherotti G: Arthroscopic anterior cruciate ligament reconstruction with patellar tendon. Arthroscopy 8:510-516, 1992.
2. Aglietti P, Buzzi R, D'Andria S, Zaccherotti G: Long-term study of anterior cruciate ligament reconstruction for chronic instability using the central one-third patellar tendon and a lateral extraarticular tenodesis. Am J Sports Med 20:38-45, 1992.
3. Barber FA: Tripled semitendinosus-cancellous bone anterior cruciate ligament reconstruction with bioscrew fixation. Arthroscopy 15:360-367, 1999.
4. Emerson RJ: Basketball knee injuries and the anterior cruciate ligament. Clin Sports Med 12:317-328, 1993.
5. Engebretsen L, Benum P, Fasting O, et al: A prospective, randomized study of three surgical techniques for treatment of acute ruptures of the anterior cruciate ligament. Am J Sports Med 18:585-590, 1990.
6. Feller J, Bartlett J, Chapman S, Delahunt M: Use of an extension-assisting brace following anterior cruciate ligament reconstruction. Knee Surg Sports Traumatol Arthrosc 5:6-9, 1997.
7. Hamner DL, Brown CH Jr, Steiner ME, et al: Hamstring tendon grafts for reconstruction of the anterior cruciate ligament: Biomechanical evaluation of the use of multiple strands and tensioning techniques. J Bone Joint Surg Am 81:549-557, 1999.
8. Harilainen A, Sandelin J, Vanhanen I, Kivinen A: Knee brace after bone-tendon-bone anterior cruciate ligament reconstruction: Randomized, prospective study with 2-year follow-up. Knee Surg Sports Traumatol Arthrosc 5:10-13, 1997.
9. Haut RC, Lancaster RL, DeCamp CE: Mechanical properties of the canine patellar tendon: Some correlations with age and the content of collagen. J Biomech 25:163-173, 1992.
10. Howell SM, Barad SJ: Knee extension and its relationship to the slope of the intercondylar roof: Implications for positioning the tibial tunnel in anterior cruciate ligament reconstructions. Am J Sports Med 23:288-294, 1995.
11. Howell SM, Berns GS, Farley TE: Unimpinged and impinged anterior cruciate ligament grafts: MR signal intensity measurements. Radiology 179:639-643, 1991.
12. Howell SM, Clark JA, Farley TE: A rationale for predicting anterior cruciate graft impingement by the intercondylar roof: A magnetic resonance imaging study. Am J Sports Med 19:276-282, 1991.
13. Howell SM, Deutsch ML: Comparison of endoscopic and two-incision techniques for reconstructing a torn anterior cruciate ligament using hamstring tendons. Arthroscopy 15:594-606, 1999.
14. Howell SM, Gittins ME, Gottlieb JE, et al: The relationship between the angle of the tibial tunnel in the coronal plane and loss of flexion and anterior laxity after anterior cruciate ligament reconstruction. Am J Sports Med 29:567-574, 2001.
15. Howell SM, Hull ML: Aggressive rehabilitation using hamstring tendons: Graft construct, tibial tunnel placement, fixation properties, and clinical outcome. Am J Knee Surg 11:120-127, 1998.
16. Howell SM, Taylor MA: Brace-free rehabilitation, with early return to activity, for knees reconstructed with a double-looped semitendinosus and gracilis graft. J Bone Joint Surg Am 78:814-825, 1996.
17. Howell SM, Wallace MP, Hull ML, Deutsch ML: Evaluation of the single-incision arthroscopic technique for anterior cruciate ligament replacement: A study of tibial tunnel placement, intraoperative graft tension, and stability. Am J Sports Med 27:284-293, 1999.
18. Jonsson H, Karrholm J: Brace effects on the unstable knee in 21 cases: A roentgen stereophotogrammetric comparison of three designs. Acta Orthop Scand 61:313-318, 1990.

6 Knee

19. Kannus P, Bergfeld J, Jarvinen M, et al: Injuries to the posterior cruciate ligament of the knee. Sports Med 12:110-131, 1991.

20. Kartus J, Stener S, Kohler K, et al: Is bracing after anterior cruciate ligament reconstruction necessary? A 2-year follow-up of 78 consecutive patients rehabilitated with or without a brace. Knee Surg Sports Traumatol Arthrosc 5:157-161, 1997.

21. Liu SH, Kabo JM, Osti L: Biomechanics of two types of bone-tendon-bone graft for ACL reconstruction. J Bone Joint Surg Br 77:232-235, 1995.

22. Magen HE, Howell SM, Hull ML: Structural properties of six tibial fixation methods for anterior cruciate ligament soft tissue grafts. Am J Sports Med 27:35-43, 1999.

23. Markolf KL, Burchfield DM, Shapiro MM, et al: Biomechanical consequences of replacement of the anterior cruciate ligament with a patellar ligament allograft. Part I. Insertion of the graft and anterior-posterior testing. J Bone Joint Surg Am 78:1720-1727, 1996.

24. Muellner T, Alacamlioglu Y, Nikolic A, Schabus R: No benefit of bracing on the early outcome after anterior cruciate ligament reconstruction. Knee Surg Sports Traumatol Arthrosc 6:88-92, 1998.

25. Nebelung W, Becker R, Merkel M, Ropke M: Bone tunnel enlargement after anterior cruciate ligament reconstruction with semitendinosus tendon using Endobutton fixation on the femoral side. Arthroscopy 14:810-815, 1998.

26. O'Brien SJ, Warren RF, Pavlov H, et al: Reconstruction of the chronically insufficient anterior cruciate ligament with the central third of the patellar ligament. J Bone Joint Surg Am 73:278-286, 1991.

27. Papageorgiou CD, Ma CB, Abramowitch SD, et al: A multidisciplinary study of the healing of an intraarticular anterior cruciate ligament graft in a goat model. Am J Sports Med 29:620-626, 2001.

28. Paulos LE, Wnorowski DC, Greenwald AE: Infrapatellar contracture syndrome: Diagnosis, treatment, and long-term followup. Am J Sports Med 22:440-449, 1994.

29. Shelbourne KD, Klootwyk TE, Wilckens JH, De Carlo MS: Ligament stability two to six years after anterior cruciate ligament reconstruction with autogenous patellar tendon graft and participation in accelerated rehabilitation program. Am J Sports Med 23:575-579, 1995.

30. Shelbourne KD, Patel DV: Timing of surgery in anterior cruciate ligament–injured knees. Knee Surg Sports Traumatol Arthrosc 3:148-156, 1995.

31. Siegel MG, Barber-Westin SD: Arthroscopic-assisted outpatient anterior cruciate ligament reconstruction using the semitendinosus and gracilis tendons. Arthroscopy 14:268-277, 1998.

32. Simmons R, Howell SM, Hull ML: Effect of the angle of the temporal and tibial tunnels in the coronal plane and incremental excision of the posterior cruciate ligament on tension of an anterior cruciate ligament graft: an in vitro study. J Bone Joint Surg Am 85:1018-1029, 2003.

33. Singhatat W, Lawhorn K, Howell S, Hull M: How four weeks of implantation affect the strength and stiffness of a tendon graft in a bone tunnel: A study of two fixation devices in an extraarticular model in ovine. Am J Sports Med 30:506-513, 2002.

34. Staubli HU, Rauschning W: Tibial attachment area of the anterior cruciate ligament in the extended knee position: Anatomy and cryosections in vitro complemented by magnetic resonance arthrography in vivo. Knee Surg Sports Traumatol Arthrosc 2:138-146, 1994.

35. To JT, Howell SM, Hull ML: Contributions of femoral fixation methods to the stiffness of anterior cruciate ligament replacements at implantation. Arthroscopy 15:379-387, 1999.

36. Tomita F, Yasuda K, Mikami S, et al: Comparisons of intraosseous graft healing between the doubled flexor tendon graft and the bone–patellar tendon–bone graft in anterior cruciate ligament reconstruction. Arthroscopy 17:461-476, 2001.

37. Wallace MP, Howell SM, Hull ML: In vivo tensile behavior of a four-bundle hamstring graft as a replacement for the anterior cruciate ligament. J Orthop Res 15:539-545, 1997.

38. Wright RW, Luhmann SJ: The effect of knee effusions on KT-1000 arthrometry: A cadaver study. Am J Sports Med 26:571-574, 1998.

Central Quadriceps Free Tendon for ACL Reconstruction

STEPHAN V. YACOUBIAN AND JOHN P. FULKERSON

CENTRAL QUADRICEPS FREE TENDON FOR ACL RECONSTRUCTION IN A NUTSHELL

History:
Traumatic episode ± "pop"; swelling, instability

Physical Examination:
Positive Lachman, pivot shift tests; hemarthrosis; rule out associated injuries

Imaging:
Radiograph: rule out associated fractures
Magnetic resonance imaging: augment physical findings

Surgical Technique:
Examination under anesthesia: range of motion, Lachman test, pivot shift
Positioning: supine; leg holder; tourniquet on proximal thigh
Diagnostic arthroscopy: assess chondral surfaces; address associated injuries
Graft harvest and preparation: incision superior to patella, midline, 3 to 5 cm; graft 10 mm wide, 8 mm deep; graft 7 to 8 cm long, whipstitches (#5 suture) each end; Endobutton knot (four strands of #5 suture) tied near graft; set for 2-cm graft in tunnel
Notchplasty: minimal notchplasty; 5.5-mm full-radius resector; identify over-the-top position
Tibial tunnel: set guide to 55 to 60 degrees; 7- to 9-mm tunnel size; use dilator as needed
Femoral tunnel: 6- to 7-mm anterior to posterior notch; 10:30 o'clock–1:30 o'clock position; use Endobutton technique
Graft passage: use #5 Ethibond on Endobutton to pull graft through femur; use #2 Ethibond to flip Endobutton
Graft fixation: place bioabsorbable screw 1 mm larger than tibial tunnel (9-mm screw, 8-mm tunnel) with knee at 10 degrees of flexion
Closure: 2-0 Vicryl for subcutaneous layers; running Prolene for subcuticular layer; Steri-Strips

Postoperative Management:
Pain control, Cryo-Cuff, range-of-motion exercises (full extension); weight bearing as tolerated in splint, crutches 7 to 10 days, then progress

Results:
84% of cases 0 to 3 mm KT-1000 at 1 year; very low morbidity, minimal pain

Case History

A healthy 19-year-old woman presents 4 weeks after a twisting injury to her left knee while playing soccer. She felt a pop during the injury and experienced immediate swelling. The swelling subsided in several days, but she began to experience giving-way episodes during her activities of daily living.

Physical Examination

The patient has full range of motion, mild effusion, a 3+ Lachman test, and a positive pivot shift.

Imaging

Anteroposterior and lateral radiographs of the left knee are unremarkable. Magnetic resonance imaging demonstrates a complete anterior cruciate ligament (ACL) tear. The meniscus signal is normal.

Indications

This young athlete has aspirations of playing soccer at the intercollegiate level. Because she has episodes of instability and a very demanding lifestyle, a central quadriceps free tendon graft is indicated.

Surgical Technique

Positioning

The patient is placed in the supine position with the left knee in an arthroscopic leg holder (Fig. 65–1). A tourni-

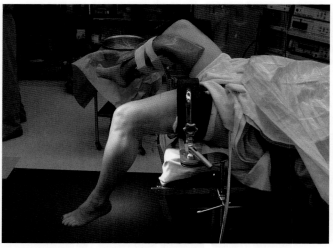

Figure 65–1 The arthroscopic leg holder and tourniquet are placed very proximally on the thigh. The contralateral knee rests in a stirrup.

quet cuff is also placed on the proximal thigh. The contralateral leg is placed on a well-padded stirrup. The foot of the table is lowered all the way, with the knee resting in flexion. This position allows the knee to be flexed up to 120 degrees, which aids in tunnel placement.

Examination under Anesthesia

Examination of the left knee reveals full range of motion, a 3+ Lachman test, and a positive pivot shift.

Diagnostic Arthroscopy

After proper prepping and draping of the extremity, a standard anterolateral arthroscopy portal is made using a number 11 blade. The arthroscope is introduced through this portal. The suprapatellar pouch is inspected first. Then the patellofemoral articulation is visualized, and any abnormality in the chondral surface or tracking is noted. The medial gutter is then visualized, followed by the medial compartment. At this point, a second arthroscopy portal is made using a spinal needle and then a blade. A probe is introduced, and the meniscus and chondral surface are probed. The notch is entered, and the ACL tear is confirmed. Next, the lateral compartment is entered, and the meniscus and chondral surfaces are inspected using a probe. Finally, the lateral gutter is visualized; any meniscal debridement or repair is done at this time.

If there is an assistant available, the ACL debridement and notchplasty can be accomplished simultaneously with graft harvest.[1,3]

Specific Surgical Steps

Graft Harvest and Preparation

We recommend a graft that is 10 to 11 mm wide by 7 to 9 mm deep by 7 to 8 cm long. The center of the quadriceps tendon is 9 mm thick on average.[2] The depth of the graft can be either full thickness (about 9 mm) or partial thickness (about 7 mm). We prefer a partial-thickness quadriceps tendon graft, as this preserves joint integrity and avoids leakage of fluid. If the suprapatellar pouch is entered during graft harvest and fluid leaks out, it should be closed to avoid loss of pressure during arthroscopy.

After the tourniquet is inflated to 250 mm Hg, a 3- to 5-cm incision is made just above the patella in the midline (Fig. 65–2). The subcutaneous tissues are carefully dissected until the tendon is visible. A self-retaining retractor is placed to expose the tendon. Two parallel cuts are made in the tendon about 10 mm apart, centered 1 to 2 mm medial to the midline of the quadriceps tendon (Fig. 65–3). These cuts are carried proximally to the point where the vastus lateralis and vastus medialis meet at the apex of the tendon insertion into the patella, and the attachment is dissected off the patella with a number 15 blade. After the cuts are made to their desired depth (at least 7 mm, the depth of a number 10 scalpel), a hemostat is placed underneath the graft about 2 cm

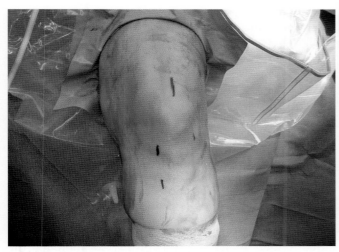

Figure 65–2   The knee is marked to orient the graft harvest site. A 3- to 5-cm incision superior to the midline of the patella is used.

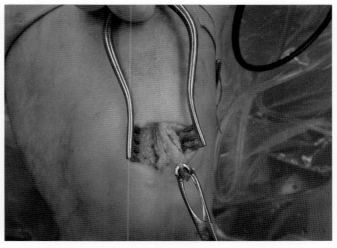

Figure 65–4   A grasping clamp facilitates proximal dissection of the graft.

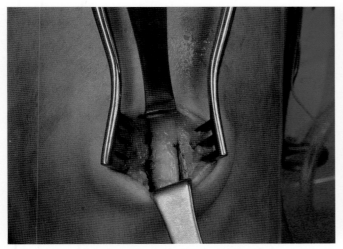

Figure 65–3   The quadriceps tendon is marked with two lines 10 mm apart. The graft is centered 1 to 2 mm medial to the midline of the quadriceps tendon.

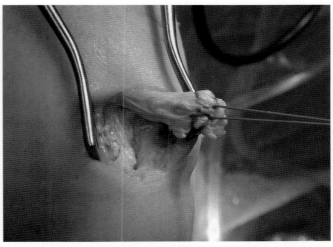

Figure 65–5   Whipstitches are placed in the distal end of the tendon, and the grasping clamp is removed.

above the patella and spread to define the back of the tendon graft. The hemostat can also be pulled proximally and distally underneath the patella to separate the graft from the remaining tendon. Careful sharp dissection then releases the tendon graft from the patella distally. Careful dissection also avoids damage to the adjacent tendon. A grasping clamp is placed on the end of the tendon (Fig. 65–4). Nonabsorbable suture (number 5 Ethibond) is used to place braided whipstitches in the distal end of the tendon (Fig. 65–5). The clamp is removed, and the tendon is lifted up using the number 5 sutures; combined gentle blunt and sharp dissection is used underneath the tendon to free it proximally. A ruler is used to mark 75 to 80 mm from the end of the tendon (Fig. 65–6). The sutures can be used to pull the tendon distally and expose the proximal attachment, where Mayo scissors are used to cut the tendon free (Fig. 65–7).

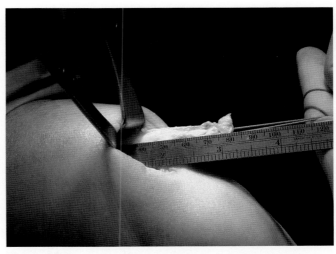

Figure 65–6   A ruler is used to determine whether adequate proximal dissection has been accomplished. A 75- to 80-mm-long tendon graft is harvested.

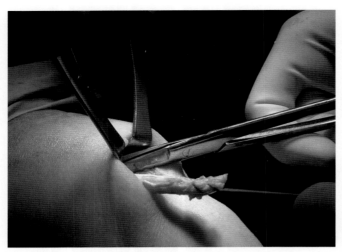

Figure 65–7 The sutures are pulled distally to expose the proximal attachment of the graft. Then Mayo scissors are used to release the graft.

Careful hemostasis is crucial, because it is possible for a geniculate artery branch to pass through the tendon. The fascia over the tendon is closed. The tendon itself does not need to be approximated. Magnetic resonance imaging studies 1 to 2 years after central quadriceps tendon harvest have shown excellent reconstitution.

After the graft is taken to the back table, the femoral side is prepared with two number 5 Ethibond braided whipstitches (four strands) tied to an Endobutton. Note that the knot is tied adjacent to the tendon graft. A number 2 Ethibond suture and a number 5 Ethibond suture are placed through the two far holes of the Endobutton. Using different size sutures helps delineate the leading end of the Endobutton during graft passage (Fig. 65–8).

A sizing block with 0.5-mm increments is used to determine the minimum tunnel size that will barely allow

passage of the free tendon graft. This ensures a tight fit when the graft is placed in the patient's knee.

The graft is placed in saline-soaked gauze and protected until the tunnels are ready.

Notchplasty

The goal of the notchplasty is to prevent impingement of the graft. To this end, we perform a minimal but adequate notchplasty, which can often be accomplished by a second surgeon while the graft is being harvested. We generally use a 5.5-mm full-radius synovectomy blade to do the notchplasty; a bur is seldom needed. Care is taken to avoid injury to the posterior cruciate ligament. When the over-the-top position is clearly visible, the notchplasty is concluded. After thorough debridement of the ACL remnants and completion of the notchplasty, a small curet is used to identify the proper location for the femoral tunnel. We recommend placing the guide pin at a point 7 to 8 mm anterior to the posterior notch edge and in the 10:30 o'clock–1:30 o'clock (right knee–left knee) position (Fig. 65–9).

Tibial Tunnel

This tunnel is drilled with an angled tibial guide set at 55 to 60 degrees. The guide is placed directly below the medial portal. The tunnel is oriented to the central posterior aspect of the tibial ACL remnant. A guide pin is then carefully placed using a power driver. Depending on the size of the graft, an appropriately sized (7 to 9 mm) reamer is used to drill the tunnel. A dilator can be used to increase the tunnel size by 0.5-mm increments. Care should be taken to avoid injury to the posterior cruciate ligament. The debris from the reaming is then debrided.

Femoral Tunnel

A small curet is used to identify the proper location for this tunnel. We recommend placing the femoral guide pin 7 to 8 mm anterior to the posterior notch and in the 10:30 o'clock–1:30 o'clock (right knee–left knee) posi-

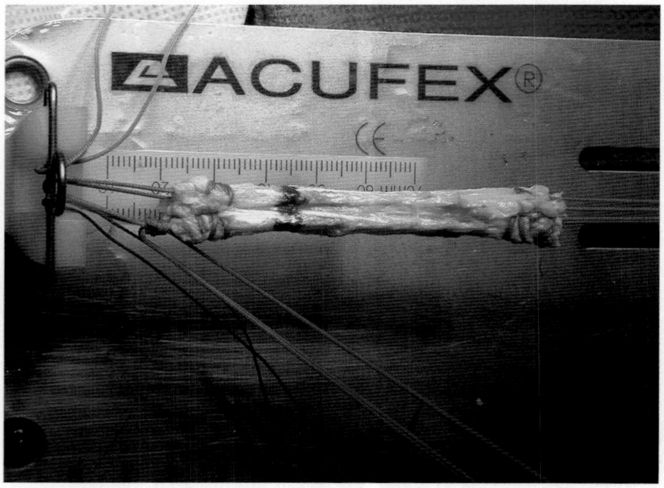

Figure 65–8 Demonstration of the "graftmaster" setup using the Endobutton. Note the knot tied adjacent to the tendon.

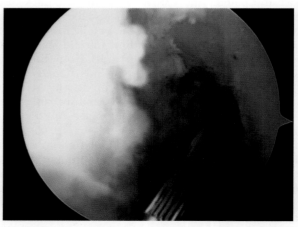

Figure 65–9 The femoral guide pin starts the femoral tunnel at the 1:30 o'clock position.

tion. The femoral guide pin is placed through the tibial tunnel with the knee at 70 to 90 degrees of flexion. Ideally, the guide pin should exit the anterolateral thigh at an angle of about 45 to 50 degrees from the axis of the femur and anterior to the iliotibial band. The tunnel is reamed to a depth of 35 to 40 mm (Fig. 65–10). Debris is cleared out. Blowing out the back wall is not a critical issue with use of an Endobutton. The Endobutton drill is then placed over the femoral guide pin, and drilling continues completely through the lateral cortex. A depth gauge is then used to measure the tunnel. Using the Endobutton "graftmaster," the distance from the Endobutton to the femoral tunnel orifice point on the graft (marked in blue) should be determined, and the suture length should be adjusted to match the measured length of the tunnel. Allow at least 2 cm of tendon graft in the tunnel. Be sure to allow room to flip the Endobutton after placement through the femoral tunnel.

Graft Passage

Using the preceding measurements, the Endobutton loop is made, with the knot tied adjacent to the graft. Be sure that the tunnel length matches the distance from the Endobutton to the tunnel exit point (2 cm minimum graft in the tunnel).

The number 5 and number 2 Ethibond sutures are now passed through the eye of the Beath pin, and the pin is pulled, taking the sutures out the lateral thigh. Then, using the number 5 Ethibond as the leading suture, the graft is pulled up into the joint (Fig. 65–11). The Endobutton is visualized through the scope as it enters the femoral tunnel (Fig. 65–12). Once the graft is seated in the femoral tunnel, the number 2 Ethibond is pulled to flip the Endobutton. A distinct click is felt as the Endobutton is properly flipped. Once this is accomplished, the Ethibond suture on the tibial side of the graft is pulled to ensure that there is solid seating of the graft on the femoral side (the graft should not move at all if the Endobutton is flipped). Remove the Endobutton leading sutures.

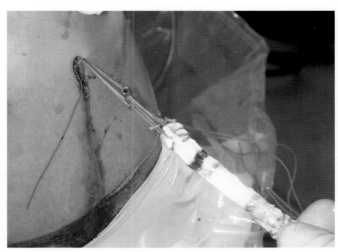

Figure 65–11   The graft is gently pulled into and through the tibial tunnel, with the Endobutton leading the way.

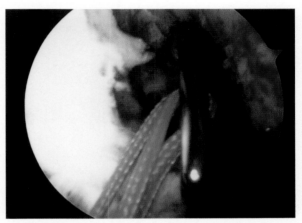

Figure 65–12   The Endobutton is pulled into the femoral tunnel using the leading number 5 sutures.

At this point, the knee is ranged several times while keeping tension on the graft (via the tibial tunnel) to ensure full range of motion and to decrease the creep in the graft (Fig. 65–13).

A guidewire is placed toward the counterclockwise side of the tibial graft; the knee is placed at 10 degrees of flexion; and, while keeping tension on the graft, a fully threaded bioabsorbable screw, 1 mm larger than the tunnel size, is placed up to the proximal end of the tunnel. The guidewire is then withdrawn. The two sutures from the tibial tunnel are tied over a button for extra security (Fig. 65–14). The knee is brought into full extension, and the graft is visualized arthroscopically to check for notch impingement.

Wound Closure

The wounds are closed in layers. The graft harvest and tibial tunnel wounds are closed with 2-0 Vicryl, followed by running subcuticular Prolene, then Steri-Strips. The Prolene is pulled out in the office after 1 week. The

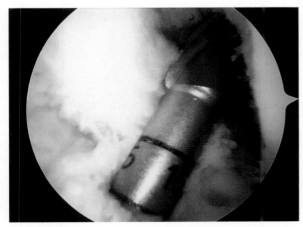

Figure 65–10   The femoral tunnel is reamed to a depth of 35 to 40 mm while carefully visualizing the depth markings on the reamer.

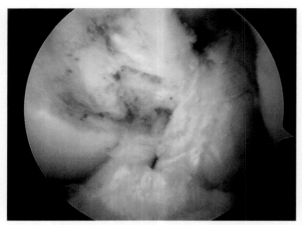

Figure 65–13 Demonstration of the quadriceps tendon graft after the Endobutton is flipped.

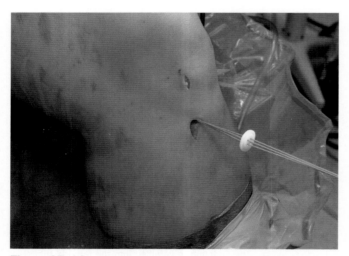

Figure 65–14 Placement of the tibial button for added tibial support.

Steri-Strips are left in place until they fall off spontaneously; we have found that this results in a lower-profile scar. We do not close the arthroscopy portals with suture; instead, we use a small piece of Xeroform and gauze. A Cryo-Cuff is also used for the first week.

Postoperative Management

Rehabilitation progresses steadily, but not aggressively, for the first 6 weeks, allowing time for graft fixation and diminished swelling. With this graft, aggressive early physical therapy is not necessary and not advised. Because there is less pain than with alternative autografts, range of motion and strength usually progress steadily and methodically. The patient is allowed toe-touch weight bearing with crutches for 2 weeks. Range of motion from 0 to 90 degrees and full extension are achieved within 2 weeks. Range of motion from 0 to 130 degrees should be established within 2 to 3 weeks. We delay straight-line running until 10 to 12 weeks, and figure-of-eight running starts at 4 months. Return to sports is allowed at 6 months following strength and functional testing.

Results

Our experience with this graft spans 6 years.[1,3] The clinical impression has been very favorable, and patients have expressed uniform satisfaction with their return to desired levels of activity. A study by Joseph et al.[4] presented at the 2002 meeting of the American Academy of Orthopaedic Surgeons showed that quadriceps tendon ACL patients have less pain postoperatively than their hamstring and bone-tendon-bone counterparts. ACL patients receiving quadriceps free tendon grafts used pain medication for an average of 5.4 days, whereas those receiving the other grafts required pain medication for an average of 19 to 22 days.

We use central quadriceps free tendons for ACL reconstruction in all patients, including two who won national championships (in gymnastics and lacrosse). We feel very comfortable recommending this technique.

Complications

There have been eight known graft ruptures related to specific postoperative injuries. To date, there have been no known quadriceps tendon ruptures in our patients undergoing ACL reconstruction with quadriceps tendon grafts. Sensitivity at the pretibial button is the most common complaint.

References

1. Fulkerson J: Central quadriceps free tendon for anterior cruciate ligament reconstruction. Oper Tech Sports Med 7:195-200, 1999.
2. Fulkerson J, Langeland R: An alternative cruciate reconstruction graft: The central quadriceps tendon. Technical note. Arthroscopy 11:252-254, 1995.
3. Fulkerson J, Mckeon B, Donahue B, et al: The central quadriceps tendon as versatile graft alternative in ACL reconstruction. Tech Orthop 13:367-374, 1998.
4. Joseph M, Fulkerson J, Nissen C, et al: A prospective comparison of function recovery and pain medication requirements in the immediate postoperative period after three different types of autograft ACL reconstructions. Poster no. 481. Presented at the annual meeting of the American Academy of Orthopaedic Surgeons, 2002.

Revision ACL Reconstruction: Indications and Technique

Bernard R. Bach, Jr.

Preoperative Planning:
Determine any associated patholaxity; assess whether tunnels are anatomic or nonanatomic, expanded or nonexpanded; decide whether tunnels need staged bone grafts; develop hardware removal strategy—remove or bypass

Surgical Technique:
Operative strategy—double incision versus endoscopic; basic principles similar to primary ACL reconstruction

Arthroscopically remove all previous ACL graft tissue to carefully assess intra-articular tunnel entrance position

Consider accessory inferomedial portal or transpatellar portal to achieve optimal tibial tunnel length

Position tibial aimer and assess medial and lateral orientation (e.g., 11 o'clock, right; 1 o'clock, left); avoid sagittal plane orientation

After drilling, assess for clearance of notch apex in extension, then advance into femoral root to stabilize

After reaming tibial tunnel, place scope retrograde up tunnel to assess for adequate tissue removal and continuity of tunnel

Define femoral "over-the-top" (OTT) position, place femoral offset aimer, assess medial and lateral orientation with knee flexed 80 to 90 degrees

Create endoscopic footprint; assess and complete tunnel

If femoral screw is vertical, remove and graft, or advance slightly to allow bypass

If anterior wall is deficient, pack with corticocancellous graft (single stage)

Once reamed, pass arthroscope retrograde to confirm intact socket and maintain OTT rim

Pass graft, assess for construct match, and secure (similar to primary ACL principles)

Consider larger-diameter screws if bone is soft; alternatively, consider stacking screws

Consider tibial "backup" fixation (button, screw or post, staple) if bone is soft

If posterior cortex is violated from index ACL, consider Endobutton femoral fixation with operative fixation,[22] or convert to two-incision technique

Remember the "funnel" concept (inverted cone and tunnel developed) to achieve accurate placement of tunnel entrance

If there is "bone mulch" or "transfix" type of index fixation, consider staged bone grafting to avoid additional stress riser (e.g., femoral fracture)

There are estimates that more than 100,000 new anterior cruciate ligament (ACL) injuries occur annually. ACL reconstruction is one of the 10 most frequently performed operative techniques in orthopedic surgery, with approximately 50,000 being done annually. Clinical follow-up studies indicate stability success rates between 85% and 90% with contemporary techniques of either patellar tendon autograft[23] or hamstring autograft reconstruction.[4,5,8,9,24] Based on these data, there may be 5000 failed ACL reconstructive surgeries in any given year. Analogous to the arthroplasty experience of the 1980s and 1990s, increasing numbers of patients are referred to our practice with failed ACL reconstructions. This chapter discusses causes of failure, indications for surgery, and surgical techniques.

There are a variety of reasons why an ACL reconstruction may fail.[7,11,19-21,27,33-37] Most authors believe that technical errors are a contributing factor in approximately 70% of failed ACL surgeries. Tunnel malpositioning is the most common reason for technical failure. There has been an evolution in tunnel malplacement from anteriorized femoral and tibial tunnels to vertically oriented femoral tunnels and posteriorized tibial tunnels (Figs. 66–1 to 66–3). If the ACL tunnels are placed too vertically on the femoral side, this can result in a normal Lachman test but inability to control rotation (see Fig. 66–3). Other technical issues that may contribute to failure include insufficient graft harvest tissue, which may include poor-quality tissue or bone blocks that are too small. The "fit and fill" relationship of the graft (tunnel–graft gap space), osteopenic bone, divergent screw placement, improper graft tensioning, and ineffective graft fixation are additional technical factors.

Loss of secondary restraints, a previous medial meniscectomy, residual medial collateral ligament laxity, or unrecognized posterolateral laxity may also affect failure rates.[25,28] In my experience, macrotraumatic retears are unusual. In nearly 1100 ACL reconstructions, fewer than 10 patients have returned for revision surgery with macrotraumatic injuries. The majority of patients (95%)

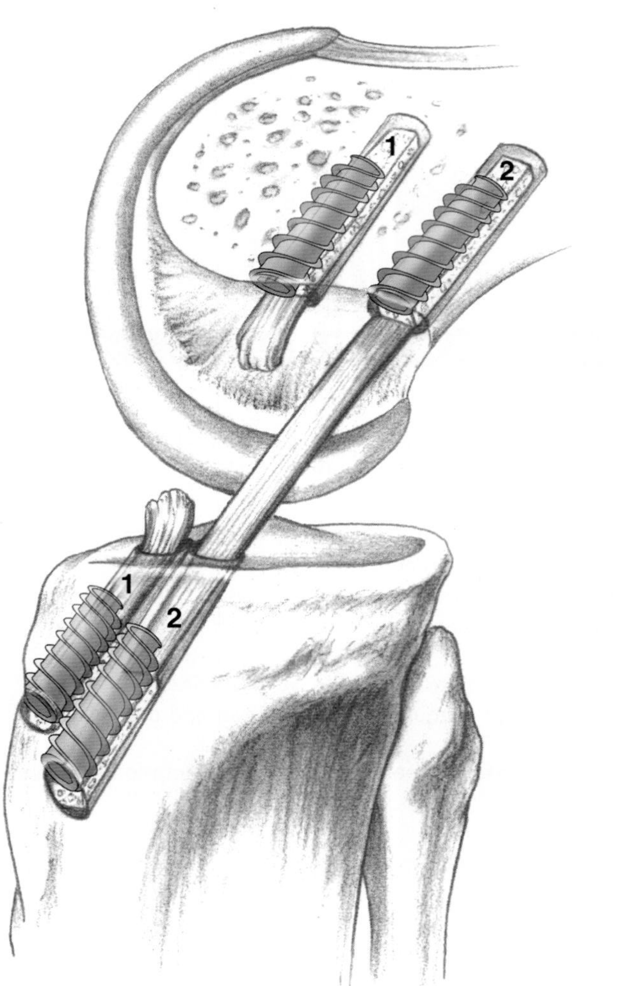

Figure 66–1   Anterior placement of the femoral and tibial tunnels (1). Revision (2) can be accomplished by reaming and reinstating the tibial screw if needed to maintain cephalad structural integrity; femoral screw removal is unnecessary. (From Bach BR, Mazzocca AD, Fox JA: Revision anterior cruciate ligament reconstruction. In Grana WA [ed]: Orthopaedic Knowledge Online. Rosemont, IL, American Academy of Orthopaedic Surgeons, 2003. Available at www.aaos.org/oko; accessed May 15, 2003.)

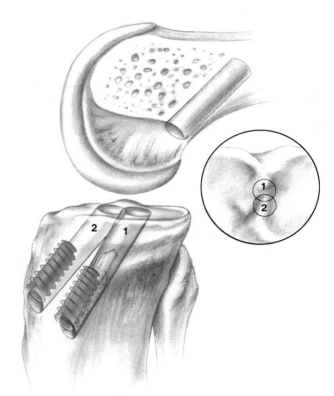

Figure 66–2   Posteriorized tibial tunnel. 1, Initial tunnel; 2, revision tunnel. Revision surgery is performed by placing the tibial tunnel more anteriorly. There will be some overlap of the intra-articular tunnel entrance site. If the index procedure used a patellar tendon graft, the index tibial bone plug provides an excellent buttress for graft fixation with the tibia. (From Bach BR, Mazzocca AD, Fox JA: Revision anterior cruciate ligament reconstruction. In Grana WA [ed]: Orthopaedic Knowledge Online. Rosemont, IL, American Academy of Orthopaedic Surgeons, 2003. Available at www.aaos.org/oko; accessed May 15, 2003.)

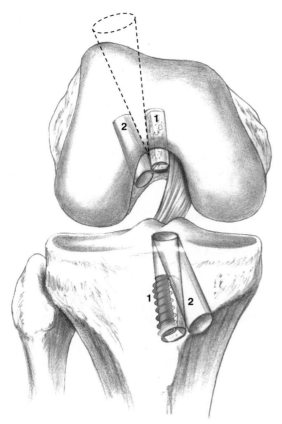

Figure 66–3 "Funnel" or divergent tunnel concept. The index procedure (1) resulted in a sagittally oriented tibial tunnel, with a resultant vertically oriented femoral tunnel. This may result in a "normal" Lachman test but does not control the pivot shift phenomenon. The revision tibial tunnel (2) maintains an intact tube of bone distally for fixation and provides an appropriate medial-to-lateral orientation for femoral tunnel revision. The index femoral tunnel can be filled with single-stage grafting, or the screw can be advanced to maintain medial wall integrity. (From Bach BR, Mazzocca AD, Fox JA: Revision anterior cruciate ligament reconstruction. In Grana WA [ed]: Orthopaedic Knowledge Online. Rosemont, IL, American Academy of Orthopaedic Surgeons, 2003. Available at www.aaos.org/oko; accessed May 15, 2003.)

who have undergone revision surgery in our practice have been referred. Patients are educated that the likelihood of a macrotraumatic event resulting in injury to the ACL graft is less than or equal to the likelihood of tearing the contralateral normal ACL. Microtraumatic injury may result in injury to the ACL graft. Graft abrasion along the intercondylar wall or the posterior cruciate ligament if the tibial tunnel is placed too laterally or medially, respectively, or intercondylar notch impingement if the graft is placed too far anteriorly, may result in microinjury and ultimate failure. A small subset of patients may have failed grafts based on biologic factors and failure of graft incorporation. Often, these individuals have hyperlaxity.

The indications for revision ACL surgery are similar to those outlined in Chapter 62. It is important for patients to understand that in many ways, revision ACL surgery should be considered a salvage procedure. In a

recent review, chondral abnormalities were noted at the time of revision ACL surgery in 75% of patients, and 50% had had previous meniscal surgery (unpublished data). Further, the results of revision surgery have been documented to be inferior to those of primary or index ACL surgery.[18–20,26,27,32,33,36,37] Less than 80% of patients had a stable knee at a minimum 2-year follow-up interval. Therefore, patient education is critical so that patients have reasonable expectations from the revision surgical procedure.

Physical Examination

Diagnosis of a failed ACL reconstruction is generally straightforward, with the physical examination findings being an abnormal Lachman test with a soft endpoint and a demonstrable pivot shift. The anterior drawer test may be more obvious than in the primary situation, as many patients have lost a meniscus and therefore have lost a component of secondary restraint. The KT-1000 arthrometer plays a role in the evaluation of ACL-reconstructed patients and the assessment of failed ACL surgery. In general, the maximum manual side-to-side difference is greater than 5 mm. This is an accepted criterion for the arthrometric determination of failure.

Imaging

Radiographic assessment is important in this patient population. I use standing full-length radiographs to assess for malalignment. For example, if a patient has had a complete meniscectomy and has medial compartment arthritis in conjunction with the failed ACL reconstruction, the focus is on realignment tibial osteotomy. If the patient has a varus alignment and loss of a meniscus with normal radiographs, I would consider meniscal transplantation in conjunction with the ACL revision procedure. Radiographic assessment is also critical to assess tunnel positioning, lucencies, and hardware placement. If patients have had soft tissue grafts, such as hamstring or Achilles tendon allograft procedures; synthetic grafts, such as Gore-Tex; or a ligament augmentation device (LAD) (3M, Minneapolis, MN), I often obtain computed tomography scans to better study the status of the femoral and tibial tunnels.[15,17,33]

Decision-Making Principles

The choice of graft for revision is dependent on which tissues were used initially.[6,14,30,31] If a hamstring reconstruction was performed at the index reconstruction, I would consider using a patellar tendon autograft. If, however, the patient has significant patellofemoral complaints in the affected knee, I would consider using a nonirradiated patellar tendon allograft or contralateral patellar tendon autograft. Shelbourne popularized the use of the contralateral patellar tendon graft for index and revision procedures. I have not been as successful in convincing my patients to use tissue from a previously unoperated knee that is considered the "normal" knee. Some surgeons who are hamstring advocates may consider using a contralateral hamstring graft for a failed hamstring reconstruction. Generally, I am not an advocate of hamstring grafts for revision situations because the tunnels are frequently enlarged, and the "fit and fill" analogy cannot be consistently achieved. If patients have had a failed hamstring graft, another option is a quadriceps tendon construct from the ipsilateral or contralateral extremity. Because the patellar tendon autograft is the most commonly used graft for index procedures in my area, it is also the most common graft seen at the time of revision surgery. The majority of these patients select a nonirradiated patellar tendon allograft reconstruction. Patients' subjective satisfaction level following revision surgery does not compare with that achieved with index procedures. These patients are generally disappointed that their initial grafts have failed, and we are trying to reduce morbidity for these patients.

Preoperative Planning

Preoperative planning generally includes graft selection and considerations of whether the operation will be performed as a single-stage or two-stage procedure. If tunnels are expanded, this may warrant a staged procedure, with removal of hardware and iliac crest bone grafting (Fig. 66–4). Harner (personal communication) is an advocate of this philosophy, but I have performed staged reconstructions infrequently. The advantages of a nonirradiated patellar tendon allograft are that bone plugs can be customized and additional bone graft is available to compensate for tunnel expansion or tunnel insufficiency issues.

Additional preoperative considerations include assessment of present hardware. The basic questions are: Does the hardware have to be removed? Can it be removed? And can it be bypassed? One should have an array of screwdrivers available, although most interference screws use a 3.5-mm hexagonal head recess. Some manufacturers use 3- or 4-mm recesses. Additionally, one manufacturer has a threaded insert for the interference screw (Instrument Makar, Okemos, MI). Screwdriver extractors should also be available, because the screw head recess may have been stripped during the initial insertion or may be stripped during the attempted removal. With two-incision index procedures, "screw and post" hardware placed on the femoral side generally does not require surgical removal. Staple removal may be problematic if the staples are covered with bone, as this may create an incompetent tibial cortex.

An additional preoperative consideration is whether the procedure can be performed as an endoscopic procedure or as a two-incision procedure (Fig. 66–5). In general, the majority of two-incision failures can be approached endoscopically, and the majority of endoscopic failures can also be revised endoscopically. The exception to the latter situation may be the case of tunnel insufficiency, with either posterior cortical blowout or overlapped tunnels that may affect graft fixation (Figs. 66–6 and 66–7). In this situation, conversion to a two-incision technique may create an intact femoral tube for rigid fixation. Preoperatively, one should have an idea whether index tunnels are anatomically or nonanatomically placed (Figs. 66–8 and 66–9) and whether they are expanded or nonexpanded. If the tunnels are nonanatomic, they may be overlapping or not (Fig. 66–10). Nonoverlapping tunnels can be easily revised (see Figs. 66–1 and 66–8), but overlapping tunnels may require a staged bone graft, conversion to a two-incision technique, or simultaneous single-stage bone grafting.

Surgical Technique

Positioning and Examination under Anesthesia

The principles of revision ACL surgery are similar to those of index ACL reconstruction.[1,12,13,16] The examination under anesthesia and patient positioning are identical to that for an index ACL reconstruction.

Specific Surgical Steps

In general, before harvesting a graft, I place the arthroscope into the knee to be absolutely certain that I feel comfortable proceeding with a revision procedure. Remnant ACL tissue is removed. The former ACL insertion region is carefully debrided so that the entrance site can be clearly delineated arthroscopically. Revision notchplasty is performed as needed with a 0.25-inch curved osteotome, metal mallet, grasper, and spherical motorized bur. The femoral socket is identified, and soft tissue is removed with an arthroscopic electrocautery, shaver, and curet to identify the interference screw. Spinal needle triangulation is generally performed with hyperflexion, and an accessory inferomedial portal is created to provide the best colinear approach to this interference screw. A probe may be used to remove soft tissue from the hexagonal head recess. A Capener gauge or small osteotome may be required to remove surrounding bone to completely expose the circumferential aspect of the interference screw. At this point, the screw is removed. An exception might be in the case of a vertically oriented femoral screw and overlapping of the tunnel at the initiation of the new femoral screw. In this situation, I might consider further recession of the index femoral screw, which would maintain continuity of the medial wall.

An accessory inferomedial portal is routinely used in revision situations. Because the tibial aimer is being inserted through an arthroscopic portal rather than through retracted skin edges, it is critical to place the aimer more distally, to allow appropriate positioning of the tibial aimer stylet; this allows the creation of a longer tibial tunnel. Occasionally, I make a transpatellar portal to ensure an appropriate medial to lateral orientation of the tibial tunnel. Once the aimer is provisionally positioned, this allows appropriate access to the surgical

Text continued on p. 683

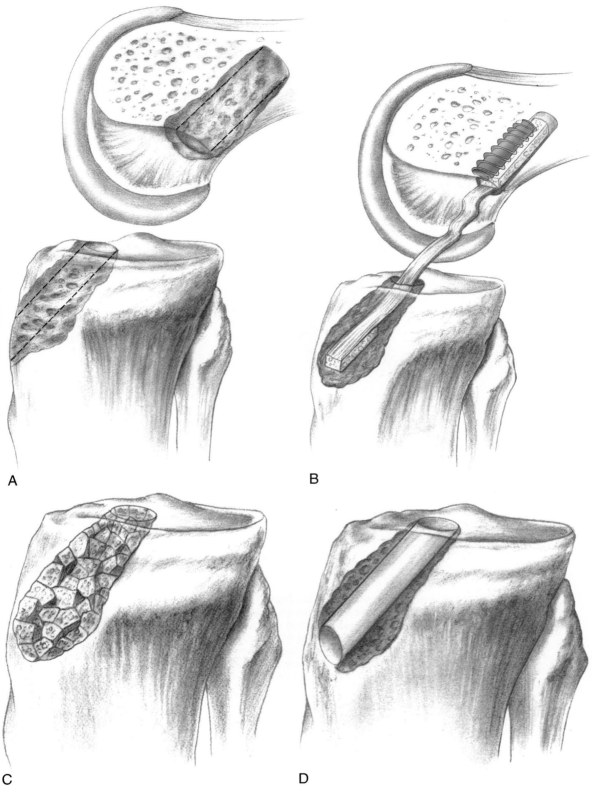

A

B

C

D

Figure 66–4   Failed anterior cruciate ligament reconstruction with marked tibial tunnel expansion (A). This is more commonly noted in Achilles tendon or hamstring grafts. In this setting, staged iliac crest cancellous grafting is performed (B), and at 4 to 6 months, a revision procedure is performed (C). D, Once the graft has healed, a revision tunnel may be redrilled without concern of tunnel overlap or loss of integrity. (From Bach BR, Mazzocca AD, Fox JA: Revision anterior cruciate ligament reconstruction. In Grana WA [ed]: Orthopaedic Knowledge Online. Rosemont, IL, American Academy of Orthopaedic Surgeons, 2003. Available at www.aaos.org/oko; accessed May 15, 2003.)

6 Knee

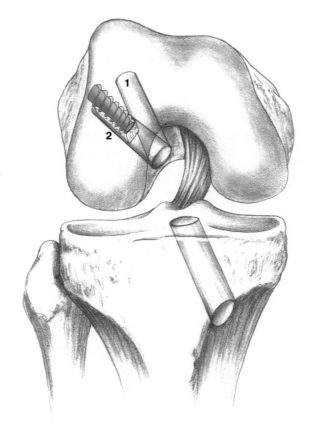

Figure 66–5 Appropriate tunnel location (1). Revision (2) may be performed by using the original tunnels if they are not expanded, or by using a two-incision technique with outside-in placement of the revision femoral screw. (From Bach BR, Mazzocca AD, Fox JA: Revision anterior cruciate ligament reconstruction. In Grana WA [ed]: Orthopaedic Knowledge Online. Rosemont, IL, American Academy of Orthopaedic Surgeons, 2003. Available at www.aaos.org/oko; accessed May 15, 2003.)

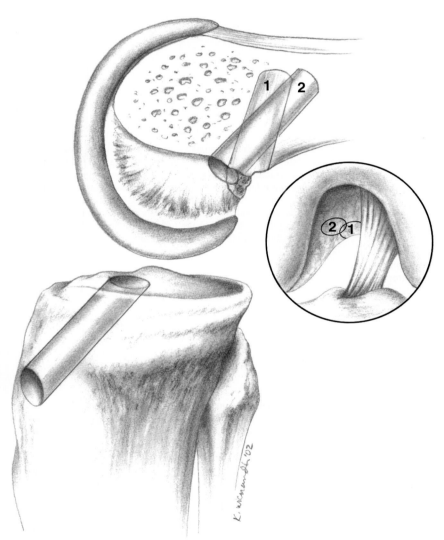

Figure 66–6   Cortical violation of the posterior femoral "over-the-top" (OTT) or "blowout" may occur during the index procedure (**1**) or at revision (**2**). (From Bach BR, Mazzocca AD, Fox JA: Revision anterior cruciate ligament reconstruction. In Grana WA [ed]: Orthopaedic Knowledge Online. Rosemont, IL, American Academy of Orthopaedic Surgeons, 2003. Available at www.aaos.org/oko; accessed May 15, 2003.)

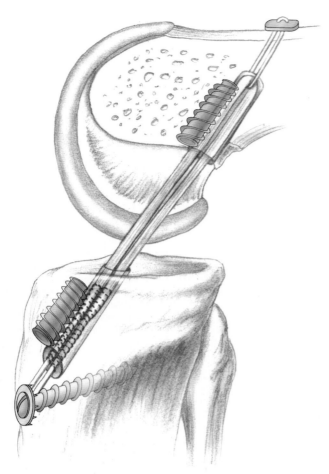

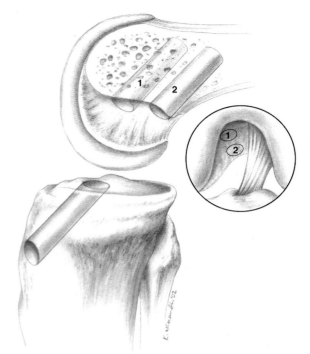

Figure 66–8 Nonoverlapping, anteriorized femoral tunnel (1) and appropriately placed femoral tunnel (2). The intact anterior "wall" allows for structural maintenance of the revision femoral tunnel. The original femoral interference screw does not necessarily require removal. (From Bach BR, Mazzocca AD, Fox JA: Revision anterior cruciate ligament reconstruction. In Grana WA [ed]: Orthopaedic Knowledge Online. Rosemont, IL, American Academy of Orthopaedic Surgeons, 2003. Available at www.aaos.org/oko; accessed May 15, 2003.)

Figure 66–7 If the posterior cortex is violated and the tunnel is incompetent, fixation options may include the use of Endobutton fixation with operative fixation. Here, a hamstring construct is depicted. (From Bach BR, Mazzocca AD, Fox JA: Revision anterior cruciate ligament reconstruction. In Grana WA [ed]: Orthopaedic Knowledge Online. Rosemont, IL, American Academy of Orthopaedic Surgeons, 2003. Available at www.aaos.org/oko; accessed May 15, 2003.)

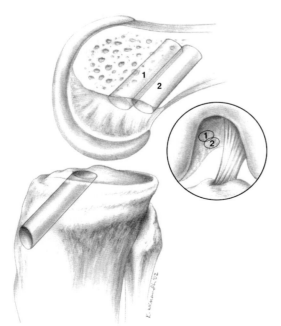

Figure 66–9 Nonanatomic femoral tunnel (1) with the revision femoral tunnel (2). The anterior wall is not intact and should be addressed by single-stage bone graft, staged bone grafting, customized femoral plug, or stacked interference screw fixation. (From Bach BR, Mazzocca AD, Fox JA: Revision anterior cruciate ligament reconstruction. In Grana WA [ed]: Orthopaedic Knowledge Online. Rosemont, IL, American Academy of Orthopaedic Surgeons, 2003. Available at www.aaos.org/oko; accessed May 15, 2003.)

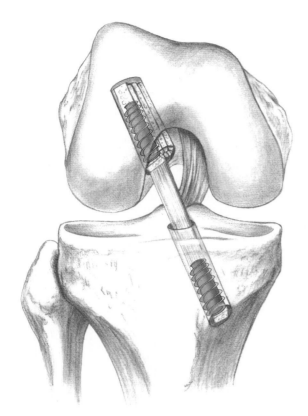

Figure 66–10   In an expanded femoral tunnel or overlapping femoral tunnels, bone grafting with corticocancellous "matchstick" grafts from the patellar allograft may avoid inadequate fixation or preclude staged grafting. (From Bach BR, Mazzocca AD, Fox JA: Revision anterior cruciate ligament reconstruction. In Grana WA [ed]: Orthopaedic Knowledge Online. Rosemont, IL, American Academy of Orthopaedic Surgeons, 2003. Available at www.aaos.org/oko; accessed May 15, 2003.)

incision. In general, a portion of the former graft harvest incision is used to access the medial metaphyseal region. If an interference screw has been placed on the tibial side and is not readily palpable or identifiable, I use a fluoroscan to help identify its placement. The goal is to minimize the amount of cortical bone removed when the tibial screw is removed. If, however, the initial tibial tunnel was placed in a more sagittally or horizontally oriented plane, I may leave the screw in place and bypass this with the new tibial tunnel. The goal of tibial pin placement is identical to that in index ACL reconstruction. When drilling the ⅗₂-inch Steinmann pin, there is generally good bone purchase with initial placement of the pin, but as it approaches the intra-articular entrance site, it usually exits within some portion of the former ACL tibial tunnel entrance. Therefore, when drilling the tibial tunnel, if this pin is appropriately positioned, I tap the pin up into the femoral roof and then further secure this with a hemostat or Kocher clamp when overreaming the pin. Before this step, I bring the knee out in complete extension to make certain that the entrance site of the pin is posterior to the apex of the intercondylar notch. This pin is generally overreamed with an 11-mm cannulated reamer. Then the arthroscope is passed ret-

rograde through the tibial tunnel to assess the continuity of the tibial tube. Additionally, this allows an assessment for remnants of soft tissue that may be within the former tibial tunnel. A shaver may be placed retrograde through the tibial tunnel and viewed from the inferolateral portal arthroscopically to clarify the adequacy of soft tissue removal. The intra-articular entrance site is also cleared of residual tissue with an arthroscopic shaver. If needed, the arthroscopic chamfer reamer and rasp are used to smooth the posterior edge. In situations in which the tibial tunnel has been placed too posteriorly with a bone-tendon-bone graft, the former tibial bone plug generally acts as an excellent buttress for placement of the new tibial tunnel. This may be more problematic with placement of a soft tissue graft, and a customized tibial plug may be necessary.

Once the tibial tunnel has been created, attention is directed toward femoral socket creation. The options are, as previously noted, endoscopic placement of this tunnel or conversion to a two-incision approach. If a two-incision approach is used, a 1.5-inch incision is made midline of the thigh, extending to the proximal pole of the patella. The skin is incised and infiltrated with dilute epinephrine solution, and the dissection is carried down to the iliotibial band. The subcutaneous tissues are reflected, the thicker portion of the iliotibial band midsubstance is palpated and identified, and a 2-inch longitudinal incision is made. One should place a finger behind the vastus lateralis and palpate the lateral intermuscular septum. A Z-retractor can then be positioned to retract the vastus lateralis anteriorly, thus exposing the lateral supracondylar region. Tissues are then incised with electrocautery, and the periosteum is incised. A subperiosteal dissection is performed with a Cobb elevator so that one can place a finger antegrade in the "over-the-top" position. At this point, a J-shaped guide passer is placed retrograde from the inferomedial portal and visualized arthroscopically as it passes the over-the-top position retrograde; this is palpated with a finger placed in the over-the-top position. The J-shaped guide passer then pops through the capsule and is delivered into the surgical wound region anterior to the intermuscular septum. The side-specific rear-entry femoral aimer is attached to the guide passer and brought intra-articularly. It is placed in the 11 o'clock position, secured to the lateral femoral condylar region, and drilled with provisional pin placement. Once this pin has been appropriately positioned, it is overreamed with a 10-mm cannulated reamer.

Some authors, myself included, advocate a "funnel" or tunnel diversion concept that is helpful with revision ACL surgical procedures (see Fig. 66–3).[8,11] If the intra-articular entrance site is properly selected, one can drill the femoral tunnel at a different angle or orientation to create an intact femoral socket. This is applicable for either a two-incision or an endoscopic approach. On occasion, I use an accessory inferomedial approach for placement of the endoscopic tunnel. O'Donnell and Scerpella[29] popularized the routine use of an accessory inferomedial portal with the knee placed in hyperflexion to drill the femoral socket. They reported a lower incidence of screw divergence with this technique than with the standard transtibial endoscopic femoral tunnel socket. Generally, if the tibial tunnel has the appropriate medial to lateral orientation, this is not problematic, and a retrograde transtibial femoral approach can usually be used. Similar to index ACL reconstructions, I generally use a 7-mm femoral offset aimer, place this in the over-the-top position with the knee flexed to 80 degrees, and drill a provisional pin placement. This pin may meet resistance as it is drilled into the former femoral bone plug if a patellar tendon graft was previously used. This is then overreamed with a cannulated 10-mm endoscopic reamer with the knee flexed at approximately 80 degrees, and an endoscopic footprint is created. If there are overlapping femoral tunnels, I frequently pack the former tunnel with cancellous graft from the patellar tendon allograft (see Fig. 66–10). This is positioned and impacted to create a firm construct. The next step is the creation of the new femoral socket. It is critical to make certain that the femoral cortex is not blown out; therefore, similar to an index ACL procedure, the provisional footprint is assessed. This is then overreamed with a cannulated 10-mm reamer to a depth of 35 mm with the knee flexed 75 to 90 degrees. The pin and reamer are then removed, and after copious irrigation of the knee, the scope is passed retrograde via the tibial tunnel up into the femoral socket to ensure that the posterior cortex is maintained and that there is no posterior cortical wall blowout (Fig. 66–11).[10]

At this point, a graft is created. If expanded tunnels were anticipated, I may customize the size of the bone plug being used on either the femoral or tibial side.

Once the graft is created, it is passed in standard fashion using a "push-in" technique, as described in Chapter 63. The graft is pushed up through the femoral socket, grasped with a hemostat, and guided up into the femoral socket. The cortex is oriented posteriorly in the coronal plane. The bone plug is left slightly prominent

initially, for subsequent placement of a nitinol hyperflex pin at the 11 o'clock position. This allows the bone plug to act as a skid, thus ensuring parallel placement of the interference screw. Once the knee is hyperflexed, the pin is advanced until it "bottoms out" within the femoral socket. The graft is then pushed flush to the articular margin and assessed for graft mismatch. Similar concepts of graft recession, graft rotation, and free bone block modification are applied to allograft situations (Fig. 66–12).[24] Once the appropriate construct match is achieved, an interference screw—generally a 7- by 25-mm metal cannulated interference screw—is used. In situations in which the bone is softer, a larger-diameter screw may be used. Some authors advocate the use of stacked screws, with an additional screw placed to reinforce fixation[2] (Fig. 66–13). I have not used this

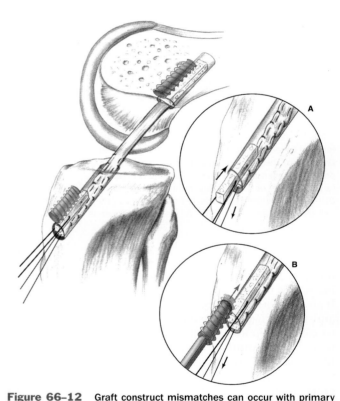

Figure 66–12 Graft construct mismatches can occur with primary or revision procedures. In a revision procedure using a patellar tendon allograft, construct mismatches may occur if a graft from a taller donor is used in a smaller recipient. Several options exist: graft advancement on the femoral side, graft rotation up to 540 degrees to shorten the construct by 6 to 8 mm, or use of a "free bone block" modification. In this situation, the graft is prepared normally, and then one bone block is sharply dissected for the graft, creating a pseudo–quadriceps tendon graft. The graft is fixed on the femoral side and tensioned, and the bone plug is placed into the tibial tunnel (A). Tension is maintained on the graft and bone plug. Interference screw fixation is then performed with the knee extended and axially loaded (B). (From Bach BR, Mazzocca AD, Fox JA: Revision anterior cruciate ligament reconstruction. In Grana WA [ed]: Orthopaedic Knowledge Online. Rosemont, IL, American Academy of Orthopaedic Surgeons, 2003. Available at www.aaos.org/oko; accessed May 15, 2003.)

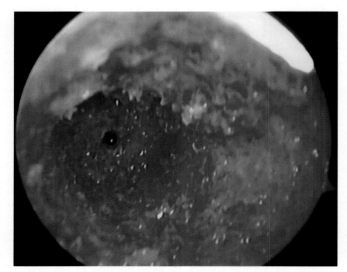

Figure 66–11 Retrograde placement of the arthroscope via the tibial tunnel into the femoral socket to ensure that the posterior wall is intact.

approach on the femoral side but have employed it on the tibial side. Once the graft is secured on the femoral side, it is multiply cycled and assessed for adequate fixation and gross isometry. The knee is then brought out into complete extension, and attention is directed toward graft fixation on the tibial side. The graft is rotated so that the cortex is in the coronal plane and oriented anteriorly. If there is some incompetence of the cortical entrance site secondary to former screw removal, stacking of screws can be helpful. Because graft fixation is generally less optimal on the tibial than the femoral side, in some situations I also consider reinforcing with a screw and post or securing over a Hewson ligament button (Richards, Memphis, TN). After fixation of the tibial side, the knee is examined, and the Lachman, anterior drawer, and pivot shift tests are performed in the operating room. The graft is inspected for impingement and for tension. A standard closure is performed, as described in Chapter 63.

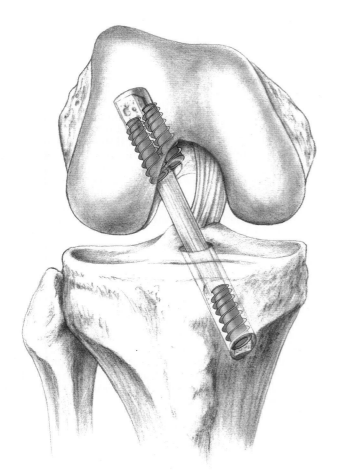

Figure 66–13 In osteopenic bone or in the case of an expanded femoral tunnel, fixation may be enhanced by placing, or "stacking," an additional interference screw. (From Bach BR, Mazzocca AD, Fox JA: Revision anterior cruciate ligament reconstruction. In Grana WA [ed]: Orthopaedic Knowledge Online. Rosemont, IL, American Academy of Orthopaedic Surgeons, 2003. Available at www.aaos.org/oko; accessed May 15, 2003.)

Postoperative Management

These procedures are performed on an outpatient basis. I use the identical rehabilitation protocol as for index ACL procedures. This protocol follows many of the principles advocated by Shelbourne and coworkers. Patients are allowed to bear weight as tolerated in extension. A drop-lock brace is not used for 6 weeks, in contrast to autografts. Once the patient has 90 degrees of flexion, is able to demonstrate excellent quadriceps control, and has complete extension, he or she is allowed to discontinue use of either the drop-lock brace or the knee immobilizer by 3 weeks. However, it is recommended that the patient use one of these braces at night to maintain extension. Postoperative follow-up intervals are identical to those for index procedures, and the criteria for return to sports are similar as well.

Results

Recently, I personally reviewed 33 ACL revisions performed with nonirradiated patellar tendon allografts for failed patellar tendon autografts using an accelerated rehabilitation program. There were 14 males and 19 females. The mean age at revision was 28 years. The mean number of surgeries was 2.8, and five patients presented for a re-revision. Chondral pathology was noted at the time of revision surgery in 70% of patients. Previous meniscal surgery had been performed in 50%. At a minimum 2-year follow-up (mean, 48 months; range, 24 to 81 months), 71% had a negative pivot shift; 82% had a 0 or 1+ pivot shift. KT-1000 arthrometry demonstrated that 81% had a maximum manual side-to-side difference of 3 mm or less, 9% ranged between 3 and 5 mm, and 9% had a greater than 5 mm difference. In this group there were no infections, pulmonary emboli, or deep vein thrombosis. Subjective satisfaction measures demonstrated that 84% of patients were completely or mostly satisfied. However, only 50% were *completely* satisfied, and the overall subjective satisfaction level was clearly less than that for index ACL patients.[3-5] The Lysholm, Tegner, Hospital for Special Surgery (HSS), and Noyes knee rating scale scores were less than those for index reconstructions.[3-5] Functional testing overall demonstrated insignificant side-to-side differences (4%).

In summary, revision ACL surgery should be considered a salvage procedure. Results are not comparable to those for index reconstructions, and ACL revision surgery presents an array of challenges to the surgeon. Preoperative planning may significantly reduce these potential intraoperative challenges.

References

1. Bach BR Jr: Arthroscopy assisted patellar tendon substitution for anterior cruciate ligament insufficiency: Surgical technique. Am J Knee Surg 2:3-20, 1989.
2. Bach BR Jr: Technical pitfalls of Kurosaka screw interference fixation. Am J Knee Surg 2:76-82, 1989.

6 Knee

3. Bach BR Jr, Jones GT, Sweet F, Hager CA: Arthroscopic assisted ACL reconstruction using patellar tendon substitution: Two year follow up study. Am J Sports Med 22:758-767, 1994.

4. Bach BR Jr, Levy ME, Bojchuk J, et al: Single-incision endoscopic anterior cruciate ligament reconstruction using patellar tendon autograft: Minimum two year follow-up evaluation. Am J Sports Med 26:30-40, 1998.

5. Bach BR Jr, Tradonsky S, Bojchuk J, et al: Arthroscopically assisted anterior cruciate ligament reconstruction using patellar tendon autograft: Five to nine year follow-up evaluation. Am J Sports Med 26:20-29, 1998.

6. Brown CH Jr, Carson EW: Revision anterior cruciate ligament surgery. Clin Sports Med 18:109-171, 1999.

7. Brown CH Jr, Sklar JH: Endoscopic anterior cruciate ligament reconstruction using quadrupled hamstring tendons and Endobutton femoral fixation. In Bach BR Jr (ed): ACL surgical techniques. Tech Orthop 13:281-298, 1998.

8. Bryan JM, Bach BR Jr, Bush-Joseph CA, et al: Comparison of "inside-out" and "outside-in" interference screw fixation for anterior cruciate ligament surgery in a bovine knee. Arthroscopy 12:76-81, 1996.

9. Bush-Joseph C, Bach BR Jr, Bryan J: Posterior cortical violation during endoscopic ACL reconstruction. Am J Knee Surg 8:130-133, 1995.

10. Clancy WG Jr, Pietropail MP: Revision anterior cruciate ligament reconstruction using the "anatomic-endoscopic" method. In Bach BR Jr (ed): ACL surgical techniques. Tech Orthop 13:391-410, 1998.

11. Dworsky B, Jewell BF, Bach BR Jr: Interference screw divergence in endoscopic anterior cruciate ligament reconstruction. Arthroscopy 12:45-49, 1996.

12. Ferrari JD, Bush-Joseph CA, Bach BR Jr: Double incision arthroscopically assisted ACL reconstruction using patellar tendon substitution. In Bach BR Jr (ed): ACL surgical techniques. Tech Orthop 13:242-252, 314-317, 1998.

13. Ferrari JD, Bush-Joseph CA, Bach BR Jr: Arthroscopically assisted ACL reconstruction using patellar tendon substitution via endoscopic technique. In Bach BR Jr (ed): ACL surgical techniques. Tech Orthop 13:262-274, 1998.

14. Fulkerson JP, McKeon BP, Donahue BJ, Tarinelli DJ: The central quadriceps tendon as a versatile graft alternative in anterior cruciate ligament reconstruction: Techniques and observations. In Bach BR Jr (ed): ACL surgical techniques. Tech Orthop 13:367-374, 1998.

15. Glousman R, Shields C, Kerlan R, et al: Gore-Tex prosthetic ligament in anterior cruciate deficient knees. Am J Sports Med 16:321-326, 1988.

16. Hardin GT, Bach BR Jr, Bush-Joseph CA, Farr J: Endoscopic single incision ACL reconstruction using patellar tendon autograft: Surgical technique. Am J Knee Surg 5:144-155, 1992.

17. Indelicato PA, Pascale MS, Huegel MO: Early experience with the Gore-Tex polytetrafluoroethylene anterior cruciate ligament prosthesis. Am J Sports Med 17:55-62, 1989.

18. Johnson D, Coen MJ: Revision ACL surgery: Etiology, indications, techniques, and results. Am J Knee Surg 8:155-167, 1995.

19. Johnson DL, Harner CD, Maday MG, Fu FH: Revision anterior cruciate ligament surgery. In Fu FH, Harner CD, Vince KG, Miller MD (eds): Knee Surgery. Baltimore, Williams & Wilkins, 1994, pp 877-896.

20. Johnson DL, Swenson TM, Irrang JJ, et al: Revision anterior cruciate ligament surgery: Experience from Pittsburgh. Clin Orthop 325:100-109, 1996.

21. Juareguito JW, Paulos LE: Why grafts fail. Clin Orthop 325:25-41, 1996.

22. Lyons PM, Graf BK: Pearls and pitfalls of Endobutton fixation. In Bach BR Jr (ed): ACL surgical techniques. Tech Orthop 13:299-305, 1998.

23. Nedeff D, Bach BR Jr: Arthroscopy assisted ACL reconstruction using patellar tendon autograft: A comprehensive review of contemporary literature. Am J Knee Surg 14:243-258, 2001.

24. Novak PJ, Williams JS, Wexler G, et al: Comparison of screw post fixation and free bone block interference fixation for anterior cruciate ligament soft tissue grafts: Biomechanical considerations. Arthroscopy 12:470-473, 1996.

25. Noyes FR, Barber S, Simon R: High tibial osteotomy and ligament reconstruction in varus angulated, anterior cruciate ligament deficient knees. Am J Sports Med 21:2-12, 1993.

26. Noyes FR, Barber-Westin SB: Revision anterior cruciate ligament surgery: Experience from Cincinnati. Clin Orthop 325:116-129, 1996.

27. Noyes FR, Barber-Westin SD, Roberts CS: Use of allografts after failed treatment of rupture of the anterior cruciate. J Bone Joint Surg Am 76:1019-1031, 1994.

28. O'Brien SJ, Warren RF, Pavlov H, et al: Reconstruction of the chronically insufficient ACL with the central third of the patellar ligament. J Bone Joint Surg Am 73:278-286, 1991.

29. O'Donnell JB, Scerpella TA: Endoscopic anterior cruciate ligament reconstruction: Modified technique and radiographic review. Arthroscopy 11:577-584, 1995.

30. Ritchie JR, Parker RD: Graft selection in anterior cruciate ligament revision surgery. Clin Orthop 325:65-77, 1996.

31. Shapiro JD, Jackson DW, Aberman HM, et al: Comparison of pullout strength of seven- and nine-millimeter diameter interference screw size as used in anterior cruciate ligament reconstruction. Arthroscopy 11:596-599, 1995.

32. Steadman JR, Saterbak AM: Revision anterior cruciate ligament reconstruction: Technique and tips—the Vail experience. In Bach BR Jr (ed): ACL surgical techniques. Tech Orthop 13:384-390, 1998.

33. Steadman JR, Seeman MD, Hutton KS: Revision ligament reconstruction of failed prosthetic anterior cruciate ligaments. Instr Course Lect 44:417-429, 1995.

34. Uribe JW, Hechtman KS, Zvijac JE, Tjin-A-Tsoi EW: Revision anterior cruciate ligament surgery: Experience from Miami. Clin Orthop 325:91-99, 1996.

35. Vergis A, Gillquist J: Graft failure in intra-articular anterior cruciate ligament reconstructions: A review of the literature. Arthroscopy 11:312-321, 1995.

36. Williams RJ III, Warren RF, Carson EW, Wickiwiecz TL: Revision anterior cruciate ligament reconstruction: The Hospital for Special Surgery experience. In Bach BR Jr (ed): ACL surgical techniques. Tech Orthop 13:375-383, 1998.

37. Wirth CJ, Kohn D: Revision anterior cruciate ligament surgery: Experience from Germany. Clin Orthop 325:110-115, 1996.

Posterior Cruciate Ligament: Diagnosis and Decision Making

Christina R. Allen, Jeffrey A. Rihn, and Christopher D. Harner

---

POSTERIOR CRUCIATE LIGAMENT: DIAGNOSIS AND DECISION MAKING IN A NUTSHELL

PCL Anatomy and Function:
Originates on the lateral border of the medial femoral condyle

Inserts 1 cm inferior to the posterior rim of the tibia in the fovea

Consists of three main portions: larger anterolateral (taut in flexion), smaller posteromedial (taut in extension), and meniscofemoral ligaments (Humphry, Wrisberg)

Primary restraint to posterior tibial translation at 30 and 90 degrees

PCL Injury Mechanisms:
Anterior blow to proximal tibia (dashboard injury)

Hyperflexion (common in sports), hyperextension

Evaluation of PCL Injury:
May occur as an isolated injury or in combination with other knee ligament injuries or pathology

Concomitant injuries, especially to posterolateral corner and neurovascular structures, should be suspected; thorough knee examination, including neurovascular status, is critical for accurate diagnosis

Isolated PCL injuries may have minimal swelling and pain

Examine gait (check for varus thrust) and alignment, and evaluate for MCL, ACL, LCL, meniscus, and posterolateral corner injury

Tests specific for PCL injury include posterior drawer, posterior Lachman, prone drawer, dynamic posterior shift, quadriceps active, and Godfrey tests

Evaluate for posterolateral corner injury using dial test and reverse pivot shift test

Radiographs may show evidence of PCL bony avulsion or concomitant injury (fibular head fracture indicating PLS injury) or may demonstrate posterior subluxation of tibia; bone scan may be useful in chronic PCL insufficiency to identify degenerative changes; MRI is useful in evaluating extent of soft tissue injury to ligaments and menisci

Examination under anesthesia and diagnostic arthroscopy are definitive diagnostic and planning tools in formulating a treatment plan

Natural History of PCL Deficiency:
Unknown whether PCL reconstruction alters the natural course of PCL deficiency

Many patients function well with PCL-deficient knees

Some studies show that chronic PCL deficiency leads to medial and patellofemoral compartment degenerative changes and meniscal tears

Continued

Management of PCL Injuries: General Guidelines:

Approach should take into account severity of injury (isolated vs. combined), timing (acute vs. chronic), symptoms (asymptomatic vs. pain or instability), and activity level (athletic vs. sedentary lifestyle)

Management of Acute PCL Injuries:

See Figure 67–8 for treatment algorithm

Most agree that avulsion fractures of the PCL should be acutely repaired

Combined injuries to the PCL and ACL, PLSs, or MCL should be surgically reconstructed, preferably within 2 weeks of injury

Isolated PCL injuries (grades I and II) can be treated nonoperatively with protected weight bearing and quadriceps muscle rehabilitation; patients are able to return to sports within 2 to 4 weeks after injury

Outcome of acute grade III PCL injuries is not as predictable, with risk of occult injury to posterolateral corner; immobilize knee in extension for 2 to 4 weeks to decrease tension on anterolateral fibers of PCL and posterolateral corner, then progress with rehabilitation; generally takes an additional 8 weeks for return to full activities

Some grade III PCL injuries may require surgical treatment because of medial or patellofemoral chondrosis or continued complaints of instability despite adequate physical therapy

Management of Chronic PCL Deficiency:

See Figure 67–9 for treatment algorithm

Chronic, isolated grade I or II PCL tears are treated with physical therapy

Chronic grade III PCL injuries are treated surgically if symptoms of pain or instability develop or persist despite therapy

Some patients with "isolated" PCL injury may have occult posterolateral corner injury; if so, PCL-PLS reconstruction is recommended, because PCL reconstruction alone may have a higher risk of failure

Perform high tibial osteotomy before PCL reconstruction if the patient has varus malalignment of the knee or dynamic varus thrust with ambulation

Patients with severe arthrosis should not undergo PCL reconstruction

PCL Reconstruction:

No "gold standard"

Difficult to reproduce tensioning patterns of AL and PM bands

Grafts may be autografts (patellar, hamstring, quadriceps tendons) or allografts (patellar, Achilles, quadriceps tendons)

PCL repair has not been consistently successful

Single-bundle transtibial PCL reconstruction is designed to simulate the stronger and larger AL bundle; femoral tunnel starting point is in the anatomic insertion site of the AL bundle

Double-bundle PCL reconstruction uses two divergent femoral tunnels in an attempt to re-create anatomy of AL and PM bundles and restore normal knee mechanics throughout the entire flexion-extension cycle

Tibial inlay technique uses a posterior approach to allow graft bone inlay to be placed in the original PCL tibial footprint; this avoids the sharp graft angle at the proximal margin of the tibial tunnel in the traditional transtibial technique, which might generate increased graft stress and friction, contributing to graft elongation or failure

Postoperative Management:

Knee braced in extension for 4 weeks, supporting the tibia to prevent posterior translation and excessive stress on the graft

Partial weight bearing as tolerated and quadriceps exercises starting on the first postoperative day

Closed chain exercises starting at approximately 6 weeks, followed by proprioceptive training at 12 weeks, increasing knee stability

Patients progress slowly through passive flexion exercises in the early postoperative period, with full flexion by 5 to 7 months

Hamstring exercises delayed for 4 months, because they stress the graft

Light jogging begins at 6 months; full activity at 9 to 12 months

Complications:

Failure to carefully position the extremities with adequate padding can lead to neurapraxia

Loss of motion (usually decreased flexion) can result from errors in graft positioning and excessive tensioning during graft fixation or from inadequate range-of-motion exercises during postoperative rehabilitation

Peroneal nerve injuries are more common in combined PCL-PLS injuries that require PLS reconstruction; neurapraxia often resolves with time (12 to 18 months), whereas complete nerve injuries have a much lower chance of recovery

Injury to popliteal vessels is an infrequent but serious complication; with the transtibial technique, great care must be taken to avoid overdrilling the posterior tibial cortex, given the close proximity of the popliteal artery and vein; during the posterior approach of the inlay technique, popliteal vessels are encountered

Surgeon should regularly palpate the patient's calf and thigh preoperatively, intraoperatively, and postoperatively to evaluate for a developing compartment syndrome caused by fluid extravasation

Avascular necrosis of medial femoral condyle can be avoided by placing the entry-exit point of the femoral tunnel proximal enough to allow preservation of subchondral bone

Injuries to the posterior cruciate ligament (PCL), once considered a rarity, reportedly have an incidence that varies between 3% of all ligament injuries in the general population and 37% of all ligament injuries in an emergency room trauma setting.[13,23,24,57] Nevertheless, research into the treatment of PCL injuries is sparse compared with studies of anterior cruciate ligament (ACL) injuries. Whereas there is an established "gold standard" for ACL reconstruction, there is no such model for the surgical treatment of PCL injuries. In fact, there is significant controversy regarding the surgical indications for PCL reconstruction. No studies to date have shown that reconstructing the PCL in isolated injuries alters the natural history of PCL deficiency.

This chapter summarizes the anatomy and biomechanics of the PCL and focuses on the principles of diagnosis and decision making related to the treatment of PCL injuries. A section on surgical techniques addresses the current methods of PCL reconstruction.

Anatomy and Biomechanics

The PCL originates on the lateral border of the medial femoral condyle at the junction of the medial wall and roof of the intercondylar notch. The footprint of the femoral attachment is 32 mm in diameter and terminates 3 mm proximal to the articular cartilage margin of the femoral condyle.[79] The ligament averages between 32 and 38 mm in length and inserts approximately 1 to 1.5 cm inferior to the posterior rim of the tibia, in a depression between the posterior medial and lateral tibial plateaus called the PCL facet or fovea.[15,29] The proximity of the PCL tibial insertion to the popliteal neurovascular bundle necessitates surgical precision during PCL reconstruction.[52] There are three main portions of the PCL, based on tensioning patterns: the larger anterolateral (AL) band, the smaller posteromedial (PM) band, and the variable anterior (ligament of Humphry) and posterior (ligament of Wrisberg) meniscofemoral ligaments.[39,45,65] The names for the AL and PM bands are based on the femoral origin and tibial insertion for each band.[29] Recently, the PCL architecture was described as four fiber regions based on their orientation and function at different degrees of knee flexion.[49] Further study is needed to evaluate the biomechanical and clinical implications of this anatomic description.

The AL bundle is two times larger in cross-sectional area than the PM bundle.[39,65] Functionally, the two components have different tensioning patterns that depend on the degree of knee flexion. The larger AL bundle is under greater tension with increasing flexion (making it the important posterior stabilizer with knee flexion), whereas the PM bundle is under greater tension with increasing extension (making it the important posterior stabilizer with knee extension).[39] Therefore, tension develops in a reciprocal fashion in each bundle during knee flexion and extension, with very few fibers of the PCL exhibiting isometric behavior. The large ligamentous insertion sites and the lack of isometry complicate the task of replicating PCL function with a single-bundle

PCL graft. As a result, new surgical techniques involving double-bundle reconstruction have been created, with an increased emphasis on determining optimal placement of the femoral tunnel during PCL reconstruction.[11,36,37,50,73]

The meniscofemoral ligaments originate from the posterior horn of the lateral meniscus, run adjacent to the PCL, and insert anteriorly (Humphry) and posteriorly (Wrisberg) to the PCL on the medial femoral condyle.[47] The presence of these ligaments is widely variable. Published studies show that both ligaments exist in 6% to 88% of knees, 4% to 71% of knees have only a ligament of Humphry, 8% to 35% of knees have only a ligament of Wrisberg, and 0% to 23% of knees lack meniscofemoral ligaments.[79] The importance of the meniscofemoral ligaments has not been fully characterized. It has been suggested that they contribute to the anteroposterior and rotatory stability of the knee.[39] No studies exist, however, that clearly define their biomechanical role.

The PCL is the primary restraint to posterior translation of the tibia. It resists 85% to 100% of a posteriorly directed knee force at 30 and 90 degrees of knee flexion. The lateral collateral ligament (LCL), posterolateral corner (including the popliteus, LCL, popliteofibular ligament, posterolateral joint capsule, and iliotibial band), and medial collateral ligament (MCL) are important secondary constraints to posterior translation of the tibia,[27,36] especially in the presence of PCL deficiency. The amount of posterior tibial translation increases dramatically when both primary and secondary restraints are disrupted, as in the case of a combined ligament injury. The PCL is also a secondary restraint to external tibial rotation, which is important when dealing with combined PCL–posterolateral corner injuries.[16,39]

Mechanism of Injury

The most common mechanism of injury to the PCL is an anterior blow to the proximal tibia (e.g., the classic "dashboard injury" in car crashes). Hyperflexion is the most common cause of PCL injury in sports, often due to a fall on the flexed knee with the foot in plantar flexion.[1,13,26] Additionally, hyperextension has been described in the literature as a mechanism that commonly results in a combined injury of the PCL and posterior capsule.[43]

Clinical Evaluation

History

Evaluation of the knee should begin with an accurate history of the original injury. The mechanism may reveal the potential severity of the injury and whether it is an isolated PCL injury or involves multiple ligaments. It is important to remember that in a trauma setting, 95% of patients with PCL injuries have associated ligamentous injuries in the same knee. The most common associated injury involves the posterolateral structures (PLSs) of the knee, which may be found in 60% of cases.[23] Therefore, a thorough examination of all structures is imperative, as is a careful neurovascular examination.[23,24] With any combined ligament injury involving the PCL, the physician must suspect a possible knee dislocation and rule out associated injuries, including injury to the peroneal nerve and vascular structures. In one study of knee dislocations, defined as combined ACL-PCL injuries, the incidence of vascular injury was 14%, regardless of whether patients presented with spontaneously reduced or dislocated knees.[32,81] Even a slightly diminished pulse should be a warning sign that vascular injury has occurred. Patients with incomplete lesions (e.g., an intimal tear of the artery) have diminished but intact pulses. If there is any uncertainty, ankle-brachial pressure measurements can be obtained. If the ratio is less than 0.8, an arteriogram should be ordered.[31]

In the case of acute isolated PCL injuries, patients may present with complaints of only mild swelling, mild discomfort, and knee stiffness. Patients with isolated PCL injuries do not usually relate a sense of knee instability. A large effusion and substantial loss of motion, instability, and significant pain should raise concerns about injuries to additional knee structures.

Physical Examination

The physical examination should begin with an evaluation of the patient's gait and standing, weight-bearing alignment. Fleming et al.[25] noted that apparent tibia vara, external rotation, and genu recurvatum are subtle signs of a PCL-deficient gait caused by posterior subluxation of the lateral tibia. The patient may ambulate with a slightly bent knee to avoid terminal extension and accentuation of external rotation of the tibia on the femur. A varus thrust gait may be an indication of a concomitant posterolateral corner injury, and the patient may attempt to compensate by walking with a flexed knee gait with the foot internally rotated.[56]

Patients with isolated PCL tears may have mild or moderate effusions. The injured knee may lack only 10 to 20 degrees of flexion compared with the noninjured knee,[36] or motion may be symmetrical. The knee should be examined for signs of MCL and posterolateral corner injuries (including the LCL). The LCL and MCL are palpated for tenderness, and varus and valgus stress testing is performed at full extension (stressing the posterolateral and posteromedial structures) and at 30 degrees of flexion (evaluating the integrity of the LCL and MCL). The joint line is palpated medially and laterally, and a flexion McMurray test is performed to rule out meniscal injury.

Special care is needed when evaluating the ACL in the setting of PCL disruption. The noninjured knee should be examined first to determine the proper relationship of the tibia to the femur, so that posterior subluxation of the tibia in the PCL-injured knee can be corrected before performing a Lachman test or anterior drawer test. Without this correction, the examiner risks falsely attributing an increase in anteroposterior laxity to a torn ACL.

The posterior drawer test, performed at 90 degrees of flexion with the tibia held in a neutral position, is considered the most accurate test for detecting a PCL injury.[13,17] While applying a posteriorly directed force to the proximal tibia, the extent of translation is evaluated by noting the change in step-off between the medial tibial plateau and the medial femoral condyle (Fig. 67–1). In a normal knee, the medial tibial plateau is usually 1 cm anterior to the medial femoral condyle. A PCL injury should be suspected if this step-off is not present, or if the application of posterior force to the proximal tibia reveals a soft endpoint. The grade of PCL injury can be determined by the amount of posterior laxity. In a grade I injury, there is still a step-off between the tibial plateau and the femoral condyle, but it is only 0 to 5 mm. Grade II injuries allow 5 to 10 mm of posterior translation, so that the tibial plateau ends up being displaced flush with the medial femoral condyle. Grade I and II injuries represent partial PCL tears. Grade III (complete) PCL injuries (>10 mm posterior translation) allow the medial tibial plateau to be displaced posterior to the medial femoral condyle and demonstrate an obvious posterior sag of the tibia.[36] Additional information can be obtained by performing the posterior drawer test with the tibia held in internal and external rotation. A decrease in translation with the tibia held in internal rotation results from tightening of one of the medial structures. It has been suggested that this decreased laxity indicates intact meniscofemoral ligaments. However, a recent biomechanical study by Bergfeld et al.[5] showed that the meniscofemoral ligaments are not responsible for the decreased posterior tibial translation noted with internal rotation. The authors suggested that the MCL or posterior oblique ligament more likely functions as a secondary restraint.

It is important to rule out injury to the PLSs when the posterior drawer is greater than 10 mm. This can be done

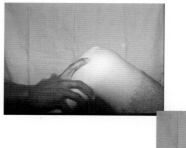
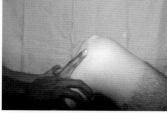

Figure 67–1   Posterior drawer test. The examiner's finger is positioned on the anteromedial joint line of the knee. When a posterior load is applied to the proximal tibia, the examiner can palpate a posterior translation of the tibial plateau in relation to the medial femoral condyle.

by assessing posterior translation at 30 degrees of flexion. A small increase in posterior translation at 30 degrees but not at 90 degrees may indicate a PLS injury; increased posterior translation at 90 and 30 degrees with maximal translation at 90 degrees suggests a PCL injury. The tibial external rotation or "dial" test is also used to evaluate the PLSs (Fig. 67–2). The test can be performed with the patient supine or prone, with the knee flexed at 30 and then 90 degrees. It is considered positive if the medial border of the foot or the tibial tubercle externally rotates 10 to 15 degrees more than the noninjured side.[22] Increased external rotation of 30 degrees is consistent with an isolated PLS injury, whereas increased external rotation at 30 and 90 degrees indicates a combined PLS-PCL injury.[16,80] The reversed pivot shift test can also be used to assess PLS injury.[15] This test is performed with the patient supine and the knee held in 90 degrees of flexion. The knee is then externally rotated and passively extended. If an injury of the PLSs is present, a shift occurs at 20 to 30 degrees of flexion as the posteriorly subluxated lateral tibia plateau reduces anteriorly. The reversed pivot shift is often difficult to elicit in the office setting because of patient guarding, but it is a useful diagnostic tool during an examination under anesthesia.

A variety of other adjunctive tests for verifying PCL injury have been described. These include the posterior Lachman, prone drawer, dynamic posterior shift, quadriceps active, and Godfrey tests.[19,30,41,67,78,82] The Godfrey test, or the posterior sag test, is performed by flexing the patient's knees and hips to 90 degrees while the patient is supine. The examiner holds both legs in the air. Gravity causes the tibia of the PCL-deficient leg to rest in a

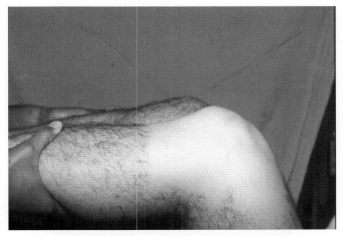

Figure 67–3 Godfrey test demonstrating displacement of the tibia posterior to the femur due to the pull of gravity in the face of posterior cruciate ligament deficiency.

posteriorly subluxated position compared with the intact knee. Posterior tibial translation of the injured leg supports the diagnosis of a PCL injury (Fig. 67–3). The quadriceps active test places the knee at 60 degrees of flexion, with the foot flat on the examination table. The tibia of the PCL-deficient leg is posteriorly subluxated in this position. The patient is asked to fire the quadriceps muscle or extend the knee by sliding the foot on the examination table. When the quadriceps contracts in a PCL-deficient knee, the posteriorly subluxated tibia visibly translates anteriorly to a reduced position. The dynamic posterior shift test is performed by slowly extending the knee from 90 degrees of flexion to full extension while the hip remains flexed at 90 degrees. The test is positive if the tibia reduces with a "clunk" near full extension.

Imaging

Radiographs should be obtained following physical examination, including flexion weight-bearing posteroanterior views and patellar views, which can be helpful in evaluating degenerative changes in chronic PCL deficiency. Radiographs should be examined carefully for evidence of tibial plateau fractures, Gerdy's tubercle avulsions, and fibular head fractures (indicative of a possible PLS injury). The lateral radiograph may provide evidence of a bony avulsion of the PCL tibial insertion, an osteochondral defect, or a posterior subluxation of the tibia in a PCL-deficient knee (Fig. 67–4). Stress radiographs may also be useful in the diagnosis of PCL injury. Recently, the utility of the "gravity sag" view, a lateral radiograph of the knee flexed to 90 degrees with the hip flexed 45 degrees, has been described in evaluating the tibia-femur step-off in PCL deficiency.[71] In patients with chronic PCL deficiency who complain of pain and instability, radionuclide imaging (bone scan) may identify early degenerative changes in the patellofemoral or medial compartment, indicating that

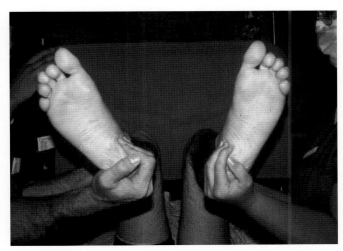

Figure 67–2 Tibial external rotation, or dial, test. This test can be performed with the patient supine or prone, with the knee flexed at 30 and then 90 degrees. The test is considered positive if the medial border of the foot or the tibial tubercle externally rotates 10 to 15 degrees more than the noninjured side. Increased external rotation of 30 degrees is consistent with an isolated posterolateral corner injury, whereas increased external rotation at 30 and 90 degrees indicates a combined posterior cruciate ligament–posterolateral structure (PCL-PLS) injury. In this case, the patient's right lower extremity demonstrates evidence of a combined PCL-PLS injury.

6 Knee

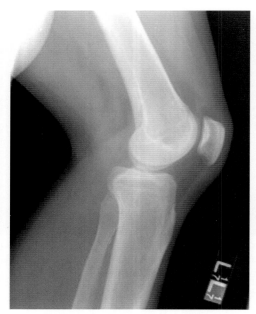

Figure 67-4 Lateral radiograph demonstrating posterior subluxation of the tibia in a posterior cruciate ligament–deficient knee.

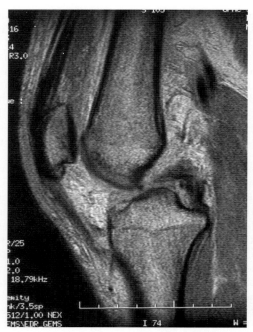

Figure 67-6 Sagittal magnetic resonance imaging view demonstrating a torn posterior cruciate ligament.

surgical stabilization may be advisable to prevent further progression.[77]

Magnetic resonance imaging (MRI) is highly sensitive and specific in the diagnosis and description of acute PCL tears, as well as being useful in identifying concomitant injuries such as to the PLSs (Figs. 67–5 and 67–6). One study demonstrated that MRI had 100% sensitivity and specificity in identifying complete tears of the PCL.[34] There is some evidence that PCL tears can heal in an elongated fashion, giving a chronic PCL tear an essentially normal signal appearance on MRI.[68] In these cases, an increase in posterior tibial translation on the

sagittal view may be the only indication of a PCL lesion. For this reason, MRI is not as sensitive in diagnosing chronic PCL injuries.

As stated previously, with any combined ligament injury involving the PCL, the physician must suspect a possible knee dislocation and rule out associated vascular injury. Patients with incomplete lesions (e.g., an intimal tear of the artery) have diminished but intact pulses. If there is any uncertainty, an arteriogram should be ordered.[31]

Examination under Anesthesia

Examination under anesthesia (EUA) is a valuable resource in diagnosing PCL and PLS injuries. PCL deficiency can be confirmed with the posterior drawer, posterior Lachman, and Godfrey (sag) tests. Further, PLS injuries that are subtle or absent on initial clinical examination can be demonstrated under anesthesia with asymmetrical external rotation (dial test), asymmetrical posterolateral drawer, and positive reversed pivot shift tests. It should be noted that many of these tests have a high false-positive rate, and comparison to the patient's contralateral knee is crucial in making an appropriate assessment.[14]

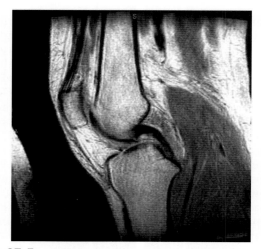

Figure 67-5 Sagittal magnetic resonance imaging view demonstrating a normal posterior cruciate ligament. The ligament has a curvilinear appearance, representative of the larger anterolateral band, which is relatively lax in full extension.

Diagnostic Arthroscopy

Diagnostic arthroscopy is carried out to document injury to the PCL and other intra-articular structures. It is a final confirmation of injury before reconstructing the PCL. Because the anterior, medial, and lateral aspects of the PCL are encased in synovium, an injury cannot be

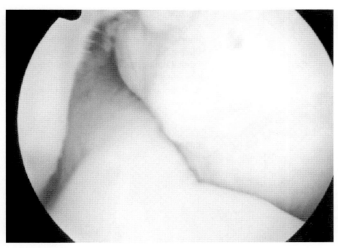

Figure 67–7   Intraoperative arthroscopy view of the "sloppy ACL" sign. Posterior subluxation of the tibia due to PCL deficiency causes pseudolaxity of the ACL and may be misinterpreted as ACL injury.

recognized until the ligament itself is visualized. Often a PCL tear is obscured by the ACL, and there is no obvious "stump," as is seen with ACL injuries.[23] Several signs can be recognized arthroscopically that support the diagnosis of a torn PCL. The native ACL appears lax in a PCL-deficient knee (Fig. 67–7). This "sloppy ACL" sign, or ACL pseudolaxity, results from posterior subluxation of the tibia. An anterior drawer can be applied to the knee to reduce the tibia and assess the native ACL. Failure to do so may result in misdiagnosis and an unnecessary ACL reconstruction. Additional arthroscopic findings in a PCL-injured knee include posterior displacement of the medial femoral condyle in relation to the medial meniscus and, in the setting of chronic PCL deficiency, chondrosis of the medial and patellofemoral compartments.[24]

Natural History

The natural history of an injury often guides decision making about the appropriate treatment options. Unfortunately, the natural history of isolated PCL injuries is the subject of continual debate. Many past studies supported the theory that isolated PCL injuries do well with nonoperative treatment.[63,77] Shelbourne and Patel[69] followed 133 patients with PCL injuries for an average of 5 years. The authors reported that nearly 50% of the patients returned to an equivalent or higher level of sports performance following nonoperative treatment. One third of the patients did not reach preinjury performance levels. Further, there was no increased radiographic evidence of osteoarthritis in the injured knees in the nonoperative treatment group. Parolie and Bergfeld[63] reported the results of 26 athletes treated nonoperatively for isolated PCL injuries. They found that 80% of the patients were subjectively satisfied with the outcome and that 68% had returned to their preinjury level of athletic performance following a nonoperative course of treatment. Favorable outcomes in this study were correlated

with maintenance of quadriceps strength. Other studies, however, have demonstrated mixed results, with patients doing well functionally but complaining of pain with activity. In a study evaluating the outcome of nonoperative treatment of PCL injury, Keller et al.[44] reported that 65% of their patients had activity limitations, with 90% reporting knee pain during activity, 43% complaining of problems while walking, and 45% reporting knee swelling. Other studies have demonstrated the development of medial compartment and patellofemoral degenerative changes with chronic PCL deficiency, as well as an increased risk of meniscal tears.[13,18,28]

More recent studies have emphasized the identification of prognostic factors that can predict outcome and assist in treatment decisions.[8,40,69] Inoue et al.[40] reported that gastrocnemius strength and medial and patellofemoral degenerative changes were predictive of functional outcome. In contrast, PCL laxity, chronicity of injury, and quadriceps strength were not predictive of outcome. Therefore, PCL injuries may not be as benign as originally thought, especially in the case of grade III injuries. One should also consider the healing potential of the PCL, which may contribute to the variable outcomes seen in PCL deficiency. A recent MRI study demonstrated that a high percentage of acutely injured PCLs are likely to heal, albeit in a somewhat elongated condition. This partial healing may establish a block to posterior translation, perhaps explaining why some patients do well functionally after PCL injury.[2]

Treatment Options: Indications and Contraindications

The approach to the treatment of PCL injuries should take into account the severity of the knee injury (isolated vs. combined), timing (acute vs. chronic), symptoms (asymptomatic vs. pain or instability), and activity level (athletic vs. sedentary lifestyle). Because of the controversy surrounding the natural history of PCL deficiency and the difficulties in accurately reconstructing the complex function of the PCL operatively, there is no consensus regarding the indications for PCL reconstruction. Most authors agree that avulsion fractures of the PCL should be acutely repaired with sutures through drill holes or screw fixation, usually with good results.[21,46,54,66] Additionally, combined injuries to the PCL and ACL, PLSs, or MCL should be surgically reconstructed, preferably within 2 weeks after injury to enable anatomic restoration and normal knee function.[23,36] Outside of these specific scenarios, the treatment decision algorithm needs to be individually tailored, taking into consideration injury severity and timing and patient expectations.

An algorithm for the treatment of acute PCL injuries is shown in Figure 67–8. In general, isolated PCL injuries (grades I and II) can be treated nonoperatively.[17,18,26,36,63,69,77] Treatment of acute grade I and II PCL injuries involves protected weight bearing and quadriceps muscle rehabilitation. The majority of patients are able to return to sports within 2 to 4 weeks after injury.

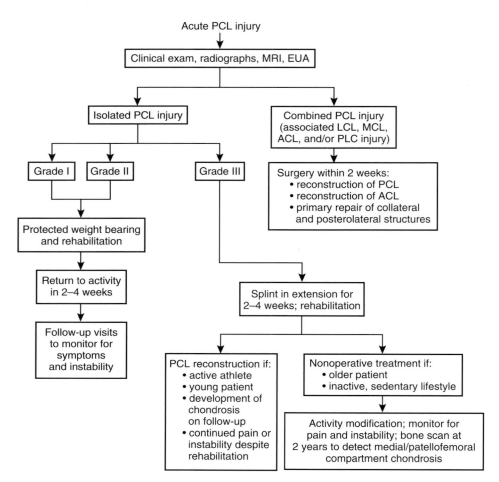

Figure 67–8 Treatment algorithm for acute posterior cruciate ligament (PCL) injury. ACL, anterior cruciate ligament; EUA, examination under anesthesia; LCL, lateral collateral ligament; MCL, medial collateral ligament; MRI, magnetic resonance imaging; PLC, posterolateral corner.

The outcome of acute grade III PCL injuries is not as predictable. Because of the risk of an occult injury to the posterolateral corner, it is recommended that the knee be splinted in extension for 2 to 4 weeks. Immobilization in extension decreases tension on the anterolateral fibers of the PCL and on the posterolateral corner, facilitating healing and minimizing posterior tibial translation secondary to hamstring tension and gravity.[36] After this period of immobilization, rehabilitation progresses as with grade I and II PCL injuries, but it generally takes an additional 8 weeks before a return to full activities. A functional brace may facilitate a return to sports in the acute postinjury setting, but it does not seem to be useful in cases of chronic PCL deficiency. Some grade III PCL injuries may require surgical treatment because of the development of medial or patellofemoral chondrosis or continuing complaints of instability despite adequate physical therapy.[13,17]

An algorithm for the treatment of chronic PCL injuries is shown in Figure 67–9. Chronic, isolated grade I or II PCL tears are treated with physical therapy. Symptomatic patients with recurrent swelling and pain are treated with activity modification, because surgical reconstruction of grade I or II injuries has not resulted in significant improvement in symptoms or function.[36] Chronic grade III PCL injuries are treated surgically if

symptoms of pain or instability develop or persist despite therapy. Some patients with "isolated" PCL injuries may in fact have occult posterolateral corner injuries, resulting in significant instability and pain. In this scenario, a PCL-PLS reconstruction is recommended, because surgical reconstruction of the PCL alone may have a higher risk of failure due to the concomitant PLS injury.[38]

When evaluating chronic PCL injuries for surgical intervention, it is important to determine whether there is varus malalignment of the knee and to evaluate the patient's gait for the presence of a dynamic varus thrust with ambulation.[55] With these findings, a high tibial osteotomy should be performed before PCL reconstruction.[60,61] A biplanar osteotomy has been used at our institution to correct varus deformity and reduce dynamic posterior tibial translation (by increasing tibial slope). Finally, patients with severe arthrosis should be excluded from consideration for PCL reconstruction.

Surgical Technique

Several different methods of PCL reconstruction have been described. However, there is no "gold standard" for PCL reconstruction that provides consistently excellent

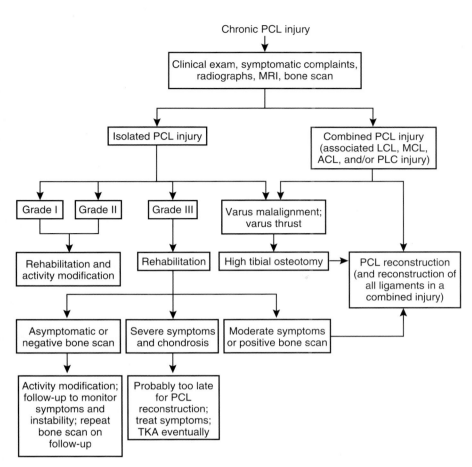

Figure 67–9   Treatment algorithm for chronic posterior cruciate ligament (PCL) injury. ACL, anterior cruciate ligament; LCL, lateral collateral ligament; MCL, medial collateral ligament; MRI, magnetic resonance imaging; PLC, posterolateral corner; TKA, total knee arthroplasty.

results. Because of the complexity of tensioning patterns in the two bands of the PCL, it is difficult to reproduce the position and function of the native ligament complex. Current reconstructive techniques include the transtibial single-bundle and double-bundle techniques and the tibial inlay technique.

Specific Surgical Steps

Graft Selection

Graft types can be divided into autografts, allografts, and synthetic grafts. In choosing a graft, one should consider graft length and cross-sectional area and to bony fixation at the ends of the graft. Autograft sources that are commonly used for PCL reconstruction include the patellar, hamstring, and quadriceps tendons.[11,13,48,73,74] The patellar tendon is the most commonly used graft for PCL reconstruction.[13] The proximal and distal bone plugs of this graft allow for rigid fixation. The hamstring tendon, although associated with relatively little donor site morbidity, provides inferior initial fixation than grafts that incorporate a bone plug.[83] The quadriceps tendon is a popular choice owing to the large graft size and the availability of tissue.[11] The large cross-sectional area and generous length of the quadriceps tendon graft allow for close approximation of the native PCL and mini-

mize problems related to graft tunnel length and size mismatch.

The allograft is an excellent alternative in PCL reconstruction, especially for knee injuries that involve multiple ligaments, for revision surgery, or for patients with general ligament laxity.[7,75] The Achilles tendon allograft is a popular choice for PCL reconstruction because of its generous cross-sectional area and calcaneal bone plug, which provides rigid bony fixation.[3,36] Advantages of using an allograft include reduced donor site morbidity and surgical time, as well as the ability to use multiple grafts when treating combined injuries or performing a double-bundle reconstruction. Concerns exist, however, regarding the increased risk of disease transmission, the delay in the remodeling process of the allograft compared with an autograft, and the excessive cost. Several studies have documented the differential delay in revascularization, cellular repopulation, and maturation of allograft versus autograft tendons.[42,59,70]

The use of synthetic grafts has been discouraged because of the poor results obtained in ACL reconstruction. Synthetic grafts are very stiff and do not simulate the biomechanical properties of ligaments and tendons. Attachment site problems, cyclic wear, foreign body reaction, and fatigue failure have drastically reduced the indications for using such grafts in knee ligament reconstruction.

6 Knee

Ligament Repair

Primary repair of midsubstance PCL tears has not been consistently successful.[6] However, PCL avulsions (bony or ligamentous) can typically be repaired with good results.[20,46] For large avulsion fragments, AO screws can be used; smaller fragments can be stabilized with Kirschner wires, tension band wiring, or suture repair through drill holes. Acute repair may have superior results compared with chronic treatment.[46]

Transtibial Tunnel Reconstruction: Single- and Double-Bundle Techniques

For both single- and double-bundle transtibial techniques for PCL reconstruction, the patient is placed in the supine position following an examination under anesthesia. A tourniquet is placed on the proximal thigh of the injured leg but is often not used, to reduce the risk of venous thrombosis. Because of the proximity of the vessels to the tibial tunnel, a qualified vascular surgeon should be immediately available in case of vascular injury. Fluid extravasation is also a potential problem in arthroscopic reconstruction of the PCL-injured knee, especially in the setting of multiple ligament injuries. The use of gravity flow through the arthroscope is recommended (rather than using a fluid pump) to reduce the risk of compartment syndrome. The surgeon should regularly palpate the calf and thigh preoperatively, intraoperatively, and postoperatively to evaluate for a developing compartment syndrome caused by fluid extravasation. If there is any concern about excessive fluid extravasation, the arthroscopic procedure should be abandoned, and an open reconstruction should be performed.

The patient is prepared and draped in the usual sterile fashion. Standard diagnostic arthroscopy is carried out to document injury to the PCL and to address any associated intra-articular pathology. Depending on graft selection, the graft is either harvested or thawed and then prepared according to the preferred technique of the surgeon.

Visualization of the tibial stump of the torn PCL is accomplished with a 70-degree arthroscope in the anterolateral portal. This scope allows adequate visualization of the tibial insertion site below the slope of the posterior tibial plateau. A posteromedial portal is used for elevation of the posterior capsule (using a curet or periosteal elevator) and debridement of the tibial PCL stump, allowing visualization of the tibial insertion site during tibial tunnel preparation. To avoid injury to the saphenous vein and nerve, the arthroscope is used to transilluminate the posteromedial corner while creating the posteromedial portal. A tibial drill guide is introduced through the anteromedial portal and positioned in the posterolateral aspect of the PCL tibial insertion site under arthroscopic visualization. The starting point for the guidewire is 4 cm distal to the joint line and 2 cm medial to the tibial tubercle. In preparation for drilling of the tibial tunnel, a 2- to 3-cm vertical skin incision is made. The guidewire is placed under arthroscopic visualization with the knee in 90 degrees of flexion (Fig.

67–10), and the position is checked using a lateral radiograph. In the lateral view, the guidewire should be placed at the level of the proximal tibia-fibula joint line and should exit the posterior tibial cortex approximately 10 mm below the tibial plateau (Fig. 67–11). A tibial tunnel of 10 or 11 mm is then drilled. The tibial tunnel must be drilled with great care, making sure to avoid overdrilling, which can perforate the posterior capsule and damage the popliteal vessels.

The single-bundle PCL reconstruction is designed to simulate the stronger and stiffer AL bundle of the PCL. The femoral tunnel starting point is positioned within the anatomic insertion site of the AL bundle of the intact PCL on the lateral wall of the medial femoral condyle. Several studies have shown that the location of the femoral tunnel has more impact on the reconstruction's ability to restore intact knee kinematics than does the position of the tibial tunnel.[10,33,72] Additionally, most authors agree that proximal to distal variation of the femoral tunnel has more effect on graft performance than does anterior to posterior variation.[33,62,72] The ideal placement of the femoral tunnel when reconstructing the AL bundle is 10 mm posterior to the articular cartilage of the medial femoral condyle and 13 mm inferior to the articular cartilage of the medial intercondylar roof (the 2 o'clock position on a right knee).[58] At our institution, we center the femoral tunnel 6 mm off the articular margin, at the 1 o'clock position in the right knee or the 11 o'clock position in the left knee. The femoral tunnel drill guide is inserted under arthroscopic visualization through the anterolateral portal. An 11-mm femoral tunnel is drilled following guidewire placement to a depth of 30 mm; then a 3.2-mm drill bit is used to complete a tunnel exit through the medial femoral condyle to allow graft passage and tensioning during fixation.

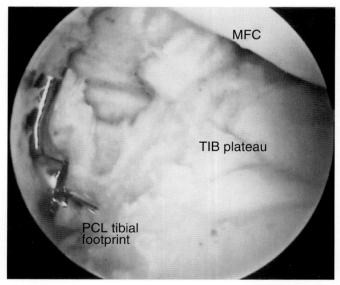

Figure 67–10 Arthroscopic view with 70-degree arthroscope showing positioning of the posterior cruciate ligament (PCL) guide on the PCL tibial footprint. MFC, medial femoral condyle; TIB, tibial.

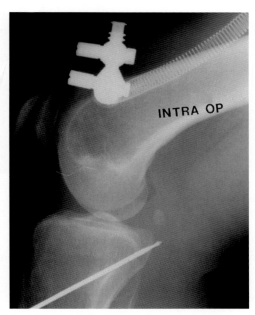

Figure 67–11 Lateral radiograph demonstrating posterior cruciate ligament tibial guide pin placement.

In the single-bundle technique, graft passage is determined by the type of graft used. When using Achilles tendon or quadriceps tendon, we recommend passing the graft from the femur to the tibia. If one elects to use a patellar tendon graft for PCL reconstruction, we recommend passing the graft from the tibia to the femur. This allows easier graft passage around the posterior corner of the tibia. At our institution, we use Achilles tendon allograft for single-bundle PCL reconstructions. An 18-gauge wire loop is placed up through the tibial tunnel into the knee joint and pulled out through the anterolateral portal. The whipstitch sutures of the soft tissue end of the Achilles allograft are then pulled into the knee and antegrade out through the tibial tunnel using the wire loop, advancing the soft tissue end of the graft into the tibial tunnel. A Beath needle is then advanced via the anterolateral portal into the femoral tunnel and out through the skin of the anteromedial thigh. The bone plug sutures of the graft are threaded through the eye of the Beath needle, and the needle and sutures are pulled retrograde out through the femoral tunnel, advancing the bone plug into the femoral tunnel.

The double-bundle PCL reconstruction uses two femoral tunnels in an attempt to re-create the functional anatomy of the AL and PM bundles of the native PCL. It has been hypothesized that double-bundle PCL reconstruction more closely restores normal knee mechanics throughout the entire flexion-extension cycle.[11,12,37,50,64,73] Harner et al.,[37] in a biomechanical study comparing single- and double-bundle PCL reconstruction techniques, reported that double-bundle reconstruction restored posterior tibial laxity equivalent to that of the intact knee, and it restored the in situ force of the PCL more closely to that of the intact knee than did single-bundle reconstruction.

Two divergent femoral tunnels are required for double-bundle reconstruction. The femoral tunnel for the AL graft is placed as discussed earlier for the single-bundle technique. The 6- or 7-mm-diameter PM tunnel is placed within the PCL footprint inferior to and slightly deeper in the intercondylar notch than the AL tunnel (3 to 4 mm of the articular margin, at the 2:30 o'clock position in the right knee or 9:30 in the left knee). A bone bridge of at least 5 mm should be preserved to avoid tunnel bridge collapse (Figs. 67–12 and 67–13). Harner and Baek[35] reported a PCL femoral insertion area of 128 mm². This large femoral footprint provides enough surface area to accommodate the two tunnels. To most

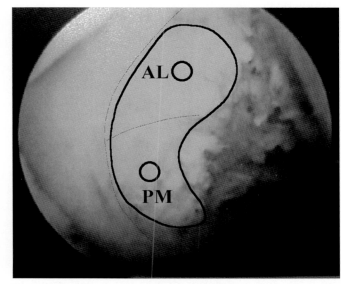

Figure 67–12 Position of the anterolateral (AL) and posteromedial (PM) femoral tunnels for double-bundle posterior cruciate ligament reconstruction.

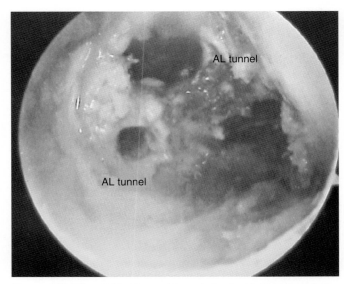

Figure 67–13 Drilled femoral tunnels for double-bundle posterior cruciate ligament reconstruction. AL, anterolateral.

6 Knee

accurately simulate the intact PCL, graft selection and tunnel size should be proportionate to the size and strength of the native AL and PM bundles. At our institution, a 10-mm Achilles allograft and a 7- to 8-mm doubled semitendinosus autograft are used to reconstruct the AL and PM bundles, respectively (Fig. 67–14).[37]

In the double-bundle technique, two separate grafts or a split graft are passed through the tibial tunnel and then fixed in separate femoral tunnels.

The method of graft fixation for single- or double-bundle reconstructions varies greatly, depending on graft selection. Bone block fixation can be achieved using an interference screw. A variety of techniques exist for fixation of the soft tissue end of a graft. Options that provide secure fixation include a soft tissue interference screw (biodegradable), a screw and spike washer, or an Endobutton. Use of an Endobutton requires modification when drilling the femoral tunnel. For patellar tendon grafts, we do not believe that fixation with an interference screw on the tibia is sufficient and suggest augmentation with a post and washer on the tibial side.[36] The graft should be preconditioned before final fixation to minimize graft elongation. This is accomplished by cycling the knee through the in situ range of motion several times while applying tension (10 pounds) to the graft.

During fixation of the graft in the single-bundle reconstruction, the knee is held in 70 to 90 degrees of flexion, and an anterior drawer force is applied to recover the normal step-off between the medial femoral condyle and the medial tibial plateau. Harner et al.[37] showed, in a biomechanical cadaveric study, that these fixation conditions are optimal for restoring intact knee biomechanics. Tension is applied to the unfixed end of the graft, and a posterior drawer test is performed to confirm that PCL stability has been restored. Final fixation is performed using one of the methods discussed earlier (Fig. 67–15).

In the double-bundle reconstruction, the AL graft is fixed under the same conditions described earlier. The PM graft is fixed while an anterior drawer is applied to the tibia near full extension and tension is held on the graft.[37] Like the AL graft, the PM graft should be preconditioned to minimize elongation following fixation. Fixing the PM graft under these conditions provides

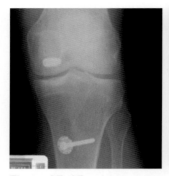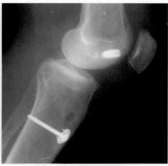

Figure 67–15   Postoperative anteroposterior and lateral radiographs of single-bundle posterior cruciate ligament reconstruction.

increased posterior stability near full extension (Fig. 67–16).

Tibial Inlay Technique

The inlay technique for PCL reconstruction was first described in Europe by Thomann and Gaechter[76] in 1994 and in the United States by Berg[4] a year later. This technique provides anatomic reconstruction of the AL bundle of the PCL. Modifications can be made using split grafts that allow for a double-bundle reconstruction. The tibial inlay technique of PCL reconstruction uses a posterior approach to the knee to allow a graft bone inlay to be secured directly to the posterior tibia in a trough placed in the original PCL footprint. This method of tibial fixation avoids the sharp angle of the graft at the proximal margin of the tibial tunnel in the traditional transtibial technique. It has been proposed that this "killer turn" generates increased graft stress and friction, which may contribute to graft elongation or failure after initial fixation.[4,55,76] Bergfeld et al.[5] performed a

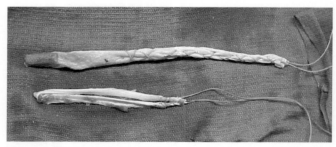

Figure 67–14   Achilles tendon allograft and doubled semitendinosus autograft used to reconstruct the anterolateral and posteromedial bundles, respectively, for double-bundle posterior cruciate ligament reconstruction.

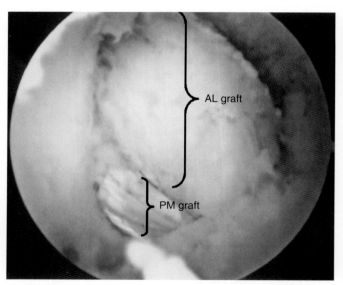

Figure 67–16   Arthroscopic view of double-bundle posterior cruciate ligament reconstruction. AL, anterolateral; PM, posteromedial.

biomechanical comparison of tibial inlay and transtibial reconstructions in cadaver knees and concluded that the tibial inlay technique results in less posterior translation and less graft degradation (caused by the sharp turn the graft makes at the back of the tibia) compared with the transtibial tunnel technique. More recent biomechanical studies, however, failed to show a significant difference in knee stability when comparing the inlay and transtibial techniques.[51,53]

For the tibial inlay technique, the patient is positioned in the lateral decubitus position with the operative leg up. From this position, a posterior approach to the tibial insertion of the PCL can be made directly. Additionally, the hip can be abducted and externally rotated 45 degrees and the knee can be flexed to 90 degrees with the foot on the operating table to perform standard arthroscopy, graft harvest, femoral tunnel placement, and graft passage. This method of positioning avoids having to turn the patient prone after performing arthroscopy.

Following examination under anesthesia, the patient is positioned in the lateral decubitus position. The hip is abducted and externally rotated, and the knee is flexed. Arthroscopy is carried out to document injury to the PCL and to address any associated intra-articular pathology. The inlay technique requires that at least one end of the graft have a bony block for fixation, limiting graft selection to the patellar tendon, quadriceps tendon, or Achilles tendon. Berg[4] originally described this technique using a bone–patellar tendon–bone graft, which remains the most commonly used graft for the inlay procedure. The bone plug that will be fixed in the tibial trough is fashioned with a flattened surface and is drilled during graft preparation to accept a 4.5-mm cortical screw. The plug to be fixed on the femoral side is contoured into a bullet-tipped cylinder shape to facilitate graft passage.

Following arthroscopic debridement of the PCL stump, a femoral drill guide is positioned in the anterior portion of the PCL footprint at its femoral insertion. The starting point is centered on the medial cortex of the medial femoral condyle. The entry point is more proximal to preserve subchondral bone and reduce the risk of avascular necrosis of the medial femoral condyle. The guide tip is placed 8 mm from the medial femoral condyle articular surface at the 11 or 1 o'clock position, and the tunnel is drilled to the appropriate size for the prepared graft. A looped 18-gauge wire or graft passer, which will be used later to pass the graft, is placed antegrade through the femoral tunnel into the joint. The injured leg of the patient is then repositioned in preparation for the posterior approach, with the knee extended and the leg abducted. Different posterior approaches used in the tibial inlay procedure have been described in the literature.[4,9] Burks and Schaffer[9] described a horizontal incision over the popliteal crease that has an extension over the medial head of the gastrocnemius. The interval between the medial head of the gastrocnemius and semitendinosus is developed bluntly to expose the posterior joint capsule. Lateral retraction of the gastrocnemius provides access to the posterior capsule of the knee and protects the neurovascular

structures of the popliteal fossa. The posterior tibial sulcus (PCL insertion site) and wire loop should be palpable, and a vertical capsule incision then exposes the PCL footprint on the tibia.

After exposing the tibial sulcus, an osteotome is used to create a unicortical bone trough at the site of tibial PCL insertion large enough to accommodate the tibial side of the graft. The size of both the bone plug and trough can be adjusted to ensure a tight fit. The tibial side of the graft is placed in the trough and fixed to the tibia. The recommended method of fixation varies; options include staple fixation or using a 6.5-mm cancellous screw and a flat washer or a 4.5-mm cortical screw with bicortical fixation. The graft is passed retrograde through the notch and into the femoral tunnel using the prepositioned 18-gauge wire. If a bone–patellar tendon–bone graft is used, the femoral bone plug is positioned in the femoral tunnel, and the graft is tensioned and preconditioned by passively cycling the knee through its full range of motion. Ideally, the bone plug is positioned flush with the articular joint surface. If the bone plug is positioned too far into the femoral tunnel, the tibial trough and tibial bone plug can be moved distally. Fixation is achieved using an interference screw in the femoral tunnel. If an Achilles or quadriceps graft is used, the soft tissue end of the graft is passed retrograde through the femoral tunnel, tensioned, preconditioned, and fixed using a screw and spiked washer. The graft is fixed in a manner similar to that described earlier for the transtibial technique: with the knee flexed 70 to 90 degrees and an anterior drawer force applied to the tibia, tension is placed on the sutures exiting the femoral tunnel. After fixation, a posterior drawer test assesses the stability of the reconstruction.

Postoperative Management

Most postoperative PCL reconstruction protocols brace the knee in extension for 4 weeks, supporting the tibia to prevent posterior translation and excessive stress on the graft. Partial weight bearing as tolerated and quadriceps exercises start on the first postoperative day. Closed chain exercises start at approximately 6 weeks, followed by proprioceptive training at 12 weeks, increasing knee stability. Range-of-motion exercises are essential to regaining full knee flexion. Patients are progressed slowly through passive flexion exercises in the early postoperative period and, in most cases, regain full flexion in 5 to 7 months. Hamstring exercises are delayed for 4 months, because they place excessive posterior loads on the tibia during the early stages of graft healing. Light jogging begins at 6 months. The patient is allowed to return to full activities 9 to 12 months after surgery, depending on the individual demands of daily activity and the progression of physical therapy. The goal of rehabilitation is to achieve adequate knee stability, full range of motion, and quadriceps strength that is symmetrical to that of the contralateral leg. A structured physical therapy program is essential to regaining motion, strength, and proprioception.

6 Knee

Complications

As with any operation, PCL reconstruction involves the risks of infection and bleeding. These risks can be minimized with appropriate draping and sterile technique, careful dissection, and hemostasis. The use of a tourniquet is controversial. Although it allows for better hemostasis during surgery, it may increase the risk of venous thrombosis and neurapraxia. Additionally, complications of PCL reconstruction can occur as a result of improper preoperative positioning, poor operative technique, intraoperative injury to neurovascular structures, and inadequate postoperative rehabilitation.

Because PCL reconstructions tend to be lengthy procedures, failure to carefully position the extremities with adequate padding can lead to neurapraxia. Loss of motion following PCL reconstruction (usually decreased flexion) can result from errors in graft positioning and excessive tensioning of the graft during fixation. Fixing the AL graft in extension may result in increased graft tension and subsequent loss of motion at positions of increased knee flexion. Further, inadequate range-of-motion exercises during postoperative rehabilitation can lead to loss of motion that requires manipulation or surgical intervention to correct.

Nerve and vascular injuries rarely occur during PCL reconstruction. Peroneal nerve injuries are more common in combined injuries that require PLS reconstruction. Neurapraxia often resolves with time (12 to 18 months), whereas complete nerve injuries have a much lower chance of recovery. Injury to the popliteal vessels is an infrequent but serious complication. In the transtibial technique, great care must be taken to avoid over-drilling, given the close proximity of the popliteal artery and vein. During the posterior approach of the inlay technique, the popliteal vessels are encountered, and care must be taken to protect these structures to avoid intraoperative injury.

Fluid extravasation is also a potential problem in arthroscopic reconstruction of the PCL-injured knee, especially in the setting of a multiple ligament injury. The surgeon should regularly palpate the calf and thigh preoperatively, intraoperatively, and postoperatively to evaluate for a developing compartment syndrome caused by fluid extravasation.

Proper operative technique when drilling the femoral tunnel is critical to avoid the risk of avascular necrosis of the medial femoral condyle. The entry-exit point of the femoral tunnel on the medial femoral condyle should be placed proximal enough to allow the preservation of subchondral bone.

The development of residual posterior laxity following PCL reconstruction can also be considered a complication of surgery. The majority of patients undergoing PCL reconstruction do develop late posterior laxity that may or may not manifest clinically. Accurate tunnel placement, anatomic fixation, and repair or reconstruction of associated ligamentous injuries may help minimize clinically significant posterior laxity following surgery.

Future Directions

PCL injuries are not as benign or rare as was once assumed. Recent studies examining the biomechanical properties and anatomy of the PCL have led to new surgical techniques in PCL reconstruction that attempt to duplicate the functional behavior of the native PCL from full flexion to full extension. Further studies are needed to fully evaluate the long-term clinical effectiveness of single-bundle PCL reconstruction compared with tibial inlay and double-bundle PCL reconstruction techniques, and whether these reconstructive techniques truly improve on or alter the clinical course of chronic PCL deficiency.

References

1. Abbott LC, Saunders JBN, Bost FC: Injuries to the ligaments of the knee joint. J Bone Joint Surg Am 26:503-521, 1944.
2. Akisue T, Kurosaka M, Yoshiya S, et al: Evaluation of healing of the injured posterior cruciate ligament: Analysis of instability and magnetic resonance imaging. Arthroscopy 17:264-269, 2001.
3. Annunziata CC, Giffin JR, Harner CD: PCL reconstruction. Curr Orthop 14:329-336, 2000.
4. Berg EE: Posterior cruciate ligament tibial inlay reconstruction. Arthroscopy 11:69-76, 1995.
5. Bergfeld JA, McAllister DR, Parker RD, et al: A biomechanical comparison of posterior cruciate ligament reconstruction techniques. Am J Sports Med 29:129-136, 2001.
6. Bianchi M: Acute tears of the posterior cruciate ligament: Clinical study and results of operative treatment in 27 cases. Am J Sports Med 11:308-314, 1983.
7. Borden PS, Nyland JA, Caborn DN: Posterior cruciate ligament reconstruction (double bundle) using anterior tibialis tendon allograft. Arthroscopy 17:E14, 2001.
8. Boynton MD, Tietjens BR: Long-term follow-up of untreated posterior cruciate deficient knees. Am J Sports Med 24:306-310, 1996.
9. Burks RT, Schaffer JJ: A simplified approach to the tibial attachment of the posterior cruciate ligament. Clin Orthop 254:216-219, 1990.
10. Burns WC, Draganich LF, Pyevich MP: The effect of femoral tunnel position and graft tensioning technique on posterior laxity of the posterior cruciate ligament–reconstructed knee. Am J Sports Med 23:424-430, 1995.
11. Chen C-H, Chen W-J, Shih C-H: Arthroscopic double-bundled posterior cruciate ligament reconstruction with quadriceps tendon-patellar bone autograft. Arthroscopy 16:780-782, 2000.
12. Clancy WG, Bisson LJ: Double bundle technique for reconstruction of the posterior cruciate ligament. Oper Tech Sports Med 7:110-117, 1999.
13. Clancy WG, Shelbourne KD, Zoellner GB, et al: Treatment of knee joint instability secondary to rupture of the posterior cruciate ligament: Report of a new procedure. J Bone Joint Surg Am 65:310-322, 1983.
14. Cooper DE: Tests for posterolateral instability of the knee in normal subjects: Results of examination under anesthesia. J Bone Joint Surg Am 73:30-36, 1991.
15. Cosgarea AJ, Jay PR: Posterior cruciate ligament injuries: Evaluation and treatment. J Am Acad Orthop Surg 9:297-307, 2001.

16. Covey DC: Current concepts review: Injuries of the posterolateral corner of the knee. J Bone Joint Surg Am 83:106-118, 2001.

17. Covey DC, Sapega AA: Injuries to the posterior cruciate ligament. J Bone Joint Surg Am 75:1376-1386, 1993.

18. Dandy DJ, Pusey RJ: The long term results of unrepaired tears of the posterior cruciate ligament. J Bone Joint Surg Br 64:92-94, 1982.

19. Daniel DM, Stone ML, Barnett P, et al: Use of the quadriceps active test to diagnose posterior cruciate ligament disruption and measure posterior laxity of the knee. J Bone Joint Surg Am 70:386-391, 1988.

20. Deehan DJ, Pinczewski LA: Technical note: Arthroscopic reattachment of an avulsion fracture of the tibial insertion of the posterior cruciate ligament. Arthroscopy 17:422-425, 2001.

21. Espejo-Baena A, Lopez-Arevalo R, Urbano V, et al: Arthroscopic repair of the posterior cruciate ligament: Two techniques. Arthroscopy 16:656-660, 2000.

22. Fanelli GC: The dislocated knee: Treatment of combined anterior cruciate ligament–posterior cruciate ligament–lateral side injuries of the knee. Clin Sports Med 19:493-502, 2000.

23. Fanelli GC, Edson CJ: Posterior cruciate ligament injuries in trauma patients. Part II. Arthroscopy 11:526-529, 1995.

24. Fanelli GC, Giannotti BF, Edson CJ: Current concepts review. The posterior cruciate ligament: Arthroscopic evaluation and treatment. Arthroscopy 10:673-688, 1994.

25. Fleming RE, Blatz DJ, McCarroll JR: Posterior problems in the knee. Am J Sports Med 9:107-113, 1981.

26. Fowler PJ, Messieh SS: Isolated posterior cruciate ligament injuries in athletes. Am J Sports Med 15:553-557, 1987.

27. Fu FH, Harner CD, Johnson DL, et al: Biomechanics of knee ligaments: Basic concepts and clinical application. J Bone Joint Surg Am 75:1716-1727, 1993.

28. Geissler WB, Whipple TL: Intraarticular abnormalities in association with posterior cruciate ligament injuries. Am J Sports Med 21:846-849, 1993.

29. Girgis FG, Marshall JL, Monajem ARSA: The cruciate ligaments of the knee joint: Anatomical, functional and experimental analysis. Clin Orthop 106:216-231, 1975.

30. Godfrey JD: Ligamentous injuries of the knee. Curr Pract Orthop Surg 5:56-92, 1973.

31. Good L, Johnson RJ: The dislocated knee. J Am Acad Orthop Surg 3:284-292, 1995.

32. Green NE, Allen BL: Vascular injuries associated with dislocation of the knee. J Bone Joint Surg Am 59:236-239, 1977.

33. Grood ES, Hefzy MS, Lindenfeld TN: Factors affecting the region of most isometric femoral attachments. Part I. The posterior cruciate ligament. Am J Sports Med 17:197-207, 1989.

34. Gross ML, Grover JS, Bassett LW, et al: Magnetic resonance imaging of the posterior cruciate ligament: Clinical use to improve diagnostic accuracy. Am J Sports Med 20:732-737, 1992.

35. Harner CD, Baek GH: Quantitative analysis of human cruciate ligament insertions. Arthroscopy 15:741-749, 1999.

36. Harner CD, Hoher J: Evaluation and treatment of posterior cruciate ligament injuries. Am J Sports Med 26:471-482, 1998.

37. Harner CD, Janaushek MA, Kanamori A, et al: Biomechanical analysis of a double-bundle posterior cruciate ligament reconstruction. Am J Sports Med 28:144-151, 2000.

38. Harner CD, Vogrin TM, Hoher J, et al: Biomechanical analysis of a posterior cruciate ligament reconstruction: Deficiency of the posterolateral structures as a cause of graft failure. Am J Sports Med 1:32-39, 2000.

39. Harner CD, Xerogeanes JW, Livesay GA: The human posterior cruciate ligament complex: An interdisciplinary study. Ligament morphology and biomechanical evaluation. Am J Sports Med 23:736-745, 1995.

40. Inoue M, Yasuda K, Ohkoshi Y: Factors that affect prognosis of conservatively treated patients with isolated posterior cruciate ligament injury. Paper presented at the 64th Annual Meeting of the American Academy of Orthopaedic Surgeons, 1997, San Francisco.

41. Insall JN, Hood RW: Bone-block transfer of the medial head of the gastrocnemius for posterior cruciate insufficiency. J Bone Joint Surg Am 64:691-699, 1982.

42. Jackson DW, Corsetti J, Simon TM: Biologic incorporation of allograft anterior cruciate ligament replacements. Clin Orthop 324:126-133, 1996.

43. Kannus P, Bergfeld JA, Jarvinen M: Injuries to the posterior cruciate ligament of the knee. Sports Med 12:110-131, 1991.

44. Keller PM, Shelbourne KD, McCarroll JR, et al: Nonoperatively treated isolated posterior cruciate ligament injuries. Am J Sports Med 21:132-136, 1993.

45. Kennedy JC, Hawkins RJ, Willis RB: Tension studies of human knee ligaments. J Bone Joint Surg Am 58:350-355, 1976.

46. Kim S-J, Shin S-J, Choi N-H, et al: Arthroscopically assisted treatment of avulsion fractures of the posterior cruciate ligament from the tibia. J Bone Joint Surg Am 83:698-708, 2001.

47. Kusayama T, Harner CD, Carlin GJ: Anatomical and biomechanical characteristics of human meniscofemoral ligaments. Knee Surg Sports Traumatol Arthrosc 2:234-237, 1994.

48. Lipscomb AB, Johnston RK, Snyder RB: The technique of cruciate ligament reconstruction. Am J Sports Med 9:77-92, 1981.

49. Makris CA, Georgoulis AD, Papageorgiou CD, et al: Posterior cruciate ligament architecture: Evaluation under microsurgical dissection. Arthroscopy 16:627-632, 2000.

50. Mannor DA, Shearn JT, Grood ES, et al: Two-bundle posterior cruciate ligament reconstruction: An in vitro analysis of graft placement and tension. Am J Sports Med 28:833-845, 2000.

51. Margheritini F, Mauro CS, Stabile KJ: Biomechanical comparison of tibial inlay and trans-tibial tunnel PCL reconstructions. Paper presented at the 10th Congress of the European Society of Sports, Traumatology, Knee Surgery and Arthroscopy, 2002, Rome, Italy.

52. Matava MJ, Sethi NS, Totty WG: Proximity of the posterior cruciate ligament insertion to the popliteal artery as a function of the knee flexion angle: Implication for posterior cruciate ligament reconstruction. Arthroscopy 16:796-804, 2000.

53. McAllister D, Markolf K, Oakes D: A biomechanical study of posterior cruciate ligament reconstruction techniques: Analysis of graft pretensions and laxities. Paper presented at the 47th annual meeting of the Orthopaedic Research Society, 2001, San Francisco, CA.

54. Meyers MH: Isolated avulsion of the tibial attachment of the posterior cruciate ligament of the knee. J Bone Joint Surg Am 57:669-672, 1975.

55. Miller MD, Bergfeld JA, Fowler PJ, et al: The posterior cruciate ligament injured knee: Principles of evaluation and treatment. Instr Course Lect 48:199-206, 1999.

56. Miller MD, Cooper DE, Fanelli GC, et al: Posterior cruciate ligament: Current concepts. Instr Course Lect 51:347-351, 2002.

6 Knee

57. Miyasaka KC, Daniel DM: The incidence of knee ligament injuries in the general population. Am J Knee Surg 4:3-8, 1991.

58. Morgan CD, Kalman VR, Grawl DM: The anatomic origin of the posterior cruciate ligament: Where is it? Reference landmarks for PCL reconstruction. Arthroscopy 13:325-331, 1997.

59. Nikolaou PK, Seaber AV, Glisson RR, et al: Anterior cruciate ligament allograft transplantation: Long-term function, histology, revascularization, and operative technique. Am J Sports Med 14:348-360, 1986.

60. Noyes FR, Barber-Westin SD: Treatment of complex injuries involving the posterior cruciate and posterolateral ligaments of the knee. Am J Knee Surg 9:200-214, 1996.

61. Noyes FR, Roberts CS: High tibial osteotomy in knees with associated chronic ligament deficiencies. In Jackson DW (ed): Reconstructive Knee Surgery. New York, Raven Press, 1995, pp 185-210.

62. Ogata K, McCarthy JA: Measurements of length and tension patterns during reconstruction of the posterior cruciate ligament. Am J Sports Med 20:351-355, 1992.

63. Parolie JM, Bergfeld JA: Long-term results of nonoperative treatment of isolated posterior cruciate ligament injuries in the athlete. Am J Sports Med 14:35-38, 1986.

64. Petrie RS, Harner CD: Double bundle posterior cruciate ligament reconstruction technique: University of Pittsburgh approach. Oper Tech Sports Med 7:118-126, 1999.

65. Race A, Amis AA: The mechanical properties of the two bundles of the human posterior cruciate ligament. J Biomech 27:13-24, 1994.

66. Richter M, Kiefer H, Hehl G, et al: Primary repair for posterior cruciate ligament injuries: An eight-year followup of fifty-three patients. Am J Sports Med 24:298-305, 1996.

67. Shelbourne KD, Benedict F, McCarroll JR, et al: Dynamic posterior shift test: An adjuvant in evaluation of posterior tibial subluxation. Am J Sports Med 17:275-277, 1989.

68. Shelbourne KD, Jennings RW, Vahey TN: Magnetic resonance imaging of posterior cruciate ligament injuries: Assessment of healing. Am J Knee Surg 12:209-213, 1999.

69. Shelbourne KD, Patel DV: The natural history of acute, isolated, nonoperatively treated posterior cruciate ligament injuries of the knee: A prospective study. Paper presented at the 64th Annual Meeting of the American Academy of Orthopaedic Surgeons, 1997, San Francisco.

70. Shino K, Inoue M, Horibe S, et al: Maturation of allograft tendons transplanted into the knee: An arthroscopic and histological study. J Bone Joint Surg Br 70:556-560, 1988.

71. Shino K, Mitsuoka T, Horibe S, et al: The gravity sag view: A simple radiographic technique to show posterior laxity of the knee. Arthroscopy 16:670-672, 2000.

72. Sidles JA, Larson RV, Garbini JL: Ligament length relationship in the moving knee. J Orthop Res 6:593-610, 1988.

73. Stahelin AC, Sudkamp NP, Weiler A: Anatomic double-bundle posterior cruciate ligament reconstruction using hamstring tendons. Arthroscopy 17:88-97, 2001.

74. Staubli HU, Schatzmann C, Brunner P: Quadriceps tendon and patellar ligament: Cryosectional anatomy and structural properties in young adults. Knee Surg Sports Traumatol Arthrosc 4:100-110, 1996.

75. Swenson TM, Harner CD, Fu FH: Arthroscopic posterior cruciate ligament reconstruction with allograft. Sports Med Arthrosc Rev 2:120-128, 1994.

76. Thomann YR, Gaechter A: Dorsal approach for reconstruction of the posterior cruciate ligament. Arch Orthop Trauma Surg 113:142-148, 1994.

77. Torg JS, Barton TM, Pavlov H, et al: Natural history of the posterior cruciate ligament–deficient knee. Clin Orthop 246:208-216, 1989.

78. Torg JS, Conrad W, Kalen V: Clinical diagnosis of anterior cruciate ligament instability in the athlete. Am J Sports Med 4:84-93, 1976.

79. VanDommelen BA, Fowler PJ: Anatomy of the posterior cruciate ligament: A review. Am J Sports Med 17:24-29, 1989.

80. Veltri DM, Warren RF: Posterolateral instability of the knee. Instr Course Lect 44:441-453, 1995.

81. Wascher DC, Dvimak PC, DeCoster TA: Knee dislocation: Initial assessment and implications for treatment. J Orthop Trauma 11:525-529, 1997.

82. Whipple TL, Ellis FD: Posterior cruciate ligament injuries. Clin Sports Med 10:515-527, 1991.

83. Yasuda K, Tsujino J, Ohkoshi Y: Graft site morbidity with autologous semitendinosus and gracilis tendons. Am J Sports Med 23:706-714, 1995.

CHAPTER

68

Transtibial Tunnel PCL Reconstruction

GREGORY C. FANELLI

TRANSTIBIAL TUNNEL PCL RECONSTRUCTION IN A NUTSHELL

History:
  Posterior blow to tibia; hyperflexion or hyperextension injury; combined injury (especially posterolateral corner)

Physical Examination:
  Posterior drawer; external rotation symmetry (dial test)

Imaging:
  Plain radiographs: patellofemoral and medial compartment degenerative joint disease if chronic; stress radiographs; magnetic resonance imaging

Indications:
  Symptomatic grade II or III injury; all combined injuries

Surgical Technique:
  Safety incision; "low" transtibial tunnel; drill tibial tunnel (use caution); create femoral tunnel; graft passage and tensioning (tensioning boot); graft fixation with backup

Postoperative Management:
  Full extension at 6 weeks; range of motion at 4 weeks; non–weight bearing, then progressive weight bearing at weeks 7 to 10; return to sports at 9 months

Results:
  Normal posterior drawer: 70%
  Grade I posterior drawer: 77%

This chapter describes my technique of arthroscopic single bundle–single femoral tunnel transtibial posterior cruciate ligament (PCL) reconstruction and presents the Fanelli Sports Injury Clinic's 2- to 10-year results using this technique. The information in this chapter has been presented elsewhere, and the reader is referred to these sources for additional information.[1-15]

Surgical Technique

Positioning, Examination under Anesthesia, and Diagnostic Arthroscopy

The patient is positioned on the operating table in the supine position, and the surgical and nonsurgical knees are examined under general anesthesia. A tourniquet is applied to the operative extremity, and the surgical leg is prepared and draped in a sterile fashion. Allograft tissue is prepared before beginning the surgical procedure, and autograft tissue is harvested before the arthroscopic portion of the procedure is begun. The inflow is inserted through the superolateral patellar portal, the arthroscope through the inferolateral patellar portal, and the instruments through the inferomedial patellar portal. The portals are interchanged as necessary. The joint is thoroughly evaluated arthroscopically, and the PCL is evaluated using the three-zone arthroscopic technique.[9] The PCL tear is identified, and the residual stump of the ligament is debrided with hand tools and the synovial shaver.

Specific Surgical Steps

Initial Incision

An extracapsular posteromedial safety incision approximately 1.5 to 2 cm long is created (Fig. 68–1). The crural fascia is incised longitudinally, taking precautions to protect the neurovascular structures. The interval is developed between the medial head of the gastrocnemius muscle and the posterior capsule of the knee joint, which is anterior. The neurovascular structures should be posterior to the surgeon's gloved finger, and the posterior aspect of the joint capsule anterior to the finger. This technique enables the surgeon to monitor surgical instruments, such as the over-the-top PCL instruments and the PCL–anterior cruciate ligament (ACL) drill guide, as they are positioned in the posterior aspect of the knee. The surgeon's finger in the posteromedial safety incision also confirms accurate placement of the guidewire before tibial tunnel drilling in the medial-lateral and proximal-distal directions (Fig. 68–2).

Posterior Capsule Elevation

The curved over-the-top PCL instruments are used to carefully lyse adhesions in the posterior aspect of the knee and to elevate the posterior knee joint capsule away from the tibial ridge on the posterior aspect of the tibia.

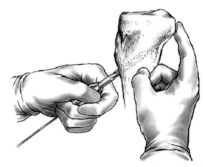

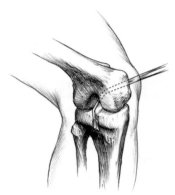

Figure 68–2 The surgeon can palpate the posterior aspect of the tibia through the extracapsular, extra-articular posteromedial safety incision. This enables the surgeon to accurately position guidewires, create the tibial tunnel, and protect the neurovascular structures. (Courtesy of Arthrotek, Inc., Warsaw, IN.)

Figure 68–3 Posterior capsular elevation using Arthrotek posterior cruciate ligament instruments. (Courtesy of Arthrotek, Inc., Warsaw, IN.)

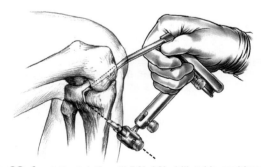

Figure 68–4 Arthrotek Fanelli PCL-ACL drill guide positioned to place the guidewire in preparation for creation of the tibial tunnel. (Courtesy of Arthrotek, Inc., Warsaw, IN.)

This capsular elevation enhances correct drill guide and tibial tunnel placement (Fig. 68–3).

Drill Guide Positioning

The arm of the Arthrotek Fanelli PCL-ACL drill guide (Arthrotek, Inc., Warsaw, IN) is inserted into the knee through the inferomedial patellar portal and positioned in the PCL fossa on the posterior tibia (Fig. 68–4). The

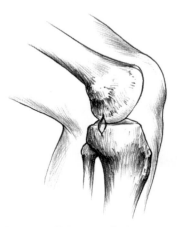

Figure 68–1 Posteromedial extra-articular, extracapsular safety incision. (Courtesy of Arthrotek, Inc., Warsaw, IN.)

bullet portion of the drill guide contacts the anteromedial aspect of the proximal tibia approximately 1 cm below the tibial tubercle, at a point midway between the tibial crest anteriorly and the posterior medial border of the tibia. This drill guide positioning creates a tibial tunnel that is relatively vertically oriented and has its posterior exit point in the inferior and lateral aspect of the PCL tibial anatomic insertion site. Thus, the angle of graft orientation is such that the graft turns with two smooth 45-degree angles on the posterior aspect of the tibia, eliminating the 90-degree "killer turn" (Fig. 68–5).

The tip of the guide in the posterior aspect of the tibia is confirmed with the surgeon's finger through the extracapsular posteromedial safety incision. Intraoperative anteroposterior and lateral radiographs, as well as arthroscopic visualization, can also be used to confirm drill guide and guide pin placement. A blunt, spade-tipped guidewire is drilled from anterior to posterior and can be visualized with the arthroscope, in addition to being palpated with the finger in the posteromedial safety incision. Having the finger in the posteromedial safety incision is the most important step for accuracy and safety.

Tibial Tunnel Drilling

A standard, appropriately sized cannulated reamer is used to create the tibial tunnel. The closed curved PCL curet may be positioned to cap the tip of the guidewire (Fig. 68–6). The arthroscope, when positioned in the posteromedial portal, visualizes the guidewire being captured by the curet. The surgeon's finger in the posteromedial safety incision monitors the position of the guidewire, thus protecting the neurovascular structures. The standard canulated drill is advanced to the posterior cortex of the tibia. The drill chuck is then disengaged from the drill, and the tibial tunnel reaming is completed by hand, providing an additional margin of safety. The tunnel edges are chamfered and rasped with the PCL-ACL system rasp (Fig. 68–7).

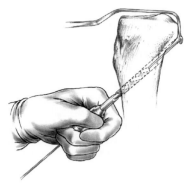

Figure 68–6 The Arthrotek posterior cruciate ligament closed curet is used to cap the guidewire during tibial tunnel drilling. (Courtesy of Arthrotek, Inc., Warsaw, IN.)

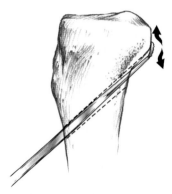

Figure 68–7 Tunnel edges are chamfered after drilling to smooth any roughness. (Courtesy of Arthrotek, Inc., Warsaw, IN.)

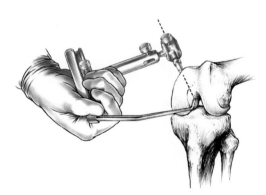

Figure 68–8 Arthrotek Fanelli PCL-ACL drill guide is positioned to drill the guidewire from outside in. The guidewire begins at a point halfway between the medial femoral epicondyle and the medial femoral condyle trochlear articular margin, approximately 2 to 3 cm proximal to the medial femoral condyle distal articular margin. It exits through the center of the anterolateral bundle of the posterior cruciate ligament stump. (Courtesy of Arthrotek, Inc., Warsaw, IN.)

Femoral Tunnel Drilling

The Arthrotek Fanelli PCL-ACL drill guide is positioned to create the femoral tunnel (Fig. 68–8). The arm of the guide is introduced into the knee through the inferomedial patellar portal and is positioned such that the guidewire will exit through the center of the stump of

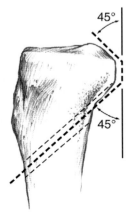

Figure 68–5 Desired turning angles of the posterior cruciate ligament graft after creation of the tibial tunnel. (Courtesy of Arthrotek, Inc., Warsaw, IN.)

the anterolateral bundle of the PCL. The blunt, spade-tipped guidewire is drilled through the guide, and just as it begins to emerge through the center of the stump of the PCL's anterolateral bundle, the drill guide is disengaged. The accuracy of the guidewire position is confirmed arthroscopically by probing and direct visualization. To ensure that the patellofemoral joint has not been violated, it is examined arthroscopically before drilling the femoral tunnel.

A standard, appropriately sized cannulated reamer is used to create the femoral tunnel. A curet is used to cap the tip of the guidewire to avoid inadvertent advancement of the guidewire, causing damage to the articular surface, the ACL, or other intra-articular structures. As the reamer is about to penetrate the wall of the intercondylar notch, it is disengaged from the drill, and the final femoral tunnel reaming is completed by hand for an additional margin of safety (Fig. 68–9). The reaming debris is evacuated with a synovial shaver to minimize the fat pad inflammatory response and the subsequent risk of arthrofibrosis. The tunnel edges are chamfered and rasped.

Tunnel Preparation and Graft Passage

The Arthrotek Magellan suture-passing device is introduced through the tibial tunnel and into the knee joint, and retrieved through the femoral tunnel with an arthroscopic grasping tool (Fig. 68–10). A 7.9-mm Gore-Tex Smoother (W. L. Gore, Inc., Flagstaff, AZ) flexible rasp is attached to the Magellan suture-passing device, and the smoother is pulled into the femoral tunnel, into the joint, and into and out of the tibial tunnel opening (Fig. 68–11). The tunnel edges are chamfered and rasped at 0, 30, 60, and 90 degrees of knee flexion. Care must be

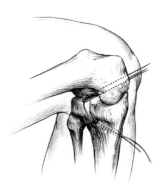

Figure 68–10   Retrieval of suture-passing wire. (Courtesy of Arthrotek, Inc., Warsaw, IN.)

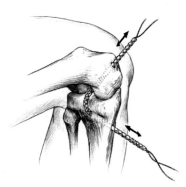

Figure 68–11   Tunnel rasping with Gore-Tex Smoother. (Courtesy of Arthrotek, Inc., Warsaw, IN.)

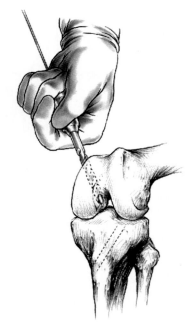

Figure 68–9   Femoral tunnel reaming is completed by hand, for an additional margin of safety. (Courtesy of Arthrotek, Inc., Warsaw, IN.)

taken to avoid excessive pressure when using the smoother, or the tunnel configuration could be altered or the bone destroyed. The traction sutures of the graft material are attached to the loop of the flexible rasp, and the PCL graft material is pulled into position.

Graft Tensioning and Fixation

Fixation of the PCL substitute is accomplished with primary and backup fixation on both the femoral and tibial sides. My preferred graft source for PCL reconstruction is the Achilles tendon allograft. Femoral fixation is accomplished with press-fit fixation of a wedge-shaped calcaneal bone plug and aperture-opening fixation using the Arthrotek Gentle Thread bioabsorbable interference screw; alternatively, one can use primary aperture-opening fixation with the Arthrotek Gentle Thread bioabsorbable interference screw and backup fixation with a ligament fixation button, screw and spiked ligament washer, or screw and post assembly. The Arthrotek Graft Tensioner is applied to the traction sutures of the graft material on its distal end, 20 pounds of tension is applied, and the knee is cycled through 25 full flexion-extension cycles for graft pretensioning and settling (Fig. 68–12). The knee is placed in approximately 70 degrees of flexion, and tibial fixation of the Achilles tendon allograft is achieved with primary aperture-opening fixation using the Arthrotek Gentle

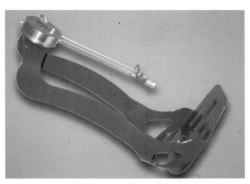

Figure 68–12 Arthrotek knee ligament Graft Tensioner boot. This mechanical tensioning device uses a ratcheted torque wrench to assist the surgeon during graft tensioning. (Courtesy of Arthrotek, Inc., Warsaw, IN.)

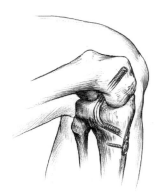

Figure 68–13 Final graft fixation using primary and backup fixation. (Courtesy of Arthrotek, Inc., Warsaw, IN.)

Thread bioabsorbable interference screw and backup fixation with a ligament fixation button, screw and post, or screw and spiked ligament washer assembly (Fig. 68–13).

Additional Surgery and Wound Closure

When multiple ligament surgeries are performed during the same operative session, the PCL reconstruction is performed first, followed by the ACL reconstruction and then collateral ligament surgery. The reader is referred to Chapters 71 and 72 for descriptions of multiple ligament surgeries of the knee.

At the completion of the procedure the tourniquet is deflated and the wounds are copiously irrigated. The incisions are closed in the standard fashion.

Postoperative Management

The knee is kept locked in a long leg brace in full extension for 6 weeks, and the patient remains non–weight bearing using crutches. Progressive range of motion occurs during weeks 4 through 6. The brace is unlocked at the end of 6 weeks, and progressive weight bearing is instituted at 25% body weight per week during postoperative weeks 7 through 10. The crutches are discontin-

ued at the end of week 10. Progressive closed kinetic chain strength training and continued motion exercises are performed. Return to sports and heavy labor occurs after 6 to 9 months, when sufficient strength, range of motion, and proprioceptive skills have returned.

Results

I performed 41 arthroscopically assisted PCL–posterolateral complex reconstructions. The patients were evaluated pre- and postoperatively using the Tegner, Lysholm, and Hospital for Special Surgery knee ligament rating scales. The knees were also evaluated using the KT-1000 arthrometer, and stress radiography was performed with the Telos device. Postoperative examinations were performed by an independent examiner to eliminate surgeon bias, and the statistical analysis was performed by an independent statistician. The range of follow-up was 24 to 120 months. The PCL reconstructions were performed as described earlier, and the posterolateral complex reconstructions were performed using biceps femoris tendon transfer procedures, posterolateral capsular shift, and primary repair.

Postoperative results demonstrated a normal posterior drawer in 29 of 41 knees (70%) and a grade I posterior drawer in 11 of 41 knees (27%). Postoperative KT-1000 arthrometer measurements demonstrated a statistically significant postoperative improvement on the PCL screen and the corrected posterior measurements ($P \leq$ .001). There was a statistically significant improvement in all three knee ligament rating scales ($P \leq$ .001). Preoperatively, 90-degree posterior tibial displacement mean stress radiographic side-to-side measurements were 10.40 mm, compared with 2.26 mm postoperatively. This was a statistically significant improvement ($P \leq$ .001).

Conclusion

The arthroscopically assisted single-bundle transtibial PCL reconstruction technique is a reproducible surgical procedure. Documented results demonstrate statistically significant improvements from preoperative to postoperative status as evaluated by physical examination, knee ligament rating scales, arthrometer measurements, and stress radiography.

References

1. Arthrotek PCL Reconstruction Surgical Technique Guide: Fanelli PCL-ACL Drill Guide System. Warsaw, IN, Arthrotek, 1998.
2. Fanelli GC: Point counter point. Arthroscopic posterior cruciate ligament reconstruction: Single bundle/single femoral tunnel. Arthroscopy 16:725-731, 2000.
3. Fanelli GC: Arthroscopic evaluation of the PCL. In Fanelli GC (ed): Posterior Cruciate Ligament Injuries: A Guide to Practical Management. New York, Springer-Verlag, 2001, pp 95-108.

4. Fanelli GC: Arthroscopic PCL reconstruction: Transtibial technique. In Fanelli GC (ed): Posterior Cruciate Ligament Injuries: A Guide to Practical Management. New York, Springer-Verlag, 2001, pp 141-156.

5. Fanelli GC: Complications in PCL surgery. In Fanelli GC (ed): Posterior Cruciate Ligament Injuries: A Guide to Practical Management. New York, Springer-Verlag, 2001, pp 291-302.

6. Fanelli GC: Arthroscopic posterior cruciate ligament reconstruction: Transtibial tunnel technique. Surgical technique and 2–10 year results. Arthroscopy 18(9) Suppl 2:44-49, 2002.

7. Fanelli GC, Edson CJ: Management of posterior cruciate ligament and posterolateral instability of the knee. In Chow J (ed): Advanced Arthroplasty. New York, Springer-Verlag, 2001, pp 545-558.

8. Fanelli GC, Edson CJ: Arthroscopically assisted combined ACL/PCL reconstruction: 2–10 year follow-up. Arthroscopy 18:703-714, 2002.

9. Fanelli GC, Giannotti B, Edson CJ: Current concepts review. The posterior cruciate ligament: Arthroscopic evaluation and treatment. Arthroscopy 10:673-688, 1994.

10. Fanelli GC, Giannotti B, Edson CJ: Arthroscopically assisted PCL/posterior lateral complex reconstruction. Arthroscopy 12:521-530, 1996.

11. Fanelli GC, Monahan TJ: Complications of posterior cruciate ligament reconstruction. Sports Med Arthrosc Rev 7:296-302, 1999.

12. Fanelli GC, Monahan TJ: Complications and pitfalls in posterior cruciate ligament reconstruction. In Malek MM (ed): Knee Surgery: Complications, Pitfalls, and Salvage. New York, Springer-Verlag, 2001, pp 121-128.

13. Fanelli GC, Monahan TJ: Complications in posterior cruciate ligament and posterolateral complex surgery. Oper Tech Sports Med 9:96-99, 2001.

14. Malek MM, Fanelli GC: Technique of arthroscopic PCL reconstruction. Orthopaedics 16:961-966, 1993.

15. Miller MD, Cooper DE, Fanelli GC, et al: Posterior cruciate ligament: Current concepts. Instr Course Lect 51:347-351, 2002.

Transtibial Double-Bundle PCL Reconstruction

Kathryne J. Stabile, Jon K. Sekiya, and Christopher D. Harner

TRANSTIBIAL DOUBLE-BUNDLE PCL RECONSTRUCTION IN A NUTSHELL

History:
  Dashboard injury

Physical Examination:
  Check limb alignment and gait; posterior drawer; external rotation at 30 and 90 degrees; varus-valgus at 0 and 30
    degrees

Indications:
  Symptomatic 3+ posterior drawer; combined posterior cruciate ligament–posterolateral corner injury

Surgical Technique:
  Positioning, examination under anesthesia; graft preparation
  Tibial tunnel: distal one third of footprint; fluoroscopic control; visualize with 70-degree scope in posteromedial portal
  Femoral tunnel: outside-in; 4- to 5-mm separation of tunnels
  Graft: Achilles anterolateral; doubled semitendinosus posteromedial

Postoperative Management:
  Extension at 4 weeks; progressive weight bearing at 4 to 6 weeks

Results:
  Restores stability and biomechanics

The double-bundle posterior cruciate ligament (PCL) reconstruction technique was devised in an attempt to anatomically reproduce the anterolateral and postero-medial bundles of the PCL.[4,12,32] Recent biomechanical cadaver studies suggest that a double-bundle PCL reconstruction more closely restores normal knee biomechanics and stability in the PCL-deficient knee.[18,32] Although a single anterolateral bundle reconstruction restores stability at mid to high knee flexion angles, residual laxity is present near full knee extension.[18] In addition, there is evidence that the posteromedial bundle reduces posterior tibial translation in knee flexion as well as extension, suggesting that this bundle plays an important role throughout the full range of knee motion.[11,18,32] For these reasons, we use a double-bundle PCL reconstruction technique for chronic PCL injuries to more closely restore normal knee biomechanics and stability.

Case History

A 39-year-old mechanic presented to our clinic with a chief complaint of right knee pain that had been increasing since he sustained an injury in a motor vehicle accident 8 months earlier when his anterior tibia struck the car's dashboard. The car had been traveling at 50 to 60 miles per hour when it struck a guardrail. He was a restrained driver, there was no airbag, and there was severe front-end damage to the car. There were no other passengers in the car, and the patient sustained no other injuries.

He complained of mostly anterior knee pain that was exacerbated with squatting and standing for long periods, which was critical for his job as a mechanic. When questioned about symptoms of instability, he noted that his knee occasionally "gave way," especially when walking downhill or downstairs. He did not play any sports, and he was relatively healthy.

Physical Examination

Patients with chronic PCL injuries suffer from pain and instability and experience a range of disability, from almost no functional limitations to severe limitations during activities of daily living. When evaluating a patient with a chronic PCL injury, it is important to assess limb alignment and gait. Ligamentous repair or reconstruction in a knee with varus malalignment, degenerative changes, and a varus or lateral thrust may have a significant risk of failure due to chronic repetitive elongation of the reconstruction over time.[5,37] In this setting, a high tibial osteotomy may be necessary to restore alignment, and this should be performed in a staged fashion before reconstruction of the PCL or posterolateral corner. In this patient, alignment and gait were normal.

He was 6 feet 2 inches tall and weighed 250 pounds. His right knee had a range of motion from 0 to 125 degrees (compared with −2 to 130 degrees on the left). He had a small effusion with 10% quadriceps atrophy. Full squatting caused pain anteriorly. He had moderate patellar crepitation without facet tenderness or apprehension. He had a 0-degree patellar tilt with equal medial and lateral glides. There was no medial or lateral joint line tenderness. A flexion McMurray test was also negative.

Part of a thorough knee examination is distinguishing between an isolated and a combined PCL injury. The most important tests for making this distinction are the posterior drawer and external rotation tests at 90 and 30 degrees, posterolateral corner tests, and varus and valgus tests at 0 and 30 degrees.[1,3,5-7,14,17,24,36,38] The posterior drawer test evaluates the distance of the medial tibial plateau from the medial femoral condyle at 90 degrees and categorizes PCL injuries into three grades. Grade I is described as a palpable but diminished step-off (0 to 5 mm); grade II has no step-off, and the medial tibial plateau cannot be pushed beyond the medial femoral condyle (5 to 10 mm); and grade III designates a complete PCL injury with a loss of the medial step-off, a medial tibial plateau that can be pushed beyond the medial femoral condyle (>10 mm), and possibly a posterior sag.[17,38] Because the posterolateral corner is the primary restraint to external rotation at both 90 and 30 degrees of flexion, evaluating passive external rotation may reveal a posterolateral corner insufficiency.[13,14,38] This is best done by reducing the knee to the "neutral" position when testing the posterolateral corner at 90 and 30 degrees of flexion.[6,28]

In this patient, ligament testing revealed a grade III posterior drawer with a grade III posterior sag. There was increased external rotation of the tibia on the femur at 90 degrees, which improved to normal at 30 degrees. The knee was stable to varus and valgus testing at 0 and 30 degrees. The Lachman test was stable, with a firm endpoint, when the tibia was reduced anteriorly before performing the maneuver.

Imaging

Plain radiographs should always be obtained. They can help assess the presence of large or small bony avulsion fractures or tibial plateau fractures, which may be indicative of a severe combined ligament injury. Flexion weight-bearing and full posteroanterior lower extremity long-cassette, lateral, and Merchant views aid in assessing any joint space narrowing, Fairbank changes, and malalignment, typically seen with chronic posterior instability.[34] Our patient showed no evidence of malalignment or joint space narrowing on any of the views obtained (Fig. 69–1).

Magnetic resonance imaging, with an accuracy between 96% and 100%, is a reliable test for evaluating PCL injuries.[10,16,20,30,35] With its sensitivity and accuracy, it can also evaluate the location of the PCL tear (femoral, midsubstance, tibial), meniscal injury, articular surfaces, and other ligaments.[15,17,22,38] In our patient, magnetic resonance imaging revealed a midsubstance isolated PCL tear (Fig. 69–2).

Bone scans can be helpful in assessing chronic PCL injuries and may reveal increased uptake, which is indicative of early medial and patellofemoral compartment chondrosis, particularly when there is no radiographic

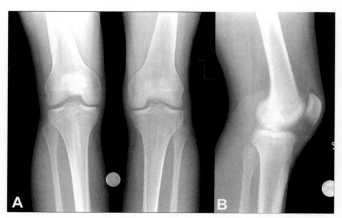

Figure 69–1 Posteroanterior (A) and lateral (B) 45-degree-flexion, weight-bearing radiographs show no evidence of malalignment or joint space narrowing. Note on the lateral view (B) that the tibia is displaced slightly posteriorly.

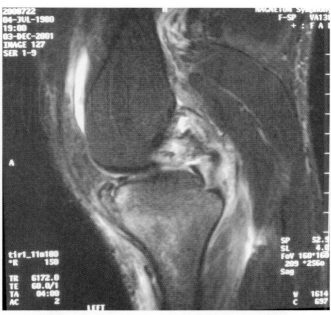

Figure 69–2 Magnetic resonance imaging clearly shows an isolated, midsubstance posterior cruciate ligament tear.

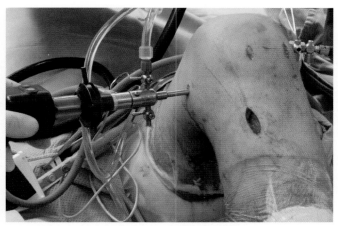

Figure 69–3 Extra-articular view of the accessory posteromedial portal.

evidence of joint space narrowing.[8] A bone scan in this patient showed an increased signal in the medial and patellofemoral compartment, indicating early chondrosis.

Surgical Technique

Positioning

For an arthroscopic transtibial technique, the patient is placed supine, with a well-padded tourniquet placed around the upper thigh. We often perform this procedure without the use of a tourniquet.

Examination under Anesthesia

Examination under anesthesia is a way to confirm the results of the posterior drawer, posterior sag, reversed pivot shift, and passive external rotation tests. Our examination confirmed isolated PCL deficiency, with no evidence of posterolateral or posteromedial insufficiency.

Diagnostic Arthroscopy

Arthroscopic evaluation is the final confirmation of a PCL injury. With the use of an accessory posteromedial portal (Fig. 69–3), the patient's PCL injury was directly visualized. The injured PCL was then debrided, leaving a remnant of the tibial and femoral attachments and preserving the meniscofemoral ligaments (when possible).

Specific Surgical Steps

Graft Harvest and Preparation

There are many graft choices for knee reconstructions, including the use of both autografts and allografts.[29] The most common autografts are patellar, hamstring, and quadriceps tendon. The most common allografts are Achilles, patellar, and tibialis anterior tendons.[25] Studies have shown histologically and arthroscopically that although transplanted allograft tendons take longer to incorporate than autografts do, they both undergo a similar process of revascularization and cellular repopulation while reaching maturity.[21,26,33] A study performed at our institution comparing the use of allografts and autografts in anterior cruciate ligament reconstruction demonstrated no difference in objective or subjective clinical outcome, with a 3- to 5-year follow-up.[19] Although there are mixed results using the various graft types, our preferred graft is the Achilles tendon allograft, owing to its high tensile strength, shorter operating time, ease of passage, and lack of donor site morbidity.[2,9,27] It also provides a remarkably large bone block and bony attachment at one end, allowing for rigid fixation and bone-to-bone healing.

An Achilles tendon allograft was prepared to fit an 11-mm tunnel and was then sutured with number 5 braided, nonabsorbable suture (Fig. 69–4). The posteromedial bundle was reconstructed using a semitendinosus or gracilis autograft. Graft harvesting was performed in a standard fashion through the anteromedial tibial incision. The graft was doubled over; sutured with number 2 braided, nonabsorbable suture; and made to fit a 6- or 7-mm tunnel (see Fig. 69–4).

Tibial Tunnel

To improve visualization, a 70-degree arthroscope was used in the accessory posteromedial portal. Using a PCL drill guide with the knee in 90 degrees of flexion, a transtibial Steinmann pin was placed from the antero-medial tibia through the distal one third of the tibial

6 Knee

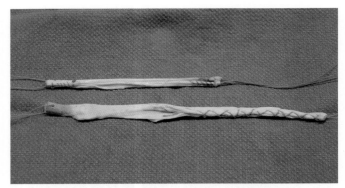

Figure 69–4　Achilles tendon allograft and semitendinosus autograft prepared on the back table for 11-mm and 7-mm tunnels, respectively.

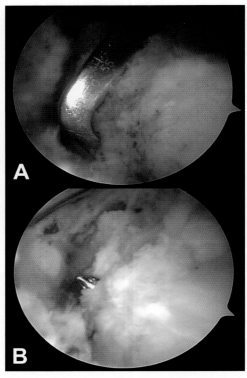

Figure 69–5　View through a 70-degree arthroscope placed in the posteromedial portal. Note the drill guide placement *(A)*, followed by placement of the Steinmann pin *(B)* in the distal one third of the tibial footprint.

footprint (Fig. 69–5). The tibial footprint is the junction of the middle and distal thirds of the posterior tibial eminence, slightly lateral to the center of the knee. A lateral radiograph was obtained to verify anatomic positioning. The tibial tunnel was prepared by hand using an 11-mm cannulated drill bit, followed by an 11-mm tunnel dilator.

Femoral Tunnel

The anterolateral tunnel was drilled first. A guide pin was placed through the anterolateral portal into the footprint of the anterolateral bundle at the 1 o'clock position (in a right knee), 6 mm off the articular margin. The anterolateral femoral tunnel was hand drilled to an 11-mm diameter and a 30-mm depth (Fig. 69–6). A drill hole of 3.2 mm was then placed through the end of the tunnel, and a Beath needle was placed through this drill hole out of the anteromedial femoral cortex and skin.

The posteromedial tunnel was drilled through the same portal (anterolateral) in the 2:30 o'clock position (in a right knee), 4 to 5 mm off the articular margin, depending on tunnel size, and at least 4 to 5 mm away from the anterolateral tunnel. The guide pin was placed divergent from the anterolateral tunnel to prevent tunnel collapse. The posteromedial tunnel was hand drilled to a 6- or 7-mm diameter and a 30-mm depth (see Fig. 69–6). A drill hole of 3.2 mm was then placed through the end of the tunnel, and a Beath needle was

placed through this drill hole out of the anteromedial femoral cortex and skin.

Graft Passage and Fixation

Before pulling the graft intra-articularly, we rasped the superior edge of the intra-articular tibial tunnel to smooth the corner. The bone plug of the Achilles tendon allograft was pulled into the anterolateral femoral tunnel using the Beath needle. The Achilles tendon bone plug was secured in the femoral tunnel using a guide pin and a 7- by 20-mm metal interference screw (Fig. 69–7). Next, the doubled end of the semitendinosus or gracilis graft was pulled into the femoral tunnel using the Beath

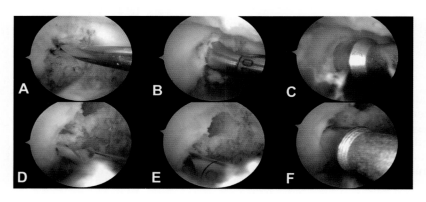

Figure 69–6　Kirschner wire placement *(A and D)*, hand drilling *(B and E)*, and tunnel dilatation *(C and F)* for the anterolateral and the posteromedial femoral tunnels, respectively.

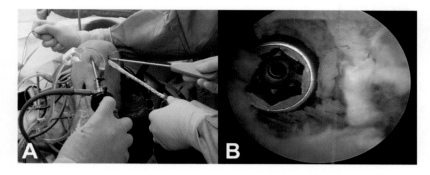

Figure 69–7 Extra-articular *(A)* and arthroscopic *(B)* views showing placement and fixation of the interference screw, with the Achilles tendon bone plug in the femoral tunnel.

needle and tied over a button through a separate anteromedial incision. Alternatively, a soft tissue biointerference screw can be placed arthroscopically.

The soft tissue end of the Achilles tendon allograft and the open end of the semitendinosus or gracilis graft were then pulled into the tibial tunnel using an 18-gauge wire loop placed through the tibial tunnel in the knee and pulled out of the anterolateral arthoscopic portal (Fig. 69–8).

The grafts were then tensioned, and the knee was put through several cycles of flexion and extension, which helped seat the sutures in the graft as well as work the graft through the tunnels. The knee was flexed to 90 degrees, and an anterior drawer was applied. While the graft was being tensioned, a screw and soft tissue washer

were used to fix the soft tissue end of the Achilles tendon to the anteromedial tibia.

Using a separate screw and soft tissue washer, the semitendinosus or gracilis graft was fixed to the tibia in a similar fashion. Tibial fixation was performed at 15 degrees of knee flexion while an anterior drawer was applied. We often supplement tibial tunnel fixation with a bioabsorbable interference screw. The knee was then examined for the presence of any residual laxity or restriction of motion. If either of these conditions is present, we reapply tibial fixation until stability and full motion are restored.

Closure

Pedal pulses were checked at this point to verify that no vascular injury had occurred. The knee was closed in layers in a standard fashion, following copious irrigation with an antibiotic solution. The periosteum over the tibial tunnels was closed with number 0 braided, absorbable suture, and the subcutaneous tissue was reapproximated with 3-0 braided, absorbable suture. The skin and arthroscopic portals were closed with staples, and the knee was bandaged in a sterile compression dressing. A cooling device and hinged knee brace locked in full extension were placed securely.

Postoperative Management

We use a formal, physical therapist–directed rehabilitation program following surgery. The knee brace is locked in full extension for 4 weeks to allow the reconstruction to heal and prevent posterior tibial subluxation. Immediately postoperatively, the patient begins quadriceps sets, straight leg raises, and calf pumps, performed 5 to 10 times a day. Partial weight bearing with crutches is initiated immediately, with a gradual return to full weight bearing over a 4- to 6-week period. If necessary, electrical stimulation is used to assist with voluntary quadriceps muscle contraction. At 4 weeks, the brace is unlocked, and the patient begins heel slides and passive flexion exercises. Isometric and light resistive exercises are continued at this point through a protected range of motion. We hope to have 90 degrees of knee flexion by 8 weeks after surgery and near full flexion by 12 weeks. Stationary bicycling is begun once knee range of motion is sufficient for this activity.

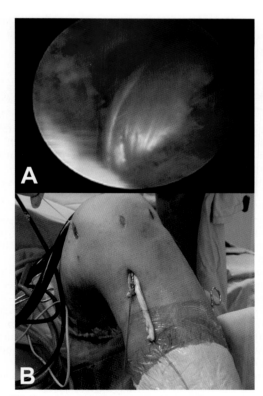

Figure 69–8 *A,* Arthroscopic view of the Achilles and semitendinosus grafts passing into the tibial tunnel. *B,* Extra-articular view of both grafts passed.

6 Knee

At 3 months, physical therapy is directed toward regaining the final degrees of full motion and focuses on a muscle strengthening program with weights. Hamstring strengthening is delayed until this point to avoid directly stressing the PCL graft. At 4 months, a walking program on a treadmill can be instituted, as well as pool running and swimming.

At 6 months, straight running can be started on even ground without any cutting or pivoting movements. By 8 to 10 months, sports-specific exercises can be performed, in anticipation of a full return to sporting activities (if the patient is an athlete) by 1 year postoperatively.

Results

Harner et al.[18] compared double-bundle PCL reconstruction with a single-bundle technique in 10 cadaver knees. They found that although single-bundle reconstruction improved posterior stability, only the double-bundle technique was able to restore knee stability and biomechanics to normal (Fig. 69–9). Additionally, they found that the posteromedial bundle contributes significantly to posterior knee stability at all the flexion angles tested (in a single-bundle technique, only the anterolateral bundle is reconstructed).

Race and Amis[31] compared double-bundle PCL reconstruction with two single-bundle techniques in cadaver knees. They found that the single-bundle techniques either (1) overconstrained the knee in extension, with laxity in flexion, or (2) restored knee stability only at lower flexion angles, losing this effect at greater knee flexion angles. Only the double-bundle graft was able to restore normal knee biomechanics across the full range of knee motion.

Mannor et al.[23] also compared single- and double-bundle PCL reconstruction in 12 cadaver knees. Inter-estingly, they did not use the classic description of anterolateral and posteromedial bundles in their reconstruction; instead, they described two shallow bundles (S1 and S2) and one deep bundle (D).[12] Regardless of this difference, they found that although a one-bundle reconstruction restored posterior knee stability, significantly higher forces were seen in this single graft than in the two-bundle reconstruction, which exhibited a reciprocal load-sharing phenomenon between the two grafts while also restoring normal knee stability. The authors postulated that the higher forces seen in the single-bundle reconstruction could lead to graft elongation, which may explain the inability of single-bundle reconstructions to restore normal posterior stability in the clinical setting.

To date, there are no clinical studies documenting the outcome of double-bundle PCL reconstruction. We need well-designed, prospective clinical studies to determine the long-term efficacy of this new PCL reconstruction technique.

Conclusion

Grade III PCL injuries are difficult to treat. However, an improved understanding of the anatomy, biomechanics, and natural history of this injury has directed our management decisions. Although surgical treatment of the PCL-deficient knee continues to be controversial, with several techniques having been described in the literature, we believe that the double-bundle PCL reconstruction most closely restores knee biomechanics and stability in vitro. Nonetheless, prospective clinical studies are needed to definitively determine the optimal treatment method for this difficult problem.

References

1. Bergfeld JA, McAllister DR, Parker RD, et al: The effects of tibial rotation on posterior translation in knees in which the posterior cruciate ligament has been cut. J Bone Joint Surg Am 83:1339, 2001.
2. Bullis DW, Paulos LE: Reconstruction of the posterior cruciate ligament with allograft. Clin Sports Med 13:581, 1994.
3. Clancy WG, Shelborne KD, Zoellner GB, et al: Treatment of knee joint instability secondary to rupture of the posterior cruciate ligament. J Bone Joint Surg Am 65:310, 1983.
4. Clancy WJ, Bisson LJ: Double tunnel technique for reconstruction of the posterior cruciate ligament. Oper Tech Sports Med 7:110-117, 1999.
5. Cooper DE: Evaluation and treatment of posterior cruciate and posterolateral knee ligament injuries. In American Orthopaedic Society for Sports Medicine: Instructional Course Lectures. Vancouver, BC, American Orthopaedic Society for Sports Medicine, 1998, p 29.
6. Covey DC, Sapega AA: Injuries of the posterior cruciate ligament. J Bone Joint Surg Am 75:1376, 1993.
7. Covey DC, Sapega AA, Sherman GM: Testing for isometry during reconstruction of the posterior cruciate ligament. Am J Sports Med 24:740, 1996.

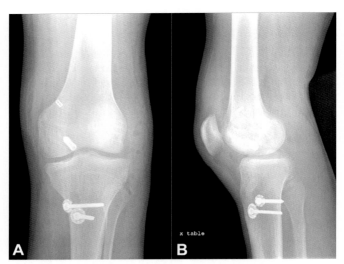

Figure 69–9 Postoperative anteroposterior (A) and lateral (B) radiographs showing the hardware and tunnel placement following a double-bundle posterior cruciate ligament reconstruction. This particular patient also underwent posterolateral corner reconstruction.

8. Dye SF: Imaging of the knee. Orthop Rev 22:901, 1993.
9. Fanelli GC, Giannotti BF, Edson CJ: The posterior cruciate ligament arthroscopic evaluation and treatment. Arthroscopy 10:673, 1994.
10. Fisher SP, Fox JM, Del Pizzo W, et al: Accuracy of diagnosis from magnetic resonance imaging of the knee. J Bone Joint Surg Br 73:452, 1991.
11. Fox RJ, Harner CD, Sakane M, et al: Determination of the in situ forces in the human posterior cruciate ligament using robotic technology—a cadaveric study. Am J Sports Med 26:395, 1998.
12. Girgis FG, Marshall JL, Al Monajem ARS: The cruciate ligaments of the knee joint: Anatomical, functional and experimental analysis. Clin Orthop 106:216, 1975.
13. Gollehon DL, Torzilli PA, Warren RF: The role of the posterolateral and cruciate ligaments in the stability of the human knee. J Bone Joint Surg Am 69:233, 1987.
14. Grood ES, Stowers SF, Noyes FR: Limits of movement in the human knee: The effects of sectioning the PCL and posterolateral structures. J Bone Joint Surg Am 70:88, 1988.
15. Gross ML, Grover JS, Bassett LW, et al: Magnetic resonance imaging of the posterior cruciate ligament: Clinical use to improve diagnostic accuracy. Am J Sports Med 20:732, 1992.
16. Grover JS, Bassett LW, Gross ML, et al: Posterior cruciate ligament: MR imaging. Radiology 174:527, 1990.
17. Harner CD, Hoeher J: Evaluation and treatment of posterior cruciate ligament injuries. Am J Sports Med 26:471, 1998.
18. Harner CD, Janaushek MA, Kanamori A, et al: Biomechanical analysis of a double-bundle posterior cruciate ligament reconstruction. Am J Sports Med 28:144, 2000.
19. Harner CD, Olson JJ, Irrgang JJ, et al: Allograft versus autograft anterior cruciate ligament reconstruction. Clin Orthop 324:134, 1996.
20. Heron CW, Calvert PT: Three-dimensional gradient echo MR imaging of the knee: Comparison with arthroscopy. Radiology 166:865, 1992.
21. Jackson DW, Corsetti J, Simon TM: Biologic incorporation of allograft anterior cruciate ligament replacements. Clin Orthop 324:126-133, 1996.
22. LaPrade RF, Gilbert TJ, Bollom TS, et al: The magnetic resonance imaging appearance of individual structures of the posterolateral knee: A prospective study of normal knees and knees with surgically verified grade III injuries. Am J Sports Med 28:191, 2000.
23. Mannor DA, Shearn JT, Grood ES, et al: Two-bundle posterior cruciate ligament reconstruction: An in vitro analysis of graft placement and tension. Am J Sports Med 28:833, 2000.
24. Markolf KL, Slauterbeck FJ, Armstrong KL, et al: Biomechanical study of replacement of the posterior cruciate ligament with a graft. J Bone Joint Surg Am 79:375-380, 1997.
25. Miller MD, Harner CD: The use of allograft: Techniques and results. Clin Sports Med 12:757, 1993.
26. Nikolaou PK, Seaber AV, Glisson RR, et al: Anterior cruciate ligament allograft transplantation: Long-term function, histology, revascularization, and operative technique. Am J Sports Med 14:348, 1986.
27. Noyes FR, Barber-Westin B: Treatment of complex injuries involving the posterior cruciate and posterolateral ligaments of the knee. Am J Knee Surg 9:200, 1996.
28. Noyes FR, Barber-Westin SD: Surgical restoration to treat chronic deficiency of the posterolateral complex and cruciate ligaments of the knee joint. Am J Sports Med 24:415, 1996.
29. Noyes FR, Butler DL, Grood ES, et al: Biomechanical analysis of human knee ligament grafts used in knee ligament repairs and reconstructions. J Bone Joint Surg Am 66:344-352, 1984.
30. Polly DW, Callaghan JJ, Sikes RA, et al: The accuracy of selective magnetic resonance imaging compared with the findings of arthroscopy of the knee. J Bone Joint Surg Am 70:192, 1988.
31. Race A, Amis AA: The mechanical properties of the two bundles of the human posterior cruciate ligament. J Biomech 27:13, 1994.
32. Race A, Amis AA: PCL reconstruction: In vitro biomechanical evaluation of isometric versus single and double bundled anatomic grafts. J Bone Joint Surg Br 80:173, 1998.
33. Shino K, Inoue M, Horibe S, et al: Maturation of allograft tendons transplanted into the knee: An arthroscopic and histological study. J Bone Joint Surg Br 70:556, 1988.
34. Shino K, Mitsuoka T, Horibe S, et al: The gravity sag view: A simple radiographic technique to show posterior laxity of the knee. Arthroscopy 16:670, 2000.
35. Turner DA, Prodromos CC, Petasnick JP, et al: Acute injuries of the ligaments of the knee: Magnetic resonance evaluation. Radiology 154:717, 1985.
36. Veltri DM, Deng XH, Torzilli PA, et al: The role of the popliteofibular ligament in stability of the human knee. Am J Sports Med 24:19, 1996.
37. Veltri DM, Warren RF: Anatomy, biomechanics, and physical findings in posterolateral knee instability. Clin Sports Med 13:599, 1994.
38. Veltri DM, Warren RF: Posterolateral instability of the knee. J Bone Joint Surg Am 64:460, 1994.

6 Knee

PCL Tibial Inlay and Posterolateral Corner Reconstruction

SANJITPAL S. GILL, STEVEN B. COHEN,
AND MARK D. MILLER

PCL TIBIAL INLAY AND POSTEROLATERAL CORNER RECONSTRUCTION IN A NUTSHELL

History:
  PCL: blow to proximal tibia; fall with foot plantar flexed
  PLC: rotational injury

Physical Examination:
  PCL: posterior drawer
  PLC: external rotation asymmetry

Imaging:
  PCL: stress radiographs, magnetic resonance imaging
  PLC: magnetic resonance imaging

Indications:
  PCL: grade III laxity; bony avulsion injury
  PLC: combined PCL-PLC injury

Surgical Technique:

PCL

1. Femoral drill guide placed in anterior portion of PCL footprint at femoral origin, with starting point centered on medial cortex of medial femoral condyle (8 mm from articular surface at 11 or 1 o'clock position)
2. Pass graft passer or 18-gauge wire into femoral tunnel and posterior aspect of knee
3. Approach posterior knee with popliteal fossa incision through interval between medial head of gastrocnemius and semimembranosus (protect neurovascular bundle with lateral retraction of gastrocnemius)
4. Retrieve preplaced graft passer through vertical capsular incision to expose posterior knee joint, and inlay tibial side of graft to sit flush with posterior tibia
5. "Toggle" patellar end of graft through femoral tunnel—first pass into notch by relaying sutures on end of graft out anteromedial portal, then pass second loop from femoral tunnel out same portal to toggle bone plug into femoral tunnel

Continued

PCL TIBIAL INLAY AND POSTEROLATERAL CORNER RECONSTRUCTION IN A NUTSHELL—cont'd

6. Tension graft after ranging knee; fix with 9- by 20-mm interference screw in femoral tunnel (may be necessary to move inlaid bone block distally on tibia to appropriately tension graft) while applying anterior drawer force to tibia and pulling on sutures exiting femoral tunnel

PLC
1. Direct repair for acute reconstruction from deep to superficial
2. Superficial layer: iliotibial band, biceps femoris tendon (peroneal nerve posterior to tendon); deep layer: popliteus, LCL, popliteofibular ligament, joint capsule
3. Femoral-sided avulsions of LCL and popliteus repaired with transosseous drill holes in bony bed on lateral femoral condyle; tibial avulsions of popliteus reattached with sutures or cancellous screw in posterolateral tibia
4. Transosseous sutures through fibular head for avulsions of LCL and arcuate ligament from fibular styloid
5. Popliteus tenodesis to posterior fibula for popliteofibular ligament reconstruction
6. Posterolateral capsular imbrication anterior to lateral head of gastrocnemius
7. Reconstruction of chronic PLC injuries—(a) augmentation procedures include biceps tenodesis to lateral femoral condyle and distally based central slip of biceps tendon secured to lateral femoral condyle for LCL reconstruction; (b) popliteus or popliteofibular ligament augmentation can be addressed with graft from lateral femoral condyle through tunnels in proximal tibia or fibula

Postoperative Management:
PCL: gravity-assisted flexion exercises to 90 degrees and closed chain quadriceps exercises in the *prone* position
PLC: protection from external rotation and varus stresses at the tibia for at least 6 to 8 weeks

Results:
PCL: less residual laxity with tibial inlay technique than with arthroscopic-assisted anterior PCL reconstruction
PLC: variable, depending on technique and chronicity

Complications:
PCL: avascular necrosis of medial femoral condyle; wound breakdown
PLC: common peroneal nerve palsy; persistent instability; arthrofibrosis

LCL, lateral collateral ligament; PCL, posterior cruciate ligament; PLC, posterolateral corner.

The posterior cruciate ligament (PCL) is the primary restraint to posterior tibial translation.[5,15] Hughston et al.[19] believe that the PCL is the fundamental stabilizer of the knee. PCL injuries account for 3% to 20% of all knee ligament injuries.[9,11] The true incidence of PCL injuries is unknown, however, because many isolated injuries to the PCL go undetected. Further, posterolateral corner (PLC) injuries are associated with concurrent ligamentous instability 43% to 80% of the time.[6] Often, the history is helpful in making the diagnosis of a PCL injury, such as when a dashboard impacts a tibia with a flexed knee. A fall onto a flexed knee with the foot in plantar flexion and even hyperflexion without a direct blow can also cause PCL injury.[7,37] The ability to differentiate isolated and combined PCL injuries is critical in deciding how to manage a patient. Other considerations when deciding between conservative and surgical options may differ, depending on the chronicity of the injury, symptoms, activity level, and degree of laxity. This chapter focuses on PCL injuries as well as injuries to the PLC, which are commonly associated with PCL-injured knees.

History

Typically, patients report a posteriorly directed force over the anterior tibia or a hyperflexion injury, such as a dashboard injury or a football tackle. The knee may be in full extension at the time of the injury. Rotational forces can create a combined PCL-PLC injury. Instability, characteristic of anterior cruciate ligament (ACL) injuries, is not the primary symptom. Patients often have pain and swelling in the knee, with the pain in the medial and patellofemoral compartments, and they complain about the knee "not being right." Initial radiographs are usually negative for a fracture or dislocation.

Physical Examination

Particular attention must be paid to posterior translation, external rotation, and varus angulation,[46] which may differ at 30 and 90 degrees of knee flexion because of an isolated injury to the PLC versus a combined PCL-PLC injury.

Varus and valgus stress testing is performed at both full knee extension and 30 degrees of flexion. Increased varus opening in full extension is significant for a combined lateral collateral ligament (LCL)–PLC injury, whereas opening at 30 degrees suggests an LCL injury and a possible PLC injury. Gross varus instability may be due to an additional ligamentous injury, such as ACL disruption.[11] Medial collateral ligament injury can also be seen with PCL injuries, so valgus stress testing must be performed at 0 and 30 degrees.

Testing for passive external rotation is done with the patient prone and is considered the sine qua non for PLC injury.[15] A finding of excessive external rotation (gauged by the medial border of the foot relative to the femur) at both 30 and 90 degrees, compared with the normal contralateral limb, is consistent with an injury to both the PCL and the PLC. Increased external rotation only at 30 degrees suggests an isolated PLC injury (Fig. 70–1).

The posterior drawer test is best performed with the knee at 90 degrees of flexion and the foot stabilized. Although the classic 0 to 5 mm (grade I), 5 to 10 mm (grade II), and greater than 10 mm (grade III) displacements are commonly used, it may be more helpful to classify PCL injuries based on the medial tibial plateau–medial femoral condyle position.[30] In this classification, grade I injuries result in some preservation of the anterior position of the tibia, grade II injuries occur when the tibia is flush with the medial femoral condyle, and grade III injuries are manifested by displacement of the anterior tibia posterior to the medial femoral condyle (Fig. 70–2). Of note, chronically PCL-deficient knees may have a stable endpoint.[46] Posterior laxity that decreases with internal rotation of the tibia may have a better prognosis for conservative management, possibly owing to an intact Humphry or Wrisberg ligament.[7] Additionally, a Lachman test must be done to assess ACL

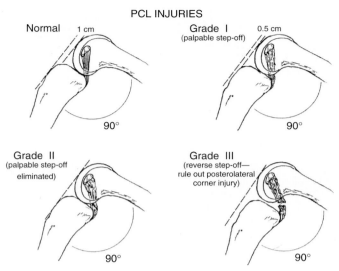

Figure 70–2 Classification of posterior cruciate ligament (PCL) injuries. Grade 0, normal; grade I, decrease in the tibiofemoral step-off; grade II, loss of the step-off, with the tibia flush with the medial femoral condyle; grade III, reverse step-off (tibia can be displaced posterior to the medial femoral condyle). Step-off is palpated on the medial side of the joint. (From Petrie RS, Harner CD: Evaluation and management of the posterior cruciate injured knee. Oper Tech Sports Med 7:93-103, 1999.)

integrity. Anterior drawer testing may give a false-positive result because of a posterior sag to the tibia.

The quadriceps active test is a useful adjunct for determining PCL deficiency.[13] The patient is placed supine on the examining table with the knee flexed 90 degrees. Quadriceps contraction normally causes posterior translation of the tibia relative to the femur, but in PCL-injured knees, anterior translation occurs. This paradoxical motion is due to the posterior resting point of the tibia in PCL-deficient knees.

Other adjunctive tests for PLC injury include the external rotation recurvatum test,[21] posterolateral drawer test,[21] and reversed pivot shift test.[23] These tests may have a high false-positive rate, and comparison with the contralateral extremity is required.[10]

Imaging

Plain radiographs should always be obtained to assess for a fracture. Additionally, if a bony avulsion can be identified, there is little controversy that these injuries need to be fixed.[29] Flexion weight-bearing posteroanterior views and patellar views can be helpful in evaluating medial compartment and patellar chondrosis in knees with chronic posterior laxity. Stress radiographs have also been useful in determining PCL integrity[18] and are helpful in objectively measuring PCL reconstruction results.

Magnetic resonance imaging has proved to be highly efficacious in confirming PCL injuries. It has demonstrated 100% sensitivity and specificity in identifying complete tears of the PCL (Fig. 70–3).[16] Also, magnetic

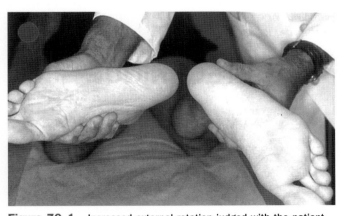

Figure 70–1 Increased external rotation judged with the patient prone and the knee flexed at 30 degrees. Asymmetry of more than 10 to 15 degrees at 30 degrees of flexion suggests an isolated posterolateral corner (PLC) injury. Asymmetry of more than 10 to 15 degrees at 90 degrees of flexion suggests a combined posterior cruciate ligament–PLC injury. (From Miller MD, Gordon WT: Posterior cruciate ligament reconstruction: Tibial inlay techniques—principles and procedures. Oper Tech Sports Med 7:127-133, 1999.)

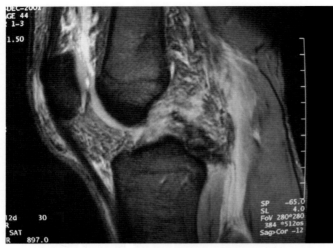

Figure 70–3 T2-weighted sagittal magnetic resonance imaging scan indicating complete rupture of the posterior cruciate ligament.

resonance imaging can be useful in evaluating chondral and meniscal damage.

Radionuclide imaging can identify the underlying chondrosis in chronic PCL injuries. These bone scans may be useful in monitoring the long-term effects of PCL deficiency in the patellar and medial compartments of the knee.

Indications and Contraindications

Significant controversy surrounds the treatment recommendations for PCL-deficient knees. There is universal agreement, however, that PCL avulsion fractures should be repaired.[39,41] Combined ligamentous injuries to the PCL and ACL, PCL and PLC, or PCL and medial collateral ligament should also be reconstructed.[38,40,44] Some authors advocate PCL reconstruction in knees with repairable meniscal and chondral lesions.[43]

Outside of these parameters, PCL reconstruction is more controversial, but authors have tried to elucidate guidelines based on the chronicity of the injury. Early reconstruction of acute PCL injuries with grade III laxity (which are often combined PCL-PLC injuries) has been advocated.[30] Other isolated PCL injuries can be treated conservatively, with an emphasis on quadriceps strengthening. In patients with symptomatic grade II or III chronic laxity, especially active, younger patients, PCL reconstruction is warranted.[32] However, when evaluating symptomatic chronic PCL injuries, attention must be given to limb alignment and arthrosis. A high tibial osteotomy may be needed in limbs with varus malalignment,[35] and knees with advanced degenerative changes should not undergo PCL reconstruction.

The site of injury to the PCL determines treatment options. Primary repair of the ligament is indicated for avulsion fractures from the origin or insertion site. Tibial avulsions are more common and require a posterior approach to the knee for reduction and fixation[29] or a modified posterior approach, similar to the approach for

a tibial inlay.[4] For larger avulsion fragments, anatomic reduction and primary repair can be performed with lag screws, and smaller fragments can be repaired with suture fixation through drill holes.

For complete, midsubstance tears, primary repair has resulted in poor outcomes and is not recommended. Historically, anterior arthroscopic procedures were used to reconstruct the PCL, but these procedures resulted in limited exposure to the PCL fossa, which led to a sharp graft angle as it exited the tibial tunnel. This angle is referred to as the "killer turn," and it may be associated with postoperative laxity and late graft failure.[30] Recent biomechanical studies have demonstrated 3 to 5 mm of laxity with cyclic testing.[3] Thus, we recommend the tibial inlay technique for PCL reconstruction because of smaller graft bending angles and improved patient outcomes.[2,31] The inlay technique, developed by Berg, is an adaptation of the method used to perform primary fixation of PCL tibial avulsion fractures.

Surgical Technique

Positioning

If the traditional arthroscopic transtibial technique is used, the patient is placed supine. For the tibial inlay technique, the patient is positioned on the operating table in the lateral decubitus position, with the operative leg up. This position allows a direct posterior approach, and the hip can be abducted, flexed to 90 degrees, and externally rotated with the foot on the table to perform arthroscopy, graft harvest, femoral tunnel placement, and graft passage. A commercially available leg holder, commonly used for total knee arthroplasty, can be helpful. An examination under anesthesia is performed before patient positioning. If graft material is to be harvested from the contralateral knee, this is also done before positioning. A tourniquet is placed on the proximal thigh, although it is not routinely elevated, and the leg is prepared and draped in the usual sterile fashion.

Examination under Anesthesia

A valuable resource in diagnosing PCL and PLC injuries is an examination under anesthesia. The PCL deficiency can be confirmed with the posterior drawer, posterior sag, and reversed pivot shift tests. The PLC injury can be demonstrated with asymmetrical external rotation, recurvatum, asymmetrical posterolateral drawer, and reversed pivot shift tests.

Diagnostic Arthroscopy

Final confirmation of the PCL injury is made before undertaking PCL reconstruction (Fig. 70–4). Because the PCL is encased in its own synovial sheath, injuries to the ligament may not be noted until the PCL is actually visualized. A modified Gillquist view or posteromedial portal view (Fig. 70–5) can directly visualize a PCL injury. LaPrade[27] demonstrated the arthroscopic drive-through sign of the knee when excessive lateral joint laxity is present.

PCL injury is often best noted with indirect signs,[14] which include the sloppy ACL sign (ACL pseudolaxity), posterior displacement of the medial femoral condyle in relation to the medial meniscus, and chondrosis of the medial femoral condyle and patellofemoral joint (late finding).[30] Pseudolaxity is assessed by providing an anterior drawer force to the knee, which restores the normal anatomic relationship between the medial femoral condyle and the medial tibial plateau. Failure to recog-

nize this pseudolaxity may lead to unnecessary ACL reconstruction in an ACL-intact knee (Fig. 70–6).

Specific Surgical Steps

Graft Selection

Autografts using bone–patellar tendon–bone or quadriceps tendon (ipsilateral or contralateral) or allografts using Achilles tendon or bone–patellar tendon–bone may be used, depending on the specific case. Consideration should be given to the necessary length of the graft

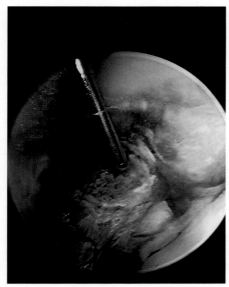

Figure 70–4 Arthroscopic image documenting a complete posterior cruciate ligament injury seen through a standard anterolateral portal.

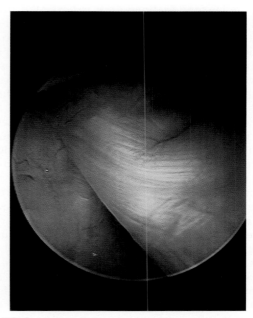

Figure 70–6 Arthroscopic view of anterior cruciate ligament pseudolaxity.

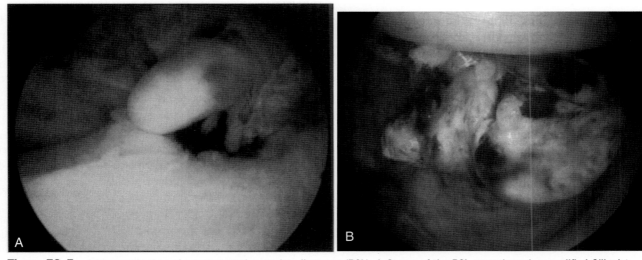

Figure 70–5 Arthroscopic view of a torn posterior cruciate ligament (PCL). *A*, Stump of the PCL seen through a modified Gillquist view. *B*, PCL remnants seen through a posteromedial portal.

6 Knee

and bony fixation at the ends of the graft. In general, we prefer ipsilateral bone–patellar tendon–bone grafts for PCL reconstruction and ipsilateral semitendinosus and gracilis grafts for PLC reconstruction.

Tibial Inlay for Posterior Cruciate Ligament Reconstruction

The tibial inlay technique provides anatomic reconstruction of the anterolateral component of the PCL. This technique can be modified for two-bundle procedures.[34] After an examination under anesthesia and diagnostic arthroscopy, a central anterior knee incision is made approximately 6 to 8 cm long (sufficient for central patellar tendon autograft harvest). An 11-mm bone–patellar tendon–bone graft is harvested from the central third of the patellar tendon, being careful to harvest a rectangular or trapezoidal bone plug from the tibial side. The tibial portion of the graft, which will be inlaid into the tibia, is fashioned with a flattened surface and prepared to accept a 4.5-mm bicortical screw by drilling and tapping. The patellar portion of the graft should be contoured in a cylindric fashion and the tip sculpted in a "bullet" shape to facilitate graft passage. We try to make this graft approximately 18 mm long and fashion it to easily pass through the femoral tunnel. Perpendicular sutures are placed in this end to avoid suture cutout during graft fixation.

Standard arthroscopy is then performed to verify PCL deficiency (this may be done before graft harvesting if there is any question) and any other intra-articular pathology (Fig. 70–7) and to identify landmarks for reconstruction. The PCL stump is debrided, and preparations for the femoral tunnel are finalized. A commercially available femoral drill guide is placed in the anterior portion of the PCL footprint at its femoral insertion. The starting point is centered on the medial cortex of the medial femoral condyle. The entry point is more proximal to preserve subchondral bone and reduce the risk of avascular necrosis of the medial femoral condyle. The guide tip should be placed 8 mm from the medial femoral condyle articular surface at the

11 or 1 o'clock position and subsequently overdrilled with a cannulated drill bit sized appropriately for the graft. An 18-gauge guidewire or commercially available graft passer is introduced into the femoral tunnel and the posterior aspect of the knee joint to facilitate graft passage. The posterior aspect of the tunnel is rasped to reduce graft abrasion.

The patient is then repositioned with the operative knee extended and the lower leg placed on a padded Mayo stand. We prefer the posterior approach, similar to that described by Burks and Schaffer.[4] A horizontal incision is made in the crease of the popliteal fossa. The interval between the medial head of the gastrocnemius and the semimembranosus is developed. Lateral retraction of the gastrocnemius provides access to the posterior capsule of the knee and simultaneously protects the neurovascular structures of the popliteal fossa (Fig. 70–8). The fascial incision is then extended distally and medially. The medial head of the gastrocnemius can be partially released to provide additional exposure, but this is rarely, if ever, necessary. The surgeon can then palpate both the posterior tibial sulcus and the prepositioned wire loop. A vertical capsular incision is made to expose the posterior knee joint and retrieve the loop.

Muscle fibers of the popliteus are split, and the posterior cortex of the tibia is exposed. It is helpful to palpate the PCL sulcus, which lies between two ridges, before exposing the sulcus. It is important to clear all soft tissue between the posterior arthrotomy and the planned bony trough. With the use of an osteotome, bur, and tamp, a unicortical window is made at the site of tibial insertion of the PCL to match the tibial side of the graft prepared earlier. The graft is inlaid in the window, and the window, bone plug, or both are adjusted so that the plug fits snugly, flush with the back of the tibia. The graft is then provisionally fixed to the back of the tibia with a staple; the staple should be left prominent, to facilitate removal if adjustment is necessary. Alternatively, the graft can be fixed with a posterior to anterior 4.5-mm bicortical screw.

The prepositioned 18-gauge wire or graft passer is used to pass the patellar end of the graft through the notch and into the femoral tunnel (Figs. 70–9 and 70–10). This maneuver sometimes requires two steps. In the first step, the graft is passed into the notch by passing the sutures from the bony end of the graft out the anteromedial portal. In the second step, a second loop is passed from the femoral tunnel out the same portal and is used to pull the bone plug up into the tunnel. It is helpful to place multiple sutures in the patellar bone block, with sutures placed near the tapered end of the block passed into the femoral tunnel, and sutures near the opposite end of the block passed through an anteromedial portal. In this manner, the graft can be manipulated into the femoral tunnel with one set of sutures and then "toggled" to line up with the tunnel with the sutures that were retrieved through the anteromedial portal.

The knee is passively taken through the full range of motion, any kinks in the graft are eliminated, and the stability of the graft is assessed. The location of the bone plug–tendon junction is carefully evaluated. It is our goal to have this junction right at the intra-articular margin

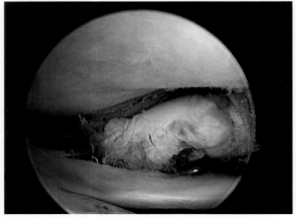

Figure 70–7 Popliteal tendon rupture viewed from an anterolateral portal.

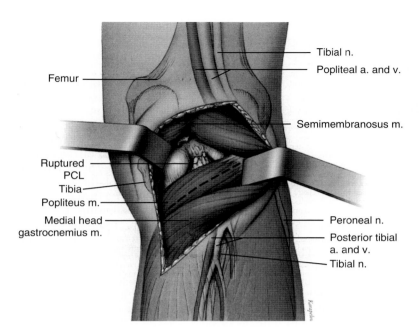

Figure 70–8   Posterior knee anatomy, with identification of the interval between the medial head of the gastrocnemius (laterally) and the semimembranosus (medially). The neurovascular structures are protected by the medial head of the gastrocnemius. a., artery; m., muscle; n., nerve; PCL, posterior cruciate ligament; v., vein. (From Miller MD, Gordon WT: Posterior cruciate ligament reconstruction: Tibial inlay techniques. Oper Tech Orthop 9:289-297, 1999.)

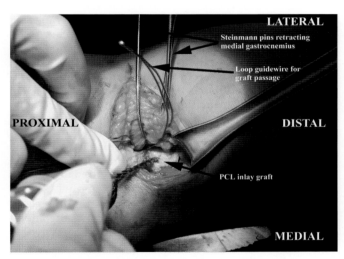

Figure 70–9   Intraoperative picture of graft passage from posterior to anterior in the knee. The loop guidewire is a preplaced 18-gauge wire (from the anterior aspect of the knee) used to pass the patellar end of the graft through the notch and into the femoral tunnel. PCL, posterior cruciate ligament.

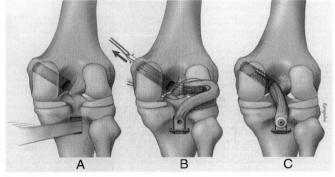

Figure 70–10   Placement of the tibial inlay posterior cruciate ligament graft and passage into the femoral tunnel. *A*, The trough is made between the medial eminence and the less prominent lateral eminence. A posterior arthrotomy is made, extending vertically from the trough. *B*, After provisional fixation with a staple, the graft is passed anteriorly either through the patellar defect or out the inferomedial portal. The suture is used to "toggle" the graft into the femoral tunnel. *C*, Once adequate graft tension is established, the tibial side of the graft is secured with a bicortical screw, and the femoral side is fixed with a 9-mm interference screw. (From Miller MD, Gordon WT: Posterior cruciate ligament reconstruction: Tibial inlay techniques—principles and procedures. Oper Tech Sports Med 7:127-133, 1999.)

of the femoral tunnel. The graft is tensioned, and the tension is assessed. If the bone plug goes too far into the femoral tunnel, the tibial window or inlaid bone block can be moved distally.

The tibial bone block is then secured using a bicortical 4.5-mm cortical screw and flat washer placed through the predrilled hole in the graft and lagged to the anterior cortex of the tibia. We frequently supplement this with a staple, usually placed distal to the screw. After ensuring that the graft is fully in the femoral tunnel, this side of the graft is fixed with a 9- by 20-mm interference screw. The knee is flexed 70 to 80 degrees, an anterior drawer force is applied to the tibia to reproduce the normal medial step-off, and tension is placed on the sutures exiting the femoral tunnel. A posterior drawer test confirms that PCL stability has been restored. Additional fixation may be used, consisting of a screw and post technique or sutures tied over a button at the extra-articular side of the femoral tunnel.

Bone graft, which is saved during graft preparation and femoral tunnel drilling, is packed into the patella and, if enough remains, into the tibial tubercle. Wounds are closed in the standard fashion, and a sterile dressing is applied. Radiographs are obtained before the patient

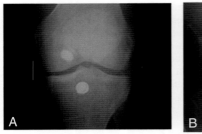 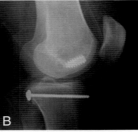

Figure 70–11 Anteroposterior *(A)* and lateral *(B)* radiographs of posterior cruciate ligament reconstruction using the tibial inlay procedure.

leaves the operating room to ensure that the graft and hardware placement is appropriate (Fig. 70–11).

Posterolateral Corner Reconstruction

Acute reconstruction of the PLC of the knee has had greater success than surgery for chronic posterolateral insufficiency.[20,26] Failure to reconstruct the PLC is also a possible source of failure of PCL reconstruction.[17] Direct, anatomic repair within the first 3 weeks of injury has demonstrated the best surgical results.[10,23] PCL reconstruction should be performed before PLC repair or reconstruction.

The PLC can be approached through a lateral hockey-stick, curvilinear, or straight incision. An understanding of the anatomy of the PLC is paramount before undertaking reconstruction. Three distinct layers can be found in the PLC: superficial, middle, and deep (Fig. 70–12).[42] The superficial layer consists of the iliotibial band and the biceps femoris tendon. The common peroneal nerve is found posterior to the biceps tendon. The middle layer consists of the patellomeniscal ligament and the quadriceps retinaculum anteriorly; this retinaculum is incomplete posteriorly and is represented by two patellofemoral ligaments. The deep layer consists of the joint capsule, LCL, fabellofibular ligament, poplite-ofibular ligament, arcuate ligament, and popliteus muscle and popliteal tendon. From a practical standpoint, two layers are important—the superficial and the deep.

Terry and LaPrade[45] described three fascial incisions and one capsular incision that enables access to repair components of the PLC. The first fascial incision is oriented parallel to the fibers of the iliotibial tract. It originates at the midpoint of Gerdy's tubercle and extends proximally, splitting the proximal portion of the iliotibial tract. Posterior retraction of the superficial layer of the iliotibial tract allows visualization of the deep and capsulo-osseous layers, which can then be dissected from the lateral intermuscular septum, allowing posterior retraction of the posterior half of the iliotibial tract for exposure of the more posterior structures on the lateral side. The second fascial incision is made in the interval between the posterior aspect of the iliotibial tract and the short head of the biceps femoris muscle, starting approximately 6 to 7 cm proximal to the lateral epicondyle. When extended distally, this incision is parallel to the femur but remains posterior to the lateral intermuscular septum. The third fascial incision is made posterior to the long head of the biceps femoris muscle and parallel to the peroneal nerve. An external neurolysis may be required to mobilize the peroneal nerve for access to the structures posterior and medial to the fibular head. In this interval, the popliteus muscle, medial and lateral limbs of the arcuate arch, fabellofibular ligament, and posterior popliteofibular ligament can be addressed. Finally, the capsular incision is made with the knee in 60 degrees of flexion with a more vertical orientation, anterior and parallel to the LCL. This window allows visualization of the middle third of the capsular ligament, the popliteal attachments, and the lateral meniscus. Of note, the medial fibers of the LCL insert into the lateral edge of the fibular head, and the lateral fibers of the LCL continue distally, medial to the long head of the biceps tendon, blending with the superficial fascia of the lateral compartment of the leg. Proximally, the LCL is covered

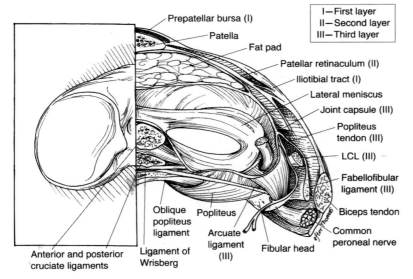

Figure 70–12 Three layers of the posterolateral aspect of the knee. LCL, lateral collateral ligament. (From Seebach JR, Inglis AE, Marshall FL, Warren RF: The structure of the posterolateral aspect of the knee. J Bone Joint Surg Am 64:536-541, 1982.)

laterally by the lateral aponeurosis of the long head of the biceps femoris.

The PLC repair should proceed from deep to superficial; direct suture repair, drill holes through bone, or suture anchors can be used.[23] The knee should be kept at 60 degrees of flexion, and the tibia should remain in neutral or slight internal rotation. Avulsions of the LCL and femoral origin of the popliteus can be repaired with suture through transosseous drill holes in a bony bed in the lateral femoral condyle.[6] The tibial attachment of the popliteus can be reattached with either sutures or a cancellous screw in the posterolateral tibia, and avulsions of the LCL and arcuate ligament from the fibular styloid can be repaired through transosseous sutures in the fibular head. The popliteal tendon can be tenodesed to the posterior aspect of the fibular head to address disruption of the fibular attachment of the popliteofibular ligament. The fabellofibular ligament, when present, can be used to reinforce the tenodesis repair. PLC repair should also include an imbrication of the posterolateral capsule anterior to the lateral head of the gastrocnemius. A severe injury may require augmentation with hamstring tendon, biceps femoris tendon, iliotibial band, or allograft.[32,48] Reconstruction of a chronic PLC injury is a much more complex problem. There is ample literature describing procedures for augmentation, advancement, and reconstruction of the PLC (Fig. 70–13).[1,8,12,20,24,33] In addition to deciding which type of PLC reconstruction is preferable, assessment of gait, limb alignment, and arthrosis is mandatory.

Clancy and Sutherland[8] showed that tenodesis of the biceps femoris tendon to the lateral femoral epicondyle can diminish the deforming force of the biceps muscle while simultaneously approximating the LCL (Fig. 70–14). In their study, 77% of patients had no restrictions in their daily activities, and 54% returned to their previous level of participation in sports. However, hardware prominence and hamstring weakness can be problems.

Veltri and Warren[47,48] support anatomic reconstruction of all injured posterolateral structures. A distally based, central slip of the biceps femoris tendon can be used to reconstruct the LCL. The graft is tubularized and then secured proximally on the lateral femoral condyle while leaving the rest of the biceps attachment intact (Fig. 70–15). Autografts or allografts are alternative graft choices for LCL reconstruction, with a proximally based

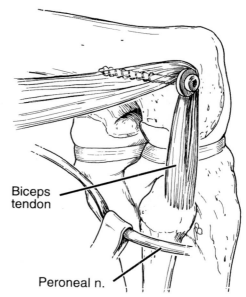

Figure 70–14   Biceps tenodesis for posterolateral corner reconstruction. (From Veltri DM, Warren RF: Treatment of acute and chronic injuries to the posterolateral and lateral knee. Oper Tech Sports Med 4:174-181, 1996.)

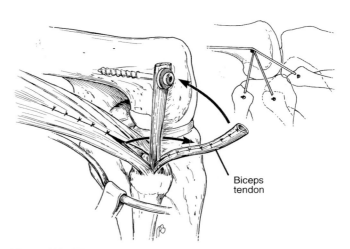

Figure 70–15   Distally based biceps tendon reconstruction of the lateral collateral ligament (LCL). The inset demonstrates isometric reconstruction of the LCL. (From Veltri DM, Warren RF: Treatment of acute and chronic injuries to the posterolateral and lateral knee. Oper Tech Sports Med 4:174-181, 1996.)

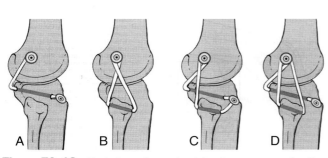

Figure 70–13   Techniques for posterolateral corner reconstruction. *A*, Popliteal bypass (Muller). *B*, Figure eight (Larsen). *C*, Two tail (Warren). *D*, Three tail (Warren and Miller).

bone plug in the lateral femoral condyle and a distal bone plug fixed to the proximal fibula. Popliteal and popliteofibular ligament reconstruction can be addressed by a single, split Achilles tendon allograft anchored in the distal lateral femoral condyle and passed through tunnels in the proximal tibia and fibula (Fig. 70–16). This theoretically reapproximates the normal anatomy of the PLC because the tibial attachment of the popliteus and the fibular attachment of the popliteofibular ligament are reconstructed. Isolated popliteofibular reconstruction can be accomplished in the same manner with a single tunnel through the proximal fibula

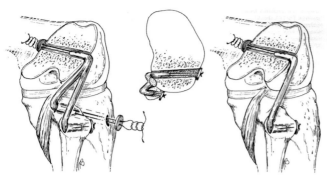

Figure 70-16   Reconstruction of the popliteus and the popliteofibular ligament with a split patellar tendon graft versus isolated reconstruction of the popliteofibular ligament. (From Veltri DM, Warren RF: Treatment of acute and chronic injuries to the posterolateral and lateral knee. Oper Tech Sports Med 4:174-181, 1996.)

instead of two tunnels in the proximal tibia and fibula. A two-strand semitendinosus and gracilis autograft can also be used to re-create the deficient popliteus-arcuate complex, with the bone plug fixed in the femoral anatomic insertion of the popliteus and the tendons fixed into the tibia and fibula (as described previously).

Latimer et al.[28] reported success reconstructing the LCL and PLC with a bone–patellar tendon–bone allograft secured in the fibular head and tibia with interference screws. Proximally, the tunnel is located at an isometric point on the lateral femoral condyle that lies 5 mm anterior to the lateral epicondyle and the femoral origin of the LCL. The graft is passed through the iliotibial tract and tensioned in 20 to 30 degrees of knee flexion while a valgus force is applied to the knee (Fig. 70–17). The large cross-sectional area of this graft could contribute to the restoration of not only the LCL but also the arcuate and popliteofibular ligaments.

Pearls and Pitfalls

Preoperative planning is an important factor in successful PCL reconstruction. If there is other associated ligamentous damage, especially to the PLC, simultaneous PCL and PLC reconstruction should be considered. A generous arthrotomy should be made to assist in graft passage, because failure to do so may result in graft laxity. Steinmann pins are used to assist in retracting the medial head of the gastrocnemius. An extra suture may be passed out of the anterior portal to help "toggle" the graft. After securing the tibial side of the graft and before proximal fixation, the knee should be cycled in flexion and extension to tension the graft.

The most serious complication of surgery is injury to the neurovascular structures during tibial tunnel drilling and graft passage. Other potential complications are infection, loss of motion, medial femoral condyle osteonecrosis, anterior knee pain, and painful hardware. The most common complication of surgery is residual laxity, which we believe occurs more commonly with arthroscopic-assisted anterior PCL reconstruction than with tibial inlay reconstruction.[30,31]

Postoperative Management

Postoperatively, the knee is braced in extension, with support to the posterior tibia to prevent posterior translation. Shortly after surgery, continuous passive motion, isometric quadriceps strengthening, and straight leg raising exercises are initiated. Weight bearing as tolerated with crutches is initiated as early as the first postoperative day. Simultaneous use of the hamstring, quadriceps, and gastrocnemius muscles during ambulation essentially unloads the cruciate ligaments.[36] Gravity-assisted flexion exercises to 90 degrees and closed chain quadriceps exercises in the *prone* position are stressed during early rehabilitation. The effect of gravity and the

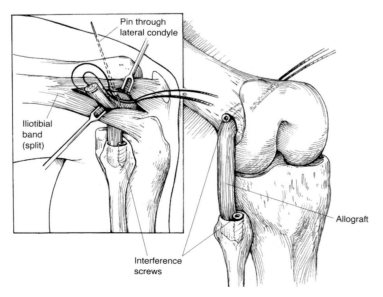

Figure 70–17   Bone–patellar tendon–bone reconstruction of the lateral collateral ligament. The isometric point on the lateral epicondyle is located 5 mm anterior to the epicondyle. Interference screws are used to anchor the bone plugs in the femur and fibula after the graft has been passed deep to the iliotibial band. (From Latimer HA, Tibone JE, ElAttrache NS, McMahon PJ: Reconstruction of the lateral collateral ligament of the knee with patellar tendon allograft: Report of a new technique in combined ligament injuries. Am J Sports Med 26:656-662, 1998.)

Pin through lateral condyle

Iliotibial band (split)

Interference screws

Allograft

tendency for posterior displacement while in the supine position must be appreciated. We prefer to teach the patient's partner to passively flex the reconstructed knee with the patient in the prone position several times per day. Bracing in extension is continued for 6 weeks, and closed chain rehabilitative exercises are started shortly after this period. Of note, when the PLC is reconstructed, patients should be protected from external rotation and varus stresses at the tibia for at least 6 to 8 weeks. Proprioceptive training, which can add further stability to the knee, is usually initiated at 12 weeks.[25] Hamstring exercises are delayed until the fourth postoperative month, and light jogging is allowed at 6 months. The patient should be able to return to full activities 9 to 12 months after surgery, provided the knee is stable, full range of motion has returned, and quadriceps strength is symmetrical to the contralateral leg.

Results

We are currently completing a follow-up study of PCL inlay reconstruction with a minimum 2-year follow-up. The preliminary results are encouraging, and we will be reporting our results in the peer-reviewed literature soon. We have found less residual laxity with the tibial inlay technique than with arthroscopic-assisted anterior PCL reconstruction.

Complications

Residual laxity can be decreased by avoiding kinking or hanging up of the graft during graft passage. Reports of avascular necrosis of the medial femoral condyle are a concern, so the tunnel should be started proximal to the articular margin. The intra-articular location of the tunnel should also be assessed, because this location affects the biomechanics of the graft. Wound breakdown of the upper medial aspect of the posterior incision has also been a concern. Usually, local wound care, with or without oral antibiotics, resolves the problem.

Complications of PLC reconstruction include common peroneal nerve palsy, especially in cases of chronic PLC reconstruction; persistent instability; arthrofibrosis; and hamstring weakness, especially in biceps tenodesis procedures. Hardware complications and infection are inherent in surgical procedures about the knee.

Conclusion

The natural history of the PCL-deficient knee is not as benign as once thought, owing to the patellofemoral and medial compartment arthrosis that can develop. Understanding the anatomy and biomechanics of the PCL and PLC can assist in postinjury management. Surgical techniques should strive to re-create normal anatomy, as with the tibial inlay technique for PCL reconstruction. With the evolution of surgical techniques and with greater knowledge of the biomechanical implications of the different components of the PLC, posterolateral reconstruction can also be performed in an anatomic manner. Postoperative rehabilitation should focus on countering the effects of gravity by incorporating prone exercises and providing posterior support. By reestablishing normal stability and kinematics to the knee, long-term success can be achieved when isolated and combined injuries to the posterior and lateral aspects of the knee are encountered.

References

1. Albright JP, Brown AW: Management of chronic posterolateral rotatory instability of the knee: Surgical technique for the posterolateral corner sling procedure. Instr Course Lect 47:369-378, 1998.
2. Berg EE: Posterior cruciate ligament tibial inlay reconstruction. Arthroscopy 11:69-76, 1995.
3. Bergfeld JA, McAllister DR, Parker RD, et al: The effects of tibial rotation on posterior translation in knees in which the posterior cruciate ligament has been cut. J Bone Joint Surg Am 83:1339-1343, 2001.
4. Burks RT, Schaffer JJ: A simplified approach to the tibial attachment of the posterior cruciate ligament. Clin Orthop 254:216-219, 1990.
5. Butler DL, Noyes FR, Grood ES: Ligamentous restraints to anteroposterior drawer in the human knee: A biomechanical study. J Bone Joint Surg Am 63:259-270, 1980.
6. Chen FS, Rokito AS, Pitman MI: Acute and chronic posterolateral rotatory instability of the knee. J Am Acad Orthop Surg 8:97-110, 2000.
7. Clancy WG Jr, Shelbourne KD, Zoellner GB, et al: Treatment of knee joint instability secondary to rupture of the posterior cruciate ligament: Report of a new procedure. J Bone Joint Surg Am 65:310-322, 1983.
8. Clancy WG Jr, Sutherland TB: Combined posterior cruciate ligament injuries. Clin Sports Med 13:629-647, 1994.
9. Clendenin MB, DeLee JC, Heckman JD: Interstitial tears of the posterior cruciate ligament of the knee. Orthopedics 3:764-772, 1980.
10. Cooper DE: Tests for posterolateral instability of the knee in normal subjects: Results of examination under anesthesia. J Bone Joint Surg Am 73:30-36, 1991.
11. Cooper DE, Warren RF, Warner JJP: The posterior cruciate ligament and posterolateral structures of the knee: Anatomy, function, and patterns of injury. Instr Course Lect 40:249-270, 1991.
12. Covey DC: Injuries of the posterolateral corner of the knee. J Bone Joint Surg Am 83:106-118, 2001.
13. Daniel DM, Stone ML, Barnett P, et al: Use of a quadriceps active test to diagnose posterior cruciate ligament disruption and measure posterior laxity of the knee. J Bone Joint Surg 70:386-391, 1988.
14. Fanelli GC, Giannotti BF, Edson CJ: The posterior cruciate ligament arthroscopic evaluation and treatment. Arthroscopy 10:673-688, 1994.
15. Gollehon DL, Torzilla PA, Warren RF: The role of the posterolateral and cruciate ligaments in the stability of the human knee: A biomechanical study. J Bone Joint Surg Am 69:233-242, 1987.
16. Gross ML, Grover JS, Bassett LW, et al: Magnetic resonance imaging of the posterior cruciate ligament: Clinical use to improve diagnostic accuracy. Am J Sports Med 20:732-737, 1992.

17. Harner CD, Vogrin TM, Hoher J, et al: Biomechanical analysis of a posterior cruciate ligament reconstruction: Deficiency of the posterolateral structures as a cause of graft failure. Am J Sports Med 28:32-39, 2000.
18. Hewett TE, Noyes FR, Lee MD: Diagnosis of complete and partial posterior cruciate ligament ruptures: Stress radiography compared with KT-1000 arthrometer and posterior drawer testing. Am J Sports Med 25:648-655, 1997.
19. Hughston JC, Bowden JA, Andrews JA, et al: Acute tears of the posterior cruciate ligament: Results of operative treatment. J Bone Joint Surg Am 62:438-450, 1980.
20. Hughston JC, Jacobsson KE: Chronic posterolateral instability of the knee. J Bone Joint Surg Am 67:351-359, 1985.
21. Hughston JC, Norwood LA Jr: The posterolateral drawer test and external rotational recurvatum test for posterolateral rotatory instability of the knee. Clin Orthop 147:82-87, 1980.
22. Jacobson KE: Technical pitfalls of collateral ligament surgery. Clin Sports Med 18:847-882, 1999.
23. Jakob RP, Hassler H, Staeubli HU: Observations on rotatory instability of the lateral compartment of the knee: Experimental studies on the functional anatomy and the pathomechanism of the true and the reversed pivot shift sign. Acta Orthop Scand Suppl 191:1-32, 1981.
24. Jakob RP, Warner JJP: Lateral and posterolateral rotatory instability of the knee. In Jakob RP, Staubli H-I (eds): The Knee and the Cruciate Ligaments: Anatomy, Biomechanics, Clinical Aspects, Reconstruction, Complications, and Rehabilitation. New York, Springer, 1992, pp 463-494.
25. Johansson H, Sjolander P, Sojka P: A sensory role for the cruciate ligaments. Clin Orthop 268:161-178, 1991.
26. Krukhaug Y, Molster A, Rodt A, et al: Lateral ligament injuries of the knee. Knee Surg Sports Traumatol Arthrosc 6:21-25, 1998.
27. LaPrade RF: Arthroscopic evaluation of the lateral compartment of knees with grade 3 posterolateral knee complex injuries. Am J Sports Med 25:596-602, 1997.
28. Latimer HA, Tibone JE, ElAttrache NS, McMahon PJ: Reconstruction of the lateral collateral ligament of the knee with patellar tendon allograft: Report of a new technique in combined ligament injuries. Am J Sports Med 26:656-662, 1998.
29. Meyers MH: Isolated avulsion of the tibial attachment of the posterior cruciate ligament of the knee. J Bone Joint Surg Am 57:669-672, 1975.
30. Miller MD, Bergfeld JA, Fowler PJ, et al: The posterior cruciate ligament injured knee: Principles of evaluation and treatment. Instr Course Lect 48:199-207, 1999.
31. Miller MD, Olszewski AD: Posterior cruciate ligament injuries: New treatment options. Am J Knee Surg 8:145-154, 1995.
32. Noyes FR, Barber-Westin SD: Treatment of complex injuries involving the posterior cruciate and posterolateral ligaments of the knee. Am J Knee Surg 9:200-214, 1996.
33. Noyes FR, Barber-Westin SD: Surgical restoration to treat chronic deficiency of the posterolateral complex and cruciate ligaments of the knee joint. Am J Sports Med 24:415-426, 1996.
34. Noyes FR, Barber-Westin SD, Grood ES: Newer concepts in the treatment of posterior cruciate ligament injuries. In Insall JN, Scott WN (eds): Surgery of the Knee. Philadelphia, WB Saunders, 2000, pp 841-877.
35. Noyes FR, Roberts CS: High tibial osteotomy in knees with associated chronic ligament deficiencies. In Jackson DW (ed): Reconstructive Knee Surgery. New York, Raven Press, 1995, pp 185-210.
36. O'Connor JJ: Can muscle co-contraction protect knee ligaments after injury or repair? J Bone Joint Surg Br 75:41-48, 1993.
37. Parolie JM, Bergfeld JA: Long-term results of nonoperative treatment of isolated posterior cruciate ligament injuries in the athlete. Am J Sports Med 14:35-38, 1986.
38. Plancher KD, Siliski JM, Ribbans W: Traumatic dislocation of the knee: Complications and results of operative and nonoperative treatment. In Proceedings of the American Academy of Orthopaedic Surgeons 56th Annual Meeting, 1989, Las Vegas, NV, p 85.
39. Richter M, Kiefer H, Hehl G, et al: Primary repair for posterior cruciate ligament injuries: An eight-year followup of fifty-three patients. Am J Sports Med 24:298-305, 1996.
40. Roman PD, Hopson CN, Zenni EJ Jr: Traumatic dislocation of the knee: A report of 30 cases and literature review. Orthop Rev 16:917-924, 1987.
41. Satku K, Chew CN, Seow H: Posterior cruciate ligament injuries. Acta Orthop Scand 55:26-29, 1984.
42. Seebacher JR, Inglis AE, Marshall JL, et al: The structure of the posterolateral aspect of the knee. J Bone Joint Surg Am 64:537, 1982.
43. Shino K, Horibe S, Nakata K, et al: Conservative treatment of isolated injuries to the posterior cruciate ligament in athletes. J Bone Joint Surg Br 77:895-900, 1995.
44. Sisto DJ, Warren RF: Complete knee dislocation: A follow-up study of operative treatment. Clin Orthop 198:94-101, 1985.
45. Terry GC, LaPrade RF: The posterolateral aspect of the knee: Anatomy and surgical approach. Am J Sports Med 24:732-739, 1996.
46. Veltri DM, Warren RF: Isolated and combined posterior cruciate ligament injuries. J Am Acad Orthop Surg 1:67-75, 1993.
47. Veltri DM, Warren RF: Anatomy, biomechanics, and physical findings in posterolateral knee instability. Clin Sports Med 13:599-614, 1994.
48. Veltri DM, Warren RF: Operative treatment of posterolateral instability of the knee. Clin Sports Med 13:615-627, 1994.

Multiligament Injuries: Diagnosis and Decision Making

GREGORY C. FANELLI

The knee with multiple ligament injuries is a complex problem in orthopedic surgery. These injuries may or may not present as acute knee dislocations, and careful assessment of the extremity's vascular status is essential because of the possibility of arterial or venous compromise. These complex injuries require a systematic approach to evaluation and treatment. Physical examination and imaging studies enable the surgeon to make the correct diagnosis and formulate a treatment plan. My colleagues and I have previously published our approach to these complex issues, and the reader is referred to these sources for additional information.[1,3-28,35,36]

Posterior cruciate ligament (PCL) injuries reportedly account for 1% to 40% of acute knee injuries. This range is dependent on the patient population, and the incidence is approximately 3% in the general population and 38% in reports from regional trauma centers.[12,13,22] In my practice at a regional trauma center, there is a 38.3% incidence of PCL tears in acute knee injuries, and 56.5% of these PCL injuries occur in multiple trauma patients. Of these PCL injuries, 45.9% are combined anterior cruciate ligament (ACL)–PCL tears, and 41.2% are PCL–posterolateral corner tears. Only 3% of acute PCL injuries seen in the trauma center are isolated.

The purpose of this chapter is to identify trends that occur with combined ACL-PCL injuries and to present a treatment strategy for these injuries.

Classification

Combined ACL-PCL injuries may or may not present as acute knee dislocations. Classification of knee dislocations is based primarily on the direction the tibia dislocates relative to the femur.[30,32] This results in five different categories: anterior, posterior, lateral, medial, and rotatory. Anteromedial and lateral dislocations and posteromedial and lateral dislocations are classified as

rotatory. Other factors to be considered include whether (1) the injury is open or closed, (2) it is due to high- or low-energy trauma, (3) the knee is completely dislocated or subluxed, and (4) there is neurovascular involvement. Further, one should be acutely aware of the fact that a complete knee dislocation may spontaneously reduce, and any triple-ligament knee injury constitutes a frank dislocation.[4-6,9,10,12,17,19-21,23,25,38,41]

Open knee dislocations are not uncommon, with a reported incidence between 19% and 35% of all dislocations.[37,39] An open knee dislocation carries a worse prognosis secondary to severe injury to the soft tissue envelope. Further, an open injury may require an open ligament reconstruction or a staged reconstruction, because arthroscopically assisted techniques cannot be performed in the acute setting with open injuries.

Distinguishing between low- and high-energy injuries is important. Low-energy or low-velocity injuries, usually associated with sports injuries, have a decreased incidence of associated vascular injury. High-energy or high-velocity injuries secondary to motor vehicle accidents or falls from heights tend to have an increased incidence of vascular compromise. Decreased pulses in an injured limb and a history of a high-energy injury indicate that vascular studies should be obtained urgently.

Mechanism of Injury

The mechanisms of injury for the two most common knee dislocation patterns—anterior and posterior—are reasonably well described. Kennedy[34] was able to reproduce anterior dislocation by a hyperextension force acting on the knee. At 30 degrees of hyperextension, the posterior capsule failed. When extended further to approximately 50 degrees, the ACL, PCL, and popliteal artery failed. There is some question whether the ACL or PCL fails first with hyperextension.[31,34]

The most frequent ACL–PCL–posterolateral corner mechanism of injury at our trauma center is forced varus, resulting in knee dislocation. The most frequent ACL–PCL–medial collateral ligament mechanism of injury is forced valgus, resulting in knee dislocation.[3,13,22]

Clinical Evaluation

Evaluation of an acute ACL-PCL injury includes a history of injury mechanism, physical examination with careful neurovascular examination (arteriogram and venogram), plain radiographs, magnetic resonance imaging studies, and examination under anesthesia and diagnostic arthroscopy. In chronic cases, bone scans may be helpful.[2]

History

When an acute ACL-PCL injury presents as a dislocated knee, a gentle closed reduction should be performed immediately, and careful assessment of the neurovascular status performed. In acute ACL-PCL injuries that present without documented dislocation, the neurovascular status of the extremity must also be carefully assessed, because a knee that was dislocated "in the field" may have undergone spontaneous reduction. Wascher et al.[41] reported a 14% incidence of arterial injury in dislocated knees, and we reported an 11% incidence of arterial injury in acute three-ligament knee injuries at our center.[20] Our recommendation is to obtain arteriograms in acute three-ligament injuries to rule out vascular damage, especially intimal flap tears that may present several days after injury. We have also experienced deep venous thrombosis associated with acute knee dislocation–three-ligament injuries and suggest venograms in these patients when clinically indicated.

Physical Examination

Physical examination features of ACL–PCL–posterolateral corner injuries include abnormal anterior and posterior translation at both 25 and 90 degrees of knee flexion. At 90 degrees of knee flexion, the tibial step-off is absent, and the posterior drawer test is 2+ or greater, indicating greater than 10 mm of pathologic posterior tibial displacement. The Lachman test and pivot shift phenomenon are positive, indicating ACL disruption.

Posterolateral instability includes at least 10 degrees of increased tibial external rotation compared with the normal knee at 30 degrees of knee flexion (positive dial test and external rotation thigh-foot angle test) and variable degrees of varus instability, depending on the injured anatomic structures.[1] We have described three types of posterolateral instability: A, B, and C.[20] Type A has increased external rotation only, corresponding to injury to the popliteofibular ligament and popliteal tendon only. Type B presents with increased external rotation and mild varus instability consisting of approximately 5 mm increased lateral joint line opening to varus

stress at 30 degrees of knee flexion. This occurs with damage to the popliteofibular ligament, popliteal tendon, and attenuation of the fibular collateral ligament. Type C presents with increased tibial external rotation and varus instability of 10 mm greater than the normal knee tested at 30 degrees of flexion with varus stress. This occurs with injury to the popliteofibular ligament, popliteal tendon, fibular collateral ligament, and lateral capsular avulsion, in addition to cruciate ligament disruption. The intact medial collateral ligament, tested with valgus stress at 30 degrees of knee flexion, is the stable hinge in a knee with an ACL–PCL–posterolateral corner injury.

The presence of a dimple sign on the anteromedial surface of the knee should be recognized. This indicates a posterolateral dislocation and is associated with a high incidence of irreducibility and potential skin necrosis. Open reduction is indicated.

Combined ACL–PCL–medial side injuries present with the same central pivot physical examination as described earlier, plus significant valgus laxity at 0 and 30 degrees of knee flexion. The patellofemoral joint must be carefully assessed in these injuries, because lateral patellar dislocation can occur (Fig. 71–1).

Imaging

Plain radiographs should include standing anteroposterior views of both knees, 30-degree anteroposterior axial views of both patellas, and intercondylar notch views. These radiographs will help document reduction of the tibiofemoral and patellofemoral joints, assess bony alignment, and evaluate for insertion site bony avulsions of the cruciates, collateral ligament complexes, and extensor mechanisms.

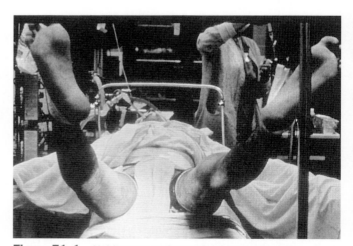

Figure 71–1 Multitrauma patient with left knee anterior cruciate ligament–posterior cruciate ligament–medial collateral ligament tear and right knee anterior cruciate ligament–posterolateral corner tears. (From Fanelli GC, Feldmann DD: Management of the dislocated/multiple ligament injured knee. Oper Tech Orthop 9:298-308, 1999.)

Magnetic resonance imaging has a high diagnostic accuracy in acute PCL injuries and is helpful in assessing tear location in the cruciate and collateral ligaments and in formulating a treatment plan.[29,33] Bone scans may be helpful for evaluating subacute and chronic cases. Increased activity in the patellofemoral joint and medial compartment may signify the onset of early degenerative arthrosis, which is an indication for surgical stabilization.[2,40]

In the presence of cyanosis, pallor, weak capillary refill, and decreased peripheral temperature following reduction, arteriography must be considered. Venography is considered when the clinical picture indicates adequate limb perfusion but obstruction of outflow (Fig. 71–2).

Diagnostic Arthroscopy

The three-zone method of PCL evaluation enhances the information gained from imaging studies and examination of the injured knee under anesthesia.[22] Zone 1 of the PCL is the femoral insertion to the middle third of the ligament, zone 2 is the middle third of the PCL, and zone 3 is the tibial insertion site area. With the use of a 30-degree arthroscope, the anterolateral patellar portal, and the posteromedial portal, the PCL and the posterolateral structures can be evaluated systematically. Direct and indirect findings are assessed, and surgical treatment decisions are made. I have found arthroscopic evaluation of the PCL to be most helpful in assessing interstitial damage to the PCL and ACL in the case of bony inser-

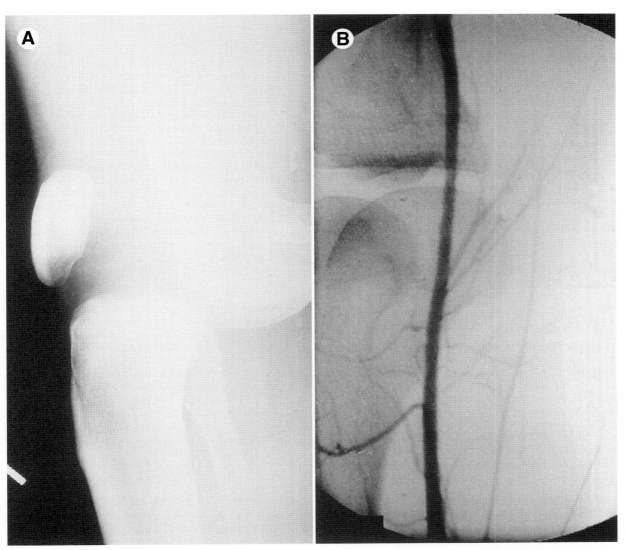

Figure 71–2 *A*, Lateral radiograph of anterior tibiofemoral knee dislocation. *B*, Arteriogram after closed reduction of dislocated knee, documenting the vascular status of the extremity. (From Fanelli GC, Feldmann DD: Management of the dislocated/multiple ligament injured knee. Oper Tech Orthop 9:298-308, 1999.)

6 Knee

tion site avulsions. Severe interstitial disruption of zone 2 indicates that reconstruction is the procedure of choice, rather than primary repair.

Other Considerations

An unreduced dislocated knee is an orthopedic emergency and requires urgent reduction. When there is suspicion of arterial injury, arteriography and vascular surgery consultation should be obtained. Popliteal vein injury is also possible, and if the clinical picture warrants, a venogram should be performed.

A state of irreducibility or vascular injury warrants immediate surgical intervention. One should consider four-compartment fasciotomy of the limb when ischemic time is greater than 2.5 hours. Inability to maintain reduction mandates early ligamentous reconstruction to stabilize the knee and avoid recurrent vascular compromise. Open dislocations and open fracture-dislocations warrant immediate surgical debridement and possibly external fixation.

Summary

Multiligament knee injuries are a complex problem in orthopedic surgery. These injuries may or may not present as acute knee dislocations, and careful assessment of the extremity's vascular status is essential because of the possibility of arterial or venous compromise. These complex injuries require a systematic approach to evaluation and treatment. History taking, physical examination, injury classification, knowledge of the injury mechanism, imaging studies, and diagnostic arthroscopy enable the surgeon to make the correct diagnosis and formulate a treatment plan.

References

1. Bleday RM, Fanelli GC, Giannotti BF, et al: Instrumented measurement of the posterolateral corner. Arthroscopy 14:489-494, 1998.
2. Clancy WG: Repair and reconstruction of the posterior cruciate ligament. In Chapman M (ed): Operative Orthopaedics. Philadelphia, JB Lippincott, 1988, pp 1651-1665.
3. Fanelli GC: Posterior cruciate ligament injuries in trauma patients. Arthroscopy 9:291-294, 1993.
4. Fanelli GC: Combined anterior and posterior cruciate ligament injuries: The multiple ligament injured knee. Sports Med Arthrosc Rev 7:289-295, 1999.
5. Fanelli GC: Treatment of combined anterior cruciate ligament–posterior cruciate ligament–lateral side injuries of the knee. Clin Sports Med 19:493-502, 2000.
6. Fanelli GC: Arthroscopic combined ACL/PCL reconstruction. In Posterior Cruciate Ligament Injuries: A Guide to Practical Management. New York, Springer-Verlag, 2001, pp 215-236.
7. Fanelli GC: Arthroscopic evaluation of the PCL. In Posterior Cruciate Ligament Injuries: A Guide to Practical Management. New York, Springer-Verlag, 2001, pp 95-108.
8. Fanelli GC: Complications in PCL surgery. In Posterior Cruciate Ligament Injuries: A Guide to Practical Management. New York, Springer-Verlag, 2001, pp 291-302.
9. Fanelli GC: Posterior Cruciate Ligament Injuries: A Guide to Practical Management. New York, Springer-Verlag, 2001.
10. Fanelli GC: Surgical treatment of the acute and chronic ACL/PCL/medial side/lateral side injuries of the knee. Sports Med Arthrosc Rev 9(3):208-218, 2001.
11. Fanelli GC: Complications in the multiple ligament injured knee. In Schenck RC Jr (ed): AAOS Monograph on Multiple Ligamentous Injuries of the Knee in the Athlete. Rosemont, IL, American Academy of Orthopaedic Surgeons, 2002, pp 101-107.
12. Fanelli GC: The Multiple Ligament Injured Knee: A Practical Guide to Management. New York, Springer-Verlag, 2004 (in press).
13. Fanelli GC, Edson CJ: Posterior cruciate ligament injuries in trauma patients. Part II. Arthroscopy 11:526-529, 1995.
14. Fanelli GC, Edson CJ: Management of combined anterior cruciate ligament/posterior cruciate ligament injuries of the knee. In Chow J (ed): Advanced Arthroplasty. New York, Springer-Verlag, 2001, pp 533-544.
15. Fanelli GC, Edson CJ: Management of posterior cruciate ligament and posterolateral instability of the knee. In Chow J (ed): Advanced Arthroplasty. New York, Springer-Verlag, 2001, pp 545-558.
16. Fanelli GC, Edson CJ: Arthroscopically assisted combined ACL/PCL reconstruction: 2–10 year follow-up. Arthroscopy 18:703-714, 2002.
17. Fanelli GC, Edson CJ, Maish DR: Management of combined ACL/PCL injuries. Tech Orthop 16:157-166, 2001.
18. Fanelli GC, Feldmann DD: The use of allograft tissue in knee ligament reconstruction. In Parisien JS (ed): Current Techniques in Arthroscopy. Philadelphia, Current Medicine, 1998, pp 47-56.
19. Fanelli GC, Feldmann DD: The dislocated/multiple ligament injured knee. Oper Tech Orthop 9:1-12, 1999.
20. Fanelli GC, Feldmann DD: Management of combined ACL/PCL/posterolateral complex injuries of the knee. Oper Tech Sports Med 7:143-149, 1999.
21. Fanelli GC, Feldmann DD, Edson CJ, Maish DR: The multiple ligament injured knee. In DeLee JC, Drez DD, Miller MD (eds): DeLee and Drez's Orthopaedic Sports Medicine, 2nd ed. Philadelphia, Elsevier, 2003, pp 2111-2121.
22. Fanelli GC, Giannotti BF, Edson CJ: Current concepts review: The posterior cruciate ligament arthroscopic evaluation and treatment. Arthroscopy 10:673-688, 1994.
23. Fanelli GC, Giannotti, B, Edson CJ: Arthroscopically assisted combined ACL/PCL reconstruction. Arthroscopy 12:5-14, 1996.
24. Fanelli GC, Larson RV: Practical management of posterolateral instability of the knee. Arthroscopy 18(Suppl 1):1-8, 2002.
25. Fanelli GC, Maish DR: Knee ligament injuries: Epidemiology, mechanism, diagnosis, and natural history. In Fitzgerald R, Kaufer H, Mallani A (eds): Orthopaedics. St Louis, CV Mosby, 2002, pp 619-636.
26. Fanelli GC, Monahan TJ: Complications of posterior cruciate ligament reconstruction. Sports Med Arthrosc Rev 7:296-302, 1999.
27. Fanelli GC, Monahan TJ: Complications and pitfalls in posterior cruciate ligament reconstruction. In Malek M (ed): Knee Surgery: Complications, Pitfalls, and Salvage. New York, Springer-Verlag, 2001, pp 121-128.
28. Fanelli GC, Monahan TJ: Complications in posterior cruciate ligament and posterolateral complex surgery. Oper Tech Sports Med 9:96-99, 2001.

29. Fowler PJ: Imaging of the posterior cruciate ligament. In Fanelli GC (ed): Posterior Cruciate Ligament Injuries. New York, Springer-Verlag, 2001, pp 77-86.

30. Ghalambor N, Vangsness CT: Traumatic dislocation of the knee: A review of the literature. Bull Hosp Jt Dis 54:19-24, 1995.

31. Girgis FG, Marshall JL, Al Monajem ARS: The cruciate ligaments of the knee joint: Anatomic, functional, and experimental analysis. Clin Orthop 106:216-231, 1975.

32. Good L, Johnson RJ: The dislocated knee. J Am Acad Orthop Surg 3:284-292, 1995.

33. Harner CD, Hoher J: Current concepts: Evaluation and treatment of posterior cruciate ligament injuries. Am J Sports Med 26:471-482, 1998.

34. Kennedy JC: Complete dislocation of the knee joint. J Bone Joint Surg Am 45:889-904, 1963.

35. Malek MM, Fanelli GC: Arthroscopically assisted posterior cruciate ligament reconstruction using Achilles tendon allograft. In Parisien JS (ed): Therapeutic Arthroscopy. New York, Raven Press, 1993, pp 47-56.

36. Miller MD, Cooper DE, Fanelli GC, et al: Posterior cruciate ligament: Current concepts. Instr Course Lect 51:347-351, 2002.

37. Myers MH, Harvey JP: Traumatic dislocation of the knee joint: A study of eighteen cases. J Bone Joint Surg Am 53:16-29, 1971.

38. Shelbourne KD, Porter DA, Clingman JA, et al: Low velocity knee dislocation. Orthop Rev 20:995-1004, 1991.

39. Shields L, Mital M, Cave EF: Complete dislocation of the knee: Experience at the Massachusetts General Hospital. J Trauma 9:192-215, 1969.

40. Skyhar MJ, Warren RF, Oritz GJ, et al: The effects of sectioning the posterior cruciate ligament and the posterolateral complex on the articular contact pressure within the knee. J Bone Joint Surg Am 75:694-699, 1993.

41. Wascher DC, Dvirnak PC, Decoster TA: Knee dislocation: Initial assessment and implications for treatment. J Orthop Trauma 11:525-529, 1997.

6 Knee

Multiligament Injuries: Surgical Technique

Gregory C. Fanelli

History:
Knee dislocation: high velocity (motor vehicle accident), low velocity (sports and vocational or avocational injuries)

Physical Examination:
Neuromuscular evaluation; Lachman (ACL); posterior drawer (PCL); varus-valgus (collateral ligaments); external rotation asymmetry (PLC)

Indications:
Severe functional instability

Surgical Technique:
PCL tunnels; ACL tunnels; PCL passage + tensioning; ACL passage + tensioning; PLC—split biceps transfer; posteromedial—posteromedial capsule shifted anteriorly

Postoperative Management:
Non–weight bearing and braced in extension for 6 weeks

Results:
Lysholm, Tegner, Hospital for Special Surgery scores of 91.2, 5.3, 86.8, respectively; stress radiographs 0 to 3 mm in 52%, 4 to 5 mm in 24%

ACL, anterior cruciate ligament; PCL, posterior cruciate ligament; PLC, posterolateral corner.

The preferred approach to combined anterior and posterior cruciate ligament (ACL-PCL) injuries is an arthroscopic ACL-PCL reconstruction using the transtibial PCL technique and single-incision arthroscopic ACL reconstruction, with collateral or capsular ligament surgery as indicated. Not all cases are amenable to an arthroscopic approach, and the operating surgeon must assess each case individually. Surgical timing is dependent on vascular status, reduction stability, skin condition, systemic injuries, open versus closed knee injury, meniscus and articular surface injuries, other orthopedic injuries, and the collateral or capsular ligaments involved.

This chapter describes my surgical technique of combined ACL-PCL and collateral ligament reconstruction and presents the Fanelli Sports Injury Clinic 2-

to 10-year results using this technique. The material in this chapter has also been presented elsewhere, and the reader is referred to these sources for additional information.[1,3-29,31-34,36]

Surgical Indications and Timing

The goals in the treatment of ACL-PCL injuries are to assess the neurovascular status, restore functional and objective stability to the injured knee, guard against progressive joint degeneration, and provide objective follow-up results regarding the treatment of these patients. Surgery is indicated for ACL-PCL injuries that result in severe functional instability. These knees are at high risk for progressive instability and the development of post-traumatic arthrosis.

Surgery should be performed as soon as it is possible to do so safely, generally 2 to 3 weeks after injury. During this period, the acute inflammatory phase subsides, and range of motion is restored. This lessens the risk of post-operative stiffness, which is high in these knees with multiligament injuries.[12,23,24,39] While awaiting surgery, the knee is protected in full extension in a long-leg, hinged range-of-motion brace. At 2 to 3 weeks after injury, enough capsular sealing has occurred to allow arthroscopic ACL-PCL reconstruction, as well as primary repair or reconstruction of the injured collateral ligament structures.

Special considerations that affect the timing of surgery include the vascular status of the extremity, reduction stability in dislocated knees, skin condition, multiple system injuries, open injuries, and other orthopedic injuries. These overriding conditions may necessitate that surgery be performed earlier or later than planned. My colleagues and I have reported excellent results with delayed reconstruction of multiligament injuries in the knee.[12,23,24]

Graft Selection

The ideal graft material is strong, provides secure fixation, is easy to pass, is readily available, and has low donor site morbidity. The available options in the United States are autograft and allograft sources. My preferred graft for the PCL is the Achilles tendon allograft because of its large cross-sectional area and strength, absence of donor site morbidity, and easy passage with secure fixation (Fig. 72–1). I prefer Achilles tendon allograft or bone–patellar tendon–bone allograft for ACL reconstruction.[19] The preferred graft material for the posterolateral corner is a split biceps tendon transfer, free autograft (semitendinosus), or allograft tissue when the biceps tendon is not available. Medial side reconstruction is performed with Achilles tendon allograft, capsular shift procedures, or a combination of both.

Surgical Technique

Positioning

The patient is positioned supine on the operating table. The surgical leg hangs over the side of the table, and the well leg is supported by the fully extended table. A lateral post is used for control of the surgical leg; I do not use a leg holder. The surgery may be done under tourniquet control. Fluid inflow is by gravity; I do not use an arthroscopic fluid pump.

Specific Surgical Steps

The inflow is placed in the superolateral portal, the arthroscope is placed in the inferolateral patellar portal, and the instruments are placed in the inferomedial patellar portal. An accessory extracapsular, extra-articular posteromedial safety incision is used to protect the neurovascular structures and to confirm the accuracy of tibial tunnel placement (Fig. 72–2).

The notchplasty is performed first and consists of ACL and PCL stump debridement, bone removal, and contouring of the medial wall of the lateral femoral condyle and the intercondylar roof. This allows visualization of the over-the-top position and prevents ACL graft impingement throughout the full range of motion. Specially curved PCL instruments (Arthrotek, Inc., Warsaw, IN) are used to elevate the capsule from the posterior aspect of the tibia (Fig. 72–3).

The PCL tibial and femoral tunnels are created with the help of the Arthrotek Fanelli PCL-ACL drill guide (Fig. 72–4). The transtibial PCL tunnel is drilled from the anteromedial aspect of the proximal tibia 1 cm below the tibial tubercle and exits in the inferolateral aspect of the PCL anatomic insertion site (Fig. 72–5). The PCL femoral tunnel originates externally between the medial femoral epicondyle and the medial femoral condyle articular surface, approximately 2 cm proximal to the distal medial femoral condyle articular surface, and emerges through the center of the stump of the PCL's anterolateral bundle (Fig. 72–6). This external position

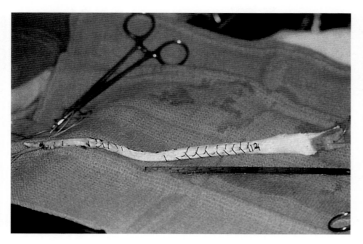

Figure 72–1 Prepared Achilles tendon allograft. The graft is tubed for easy passage and for filling of the bone tunnels. Number 5 braided permanent sutures are woven through the ends of the graft for traction or fixation. (From Fanelli GC, Feldman DD: Management of the dislocated/multiple ligament injured knee. Oper Tech Orthop 9:298-308, 1999.)

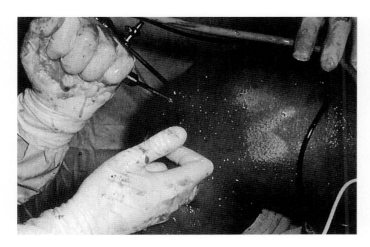

Figure 72–2 A 1- to 2-cm extracapsular, extra-articular posteromedial safety incision allows the surgeon's finger to protect the neurovascular structures, confirm the position of the posterior cruciate ligament (PCL) instruments and drill guide on the posterior aspect of the proximal tibia, and ensure the accuracy of PCL tibial tunnel placement in both the medial-lateral and proximal-distal planes. (From Fanelli GC: Oper Tech Orthop 9:298-308, 1999.)

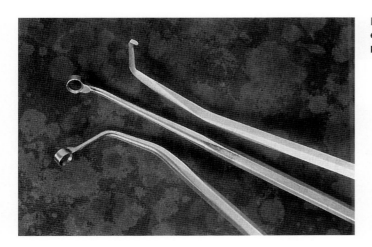

Figure 72–3 Curved posterior cruciate ligament instruments enable the surgeon to elevate the capsule from the posterior proximal tibia. (Courtesy of Arthrotek, Inc., Warsaw, IN.)

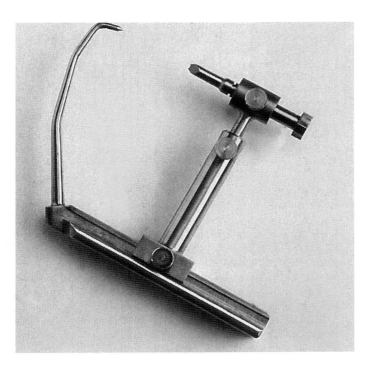

Figure 72–4 The posterior cruciate ligament (PCL)–anterior cruciate ligament (ACL) drill guide enables the surgeon to drill the PCL and ACL tibial and femoral tunnels. (Courtesy of Arthrotek, Inc., Warsaw, IN.)

6 Knee

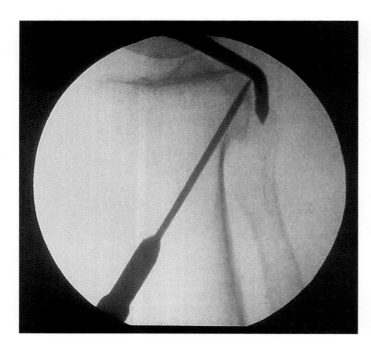

Figure 72–5 The posterior cruciate ligament tibial tunnel should exit at the inferior and lateral aspect of the ligament's anatomic insertion site. (From Fanelli GC: Oper Tech Orthop 9:298-308, 1999.)

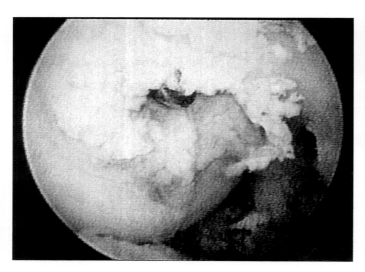

Figure 72–6 The posterior cruciate ligament (PCL) femoral tunnel enters the joint through the center of the anterolateral fiber region, or bundle, of the ligament's anatomic insertion site. The single-bundle PCL reconstruction technique reproduces the PCL's anterolateral bundle. The femoral drill hole is in the center of the anterolateral bundle of the PCL. (From Fanelli GC: Oper Tech Orthop 9:298-308, 1999.)

of the femoral tunnel minimizes the chance of avascular necrosis or subchondral fracture of the medial femoral condyle. The PCL graft is positioned and anchored on the femoral side and is left free on the tibial side.

The ACL tunnels are created using the single-incision technique.[14,22,33] The tibial tunnel begins externally at a point 1 cm proximal to the tibial tubercle on the anteromedial surface of the proximal tibia and emerges through the center of the stump of the ACL tibial footprint. The femoral tunnel is positioned next to the over-the-top position on the medial wall of the lateral femoral condyle near the ACL anatomic insertion site. The tunnel is created to leave a 1- to 2-mm posterior cortical wall so that interference fixation can be used. The ACL graft is positioned and anchored on the femoral side, with the tibial side left free.

My preferred technique for posterolateral reconstruction is the split biceps tendon transfer to the lateral femoral epicondyle.[2,3,5,6,9-11,15-18,20-22,24-26,36,40] The requirements for this procedure include an intact proximal tibiofibular joint, intact posterolateral capsular attachments to the common biceps tendon, and intact biceps femoris tendon insertion into the fibular head. This technique reproduces the function of the popliteofibular ligament and lateral collateral ligament, tightens the posterolateral capsule, and provides a post of strong autogenous tissue to reinforce the posterolateral corner.

A lateral hockey-stick incision is made. The peroneal nerve is dissected free and protected throughout the procedure. The long head and common biceps femoris tendon are isolated, and the anterior two thirds is separated from the short head muscle. The tendon is detached proximally and left attached distally to its anatomic insertion site on the fibular head. The strip of biceps tendon should be 12 to 14 cm long. The iliotibial band is incised in line with its fibers, and the fibular collateral ligament and popliteal tendon are exposed. A drill hole is made 1 cm anterior to the fibular collateral ligament's femoral insertion. A longitudinal incision is made in the lateral capsule just posterior to the fibular collateral ligament. The split biceps tendon is passed medial to the iliotibial band and secured to the lateral femoral epicondylar region with a screw and spiked ligament washer at the above-mentioned point. The residual tail of the transferred split biceps tendon is passed medial to the iliotibial band and secured to the fibular head. The posterolateral capsule that had been incised previously is shifted and sewn into the strut of the transferred biceps tendon to eliminate posterolateral capsular redundancy (Fig. 72–7).

Posteromedial and medial reconstructions are performed through a medial hockey-stick incision. Care is taken to maintain adequate skin bridges between incisions. The superficial medial collateral ligament (MCL) is exposed, and a longitudinal incision is made just posterior to the posterior border of the MCL. Care is taken

not to damage the medial meniscus during the capsular incision. The interval between the posteromedial capsule and the medial meniscus is developed, and the posteromedial capsule is shifted anterosuperiorly. The medial meniscus is repaired to the new capsular position, and the shifted capsule is sewn into the MCL. When superficial MCL reconstruction is indicated, this is performed with allograft tissue or semitendinosus autograft. This graft material is attached at the anatomic insertion sites of the superficial MCL on the femur and tibia. The posteromedial capsule is advanced and sewn into the newly reconstructed MCL (Fig. 72–8).

The PCL is reconstructed first, followed by the ACL, the posterolateral complex, and the medial ligament complex. Tension is placed on the PCL graft distally using the Arthrotek knee ligament tensioning device, with the tension set for 20 pounds (Fig. 72–9). This restores the anatomic tibial step-off. The knee is cycled through a full range of motion 25 times to allow pretensioning and settling of the graft. The knee is placed in 0 or 70 degrees of flexion, and fixation is achieved on the tibial side of the PCL graft with a screw and spiked ligament washer and a bioabsorable interference screw. The knee is then placed in 30 degrees of flexion, the tibia is

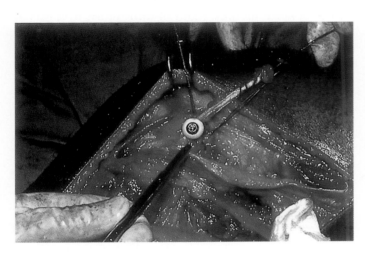

Figure 72–7 The posterolateral reconstruction is performed using a split biceps tendon transfer combined with a posterolateral capsular shift. This technique re-creates the function of the popliteofibular and lateral collateral ligaments and eliminates the posterolateral capsular redundancy. The anterior two thirds of the long head and common biceps femoris tendon is isolated from the short head muscle. The tendon is detached proximally and left attached distally to its anatomic insertion site. The peroneal nerve is protected. The split biceps tendon is passed medial to the iliotibial band and secured to the lateral femoral epicondyle approximately 1 cm anterior to the fibular collateral ligament's femoral insertion using a cancellous screw and spiked ligament washer. (From Fanelli GC: Oper Tech Orthop 9:298-308, 1999.)

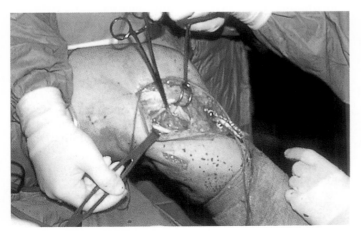

Figure 72–8 Posteromedial reconstruction is performed through a medial hockey-stick incision using the posteromedial capsular shift procedure. (From Fanelli GC: Oper Tech Orthop 9:298-308, 1999.)

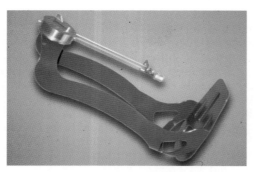

Figure 72–9 A mechanical tensioning device is used to precisely tension posterior cruciate ligament (PCL) and anterior cruciate ligament (ACL) grafts. During PCL reconstruction, the tensioning device is attached to the tibial end of the graft, and the torque wrench ratchet is set to 20 pounds. The knee is cycled through 25 full flexion-extension cycles. Then, with the knee at 0 degrees of flexion, final PCL tibial fixation is achieved with a Lactosorb resorbable interference screw and a screw and spiked ligament washer for backup fixation. The tensioning device is set to 20 pounds and applied to the ACL graft with the knee in 70 degrees of flexion. Final ACL fixation is achieved with Lactosorb bioabsorbable interference screws and a spiked ligament washer for backup fixation. The mechanical tensioning device ensures consistent graft tensioning and eliminates graft advancement during interference screw insertion. It also restores the anatomic tibial step-off during PCL graft tensioning and applies a posterior drawer force during ACL graft tensioning. (Courtesy of Arthrotek, Inc., Warsaw, IN.)

internally rotated, slight valgus force is applied to the knee, and final tensioning and fixation of the posterolateral corner is achieved. The Arthrotek knee ligament tensioning device is applied to the ACL graft and set to 20 pounds. The knee is placed in 70 degrees of flexion, and final fixation of the ACL graft is achieved with a bioabsorbable interference screw and spiked ligament washer backup fixation. The MCL reconstruction is tensioned with the knee in 30 degrees of flexion with the leg in a figure-four position. Full range of motion is confirmed on the operating table to ensure that the knee is not "captured" by the reconstruction.

Pearls and Pitfalls

The posteromedial safety incision protects the neurovascular structures, confirms accurate tibial tunnel placement, and allows the surgical procedure to be done at an accelerated pace. The single-incision ACL reconstruction technique prevents lateral cortex crowding and eliminates multiple through-and-through drill holes in the distal femur, reducing the stress riser effect. It is important to be aware of the two tibial tunnel directions and to have a 1-cm bone bridge between the PCL and ACL tibial tunnels. This reduces the possibility of fracture. I have found it useful to use primary and backup fixation—primary fixation with resorbable interference screws, and backup fixation with a screw and spiked ligament washer. Secure fixation is critical to the success of this surgical procedure.

Postoperative Management

Rehabilitation following multiple ligament reconstruction is an ever-evolving process, with principles based on existing knowledge and scientific rationale. Rehabilitation guidelines should consider surgical technique and the natural alignment of the lower extremity. The first 6 postoperative weeks constitute the maximum protection phase. During weeks 1 through 6, the patient is non–weight bearing, and the surgical extremity is braced in full extension. During weeks 4 through 6, range of motion is progressed. Beginning at postoperative week 7, the patient increases weight bearing by one third body weight per week and should be fully weight bearing with crutches at the end of week 10. Varus and valgus forces are avoided during range-of-motion exercises to protect the collateral ligaments that have been reconstructed. Brace protection is continued through weeks 10 to 12. Range-of-motion exercises are progressed using a stationary bicycle, and closed chain exercises are performed with stair-stepping machines. Proprioceptive skill training is also advanced. Straight-line jogging is initiated between postoperative months 3 and 4, depending on the patient's strength and proprioception.

Sports-specific exercises and training begin between postoperative months 4 and 5, with return to sports at the end of months 6 to 9 if the following criteria are met: quadriceps and hamstring strength is 90% or greater than that of the uninvolved extremity, the patient is able to perform all necessary skills without pain or restriction, and a functional (combined instability) brace is obtained. It should be noted that a loss of 10 to 15 degrees of terminal flexion can be expected in these complex knee ligament reconstructions. This does not cause a functional problem and is no reason for alarm.

Results

My colleagues and I previously published the results of our arthroscopically assisted combined ACL-PCL and PCL–posterolateral complex reconstructions using the technique described in this chapter.[3,5,6,9,15,17,18,20-24,36] More recently, Ibrahim[30] reported the results of 41 traumatic knee dislocations treated with ACL and PCL reconstruction at a mean follow-up of 39 months. In these young patients (mean age 26.3 years), early mobilization with continuous passive motion and active range-of-motion exercises was started on postoperative day 2. Based on these results, he recommended early reconstruction of the cruciate ligaments, early repair of the collateral ligaments, and aggressive rehabilitation in young, active patients.

Other studies that evaluated results based on arthrometric data support early reconstruction of the cruciate ligaments and early repair of the collateral ligaments. Although results vary, they all demonstrate that residual laxity is present in a certain portion of reconstructed knees.[35,37,38]

Yeh et al.[41] reported on the results of PCL reconstruction with ACL debridement. This study did not report mean side-to-side difference in anteroposterior laxity, but the authors reported good range of motion and a mean Lysholm score of 84 at a follow-up of 27 months.

Fanelli Sports Injury Clinic Results

This section presents the 2- to 10-year results of 35 arthroscopically assisted combined ACL-PCL reconstructions evaluated pre- and postoperatively using the Lysholm, Tegner, and Hospital for Special Surgery (HSS) knee ligament rating scales; KT-1000 arthrometer testing; stress radiography; and physical examination.[11,17,18]

The study population comprised 26 males and 9 females with 19 acute and 16 chronic knee injuries. The ligament injuries consisted of 19 ACL-PCL-posterolateral instabilities, 9 ACL-PCL-MCL instabilities, 6 ACL-PCL-posterolateral-MCL instabilities, and 1 ACL-PCL instability. All knees had grade III laxity preoperatively. Arthroscopically assisted combined ACL-PCL reconstructions were performed using the single-incision endoscopic ACL technique and the single femoral tunnel–single-bundle transtibial tunnel PCL technique. PCLs were reconstructed with Achilles tendon allograft (26), bone–tendon–bone (BTB) autograft (7), and semitendinosus-gracilis autograft (2). ACLs were reconstructed with BTB autograft (16), BTB allograft (12), Achilles tendon allograft (6), and semitendinosus-gracilis autograft (1). MCL injuries were treated with bracing or open reconstruction. Posterolateral instability was treated with biceps femoris tendon transfer, with or without primary repair, and with posterolateral capsular shift procedures as indicated.

Postoperative physical examination revealed normal posterior drawer–tibial step-off in 16 of 35 knees (46%). Lachman and pivot shift tests were normal in 33 of 35 knees (94%). Posterolateral stability was restored to normal in 6 of 25 knees (24%) and was tighter than the normal knee in 19 of 25 knees (76%) evaluated with the external rotation thigh-foot angle test. Thirty-degree varus stress testing was normal in 22 of 25 (88%) and revealed grade I laxity in 3 (12%). Thirty-degree valgus stress testing was normal in 7 of 7 (100%) surgically treated MCL tears and was normal in 7 of 8 (87.5%) brace-treated knees. Postoperative KT-1000 arthrometer measurements of mean side-to-side difference were 2.7 mm (PCL screen), 2.6 mm (corrected posterior), and 1 mm (corrected anterior). On postoperative stress radiographs, the mean side-to-side differences at 90 degrees of knee flexion and 32 pounds of posteriorly directed proximal force were 0 to 3 mm in 11 of 21 knees (52.3%), 4 to 5 mm in 5 of 21 (23.8%), and 6 to 10 mm in 4 of 21 (19%). Postoperative Lysholm, Tegner, and HSS mean values were 91.2, 5.3, and 86.8, respectively. These objective assessments demonstrated statistically significant differences from preoperative values ($P \leq .001$).

Complications

Potential complications in the treatment of combined ACL–PCL–posterolateral corner injuries include failure to recognize and treat vascular injuries (both arterial and venous), iatrogenic neurovascular injury at the time of reconstruction, iatrogenic tibial plateau fractures at the time of reconstruction, failure to recognize all components of the instability, medial femoral condyle osteonecrosis, knee motion loss, and postoperative anterior knee pain.[8,13,27-29] Our complications included postoperative adhesions requiring arthroscopic lysis and manipulation in three patients and removal of painful hardware in five patients.

Conclusion

ACL-PCL injuries are most frequently seen in multiple trauma patients, but they do occur in the athletic population as well. Acute three-ligament injuries of the knee may have been tibiofemoral dislocations with spontaneous reduction in the field. Therefore, careful documentation of the neurovascular status is essential to avoid the complications associated with limb ischemia. Systematic evaluation of these patients, including a history, physical examination, imaging studies, examination under anesthesia, and diagnostic arthroscopy, can aid in correct diagnosis and treatment plan formulation. Combined ACL-PCL instabilities can be treated successfully with arthroscopic reconstruction and the appropriate collateral ligament surgery. Statistically sifnificant improvement from the preoperative condition has been noted at 2- to 10-year follow-up using the objective parameters of knee ligament rating scales, arthrometer testing, stress radiography, and physical examination. Postoperatively, these knees are not normal, but they are functionally stable. Continuing technical improvements will likely improve future results.

References

1. Bleday RM, Fanelli GC, Giannotti BF, et al: Instrumented measurement of the posterolateral corner. Arthroscopy 14:489-494, 1998.
2. Clancy WG: Repair and reconstruction of the posterior cruciate ligament. In Chapman M (ed): Operative Orthopaedics. Philadelphia, JB Lippincott, 1988, pp 1651-1665.
3. Fanelli GC: Combined anterior and posterior cruciate ligament injuries: The multiple ligament injured knee. Sports Med Arthrosc Rev 7:289-295, 1999.
4. Fanelli GC: Point counter point. Arthroscopic posterior cruciate ligament reconstruction: Single bundle/single femoral tunnel. Arthroscopy 16:725-731, 2000.
5. Fanelli GC: Treatment of combined anterior cruciate ligament–posterior cruciate ligament–lateral side injuries of the knee. Clin Sports Med 19:493-502, 2000.
6. Fanelli GC: Arthroscopic combined ACL/PCL reconstruction. In Posterior Cruciate Ligament Injuries: A Guide to

Practical Management. New York, Springer-Verlag, 2001, pp 215-236.

7. Fanelli GC: Arthroscopic PCL reconstruction: Transtibial technique. In Posterior Cruciate Ligament Injuries: A Guide to Practical Management. New York, Springer-Verlag, 2001, pp 141-156.

8. Fanelli GC: Complications in PCL surgery. In Posterior Cruciate Ligament Injuries: A Guide to Practical Management. New York, Springer-Verlag, 2001, pp 291-302.

9. Fanelli GC: Posterior Cruciate Ligament Injuries: A Practical Guide to Management. New York, Springer-Verlag, 2001.

10. Fanelli GC: Posterior cruciate ligament, posterolateral reconstruction, meniscus transplant procedures. In Poehling GC (ed): Masters in Arthroscopy. CD-ROM. St Louis, Mosby.

11. Fanelli GC: Surgical treatment of the acute and chronic ACL/PCL/medial side/lateral side injuries of the knee. Sports Med Arthrosc Rev 9:208-218, 2001.

12. Fanelli GC: Arthroscopic posterior cruciate ligament reconstruction: Transtibial tunnel technique. Surgical technique and 2–10 year results. Arthroscopy 18(9) Suppl 2:44-49, 2002.

13. Fanelli GC: Complications in the multiple ligament injured knee. In Schenck RC (ed): AAOS Monograph on Multiple Ligamentous Injuries of the Knee in the Athlete. Rosemont, IL, American Academy of Orthopaedic Surgeons, 2002, pp 101-107.

14. Fanelli GC, Desai B, Cummings PD, et al: Divergent alignment of the femoral interference screw in single incision endoscopic reconstruction of the ACL. Contemp Orthop 28:21-25, 1994.

15. Fanelli GC, Edson CJ: Management of combined anterior cruciate ligament/posterior cruciate ligament injuries of the knee. In Chow J (ed): Advanced Arthroplasty. New York, Springer-Verlag, 2001, pp 533-544.

16. Fanelli GC, Edson CJ: Management of posterior cruciate ligament and posterolateral instability of the knee. In Chow J (ed): Advanced Arthroplasty. New York, Springer-Verlag, 2001, pp 545-558.

17. Fanelli GC, Edson CJ: Arthroscopically assisted combined ACL/PCL reconstruction: 2–10 year follow-up. Arthroscopy 18: 2002, pp 703-714.

18. Fanelli GC, Edson CJ, Maish DR: Management of combined ACL/PCL injuries. Tech Orthop 16:157-166, 2001.

19. Fanelli GC, Feldman DD: The use of allograft tissue in knee ligament reconstruction. In Parisien JS (ed): Current Techniques in Arthroscopy. Philadelphia, Current Medicine, 1998, pp 47-56.

20. Fanelli GC, Feldmann DD: The dislocated/multiple ligament injured knee. Oper Tech Orthop 9:1-12, 1999.

21. Fanelli GC, Feldmann DD: Management of combined anterior cruciate ligament/posterior cruciate ligament/posterolateral complex injuries of the knee. Oper Tech Sports Med 7:143-149, 1999.

22. Fanelli GC, Feldmann DD, Edson CJ, Maish DR: The multiple ligament injured knee. In DeLee JC, Drez DD, Miller MD (eds): DeLee and Drez's Orthopaedic Sports Medicine, 2nd ed. Philadelphia, Elsevier, 2003, pp 2111-2121.

23. Fanelli GC, Giannotti BF, Edson CJ: Current concepts review. The posterior cruciate ligament: Arthroscopic evaluation and treatment. Arthroscopy 10:673-688, 1994.

24. Fanelli GC, Giannotti BF, Edson CJ: Arthroscopically assisted combined ACL/PCL reconstruction. Arthroscopy 12:5-14, 1996.

25. Fanelli GC, Giannotti BF, Edson CJ: Arthroscopically assisted PCL/posterior lateral complex reconstruction. Arthroscopy 12:521-530, 1996.

26. Fanelli GC, Larson RV: Practical management of posterolateral instability of the knee. Arthroscopy 18(Suppl 1):1-8, 2002.

27. Fanelli GC, Monahan TJ: Complications of posterior cruciate ligament reconstruction. Sports Med Arthrosc Rev 7:296-302, 1999.

28. Fanelli GC, Monahan TJ: Complications and pitfalls in posterior cruciate ligament reconstruction. In Malek M (ed): Knee Surgery: Complications, Pitfalls, and Salvage. New York, Springer-Verlag, 2001, pp 121-128.

29. Fanelli GC, Monahan TJ: Complications in posterior cruciate ligament and posterolateral complex surgery. Oper Tech Sports Med 9:96-99, 2001.

30. Ibrahim SA: Primary repair of the cruciate and collateral ligaments after traumatic dislocation of the knee. J Bone Joint Surg Br 81:987-990, 1999.

31. Malek MM, Fanelli GC: Arthroscopically assisted posterior cruciate ligament reconstruction using Achilles tendon allograft. In Parisien JS (ed): Therapeutic Arthroscopy. New York, Raven Press, 1993, pp 47-56.

32. Malek MM, Fanelli GC: Technique of arthroscopic PCL reconstruction. Orthopaedics 16:961-966, 1993.

33. Malek MM, Fanelli GC, Deluca JV: Intra-articular and extra-articular anterior cruciate ligament reconstruction. In Scott WN (ed): The Knee. St Louis, Mosby, 1994, pp 791-812.

34. Malek MM, Fanelli GC, Golden MD: Combined intra-articular and extra-articular anterior cruciate ligament reconstruction. In Scott WN (ed): Ligament and Extensor Mechanism Injuries of the Knee. St Louis, Mosby, 1991, pp 267-284.

35. Martinek V, Imhoff AB: Combined anterior cruciate ligament and posterior cruciate ligament injury—technique and results of simultaneous arthroscopic reconstruction. Zentralbl Chir 123:1027-1032, 1998.

36. Miller MD, Cooper DE, Fanelli GC, et al: Posterior cruciate ligament: Current concepts. Instr Course Lect 51:347-351, 2002.

37. Noyes FR, Barber-Westin SD: Reconstruction of the anterior and posterior cruciate ligaments after knee dislocation: Use of early protected motion to decrease arthrofibrosis. Am J Sports Med 25:769-778, 1997.

38. Wascher DC, Becker JR, Dexter JG, Blevins FT: Reconstruction of the anterior and posterior cruciate ligaments after knee dislocation: Results using fresh frozen nonirradiated allografts. Am J Sports Med 27:189-196, 1999.

39. Wascher DC, Dvirnak PC, Decoster TA: Knee dislocation: Initial assessment and implications for treatment. J Orthop Trauma 11:525-529, 1997.

40. Wascher DC, Grauer JD, Markoff KL: Biceps tendon tenodesis for posterolateral instability of the knee: An in vitro study. Am J Sports Med 21:400-406, 1993.

41. Yeh WL, Tu YK, Su JY, Hsu RW: Knee dislocation: Treatment of high velocity knee dislocation. J Trauma 46:693-701, 1999.

CHAPTER

73

Lateral Release and Medial Repair for Patellofemoral Instability

JACK FARR

LATERAL RELEASE AND MEDIAL REPAIR FOR PATELLOFEMORAL INSTABILITY IN A NUTSHELL

History:
Is the pain or instability the main problem, and what incites this problem? How localized are symptoms, and how do they correlate to pathoanatomy?

Physical Examination:
Lateral release candidates: pain localized to lateral retinaculum, patellar tilt, no abnormal laxity
Medial repair candidates: abnormal laxity of medial structures, apprehension with lateral displacement

Imaging:
Axial view in 30 to 45 degrees of knee flexion, true lateral, standing flexed posteroanterior; supplemental computed tomography, magnetic resonance imaging, bone scan

Indications and Contraindications:
Lateral release indicated for focal lateral retinacular pain associated with tilt and failed conservative management; contraindicated for global pain
Medial repair indicated for laxity of medial supporting structures resulting in functional lateral patellar instability; contraindicated when tightening medially would overload articular cartilage or when pain is primary complaint

Surgical Technique:
Lateral release: conservative release approximately to level of superior pole; attention to hemostasis—tourniquet down (under-release is better than medial subluxation secondary to over-release)
Medial repair: attempt to re-create normal tension in medial retinaculum and defined medial patellar ligaments; mini-arthrotomy preferred to distorting anatomometric-physiometric position of medial tissues

Pearls:
Correct pathoanatomy to "normal" anatomy, not to "overcorrected" or "invented" anatomy; consider entire kinetic chain; goal is to restore function by allowing the knee to reenter a zone of homeostasis through integration of surgery and rehabilitation

Pitfalls:
Overzealous release or tightening; failure to identify true pathoanatomy; failure to consider entire knee and kinetic chain when selecting treatment

Postoperative Management:
Early strengthening and protected range of motion; prevention of adhesions

Results:
Highly dependent on proper patient selection, avoidance of creating abnormal anatomy or forces, functional rehabilitation

---

With more than 100 surgeries described to treat patellofemoral problems, two observations are apparent: most surgeries are successful to some extent, but no one surgical approach has had such an overwhelming positive outcome that it supersedes all other options.[22] Underlying this dilemma is the multifactorial nature of the causes of patellofemoral pain and instability and the unique patient population.

When considering treatment options, keep in mind that the least invasive should be contemplated first. This is especially true in cases of patellofemoral medial and lateral soft tissue intervention. It is imperative to appreciate the delicate nature of the patellofemoral system and to remember that any intervention may be considered extensive by the patient. An arthroscopic lateral release through two small portals should not be thought of as minimally invasive. Many patients can tolerate only one intervention from both a physical and mental standpoint.

As the evolution of patellofemoral surgery continues, it is being guided by a renewed appreciation of anatomic variants (and associated pathoanatomy) that predispose a patient to patellofemoral problems. For lateral patellar instability, subluxation and dislocation are two points on a continuum and are treated in a similar manner, with attention to the magnitude of forces associated with the occurrence. Exhaustive groundwork initially focused on the bony anatomy and patellofemoral alignment, because these can be measured clinically and radiographically; however, the common denominator among pathology resulting in lateral patellar instability is inadequate medial restraint.[7,16,17,29,31] Early approaches to this pathology included a variety of advances, reefs, and imbrications designed to remove excessive laxity from the medial structures that were allowing abnormal lateral movement. These procedures in most cases did restrain the patella, but patellofemoral pain has been reported over the long term, perhaps related to increased medial stress.[31]

Similar to the learning curve for shoulder instability, patellar instability has now been directly linked to injuries of specific anatomic structures. The most important restraint to abnormal lateral patellar movement is the medial patellofemoral ligament (MPFL) (Fig. 73–1); however, the importance of the patellotibial and patellomeniscal ligaments should not be underestimated, especially given reports of MPFL variants.[5,7,8,11,16,23] To expand the shoulder analogy, the goal in patellar instability surgery should be to reestablish anatomy, rather than to make new surgeon-created anatomy. Thus, the current treatment of an isolated anterior shoulder dislocation is repair of the specific pathoanatomic lesion, rather than the multiple muscle transfers of the past. Debate remains about the incidence and position of MPFL disruption, but most studies point to avulsion from the medial epicondyle as being most common, with the "double-tear" site (adjacent to the patella) less commonly reported.[3,6,31] By focusing on the pathoanatomy of the MPFL and the remaining intact restraints, it is possible to plan MPFL repair and reconstruction techniques rationally.

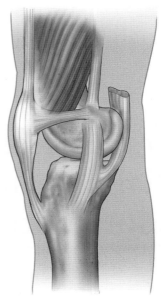

Figure 73–1   Medial patellofemoral ligament attachments.

Sequential sectioning of medial and lateral patellar structures has allowed an interesting observation, which, at least initially, is counterintuitive: the lateral retinaculum plays a role in limiting lateral patellar displacement.[11] Thus, there must be extensive justification for using lateral release in patients with lateral patellar instability. In fact, overzealous use of lateral release may not only lead to new medial instability but also exacerbate the initial problem of lateral patellar instability. Nevertheless, Merchant and Mercer[27] demonstrated that with thorough screening and proper patient assessment, in certain circumstances, lateral release may decrease subsequent lateral patellar instability. With the present appreciation of pathoanatomy, this approach must be viewed with caution and invites a quest for an explanation of its success. Certainly, it appears that patient selection is crucial. One question to be considered: Are successful patients those with otherwise normal anatomy in which the lateral release decreased stress on the MPFL tear site during healing? This line of questioning emphasizes the importance of determining the precise role of lateral release.[2,18] It would also help to explore the differences in approach and recommendations of those adamantly for or against isolated lateral release for the treatment of lateral patellar instability.

In each case, it is the surgeon's responsibility to justify the treatment based on the pathoanatomy. This attention to pathoanatomy requires a thorough investigation to evaluate the most commonly reported pathology in lateral patellar instability, that is, avulsion of the patellofemoral ligament from its attachment to the femoral medial epicondyle. At present, the isolated lateral release is typically used only in cases of lateral retinacular pain associated with tilt.[14,19]

Case History

A 25-year-old woman treated 10 years earlier with lateral release and tibial tubercle medialization developed worsening symptoms of patellar pain and lateral subluxation. Her subluxation was not responsive to conservative management. The examination was notable for reversible tilt and increased lateral displacement of the patella. The Merchant view demonstrated a central patellar position without joint space narrowing (Fig. 73–2). At surgery, the articular surfaces were intact, and the MPFL was retracted with scar proximally and laterally. The MPFL was mobilized, secured in a physiometric position, and augmented with a Restore biopatch (DePuy, a Johnson & Johnson Company, Warsaw, IN). Patellar mobility was symmetrical, and there was no excessive tension on the reconstructed tissues, which allowed early range of motion. The patient regained full pain-free motion in 6 weeks and continues to be free of patellar subluxation. The postoperative Merchant view demonstrated that the patella remained central; that is, overmedialization was avoided (Fig. 73–3).

History

See Table 73–1 for common patient histories of medial repair and lateral release candidates.

Physical Examination

Table 73–2 lists the findings for candidates for lateral release and medial repair.

Figure 73–2   Patellofemoral Merchant view.

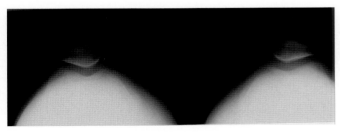

Figure 73–3   Merchant view of the central patella with nonpathologic morphology.

Table 73–1   **Patient History of Lateral Release and Medial Repair Candidates**

Lateral Release Candidates

High level of use
Failure of prolonged therapy
Focal lateral patellar pain, not global pain
Giving way from pain, not patellar instability

Medial Repair Candidates

Acute episode with internal rotation of the body (femur) on a fixed foot with lateral patellar subluxation or dislocation or, less likely, external lateral forces directed to the patella
Often, effusion after instability and possible loose body sensation
Pain medially
Possible recurrent episodes, with less energy needed to cause each subsequent episode
Possible recurrent episodes of lateral patellar instability after technically correct prior lateral release or tibial tubercle medialization

Table 73–2   **Physical Examination Findings of Lateral Release and Medial Repair Candidates**

Lateral Release Candidates

Tight lateral retinaculum expressed as tilt and decreased medial patellar displacement
Focused lateral retinaculum pain
Normal alignment, strength, flexibility

Medial Repair Candidates

Acutely, medial pain along the medial patellofemoral, patellotibial, and patellomeniscal ligaments
Increased distal lateral displacement
Apprehension with lateral displacement
Vastus medialis obliquus assessment

These are focused points for the considered procedures. See the complete patellofemoral physical examination by Post.[30]

Imaging

The workhorse of patellofemoral imaging is the axial view most commonly referred to as the Merchant view (Table 73–3; see Fig. 73–3). For patients with instability, this allows the evaluation of morphology, dysplasia, position, and subluxation (Fig. 73–4). For lateral release candidates, the goal is to rule out all other potential causes of pain, and the Merchant view may allow assessment of the tilt noted on clinical examination.[21] Magnetic resonance imaging may help confirm the site of injury to medial restraints and may detect medial articular cartilage damage to the patella. In candidates for both lateral release and medial repair, a bone scan may be helpful when marked overloading stress or sympathetic pain

6 Knee

Table 73–3
Patellofemoral-Specific Imaging

Plain Radiographs

Axial view with knee in 30 to 45 degrees of flexion (Merchant view)[28]
  Patellar position, morphology, dysplasia[1,25]
  Patellar tilt, per Grelsamer et al.[21]
True lateral view, as interpreted by Malghem and Maldague[26] and Dejour et al.[9,10]
  Tilt and trochlear dysplasia

Computed Tomography

Tilt and relation of patella to trochlea with flexion, per Schultzer et al.[33,34]
Patella, sulcus, and tubercle to entire extremity

Magnetic Resonance Imaging

True articular surface relative positions, per Staubli et al.[35]
Status of articular cartilage and subchondral bone and soft tissues (site of medial patellofemoral ligament tear)

Bone Scan

Evidence of homeostasis of patellofemoral joint, per Dye et al.[12,13]

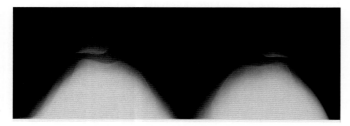

Figure 73–4   Merchant view showing dysplasia with chronic patellar subluxation.

Table 73–4   **Indications and Contraindications for Lateral Release and Medial Repair Procelures**

Lateral Release

Indicated for focal lateral patellar facet or retinacular pain and tight lateral retinaculum, as documented by clinical examination with possible imaging confirmation
Contraindicated for nonspecific pain, incomplete conservative management

Medial Repair

Indicated for laxity of medial patellar restraints causing lateral patellar dislocations or subluxations
Contraindicated for nonspecific pain, and relatively contraindicated in cases of medial patellar chondrosis

patterns are present, both of which require unique attention and may preclude surgery.

Indications and Contraindications

Table 73–4 lists the indications and contraindications for lateral release and medial repair procedures.

Surgical Technique

From an arthroscopic standpoint, the initial focus is on the medial border of the patella, where there is often a chondral fracture or hemorrhage in the synovium or MPFL. Although superficial chondral fragments may be loose, the deep bony attachments usually remain intact. It is possible to visualize the MPFL arthroscopically along most of its course (external to the synovium; Fig. 73–5), except in the area where the avulsion injury usually occurs, near the medial epicondyle. Hemorrhage in the medial gutter is often not visible because the disruption is usually superficial to the synovium, thus evading arthroscopic inspection.

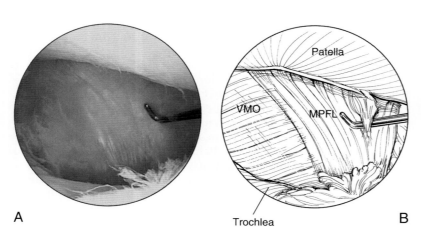

Figure 73–5   *A,* Arthroscopic view of the medial patellofemoral ligament (MPFL). *B,* Illustration of the MPFL. VMO, vastus medialis obliquus.

A

B

In the past, the extent of abnormal laxity in the MPFL was determined either before or during surgery by direct lateral and distal-lateral displacement. This emphasizes that in addition to the MPFL being avulsed from the medial epicondyle, the injury extends proximally to a varying degree as the injury disrupts the fascial attachment to the adductor. The result is repositioning of the avulsed MPFL edge both laterally (anteriorly) and proximally. This is a key concept regardless of the type of repair. *If the broad edge of the torn tissue is repositioned to the medial epicondyle, it will not be anatomic* (Fig. 73–6). Only one site of this broad tear surface (that avulsed from the medial epicondyle) is appropriate for repositioning— that is, specific anatomometric-physiometric reapproximation. This involves both a distal and a medial (posterior) transposition to the medial epicondyle. This concept is similar to how rotator cuff tears are repaired. The visible, free edge of the tear is not merely pulled directly to bone; first, the margins are "puzzle fitted" back together (often side to side) and then attached to bone. Thus, rotator cuff tears that appeared to be irreparable turned out to be quite amenable to repair, and in the case of the MPFL, the concept allows physiometric positioning. As with the shoulder, one should avoid overconstraining or abnormally constraining the patella, as this may cause abnormal stress, which could lead to chondrosis or pain.[31]

With this attention to reestablishing anatomy, it is now obvious that the full extent of the medial injury needs to be evaluated. If, for example, the trauma was low energy and a minimal avulsion from the adductor has healed in that position, classic surgeries directed at straight medial tightening may be successful. These tightening procedures usually approach the medial retinaculum as a single structure and may combine advancement of the vastus medialis obliquus with medial reefing or plication (Fig. 73–7*A*). Open advancements, reefs, and imbrications have been adapted to arthroscopic approaches. The early arthroscopic approach[24] (Fig. 73–7*B*) developed a plane between the medial subcutaneous tissues and the medial retinaculum. Large, curved needles are introduced through the skin and retinaculum and then spanned across the amount of retinaculum to be reefed. The needle then follows its curved course outward through the retinaculum and skin. By redirecting the needle through the plane between the subcutaneous tissue and retinaculum, it exits from the original entrance hole. The amount of imbrication is determined by both the grasped loop of retinaculum and the amount of retinaculum removed sharply or electrothermally. This typically involves two to four sutures. Tracking of the patella may be observed during this process, but one must be careful not to overinterpret this tracking in relation to what will occur clinically. This technique has been modified by Fulkerson[18] to better appreciate the MPFL and avoid overtightening.

With the current enthusiasm for minimally invasive surgery, thermal capsular shrinkage using laser, heat probe, or other radiofrequency electrothermal device may be applied to the medial patellar restraints (Fig. 73–8), with the same cautions, warnings, and concerns extrapolated from experience in the shoulder. Barber[4] cautioned that the medial retinaculum must heal before thermal shrinkage. In his early series, there were 2 redislocations in 20 patients, with a minimum follow-up of 12 months.

The literature demonstrates that reefing the medial retinaculum may achieve the desired initial goal of halting further lateral patellar instability. However, the ultimate goal is to accomplish this without long-term injury to the chondral surface and to allow the return of full function, strength, and physiometric motion of the patellofemoral joint. Theoretical concerns are based on the possibility of overconstraint or unbalanced, nonphysiometric constraint. This abnormal constraint may occur if it is necessary to tighten the medial structures sufficiently to normalize tracking and those structures are not the true pathology. That is, if the true pathology is the medial epicondylar loss of attachment, then more aggressive reefing of the loose, scarred, now nonanatomic MPFL may be necessary to centralize the patellar. Although the patella may appear centralized, it is central only through "new" kinematics (Fig. 73–9). If

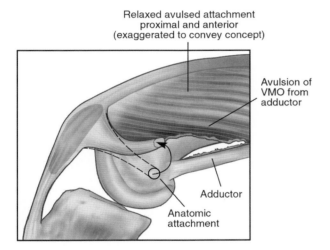

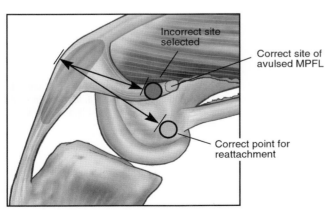

Figure 73–6 Medial patellofemoral ligament (MPFL) injury pattern. The repair site affects the length of the MPFL. VMO, vastus medialis obliquus.

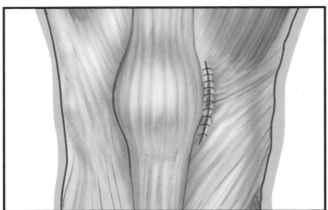

A

Figure 73–7 *A*, Classic open reef. *B*, Arthroscopic adaptation. This example does not address the medial epicondylar attachment.

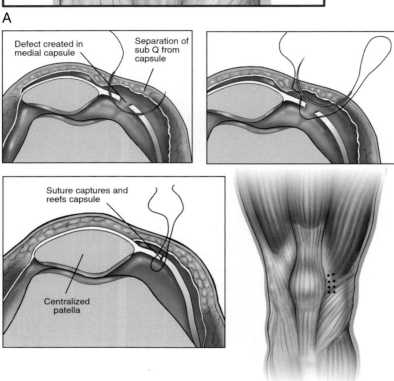

B

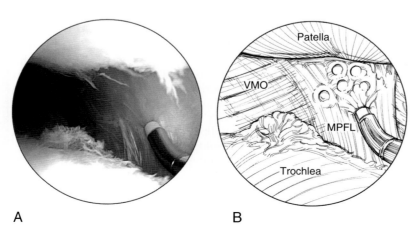

A   B

Figure 73–8 *A*, Arthroscopic view of thermal capsular shrinkage of the medial retinaculum. *B*, Illustration of the view in *A*. MPFL, medial patellofemoral ligament; VMO, vastus medialis obliquus.

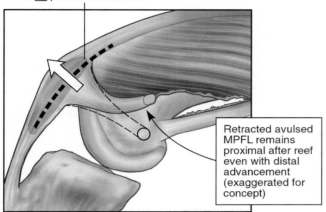

"Reefing" (open or thermal) may not reestablish MPFL unless there is <u>no</u> proximal retraction

Retracted avulsed MPFL remains proximal after reef even with distal advancement (exaggerated for concept)

Figure 73–9   Potential nonanatomic position of the medial patellofemoral ligament (**MPFL**), with a reef adjacent to the patella.

the avulsion from the adductor is extensive, this reefing might fail to restrict lateral displacement, and the altered kinematics may in fact be detrimental to the patellofemoral joint. To avoid this complication and to specifically address the patient's unique pathology, I combine arthroscopic and clinical assessment of the MPFL pathology and then perform mini–open reconstruction or repair of the MPFL with or without arthroscopic limited lateral release.

Specific Surgical Steps

Lateral Release

Patellar tilt is assessed clinically with the tilt test and medial-lateral displacement. Unless there is abnormal tilt and markedly diminished medial translation, a lateral release is typically not necessary in the subacute setting. Some patients with more chronic patholaxity of the MPFL may have developed gradual contracture of the lateral retinaculum, which suggests that release would be appropriate to relax tension on the repaired or reconstructed MPFL. The lateral release is performed arthroscopically, with minimal inflow pressure and without a tourniquet. The release is performed from approximately the superior pole of the patella to the anterolateral portal (Fig. 73–10). Thermal devices are used cautiously and in a systematic manner to allow coagulation and cutting at the same time. This is a gradual process from the synovial layer to the subcutaneous fat. Proximally, the superolateral geniculate is typically encountered and should be searched for and coagulated if cut. This is, by definition, a limited lateral release biomechanically. It can be converted to a complete release by continuing the release distally, immediately adjacent to the lateral border of the patellar tendon. Superiorly, it is important not to enter the quadriceps tendon or violate the vastus lateralis. Without the use of a tourniquet, adequate homeostasis is achieved and verified. Without tethering of the lateral retinaculum, patellar position with minimal inflow pressure is determined by the laxity of the medial structures and the position of the tibial tubercle. It is important to remember that if the

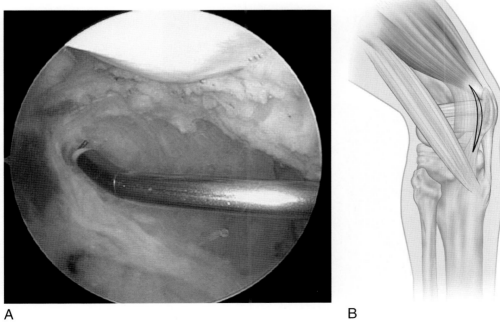

A   B

Figure 73–10   *A,* Arthroscopic view of a lateral release. *B,* Anatomic representation of a lateral release.

6 Knee

tubercle-sulcus angle is excessive, continued dynamic pull of the quadriceps may gradually stretch out an otherwise successful medial repair or reconstruction.

Medial Repair or Reconstruction

At this point in the surgery, lateral tension or passive medial displacement is optimal. If the MPFL is absent, it can be reconstructed using a hamstring.[32] Attention is now focused on reestablishing proper medial restraint to lateral patellar displacement. In the majority of cases, the primary MPFL pathology is at the medial epicondyle; less commonly, it involves more lateral (anterior) portions of the ligament. Therefore, although the course of the ligament is traced on the skin obliquely from the medial epicondyle to the medioproximal one third of the patella, only the distal aspect of the skin is incised initially. Typically, the incision is centered over the medial epicondyle (Fig. 73–11A). The skin and subcutaneous layer are bluntly dissected from the superficial fascia of the knee. This thin fascia is incised with scissors dissec-

tion in line with the skin excision. With loop retractors, it is possible to move this fascia to fully expose the course of the ligament from the medial epicondyle to the medial border of the patella. The vastus medialis obliquus usually bulges over (hides) the proximal margin of the MPFL; distally, the MPFL is confluent with the capsule. However, at the distal extent of the MPFL, the fiber course can be delineated from the more distal retinaculum and from the more dense fibers forming the patellomeniscal and patellotibial ligaments.

In chronic tears, or those with marked avulsion from the adductor, the site to be reapproximated is markedly anterior (lateral) and proximal. It is important to temporarily identify this tissue and mark it with a suture or clamp. In these chronic cases, it may also be necessary to sharply free the distal border of the MPFL from the remainder of the retinaculum. This is possible without entering the synovium and will be repaired side to side at the end of the reconstruction. The anatomy of the adductor, MPFL, and medial collateral ligament as they relate to the medial epicondyle is kept in mind as the

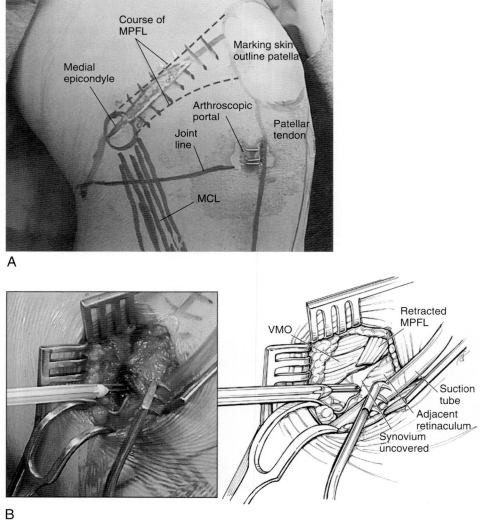

Figure 73–11 *A,* Photograph of a planned approach to the medial patellofemoral ligament (MPFL). *B,* Suture anchor insertion into the medial epicondyle–MPFL attachment site.

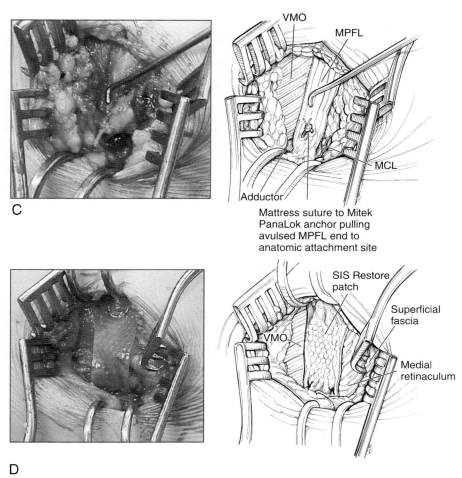

C

Mattress suture to Mitek
PanaLok anchor pulling
avulsed MPFL end to
anatomic attachment site

D

Figure 73–11, cont'd. *C,* Suture in place, securing the MPFL to the suture anchor.
D, Restore patch overlying the MPFL reconstruction. MCL, medial collateral ligament; SIS,
small intestine submucosa; VMO, vastus medialis obliquus.

clamp approximates the presumed avulsion site of the MPFL to the medial epicondyle. The knee is then put through its range of motion. In a manner similar to anterior cruciate ligament reconstruction, the objective is not to place the ligament isometrically but rather to place it anatomometrically and physiometrically. That is, the goal is to reproduce the strain of the natural MPFL. The ligament is usually mildly lax in full extension, tightens gently in early flexion, and loosens in deeper flexion, which corresponds to function as it relates to the positions in which the patella is at maximal risk for instability. This technique of securing a properly tensioned MPFL allows early range of motion, which is known to aid in strengthening soft tissue repairs. Once this desired position on the medial epicondyle is documented, it is marked. The site is then drilled, creating a blind tunnel into which a bioabsorbable anchor (PanaLok, Mitek, Inc., Somerville, NJ) is positioned (Fig. 73–11*B*). A mattress suture secures the MPFL in this position (Fig. 73–11*C*), and through range of motion, optimal physiometric position is confirmed. The repair is then augmented with figure-of-eight number 1 PDS; each suture is tested by range of motion to ensure that phys-

iometric position is not altered. At this point, a firm endpoint to lateral patellar displacement is appreciated and should be balanced. The patella should track smoothly, without abnormal shifts. If tracking is not smooth, the repair should be reassessed or even repositioned.

In many cases, the tissues are dysplastic or atrophic, which may have caused the propensity for instability or developed as a sequela of repeated instability. When the reconstructed tissues appear marginal, some authors have suggested augmentation with a variety of structures, including a portion of the adductor, a free or attached hamstring, or allograft. Currently, in a "fresh" reconstruction, it is usually possible to identify and properly position host tissues, avoiding the morbidity of autograft. To accelerate the healing response and supplement soft tissue repair, I custom-cut a rectangular section of Restore biopatch (DePuy Orthopaedics, Inc., a Johnson & Johnson Company, Warsaw, IN) to be sutured in tension directly over the reconstruction (Fig. 73–11*D*). The distal edge of the MPFL is then repaired side to side if it was released during the exploratory portion of the dissection. The fascia of the knee is reapproximated over the MPFL reconstruction, as are the subcutaneous tissues

Table 73–5

Complications of Lateral Release and Medial Repair or Reconstruction

Lateral Release	Medial Repair or Reconstruction
Early	**Early**
Hemarthrosis—early aspiration to allow improved quadriceps function	As above and, in addition, loss of flexion:
Quadriceps "shut down"—physical therapy for retraining, functional electrical stimulation	If repair was nonanatomic, revision may be needed
Sympathetic pain—early sympathetic blocks and desensitization	If repair or reconstruction was documented to be physiometric, consider standard early measures for arthrofibrosis; if no evidence of generalized arthrofibrosis, increase physical therapy and consider dynamic bracing
Late	**Late**
Giving way secondary to weakness—physical therapy	Giving way secondary to weakness—patellar stabilizing brace and physical therapy
Lateral subluxation—consider that the original problem was laxity of medial restraints, which is corrected with medial patellofemoral surgery, rather than tightness of lateral retinaculum	Recurrence of subluxation or dislocation—evaluate tubercle-sulcus distance to note effect of lateral vector on initial surgery[20]; secondary surgery may require grafting, applying the same physiometric principles
Medial subluxation—test with Fulkerson examination[18]; if problem persists, consider repair or reconstruction of lateral release site	Pain, which may be related to stress or chondrosis development or progression—measures to decrease stress medially, such as Fulkerson anterolateralization; restoration of cartilage per standard algorithms
Pain related to underlying malalignment or articular cartilage pathology—realignment using principles of Fulkerson[18] or principles of cartilage restoration	

and skin in layers. Because the repair has been shown not to have abnormal tension, bracing is not necessary during postoperative wound healing.

Postoperative Management

Lateral release patients are managed with a compressive dressing. Aggressive rehabilitation is delayed until swelling is controlled. Weight bearing and motion are based on patient comfort, with a focus on reestablishing quadriceps strength and function and maintaining patellar mobility.

Medial repair or reconstruction patients are encouraged to begin early quadriceps strengthening. Weight bearing is allowed as tolerated with two crutches to prevent limping. Early active range of motion is initiated at the surgeon's discretion, based on his or her interpretation of the observed physiometric tension of the repair or reconstruction at surgery. If the repair or reconstruction is physiometric and the repair is augmented with healing stimulators, early motion is important to prevent excessive scarring or block to flexion. When the incisions are healed, a soft patellar tracking knee brace can provide improved security as the patient is weaned from crutches. Standard patellar protection rehabilitation continues until optimal comfort and function are achieved. For sports participation, in addition to bracing, it is important to achieve full endurance, proprioception, and skill. The final return to sports is monitored through completion of a functional progression program.

Results

Since 2000, I have treated more than 25 patients (severe patellofemoral dysplasias were not included in this series) with repair or reconstruction of the MPFL using minor variations of this technique, with or without limited lateral release. Peer-review presentation will require additional follow-up, but to date, no patient has had a recurrence of dislocation, and none has required surgery for arthrofibrosis. For a review of the literature results up to 2002, see Fulkerson's article.[18]

Complications

Complications of the lateral release and medial repair or reconstruction procedures are listed in Table 73–5.

References

1. Aglietti P, Insall JN, Cerulli G: Patellar pain and incongruence. I. Measurements of incongruence. Clin Orthop 176:217-224, 1983.
2. Arendt EA: Management of patellofemoral disorders. Orthopedics Special Edition 7:1-7, 2001.
3. Avikainen VJ, Nikku RK, Seppanen-Lehmonen TK: Adductor magnus tenodesis for patellar dislocation: Technique and preliminary results. Clin Orthop 297:12-16, 1993.

4. Barber FA: Patellofemoral surgery: My techniques, pearls and pitfalls. Arthroscopy Association of North America fall course, 2001.

5. Boden BP, Pearsall AW, Garrett WE Jr, et al: Patellofemoral instability: Evaluation and management. J Am Acad Orthop Surg 5:47-57, 1997.

6. Burks RT, Desio SM, Bachus KN, et al: Biomechanical evaluation of lateral patellar dislocations. Am J Knee Surg 10:24-31, 1997.

7. Burks RT, Desio SM, Bachus KN, et al: Biomechanical evaluation of lateral patellar dislocations. Am J Knee Surg 11:24-31, 1998.

8. Conlan T, Garth WP Jr, Lemons JE: Evaluation of the medial soft tissue restraints of the extensor mechanism of the knee. J Bone Joint Surg Am 75:682-693, 1993.

9. Dejour H, Walch G, Neyret PH, et al: Dysplasia of the femoral trochlea [French]. Rev Chir Orthop Reparatrice Appar Mot 76:45-54, 1990.

10. Dejour H, Walch G, Nove-Josseraqnd L, et al: Factors of patellar instability: An anatomic radiographic study. Knee Surg Sports Traumatol Arthrosc 2:19-26, 1994.

11. Desio SM, Burks RT, Bachus KN: Soft tissue restraints to lateral patellar translation in the human knee. Am J Sports Med 26:59-65, 1998.

12. Dye SF, Chew MH: The use of scintigraphy to detect increased osseous metabolic activity about the knee. J Bone Joint Surg Am 75:1388-1406, 1993.

13. Dye SF, Staubli H-U, Biedert RM, et al: The mosaic of pathophysiology causing patellofemoral pain: Therapeutic implications. Oper Tech Sports Med 7:46-54, 1999.

14. Farahmand F, Senavongse W, Amis AA: Quantitative study of the quadriceps muscles, trochlear groove geometry related to instability of the patellofemoral joint. J Orthop Res 16:136-143, 1998.

15. Farr J: Anteromedialization of the tibial tubercle for treatment of patellofemoral malpositioning and concomitant isolated patellofemoral arthrosis. Tech Orthop 12:151-164, 1997.

16. Fithian DC, Meier SW: The case for advancement and repair of the medial patellofemoral ligament in patients with recurrent patellar instability. Oper Tech Sports Med 7:81-89, 1999.

17. Fithian DC, Normura E, Arendt E: Anatomy of patellar dislocation. Oper Tech Sports Med 9:102-111, 2001.

18. Fulkerson JP: Diagnosis and treatment of patients with patellofemoral pain. Am J Sports Med 30:447-455, 2002.

19. Garth WP Jr, DiChristina DG, Holt G: Delayed proximal repair and distal realignment after patellar dislocation. Clin Orthop 377:132-144, 2000.

20. Grelsamer RP: Current concepts review: Patellar malalignment. J Bone Joint Surg Am 82:1639-1650, 2000.

21. Grelsamer RP, Bazos AN, Proctor CS: Radiographic analysis of patellar tilt. J Bone Joint Surg Br 75:822-824, 1993.

22. Handy MH, Miller MD: Surgical treatment of acute patellar dislocation. Oper Tech Sports Med 9:164-168, 2001.

23. Hautamaa PV, Fithian DC, Kaufmann KR, et al: Medial soft tissue restraints in lateral patellar instability and repair. Clin Orthop 349:174-182, 1998.

24. Johnson LL: Arthroscopic Surgery: Principles and Practice, 3rd ed. St Louis, CV Mosby, 1986.

25. Laurin CA, Dussault R, Levesque HP: The tangential x-ray investigation of the patellofemoral joint: X-ray technique, diagnostic criteria and their interpretation. Clin Orthop 144:16-26, 1979.

26. Malghem J, Maldague B: Le profil du genou. Anatomie radiologique differentielle des surfaces articulaires. J Radiol 67:725-735, 1986.

27. Merchant AC, Mercer RL: Lateral release of the patella: A preliminary report. Clin Orthop 103:40-45, 1974.

28. Merchant AC, Mercer RL, Jacobsen RH, et al: Radiographic analysis of patellofemoral congruence. J Bone Joint Surg Am 56:1391-1396, 1974.

29. Nomura E: Classification of lesions of the medial patellofemoral ligament in patellar dislocation. Int Orthop 23:260-263, 1999.

30. Post WR, Teitge R, Amis A: Patellofemoral malalignment: looking beyond the viewbox. Clin Sports Med 21:521-546, 2002.

31. Sallay PI, Poggi J, Speer KP, et al: Acute dislocation of the patella: A correlative pathoanatomic study. Am J Sports Med 24:52-60, 1996.

32. Schock EJ, Burks RT: Medial patellofemoral ligament reconstruction using a hamstring graft. Oper Tech Sports Med 9:169-175, 2001.

33. Schultzer SF, Ramsby GR, Fulkerson JP: Computed tomographic classification of patellofemoral pain patients. Orthop Clin North Am 17:235-248, 1986.

34. Schultzer SF, Ramsby GR, Fulkerson JP: The evaluation of patellofemoral pain using computerized tomography: A preliminary study. Clin Orthop 204:286-293, 1986.

35. Staubli H-U, Porcellini B, Rauschning W: Anatomy and surface geometry of the patellofemoral joint in the axial plane. J Bone Joint Surg Br 81:452-458, 1999.

6 Knee

Arthroscopically Assisted Fracture Repair for Intra-articular Knee Fracture

MARK J. BERKOWITZ AND CRAIG R. BOTTONI

ARTHROSCOPICALLY ASSISTED FRACTURE REPAIR FOR INTRA-ARTICULAR KNEE FRACTURE IN A NUTSHELL

	Tibial Plateau	Tibial Spine	Patella	Distal Femur
History:	Axial load; valgus movement	Adolescent biking/ roller-blading	Fall or near fall	Trauma/fall
Physical Examination:	Tense effusion; valgus alignment; check for compartment syndrome	Effusion; loss of motion	Painful effusion; defect; loss of extension	Painful effusion; loss of motion
Imaging:	Plain radiograph with 10- to 20-degree caudal tilt; computed tomography	Radiographs	Posteroanterior, lateral, Merchant views	Plain radiographs; computed tomography
Indications:	Schatzker type I to III; delay 5 to 7 days	Displaced irreducible fragment	Transverse fracture displacement > 3 mm; step-off > 2 mm	Displaced type AO, B1, B2, C1 without comminution
Surgical Technique:	Examination under anesthesia; no pump; reduction; bone grafting; 6.5-mm cannulated screw fixation; buttress if comminuted	Bed debrided; ORIF— screw (antegrade or retrograde suture)	Debridement reduction; ORIF—two 4-mm cannulated screws ± cerclage augmentation	Debridement reduction; ORIF— 6.5-mm cannulated screws
Postoperative Management:	Immobilizer 2 to 5 days; cryotherapy; non–weight bearing for 3 months	Extension 3 to 4 weeks; partial weight bearing; range of motion 0 to 70 degrees for 4 weeks	Weight bearing; full extension; early range of motion	Non–weight bearing for 3 months
Results:	90% good to excellent	Depends on accuracy of reduction	Good union; less morbidity	Good union

ORIF, open reduction and internal fixation.

The views expressed herein are those of the authors and should not be construed as official policy of the Department of the Army or the Department of Defense.

Intra-articular fractures pose a unique challenge to the orthopedic surgeon. Sir John Charnley noted that anatomic reduction and restoration of free joint movement could be obtained only by rigid internal fixation. Failure to achieve these goals often results in the undesirable effects of both closed and open treatment: the risks of open reduction and stiffness from prolonged immobilization. Improved implants, more careful soft tissue handling, antibiotic prophylaxis, and better rehabilitation protocols have greatly enhanced our ability to treat articular fractures. On this basis, Schatzker et al.[33] delineated several essential principles of treating articular fractures (Table 74–1).

Arthroscopic principles have improved our ability to treat intra-articular fractures about the shoulder, wrist, elbow, hip, knee, and ankle. Tibial plateau fractures, avulsions of the intercondylar tibial eminence, and patellar fractures have all been treated with arthroscopically assisted techniques. Arthroscopic management of these fractures offers several distinct advantages compared with open treatment (Table 74–2).

The orthopedic literature is replete with innovative arthroscopic techniques for the treatment of fractures about the knee. This chapter reviews fractures of the tibial plateau, tibial eminence, and patella and describes arthroscopic treatment techniques. We also highlight new and potential applications of arthroscopy in the treatment of these fractures.

Table 74–1	
Principles of Articular Fracture Treatment	

Prolonged immobilization after open reduction and internal fixation of articular fractures produces stiffness
Depressed articular fragments are impacted and will not reduce closed
Major articular depressions create permanent instability
Anatomic reduction and stable fixation of articular fragments are necessary to restore joint congruity
Metaphyseal defects must be bone grafted to prevent articular redisplacement
Immediate range of motion is necessary to prevent joint stiffness and encourage articular healing

Table 74–2	**Advantages of Arthroscopic Treatment of Fractures about the Knee**

Allows direct evaluation of articular cartilage
Permits more accurate assessment of articular reduction
Provides ability to evaluate and treat concomitant meniscal, chondral, and ligamentous injuries
Enables lavage of hemarthrosis and intra-articular debris
Decreases soft tissue stripping, dissection
Avoids morbidity of arthrotomy
Facilitates early rehabilitation and range of motion

Tibial Plateau Fracture

Fractures of the tibial plateau are some of the most challenging periarticular injuries to treat. Anatomic restoration of the articular surface with rigid internal fixation, allowing immediate range of motion, is critical to a successful, functional outcome. Classically, this has been accomplished using standard open surgical approaches and arthrotomy. Surgical principles include detachment and elevation of the lateral meniscus, restoration of depressed articular fragments, buttress of the articular surface via bone grafting of the metaphyseal defect, and rigid internal fixation. These goals are now increasingly being achieved using arthroscopically assisted techniques.

Arthroscopic techniques possess several advantages over conventional open reduction and internal fixation performed through an arthrotomy (Table 74–3). Most notably, arthroscopically assisted techniques allow excellent visualization of the articular surface and confirmation of anatomic reduction through much smaller incisions, with the expectation of decreased postoperative stiffness and morbidity often associated with arthrotomy. In addition, the arthroscopic approach preserves the soft tissue envelope of the proximal tibia and potentially decreases the risk of infection. Arthroscopy also allows for simultaneous diagnosis and treatment of associated chondral, meniscal, and ligamentous injuries, which are found in up to 50% of patients with tibial plateau fractures.[5,31]

Mechanism of Injury

Fractures of the tibial plateau result from axial loads applied to the lower limb with varying degrees of varus or, more commonly, valgus moment.[9] Mechanisms of injury include both high-energy trauma, such as motor vehicle and motorcycle accidents, and athletic injuries. Patients frequently present with a tense effusion and are unable to ambulate (Table 74–4). Arthrocentesis reveals a hemarthrosis with fat globules. The lower limb may appear to be in valgus malalignment. Often bony tenderness localizes to the lateral aspect of the proximal tibia, with varying degrees of medial tenderness along the medial collateral ligament. Signs and symptoms of compartment syndrome or neurovascular compromise must be elicited. Assessment of ligamentous stability is critical to the evaluation of tibial plateau fractures. However, this is often better accomplished under general anesthesia in the operating room.

Table 74–3	**Advantages of Arthroscopic Treatment of Tibial Plateau Fractures**

Facilitates visualization of articular surface
Confirms anatomic reduction
Decreases soft tissue stripping
Allows assessment and treatment of concomitant soft tissue injuries

Table 74–4

Clinical Findings in Tibial Plateau Fractures

Inability to ambulate
Tense effusion
Lipohemarthrosis
Valgus malalignment
Neurovascular status: intact or compromised
Ligamentous integrity: stable or unstable

Imaging

Successful treatment of any complex injury requires careful preoperative planning. In the treatment of plateau fractures, this begins with meticulous evaluation of the radiographs to accurately characterize the fracture. Standard anteroposterior and lateral radiographs and a 10- to 20-degree caudal tilt view are recommended to accurately visualize the tibial articular surface.[33] As in most periarticular fractures, computed tomography (CT) can greatly enhance the surgeon's understanding of the fracture pattern and aid in preoperative planning. For this reason, we routinely perform preoperative CT scans in all patients with fractures of the tibial plateau. Magnetic resonance imaging, although a useful adjunct

for assessing the presence of concomitant soft tissue injuries, is not routinely obtained.

Classification

Accurate classification of the fracture is important in determining the operative approach. Schatzker's classification of tibial plateau fractures is extremely useful owing to its simplicity and familiarity among orthopedic surgeons (Fig. 74–1; Table 74–5).

Indications

We routinely use arthroscopic techniques only for Schatzker fracture types I to III (Table 74–6).[14] Although arthroscopic treatment of types IV to VI has been described,[27] these patterns frequently represent more complex, higher-energy injuries with greater compromise of the soft tissue envelope. We approach these significant injuries using standard open techniques, often in combination with external or hybrid fixation.[9] Other factors to consider in determining the need for operative intervention include articular incongruity, displacement, alignment, and stability.[1] The ideal time for arthroscopic fixation is 5 to 7 days after injury.

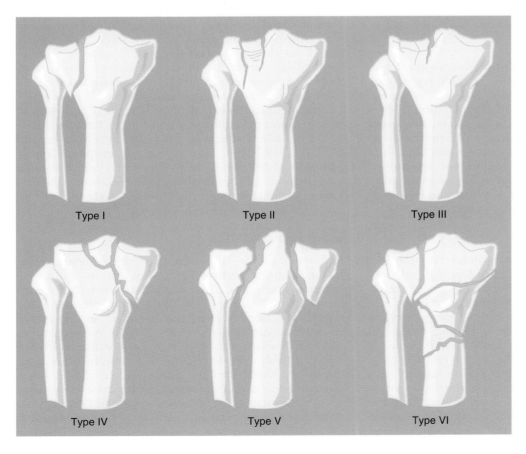

Figure 74–1 **The Schatzker classification for tibial plateau fractures.** (From Insall JN, Scott WN: Surgery of the Knee, 2nd ed. Philadelphia, Churchill Livingstone, 2001, p 1268.)

Type I Type II Type III

Type IV Type V Type VI

6 Knee

Table 74–5 Schatzker's Classification of Tibial Plateau Fractures

Type	Patient Profile	Mechanism
I—split lateral tibial condyle	Young	Medium-energy trauma (motor vehicle accident, sports)
II—split depression	Older	Medium-energy trauma
III—depression	Older, osteopenic	Low-energy trauma (fall)
IV—medial condyle split or depressed	Young	Medium-energy trauma
V—bicondylar	Older	High-energy trauma
VI—bicondylar with metaphyseal-diaphyseal dissociation	Young	Extremely high-energy trauma, significant soft tissue compromise

Table 74–6 Indications for Arthroscopic Treatment of Tibial Plateau Fractures

Schatzker types I, II, or III
Articular step-off > 3 mm
Articular displacement > 5 mm
Valgus malalignment
Valgus laxity with knee in extension > 10 degrees

Surgical Technique

Positioning

The patient is placed supine with the contralateral leg in a standard well leg holder, and the affected leg is stabilized in an arthroscopic leg holder. The table is broken at 90 degrees, and the leg can be supported on a Mayo stand (Fig. 74–2). A tourniquet is placed on the upper part of the thigh but is used sparingly. We prefer not to use a pump for fluid inflow owing to potential fluid extravasation and resultant compartment syndrome.[3] Alternatively, a pump can be used at low pressures after exposing the metaphyseal fracture site and routinely evaluating the calf for increased pressure.[9]

Examination under Anesthesia

General endotracheal anesthesia is preferred. Spinal or epidural anesthesia has the benefit of prolonged postoperative analgesia; however, the ability to accurately assess the postoperative neurovascular status is lost.

The surgical approach begins with a thorough examination under anesthesia in the operating room. All major ligaments are tested in standard fashion using Lachman, posterior drawer, and varus and valgus testing, as well as specialized tests of posterolateral stability such as the varus recurvatum and dial test. Particular attention is paid to knee stability during valgus stress with the knee extended. The pivot shift should be avoided because of potential damage to the lateral plateau.[16]

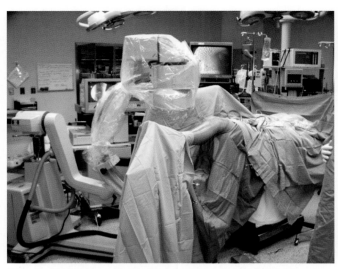

Figure 74–2 The operating room setup for arthroscopically assisted treatment of tibial plateau fractures. (Courtesy of Don Johnson.)

Diagnostic Arthroscopy

Standard three-portal diagnostic arthroscopy is then performed. The anterolateral portal should be at the inferior pole of the patella so that the plateau can be visualized from above.[9] Initially, the joint should be lavaged thoroughly for several minutes to evacuate the hematoma and any intra-articular debris. A thorough evaluation of the meniscus, ligaments, and associated chondral surfaces is then performed and documented with arthroscopic pictures.[5] An arthroscopic shaver introduced via the anteromedial portal is used to remove residual clots from the joint. Alternatively, the arthroscope can be replaced through the anteromedial portal to better view the lateral plateau and lateral meniscus.[16] Lateral meniscal tears may be present in 20% to 40% of patients and can be interposed within the fracture site.[5,36] If a repairable meniscal tear is found, it is reduced and then stabilized using one of several acceptable repair techniques.[8] We prefer the inside-out technique using a combination of absorbable and nonabsorbable 2-0 sutures on long, straight needles passed via curved cannulas for body or posterior horn tears.

Specific Surgical Steps

Reduction of the displaced plateau fragment is performed under arthroscopic visualization from the anteromedial portal. Split fragments are reduced with direct manual pressure or using a pointed reduction clamp. Depressed fracture fragments are also amenable to arthroscopic reduction (Fig. 74–3). We employ an anterior cruciate tibial guide to localize the depressed fragment with a guide pin. An 8- to 10-mm cannulated reamer is placed over the guidewire, creating a metaphyseal defect directly beneath the depressed fragment. A curved impactor is then used to elevate the subchondral bone and articular surface (Figs. 74–4 to 74–7). A 1-mm overreduction is recommended in anticipation of

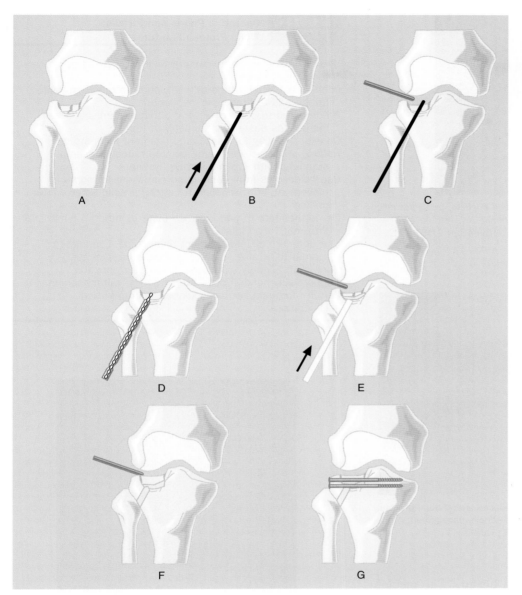

Figure 74–3 Technique for reduction and stabilization of lateral tibial plateau fractures. (From Insall JN, Scott WN: Surgery of the Knee, 2nd ed. Philadelphia, Churchill Livingstone, 2001, p 1280.)

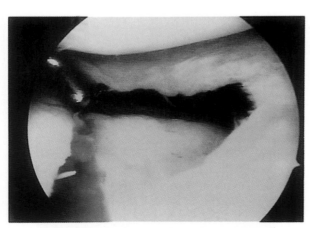

Figure 74–4 Arthroscopic view of lateral tibial plateau fracture. (From Guanche CA, Markman AW: Arthroscopic management of tibial plateau fractures. Arthroscopy 9:467-471, 1993.)

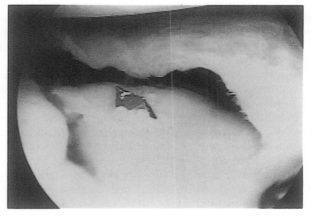

Figure 74–5 Arthroscopic view of guidewire in central portion of lateral tibia. (From Guanche CA, Markman AW: Arthroscopic management of tibial plateau fractures. Arthroscopy 9:467-471, 1993.)

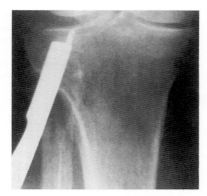

Figure 74–6 Fluoroscopic view of bone impactor being advanced over guidewire. (From Guanche CA, Markman AW: Arthroscopic management of tibial plateau fractures. Arthroscopy 9:467-471, 1993.)

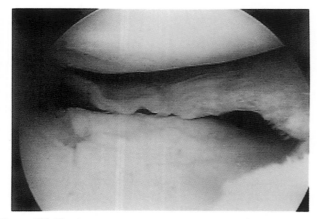

Figure 74–7 Arthroscopic view of reduced lateral tibial plateau. (From Guanche CA, Markman AW: Arthroscopic management of tibial plateau fractures. Arthroscopy 9:467-471, 1993.)

Table 74–7	Operative Pearls and Pitfalls: Tibial Plateau Fractures

Use arthroscopic leg holder, gravity inflow—avoid pump, tourniquet, flexion

Position anterolateral portal high, perform thorough joint lavage and arthroscopic inspection

Be prepared to perform several different meniscal repair techniques based on geometry of tear

Consider staging for associated ligament reconstruction

Reduce split fractures using pointed reduction clamp, stabilized with 6.5-mm screws/washers

Use guidewires from cannulated screw set for screw placement, but exchange for stronger solid screws after drilling

Do not hesitate to add buttress plate (Synthes 4.5-mm LCP Proximal Tibia Plate)

Use anterior cruciate ligament tibial guide, cannulated reamer to localize, elevate depressed fragments

Bone graft liberally to achieve 1-mm overreduction

Support subchondral bone with 4.5-mm "rafter" screws

Perform frequent neurovascular and compartment evaluations

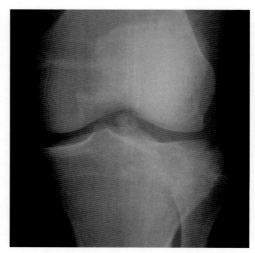

Figure 74–8 Anteroposterior radiograph of Schatzker type I lateral tibial plateau fracture.

some degree of subsidence with healing. The metaphyseal defect is then packed densely with bone graft. In older patients with less stout bone, we prefer autogenous iliac crest bone graft. Bone substitutes such as hydroxyapatite may also be considered.[17] If the final anatomic reduction is difficult to assess arthroscopically, it should be confirmed using fluoroscopy. Our operative technique and key elements are outline in Table 74–7.

Split fractures are stabilized using 6.5-mm Synthes cancellous screws with washers (Figs. 74–8 and 74–9). We use guidewires from the cannulated screw set to ensure proper placement and orientation of the screws. However, after drilling with the appropriate cannulated reamer, the guidewire is removed and a solid 6.5-mm partially threaded screw is placed, owing to its improved mechanical strength. To support depressed fragments, smaller screws placed in "rafter" fashion provide the best results. We routinely use four 3.5- or 4.5-mm fully threaded cancellous screws for stabilization of type III plateau fractures.[19,37]

In comminuted fractures or in patients with poor bone quality, the addition of a lateral buttress plate is

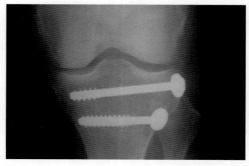

Figure 74–9 Postoperative anteroposterior radiograph after screw fixation.

strongly advised. Our current preference is the locking proximal tibial periarticular plate, which can be inserted simply by extending the incision used to bone graft the metaphyseal defect.

Pearls and Pitfalls

See Table 74–7.

Postoperative Management

The patient remains hospitalized for 2 to 5 days. The knee is splinted using a standard knee immobilizer. Cryotherapy begins immediately with placement of an Aircast Cryo-Cuff in the operating room. We do not routinely use continuous passive motion devices. The dressing is changed in 2 to 3 days, at which time supervised active and passive range-of-motion exercises are begun. Non–weight bearing with crutches is strictly enforced. Isometric quadriceps strengthening is started at 2 weeks. Stationary bicycling can begin as early as 3 to 4 weeks. Progressive partial weight bearing is allowed at 3 months if radiographs show evidence of healing.

Results

Arthroscopic and arthroscopically assisted techniques can be highly effective in restoring the anatomy of the proximal tibia in a minimally invasive manner (Table 74–8). Caspari et al.[11] and Jennings[18] in 1985 were the first to report their experience treating tibial plateau fractures arthroscopically. Caspari treated 20 patients and Jennings 21. Despite these relatively small numbers, both authors reported good results, with early return to functional range of motion and minimal complications.

Subsequent experience by multiple authors has confirmed these findings (see Table 74–8). Fowble et al.[12] presented their experience treating 23 tibial plateau fractures; 12 underwent arthroscopically assisted reduction, and 11 underwent formal open reduction and internal fixation. The arthroscopically managed group had superior results in terms of duration of hospitalization, time to full weight bearing, and ability to achieve anatomic reduction. Lobenhoffer et al.[22] prospectively compared 10 lateral tibial plateau fractures treated using arthroscopic reduction with 16 fractures treated using fluoroscopic reduction. Nine of 10 arthroscopically treated patients and 15 of 16 in the fluoroscopic group achieved excellent or good results, suggesting that equivalent results without exposure to radiation are possible using arthroscopy. The authors cautioned, however, that this procedure is efficient only in the hands of surgeons who are familiar with arthroscopic techniques and that fluoroscopic reduction is an excellent option for surgeons who are more familiar with that method.

Mazoue et al.[27] reported a high percentage of good and excellent results using arthroscopic techniques in the treatment of unselected plateau fractures, including Schatzker types IV, V, and VI. Although we are still hesitant to employ arthroscopic techniques in these higher-energy injuries, this work demonstrates that the role of arthroscopy in managing proximal tibia fractures continues to expand.

Complications

The rate of complications following arthroscopic management of tibial plateau fractures is extremely low (Table 74–9). Compartment syndrome has been sporadically reported following various arthroscopic procedures and represents the most serious potential complication of arthroscopic tibial plateau surgery; use of an infusion pump has been implicated in several of these cases.[7] To minimize the risk of compartment syndrome, we limit our indications for arthroscopic management to type I to III fractures, owing to the greater metaphyseal exposure in higher-energy injuries. Buchko and Johnson[9] recommend the creation of a metaphyseal window to allow the egress of arthroscopic fluid, which might otherwise

6 Knee

Table 74–8

Results of Arthroscopic Treatment of Tibial Plateau Fractures

Author (Date)	No. of Patients	Age (yr)	Follow-up	Outcome
Guanche and Markman (1993)[14]	5	21–56	Fracture union	Full return to activities
Caspari et al. (1985)[11]	20	14–85	Fracture union	100% good to excellent
Jennings (1985)[18]	21	13–62	12–60 mo	17 of 20 return to activity without limitation
Lobenhoffer et al. (1999)[22]	10	15–66	52 mo	9 of 10 good to excellent
Itokazu and Matsunaga (1993)[17]	13	18–77 (47)*	66 mo	Full range of motion, good pain relief
Fowble et al. (1993)[12]	12	17–81 (38.4)	6.6 mo	100% anatomic reduction, full range of motion, 1 of 12 with residual pain
Gill et al. (2001)[13]	25	17–74 (45.2)	24 mo	92% good to excellent
Mazoue et al. (1999)[27]	14	25–65 (43)	14.6 mo	79% good to excellent
Bernfeld et al. (1996)[6]	9	38–63 (50.2)	10.6 mo	100% return to activity by 7 mo
Holzach et al. (1994)[16]	15	28–69 (51.4)	35.3 mo	14 of 15 excellent

*Numbers in parentheses indicate mean age.

Table 74–9

Potential Complications of Arthroscopic Treatment of Tibial Plateau Fractures

Complication	Timing	Cause	Prevention/Treatment
Compartment syndrome	Acute	Extravasation of arthroscopic fluid	Avoid pump, flexion, minimize tourniquet, frequent examination, fasciotomy
Hardware failure	Early	Failure to add buttress plate	Lateral locking buttress plate
Loss of reduction	Early	Premature weight bearing, poor choice of hardware	Minimum 3 mo non–weight bearing, "rafter" screws, bone graft
Arthrofibrosis	Early	Prolonged immobilization, noncompliance with therapy	Aggressive supervised physical therapy, continuous passive motion devices
Post-traumatic arthritis	Late	Articular incongruity, chondral damage, ligament instability, mechanical malalignment	Accurate articular reduction, restoration of alignment, stability

extravasate into the soft tissues. Most importantly, the condition of the soft tissues must be evaluated often so that an impending compartment syndrome can be aborted or released promptly.

Complications occurring in the early postoperative period after arthroscopically assisted plateau surgery include hardware failure, loss of reduction, and arthrofibrosis. Hardware complications most frequently result from errors in judgment or application. One should not hesitate to add a buttress plate if the stability of screw-only fixation is uncertain. Likewise, patients must repeatedly be counseled about the need for prolonged protected weight bearing. Patients treated arthroscopically frequently regain motion and have resolution of swelling sooner than those treated with standard open techniques. For this reason, they may be at greater risk for complications due to premature weight bearing.[1]

The most common complication of tibial plateau fractures is post-traumatic arthritis. It may result from a combination of residual articular incongruity, direct chondral injury, ligamentous insufficiency, and mechanical malalignment.[26] Because of its complex cause, no single technique can completely eliminate the risk of late arthritis. However, arthroscopic techniques allow direct visualization of the articular surface at the time of reduction. By maximizing the potential for accurate articular reduction, arthroscopic management optimizes the patient's chance for a good long-term functional outcome.

Tibial Spine Fracture

Although occasionally seen in adults, tibial eminence or spine fracture is considered an injury of children and adolescents. These injuries typically occur after a bicycling or in-line skating fall. The tibial insertion of the adolescent anterior cruciate ligament (ACL) fails before ligament disruption, resulting in an intra-articular fragment. Meyers and McKeever[30] classified these injuries into four types based on the amount of displacement (Fig. 74–10, Table 74–10).

The patient typically presents with an acutely swollen, painful knee with severely restricted motion. Routine radiographs of the knee usually demonstrate the avulsion fracture, although the amount of displacement is not always easily ascertained.

Table 74–10

Classification of Tibial Spine Fractures

Type	Description
I	Minimally displaced
II	Hinged posteriorly
III	Complete separation
IV	Comminuted/rotated

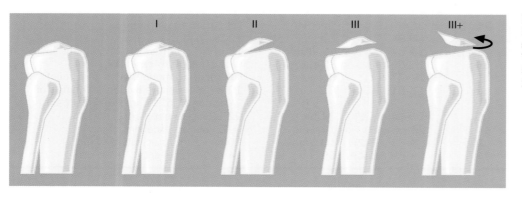

Figure 74–10 Meyers and McKeever[29] classification of tibial spine fractures. (From Herring JA: Tachkijian's Pediatric Orthopaedics, 3rd ed. Philadelphia, Elsevier, 2002, p 2355.)

Treatment of type I and II fractures is usually nonoperative. Any displacement is reduced by extending the knee after arthrocentesis and hemarthrosis evacuation. Intra-articular, intravenous, or even general anesthesia may be required to effect a reduction. Following successful reduction, extension casting or splinting is required for at least 6 weeks. Several long-term follow-up studies of patients treated with closed management have demonstrated increased tibial translation and symptomatic ACL laxity. For irreducible or severely displaced fractures, arthroscopically assisted fixation is possible. The fragment can be fixated with screws placed either antegrade or retrograde, Kirschner wires, or transtibial sutures. If the fracture fragment is large enough, Kirschner wire or screw fixation is recommended. To avoid crossing the proximal tibial physis, the screws or K-wires can be directed obliquely in the epiphysis.

Surgical Technique

Standard knee positioning and portals can be used to evaluate the fracture. The hemarthrosis is evacuated, and the fracture fragment with the ACL insertion is lifted, allowing the removal of clots and interposed soft tissue. A small amount of cancellous bone can be removed from the tibial insertion to allow countersinking of the fragment. If the fragment is large enough to allow interfragmentary fixation, the screw can be passed antegrade from a superomedial portal to secure the fragment. Alternatively, a cannulated screw can be passed from distally into the fragment over a guidewire. The ACL tibial guide can be used to reduce the fragment and allow accurate passage of the guidewire into the fragment (Figs. 74–11 and 74–12).

For fragments that are too small to allow screw fixation, or if comminution occurs while attempting to pass the screw through the fragment, transtibial suture fixation is a possibility. Using the ACL tibial guide, two parallel guidewires are passed from the proximal medial tibia into the avulsion fragment and through the distal aspect of the ACL. A cannulated 4.5-mm drill is passed over the guidewires. A suture retrieval instrument is then passed up each hole to allow a number 5 nonabsorbable suture to be pulled down over the fragment. The suture ends are tied over the bony bridge of the tibia or a post (Figs. 74–13 and 74–14).

Pearls and Pitfalls

Arthroscopic fixation of tibial eminence fractures can be fraught with complications. The anterior position of the ACL tibial insertion and the hemarthrosis can make visualization difficult. The lateral portal should be made 10 to 15 mm more lateral than normal to avoid the fat pad and improve anterior visualization. In addition, a 70-degree arthroscope should be available. Blood from the cancellous bone of the fracture can impair visualization; therefore, an arthroscopic fluid pump is recommended.

To reduce the fracture, extension of the knee is typically required. Closed reduction often fails because of interposed soft tissue or menisci. Mah et al.[24] reported

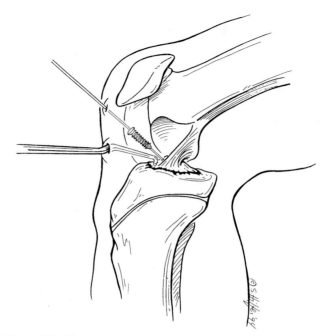

Figure 74–11 Diagram demonstrating anterior cruciate ligament tibial guide used to reduce tibial eminence fracture and placement of cannulated screw through separate anterosuperior stab incision. (From Berg EE: Pediatric tibial eminence fractures: Arthroscopic cannulated screw fixation. Arthroscopy 11:328-331, 1995.)

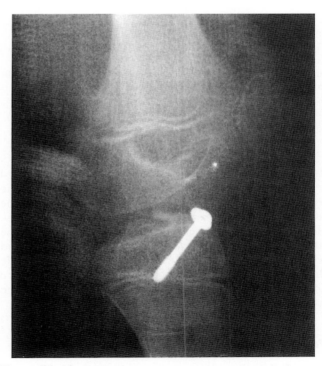

Figure 74–12 Postoperative anteroposterior radiograph after screw fixation of tibial spine. (From Berg EE: Pediatric tibial eminence fractures: Arthroscopic cannulated screw fixation. Arthroscopy 11:328-331, 1995.)

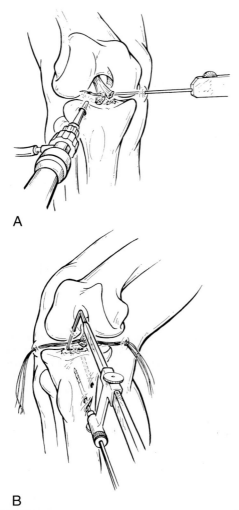

Figure 74–13 Diagram demonstrating technique for suture fixation of tibial eminence fracture. *A,* Arthroscopic passage of sutures through the ACL and tibial eminence. *B,* Use of the ACL guide to create a bone tunnel for suture passage. (From Berg EE: Comminuted tibial eminence anterior cruciate ligament avulsion fractures: Failure of arthroscopic treatment. Arthroscopy 9:446-450, 1993.)

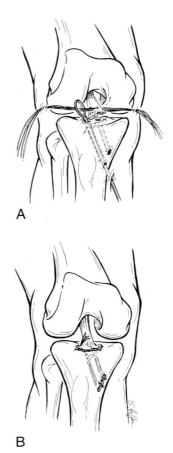

Figure 74–14 Diagram demonstrating technique for suture fixation of tibial eminence fracture. *A,* Retrieval of sutures through the tibial tunnel. *B,* Sutures tied down through tibial tunnels over the bone bridge. (From Berg EE: Comminuted tibial eminence anterior cruciate ligament avulsion fractures: Failure of arthroscopic treatment. Arthroscopy 9:446-450, 1993.)

that 9 of 10 type III eminence fractures failed closed reduction because of meniscal interposition. To hold the fracture fragment in place, a cannulated guide from the ACL set can be passed either from the medial portal, allowing an oblique screw to be placed, or from the superomedial portal, allowing a more vertically oriented screw. For retrograde guidewire insertion, an ACL guide that has a sharp tip or two prongs is best used to reduce and hold the fragment in place while the guidewires are passed through the tibia into the fragment.

Postoperative Management

Following fixation, thve knee is maintained in extension for 3 to 4 weeks. Crutch-assisted partial weight bearing is allowed as soon as tolerated. Active range of motion from 0 to 70 degrees is allowed for the next 4 weeks. Quadri-ceps rehabilitation is emphasized, similar to the standard ACL protocol.

Results

Although most series involving the arthroscopic treatment of eminence fractures are small, the accuracy and maintenance of reduction seem to correlate with the clinical results.[5,20,24,25,29] Mah et al.[24] reported that all nine of their patients had excellent subjective knee function and no laxity detected by examination after arthroscopically assisted reduction and suture fixation. In a small series, McLennan[29] reported KT-1000 measurements greater than 6 mm in four patients treated with closed immobilization, compared with less than 2 mm sagittal translation in three patients treated with arthroscopic reduction and internal fixation.

Complications

The complications associated with the treatment of tibial eminence fractures include those directly related to the procedure and long-term complications associated with failure to achieve knee stability after treatment. The intraoperative problems are similar to those found in other technically difficult arthroscopic procedures and include lack of visualization, inability to adequately reduce or stabilize the fragment, and fluid extravasation leading to potential compartment syndrome. The arthroscopically assisted procedure can and should be aborted if insurmountable difficulties are encountered or the procedure is taking an inordinate amount of time. A medial parapatellar arthrotomy can easily be made, allowing direct visualization, reduction, and stabilization of the tibial spine.

Patellar Fracture

Although traditionally treated with open reduction and internal fixation, selected fractures of the patella are amenable to arthroscopic management. The goal is to anatomically restore the articular surface of the patella with stable percutaneous fixation without the morbidity of a formal open approach. The final construct must be strong enough to restore the critical function of the extensor apparatus of the knee while allowing early rehabilitation.

Transverse fractures of the patella are typically stabilized using a Kirschner wire and tension band technique. However, biomechanical studies have demonstrated that cannulated screws and tension band wire or compression screws alone are also adequate.[4,10] It is therefore possible to insert screws percutaneously under arthroscopic visualization across transverse patellar fractures and achieve fixation that is stable enough to allow early range of motion. This approach offers several advantages over the open technique (Table 74–11).

History

The history frequently includes a fall, a direct blow to the front of the knee, or a near fall averted by strong contraction of the quadriceps muscle. Immediate pain followed by the development of a painful effusion and inability to ambulate is common (Table 74–12).

Table 74–11 **Advantages of Arthroscopic Fixation of Displaced Patellar Fractures**

Avoids long incision, soft tissue disruption
Avoids traumatized anterior skin
Improved cosmesis
Preserves blood supply to patella
Shortens anesthesia and operative time
Improves postoperative pain control
Allows perfect articular reduction without arthrotomy
Facilitates early range of motion, prevents intra-articular adhesions

---

Table 74–12 **Clinical Findings in Patellar Fractures**

History of fall or near-fall
Inability to ambulate
Anterior skin abrasion, laceration
Palpable defect in patella
Ability to perform straight leg raise after aspiration, injection of lidocaine

---

Physical Examination

The physical examination begins with close inspection of the skin for abrasion, laceration, blunt contusion, or evidence of open fracture. The entire anterior aspect of the knee is palpated for the presence of a defect in the patellar tendon, patella, or quadriceps tendon. The knee joint is then aspirated to evacuate the hematoma. One percent lidocaine is injected to aid in assessing extensor mechanism integrity. Inability to perform a straight leg raise in the presence of a patellar fracture should alert the surgeon to the presence of significant medial and lateral retinacular disruption.

Imaging

Radiographic evaluation is then performed, consisting of orthogonal posteroanterior and lateral views of the knee, as well as a tangential view. The Merchant tangential view, with the knee flexed 45 degrees and the x-ray beam angled 30 degrees from the horizontal, is the most convenient to obtain in a patient with a painful, traumatized knee.

Classification

Good plain radiographs allow the classification of patellar fractures based on the orientation of the fracture pattern. The transverse pattern is most frequently encountered and represents the fracture most conducive to arthroscopic treatment. Occasionally, patellar fractures with significant sagittal fracture lines are encountered, which also may be amenable to arthroscopically assisted stabilization using mediolateral screws.

Indications

Arthroscopic management should be considered for transverse fractures of the patella when fracture fragments are displaced more than 3 mm or when the articular step-off exceeds 2 mm (Table 74–13). Comminution should be minimal and the patient's bone of good quality to use lag screw fixation only. Fractures located at either the proximal or distal poles of the patella are not ideal for this type of fixation. Although some authors have reported success using the arthroscopic technique even when the medial and lateral retinacula are disrupted, we perform arthroscopically assisted patellar surgery only when the extensor mechanism is intact. If the retinacula

6 Knee

Table 74–13	Indications for Arthroscopic Treatment of Patellar Fractures

Displacement > 3 mm, step-off > 2 mm (displacement < 8 mm)
Transverse fractures (rarely sagittal split fractures)
Noncomminuted
Good-quality bone
Intact extensor mechanism (ability to perform straight leg raise)

are significantly disrupted, as indicated by failure to perform a straight leg raise or fracture displacement greater than 8 mm, we perform an open approach to facilitate direct retinacular repair. Surgery should be performed emergently for open fractures and urgently for knees with significant abrasions in order to prevent colonization. The arthroscopic technique is best performed within 3 days of the injury.

Surgical Technique

Positioning

The procedure is performed on a radiolucent table. A tourniquet is placed on the thigh but is inflated only if visualization is severely hampered. No leg holder is used. A bump is placed under the ipsilateral hip to prevent external rotation of the limb.

Specific Surgical Steps

Standard superolateral, anterolateral, and anteromedial portals are created. A pump is not used, but a high-inflow cannula is useful. Thorough joint lavage is performed, and all intra-articular debris is evacuated from the knee using a full-radius shaver. The knee is then inspected arthroscopically, with particular attention paid to the status of the articular cartilage of the patella and trochlea.

Using an arthroscopic probe in the superolateral portal, the transverse patellar fracture is manipulated into the reduced position. Manual external pressure aids in this reduction maneuver. The reduction is confirmed arthroscopically and held using standard pointed reduction forceps. Lateral C-arm fluoroscopy can be used to confirm the reduction. Alternatively, the anteromedial portal can be enlarged to allow digital confirmation of the articular reduction (Fig. 74–15).

Two guidewires from the 4-mm cannulated screw set are placed percutaneously from proximal to distal across the fracture site. The guidewires should be parallel and separated by approximately 2 cm. Reduction is then rechecked arthroscopically, and accurate placement of the guidewires is confirmed fluoroscopically. The skin is then incised at the entry site of the K-wires, and screw length is determined using a cannulated depth gauge. The wires are overdrilled using a 2.5-mm cannulated drill, and partially threaded 4-mm cannulated cancellous screws are inserted over the guidewires. The 16-mm threads are used to ensure that all threads cross the frac-

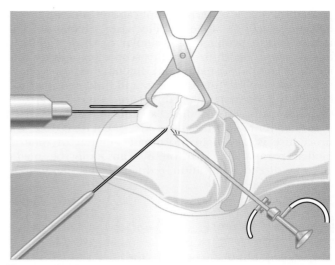

Figure 74–15 Diagram demonstrating arthroscopically assisted reduction and cannulated screw fixation of a transverse patellar fracture. (From Tandogan RN, Demirors H, Tuncay CI, et al: Arthroscopic-assisted percutaneous screw fixation of select patellar fractures. Arthroscopy 18:156-162, 2002.)

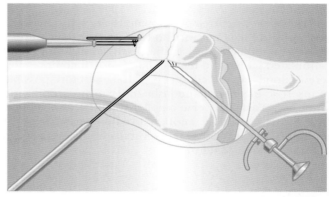

Figure 74–16 Diagram demonstrating arthroscopically assisted reduction and cannulated screw fixation of a transverse patellar fracture. (From Tandogan RN, Demirors H, Tuncay CI, et al: Arthroscopic-assisted percutaneous screw fixation of select patellar fractures. Arthroscopy 18:156-162, 2002.)

ture site. If the transverse fracture is relatively distal, the guidewires and screws can be placed in retrograde fashion to ensure that the screw threads engage the larger fragment (Fig. 74–16).

Stability of the construct is then assessed with gentle flexion and extension with the arthroscope in the superolateral portal. Approximately 90 degrees of gentle flexion should be possible without discernible motion at the fracture site. Alternatively, the construct can be augmented with cerclage wire without converting to an open repair. An 18-gauge wire is passed from proximal to distal via one of the cannulated screws and retrieved through a distal stab incision. The wire is then passed subcutaneously in the coronal plane and eventually passed distal to proximal via the second cannulated screw. The wire is tensioned proximally using one of the previously created stab wounds. Portals and stab wounds are then closed using absorbable monofilament suture, and the knee is immobilized in a standard range-of-motion brace (Figs. 74–17 to 74–19).

Pearls and Pitfalls

See Table 74–14.

Postoperative Management

The patient is hospitalized for 24 to 48 hours. Continuous passive motion devices are not routinely used but are recommended if the patient is deemed at high risk for arthrofibrosis. The patient may bear weight as tolerated using crutches with the brace locked in extension. The brace is worn continuously for 4 to 6 weeks. Isometric quadriceps strengthening exercises are performed in the brace as soon as tolerated.

On postoperative day 3, supervised physical therapy is begun, concentrating on achieving flexion range of motion. It is desirable to achieve a minimum of 100 degrees of flexion by 4 weeks. Active knee extension is avoided for the first 6 weeks, at which time it can be performed against gravity. Resisted knee extension is avoided until radiographic evidence of union is observed. As motion improves, the brace can be adjusted to allow greater degrees of flexion. The brace can be discontinued when radiographs reveal signs of union and quadriceps strength allows the patient to perform a single bent leg stance.

Results

Leung et al.[21] and Ma et al.[23] described percutaneous cerclage wiring of patellar fractures. However, Leung's

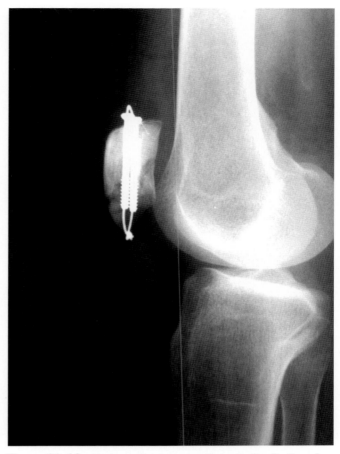

Figure 74–18   Postoperative lateral radiograph after fixation of a transverse patellar fracture. (From Tandogan RN, Demirors H, Tuncay CI, et al: Arthroscopic-assisted percutaneous screw fixation of select patellar fractures. Arthroscopy 18:156-162, 2002.)

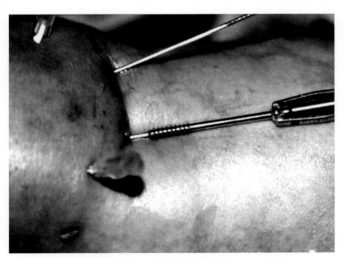

Figure 74–17   Intraoperative image of percutaneous insertion of screws after reduction of patellar fracture. (From Tandogan RN, Demirors H, Tuncay CI, et al: Arthroscopic-assisted percutaneous screw fixation of select patellar fractures. Arthroscopy 18:156-162, 2002.)

group performed the procedure on nondisplaced fractures, and a significant percentage of Ma's patients failed to achieve anatomic reduction.

Appel and Seigel[2] were the first to describe the benefits of arthroscopically assisted stabilization of patellar fractures. They reported improved cosmesis, decreased adhesion formation and stiffness, less discomfort, shorter hospitalization, and accelerated recovery using this approach.

Turgut et al.[35] reported their results treating 11 patients with transverse patellar fractures using arthroscopically assisted placement of crossed Kirschner wires. At nearly 3 years follow-up, all patients achieved solid union and good results with painless limited activity, no quadriceps atrophy, and no subjective knee disability.

Most recently, Tandogan et al.[34] reported their results treating five patients with transverse patellar fractures using a technique similar to that described by Appel and Seigel.[2] In this series, all fractures healed uneventfully without complication. Only one patient (an elderly patient with senile dementia) failed to achieve full motion. Two athletes returned to full sporting activity without restriction at 3 months.

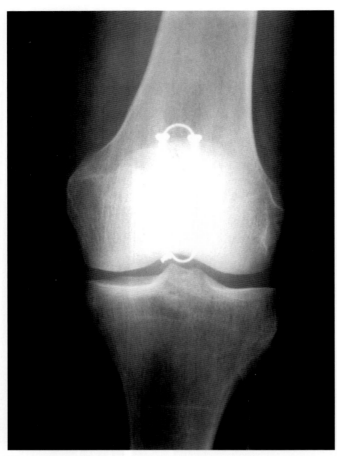

Figure 74–19 Anteroposterior radiograph after fixation of a transverse patellar fracture. (From Tandogan RN, Demirors H, Tuncay CI, et al: Arthroscopic-assisted percutaneous screw fixation of select patellar fractures. Arthroscopy 18:156-162, 2002.)

Complications

Arthroscopically assisted treatment of patellar fractures avoids many of the complications associated with the open approach. However, certain potential complications bear mentioning (Table 74–15).

Guidewires included in cannulated screw sets are not rigid and are at risk for breakage. To prevent guidewire breakage, the reduction should be held continuously using pointed reduction forceps until both screws are fully inserted. This prevents bending of the wires. Bent wires are extremely susceptible to breakage during drilling using the cannulated drill. Resistance encountered during drilling should alert the surgeon to the possibility of a bent guidewire, which can simply be exchanged for a new wire.

Fracture site distraction can also occur during cannulated screw insertion. Care should be taken when drilling both proximal and distal cortices. Again, compression should be maintained during screw insertion using the reduction forceps.

Loss of reduction is usually the result of inadequate internal fixation. As previously stated, no motion should be present at the fracture site during intraoperative flexion and extension when viewed arthroscopically. If stability is in doubt, a cerclage wire should be added. If this too proves inadequate, conversion to an open approach should be considered.

Early range of motion should not be sacrificed to make up for tenuous fixation. Prolonged immobilization in extension may result in persistent extension contracture. Again, alternative fixation should be employed if stable flexion is not achievable.

Table 74–14 Operative Pearls and Pitfalls: Patellar Fractures

Use radiolucent flat-top table
Perform thorough joint lavage; use gravity inflow, standard portals
Obtain reduction with arthroscopic probe in superolateral portal
Maintain reduction using pointed reduction clamp
Confirm reduction both fluoroscopically and digitally
Place two guidewires from cannulated screw set parallel across fracture site
Drill both cortices with cannulated drill
Do not bend guidewires
Place partially threaded 4-mm screws over guidewires: retrograde for distal fractures, antegrade for midportion or proximal fractures
Do not release reduction clamp until both screws have been inserted
Assess stability under direct arthroscopic visualization
Do not hesitate to add modified cerclage wire

Table 74–15 Potential Complications of Arthroscopic Treatment of Patellar Fractures

Complication	Cause	Prevention/Treatment
Guidewire breakage	Premature release of reduction clamp, drilling over bent guidewire	Maintain clamp until both screws inserted, replace guidewire if any resistance during drilling
Fracture site distraction	Failure to drill both cortices	Fully drill both cortices
Loss of reduction	Inadequate fixation	Confirm stable fixation arthroscopically; consider augmentation with cerclage wire; convert to open procedure if needed
Extension contracture	Prolonged immobilization	Ensure stable fixation to allow aggressive supervised physical therapy; use continuous passive motion devices

Distal Femur Fracture

Supracondylar and distal femur fractures can present a significant challenge to the orthopedic surgeon. Numerous treatment options have emerged, including the condylar blade plate, dynamic condylar screw, lateral condylar buttress plate, and supracondylar nail. Arthroscopic techniques that are useful in the treatment of these fractures have also been described. As in other fractures about the knee, arthroscopically assisted treatment of distal femur fractures offers several distinct advantages (Table 74–16).

Mechanism of Injury

Patients with fractures of the distal femur present in a manner similar to those with other fractures about the knee. Inability to ambulate, effusion, and painful restricted range of motion are the rule. When the mechanism is high-energy trauma, such as a motor vehicle accident, particular attention should be paid to the neurovascular status of the leg and the presence or absence of an open fracture.

Imaging

High-quality anteroposterior and lateral radiographs of the femur and knee are a prerequisite to treatment of these injuries (Fig. 74–20). Intra-articular fracture extensions are best visualized using CT scans (Fig. 74–21). We

Table 74–16	Advantages of Arthroscopic Treatment of Distal Femur Fractures

Allows magnification and illumination of articular disruption
Permits confirmation of anatomic articular reduction
Maximizes accuracy of intra-articular insertion of retrograde nails while minimizing unnecessary damage
Decreases soft tissue stripping and avoids arthrotomy
Decreases operative time and blood loss
Allows assessment and treatment of concomitant soft tissue injuries
May be performed as outpatient procedure

obtain CT scans in virtually every patient with a distal femur fracture unless we are completely certain about the extra-articular nature of the fracture.

Classification

Muller has provided a useful alphanumeric classification of distal femur fractures[32] (Fig. 74–22). Key elements are the amount of comminution present and the extent of intra-articular involvement.

Indications

Arthroscopic reduction and internal fixation are most appropriate for types B1, B2, and C1 displaced fractures

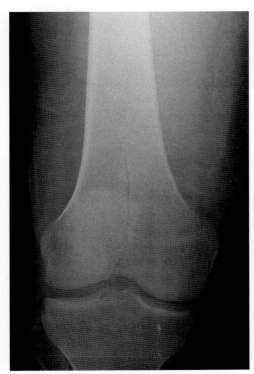

Figure 74–20 Anteroposterior radiograph of an intra-articular distal femoral condylar fracture.

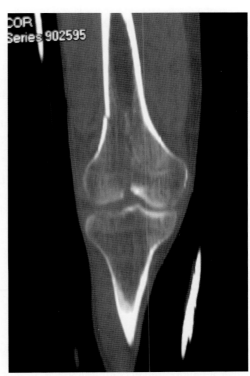

Figure 74–21 Computed tomography scan of an intra-articular distal femoral condylar fracture.

6 Knee

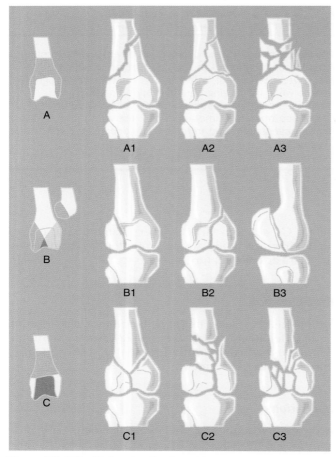

Figure 74–22 **Muller classification of fractures of the distal femur.** (From McCarthy JJ, Parker RD: Arthroscopic reduction and internal fixation of a displaced intraarticular lateral femoral condyle fracture of the knee. Arthroscopy 12:224-227, 1996.)

(Table 74–17). The large fragments present in these types of fractures are frequently amenable to screw-only fixation, which can be performed percutaneously after arthroscopically assisted reduction. Fractures with significant comminution or metaphyseal involvement most likely require plate stabilization and are best treated with a formal open approach.

Extra-articular type A fractures do not require articular reduction. These can often be successfully treated using a retrograde intramedullary nail. In this instance, arthroscopic localization of the intra-articular start point for the nail is extremely useful.

Table 74–17 **Indications for Arthroscopic Treatment of Distal Femur Fractures**

Type B1, B2, C1 fractures
Noncomminuted
Good-quality bone
Large fragments without metaphyseal involvement requiring
  plate stabilization
Extra-articular fractures treated with retrograde intramedullary
  nailing

Surgical Technique

The procedure for arthroscopic reduction and internal fixation is performed with the leg draped free on a radiolucent table. As in the previously described cases, gravity inflow is used, and the tourniquet is largely avoided. A thorough arthroscopic evaluation is performed using a standard three-portal technique. The intra-articular fracture site is identified and debrided of all adherent clot using an arthroscopic shaver. A standard arthroscopic probe can be used to disengage the articular fragments. Reduction is then generally performed using a large, pointed reduction clamp to achieve provisional interfragmentary compression. The adequacy of the reduction is determined using direct arthroscopic visualization. It should not be possible to insert the arthroscopic probe into the fracture site (Figs. 74–23 and 74–24).

Once reduction is confirmed, guidewires from the 6.5-mm cannulated screw set are inserted via percutaneous stab wounds from lateral to medial across the fracture site. Fluoroscopic visualization is used to confirm accurate wire placement. Partially threaded 6.5-mm screws

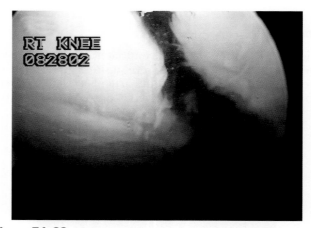

Figure 74–23 Arthroscopic image of the lateral femoral condyle before reduction.

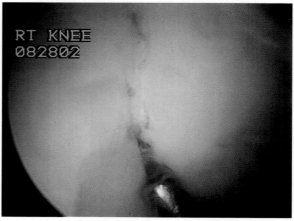

Figure 74–24 Arthroscopic image of the lateral femoral condyle after reduction.

and washers are then inserted over the guidewires, compressing and stabilizing the fracture site. Final fluoroscopic and arthroscopic confirmation of reduction is then obtained (Fig. 74–25).

When retrograde supracondylar nailing is chosen to stabilize a fracture of the distal femur, the operating room setup is similar. Supine positioning on a radiolucent table is again employed. A commercially available radiolucent "triangle" can be used to support the femur. An initial reduction is performed using longitudinal traction and confirmed fluoroscopically. Diagnostic arthroscopy is then performed using the same three standard portals. An arthroscopic shaver is used to remove the ligamentum mucosum overlying the ACL to better visualize the intercondylar notch. A 3-cm longitudinal incision based just medial to the patellar tendon is made. Sharp dissection reveals the anterior fat pad, which can be partially debrided. A guidewire is then placed under arthroscopic visualization in the intercondylar notch just anterior to the femoral insertion of the posterior cruciate ligament (Figs. 74–26 and 74–27). The guidewire is advanced, and accurate position is confirmed fluoroscopically. The canal is then opened using a cannulated reamer. A flexible guidewire is inserted into the intramedullary canal, and standard nailing is performed. After completion of the procedure, the knee is copiously lavaged. The arthroscope allows confirmation that the

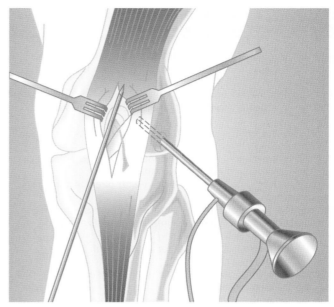

Figure 74–26 Diagram depicting arthroscopically assisted guidewire insertion in retrograde femoral nailing. (From Guerra JJ, Della Valle CJ, Corcoran TA, et al: Arthroscopically assisted placement of a supracondylar intramedullary nail: Operative technique. Arthroscopy 11:239-244, 1995.)

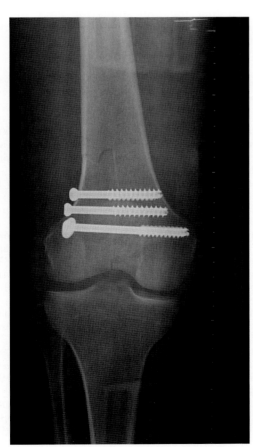

Figure 74–25 Postoperative anteroposterior radiograph after cannulated screw fixation of a distal femoral fracture.

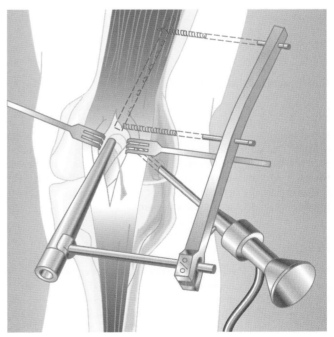

Figure 74–27 Diagram depicting arthroscopically assisted guidewire insertion in retrograde femoral nailing. (From Guerra JJ, Della Valle CJ, Corcoran TA, et al: Arthroscopically assisted placement of a supracondylar intramedullary nail: Operative technique. Arthroscopy 11:239-244, 1995.)

6 Knee

Table 74–18 Operative Pearls and Pitfalls: Distal Femur Fractures

For intra-articular distal femur fractures, accurately define fracture fragments using preoperative computed tomography scan
Use supine position on radiolucent table
Disengage articular fracture fragments using arthroscopic probe
Manipulate fragments into reduced position using probe, and hold with large, pointed reduction clamps
Place guidewires across fracture under fluoroscopic control
Use 6.5-mm cannulated screws with washers
Confirm anatomic articular reduction with direct arthroscopic visualization
When using retrograde nails, remove ligamentum mucosum using arthroscopic shaver to improve visualization of intercondylar notch
Use medial parapatellar portal for insertion of instrumentation
Position guidewire just anterior to femoral insertion of posterior cruciate ligament
After reaming and nail insertion, lavage the knee and remove all debris using shaver

nail is adequately countersunk. The arthroscopic shaver is used to remove metallic and other debris from within the joint.

Pearls and Pitfalls

See Table 74–18.

Postoperative Management

Postoperative care is similar to that described previously. A knee immobilizer is used for 2 to 4 days, followed by supervised active and passive range of motion. Isometric quadriceps exercises are performed as soon as tolerated. Strict non–weight bearing is enforced for the first 3 months for articular fractures. Extra-articular fractures stabilized with intramedullary nails may progress to partial weight bearing more quickly.

Results

McCarthy and Parker[28] described arthroscopic reduction and internal fixation of a Muller type B1 lateral condylar fracture using two 6.5-mm screws. Postoperative CT scan revealed anatomic fracture reduction and accurate screw placement. The patient, a 42-year-old woman, was healed by 3 months, and at 4-year follow-up, she had experienced no change in pain, level of activity, or range of motion. Radiographs revealed no loss of reduction.

Guerra et al.[15] described arthroscopically assisted placement of a retrograde intramedullary nail in 1995. A 19-year-old woman with a type A3 extra-articular distal femur fracture caused by a gunshot wound was treated using this technique. She achieved 110 degrees of knee flexion by postoperative day 5 and progressed to uneventful union. The authors emphasized the greater

safety of this nail insertion technique compared with the "blind" method, without the attendant morbidity of formal arthrotomy.

Complications

Potential complications are identical to those outlined previously. Loss of reduction in intra-articular fractures is frequently the result of inadequate or inappropriate fixation. The surgeon should not hesitate to augment stability with a buttress plate or convert to a formal open reduction. Range of motion should be emphasized, and physical therapy implemented rapidly.

Summary

Various arthroscopic techniques can be used to assist in managing complex fractures about the knee that were conventionally treated with direct visualization via an arthrotomy. Although the procedure is technically demanding, the smaller incisions required for arthroscopically assisted reduction and definitive stabilization afford many advantages over larger arthrotomies. A surgeon's comfort with advanced arthroscopic techniques is a prerequisite. These techniques, when applied correctly and in the appropriate setting, have the potential to decrease morbidity and speed recovery. It is anticipated that the indications for these and other arthroscopically assisted techniques will continue to expand in the future.

References

1. Ali AM, El-Shafie M, Willett KM: Failure of fixation of tibial plateau fractures. J Orthop Trauma 16:323-329, 2002.
2. Appel MH, Seigel H: Treatment of transverse fractures of the patella by arthroscopic percutaneous pinning. Arthroscopy 9:119-121, 1993.
3. Belanger M, Fadale P: Compartment syndrome of the leg after arthroscopic examination of a tibial plateau fracture: Case report and review of the literature. Arthroscopy 13:646-651, 1997.
4. Benjamin J, Bried J, Dohm M, McMurtry M: Biomechanical evaluation of various forms of fixation of transverse patellar fractures. J Orthop Trauma 1:219-222, 1987.
5. Bennett WF, Browner B: Tibial plateau fractures: A study of associated soft tissue injuries. J Orthop Trauma 8:183-188, 1994.
6. Bernfield B, Kligman M, Roffman M: Arthroscopic assistance for unselected tibial plateau fractures. Arthroscopy 12:598-602, 1996.
7. Bomberg BC, Hurley PE, Clark CA, McLaughlin CS: Complications associated with the use of an infusion pump during knee arthroscopy. Arthroscopy 8:224-228, 1992.
8. Bottoni CR, Arciero RA: Conventional meniscal repair techniques. Oper Tech Sports Med 10:194-208, 2000.
9. Buchko GM, Johnson DH: Arthroscopy assisted operative management of tibial plateau fractures. Clin Orthop 332:29-36, 1996.
10. Carpenter JE, Kasman R, Matthews LS: Fractures of the patella. Instr Course Lect 43:97-108, 1994.

11. Caspari RB, Hutton PM, Whipple TL, Meyers JF: The role of arthroscopy in the management of tibial plateau fractures. Arthroscopy 1:76-82, 1985.

12. Fowble CD, Zimmer JW, Schepsis AA: The role of arthroscopy in the assessment and treatment of tibial plateau fractures. Arthroscopy 9:584-590, 1993.

13. Gill TJ, Moezzi DM, Oates KM, Sterett WI: Arthroscopic reduction and internal fixation of tibial plateau fractures in skiing. Clin Orthop 383:243-249, 2001.

14. Guanche CA, Markman AW: Arthroscopic management of tibial plateau fractures. Arthroscopy 9:467-471, 1993.

15. Guerra JJ, Della Valle CJ, Corcoran TA, et al: Arthroscopically assisted placement of a supracondylar intramedullary nail: Operative technique. Arthroscopy 11:239-244, 1995.

16. Holzach P, Matter P, Minter J: Arthroscopically assisted treatment of lateral tibial plateau fractures in skiers: Use of a cannulated reduction system. J Orthop Trauma 8:273-281, 1994.

17. Itokazu M, Matsunaga T: Arthroscopic restoration of depressed tibial plateau fractures using bone and hydroxyapatite grafts. Arthroscopy 9:103-108, 1993.

18. Jennings JE: Arthroscopic management of tibial plateau fractures. Arthroscopy 1:160-168, 1985.

19. Karunakar MA, Egol KA, Peindl R, et al: Split depression tibial plateau fractures: A biomechanical study. J Orthop Trauma 16:172-177, 2002.

20. Kogan MG, Marks P, Amendola A: Technique for arthroscopic suture fixation of displaced tibial intercondylar eminence fractures. Arthroscopy 13:301-306, 1997.

21. Leung PC, Mak KH, Lee SY: Percutaneous tension band wiring: A new method of internal fixation for mildly displaced patella fracture. J Trauma 23:62-64, 1983.

22. Lobenhoffer P, Schulze M, Gerich T, et al: Closed reduction/percutaneous fixation of tibial plateau fractures: Arthroscopic versus fluoroscopic control of reduction. J Orthop Trauma 13:426-431, 1999.

23. Ma YZ, Zhang YF, Qu KF, Yeh YC: Treatment of fractures of the patella with percutaneous suture. Clin Orthop 191:235-241, 1984.

24. Mah JY, Adili A, Otsuka NY, Ogilvie R: Follow-up study of arthroscopic reduction and fixation of type III tibial-eminence fractures. J Pediatr Orthop 18:475-477, 1998.

25. Mah JY, Otsuka NY, McLean J: An arthroscopic technique for the reduction and fixation of tibial-eminence fractures. J Pediatr Orthop 16:119-121, 1996.

26. Marsh JL, Buckwalter J, Gelberman R, et al: Articular fractures: Does an anatomic reduction really change the result? J Bone Joint Surg Am 84:1259-1271, 2002.

27. Mazoue CG, Guanche CA, Vrahas MS: Arthroscopic management of tibial plateau fractures: An unselected series. Am J Orthop 28:508-515, 1999.

28. McCarthy JJ, Parker RD: Arthroscopic reduction and internal fixation of a displaced intraarticular lateral femoral condyle fracture of the knee. Arthroscopy 12:224-227, 1996.

29. McLennan JG: Lessons learned after second-look arthroscopy in type III fractures of the tibial spine. J Pediatr Orthop 15:59-62, 1995.

30. Meyers MH, McKeever FM: Fracture of the intercondylar eminence of the tibia. J Bone Joint Surg Am 52:1677-1684, 1970.

31. Reiner MJ: The arthroscope in tibial plateau fractures: Its use in evaluation of soft tissue and bony injury. J Am Osteopath Assoc 81:704-707, 1982.

32. Ruedi TP, Murphy WM: AO Principles of Fracture Management. New York, AO Publishing, 2000, p 53.

33. Schatzker J, McBroom R, Bruce D: The tibial plateau fracture: The Toronto experience 1968–1975. Clin Orthop 138:94-104, 1979.

34. Tandogan RN, Demirors H, Tuncay CI, et al: Arthroscopic-assisted percutaneous screw fixation of select patellar fractures. Arthroscopy 18:156-162, 2002.

35. Turgut A, Gunal I, Acar S, et al: Arthroscopic-assisted percutaneous stabilization of patellar fractures. Clin Orthop 389:57-61, 2001.

36. Vangsness CT Jr, Ghaderi B, Hohl M, Moore TM: Arthroscopy of meniscal injuries with tibial plateau fractures. J Bone Joint Surg Br 76:488-490, 1994.

37. Westmoreland GL, McLaurin TM, Hutton WC: Screw pullout strength: A biomechanical comparison of large-fragment and small-fragment fixation in the tibial plateau. J Orthop Trauma 16:178-181, 2002.

6 Knee

ARTHROSCOPY OF THE ANKLE

Ankle: Patient Positioning, Portal Placement, and Diagnostic Arthroscopy

JOHN G. KENNEDY, GORDON SLATER, AND MARTIN J. O'MALLEY

In 1931, Burman from the Hospital for Joint Diseases established that arthroscopy was possible in small joints in cadavers.[1] Since then, advances have been made in both instrumentation and techniques that facilitate safe and easy arthroscopic procedures in the ankle joint. This chapter describes current patient positioning techniques and typical portal anatomy. In addition, a stepwise approach to normal and diagnostic arthroscopy is described.

Positioning

Three standard patient positions are used in ankle arthroscopy. The lateral decubitus position and the supine position with the table broken at 90 degrees are useful methods, but our preferred method is supine positioning with a thigh holder and ankle distractor.

A thigh tourniquet is applied to the upper leg before it is prepared and draped. A thigh holder is used to secure the femur in approximately 60 degrees of hip flexion. Attention to correct placement of the thigh holder is important to prevent pressure in the popliteal space and the neurovascular structures. A gel pad is placed on the holder, and the leg is secured in the holder with an elastic bandage (Fig. 75–1). The patient is supported with a sandbag under the contralateral hip until the knee and ankle are straight on the operating table. Failure to correctly position and secure the limb at this stage can cause problems intraoperatively when ankle distraction is used.

Both invasive and noninvasive distraction techniques have been used to facilitate joint visualization. Noninva-

sive methods of distraction can be used in the overwhelming majority of cases. If adequate visualization of the joint cannot be achieved because of severe arthrosis or arthrofibrosis, a medially or laterally placed distraction device can be used.

In the standard noninvasive distractor technique, a sterile clamp is used over a single layer of draping. To this is attached a bar and ankle strap. The strap is placed around the heel and dorsum of the foot in such a manner as to avoid injury to the anterior neurovascular structures. The distractor is set at minimal distraction, and the tension in the soft tissues is set with the clamp and bar initially. This facilitates maximal intraoperative distraction once the case begins. Initial distraction should be just 4 to 5 mm. After 2 to 3 minutes, another 4 to 5 mm of distraction can be applied. This slow distraction requires consideration of the length-tension curve of tendon collagen. Slower distraction provides greater length in the soft tissues than rapid distraction does.

Care must be paid to any predistraction anatomic skin markings. The joint line will have changed from the original skin marking, and this should be checked again once the desired tension on the joint is achieved (Fig. 75–2).

If visualization cannot be achieved with noninvasive distraction techniques, a medially or laterally based external distracter can be used. Our current technique involves use of a lateral distractor as originally described by Guhl.[3]

A $\frac{3}{16}$-inch calcaneal Steinmann pin is placed 2.5 cm anterior and 2.5 cm superior to the posteroinferior calcaneal margin. The peroneal tendons and subtalar joint are avoided. The angle of entry from lateral to medial is 20 degrees cephalad in the coronal plane. This

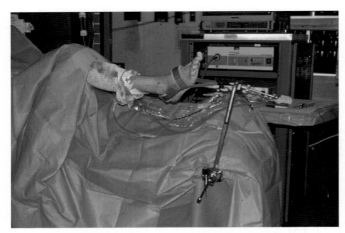

Figure 75–1 Standard setup for noninvasive distraction, with the thigh and ankle holder in place. Care must be taken to ensure that the leg holder is well padded.

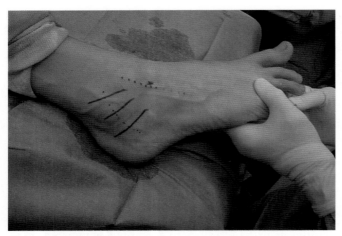

Figure 75–2 Skin markings should be drawn before placement to allow full access to all portals, avoiding the superficial peroneal nerve.

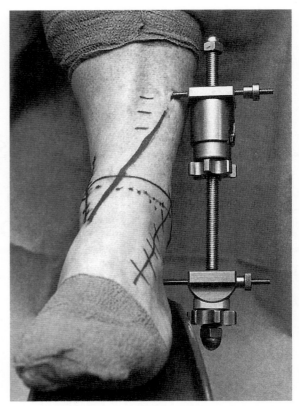

Figure 75–3 Typical invasive distractor in situ. (From Ferkel RD: Operating room environment and the surgical team. In Ferkel RD: Arthroscopic Surgery: The Foot and Ankle. Philadelphia, Lippincott, 1996, p 79.)

The potential advantages of invasive distraction are that articular damage to a tight joint can be minimized and that access to the posterior portals is easier. However, the potential for neurovascular injury and mechanical failure offsets any advantage this system has for routine use, and the noninvasive distraction system is favored in most cases.

Portal Placement

The primary utilitarian arthrotomy portals in ankle arthroscopy are the anterior portals, particularly the anteromedial and anterolateral portals. The anterior anatomic structures at the joint line include the deep peroneal nerve and dorsalis pedis artery, running between the extensor hallucis longus and extensor digitorum longus tendons. They are deep structures and are not at significant risk during portal placement. The deep peroneal nerve supplies a sensory dermatome between the first and second toes, and injury to this nerve may compromise this area as well as the motor supply to the extensor digitorum brevis. The greater saphenous vein and saphenous nerve run on the medial side of the joint and should be avoided when making the anteromedial portal. The vein can be traced out before exsanguination. The most commonly injured structure in ankle

angulation diminishes when distraction is applied, and the pins should then line up parallel. The pin is advanced to the medial calcaneal cortex but should not transgress it. The tibial Steinmann pin is placed 6 to 8 cm above the lateral joint line.

Once a stab incision is made, a small arterial clamp is tunneled anterior to the tibialis anterior muscle, through the subcutaneous tissue to the bone. A tissue protector is then placed through this tunnel to allow drilling of the lateral cortex. The pin is advanced once again to the medial cortex but not through it, to prevent a stress fracture. Once the pins are in place, the fixator is distracted (Fig. 75–3). Slow distraction allows the tendon and capsule to lengthen more than is possible when rapid distraction is used. A total of 30 to 60 pounds of traction should be sufficient for adequate visualization, with 30 pounds for a total of 60 minutes being the standard rule. After that time, the risk of neurovascular injury increases.

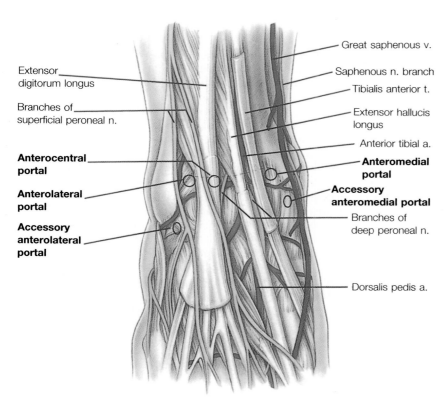

Extensor digitorum longus

Branches of superficial peroneal n.

Anterocentral portal

Anterolateral portal

Accessory anterolateral portal

Great saphenous v.

Saphenous n. branch

Tibialis anterior t.

Extensor hallucis longus

Anterior tibial a.

Anteromedial portal

Accessory anteromedial portal

Branches of deep peroneal n.

Dorsalis pedis a.

Figure 75–4 Anterior portals, demonstrating the proximity of important anatomic structures. a., artery; n., nerve; t., tendon; v., vein. (From Ferkel RD: Diagnostic arthroscopic examination. In Ferkel RD: Arthroscopic Surgery: The Foot and Ankle. Philadelphia, Lippincott, 1996, p 104.)

arthroscopy is the superficial peroneal nerve. This divides above the ankle joint into the dorsolateral and dorsomedial cutaneous branches. These branches supply the dorsum of the foot, and their injury from inadvertent anterolateral portal placement can be problematic for the patient.

Before portal placement, it is essential that these anterior structures be marked. The superficial peroneal nerve can be identified easily, particularly in slim patients, by placing pressure on the fourth metatarsal head. This makes the nerve become more prominent, and it can be drawn on the skin.

The ankle joint should initially be injected with 30 mL of fluid using an 18-gauge spinal needle. The foot will dorsiflex slightly as the joint distends.

Anteromedial Portal

The anteromedial portal is best placed close to the tibialis anterior tendon in the "soft spot" of the ankle, which is between the tendon and the saphenous vein. By keeping adjacent to the tendon, injury to the saphenous nerve is almost certainly avoided. A small 5-mm linear incision is made immediately adjacent to the tibialis anterior tendon, and a pair of blunt dissecting scissors is used to dissect down to the anterior joint line capsule. With the ankle in a dorsiflexed position to avoid damaging the talar dome, a blunt trocar is used to gain entry to the ankle joint. The trocar is inserted, and the joint is infused with fluid. The portal should not be too medial, because this will prevent visualization of the medial gutter (Figs. 75–4 and 75–5).

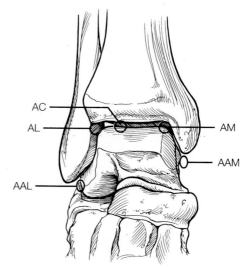

AC

AL

AAL

AM

AAM

Figure 75–5 Anterior portals and adjacent anatomic landmarks, as well as accessory portals for access to the medial and lateral gutters. AAL, accessory anterolateral; AAM, accessory anteromedial; AC, anterocentral; AL, anterolateral; AM, anteromedial. (From Ferkel RD: Diagnostic arthroscopic examination. In Ferkel RD: Arthroscopic Surgery: The Foot and Ankle. Philadelphia, Lippincott, 1996, p 104.)

Anterolateral Portal

The anterolateral portal is made under direct vision from the arthroscope in the anteromedial portal. The landmarks used are the lateral border of the peroneus tertius and the anterior joint line. Protection of the peroneus tertius and the dorsal cutaneous branch of the superfi-

7 Ankle

cial peroneal nerve is important and can be facilitated by transilluminating the skin over the proposed portal site. A spinal needle is inserted from the lateral side. Once the position is confirmed arthroscopically, a number 15 blade is used to make a skin incision, followed by blunt dissection down to the joint capsule. The blunt trocar is inserted again, with the ankle in a dorsiflexed position. Care should be taken to avoid a far lateral portal, as this will hinder visualization of the lateral gutter (see Figs. 75–4 and 75–5).

It is possible to make a central-anterior portal between the tendons of the extensor digitorum communis. We do not use this portal and consider it dangerous because the possibility of neurologic or arterial damage is high.

Posterolateral Portal

The posterolateral portal is made just lateral to the Achilles tendon. The lateral aspect of the joint is visualized arthroscopically, and an 18-gauge spinal needle is placed into the posterior aspect of the joint under direct vision. The direction of the needle is usually from distal to proximal; however, this may change, depending on the curvature of the distal tibia. Inspection of the preoperative radiograph can help in determining needle placement.

This portal can be difficult to create, and it is best made by internally rotating the ankle to allow access to the lateral part of the ankle joint. If it is suspected that this portal will be used, one should ensure during setup that the knee is flexed to allow the ankle to be well off the bed. We use this as the standard outflow arthrotomy

portal, keeping the 18-gauge spinal needle in place throughout the procedure. It is also useful for the removal of loose bodies and synovitic material and for visualizing posteromedial osteochondritis dissecans (Fig. 75–6). The anatomic structures at risk are the sural nerve and the Achilles tendon. Laceration of the tendon is unlikely; however, the nerve branches at this level and can be injured. Careful blunt dissection, keeping just lateral to the tendon, should avoid neurologic injury.

Two additional portals are possible—an accessory medial portal, which is made approximately 5 mm anterior to the distal tip of the medial malleolus, and an accessory lateral portal, which is made approximately 5 mm proximal and anterior to the tip of the fibula. Accessory portals can be useful for the removal of pathology in the medial and lateral gutters.

Posteromedial and posterocentral portals have also been described. We do not routinely use these portals. The posterocentral portal passes through the body of the Achilles tendon, making it difficult to maneuver instruments. The posteromedial portal carries a significant risk of injury to the posterior tibial nerve and artery.

Once access to the joint has been obtained, the first technical step is to remove the localized synovitis at the lateral aspect of the joint surface. This is invariably present when there is pathology within the ankle, at the trifurcation point. Marked synovial tissue occurs here owing to the infolding of the capsule. If this synovitic material is not removed almost immediately, it will become edematous, rendering further visualization of the joint very difficult. Once this is removed, the joint can be inspected. Resection of this material is facilitated by using a 2.9-mm full-radius chondrotome.

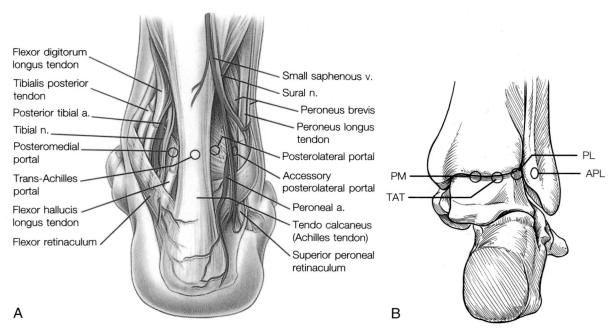

A

B

Figure 75–6 Posterior portals and adjacent anatomic landmarks. a., artery; APL, accessory posterolateral; n., nerve; PL, posterolateral; PM, posteromedial; TAT, trans–Achilles tendon; v., vein. (From Ferkel RD: Diagnostic arthroscopic examination. In Ferkel RD: Arthroscopic Surgery: The Foot and Ankle. Philadelphia, Lippincott, 1996, p 106.)

Normal Arthroscopic Anatomy

The ankle joint can be divided into the anterior, central, and posterior sections. Each division can be further subdivided so that a standard 21-point arthroscopic examination can be performed on all patients.[2]

Eight-Point Anterior Examination (Areas 1 to 8)

1. The first structure visualized during the anterior examination is the anterior part of the deltoid ligament (Fig. 75–7, area 1).
2. The next area seen is the articular surface of the medial malleolus and the talus, as well as the posterior recess and posterior ligaments (area 1).
3. The medial gutter extends from the deltoid ligament to below the dome of the talus (area 2).
4. The talar dome on the medial side is designated area 3. As the articular surface becomes more convex in the coronal plane, it is named the notch of Harty, or area 3. The scope should move easily here, because the joint space is maximal.
5. As the scope moves from medial to lateral, sweeping across the top of the talus in the sagittal groove, area 4 can be inspected. Area 4 is the sagittal groove itself and the anterior tibial articular lip.
6. Area 5 is the lateral talar shoulder, and area 6 is the lateral talofibular articulation. This area is known as the *trifurcation*, because it represents the confluence of the lateral talar articulation, the fibula, and the lateral tibial plafond. Superiorly, this area is bounded by the anteroinferior tibiofibular ligament. This is a key area in the arthroscopic examination, particularly in patients suspected of having soft tissue injuries. Synovitis is usually present in the synovial recess posterior to the ligament and can be resected at this point. In addition, any lesion of the anterolateral talar dome can be seen and probed at this time.
7. Area 7 is the lateral gutter, extending from the inferior tibiofibular ligament to the anterior talofibular ligament. This is often the site of soft tissue impingement following soft tissue injury. It may also be the site of chondromalacia.
8. The anterior gutter represents area 8 of the examination. It is a capsular reflection on the talar neck. This area is the site of tibiotalar *kissing lesions.*

Six-Point Central Examination (Areas 9 to 14)

The convex portion of the talus is inspected next (Fig. 75–8).

1. Area 9 is the medial dome of the talus, which is particularly prone to osteochondral lesions and chondromalacia.
2. Area 10 represents the central articular surface of the talus.
3. Area 11 is the lateral central articular surface of the talus and corresponds to the area bounded by the lateral talar dome, distal tibia, fibula, and syndesmotic articulation. Like the trifurcation, this area often has

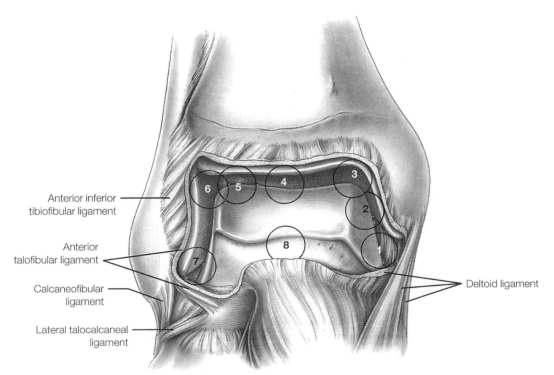

Anterior inferior tibiofibular ligament

Anterior talofibular ligament

Calcaneofibular ligament

Lateral talocalcaneal ligament

Deltoid ligament

7 Ankle

Figure 75–7   **Anterior examination areas.** (From Ferkel RD: Diagnostic arthroscopic examination. In Ferkel RD: Arthroscopic Surgery: The Foot and Ankle. Philadelphia, Lippincott, 1996, p 110.)

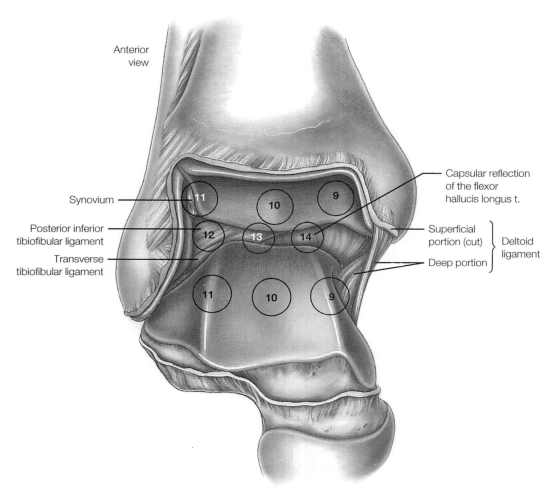

Figure 75–8 **Central examination areas.** (From Ferkel RD: Diagnostic arthroscopic examination. In Ferkel RD: Arthroscopic Surgery: The Foot and Ankle. Philadelphia, Lippincott, 1996, p 112.)

significant synovitis that can be removed at this time. Generally, the tibiofibular joint should not be visible, as it is covered by capsule and strong ligamentous structures.

4. From lateral to medial, area 12 is the inferior tibiofibular ligament, running obliquely from the posterior tibia to the fibula.
5. Area 13 corresponds to the transverse tibiofibular ligament.
6. The capsular reflection of the extensor hallucis longus tendon is area 14.

Seven-Point Posterior Examination (Areas 15 to 21)

To gain access to the posterior aspect of the joint (Fig. 75–9), the 2.7-mm arthroscope may need to be exchanged with a 1.9-mm arthroscope. First, however, tightening of the distractor apparatus is usually required, as it tends to loosen during the course of the procedure.

1. The scope is changed to the posterolateral portal, and the posteromedial recess and posterior aspect of the deltoid ligament are visualized (area 15).
2. Area 16 is the posterior medial talar dome and posterior tibial plafond.
3. Area 17 corresponds to the central talus and tibial articulation.
4. Area 18 is the posterolateral talar dome.
5. Area 19 is the posterior tibiofibular articulation.
6. Area 20 is the posterolateral gutter at the site of the most posterior and distal talofibular articulation.
7. Area 21 is the posterior gutter. Occasionally, intra-articular bodies are found in this recess. The posterolateral portal is useful for removing loose bodies from this area.

Diagnostic Arthroscopy

Ankle arthroscopy can be used to diagnose both acute and chronic soft tissue and bony pathology. These conditions are described in other chapters of this book, and

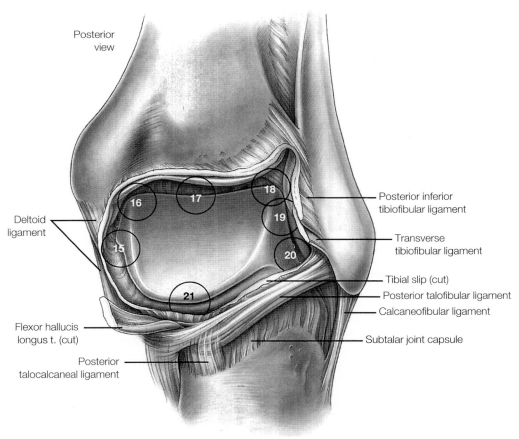

Figure 75–9   **Posterior examination areas.** (From Ferkel RD: Diagnostic arthroscopic examination. In Ferkel RD: Arthroscopic Surgery: The Foot and Ankle. Philadelphia, Lippincott, 1996, p 114.)

their pathology and treatment are not discussed here. The diagnosis of soft tissue and bony ankle pathology should not rely on arthroscopy alone. A careful patient history and physical examination will yield the most reliable diagnosis. This can be supplemented with conventional radiographs and other techniques, including computed tomography and magnetic resonance imaging. Arthroscopy is most useful for confirming clinical and radiographic suspicions and determining the degree or stage of intra-articular pathology.

The cause of chronic ankle pain following varying degrees of trauma can be difficult to diagnose, and even the most accurate magnetic resonance coils may not yield images that are sensitive or specific enough to identify the soft tissue pathology.[4] In patients with degenerative arthrosis, ankle arthroscopy may yield information on the extent and degree of arthrosis that is not evident radiographically and that may direct treatment paradigms. This is true also in the diagnosis and management of osteochondral lesions. Radiographic or computed tomographic staging may not correlate with intraoperative findings, and the final treatment is decided by direct visualization (Fig. 75–10).

In acute injuries to the ankle joint, diagnostic arthroscopy is becoming more widespread. Outcome after ankle fracture is related to the degree of articular

compromise at the time of the injury. This can be assessed by direct visualization following fracture reduction and may prove to be a more reliable indicator of arthrosis than the type of fracture pattern on conventional radiographs. In addition, injury to the talar dome can be seen, which also has an impact on outcome.

The use of a syndesmotic screw in certain ankle fracture patterns is controversial, and there are several methods of assessing the tibiofibular joint both clinically and radiographically. Direct visualization of the syndesmotic ligaments and the joint can eliminate any doubt about joint stability in such cases.

Nonspecific Synovitis

Following any traumatic episode, the joint may react with generalized or focal synovitis. This may progress to fibrous bands, adhesions, and hemosiderin deposition within the joint, which can be diagnosed arthroscopically. Associated with long-standing synovitis may be areas of chondromalacia, which can be appreciated only by arthroscope. This initial inflammatory response may progress to soft tissue impingement or may be the harbinger of degenerative arthritis or arthrofibrosis.

7 Ankle

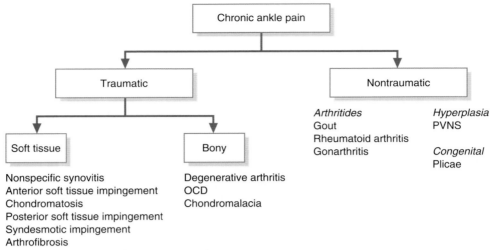

Figure 75–10   Diagnosis of chronic ankle pain. OCD, osteochondritis dissecans; PVNS, pigmented villonodular synovitis.

Anterior Soft Tissue Impingement

Anterior soft tissue impingement is typically the result of an inversion injury. The inflammatory response progresses to one of hypertrophied synovial tissue, in addition to a redundant anterior talofibular ligament or anteroinferior tibiofibular ligament. The superior part of the inflamed ligaments may correspond to a chondral lesion in the talus or fibula seen under direct visualization. A meniscus-like lesion may be seen at arthroscopy, whereby the hypertrophied ligaments become hyalinized and protrude into the anterior part of the joint, similar to a torn meniscus of the knee. Typically, these lesions are not appreciated on plain radiographs, and magnetic resonance imaging has a low specificity and sensitivity compared with arthroscopic examination.

Posterior Soft Tissue Impingement

Several ligaments may be involved either alone or in combination. Typically, the posteroinferior tibiofibular ligament or posterior talofibular ligament are hypertrophied; however, the transverse tibiofibular ligament or tibial slip may also be involved. In ballet dancers, a posterior tibiolabral tear can be seen. These injuries manifest arthroscopically as areas of synovitis, fibrosis, and posterior capsulitis. Direct visualization of these posterior structures is often difficult, and the posterolateral portal provides the best access to optimize diagnosis. When this portal is used, the manual distractor should be increased to improve the space for the arthroscope at the back of the joint.

Syndesmotic Impingement

Syndesmotic impingement is typically seen in athletes who complain of prolonged ankle pain that does not respond to conventional therapy. It may occur in combination with anterior impingement, posterior impingement, or both. Arthroscopically, this may manifest as synovitis of the anterior tibiofibular ligament as well as the posterior ligamentous structures. Up to 20% of the syndesmotic ligament is intra-articular, and this can help not only in arthroscopic diagnosis but also in treatment.

Summary

Ankle arthroscopy is an evolving art and a developing science. As newer arthroscopes are developed and distraction equipment improves, the indications for diagnostic and therapeutic arthroscopic intervention will expand.

References

1. Burman MS: Arthroscopy, a direct visualization of joints: An experimental cadaver study. J Bone Joint Surg Am 13:669, 1931.
2. Ferkel RD, Fischer SP: Progress in ankle arthroscopy. Clin Orthop 240:210, 1989.
3. Guhl JF: New concepts: Distraction in ankle arthroscopy. Arthroscopy 4:160, 1988.
4. Liu SH, Nuccion SL, Finerman G: Diagnosis of anterolateral ankle impingement: Comparison between magnetic resonance imaging and clinical examination. Am J Sports Med 25:389, 1997.

Ankle Arthrodesis and Anterior Impingement

John G. Kennedy, Gordon Slater, and Martin J. O'Malley

ANKLE ARTHRODESIS AND ANTERIOR IMPINGEMENT IN A NUTSHELL

	Arthrodesis	Impingement
History:	Prior trauma, arthropathy	Activity related; anterior ankle pain
Physical Examination:	Antalgic gait; tenderness; painful, restricted range of motion; crepitus; check alignment and for gross instability	Small effusion; limited dorsiflexion
Imaging:	Radiographs—rule out Charcot joint; computed tomography	Lateral dorsiflexion stress radiographs
Indications:	Painful arthrosis without significant bone loss or avascular necrosis	Failed conservative management for longer than 3 months
Surgical Technique:	Diagnostic arthroscopy; cartilage removal; osteophyte removal; guide pin placement; cannulated screw placement	Diagnostic arthroscopy; shaver, bur, osteotome used for spur removal; talar spur removal
Postoperative Management:	Cast; non–weight bearing for 3 weeks, then progressive weight bearing	Splint or boot for 3 to 5 days; physical therapy—range of motion
Results:	91% to 96% fusion at a mean of 9 weeks	64% good, 22% fair; best results in patients without arthrosis

Arthroscopic Ankle Arthrodesis

Despite recent advances in ankle arthroplasty, ankle arthrodesis remains the benchmark for the treatment of painful, unstable ankle joints. Several methods of open tibiotalar fusion have been reported, with an overall complication rate of up to 60%. In an effort to reduce this complication rate—caused, theoretically, by compromised vasculature from extensive open exposure—arthroscopic and minimally invasive techniques of ankle fusion have been investigated. In 1983, arthroscopic ankle debridement was reported by Schneider.[17] The technique has become more widespread as surgical instrumentation and techniques have improved. In a comparative study of open and arthroscopic ankle arthrodesis, Myerson and Quill[12] reported that the mean time for bony union in the arthroscopic cohort was 8.7 weeks, whereas the time to union in those treated with an open procedure was 14.5 weeks. Further, the high complication rate associated with open procedures has dropped since the introduction of the arthroscopic technique, making this an attractive procedure in a select cohort of patients.[2-5,7,15]

History

Typically, patients requiring arthroscopic ankle fusion have a history of ankle trauma. Other indications for this technique include patients with ankle arthrosis following hemophilic arthropathy or with talar osteochondral lesions. Patients with rheumatoid arthritis are also potential candidates for this surgery. Patients generally report severe mechanical ankle pain that is increasing and interfering with activities of daily living. The pain is usually characterized as dull and is exacerbated by physical activity and relieved by rest.

The implications of a fused ankle joint should be discussed with the patient. It may be beneficial to inject the joint with a local anesthetic to establish the location of the pathology. This can be followed with a period of immobilization in an Arizona brace or cast to demonstrate the position of the ankle and establish the limits of motion that will be imposed by a fusion. The level of function desired by the patient should be discussed in relation to the level of function that can be expected after ankle fusion.

Physical Examination

The three basic principles of evaluating any joint are applicable to the ankle: inspection, palpation, and motion.

Inspection

The patient typically walks with an antalgic gait, and the foot may have an increased foot progression angle secondary to external rotation to avoid painful dorsiflexion–plantar flexion. The overall alignment of the lower limb is assessed, and any knee malalignment noted. The attitude and position of the foot when in swing phase and when weight bearing are also assessed. Gross deformity should not be apparent on clinical examination, as this precludes arthroscopic fusion. Mild ankle swelling may be an indication of ankle joint effusion, and in patients with rheumatoid arthritis, typical rheumatoid changes in the forefoot may be apparent. Mild calf atrophy may be present from inactivity and protection of the ipsilateral limb.

The position of the heel in relation to the midline of the calf is assessed; it is normally 5 to 10 degrees of valgus. Excessive valgus can occur following calcaneal fractures, as a result of advanced degenerative or rheumatoid disease, or from a neuroarthropathy. A varus inclination of the heel is typically seen following calcaneal fractures but is more commonly associated with a neuropathy rather than degenerative disease. A varus or valgus angulation greater than 15 degrees precludes arthroscopic fusion. The condition of the skin over the ankle and at the arthrotomy portals should also be checked.

Palpation

The ankle joint is palpated anteriorly, noting any joint line tenderness or bony spurs. The subtalar joint and sinus tarsi are also palpated for pain. The arterial pulse should be established, and a sensory and motor evaluation of the foot and ankle should be performed.

Motion

The ankle joint is painful when ranged through an arc of active and passive motion. Crepitus may be evident, indicating generalized arthrosis or an old osteochondral defect. Any mechanical blocks to dorsiflexion and plantar flexion should be elicited. The knee should be at 90 degrees and in neutral to establish whether a gastrocnemius-soleus contracture exists.

Overall ankle stability is assessed. An anterior draw demonstrating ligamentous instability does not preclude an arthroscopic fusion. However, gross rotatory instability, indicative of syndesmotic disruption, is a relative contraindication to arthroscopic arthrodesis.

Imaging

Standard plain weight-bearing radiographs are invaluable in establishing the overall alignment of the joint (Fig. 76–1) and determining whether the destruction of the tibiotalar surfaces may preclude arthroscopic fusion. Gross bony destruction and bone loss are contraindications to arthroscopic fusion. Plain radiographs may also aid in establishing whether preexisting contraindications to arthroscopic fusion exist, including neuroarthropathy, active infection, or the presence of an occult lesion. Anterior bony osteophytes causing mechanical impingement that may require resection to achieve a neutral ankle fusion can also be seen on plain radiographs.

Computed tomography (CT) may be useful in establishing the bony anatomy of the ankle joint. Gross osteonecrosis of the talar joint that is not manifest on plain radiographs can be elicited on CT. The tibiotalar mortise can be more accurately visualized on CT, and the congruency of the joint can be evaluated. This is important for determining whether sufficient congruency exists to achieve a fusion by minimal resection or whether an open procedure facilitating greater resection is required. CT may also be useful in establishing the position and size of osteophytes, particularly large anterior lip osteophytes that may block reduction of the talus on the tibia. The joints of the subtalar complex should also be visualized to rule out significant athrosis. Morgan et al.[10] showed that after ankle fusion, motion in the subtalar complex increases by 11 degrees in the first year.[10] If significant arthrosis is seen in these joints, consideration should be given to fusion of more than the ankle joint.

Indications and Contraindications

Table 76–1 lists the indications for arthroscopic ankle fusion, and Table 76–2 the contraindications.

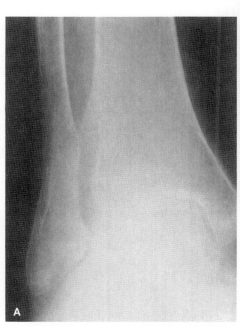
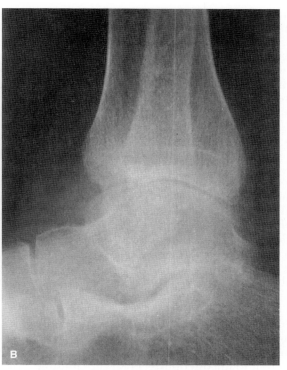

Figure 76–1   Anteroposterior *(A)* and lateral *(B)* radiographs of ankle showing minimal architectural changes but loss of joint space. The patient has rheumatoid arthritis. (From Glick JM, Ferkel RD: Arthroscopic ankle arthrodesis. In Ferkel RD: Arthroscopic Surgery: The Foot and Ankle. Philadelphia, Lippincott-Raven, 1996, p 223.)

Table 76–1

Indications for Arthroscopic Ankle Fusion

Unrelenting ankle joint pain, not responding to conservative management
Elderly patient unable to tolerate prolonged postoperative immobilization
Idiopathic or post-traumatic tibiotalar arthrosis
Rheumatoid arthritis of tibiotalar joint
Talar osteonecrosis less than 30%
Hemophilic arthropathy
Congenital deformity
Joint destruction secondary to "burned out" septic joint
Patients with poor-quality skin coverage for standard open procedure

---

Table 76–2   **Contraindications to Arthroscopic Ankle Fusion**

Significant bone loss from either bone
Rotatory malalignment
Varus or valgus angulation greater than 15 degrees
Active infection
Excessive anteroposterior translation of tibiotalar joint surfaces
Reflex sympathetic dystrophy

Surgical Technique

Positioning

The patient is placed supine on the operating table. The ankle is positioned so that the distractor can be used without impinging on the arthroscope or fluoroscope for intraoperative imaging. Local or regional anesthesia can be used.

Specific Surgical Steps

The portals are identified before the distractor is used, and the joint is infused with normal saline. Once the distractor is used, the point of infiltration will have moved, so palpation of the portal sites is necessary again. An 18-gauge needle is used to establish the joint line and arthrotomy portals. Three standard portals are used: anteromedial, anterolateral, and posterolateral.

The anterolateral portal is used first to visualize the joint. It is made with a number 11 blade just lateral to the peroneus tertius at the joint line. An arterial clamp is used to penetrate the deep layers, and a blunt obturator is used to gain access to the joint. An outflow portal is placed in the posterolateral portal. A standard

7 Ankle

21-point arthroscopic survey should be performed to determine the articular surface and viability of arthroscopic fusion.

Alternating between the two anterior portals, the articular cartilage of the tibial plafond, the talar dome, and the medial and lateral talomalleolar surfaces are removed. Care should be taken when removing cartilage so that no deep troughs are made. This can be visualized periodically under intraoperative fluoroscopy. A motorized shaver is alternated with both ring and cup curets. A grasper or shaver is used to remove floating articular cartilage.

Debridement is continued until viable, bleeding subchondral bone is seen. Excessive resection or squaring off of joint surfaces should be avoided to prevent a varus or valgus fusion (Fig. 76–2). The anterior portals are usually sufficient to visualize and abrade the posterior compartment and transmalleolar spaces. The posterior portal can be used if these areas are inaccessible.

The lateral part of the joint is usually debrided with the arthroscope in the medial portal and the debrider in the lateral portal. The converse is applicable for the medial half of the joint. An anterior lip osteophyte should be removed from the front of the joint to facilitate congruent tibiotalar fusion surfaces. If the anterior capsule is adherent to the osteophyte, great care must be exercised in creating a plane between the osteophyte and the capsule. The neurovascular bundle lies just anterior to the capsule. Occasionally, it may be necessary to make a small incision directly over the osteophyte to facilitate its removal. The posterolateral portal is best to visualize the anterior capsule when this is being carried out.

Following arthroscopic debridement, the anterolateral portal is extended proximally for 2 cm to allow direct visualization and to further facilitate osteophyte removal. It is important that this arthrotomy portal be limited to 2 cm; any greater extension can compromise the superficial peroneal nerve. Guide pins for the 6.5- or 7-mm cannulated screw set are placed from the lateral and medial malleoli until the tips of the pins can be seen arthroscopically just penetrating the bone (Fig. 76–3). The angle of entry of both pins is 45 degrees inferior and 45 degrees anterior from a posterior starting position on the malleoli (Fig. 76–4). The final fusion position is established, and the final position of the pins in the talus is estimated from their intra-articular position.

The standard ankle fusion position is neutral flexion, 5 degrees valgus, and 5 degrees external rotation. The distractor is released, and the arthroscopic instruments are removed from the joint. The fluoroscope is used to aid in the final positioning of the fusion construct. The medial pin is advanced under fluoroscopy to ensure that it does not penetrate the subtalar joint. The pin is measured, and a self-taping partially threaded cancellous screw is advanced. Minor medial translation is afforded by placing the medial screw initially. The lateral pin is advanced, screw length is measured, and the second

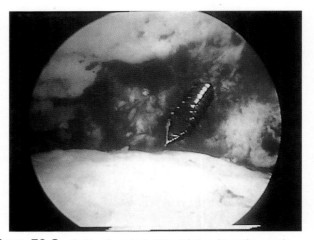

Figure 76–3　Guide pin entering the joint under arthroscopic guidance. Once the position is deemed satisfactory, the distractor is released, and the pin is advanced into the talus. (From Glick JM, Ferkel RD: Arthroscopic ankle arthrodesis. In Ferkel RD: Arthroscopic Surgery: The Foot and Ankle. Lippincott-Raven, 1996, p 226.)

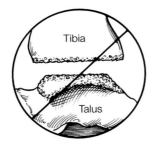

Figure 76–2　Surfaces of the tibiotalar joint should be shaved down to bleeding subchondral bone. Congruent bony surfaces rather than squared-off surfaces are critical to obtain neutral alignment. (From Glick JM, Ferkel RD: Arthroscopic ankle arthrodesis. In Ferkel RD: Arthroscopic Surgery: The Foot and Ankle. Lippincott-Raven, 1996, p 224.)

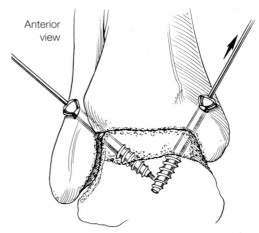

Anterior view

Figure 76–4　The angle of entry of the two malleolus screws. From a posterior starting position, the most effective angle of entry is 45 degrees anterior and 45 degrees inferior. (From Glick JM, Ferkel RD: Arthroscopic ankle arthrodesis. In Ferkel RD: Arthroscopic Surgery: The Foot and Ankle. Lippincott-Raven, 1996, p 227.)

screw is advanced across the fusion site. The final position is checked in both the anteroposterior and lateral planes under image intensification.

If an additional screw is necessary because of suboptimal bone quality and screw purchase, a third screw can be placed from the medial side and angled 25 degrees anteriorly. Preoperative assessment should have established whether a neutral flexion position of the ankle could be achieved or whether the gastrocnemius or gastrocnemius-soleus complex would prevent reduction. In the latter case, either an open gastrocnemius slide or a percutaneous Achilles tendon lengthening can be performed.

Meticulous wound closure is essential, because the ankle does not have the wound-sealing ability of other joints that are routinely arthroscoped. A 4.0 nylon suture should be used to close the arthrotomy portals; Steri-strips should not be used.

Postoperative Management

A posterior splint is worn for the first week, and the patient is encouraged not to bear weight (Table 76–3). In patients with rheumatoid disease, the period of protected weight bearing may continue for an additional 3 weeks. In cases in which excellent fixation was achieved and the patient is compliant, a removable cast boot with the hinges locked in neutral can be used as early as 2 weeks after surgery. In all cases, protection is continued until union is confirmed both radiographically and clinically.

Results

In a multicenter report of 75 patients undergoing arthroscopic ankle fusion, the overall fusion rate was 91%. When abandoned techniques were excluded from the study, this number improved to 96%. The mean time to fusion was 9 weeks, compared with 13 weeks in patients undergoing open fusion. The reported nonunion rate was 8%, and the complication rate was 5%.[5] More recent studies have confirmed this report and other earlier investigations, with good to excellent results in approximately 90% of patients. Faster fusion times and fewer complications are also universally reported with arthroscopically fused ankle joints compared with open procedures.[2-5,9,15] In the most recent study of 31 patients treated with arthroscopic ankle fusion, 30 patients achieved a solid union at a mean of 8.9 weeks. The single failure in this reported series was related to extensive avascularity of the talus. The authors recommended that greater than 30% osteonecrosis should be considered a contraindication to arthroscopic fusion.[22] Table 76–4 lists the advantages and disadvantages of arthroscopic fusion.

Anterior Bony Ankle Impingement

Anterior bony ankle impingement is a condition in which a bony prominence on the tibia impinges on a corresponding area on the neck of the talus. The exostosis is usually extra-articular but intracapsular. First described by Morris[11] in 1943, the condition was called the "athletes ankle" because it occurred in athletes in extremes of plantar flexion. No operative intervention was recommended at that time. McMurray[8] reported three cases of impingement in football players in 1958, all of whom were treated with anterior capsulotomy and excision of the bony prominence. Since then, surgical excision has been the mainstay of definitive treatment; currently, arthroscopic resection provides an excellent surgical outcome and a rapid return to activities.

Anterior bony ankle impingement is one of the most common diagnoses during ankle arthroscopy for joint pain. O'Donoghue[13] described the condition in more than 45% of football players. In ballet dancers, an incidence of greater than 59% was reported by Stoller et al.[19] The reason for the occurrence of this condition is not fully understood. It is thought to be a result of direct

---

Table 76–3 Postoperative Management of Patients Undergoing Arthroscopic Ankle Fusion

Time Frame	Care
Initial postoperative period	Well-padded posterior splint for 1 wk; patient encouraged not to bear weight
7–10 days	Sutures removed; short leg cast applied for additional 2 wk of non–weight bearing
3 wk	Cast removed and radiograph obtained; if healing is progressing well, walking cast is applied for additional 3 wk; weight bearing advanced as tolerated until bony union is seen radiographically

---

Table 76–4 Advantages and Disadvantages of Arthroscopic Ankle Fusion

Advantages

High fusion rate
Less time to bony fusion
Lower patient morbidity
Lower cost

Disadvantages

Lengthy learning curve
Not universally applicable, with a restricted cohort of suitable patients
Neurologic injury, neuroma
Superficial peroneal nerve is injured more commonly than sural, greater saphenous, and deep peroneal nerves
Wound complications
Symptomatic hardware

7 Ankle

trauma. The marginal exostosis may be an outgrowth from sclerotic bone beneath the articular cartilage; however, it is likely that repetitive dorsiflexion and plantar flexion contribute to the development of this exostosis. Forced plantar flexion causes capsular avulsion, and forced dorsiflexion causes direct impingement trauma. Repetitive microfractures of the trabecular bone from impaction heal with sclerotic bone formation and cartilage destruction.

History and Physical Examination

Patients generally complain of pain at the anterior aspect of the ankle when walking up stairs or hills, squatting, or running. Pain is chiefly activity related. Ballet dancers may complain of pain on landing from a jump.

A small anterior joint effusion may be seen or palpated on physical examination. Passive range of motion may demonstrate limited dorsiflexion with pain at the extreme arc of motion. The osteophyte can occasionally present in an anterolateral position, causing pain between the talus and fibula in athletes. In addition, medial malleolar osteophytes cause pain on abutment of the talus. Rarely, posterior osteophytes are encountered, causing symptoms in the plantarflexed ankle.

Imaging

The most important imaging technique in the diagnosis of this disorder is a lateral dorsiflexion stress radiograph. The patient stands with the knee flexed 30 degrees and the ankle maximally dorsiflexed in this position. The normal talocrural angle is 60 degrees or greater (Fig. 76–5). Any decrease in this angle is redundant bone that should be considered for removal. The anteroposterior

radiograph is useful for identifying a hidden anteromedial osteophyte. This occurs when the bony exostosis arises from the medial aspect of the talus and is not seen on the lateral radiograph. If the lesion is suspected clinically by palpating along the medial neck of the talus, an internal rotation or oblique radiograph can identify its position more clearly. Recent work has suggested that both a lateral radiograph and an anteromedial impingement or oblique radiograph should be obtained routinely to differentiate between an anteromedial and a medial spur.[21] The lateral radiograph remains the diagnostic modality of choice and is used in the classification of this disorder.

Classification

A four-grade classification system was devised by Scranton and McDermott[18] (Fig. 76–6):

Grade I: synovial impingement; less than 3 mm of spur formation
Grade II: osteochondral reaction with a spur greater than 3 mm; no talar spurs
Grade III: significant anterior exostosis; secondary talar spur formation
Grade IV: pantalocrural impingement and degenerative arthritis

CT can localize the lesion and is useful in ruling out alternative or concomitant pathology, including chondral injury or loose bodies. The precise location of the osteophyte may be determined by CT. The more common anteromedial location can be differentiated from an anterolateral exostosis, which aids in preoperative planning.

Magnetic resonance imaging currently has no advantage over CT in the diagnosis of anterior impingement.

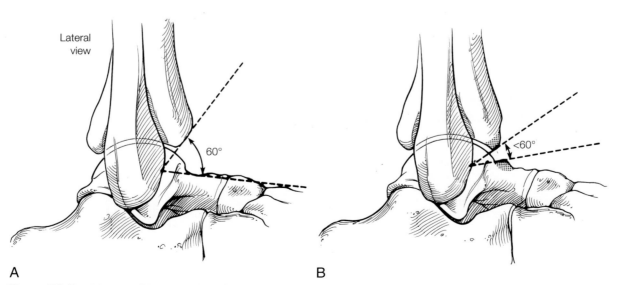

Lateral view

60°

<60°

A   B

Figure 76–5 *A,* Normal tibiotalar angle of 60 degrees. *B,* Angles less than normal indicate impingement. (From Stone JW, Guhl JF, Ferkel RD: Osteophytes, loose bodies and chondral lesions of the ankle. In Ferkel RD: Arthroscopic Surgery: The Foot and Ankle. Lippincott-Raven, 1996, p 175.)

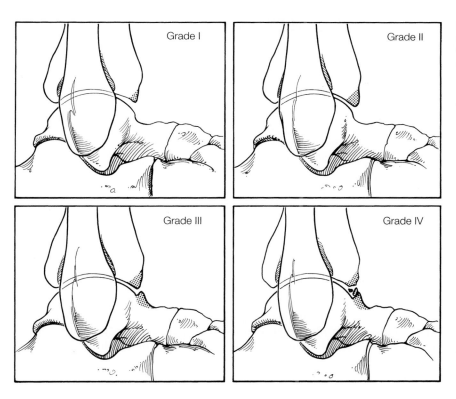

Grade I

Grade II

Grade III

Grade IV

Figure 76–6   Scranton and McDermott's[18] classification of anterior impingement based on the lateral weight-bearing dorsiflexion radiograph. (From Stone JW, Guhl JF, Ferkel RD: Osteophytes, loose bodies and chondral lesions of the ankle. In Ferkel RD: Arthroscopic Surgery: The Foot and Ankle. Lippincott-Raven, 1996, p 179.)

However, concomitant cartilaginous and soft tissue injuries may be diagnosed with this modality. Magnetic resonance imaging may also be useful in the differential diagnosis in patients with anterolateral instability.[6]

Indications

Treatment of this disorder is initially conservative. Heel lifts, nonsteroidal anti-inflammatory medication, and occasional intra-articular steroid injections may provide symptomatic relief. If symptoms persist after 3 months of conservative therapy, surgery is indicated.

Indications for open or arthroscopic resection are related to the lesion's grade. Grade I to II lesions respond very well to arthroscopic resection. Grade III lesions are less predictable and can be treated either arthroscopically or by open debridement. Grade IV lesions often require open debridement owing to their size.

Surgical Technique

A standard arthroscopy technique is used, similar to that described earlier for arthroscopic ankle fusion. The ankle is held in neutral by a clove hitch noninvasive distractor. Standard portals are made, and a 21-point inspection of the joint is performed before resection of the spur. A 3.5-mm shaver may be required initially to visualize the spur. The anterior spur is usually removed with either a rosebud bur or an acromionizer-type shaver.

Small 5- to 8-mm straight and curved osteotomes are helpful in removing the anterior tibial spurs and can easily be placed through one of the portals. Adequate visibility is essential, and extreme care should be exercised to avoid injuring the neurovascular structures. Shaver blades must never be directed dorsally toward the neurovascular bundle. The soft tissue must be peeled off the anterior osteophyte; this is best done with the shaver, with the cutting edge facing away from the soft tissue. If the capsule becomes tight with distraction, impeding resection, letting off some traction and alternating between the anteromedial and anterolateral portals can be useful.

An intraoperative radiograph is useful to determine the amount of resection; however, radiographs tend to underestimate the size of the lesion, and careful inspection of the medial extent of the osteophyte using the anterolateral portal is crucial. This medial extension of the osteophyte is often unappreciated initially, and it must be resected to prevent symptomatic bony impingement.

Attention is then focused on the talar spur. We believe that a talar spur should be removed if it measures more than 3 mm. The anterior ankle capsule, covering the spur, is debrided with a shaver. The spur is most easily seen with the ankle in dorsiflexion. It is almost impossible to remove the talar spur while the ankle is held in plantar flexion, because the anterior capsule becomes taut, making access difficult. If a large spur is encountered, an intraoperative radiograph should be used to confirm complete removal of the osteophyte. Hidden osteophytes on the medial aspect of the joint are best removed with a mini-arthrotomy. Because of their location inferior to the medial portal, they are not well visualized.

7 Ankle

Postoperative Management

The patient is placed in a posterior splint in neutral and a removable walker boot for 3 to 5 days. Physical therapy emphasizes the use of tilt-board range-of-motion exercises and anteroposterior strengthening of the calf musculature.

Results

Treatment of anterior bony ankle impingement has evolved over the past decades. Scranton and Mc-Dermott[18] published a series comparing arthroscopic and open treatment. Outcomes were similar for both treatment groups; however, hospital stay and recovery time were less in patients treated arthroscopically. The authors concluded that patients with grade I, II, and III spurs are good candidates for arthroscopic resection. Patients with grade IV spurs can be treated by either modality, but the outcome is not predictable.

Ogilvie-Harris et al.[14] reported on 17 patients who underwent arthroscopic resection for anterior bony ankle impingement. All patients had painful limitation of range of motion. An average follow-up of 39 months showed significant improvement in levels of pain, swelling, stiffness, limping, and activity. One poor result was caused by superficial infection, and two other patients had residual numbness of the foot that eventually resolved. Ankle dorsiflexion increased from a mean of 3 degrees to a mean of 12 degrees.

In the largest series to date, Brancas et al.[1] reviewed 133 patients with ankle impingement, 58 of whom were treated with ankle arthroscopy. Preoperative classification showed 15 grade I, 23 grade II, 13 grade III, and 7 grade IV lesions. Follow-up ranged from 8 to 62 months. Based on a modified ankle scoring system, there were 37 good, 13 fair, and 8 poor outcomes. Recurrent impingement was noted in four patients. The authors stated that arthroscopic debridement may defer eventual arthrodesis, even in patients with late grade III and IV disease.

Rasmussen and Hjorth Jensen[16] reported on a consecutive series of 105 patients with ankle impingement, 44 of whom had anterior bony impingement treated with arthroscopic resection without distraction. All patients complained of painful dorsiflexion and had failed to respond to conservative treatment. At 2-year follow-up, 65 patients were pain free, and 28 had experienced a reduction in pain. Gait was improved in 30 of 41 patients. The results were graded excellent in 67, good in 25, fair in 6, and poor in 7 patients. There were four deep infections and one synovial fistula reported. The deep infections all responded well to arthroscopic synovectomy and intravenous antibiotics. Persistent symptoms were recorded in a single patient. The authors concluded that ankle arthroscopy yielded good results in the treatment of anterior impingement of the ankle, effectively reducing pain and enhancing function.

Van Dijk et al.[20] showed that the presence of arthrosis is a better prognostic indicator than the size of the spur itself. In a series of 62 consecutive patients who underwent arthroscopic surgery, the most important prognostic indicator was the presence of joint arthrosis. At 2-year

Table 76–5	Complications of Arthroscopic Treatment of Anterior Impingement

Postoperative effusion
Osteophyte recurrence
Inadequate resection
Loose bodies
Infection
Neurologic injury
Tendon injury
Vascular injury
Reflex sympathetic dystrophy

follow-up, 90% of patients with no joint space narrowing had good or excellent outcomes; in contrast, just 50% of those with joint space narrowing had good or excellent results.

In summary, patients should achieve good pain relief from this procedure, but in general, only 5 to 10 degrees of increased motion will be obtained following resection of most anterior osteophytes.

Complications

Complications of arthroscopic treatment of anterior bony ankle impingement are listed in Table 76–5.

References

1. Brancas A, DiPalma L, Bucca C: Arthroscopic treatment of anterior ankle impingement. Foot Ankle Int 18: 418-424, 1997.
2. Corso SJ, Zimmer TJ: Technique and clinical evaluation of arthroscopic ankle arthrodesis. Arthroscopy 11:585-590, 1995.
3. De Vries L, Dereymaeker G, Fabry G: Arthroscopic ankle arthrodesis: Preliminary report. Acta Orthop Belg 60:389-392, 1994.
4. Fischer RL, Ryan WR, Dugdale TW, Zimmermann GA: Arthroscopic ankle fusion. Conn Med 61:643-646, 1997.
5. Guhl JF: New concepts on ankle arthroscopy. Arthroscopy 4:160, 1988.
6. Jordan LK 3rd, Helms CA, Cooperman AE, Speer KP: Magnetic resonance imaging findings in anterolateral impingement of the ankle. Skeletal Radiol 29:34-39, 2000.
7. Mann JA, Glick JM, Morgan CD, et al: Arthroscopic ankle arthrodesis: Experience with 78 cases. Paper presented to the American Academy of Orthopaedic Surgeons, 1995, Orlando, FL.
8. McMurray TP: Footballers ankle. J Bone Joint Surg Br 32:68-70, 1958.
9. Morgan CD: Arthroscopic tibiotalar arthrodesis. In McGinty JB (ed): Operative Arthroscopy. New York, Raven Press, 1991, pp 695-701.
10. Morgan CD, Henke JA, Bailey RW, Kaufer H: Long term results of tibio-talar arthrodesis. J Bone Joint Surg Am 67:546-550, 1985.
11. Morris LH: Report of cases of athletes ankle. J Bone Joint Surg Am 25:220, 1943.

12. Myerson MS, Quill G: Ankle arthrodesis: A comparison of an arthroscopic and an open method of treatment. Clin Orthop 268:84-89, 1991.

13. O'Donoghue EH: Impingement exostoses of the talus and tibia. J Bone Joint Surg Am 39:835-838, 1957.

14. Ogilvie-Harris DJ, Mahomes N, Demazire A: Anterior impingement of the ankle treated by arthroscopic removal of bony spurs. J Bone Joint Surg Br 75:437-440, 1993.

15. Ogilvie Harris DJ, Reed SC: Disruption of the ankle syndesmosis: Diagnosis and treatment by arthroscopic surgery. Arthroscopy 10:561, 1994.

16. Ramussen S, Hjorth Jensen C: Arthroscopic treatment of impingement of the ankle reduces pain and enhances function. Scand J Med Sci Sports 12:69-72, 2002.

17. Schneider A: Arthroscopic ankle fusion. Arth Video 3, 1983.

18. Scranton PE Jr, McDermott JE: Anterior tibiotalar spurs: A comparison of open versus arthroscopic debridement. Foot Ankle 13:125-129, 1992.

19. Stoller SM, Helimatt F, Kleigeer B: A comparative study on anterior impingement exostoses of the ankle in dancers and non-dancers. Foot Ankle 4:201, 1984.

20. van Dijk CN, Tol J, Verheyer CC: A prospective study of prognostic factors concerning the outcome of arthroscopic surgery for anterior ankle impingement. J Sports Med 25:737-745, 1997.

21. van Dijk CN, Wessel RN, Tol JL, Maas M: Oblique radiograph for the detection of bone spurs in anterior ankle impingement. Skeletal Radiol 31:214-221, 2002.

22. Zvijac JE, Lemak L, Schurhoff MR, et al: Analysis of arthroscopically assisted ankle arthrodeses. Arthroscopy 18:70-75, 2002.

77

Arthroscopic Subtalar Arthrodesis

James P. Tasto

History, Physical Examination, and Imaging:
  Pain laterally over subtalar joint, limitation of motion, response to subtalar injections, radiographic evidence of arthritis

Indications:
  Intractable subtalar pain secondary to rheumatoid arthritis, osteoarthritis, or post-traumatic arthritis, as well as posterior tibial tendon dysfunction

Surgical Technique:
  Lateral decubitus position with high thigh tourniquet and two- or three-portal technique; nick and spread technique used to establish all portals; diagnostic arthroscopy carried out through anterior portal; posterolateral portal used for majority of debridement, accessory anterior portal for some debridement; small shaver and bur used to remove all articular cartilage and decorticate 1 to 2 mm below subchondral plate; spot-weld vascular channels established; subtalar joint thoroughly irrigated; fixation accomplished with one 7.3-mm cannulated screw from anteromedial to posterolateral

Postoperative Management:
  Immobilization in bivalve cast; full weight bearing in ankle-foot orthosis 1 week postoperatively; orthosis removed when clinical and radiographic fusion accomplished

Results:
  Decreased morbidity and increased fusion rate, as well as reduced time until fusion

Complications:
  Minimal

Operative procedures for subtalar fusion have been in existence for more than 90 years. Nieny performed the first subtalar arthrodesis in 1905. Numerous techniques have been reported in the literature, using both intra-articular and extra-articular methods.[1,6,7,9,10,12,13,20,21] Results have generally been favorable, with a variety of complications reported.[11,14,15] Data on the rate of fusion, time until union, complications, and long-term follow-up are noticeably missing in both the older and the more recent literature. A number of other procedures for subtalar pathology have been described, including arthroscopy, arthroplasty, triple arthrodesis, and sinus

tarsi exploration. Open surgical reduction of calcaneal fractures has gained acceptance when attempting to restore the normal anatomic alignment of the joint surfaces in an effort to avoid the sequelae of post-traumatic degenerative arthritis of the subtalar joint. Both operative and conservative care of calcaneal fractures continues to be plagued with long-term symptomatic degenerative changes in the subtalar joint.

Arthroscopic subtalar arthrodesis was developed in 1992, and a preliminary review was reported at the annual meeting of the Arthroscopy Association of North America in 1994. The procedure was designed to improve traditional methods by using a microinvasive technique. The decision to attempt this surgical technique grew out of the success with arthroscopic ankle arthrodesis.[19] Subtalar arthroscopy has been described by a number of authors, but few cases or attempts at arthroscopic subtalar fusion have been published.[2] Work by Solis (personal communication, 1996) has paralleled some of this earlier work.

Use of an arthroscopic technique was intended to decrease morbidity if the procedure could not be performed using the same techniques and principles as an arthroscopic ankle fusion. It was hypothesized that perioperative morbidity could be reduced, blood supply preserved, and proprioceptive and neurosensory input enhanced. A prospective study was initiated to document the effectiveness of the procedure and determine the time until complete fusion, the incidence of delayed union and nonunion, and the prevalence of complications (see Results).

Anatomy

The subtalar joint is composed of three articulations: the posterior, middle, and anterior joints or facets (Figs. 77–1 and 77–2). There are numerous extra-articular ligaments

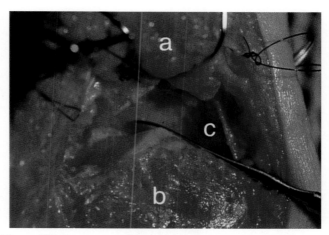

Figure 77–2 Anatomic dissection of lateral posterior subtalar joint: (a) talus, (b) calcaneus, (c) subtalar joint. (From McGinty JB: Ankle arthroscopy. In McGinty JB, Burkhark SS, Jackson RW, et al [eds]: Operative Arthroscopy, 3rd ed. New York, Lippincott Williams & Wilkins, 2002.)

that stabilize the subtalar joint. The major ligaments encountered during subtalar arthroscopy are the intra-articular components, which consist of the interosseous talocalcaneal ligament, the lateral talocalcaneal ligament, and the anterior talocalcaneal ligament (Fig. 77–3). These coalesce to form the division between the posterior and middle facets of the subtalar joint. The interosseous ligament is a broad, stout structure measuring approximately 2.5 cm in breadth from medial to lateral. It is an important landmark and marks the arthroscopic boundary for posterior subtalar arthroscopy.

History

Patients usually complain of lateral hindfoot pain that can easily be confused with ankle pathology. Increased symptoms with weight bearing on uneven ground is a classic complaint. History of a previous calcaneal fracture should immediately alert one to the possibility of subtalar pathology.

Physical Examination

The clinical findings consist of pain over the sinus tarsi and the posterolateral subtalar joint. Patients also report a reproduction of symptoms on inversion and eversion of the subtalar joint with the ankle locked in dorsiflexion.

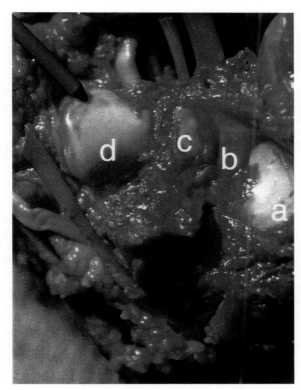

Figure 77–1 Topographic view of a prosected anatomic specimen of the posterior subtalar joint: (a) undersurface of talus, (b) middle facet of talus, (c) anterior facet of talus, (d) superior surface of calcaneus. (From McGinty JB: Ankle arthroscopy. In McGinty JB, Burkhark SS, Jackson RW, et al [eds]: Operative Arthroscopy, 3rd ed. New York, Lippincott Williams & Wilkins, 2002.)

Imaging

On occasion, computed tomography or magnetic resonance imaging may be necessary.[18] There is little need for a bone scan or arthrography.[8]

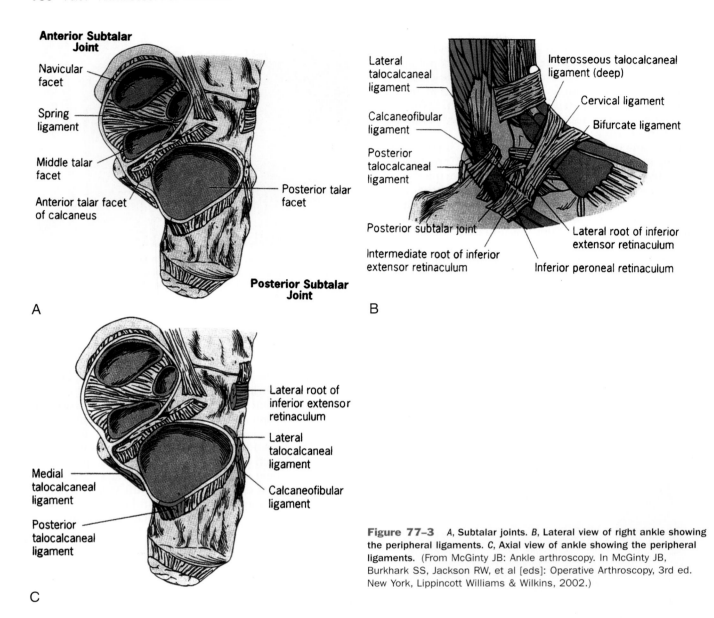

Figure 77–3 *A,* Subtalar joints. *B,* Lateral view of right ankle showing the peripheral ligaments. *C,* Axial view of ankle showing the peripheral ligaments. (From McGinty JB: Ankle arthroscopy. In McGinty JB, Burkhark SS, Jackson RW, et al [eds]: Operative Arthroscopy, 3rd ed. New York, Lippincott Williams & Wilkins, 2002.)

Indications and Contraindications

The indications for arthroscopic subtalar arthrodesis are intractable subtalar pain secondary to rheumatoid arthritis, osteoarthritis, or post-traumatic arthritis. Other indications include neuropathic conditions, gross instability, paralytic conditions, and posterior tibial tendon rupture. Whereas most of the earlier literature on subtalar surgery focused on the stabilization of paralytic deformities secondary to poliomyelitis, the majority of today's patients have post-traumatic and arthritic disorders. A small segment of the population requiring this procedure presents with posterior tibial tendon dysfunction or a talocalcaneal coalition.

Patients must have failed conservative management to qualify for arthroscopic subtalar fusion. Conservative treatment includes a variety of modalities, including orthotics, nonsteroidal anti-inflammatory drugs, activity modification, and occasional cortisone injections into the subtalar joint. Patients must also be apprised that an open procedure may be required should this technique prove to be technically unfeasible.

Contraindications to this procedure are previously failed subtalar fusion, gross malalignment requiring correction, infection, and significant bone loss. The subtalar joint is a relatively tight joint, and access is not always easy. Previous fracture and restricted joint access with concomitant arthrofibrosis may be a relative contraindication to an arthroscopic procedure, particularly if the articular surfaces are malaligned. The presence of internal fixation devices may obscure either the anterior portals or the posterior portal, making an arthroscopic procedure impossible.

On occasion, a patient with moderate malalignment is a candidate for in situ stabilization. Significant bone loss is encountered rarely and has not presented a serious problem in our personal experience with arthroscopic ankle arthrodesis.

Surgical Technique

Positioning, Setup, and Diagnostic Arthroscopy

The technique for subtalar arthroscopy has been described by Parisien[16,17] and Frey et al.[5] The patient is placed in the lateral decubitus position with the legs and hips appropriately padded. The operative procedure is generally done with the aid of an inflated thigh tourniquet. No traction is applied to the extremity, unlike in ankle arthrodesis. The application of a soft tissue distraction device actually obliterates the portal. Only a slight amount of inversion is allowed on the ankle; if extreme inversion is applied, the surrounding soft tissues can obliterate the portals and make the arthroscopic procedure more difficult.

Should an ankle arthroscopy be contemplated at the same time, the subtalar arthroscopy is performed first, because the normal extravasation that occurs with ankle arthroscopy would hinder a subsequent subtalar arthroscopy. A marking pen is used to delineate the fibula, superficial peroneal nerve, and sural nerve. All three portals are marked (Fig. 77–4).

The subtalar joint is preinjected with about 7 mL of saline, being careful not to inject into the subcutaneous tissue. This also reassures the surgeon, if a large-bore needle is used, that he or she has entered the joint and provides an appropriate angle for initial placement of the arthroscopic sheath and trocar.

The anterolateral portal is established first, using a number 11 blade and a nick and spread technique. It is usually located in the region of the sinus tarsi and approximately 1.5 to 2 cm anterior and 1 cm distal to the tip of the lateral malleolus. Only the skin is incised; further dilation and spreading are done with a small mosquito clamp. The 2.7-mm dull trocar and sheath are then placed in the anterior portal. The arthroscope should be located posterior to the interosseous ligament. If better visualization is required initially, an 18-gauge needle can be placed in juxtaposition to this to establish appropriate flow. The posterolateral portal is established next by palpating the soft tissues and establishing the entry site with an 18-gauge needle, using an outside-in technique while visualizing through the anterior portal. This portal is usually located approximately 1 cm proximal and 1 cm posterior to the distal tip of the fibula. Care is taken to avoid the sural nerve and the small saphenous vein when making this portal. The nick and spread technique is used in a vertical fashion to avoid damaging these structures. If a large amount of synovium and scar is encountered in the anterior portal and visualization is impaired, an accessory portal is established (Figs. 77–4 and 77–5), and a small shaver is used to debride this area.

Initially, visualization is obtained through the anterolateral portal, with outflow established in the posterior portal. Later in the case, these portals may be reversed. A pump is employed to control the pressure and avoid excessive extravasation and a potential compartment syndrome. The pressure is usually maintained around 35 mm Hg.

A complete diagnostic subtalar arthroscopy is carried out. Distal to the anterolateral portal is the interosseous talocalcaneal ligaments, and proximal is the talocalcaneal joint (Fig. 77–6). One can now visualize the lateral recess, reflection of the calcaneofibular ligament, lateral talocalcaneal ligament, os trigonum, and lateral process

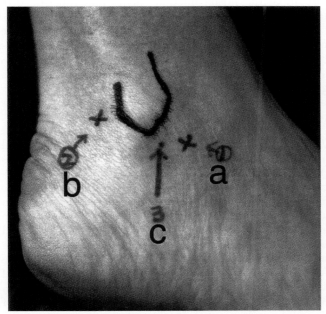

Figure 77–4 Portal sites for subtalar arthrodesis: (a) anterolateral portal, (b) posterolateral portal, (c) accessory lateral portal. (From McGinty JB: Ankle arthroscopy. In McGinty JB, Burkhark SS, Jackson RW, et al [eds]: Operative Arthroscopy, 3rd ed. New York, Lippincott Williams & Wilkins, 2002.)

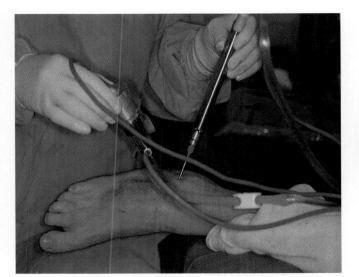

Figure 77–5 Surgical positioning for subtalar arthroscopy with the camera in the anterolateral portal and the shaver in the accessory portal. (Courtesy of C. Frey, MD, October 2002.)

7 Ankle

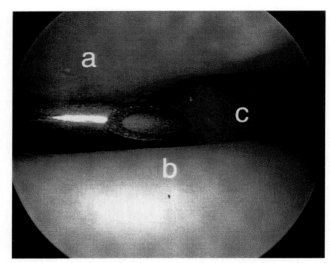

Figure 77–6 Arthroscopic view of a right posterior subtalar joint: (a) talus, (b) calcaneus, (c) posteromedial corner. (From McGinty JB: Ankle arthroscopy. In McGinty JB, Burkhark SS, Jackson RW, et al [eds]: Operative Arthroscopy, 3rd ed. New York, Lippincott Williams & Wilkins, 2002.)

of the talus (Fig. 77–7). Through this portal, one can visualize the posterior compartment but cannot see the anterior and middle facets or the anterior compartment of the subtalar joint. If there is complete disruption of the interosseous ligaments, however, the anterior compartment can be visualized. It is possible to perform arthroscopy in these compartments if a portal is extended through the interosseous ligament going distally.

As with most arthroscopic surgeries, the procedure can be done for diagnostic purposes if there are clinical indications that the disorder is isolated to this joint. Some of the more common indications include synovitis and partial disruption of the interosseous ligament in the sinus tarsi. Other indications include arthrofibrosis, residual post-traumatic scar formation, and unstable chondral or osteochondral lesions. It may also be useful in the treatment of fractures of the lateral process of the talus, loose bodies, subtalar impingement, and subtalar arthrodesis. It can be used in combination with an ankle arthroscopy in the evaluation and treatment of combined ankle and subtalar instability.[4,5,16,17]

Specific Surgical Steps

The anterolateral and posterolateral portals are the two conventional portals. If necessary, an accessory portal may be established approximately 1 cm posterior to the anterolateral portal. This portal can be used for debridement or for outflow enhancement. It can also be used for visualization on occasion. Both the anterolateral and posterolateral portals are used in an alternating fashion during the case for viewing and for instrumentation. Occasionally, significant arthrofibrosis makes entry and visualization difficult; in these cases, the accessory anterolateral portal is useful.

It is important to be certain that the arthroscope is in the subtalar joint and that the ankle joint or the fibular talar recess has not been entered inadvertently. All debridement and decortication are done posterior to the interosseous ligament, because only the posterior facet is fused. The middle and anterior facets are not visualized under normal circumstances unless the interosseous ligament has been torn or resected. The majority of the procedure is done with the arthroscope in the anterolateral portal and the instruments in the posterolateral portal. The final debridement is accomplished by alternating these two portals.

A primary synovectomy and debridement are necessary for visualization, as with other joints. The articular surface is debrided, which makes the joint more capacious and allows easier instrumentation. Complete removal of the articular surface down to subchondral bone is the next phase of the procedure (Fig. 77–8). The talocalcaneal geometry is unique and requires a variety of instruments. In general, multiangular curets and a complete set of burs and shavers will suffice.

Once the articular cartilage has been removed, approximately 1 to 2 mm of subchondral bone is removed to expose the highly vascular cancellous bone. Care must be taken not to alter the geometry and not to remove excessive bone, which would lead to poor coaptation of the joint surfaces. Once the subchondral plate is removed, small "spot-weld" holes measuring approximately 2 mm deep are made on the surface of the calcaneus and talus to create vascular channels (Fig. 77–9). The posteromedial corner must be carefully assessed, because residual bone and cartilage left there can interfere with coaptation. Often the curet safely breaks down this corner and provides the surgeon with additional tactile feedback. The neurovascular bundle is located directly at the posteromedial corner and must be protected at all times.

After the surgeon views from both portals to ensure complete debridement and decortication, the tourniquet is released and the vascularity of the calcaneus and talus is assessed. The joint is then thoroughly irrigated to remove bone fragments and debris. No autogenous bone graft or bone substitute is needed for this procedure.

Fixation of the fusion is done with a large, cannulated 7.3-mm screw. The guide pin is started at the dorsal anteromedial talus and angled posterior and inferior to the posterolateral calcaneus but does not violate the calcaneal cortical surface. Under fluoroscopy, the guidewire is placed with the ankle in maximum dorsiflexion to avoid screw head encroachment or impingement on the anterior lip of the tibia. Once the guidewire is placed under these conditions, the ankle can be relaxed, the screw inserted under fluoroscopic control, and the fusion site compressed. The screw runs along the natural axis of rotation of the subtalar joint using this technique. Starting the screw from the dorsal and medial aspect of the talus avoids painful screw head prominence over the calcaneus and avoids complications or the need for a second procedure (Figs. 77–10 and 77–11).

Steri-Strips are used instead of sutures to allow adequate drainage. A bulky dressing and a short-leg bivalve

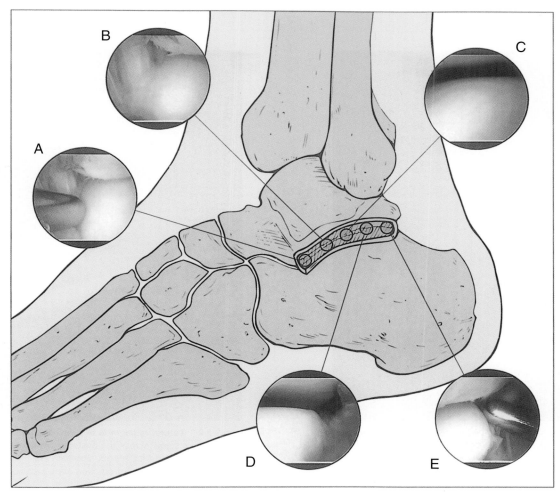

Figure 77-7 Arthroscopic visualization of areas of the posterior subtalar joint in a patient with subtalar instability: **(A)** interosseous ligament area, **(B)** anterior aspect of the joint, **(C)** midaspect of the joint, **(D)** posterior aspect of the joint, **(E)** posterior pouch of the subtalar joint. (From Parisien JS: Arthroscopy of the posterior subtalar joint. In Parisien JS [ed]: Current Techniques in Arthroscopy. New York, Thieme, 1998, pp 161-168. Adapted from Ferkel RD: Subtalar arthroscopy. In Ferkel R [ed]: Arthroscopy Surgery: The Foot and Ankle. Philadelphia, Lippincott-Raven, 1996, pp 231-254.)

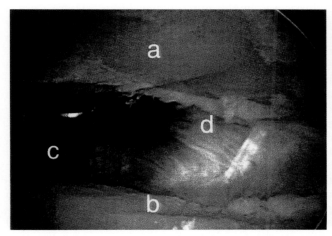

Figure 77-8 Posterior subtalar joint, viewed from the posterolateral portal: (a) talus, (b) calcaneus, (c) sinus tarsi, (d) interosseous ligament. (From McGinty JB: Ankle arthroscopy. In McGinty JB, Burkhark SS, Jackson RW, et al [eds]: Operative Arthroscopy, 3rd ed. New York, Lippincott Williams & Wilkins, 2002.)

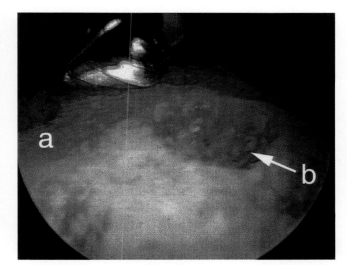

Figure 77-9 Superior surface of calcaneus (a) following removal of articular surface, decortication, and "spot-welding" (b). (From McGinty JB: Ankle arthroscopy. In McGinty JB, Burkhark SS, Jackson RW, et al [eds]: Operative Arthroscopy, 3rd ed. New York, Lippincott Williams & Wilkins, 2002.)

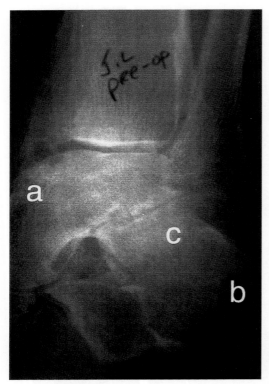

Figure 77–10 Browden view of an arthritic posterior subtalar joint: (a) talus, (b) calcaneus, (c) subtalar joint. (From McGinty JB: Ankle arthroscopy. In McGinty JB, Burkhark SS, Jackson RW, et al [eds]: Operative Arthroscopy, 3rd ed. New York, Lippincott Williams & Wilkins, 2002.)

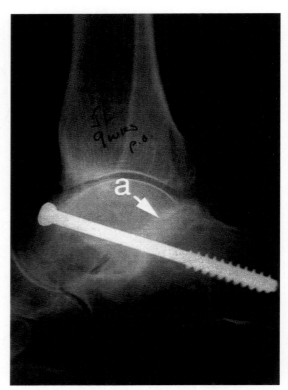

Figure 77–11 Lateral radiograph of a fused subtalar joint (a) with a single cancellous screw across the posterior facet. (From McGinty JB: Ankle arthroscopy. In McGinty JB, Burkhark SS, Jackson RW, et al [eds]: Operative Arthroscopy, 3rd ed. New York, Lippincott Williams & Wilkins, 2002.)

cast are applied. The patient is discharged home after appropriate circulatory checks in the recovery room.

Postoperative Management

The first clinical evaluation takes place in the office within 48 hours. In approximately 1 week, the cast is removed, and the patient is immediately fitted with an ankle-foot orthosis if the swelling is minimal. Full weight bearing is allowed as tolerated any time after surgery, but in general, patients can tolerate full weight bearing without crutch support within 7 to 14 days. Although patients wear the orthosis almost 24 hours a day, they are able to bathe and take the ankle and foot through a range of motion without the brace. It is removed when full union has been achieved. The standard three views of the ankle plus a Browden view are the radiographs of choice for follow-up assessment.

Results

Since September 1992, 25 patients have undergone arthroscopic subtalar fusion with sufficient follow-up time to determine the effectiveness of this procedure. Fusion rate, time until complete union, surgical tech-

nique, and complications were analyzed. One standard surgical procedure was used, and the method of internal fixation was not altered during this series. The posterior subtalar joint was the only joint fused during this procedure. Three of the 25 patients underwent a combined arthroscopic ankle and subtalar fusion. There were 8 patients with osteoarthritis, 10 with post-traumatic arthritis, 4 with posterior tibial tendon dysfunction, 2 with rheumatoid arthritis, and 1 with a talocalcaneal coalition. Each patient had a radiographic evaluation at 2-week intervals to determine the rate and quality of fusion. For an arthrodesis to be considered completely fused, both clinical and radiographic evidence were required. The parameters of a successful arthrodesis were as follows: evidence of bone consolidation across the subtalar joint, no motion or radiolucency at the screw tract, the clinical absence of pain with weight bearing, and pain-free forced inversion and eversion. The average mean follow-up time was 22 months (range, 6 to 92 months). All 25 patients exhibited union both clinically and radiographically; the average time until complete fusion was 8.9 weeks (range, 6 to 16 weeks).

All reported arthroscopic procedures have a lower infection rate compared with open procedures, and one assumes that the same is true of this procedure; however, there have been insufficient cases to validate this hypothesis. Most open series also show a longer time until union, with some prevalence of nonunion. Preliminary observations indicate a more rapid union with arthroscopic subtalar arthrodesis, as well as an increased rate of union; again, however, the series was too small to validate this hypothesis. There is a paucity of literature on isolated open subtalar arthrodesis with adequate follow-up statistics over the last 25 years.

Complications

There have been no reoperations, with the exception of one screw removal. That patient had pain at the posterolateral calcaneus where the screw penetrated the cortex, and the possibility of a stress fracture was entertained. Symptoms resolved after screw removal. Two patients had residual anterolateral pain, with some radiographic and clinical evidence of minor degenerative joint disease in the ankle. These findings had been noted on preoperative films. One patient obtained complete relief from a diagnostic and therapeutic steroid and lidocaine (Xylocaine) injection into the ankle joint. One patient eventually underwent ankle arthrodesis because of preexisting osteoarthritis of the ankle. Valgus tilting of the ankle joint following subtalar arthrodesis has been reported, but it is unclear whether this is secondary to the fusion or merely a natural progression of the disease.[3] Two cases not included in this series could not be completed arthroscopically because of significant malformation of the calcaneus and arthrofibrosis of the subtalar joint. These patients underwent a modified mini-open posterior subtalar arthrodesis. Identical screw fixation and postoperative protocols were used in these two patients. Skin problems about the hindfoot can be catastrophic and are avoided using this technique. There were no superficial or deep infections in this series

Summary

The advantages of arthroscopic subtalar arthrodesis are obvious and quite dramatic, with early weight bearing and ankle-foot orthosis immobilization allowing patients a rapid return to work. Outpatient surgery is a cost-effective benefit. Patient satisfaction and comfort are greatly enhanced, with only oral pain medication required. All patients have tolerated the postoperative regimen and same-day discharge.

Arthroscopic subtalar arthrodesis is a technically demanding procedure that requires advanced arthroscopic skills. Joint access is tight and restricted, requiring small instrumentation. Because deformities cannot be corrected at this stage, this must be considered a fusion in situ. The learning curve is steep owing to the small patient population available for enhancing one's surgical skills.

Overall, this procedure has stood the test of time and follow-up. The results appear to be excellent in terms of patient satisfaction, fusion rate, time until union, and postoperative morbidity. The recognition and enhancement of this technique, as well as the development of more advanced technology, will certainly allow this arthroscopic subtalar arthrodesis technique to mature over time.

References

1. Dick IL: Primary fusion of the posterior subtalar joint and the treatment of fractures of the calcaneus. J Bone Joint Surg Br 35:375, 1953.
2. Ferkel RA: Arthroscopic Surgery: The Foot and Ankle. Philadelphia, Lippincott-Raven, 1996.
3. Fitzgibbons TC: Valgus Tilting of the Ankle Joint Following Subtalar Arthrodesis. Dublin, Ireland, International Society of Foot and Ankle Surgery, 1995.
4. Frey C, Feder S, DiGiovanni D: Arthroscopic evaluation of the subtalar joint: Does sinus tarsi syndrome exist? Foot Ankle Int 20:185, 1999.
5. Frey C, Gasser S, Feder K: Arthroscopy of the subtalar joint. Foot Ankle Int 15:424, 1994.
6. Gallie WE: Subastragalar arthrodesis and fractures of the os calcis. J Bone Joint Surg Am 25:731, 1943.
7. Geckler EO: Comminuted fractures of the os calcis. Arch Surg 61:469, 1943.
8. Goosens M: Posterior subtalar joint arthrography: A useful tool in the diagnosis of hindfoot disorders. Clin Orthop 12:248, 1989.
9. Grice DS: An extra-articular arthrodesis of the subastragalar joint for correction of paralytic flat feet in children. J Bone Joint Surg Am 35:927, 1952.
10. Grice DS: Further experience with extra-articular arthrodesis of the subtalar joint. J Bone Joint Surg Br 42:335, 1960.
11. Gross RH: A clinical study of bachelor subtalar arthrodesis. J Bone Joint Surg Am 58:343, 1976.
12. Hall MC, Pennal GF: Primary subtalar arthrodesis in the treatment of severe fractures of the calcaneus. J Bone Joint Surg Br 42:336, 1960.
13. Harris RI: Fractures of the os calcis. Ann Surg 124:1082, 1946.
14. Mallon WJ, Nunley JA: The Grice procedure, extra-articular subtalar arthrodesis. Orthop Clin North Am 20:649, 1989.
15. Moreland JR, Westin GW: Further experience with Grice subtalar arthrodesis. Clin Orthop 207:113, 1986.
16. Parisien JS (ed): Arthroscopy Surgery. New York, McGraw-Hill, 1988.
17. Parisien JS, Vangsness T: Arthroscopy of the subtalar joint: An experimental approach. Arthroscopy 1:53, 1985.
18. Seltzer SE, Weisman B: CT of the hindfoot with rheumatoid arthritis. J Arthritis Rheumatol 28:12, 1985.
19. Tasto JP: Arthroscopic ankle arthrodesis: A seven year follow up. Paper presented at the annual meeting of the American Academy of Orthopaedic Surgeons, 1997, Rosemont, IL.
20. Thomas FB: Arthrodesis of the subtalar joint. J Bone Joint Surg 2:93, 1967.
21. Wilson PD: Treatment of fractures of the os calcis by arthrodesis of the subtalar joint. JAMA 89:1676, 1927.

7 Ankle

78

Arthroscopy of the First Metatarsophalangeal Joint

MARTIN J. O'MALLEY AND ANDREW J. ELLIOTT

ARTHROSCOPY OF THE FIRST METATARSOPHALANGEAL JOINT IN A NUTSHELL

Indications:
Pain, swelling, mechanical symptoms

Contraindications:
Infection, poor vascular status, severe degenerative joint disease

Anatomic Considerations:
Review anatomy of extensor hallucis longus and abductor hallucis tendons, as well as medial plantar hallucis, dorsomedial cutaneous, and dorsolateral nerves

Portals:
Dorsomedial, dorsolateral, medial

Equipment:
Toe traction setup, 1.9- and 2.7-mm 30-degree scopes, small joint instruments, 2- and 2.7-mm shaver, 2-mm bur, syringe with saline, two 23-gauge needles

Surgical Technique:
Traction applied and joint insufflated from dorsolateral position with 23-gauge needle placed just medial to extensor hallucis longus to ensure free flow; portals established with blunt trocars; inspection of 13 dorsolateral views and 5 medial views; when finished, remove distraction, range joint, and do one final inspection for possible loose material

Postoperative Management:
Compression dressing for 7 days with heel weight bearing; day 10, active and passive motion started; day 14, sutures removed

Results:
73% to 100% good to excellent

Complications:
Nerve or tendon injury; distraction-related injuries and instrument breakage

The arthroscope gives one the ability to inspect and perform procedures in joints without large arthrotomies, allowing earlier motion and ultimately leading to less scarring and fewer wound complications. Improvements in arthroscopic technology have led to excellent image quality through 1.9- and 2.7-mm arthroscopes, allowing their use in small joints such as the ankle and foot. Ankle arthroscopy has become a fairly familiar technique, but subtalar and first metatarsophalangeal joint (MTPJ) arthroscopy is performed less frequently. In the MTPJ, a thorough understanding of the anatomy (normal and pathologic), technique, postoperative rehabilitation, and possible complications is necessary for successful arthroscopic surgery.

Indications and Contraindications

The indications for first MTPJ arthroscopy include pain, swelling, stiffness, locking, or grinding refractory to conservative measures.[4,5,8] Chondromalacia, synovitis, osteochondral lesions, loose bodies, and early hallux rigidus may be treated arthroscopically. Contraindications include infection, poor vascular status, and severe edema. Advanced degenerative joint disease is a relative contraindication, dependent on the surgeon's experience and the preoperatively determined ability to distract the joint. There are no reports of arthroscopically assisted arthrodesis in the literature.

Anatomy

The first MTPJ is a shallow ball-and-socket joint comprising the proximal phalanx and metatarsal head. The metatarsal head also articulates with the medial and lateral sesamoids plantarly. The stout metatarsophalangeal collateral ligaments, metatarsosesamoidal ligaments, and plantar plate provide most of the static stability of the joint. Dynamic stability is effected by the abductor, adductor, flexor brevis, and extensor hallucis brevis tendons. The extensor hallucis brevis tendon blends into the dorsal capsule; the abductor and adductor tendons help support the medial and lateral capsule. The flexor brevis muscle sends a tendinous slip to each sesamoid, the plantar plate, and ultimately the proximal phalanx. The flexor hallucis longus tendon runs between the sesamoids and deep to the plantar plate. Dorsally, the extensor hallucis longus (EHL) tendon forms an important landmark lying in the dorsal midline, and fibers of its sagittal hood add strength to the capsule.

Sensation to the great toe is provided by the medial plantar hallucis nerve, dorsomedial cutaneous nerve (joined by branches of the saphenous nerve at the level of the MTPJ), dorsolateral branch of the deep peroneal nerve, and lateral plantar digital nerve. The first three are at risk of injury from the portals used during first MTPJ arthroscopy. The dorsomedial cutaneous branch is at the greatest risk and lies 2 to 5 mm plantar and medial to the EHL tendon.

Portals

Three portals are used to visualize the first MTPJ: dorsolateral, dorsomedial, and medial (Fig. 78–1). The dorsomedial and dorsolateral portals are placed just medial and lateral to the EHL tendon, just distal to the joint line. The medial portal is placed at the joint line midway between the plantar and dorsal aspects of the joint. The portal is above the abductor hallucis tendon, whereas the

medial plantar hallucis nerve is plantar to the abductor tendon.

Equipment

The following equipment is required:

- Tourniquet (ankle or thigh)
- Wrist arthroscopy traction tower or sterile Chinese finger trap on shoulder holder with counterweight
- 1.9- and 2.7-mm 30-degree arthroscopes
- Small joint instrument set (probe, 2-mm curet, grasper)
- Small joint shaver (2 and 2.7 mm)
- Small hood-protected bur (2 mm)
- 10-mL syringe with normal saline
- Two 23-gauge needles

Surgical Technique

The patient is positioned supine. Ankle block anesthesia is administered, and the foot is exsanguinated with a Martin bandage used as a tourniquet at the level of the ankle over sterile padding.

The toe is distracted with a sterile Chinese finger trap attached to the wrist arthroscopy traction tower (Linvatec; Fig. 78–2) or to the shoulder tower with a counterweight (5 to 10 pounds). The EHL tendon is identified; a 23-gauge needle on the syringe is introduced just lateral to the EHL tendon at the level of the joint and advanced into the joint. The joint is distended with saline, and the second 23-gauge needle is introduced just medial to the EHL tendon. A free flow of fluid indicates that both needles are in the joint. The lateral needle is removed, and a 4-mm skin incision is made with a number 15 blade, followed by blunt dissection with a mosquito clamp to the level of the capsule. A blunt-tipped obturator in a 2-mm cannula is introduced into the joint. The 1.9-mm scope is inserted, and orientation is obtained by visualizing the metatarsal head, the proximal phalanx base, and the outflow needle. By looking dorsomedially with the room lights dimmed, the dorsomedial nerve can be visualized by transillumination and thus avoided when establishing the dorsomedial portal. A needle is used to determine the proper location for the medial portal (see Fig. 78–1A). Inflow can be via the scope cannula or via a cannula placed in one of the other nonutilized portals. Systematic inspection of the joint from the lateral (13 points) and medial (5 points) portals has been advocated by Ferkel[5] and ensures that pathology is not missed (Fig. 78–3).

At the end of the procedure, the joint is irrigated and taken through a range of motion with the distraction off and then placed back into distraction. A final look is performed to make sure that all debris has been flushed out, because motion occasionally dislodges additional material. The portals are closed with nylon sutures, and a bulky compressive dressing is applied for 7 days to allow resynovialization of the joint and decrease the chance of a synovial fistula.

7 Ankle

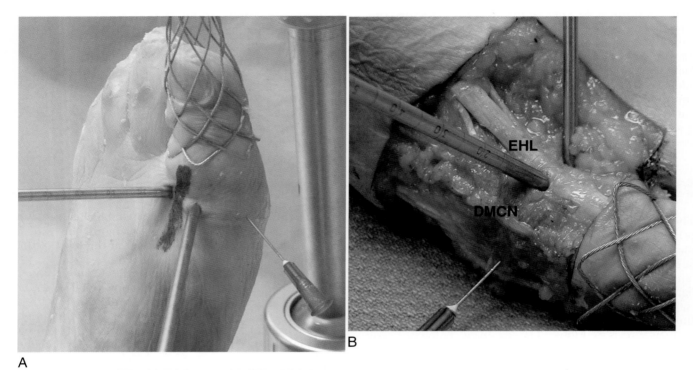

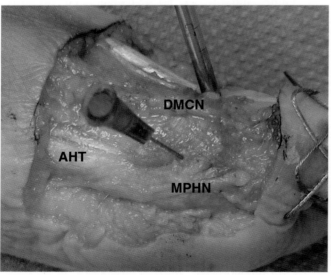

Figure 78–1 *A,* Cannulas are in the dorsomedial and dorsolateral portals on either side of the extensor hallucis longus (EHL; *dark line*), and a needle is in the proposed medial portal. *B,* Dissected specimen showing dorsolateral and dorsomedial portals, proposed medial portal (needle), EHL tendon, and dorsomedial cutaneous nerve (DMCN). *C,* Dissected specimen showing proposed medial portal (needle), abductor hallucis tendon (AHT), and medial plantar hallucis nerve (MPHN).

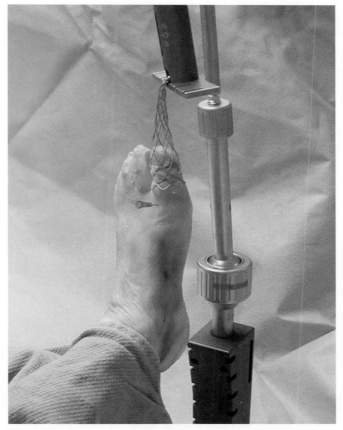

Figure 78–2   Great toe with gravity distraction in finger trap of wrist arthroscopy traction tower.

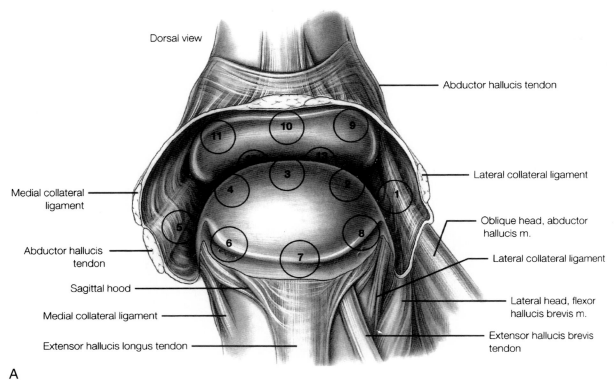

Dorsal view

Abductor hallucis tendon

Lateral collateral ligament

Medial collateral ligament

Oblique head, abductor hallucis m.

Lateral collateral ligament

Abductor hallucis tendon

Sagittal hood

Medial collateral ligament

Extensor hallucis longus tendon

Lateral head, flexor hallucis brevis m.

Extensor hallucis brevis tendon

A

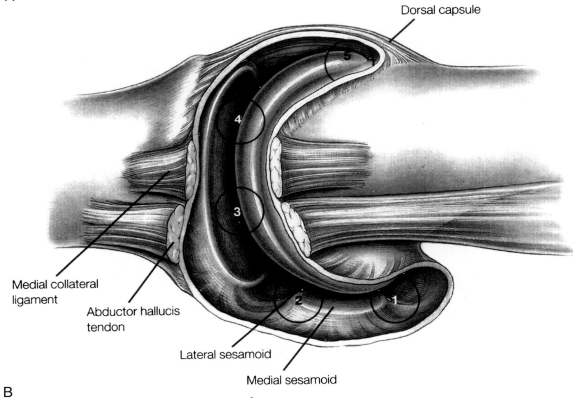

Dorsal capsule

Medial collateral ligament

Abductor hallucis tendon

Lateral sesamoid

Medial sesamoid

B

Figure 78–3 *A*, Thirteen-point examination via dorsolateral portal: (1) lateral gutter, (2) lateral corner of metatarsal head, (3) central portion of metatarsal, (4) medial corner of metatarsal head, (5) medial gutter, (6) medial capsular reflection, (7) central bare area, (8) lateral capsular reflection, (9) medial portion of proximal phalanx, (10) central portion of proximal phalanx, (11) lateral portion of proximal phalanx, (12) medial sesamoid, (13) lateral sesamoid. *B*, Five-point examination via medial portal: (1) posterior plantar capsule, (2) medial and lateral sesamoids, (3) central metatarsal head, (4) superior metatarsal head, (5) dorsal capsular structures.

Table 78-1

Results of First Metatarsophalangeal Joint Arthroscopy

	Ferkel[5]	Davies & Saxby[3]
Cases (no. of patients)	22 (22)	12 (11)
Male (M)–female (F)	7 M, 15 F	7 M, 4 F
Age (yr)	18-70 (mean, 40)	15-58 (mean, 30)
Mean duration of symptoms (mo)	37	8
Prior surgery (no. of patients)	9	1
Mean follow-up (mo)	54 (range, 13-70)	19.3 (range, 6-62)
Outcome		
Good	73%	11 patients
Fair	13.5% (all DJD)	0
Poor	13.5% (all DJD)	0
Complications	0	1 (superficial wound infection)
Eventual arthrodesis	6	0
Mini-arthrotomy at time of surgery	0	3
Diagnosis at surgery		
DJD	5	1
Arthrofibrosis	4	0
Synovitis	3	2
Osteophytes	3	0
Osteochondral lesion	3	3
Loose bodies	2	1
Chondromalacia	2	1
Proximal phalangeal cyst	0	1
Meniscoid lesion	0	0
Chondral lesion	0	1
PVNS	0	1

DJD, degenerative joint disease; PVNS, pigmented villonodular synovitis.

Postoperative Management

The patient is allowed to ambulate in a postoperative shoe with heel weight bearing. At 10 days, the patient is allowed to begin active and passive range of motion as tolerated. The sutures are left in until day 14. The patient progresses into regular shoes as the pain and swelling allow.

Results

There has been a handful of papers describing the technique and indications[4,5,7-9] and case reports[1,2] of first MTPJ arthroscopy. There are only two series with clinical results in the orthopedic literature.[3,5] The results of both are listed for comparison in Table 78–1.

Complications

Complications can arise with any surgery; however, there have been no direct reports of complications of first MTPJ arthroscopy in the literature. Ferkel et al.[6] extensively reviewed the complications of arthroscopy of the foot and ankle without mentioning actual complications

of first MTPJ arthroscopy. Possible complications include the following:

- Wrong extremity
- Tourniquet complications
- Neurovascular (dorsomedial or lateral hallucis nerve) injury
- Tendon (EHL, extensor hallucis brevis, abductor hallucis) injury
- Ligament injury
- Wound complications
- Infection
- Articular cartilage damage
- Hemarthrosis
- Effusion
- Chronic regional pain syndrome
- Distraction-related (neurovascular or skin necrosis) complications
- Instrument breakage

Future Directions

With meticulous attention to detail and a thorough understanding of the intra- and extra-articular anatomy, arthroscopy of the first MTPJ is a useful diagnostic and therapeutic procedure. As surgeons become familiar

7 Ankle

with the procedure and durable small joint equipment is developed, more result-based series will be published, and new applications will be added. Arthrodesis of the first MTPJ has been mentioned in other reviews but has yet to be performed. With advances in cartilage repair, it may become feasible to repair osteochondral lesions of the metatarsal head with arthroscopic assistance.

References

1. Bartlett DH: Arthroscopic management of osteochondritis of the first metatarsal head. Arthroscopy 4:51-54, 1998.
2. Borton DC, Peereboom J, Saxby TS: Pigmented villonodular synovitis in the first metatarsophalangeal joint: Arthoscopic treatment of an unusual condition. Foot Ankle Int 18:505-506, 1997.
3. Davies MS, Saxby TS: Arthroscopy of the first metatarsophalangeal joint. J Bone Joint Surg Br 81:203-206, 1999.
4. Davies MS, Saxby TS: Arthroscopy of the hallux metatarsophalangeal joint. Foot Ankle Clin 5:715-724, 2000.
5. Ferkel RD: Arthroscopic Surgery: The Foot and Ankle. Philadelphia, Lippencott-Raven, 1996, pp 255-272.
6. Ferkel RD, Small HN, Gittins JE: Complications in foot and ankle arthroscopy. Clin Orthop 391:89-104, 2001.
7. Ferkel RD, Van Buecken K: Great toe arthroscopy: Indications, technique and results. Paper presented at a meeting of the Arthroscopy Association of North America, Apr 1991, San Diego, CA.
8. Frey C, Niek van Dijk C: Arthroscopy of the great toe. Instr Course Lect 41:343-346, 1999.
9. Watanabe M, Ito K, Fuji S: Equipment and procedures of small joint arthroscopy. In Watanabe M (ed): Arthroscopy of Small Joints. Tokyo, Igaku-Shoin, 1986, p 3.

PART

8

ARTHROSCOPY OF THE SPINE

79

Posterior Endoscopic Lumbar Surgery

FRANCIS H. SHEN AND D. GREG ANDERSON

POSTERIOR ENDOSCOPIC LUMBAR SURGERY IN A NUTSHELL

History, Physical Examination, and Imaging:
Variable, related to the location and nature of the lesion

Indications:
Excision of a symptomatic herniated disk, particularly a far lateral disk; decompression for spinal stenosis

Advantages:
Less muscle dissection and lower potential for destabilizing the spine; direct visualization and access to spinal pathology

Anatomy:
Understanding the concept of the triangular working space is crucial to safe and accurate posterior endoscopic procedures; the triangular working space is surrounded superiorly by the exiting spinal nerve root, medially by the superior articular process, and inferiorly by the end plate of the inferior vertebra

Approaches:
Posterolateral, paramedian, midline (direct posterior), transforaminal

Surgical Technique:
If the patient history, examination, and imaging are consistent with a single-root unilateral lesion, a uniportal technique is often sufficient; large central or paramedian disk herniations may require a biportal technique
Tubular lumbar microdiskectomy techniques combine minimally invasive muscle-splitting approaches with conventional microdiskectomy techniques

Complications:
Uncommon, but can include infection, postdecompression instability, dural leak, recurrent herniation, and nerve root injury

---

Patients who would benefit from posterior endoscopic lumbar techniques are similar to those who would benefit from open posterior lumbar spine procedures.[1,3,8,10,12-14,26,31,50,56,60] Patient identification and selection are therefore the same for either type of procedure. Currently, the main indications for posterior endoscopic lumbar surgery are excision of a symptomatic herniated disk,[5,15,22,51] particularly the "far lateral" disk,[1,7,11-15,37] and decompression for lateral recess and spinal stenosis.[30,41,50]

Traditionally, posterior surgical management of these disorders required open procedures, resulting in extensive muscle dissection and potential destabilization of the spine.[8,18,19,21,25,29,44] Endoscopic procedures minimize paraspinal muscle stripping and trauma while allowing direct visualization and access to spinal pathology.[1,8,12-14,26,56] By minimizing the resection of normal stabilizing structures, endoscopic techniques can reduce the risk of creating spinal instability.[1,7,11-15,37,51]

Background

Posterior endoscopic diskectomy is different from microdiskectomy, in that endoscopic techniques approach the pathology from outside the spinal canal.[10,13,14,32] Microdiskectomy, which refers to disk excision with the aid of either a surgical microscope or loupe magnification through a small "open" incision, has been performed for decades. Endoscopic diskectomy is performed with the aid of an endoscope and uses an incision just large enough to allow its insertion; the operation is monitored by viewing a video screen.[30,34]

One of the first descriptions of the percutaneous posterolateral approach to the spine, for a vertebral body biopsy, was published in 1956.[6] By 1983, an arthroscopic technique for posterior and posterolateral disk removal through an intradiskal approach had been described by Kambin,[31] who is credited with popularizing the posterior endoscopic technique in the United States.

History

Currently, posterior endoscopic procedures are best used to treat symptomatic herniated disks (especially far lateral disks) and spinal stenosis. A careful history should help differentiate these diagnoses from other causes of back pain (Table 79–1). The surgeon should determine whether the pain is predominantly low back, with referred leg pain, or true radicular pain; the latter is most amenable to decompressive surgery.

Radicular pain secondary to a symptomatic disk herniation is typically described as a well-defined stabbing or

Table 79–1

Causes of Radicular Leg Pain and Segmental Sensory Disturbances: An Anatomic Classification

Myelogenic

Spinal cord tumor
  Ependymoma
  Astrocytoma
  Hemangioblastoma
Multiple sclerosis

Root

Spondylogenic
  Prolapsed disk
  Spinal stenosis
  Foraminal stenosis, lateral recess syndrome
  Spondyloarthropathies
  Achondroplasia
Metabolic
  Paget disease
  Osteoporosis
  Extramedullary hematopoiesis
Bone lesions
  Chordoma
  Chondrosarcoma
  Aneurysmal bone cyst
  Osteoma
  Osteogenic sarcoma
  Eosinophilic granuloma
  Other bone tumors
  Sacral cyst
Infectious
  Osteomyelitis
  Diskitis
Pyogenic
Nonpyogenic (tuberculous, fungal)
Nonbony tumors
  Neurofibroma, schwannoma
  Meningioma
  Ependymoma
  Lipoma
  Metastasis (breast, lung, thyroid, prostate, renal cell, multiple myeloma)

Infection, inflammation
  Herpes
  Syphilis
  Arachnoiditis
Trauma
  Fracture-dislocation
  Epidural hematoma
Miscellaneous
  Subarachnoid hemorrhage
  Aneurysm
  Perineural root cyst
  Extradural meningeal root cyst

Plexus

Abdominal tumor
Endometriosis
Appendiceal abscess, retroperitoneal infection
Retroperitoneal hematoma
Pelvic fracture

Peripheral

Diabetes mellitus
Trauma
  Intramuscular injection
  Posterior dislocated femur
  Inferior gluteal artery aneurysm
Entrapment
  Meralgia paresthetica
  Obturator syndrome
  Piriformis syndrome
  Common peroneal palsy
  Tarsal tunnel syndrome
Wartenberg neuritis
Tumor

Miscellaneous

Primary sciatica

From Wisneski RJ, Garfin SR, Rothman RH, Lutz GE: Lumbar disc disease. In Herkowitz HN, Garfin SR, Balderston RA, et al (eds): Rothman-Simeone The Spine, 4th ed. Philadelphia, WB Saunders, 1999, p 621.

shooting pain in the back or buttocks that radiates into the lower extremity, extending below the knee following a specific dermatomal distribution.[5,11,24,49,52] Activities that increase intradiskal pressure, such as bending, lifting, straining, or sneezing, are noted to aggravate the pain; activities that relieve intradiskal pressure, such as recumbency, decrease the pain. Far lateral disk herniations reportedly constitute approximately 0.7% to 12% of all lumbar herniations.[1,11,12,37] Generally, they involve the more proximal lumbar levels, with involvement of L3-4 and L4-5 in up to 60% of cases.[7,11] These patients often complain of radicular symptoms following the distribution of the femoral nerve.

The surgeon should also look for signs and symptoms of spinal stenosis. These patients typically present in the seventh decade of life (compared with the fifth decade for patients with herniated disks) and complain of insidious back, buttock, and thigh pain.[47,50,52,58] This pain is generally worse when standing or walking and improves with hip and spine flexion, which functionally increases the size of the lumbar canal. Care must be taken to differentiate these complaints from hip pathology and vascular claudication.[58]

Physical Examination

It is important to correlate the physical examination with the patient history. Symptoms referable to spinal stenosis or disk herniation should be elicited. In the case of a herniated disk, a careful reflex, sensory, and motor examination can help localize the involved lumbar level.[13,26,52] Typically, the herniated disk compresses the traversing nerve root while sparing the more proximal exiting nerve root. Therefore, in an L4-5 posterolateral disk herniation, the traversing L5 nerve root is compressed, and the L4 root is spared. However, in the case of an L4-5 far lateral disk herniation, the proximally exiting L4 nerve root is compressed and symptomatic. Maneuvers that place tension on the nerve root (straight leg raise) can aggravate or reproduce leg symptoms in patients with intervertebral disk herniation, and in those with proximal lumbar root compression (L1, L2, L3), the femoral tension sign may also be positive.

The physical examination is often less revealing in patients with spinal stenosis.[7,50,52,58] They generally have an absence of specific nerve root signs, and passive nerve stretch tests may be negative. Sensory changes may be minimal or nondermatomal. These patients, however, often demonstrate flattening of the lumbar lordosis and decreased range on forward flexion. Provocative testing by vigorous ambulation or stair climbing may help expose mild lower extremity weakness.[52,54,58]

Imaging

Although there has been debate about the relationship between radiographic evidence of arthritis and back pain,[16,17,23,24,36] plain radiographs should be obtained before surgery and evaluated for degenerative disk changes,[16,53] facet hypertrophy,[16] spondylolisthesis,[23,53] degenerative scoliosis, and coexisting spinal instability.[43] Decreased interpedicular distance on anteroposterior or lateral radiographs can be suggestive of spinal stenosis. Flexion, extension, and oblique radiographs are obtained on an individual basis as needed.

A symptomatic herniated disk is frequently suspected based on history and physical examination alone, but this should be confirmed with an advanced imaging study. Myelography, computed tomography (CT), or magnetic resonance imaging (MRI) may corroborate the diagnosis and help with preoperative planning.[2,9,16,20,28,35,38]

Myelography with a postmyelographic CT scan is helpful to confirm nerve root compression due to disk herniation or bony stenosis.[8,22,51] Myelography and CT-myelography, however, can miss pathology from a far lateral disk herniation,[26,28] due to the fact that the subarachnoid space extends only along the proximal nerve root sleeve and ends in the neural foramen, proximal to the site of far lateral herniation.[37]

In most cases of lumbar pathology, MRI is now the imaging modality of choice. Unlike myelography, MRI is noninvasive and can provide significant information about both bony and soft tissue structures. MRI provides details about the quality of the disk, size of the canal, presence of lateral recess stenosis, and presence or absence of a far lateral disk.[4,5,9,38,42] It is important to correlate imaging findings with the patient's history and physical examination, because up to 30% of patients can have asymptomatic degenerative lumbar changes on MRI.[4,27,38,42,59]

CT, though not as accurate as MRI with regard to soft tissue structures, can provide excellent information about the bony architecture of the spine (e.g., bony compression from facet joint hypertrophy).[2,20]

Indications

At this time, the main indications for posterior endoscopic lumbar surgery are excision of a symptomatic herniated disk and decompression for spinal stenosis.

With traditional techniques, the surgical management of a symptomatic far lateral disk can be challenging. Midline,[11] direct intermuscular, and extraforaminal approaches have been described,[7,52,57] as well as combined medial and lateral approaches to the neuroforamen.[1,11] Unfortunately, these open procedures require extensive muscle dissection and risk destabilizing the spine.

With a posterior endoscopic technique, soft tissue trauma and stripping of the paraspinal musculature are avoided, but direct visualization and access to the spinal pathology can still be achieved. By treating only the offending disk, partial facet removal is not required, in contrast to open techniques. Excessive facet resection can lead to spinal instability. Iatrogenic spondylolisthesis complicates approximately 2% of decompressions for spinal stenosis[21,44,47,48,55,57] and may lead to recurrent back and leg pain. By avoiding facet resection, endoscopic techniques allow the removal of only the offending pathology and avoid the unnecessary removal of stabilizing structures to achieve exposure. Depending on the technique employed, the disk capsule and facet hypertrophy can be directly visualized and addressed with an endoscopic approach.

Surgical Technique

Positioning

The patient is positioned prone, with the abdomen free and the spine flexed to aid in intraoperative exposure of the interlaminar space. The table and frame should be compatible with lateral fluoroscopy. Fluoroscopy images should be obtained before preparation and draping to ensure that the site of pathology can be visualized.

Diagnostic Endoscopy

Triangular Working Zone

The operation begins by placing a needle in the "triangular working zone." Understanding the anatomy of this zone is critical for the safe and accurate execution of posterior endoscopic procedures.[31] Defined by Kambin and Gellman,[31] the triangular working zone is bordered superiorly by the exiting spinal nerve root, medially by the proximal articular process (and dural sac), and inferiorly by the end plate of the inferior vertebra (Fig. 79–1).

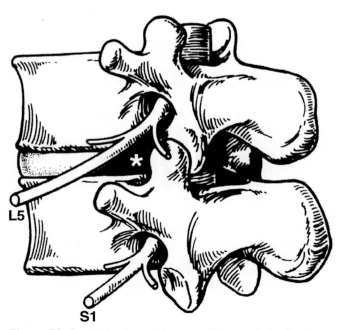

Figure 79–1 Triangular working zone. This zone is bordered superiorly by the exiting spinal nerve root, medially by the superior articular process, and inferiorly by the end plate of the inferior vertebra. (From Schaffer JL, Kambin P: Alternative forms of disk excision: Minimally invasive spine surgery. In Herkowitz HN, Garfin SR, Balderston RA, et al [eds]: Rothman-Simeone The Spine, 4th ed. Philadelphia, WB Saunders, 1999, p 729.)

Studies have demonstrated that cannulas up to 6.5 mm in diameter can be inserted safely into this zone.[31,49]

The vertebromedullary branches of the segmental arteries and the sinuvertebral nerve are superior to the triangular working zone and are usually not at risk. However, several venous structures can often be seen arthroscopically crossing the working zone and should be avoided or coagulated.[46]

Posterolateral Portal

The posterolateral approach is the classic endoscopic approach.[30,31,49] It allows access to the annulus, disk, lateral recess, foramen, and far lateral spine. The skin incision for the portal is located approximately 8 to 12 cm from the midline, and the path for the instruments is established with a needle. Once the location is confirmed with fluoroscopy, the cannula is placed within the triangular working zone.

This portal is by far the major entry site for most posterior endoscopic lumbar procedures. Other portals have been described and may be useful in special circumstances.

Paramedian Portal

The paramedian portal is typically a supplement to the posterolateral portal.[13,50] It serves as an accessory channel to the triangular working zone and allows access to the lateral recess. The skin incision is made on the contralateral side from the posterolateral portal, approximately 1 cm from the midline. The needle is inserted through the interspinous ligament and ligamenta flava, just medial to the inferior articulating facet.

Midline (Direct Posterior) Portal

The midline portal establishes entry into the posterior or lateral epidural space and provides access to the central and paracentral portions of the intervertebral disk.[30,37,50] By advancing the endoscope into the lateral recess from this portal, pathology directly under the pars can be addressed.

Transforaminal Approach

With the advent of smaller and more flexible endoscopes, transforaminal approaches have been described.[10] These endoscopes can be passed into or through the neuroforamen and provide access not only to epidural and intradiskal lesions but also to pathology from the axilla of the nerve root to the lateral pedicle. This allows for the management of both contained and uncontained disks.

Specific Lumbar Pathology

Endoscopic Posterolateral Diskectomy

Uniportal Technique

This technique is best used when the patient history and physical examination are consistent with a single root lesion and imaging studies confirm a paramedian, foraminal, or extraforaminal disk herniation.[1,7,30,50] In these cases of unilateral pathology, a single-portal technique is usually sufficient.

The patient is positioned prone on a well-padded radiolucent table. The table is flexed to help separate the spinous processes and increase the disk space. On the symptomatic side, a mark is made approximately 8 to 12 cm from the midline at the level of the involved disk.

If the surgeon is experienced and familiar with the endoscopic appearance of the periannular structures, either regional or general anesthesia can be considered. However, the uniportal technique can often be performed with the patient under local anesthesia. A skin wheal is raised, and local anesthesia is infiltrated down through the muscle layers to the fascia. Do not anesthetize the nerve root, because this may increase the likelihood of nerve injury during endoscope passage.[30,40,49,50]

Under fluoroscopic guidance, insert a spinal needle into the annular fibers parallel to the vertebral end plate (Fig. 79–2). Correct needle position is crucial to the success of this procedure, because the remaining instruments will follow the path of the spinal needle. Attempt to place the needle in the midportion or slightly medial to the middle of the triangular working zone, and penetrate the annulus in this region.

Remove the stylet and introduce a guidewire through the needle into the disk. Leave the guidewire in place and remove the needle. Insert a dilator over the guidewire and advance it to the annulus. Finally, insert a cannula over the dilator and dock the cannula with the disk.

While holding the cannula firmly against the annulus, remove the wire and dilator and insert the arthroscope with an attached irrigation sheath. Connect the cannula

to suction, and inspect the triangular working zone under direct vision to ensure that the entry site into the disk is devoid of neural and vascular tissue. Periannular veins should be avoided or coagulated under direct endoscopic vision to prevent bleeding. Resection of small marginal osteophytes from the vertebral end plates may be necessary to allow passage into the disk. Once the triangular working zone is cleared, a trephine can be used to create a hole into the disk. The trephine is removed, and the cannula and endoscope are advanced into the disk.

Within the disk, the herniated material is removed under direct endoscopic control using a combination of instruments, including forceps, punches, shavers, and resection burs. Various angled endoscopes (0-, 20-, and 70-degree) are available and can assist with visualization. In addition, articulated instruments optimize intradiskal work. At the conclusion of the procedure, the surrounding neural structures are inspected and carefully probed to ensure that a complete decompression has been performed.

Biportal Technique

In the case of large central or paramedian herniations, failures have been reported with a uniportal technique.[32] In these cases, a biportal approach using two cannulas, inserted into the intervertebral disk posterolaterally from both the right and left sides, can improve access to the pathology. This allows for triangulation of the pathology and continuous visualization during extraction of the herniated fragment. It also facilitates proper fluid management and improves depth perception. However, a biportal technique is generally more time-consuming.

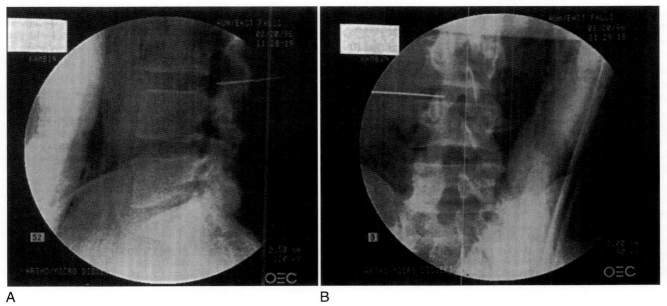

A   B

Figure 79–2 *A* and *B*, **Intraoperative fluoroscopic images demonstrating proper needle position in both the anteroposterior and lateral projections.** (From Schaffer JL, Kambin P: Alternative forms of disk excision: Minimally invasive spine surgery. In Herkowitz HN, Garfin SR, Balderston RA, et al [eds]: Rothman-Simeone The Spine, 4th ed. Philadelphia, WB Saunders, 1999, p 730.)

8 Spine

Begin the procedure by placing both the right and left spinal needles in the midportion of their respective triangular working zones. Confirm the position of both needles radiographically, and establish the working cannulas as described earlier. Two straight punch forceps can be used to develop a communication between the two portals if necessary.

Using intradiskal triangulation techniques, proceed with the diskectomy in a fashion similar to the uniportal technique. Owing to the close proximity of the dura, tears can occur. Therefore, excision of disk fragments should be performed only under direct visualization, with fluoroscopy used as needed to confirm instrument position.

Tubular Lumbar Microdiskectomy

Although somewhat different from traditional endoscopic techniques, tubular techniques have become popular and combine the advantages of both open and minimally invasive surgery.[13,14] These systems use a tubular retractor placed through a small incision centered over the lumbar pathology. By using a muscle-splitting approach and sequential dilators, a working channel is established with minimal soft tissue trauma. This working channel allows for the passage of instruments and the use of either an endoscope or microscope for visualization of the lumbar pathology.

The patient is positioned prone and is prepared and draped in the usual manner. Using a spinal needle, the disk level is located and confirmed with lateral fluoroscopy. A vertical incision, just large enough to fit the tubular retractor, is made at the puncture site.

Sequential dilators are then introduced to the level of the spine under fluoroscopic control. The usual docking site is the inferior aspect of the superior lamina, which is confirmed with fluoroscopic images. Care should be taken to avoid penetration of the ligamenta flava so that inadvertent dural tears and nerve root injuries can be avoided.

The tip of the dilator can be used to dissect soft tissue from the lamina. By adjusting the position of the dilator beneath the skin, different areas of the spine can be reached. This technique is known as "wanding."[13]

Once the dilators are placed, the tubular retractor is applied over the largest dilator. This retractor can be secured to the table to help maintain its position, and the dilators are removed. The final position should be confirmed by fluoroscopy.

By removing soft tissue, the inferior edge of the lamina is easily visualized, and the endoscope can be placed to assist with lighting and visualization. A hemilaminotomy or medial facetotomy can now be performed through this tubular corridor. The amount of decompression performed is based on the patient's pathology.

The ultimate technique is similar to traditional open disk surgery. If a diskectomy is being performed, resect the ligamenta flava with a Kerrison punch and identify the dura. Retract the traversing nerve root medially.

Identify the disk herniation, and perform an annulotomy and diskectomy using traditional instruments.[52]

Hemostasis can be achieved with a combination of cotton patties and bipolar forceps. When the tubular retractor is removed, the muscle tends to close around the retractor path, eliminating dead space. Skin closure is performed using standard techniques.

If contralateral exposure is required, the tubular retractor can be moved medially, and the spinous process and contralateral lamina can be removed sequentially. Alternatively, a separate incision from the opposite side can be used.

Pearls and Pitfalls

Table 79–2 lists the pearls and pitfalls of posterior endoscopic lumbar surgery.

Postoperative Management

Postoperative management is tailored to the patient and the procedure performed. In the majority of cases in which a simple diskectomy and decompression were performed, ambulation is allowed and encouraged on the day of surgery. Most procedures are performed on an outpatient basis. Symptomatic care, including anti-inflammatory drugs, ice, and analgesics, is provided as necessary.

Patient follow-up generally occurs 7 to 10 days after surgery, when the dressing is removed. Patients are allowed to return to work as tolerated (typically by the second week), but heavy labor and contact sports are restricted for 3 months. Physical therapy may be used on an individualized basis.

Table 79–2 Pearls and Pitfalls of Posterior Endoscopic Lumbar Surgery

Fluoroscopic confirmation of correct needle placement at the start of the case is crucial to success, because the remaining instruments follow the path of the needle

Fluoroscopic monitoring of the dilator and cannula is advised for surgeons unfamiliar with endoscopic procedures

Understanding the concept of the "triangular working zone" is crucial to safe and accurate procedures

The bony landmarks (medial and inferior border) of the triangular working zone are often easier to identify than is the superior border, which is defined by the exiting nerve root; this nerve typically travels at a 40-degree angle laterally, anteriorly, and inferiorly in relationship to the foramen from which it exits

If visualization of the spinal nerve is required, it should be undertaken after the herniated disk is resected

In the biportal technique, establish the position of both needles before inserting the cannula; this decreases the chance of the contralateral cannula obscuring the exact position of the needle tip during lateral fluoroscopy

Use of a 70-degree endoscope may improve visualization within the disk space

Complications

Complications after posterior endoscopic surgery are uncommon. Careful patient selection and surgical technique are imperative to a good outcome. The surgeon should possess a thorough understanding of the endoscopic anatomy and be aware of the limitations of each technique.

Compared with open procedures, the incidence of infection is lower with posterior endoscopic procedures.[30,49,50] However, to avoid the morbidity associated with diskitis or vertebral osteomyelitis, prophylactic antibiotics are typically used.[45,49,50]

Although not yet reported, large vessel injury is possible. Particular care should be exercised to avoid leaving the disk space when performing L5-S1 diskectomies using endoscopic techniques.[30] Instruments passed inadvertently through the anterior annulus can enter the abdominal cavity and cause iatrogenic iliac artery and vein injury. Although vascular injuries to large vessels are rare, postoperative hematomas from venous bleeding have been reported.[33] Careful intraoperative hemostasis, routine visualization of the periannular vessels, and a layered closure should be used to minimize bleeding-related complications.

The risk of nerve root injury during posterior endoscopic procedures can be reduced through several measures. First, the surgeon should have a thorough understanding of the triangular working zone and endoscopic anatomy. Second, adequate intraoperative visualization of the annulus is necessary before proceeding with the diskectomy and decompression. Third, consideration should be given to the use of local anesthesia so that the patient can alert the surgeon to nerve contact.[13,14,31,32]

Instability after decompression is a known risk of spinal surgery.[21,25,29,39,48] During open procedures, this is more likely to occur during decompression of far lateral herniations through a midline approach.[13] Depending on the location of the herniated fragment, attempts to expose this fragment from the midline require varying degrees of resection of the pars and facet, with resulting instability. Properly and carefully performed endoscopic procedures minimize this risk by using posterolateral or combined medial lateral or transforaminal portals to obtain direct visualization of and access to these fragments.[13,30,52]

Summary

In properly selected patients, posterior endoscopic techniques have decreased the need for extensive muscle dissection. Simultaneously, visualization of lumbar pathology has been maintained and in some instances enhanced. Appropriate patient selection, careful preoperative planning, and a thorough understanding of the endoscopic anatomy will improve outcome and decrease complications.

References

1. Abdullah AF, Wobler PGH, Warfield JR, et al: Surgical management of extreme lateral lumbar disc herniations: Review of 138 cases. Neurosurgery 22:648-653, 1988.
2. Bell GR, Modic MT: Radiology of the lumbar spine. In Herkowitz HN, Garfin SR, Balderston RA, et al (eds): Rothman-Simeone The Spine, 4th ed. Philadelphia, WB Saunders, 1999, pp 109-134.
3. Blumenthal SL, Baker J, Dossett A, Selby DK: The role of anterior lumbar fusion for internal disc disruption. Spine 13:566-569, 1988.
4. Boden SD, Davis DO, Dina TS, et al: Abnormal magnetic resonance scans of the lumbar spine in asymptomatic subjects. J Bone Joint Surg Am 72:403-408, 1990.
5. Bozzao A, Gallucci M, Masciocchi C, et al: Lumbar disc herniation: MR imaging assessment of natural history in patients treated without surgery. Radiology 185:135-141, 1992.
6. Craig F: Vertebral body biopsy. J Bone Joint Surg 38:93, 1956.
7. Darden BV II, Wade JF, Alexander R, et al: Far lateral disc herniations treated by microscopic fragment excision: Techniques and results. Spine 20:1500-1515, 1995.
8. Deckler R, Hamburger C, Schmiedek P, et al: Surgical observations in extremely lateral lumbar disc herniation. Neurosurg Rev 15:255-258, 1992.
9. deRoos A, Kressel H, Spritzer C, Dalinka M: MR imaging of marrow changes adjacent to end plates in degenerative lumbar disk disease. AJR Am J Roentgenol 149:531-534, 1987.
10. Ditsworth DA: Endoscopic transforaminal lumbar discectomy and reconfiguration: A posterolateral approach into the spinal canal. Surg Neurol 49:488-498, 1998.
11. Epstein NE: Evaluation of varied surgical approaches used in the management of 170 far lateral lumbar disc herniations: Indications and results. J Neurosurg 83:648-656, 1995.
12. Epstein NE, Epstein JA, Carras R, et al: Far lateral lumbar disc herniations and associated structural abnormalities: An evaluation in 60 patients of the comparative value of CT, MRI, and myelo-CT in diagnosis and management. Spine 15:534-539, 1990.
13. Foley KT, Smith MM: Microendoscopic discectomy. Tech Neurosurg 3:301-307, 1997.
14. Foley KT, Smith MM, Rampersaud YR: Microendoscopic approach to far-lateral lumbar disc herniation. Neurosurg Focus 7:article 5, 1999.
15. Frank E: Endoscopically assisted open removal of laterally herniated lumbar discs. Surg Neurol 48:430-434, 1997.
16. Frymoyer JW, Newberg A, Pope MH, et al: Spine radiographs in patients with low-back pain. J Bone Joint Surg Am 66:1048-1099, 1984.
17. Fullenlove TM, Willliams AJ: Comparative roentgen findings in symptomatic and asymptomatic backs. Radiology 68:572-574, 1957.
18. Garrido E, Connaughton PN: Unilateral facetectomy approach for lateral lumbar disc herniation. J Neurosurg 74:754-756, 1991.
19. Goldner J, Urbaniak JR, McCollum D: Anterior disc excision and interbody spinal fusion for chronic low back pain. Orthop Clin North Am 2:544-568, 1971.
20. Haughton VM, Eldevik OP, Magnases B, Amundsen P: A prospective comparison of computed tomography and myelography in the diagnosis of herniated lumbar disks. Radiology 142:103-110, 1982.

21. Hazlett JW, Kinnard P: Lumbar apophyseal process excision and spinal instability. Spine 7:171, 1982.

22. Hirsch C, Nachemson A: The reliability of lumbar disk surgery. Clin Orthop 29:189-195, 1963.

23. Horal J: The clinical appearance of low back disorders in the city of Gothenburg, Sweden. Acta Orthop Scand Suppl 118:7-109, 1969.

24. Hult L: Cervical dorsal and lumbar spinal syndromes. Acta Orthop Scand 24:174-175, 1954.

25. Jackson RK: The long-term effects of wide laminectomy for lumbar disc excision: A review of 130 patients. J Bone Joint Surg Br 53:609-616, 1971.

26. Jackson RP, Glah JJ: Foraminal and extraforaminal lumbar disc herniation: Diagnosis and treatment. Spine 12:577-585, 1987.

27. Jensen MC, Brant-Zawadzki MN, Obuchowski N, et al: Magnetic resonance imaging of the lumbar spine in people without back pain. N Engl J Med 2:69-73, 1994.

28. Johansen J: Computed tomography in assessment of myelographic nerve root compression in the lateral recess. Spine 11:492-495, 1986.

29. Johnsson KE, Willner S, Johnsson K: Postoperative instability after decompression for lumbar spinal stenosis. Spine 11:107-110, 1986.

30. Kambin PK: Posterolateral percutaneous lumbar discectomy and decompression: Arthroscopic microdiscectomy. In Kambin PK (ed): Arthroscopic Microdiscectomy: Minimal Intervention in Spinal Surgery. Baltimore, Urban & Schwarzenberg, 1991, pp 67-100.

31. Kambin P, Gellman H: Percutaneous lateral discectomy of the lumbar spine: A preliminary report. Clin Orthop 174:127, 1983.

32. Kambin P, O'Brien E, Zhou L, et al: Arthroscopic microdiscectomy and selective fragmentectomy. Clin Orthop 347:150-167, 1998.

33. Kambin P, Schaffer JL: Percutaneous lumbar discectomy: Review of 100 patients and current practice. Clin Orthop 238:24-34, 1989.

34. Kambin P, Zhou L: History and current status of percutaneous arthroscopic disc surgery. Spine 245:575-615, 1996.

35. Knox BD, Chapman TM: The anterior lumbar interbody fusion for discogram concordant pain. J Spinal Disord 6:242-244, 1993.

36. Magora A, Schwartz A: Relation between the low back pain syndrome and x-ray findings. I. Degenerative osteoarthritis. Scand J Rehabil Med 8:115-125, 1976.

37. Maroon JC, Kopitnick TA, Schulhof LA, et al: Diagnosis and microsurgical approach to far-lateral disc herniation in the lumbar spine. J Neurosurg 72:378-382, 1990.

38. Masaryk TJ, Ross JS, Modic MT, et al: High resolution MR imaging of sequestered lumbar intervertebral disks. AJNR Am J Neuroradiol 9:351-358, 1988.

39. Mathews HH, Evans MT, Molligan HJ, Long BH: Laparoscopic discectomy with anterior lumbar interbody fusion. Spine 20:1791-1802, 1995.

40. McAfee PC, Regan JR, Zdeblick TA, et al: The incidence of complications in endoscopic anterior thoracolumbar spinal reconstructive surgery. Spine 20:1624-1632, 1995.

41. Modic MT, Masaryk TJ, Boumphrey F, et al: Lumbar herniated disc disease and canal stenosis: Prospective evaluation by surface coil MR, CT and myelography. AJNR Am J Neuroradiol 7:709-727, 1986.

42. Modic MT, Steinberg PM, Ross JS, et al: Degenerative disc disease: Assessment of changes in vertebral body marrow with MR imaging. Radiology 166:193-199, 1988.

43. Nachemson A: Towards a better understanding of low-back pain: A review of the mechanics of the lumbar disc. Rheum Rehab 14:129-143, 1975.

44. Natelson SE: The injudicious laminectomy. Spine 11:966, 1986.

45. Osti OL, Fraser RD, Vernon-Roberts B: Discitis after discography: The role of prophylactic antibiotics. J Bone Joint Surg Br 72:271-274, 1990.

46. Parke WW: Clinical anatomy of the lower lumbar spine. In Kambin P (ed): Arthroscopic Microdiscectomy: Minimal Intervention in Spinal Surgery. Baltimore, Urban & Schwarzenberg, 1991, pp 11-29.

47. Postacchini F, Cinotti G, Gumina S, Perugia D: Long-term results of surgery in lumbar stenosis: Eight year review of 64 patients. Acta Orthop Scand Suppl 251:78, 1993.

48. Robertson PA, Grobler LJ, Novonty JE, et al: Postoperative spondylolisthesis at L4-5: The role of facet joint morphology. Spine 18:1483, 1993.

49. Schaffer JL, Kambin P: Percutaneous posterolateral lumbar discectomy and decompression with a 6.9-millimeter cannula: Analysis of operative failures and complications. J Bone Joint Surg Am 73:822-831, 1991.

50. Schaffer JL, Kambin P: Alternative forms of disk excision: Minimally invasive spine surgery. In Herkowitz HN, Garfin SR, Balderston RA, et al (eds): Rothman-Simeone The Spine, 4th ed. Philadelphia, WB Saunders, 1999, pp 725-737.

51. Spangfort, E: The lumbar disc herniation. Acta Orthop Scand Suppl 142:4-95, 1972.

52. Spencer DL, Bernstein AJ: Lumbar intervertebral disc surgery. In Bridwell KH, DeWald RL (eds): Textbook of Spinal Surgery, vol 2, 2nd ed. Philadelphia, Lippincott-Raven, 1997, pp 1547-1560.

53. Torgerson WR, Dotter WE: Comparative roentgenographic study of the asymptomatic and symptomatic lumbar spine. J Bone Joint Surg Am 58:850-853, 1976.

54. Wetzel FT, LaRocca SH, Lowery GL, Aprill CN: Treatment of lumbar spinal pain syndromes diagnosed by discography. Spine 19:792-800, 1994.

55. White AA, Wiltse LL: Spondylolisthesis after extensive lumbar laminectomy. Paper presented at the annual meeting of the American Academy of Orthopaedic Surgeons, 1976, New Orleans.

56. Wiltse LL, Kirkaldy-Willis WH, McIvor GWD: The treatment of spinal stenosis. Clin Orthop 115:83, 1976.

57. Wiltse L, Spencer CW: New uses and refinements of the paraspinal approach to the lumbar spine. Spine 13:696, 1988.

58. Wisneski RJ, Garfin SR, Rothman RH, Lutz GE: Lumbar disc disease. In Herkowitz HN, Garfin SR, Balderston RA, et al (eds): Rothman-Simeone The Spine, 4th ed. Philadelphia, WB Saunders, 1999, pp 613-679.

59. Yu S, Sether LA, Ho PSP, et al: Tears of the annulus fibrosus: Correlation between MR and pathologic findings in cadavers. AJNR Am J Neuroradiol 9:367-370, 1988.

60. Zucherman JF, Zdeblick TA, Bailey SA, et al: Instrumented laparoscopic spinal fusion: Preliminary results. Spine 20:2029-2035, 1995.

Thoracoscopic Surgery of the Spine

Francis H. Shen and D. Greg Anderson

History, Physical Examination, and Imaging:
Variable; related to the location and nature of the lesion

Indications:
Excision of herniated disk; biopsy and debridement of infections and tumors; assistance in managing spinal deformities
Patients must be able to tolerate single-lung ventilation and lateral decubitus position

Surgical Technique:
Position, prepare, and drape the patient in a manner that allows conversion to an open thoracotomy if necessary
The surgeon should be familiar with intrathoracic anatomy and landmarks or perform the surgery with another surgeon familiar with thoracoscopic techniques
Fluoroscopy can be helpful for identifying appropriate levels and should be used intraoperatively as needed
Preserve segmental vasculature when possible; however, ligate if necessary to improve exposure or decrease risk of inadvertent injury
Removal of 2 to 3 cm of rib head, and occasionally the entire pedicle, may be necessary to perform adequate and safe decompression
Anterior or posterior fusion (or both) with or without instrumentation should be considered when extensive debridement or decompression is performed to prevent instability
Thoracoscopic anterior releases combined with posterior procedures can increase both sagittal and coronal corrections in spinal deformity

Complications:
Pulmonary complications, particularly atelectasis, are common and should be identified and managed early

The clinical presentation of patients with thoracic spine pathology is variable.[2,5,6] Presenting signs and symptoms are dependent on the location[1,27] and nature of the spinal pathology[39,56]; however, factors such as the size of the lesion,[10] the duration of compression,[16,56] and the degree of neural compromise[18,21] contribute to the possibility of different clinical findings in patients with lesions in similar locations.[1,4,9,16,58]

It is beyond the scope of this chapter to discuss the management of all these lesions. We present here an overview of conditions that are amenable to management with thoracoscopic techniques. We emphasize the importance of careful patient selection and believe that in some cases, both nonoperative and open surgical techniques may be appropriate. At this time, thoracoscopic techniques are indicated for excision of herniated disks,[12,19,29] biopsy and debridement of vertebral abscesses[42] and spinal tumors,[39] and assistance in the management of thoracic spine deformities.[14,55,61]

Background

Thoracoscopy has steadily gained acceptance since its introduction in 1910.[30] The applications of video-assisted thoracoscopic surgery have expanded to include the treatment of spinal disorders. Mack et al.[42] published the first thoracoscopic spine series in 1993, which led to the development of equipment capable of performing biopsies and drainage of paravertebral abscesses.[52]

Currently, excision of herniated thoracic disks,[54] corpectomy for vertebral body tumors,[44] and anterior release for spinal deformity[13,14,55] are routinely performed thoracoscopically. Thoracoscopic bone grafting, fusion, and instrumentation are now being performed at specialized centers.[13,19,52,53]

Table 80–1

Differential Diagnosis of Thoracic Pathology

Spinal Pathology

Thoracic herniated disk
Tumor
    Spinal
    Paraspinal
Infection
Ankylosing spondylitis
Scheuermann kyphosis
Vertebral body fracture
Kyphoscoliosis

Nonspinal Pathology

Intercostal neuralgia
Herpes zoster
Central nervous system
    Cerebrovascular accident
    Multiple sclerosis
    Brain tumor
Cardiac
    Angina
    Myocardial infarction
    Pericarditis
Lung
    Pleurisy
    Pneumonia
Gastrointestinal
    Gastroesophageal reflux disease
    Cholecystitis
Tumor
    Lung
    Cardiac
    Breast
    Gastrointestinal
    Mediastinal
        Thyroid
        Thymus
        Lymphoma

History

The clinical presentation of patients with thoracic spine pathology is variable[2,5,6,35,41] and dependent on the location and nature of the lesion. Categorizing the causes into spinal and extraspinal disorders helps organize the various pathologies (Table 80–1). Questions that focus on the character, location, radicular pattern, and intensity of the symptoms help distinguish among these causes.[4,9,16,57] For example, if a patient is suspected of having a herniated thoracic disk, questions about motor, sensory, and radicular symptoms, as well as bowel and bladder dysfunction, are important (Table 80–2).[3,16,58] Certain "red flag" symptoms can alert the physician to the possibility of tumor or infection (Table 80–3).

Physical Examination

The physical examination should include thorough motor (Table 80–4) and sensory (Fig. 80–1) examinations. It should also include reflex testing (Table 80–5) and evaluation for radicular and myelopathic signs, sphincter dysfunction, and gait abnormalities.[3,57]

Imaging

Imaging techniques depend on the pathology being treated. Good-quality plain radiographs are essential and can help localize the level of involvement, depict overall spinal alignment, and identify associated lung and chest pathology. If thoracoscopy is being performed for

Table 80–2 Presenting Symptoms of Thoracic Disk Herniation

Symptom	No. of Patients	Percentage
Motor and sensory	131	61
Brown-Séquard syndrome	18	9
Sensory only	33	15
Motor only	13	6
Radicular pain only	20	9
Bladder or sphincter	65	30

From Arce CA, Dohrmann GJ: Herniated thoracic discs. Neurol Clin 3:383-392, 1985.

Table 80–3

"Red Flag" Symptoms of Infection or Tumor

Night pain
Pain at rest
Unexplained weight loss
Fever and chills
Night sweats

Table 80–4
Major Motor Levels

Level	Muscle Group	Action	Deep Tendon Reflex
C5	Deltoid, internal and external shoulder rotators	Abduction of shoulder, external rotation of arm	Biceps jerk (C5-6)
C6	Biceps, brachialis, wrist extensors	Flexion of elbow	Brachioradialis jerk (C5-6)
C7	Triceps, wrist flexors	Extension of elbow, wrist	Triceps jerk
C8	Intrinsic hand muscles	Abduction, adduction of fingers	
L2-3	Iliopsoas	Hip flexion	
L4	Quadriceps	Extension of knee	Knee jerk
L5	Tibialis anterior and posterior, extensor hallucis longus	Dorsiflexion of foot and big toe	
S1	Gastrocnemius	Plantar flexion of foot	Ankle jerk
S4-5	Anal sphincter	Voluntary contraction of anal sphincter	

From Levine AM, Eismont FJ, Garfin SR, Zigler JE (eds): Spinal Trauma. Philadelphia, WB Saunders, 1998, p 23.

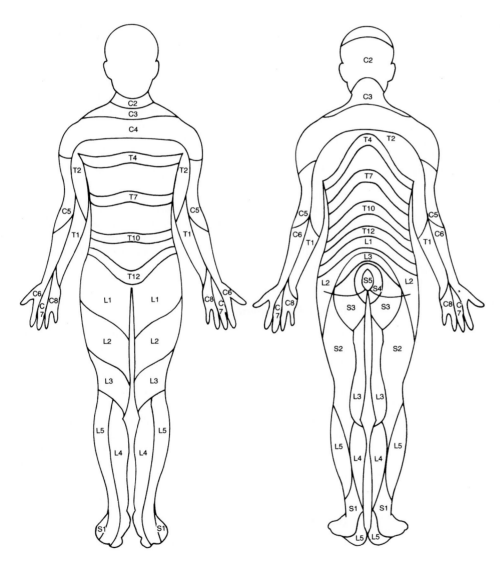

Figure 80–1   Dermatomes. (From Keenen TL, Benson DR: Initial evaluation of the spine injured patient. In Browner BD, Jupiter JB, Levine AM, et al [eds]: Skeletal Trauma: Fractures, Dislocations, Ligamentous Injuries, vol 1. Philadelphia, WB Saunders, 1992, p 595.)

Table 80–5
Segmental Reflexes

Reflex	Level
Biceps	C6
Triceps	C7
Upper abdominal*	T7-10
Lower abdominal*	T10-12
Cremasteric*	L1
Knee jerk	L4
Posterior tibial jerk	L5
Ankle jerk	S1
Bulbocavernosus†	S2-4
Anocutaneous†	S4-5

*Cutaneous reflexes; decreased in upper motor neuron lesion.
†Contraction of bulbocavernosus muscle after stimulation of glans penis.
†Contraction of anal sphincter after stroking perineal skin.
From Levine AM, Eismont FJ, Garfin SR, Zigler JE (eds): Spinal Trauma. Philadelphia, WB Saunders, 1998, p 25.

deformity, long cassette films with the patient standing, as well as bending films, are beneficial.

Preoperative magnetic resonance imaging or computed tomography is also helpful in the management of herniated thoracic disks, tumors, and infections.[25,59,63] These studies help identify the size and location of the pathology and the involvement of surrounding structures (e.g., great vessels and spinal cord). However, it is important to note that asymptomatic thoracic disk herniations have been reported in up to 15% of patients having these imaging studies performed for unrelated reasons.[5,63]

Additional studies such as diskography, myelography, and arteriography may be necessary in selected cases. These should be performed as indicated to help the surgeon characterize the pathology.

Indications and Contraindications

Thoracoscopic techniques are used for many of the same pathologic conditions that were traditionally managed with open thoracotomies.[13,19,42,44,52] In patients with associated cardiovascular or pulmonary risk factors, thoracoscopy has lower morbidity and mortality compared with traditional open procedures.[13,29,40,44] In properly selected patients, thoracoscopy can reduce incisional pain,[40] decrease chest tube drainage,[16] minimize respiratory difficulties,[37,65] and improve shoulder girdle function.[16,44]

Despite these advantages, thoracoscopy requires that a patient be able to tolerate lateral positioning and single-lung ventilation.[16,65] In patients with severe comorbidities, even thoracoscopy may not be an option.[16,24,26,60] Patients with significant pleural adhesions from previous thoracic disease or surgery are also poor candidates because of the risk of iatrogenic pulmonary injury.[16,26,37,60]

Spinal conditions amenable to a thoracoscopic approach include herniated disks,[12,19,29] vertebral abscesses,[42] spinal tumors,[39] and deformities in the thoracic spine.[14,55,61] Anterior spinal instrumentation that is currently under development and being investigated at certain centers may improve deformity correction or spinal stabilization through a less invasive thoracoscopic approach.[13,14,16,23,55]

Surgical Technique

Anesthesia, Positioning, and Setup

Thoracoscopy is performed with the patient under general anesthesia and with the use of a double-lumen endotracheal tube. This allows for ventilation of the contralateral lung and active deflation of the ipsilateral lung.[12,13,19,24]

The patient is positioned in a lateral decubitus position, and the table is flexed to widen the intercostal spaces. The extreme jackknife position should be avoided to prevent stretching an already compromised spinal cord.[19,37,42] Flexion of the arm slightly above 90 degrees and use of an axillary roll minimize the risk of compression of the neurovascular structures.[13,42,52]

Surgical instrumentation for an open thoracotomy should be available in the room, and the chest should be prepared and draped in a manner that allows easy conversion to an open procedure if necessary. The ipsilateral iliac crest should be prepared if additional bone graft is needed.

If the operating surgeons and assistants are on opposite sides of the operating table, consideration should be given to using two separate video monitors (Fig. 80–2). This will improve viewing and eliminate mirror imaging (see Table 80–6).

Portal Placement

Typically, four trocars are required. The viewing portal for the thoracoscope is created first, and the remaining portals are placed under direct vision. They are positioned in a manner that best addresses the pathology, while allowing easy instrument manipulation and dissection within the pleural cavity.

The working instrument portals are positioned over the level of the lesion along the anterior axillary line; the trocar for the thoracoscope is inserted more posteriorly along the midaxillary line. A fourth trocar can be created for retraction of the lung or diaphragm as needed.

Diagnostic Thoracoscopy

Before trocar placement, the lung on the operative side is collapsed by the anesthesiologist. The viewing portal is created in the midaxillary line between the fifth and sixth intercostal spaces. A 1-cm incision is made through the skin, and the intercostal muscles are spread with a hemostat over the rib, avoiding the intercostal

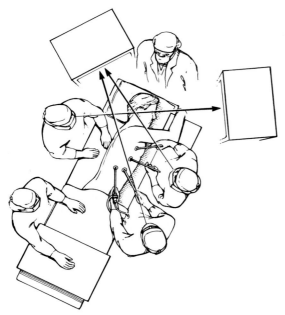

Figure 80–2   Operating room setup for thoracoscopic spine surgery. (From Regan JJ, Jarolem KL: Thoracoscopy of the spine. In Herkowitz HN, Garfin SR, Balderston RA, et al [eds]: Rothman-Simeone The Spine, 4th ed. Philadelphia, WB Saunders, 1999, p 601.)

neurovascular bundle. Blunt finger dissection is used to release pleural adhesions and allow entry into the pleural space. It is important to ensure that the lung and pleura are free from the chest wall before inserting instruments or trocars into the chest cavity. A standard portal configuration results in an inverted L-shaped pattern.

A 1-cm, rigid, 0- or 30-degree thoracoscope is introduced through the cannula to visualize the thoracic cavity. Tilting the operating table forward and using either the Trendelenburg or reverse Trendelenburg position will enable gravity will assist with lung retraction. A fan retractor inserted through a dedicated portal can also help in retracting the lung or diaphragm.

The thoracic spine can be divided into three regions, based on intrathoracic anatomy.[19,29,43] The upper region includes the T1 to T5 vertebral levels and is distinguished by the location of the segmental vertebral vascular anatomy. On the right side, the second, third, and fourth intercostal veins empty into a common superior intercostal vein, which subsequently empties into the azygos vein. The fifth intercostal vein is the first vessel to empty directly into the azygos vein.

The middle region includes the T6 to T9 vertebral levels and is distinguished by the location of the rib heads, which overlie the disk spaces, and the segmental vessels, which run in the middle of the vertebral bodies. In this region, the esophagus and mediastinal structures are just anterior to the thoracic spine.

The lower region includes the T10 to T12 vertebral segments. Here, the rib heads are generally found just below the disk space on the correspondingly numbered vertebral body.

Closure and Drainage

After completion of the surgical procedure, the chest cavity and wound are irrigated with warm saline. A thoracic chest tube is placed in the costodiaphragmatic recess, and the lung is reinflated. The thoracoscope is then slowly removed, and the portal entry sites are checked for excessive bleeding. The wounds are reapproximated in the standard layered manner.

Specific Thoracic Pathology

Biopsy and Culture

One of the best indications for thoracoscopic spine surgery is biopsy and culture of vertebral tumors, osteomyelitis, and paravertebral abscesses.[39,42] In this setting, thoracoscopic surgery is often quicker and less morbid than traditional open procedures.[12,13,19,24,26,37,52,64] It allows direct inspection of the pathology and the opportunity to obtain larger amounts of tissue than can be achieved with image-guided techniques. This improves diagnostic accuracy by providing adequate tissue for culture, histology, and special stains.[13,19,33]

Some spinal infections can be treated definitively with thoracoscopic drainage.[11,16,38,50] If significant bony destruction is present in the form of osteomyelitis, a spinal defect may be present after debridement. Autologous bone can be used to graft the defect to help promote a stable spinal fusion.[15-17,47] Large defects with significant potential for spinal instability should also undergo posterior instrumentation through a separate approach to keep hardware out of the zone of infection. A chest tube should be placed for drainage to decrease the incidence of recurrent infection.[38,50]

Herniated Thoracic Disk Disease

Thoracic disk herniations are uncommon, with the majority occurring between T8 and L1. The reported incidence of symptomatic herniated disks is 2% to 4%.[1,3,6,9,16,32,43,49,53,58] Most are central or paracentral herniations in direct contact with the cord, because the spinal canal is narrower at this level.[3,6,25,63] Before beginning any spinal resection, the correct vertebral levels should be identified by counting ribs and then confirmed with a radiograph. The disk can be approached from either the left or right side, depending on the location of the lesion (see Table 80–6). Using the endoscope, a clear view to the opposite side can be obtained if necessary to ensure complete decompression.[12,29,43,51]

The portals are established and the chest is entered as previously described. The parietal pleura is divided using electrocautery, sparing the segmental vessels if possible. If the vessels lie within the field of dissection, they can be divided to avoid accidental injury and to increase exposure.

To access the disk, the rib head and 2 to 3 cm of proximal rib should be resected using an osteotome or high-speed drill. The resected rib corresponds to the lower number vertebral body (e.g., the ninth rib head is removed to access the T8-9 disk). At the thoracolumbar junction, this may not be necessary, because the rib heads lie below the disk space. To reach the T12-L1 disk, the pleural reflection of the diaphragm should be divided to allow visualization of the L1 pedicle.

Dissecting the rib head free from the costovertebral and costotransverse ligaments allows visualization of the pedicle, posterior aspect of the disk, and spinal canal. In some cases, removal of the superior portion of the pedicle is also necessary to better visualize the posterior aspect of a herniated disk fragment.

Once exposed, the herniated disk fragment can be removed. Epidural bleeding is common and can be controlled with suction, Gelfoam, and bipolar cautery. If the majority of the disk remains following decompression, instability will not be created, and a fusion is not necessary. However, fusion should be considered when a large amount of the disk is removed. In addition, the biomechanical forces at the thoracolumbar junction are high, and it is often wise to proceed with a structural fusion when addressing disk disease below the T10 level. Fusion options include morcelized rib graft or allograft placed into the interspace or the use of a threaded fusion cage. If required, instrumentation can be applied using the same minimally invasive approach.

Corpectomy

A corpectomy generally requires removal of the entire pedicle to ensure adequate visualization of the dura. Complete diskectomies are performed above and below the level of interest, and the vertebral body is removed with a combination of osteotomes, curets, and rongeurs.

After decompression, strut allograft, autologous tricortical iliac crest, or a corpectomy cage must be placed to reconstruct the defect. After proper sizing, the structural strut graft is impacted into the corpectomy defect so that it rests firmly on the preserved end plates of the vertebrae above and below. Instrumentation should be considered to add stability to the construct and minimize the risk of graft dislodgment. Depending on the situation, anterior instrumentation may be applied through the same minimally invasive approach, or the patient may undergo posterior instrumentation through a separate surgical approach.

Spinal Deformity: Anterior Release

Anterior release with or without anterior fusion is a well-established adjuvant to posterior deformity correction in both children and adults.[36,48,55,61] Pediatric patients affected by neuromuscular scoliosis are often good candidates for the less traumatic thoracoscopic approach, owing to the pulmonary complications associated with open surgery in this group.[13,61] Anterior epiphysiodesis can also be performed thoracoscopically in skeletally immature patients at risk for developing crankshaft phenomenon following an isolated posterior fusion.[20,22,28]

Patients with rigid spinal deformities and curve magnitudes greater than 75 degrees should be considered for anterior release.[7] Adult patients may also benefit from anterior release and fusion, owing to the rigidity of the deformity and the higher risk of pseudarthrosis with posterior-only surgery.[7,14]

Traditional anterior release and fusion procedures carry the risks and morbidities of any major intrathoracic procedure. For this reason, thoracoscopic release can offer significant advantages, especially in patients with suboptimal pulmonary function, for whom thoracotomy carries the greatest risk. The anterior release is generally performed before the posterior procedure to maximize deformity correction and improve sagittal and coronal plane balance.[13,55,61]

To perform an anterior release for spinal deformity correction, portals are established on the convex side of the thoracic curve using the previously described techniques. If possible, segmental vessels should be preserved to minimize the theoretical risk of a vascular injury to the spinal cord. The disk spaces are identified, and disk excision is carried out, allowing progressive mobility of the spinal segment.

Unlike in a herniated disk procedure, the rib heads are generally not resected because it is not necessary to decompress the disk behind the level of the posterior longitudinal ligament. At least 50% of the disk should be removed to allow adequate mobility of the disk space.[13,16,55,61] To improve curve correction, an internal thoracoplasty procedure can be performed by removing or cutting multiple ribs over the apex of the curve.[46]

Morcelized rib or iliac crest graft or allogeneic bone can be placed in the disk space to promote arthrodesis. The parietal pleura can be repaired using endoscopic suturing techniques to help maintain the graft within the disk space.

Pearls and Pitfalls

Table 80–6 lists the pearls and pitfalls of thoracoscopic spine surgery.

Postoperative Management

Radiographs should be obtained daily to verify the placement of the chest tube and the absence of pleural effusion or pneumothorax. The chest tube is typically removed on the second postoperative day, when the output has decreased to less than 50 to 80 mL per 8-hour shift.[33] Intravenous antibiotics are routinely given for 24 to 48 hours postoperatively. The need for bracing depends on the pathology addressed and the procedure performed.

Complications

Despite careful and proper trocar placement, a transient intercostal neuralgia has been reported in up to 8% of patients.[45] Because the neurovascular bundle travels on the inferior aspect of the rib, this complication can be

Table 80–6	**Pearls and Pitfalls of Thoracoscopic Spine Surgery**

Careful patient positioning in the true lateral position minimizes intraoperative confusion about the orientation of the spine; this is especially important when working within the spinal canal

Orientation of both the surgeon and the thoracoscopic camera toward the video monitor eliminates mirror imaging

Trocar sites should be far enough from the pathology to allow a panoramic view and room for instrument manipulation

If visibility is inhibited by incomplete lung collapse, temporary carbon dioxide insufflation can expedite and enhance lung collapse

When performing revision herniated disk surgery, an approach from the opposite side avoids dissecting through scar tissue; the thoracoscope can be progressively advanced into the diskectomy site to ensure complete decompression

With large herniated disks, removing disk tissue within the disk space first may allow the herniated fragment to be gently teased away from the spinal cord into the newly created space

decreased by careful placement of the trocar superior to the rib.

Pulmonary complications are common and can occur in up to 15% of patients.[60,65] The most common complication is atelectasis, which can be managed with physiotherapy[43] and adequate pain control in the immediate postoperative period to prevent and decrease chest wall splinting.

Pleural effusions are uncommon, and they are generally tolerated and require no special treatment. Occasionally, if the effusion is sufficiently large or located in the costodiaphragmatic recess, reinsertion of a temporary thoracoscopy tube may be necessary.[26,33,37] This complication can be avoided with careful intraoperative hemostasis of the trocar sites at the end of the case and systematic evaluation of the daily chest radiographs before removal of the chest tube.

Dural tears may occur, especially if the pathology is adjacent or adherent to the dura mater. If the dura is torn, a primary repair should be performed. Persistent dural leaks can lead to cerebrospinal fluid fistulas and meningitis.[8,62] If the tear cannot be repaired thoracoscopically, conversion to an open thoracotomy should be considered. A drain should be left in the pleural cavity and in the subarachnoid space to help expand the lung against the thoracic wall and decrease cerebrospinal fluid pressure, respectively.[16,33,34,62]

Vascular lesions from incidental injury can occur to intercostal arteries, veins, or the azygos system.[16,31,37] These structures should be identified and isolated at the start of the case whenever possible. In most instances, these injuries can be controlled with a combination of electrocautery and endoscopic vascular clips. Aortic lesions, which are extremely rare, require immediate thoracotomy.

Neurologic deterioration is a devastating complication and can occur for a variety of reasons. Injury to the artery of Adamkiewicz or direct neurologic injury can occur with thoracoscopic procedures.[16,21,26,31,37] These complications can be minimized by careful preoperative planning, intraoperative electrophysiologic monitoring, and a thorough understanding of the thoracoscopic anatomy and surrounding landmarks. Intraoperative fluoroscopy should be used when necessary.

Summary

In carefully selected patients, thoracoscopic spine surgery is an accepted and safe surgical technique. The thoracoscopic anatomy and the indications and limitations of each technique should be well understood by the surgeon before undertaking such an approach. Complications of thoracoscopic spine surgery are uncommon, but they can occur. The patient should be positioned and draped in a manner that allows easy and quick conversion to an open procedure if necessary. As advances in technique and improvements in instrumentation occur, the indications will continue to expand.

References

1. Alberico A, Sahni KS, Hall JA Jr, Young H: High thoracic disc herniation. J Neurosurg 19:449-451, 1986.
2. Albrand OW, Corkill G: Thoracic disc herniation: Treatment and prognosis. Spine 4:41-46, 1979.
3. Arce CA, Dohrmann GJ: Herniated thoracic discs. Neurol Clin 3:383-392, 1985.
4. Arseni C, Nash F: Thoracic intervertebral disc protrusion: A clinical study. J Neurosurg 17:418-430, 1960.
5. Awwad EE, Margin DS, Smith KR, Baker BK: Asymptomatic versus symptomatic herniated thoracic discs: Their frequency and characteristics as detected by computed tomography after myelography. Neurosurgery 28:180-185, 1991.
6. Bohlman HH, Zdeblick TA: Anterior excision of herniated thoracic discs. J Bone Joint Surg Am 70:1038-1047, 1988.
7. Byrd JAI, Scoles PV, Winter RB, et al: Adult idiopathic scoliosis treated by anterior and posterior spinal fusion. J Bone Joint Surg Am 58:843-850, 1987.
8. Cammisa FP Jr, Girardi FP, Sangani PK, et al: Incidental durotomy in spine surgery. Spine. 25:2663-2667, 2000.
9. Carson J, Gumpert J, Jefferson A: Diagnosis and treatment of thoracic intervertebral disc protrusions. J Neurol Neurosurg Psychiatry 34:68-77, 1971.
10. Chesterrman PJ: Spastic paraplegia caused by sequestered thoracic intervertebral disc. Proc R Soc Med 57:87-88, 1964.
11. Chung DA, Ritchie AJ: Videothoracoscopic drainage of mediastinal abscess: An alternative to thoracotomy. Ann Thorac Surg 69:1573-1574, 2000.
12. Coltharp WH, Arnold JH, Alford WC, et al: Videothoracoscopy: Improved technique and expanded indications. Ann Thorac Surg 53:776-779, 1988.
13. Crawford AH, Wall EJ, Wolf R: Video-assisted thoracoscopy. Orthop Clin North Am 30:367-385, 1999.
14. Cunningham BW, Kotani Y, McNulty PS, et al: Video-assisted thoracoscopic surgery versus open thoracotomy for anterior thoracic spinal fusion: A comparative radiographic, biomechanical, and histologic analysis in sheep model. Spine 23:1333-1340, 1998.

15. Currier BL, Eismont FJ, Green BA: Transthoracic disc excision and fusion for thoracic herniated discs. Spine 3:323-328, 1994.

16. Currier BL, Slucky AV, Eismont FJ, Green BA: Thoracic disc disease. In Herkowitz HN, Garfin SR, Balderston RA, et al (eds): Rothman-Simeone The Spine, 4th ed. Philadelphia, WB Saunders, 1999, pp 581-595.

17. DeOliveira JC: Bone grafts and chronic osteomyelitis. J Bone Joint Surg Br 53:672-683, 1971.

18. DiChiro G, Fried LC, Doppman JL: Experimental spinal cord angiography. Br J Radiol 43:19-30, 1970.

19. Dickman CA, Karahalios DG: Thoracoscopic spinal surgery. Clin Neurosurg 43:392-422, 1996.

20. Dohin B, Dubousset JF: Prevention of the crankshaft phenomenon with anterior spinal epiphysiodesis in surgical treatment of severe scoliosis of the younger patient. Eur Spine J 3:165-168, 1994.

21. Dommisse GF: The blood supply of the spinal cord: A critical vascular zone in spinal surgery. J Bone Joint Surg Br 56:225-235, 1974.

22. Dubousset J, Herring JA, Shufflebarger H: The crankshaft phenomenon. J Pediatr Orthop 9:541-550, 1989.

23. Ebara S, Kammimura M, Itoh H, et al: A new system for the anterior restoration and fixation of thoracic spinal deformities using an endoscopic approach. Spine 25:876-883, 2000.

24. Fischel R, McKenna R: Video-assisted thoracic surgery for lung volume reduction surgery. Chest Surg Clin N Am 4:789-807, 1998.

25. Francavilla TL, Powers A, Dina T, Rizzoli HV: MR imaging of thoracic disk herniations. J Comput Assist Tomogr 11:1062-1065, 1987.

26. Fujita RA, Barnes GB: Morbidity and mortality after thoracoscopic pneumoplasty. Ann Thorac Surg 62:251-257, 1996.

27. Gelch MM: Herniated thoracic disc at T1-2 level associated with Horner's syndrome. J Neurosurg 48:128-130, 1978.

28. Gonzalez BI, Fuentes CS, Avila JMM: Anterior thoracoscopic epiphysiodesis in the treatment of a crankshaft phenomenon. Eur Spine J 4:343-346, 1995.

29. Horowitz MB, Moossy JJ, Julian T, et al: Thoracic discectomy using video assisted thoracoscopy. Spine 19:1082-1086, 1994.

30. Jacobaeus HC: Possibility of the use of cystoscope for the investigation of the serous cavities. Munch Med Wochenschr 57:3090-3092, 1910.

31. Jancovici R, Lang-Lazdunski L, Pons F, et al: Complication of video-assisted thoracic surgery: A five-year experience. Ann Thorac Surg 61:533-537, 1996.

32. Jefferson A: The treatment of thoracic intervertebral disc protrusion. Clin Neurol Neurosurg 78:1-9, 1975.

33. Johnson JP: Thoracoscopic sympathectomy. In Schmideck HH (ed): Operative Neurosurgical Techniques: Indications, Methods, and Results, vol 2, 4th ed. Philadelphia, WB Saunders, 2000, pp 2341-2346.

34. Jones AA, Stambough JL, Balderston RA, et al: Long-term results of lumbar spine surgery complicated by unintended incidental durotomy. Spine 14:443-446, 1989.

35. Kite WC Jr, Whitfield RD, Campbell E: The thoracic herniated intervertebral disc syndrome. J Neurosurg 14:61-67, 1957.

36. Kokoska ER, Gabriel KR, Silen ML: Minimally invasive anterior spinal exposure and release in children with scoliosis. J Soc Laparoendo Surg 2:255-258, 1998.

37. Krasna MJ, Deshmukh S, McLaughlin JS: Complications of thoracoscopy. Ann Thorac Surg 61:1066-1069, 1996.

38. Laisaar T: Video-assisted thoracoscopic surgery in the management of acute purulent mediastinitis and pleural empyema. Thorac Cardiovasc Surg 46:51-54, 1998.

39. Landreneau RJ, Dowling RD, Ferson PF: Thoracoscopic resection of a posterior mediastinal neurogenic tumor. Chest 102:1288-1290, 1992.

40. Landreneau RJ, Hazelrigg SR, Mack MJ: Postoperatvie pain-related morbidity: Video-assisted thoracic surgery versus thoracotomy. Ann Thorac Surg 54:800-807, 1993.

41. Logue V: Thoracic intervertebral disc prolapse with spinal cord compression. J Neurol Neurosurg Psychiatry 15:227-241, 1952.

42. Mack MJ, Regan JJ, Bobechko WP, Acuff TE: Application of thoracoscopy for diseases of the spine. Ann Thorac Surg 56:736-738, 1993.

43. Mangione P: Endoscopic approach to the thoracic spine for removal of thoracic disk herniation. In Schmidek HH (ed): Operative Neurosurgical Techniques: Indications, Methods, and Results, vol 2, 4th ed. Philadelphia, WB Saunders, 2000, pp 2132-2140.

44. McAfee PC, Regan JJ, Fedder IL, et al: Anterior thoracic corpectomy for spinal cord decompression performed endoscopically. Surg Laparosc Endosc 5:339-348, 1995.

45. McAfee PC, Regan JJ, Zdeblick T, et al: The incidence of complications in endoscopic anterior throacolumbar spinal reconstructive surgery: A prospective multicenter study compring the first 100 consecutive cases. Spine 20:1624-1632, 1995.

46. Mehlman CT, Crawford AH, Wolf RK: Video-assisted thoracoscopic surgery (VATS): Endoscopic thoracoplasty technique. Spine 22:2178-2182, 1997.

47. Nakamura H, Yamano Y, Seki M, et al: Use of folded vascularized rib graft in anterior fusion after treatment of thoracic and upper lumbar lesions: Technical note. J Neurosurg 94(2 Suppl):323-327, 2001.

48. Newton PO, Wenger DR, Mubarak SJ, et al: Anterior release and fusion in pediatric spinal deformity: A comparison of early outcome and cost of thoracoscopic and open thoracotomy approaches. Spine 22:1398-1406, 1997.

49. Otani K, Nakai S, Fujimura Y, et al: Surgical treatment of thoracic disc herniation using the anterior approach. J Bone Joint Surg Br 64:340-343, 1982.

50. Parker LM, McAfee PC, Fedder IL, et al: Minimally invasive surgical techniques to treat spine infections. Orthop Clin North Am 27:183-199, 1996.

51. Regan JJ: Percutaneous endoscopic thoracic discectomy. Neurosurg Clin N Am 7:87-98, 1996.

52. Regan JJ, Jarolem KL: Thoracoscopy of the spine. In Herkowitz HN, Garfin SR, Balderston RA, et al (eds): Rothman-Simeone The Spine, 4th ed. Philadelphia, WB Saunders, 1999, pp 597-611.

53. Rosenthal D: Endoscopic approaches to the thoracic spine. Eur Spine J Suppl 9:S8-S16, 2000.

54. Rosenthal D, Dickman CA: Thoracoscopic microsurgical excision of herniated thoracic discs. J Neurosurg 89:224-235, 1998.

55. Rothenberg S, Erickson M, Eilert R, et al: Thoracoscopic anterior spinal procedures in children. J Pediatr Surg 33:1168-1170, 1998.

56. Ryan RW, Lally JF, Kozic Z: Asymptomatic calcified herniated thoracic disks: CT recognition. AJNR Am J Neuroradiol 9:363-366, 1988.

57. Stillerman CB, Weiss MH: Management of thoracic disc disease. Clin Neurosurg 38:325-352, 1992.

58. Tovi D, Strang RR: Thoracic intervertebral disk protrusions. Acta Chir Scand Suppl 267:6-41, 1960.

59. Vanichkachorn JS, Vaccaro AR: Thoracic disk disease: Diagnosis and treatment. J Am Acad Orthop Surg 8:159-169, 2000.

60. Vollmar B, Olinger A, Hildebrandt U, et al: Cardiopulmonary dysfunction during minimally invasive thoracolumboendoscopic spine surgery. Anesth Analg 88:1244-1251, 1999.

61. Waisman M, Saute M: Thoracoscopic spine release before posterior instrumentation in scoliosis. Clin Orthop 336:130-136, 1997.

62. Wang JC, Bohlman HH, Riew KD: Dural tears secondary to operations on the lumbar spine: Management and results after a two-year-minimum follow-up of eighty-eight patients. J Bone Joint Surg Am 80:1728-1732, 1998.

63. Williams MP, Cherryman GR, Husband JE: Significance of thoracic disc herniation demonstrated by MR imaging. J Comput Assist Tomogr 13:211-214, 1989.

64. Wimmer C, Gluch H, Franzreb M, et al: Predisposing factors for infection in spine surgery: A survey of 850 spinal procedures. J Spinal Disord 11:124-128, 1998.

65. Wolfer RS, Krasna MJ, Hasnain JU, et al: Hemodynamic effects of carbon dioxide insufflation during thoracoscopy. Ann Thorac Surg 58:404-407, 1994.

81

Laparoscopic Surgery of the Spine

FRANCIS H. SHEN AND D. GREG ANDERSON

LAPAROSCOPIC SURGERY OF THE SPINE IN A NUTSHELL

History, Physical Examination, and Imaging:
  Variable; related to the location and nature of the lesion

Indications:
  Biopsy and debridement of infection and tumor; fusion for pseudarthrosis, deformity, or instability; diskectomy for herniated or degenerative disks

Advantages:
  Less muscle denervation and lower risk of postoperative hernia formation; potential for quicker recovery and return to work

Surgical Technique:
  Position, prepare, and drape the patient in a manner that allows for conversion to open laparotomy if necessary
  Trocar sites can be established with either a direct technique (Hasson) or percutaneous access (Veres)
  Transperitoneal technique uses a pneumoperitoneum to insufflate the intraperitoneal space and is ideal for visualization and management of L5-S1 pathology
  Retroperitoneal technique eliminates the need for a pneumoperitoneum and improves access to the entire lumbar spine
  Endoscopically assisted mini-laparotomy combines standard open spine surgery with endoscopically assisted surgical exposure

Complications:
  Occur in less than 1% of all laparoscopic surgeries; include intestinal, urinary, and vascular injuries

Patients who would benefit from laparoscopic spine techniques are similar to those who would benefit from open anterior lumbar spine procedures.[2,9,15,17,35,39,45,49,52,68] Identification and selection of appropriate patients are therefore the same for both techniques. Laparoscopic procedures are generally indicated to manage anterior lumbar spine pathology (i.e., the vertebral body and intervertebral disk).[13,18,23,30] Specific applications include biopsy and debridement of tumor and infection[17,19,52]; fusion for pseudarthrosis, deformity, or instability[6,12,28,33,34,37]; and diskectomy for herniated or degenerative disks.[2,15,68] The technical aspects of these procedures

are similar, and we focus mainly on the laparoscopic techniques used during diskectomy and fusion because they illustrate the major skills needed for the laparoscopic management of lumbar spine pathology.

Background

The modern era of endoscopy began in 1987 when DuBois[24] performed the first laparoscopic cholecystectomy in France. Once endoscopic techniques became accepted in general surgery, attempts were made to use them in spinal surgery.[2,6,12,37,68] Obenchain[47] is credited with the first reported successful spinal endoscopic procedure.

Traditional anterior laparoscopic approaches in the lumbar spine were originally performed transperitoneally.[12,13,39,48] However, surgeons from multiple fields, including general surgery, gynecology, and urology, eventually developed techniques allowing for a retroperitoneal approach.[24-27,53,61] Initially developed for laparoscopic nephrectomies,[26,43] this approach uses a gasless environment and provides access to the entire lumbar spine by entering and developing the retroperitoneal potential space.

Recently, a third approach called endoscopically assisted mini-laparotomy[8] has evolved that combines the benefits of open and endoscopic surgery. Though not a completely endoscopic procedure, it uses laparoscopic techniques to mobilize the retroperitoneal space to gain access to the lumbar spine. Once the spine is exposed, a mini-laparotomy is performed, and the surgery is carried out with standard open techniques.[8,38,57,58,67]

History

Diskogenic pain syndrome encompasses a continuum of diagnostic entities that involve the intervertebral disk.[7,20,21,62,66] This condition is characterized by alterations in the internal structure and metabolic function of the intervertebral disk.[21] A complete characterization and description of these disorders is beyond the scope of this book; however, they range from internal disk disruption to degenerative disk disease.[20,21]

Patients with diskogenic back pain often present with complaints of disabling midline back pain that may be referred to the sacroiliac joints, iliac crest, or posterior thigh.[21] Patients may relate a history of significant trauma before the onset of symptoms. Axial compression and flexion activities, such as bending and lifting, typically aggravate the pain. The pain is thought to arise from free nerve endings in the outer annulus, which may be stimulated by mechanical or chemical irritants.[7] In more advanced conditions, foraminal narrowing and segmental instability can develop and produce radicular symptoms from direct mechanical nerve impingement.[66]

Physical Examination

In addition to obtaining a careful history, a thorough physical examination should be performed. A neurologic examination should also be included, looking for motor, sensory, or reflex changes. In cases of associated nerve root compression, a specific nerve root pattern may be suggested by the examination (Table 81–1); generally, however, the findings are inconclusive for a single radicular pattern. Provocative maneuvers that place the sciatic nerve and its various components on stretch can also help with the diagnosis.

Often, lower extremity pain and low back pain are secondary to nonspinal pathology. The physical exami-

Table 81–1
Nerve Root Patterns

L4 Nerve Root

Pain and numbness: L4 dermatome, posterolateral aspect of thigh, across patella, anteromedial aspect of leg
Weakness and atrophy: weak extension of knee and quadriceps muscle atrophy
Reflex: depression of patellar reflex

L5 Nerve Root

Pain and numbness: L5 dermatome, posterior aspect of thigh, anterolateral aspect of leg, medial aspect of foot and great toe
Weakness and atrophy: weak dorsiflexion of foot and toes and atrophy of anterior compartment of leg
Reflex: none, or absent posterior tibial tendon reflex

S1 Nerve Root

Pain and numbness: S1 dermatome, posterior aspect of thigh, posterior aspect of leg, posterolateral aspect of foot, lateral toes
Weakness and atrophy: weak plantar flexion of foot and toes and atrophy of posterior compartment of leg
Reflex: depression of Achilles reflex

From Wisneski RJ, Garfin SR, Rothman RH, Lutz GE: Lumbar disc disease. In Herkowitz HN, Garfin SR, Balderston RA, et al (eds): Rothman-Simeone The Spine, 4th ed. Philadelphia, WB Saunders, 1999, p 629.

nation should include a peripheral vascular examination to rule out vascular insufficiency and a hip joint examination to rule out intra-articular pathology.

Imaging

Once the decision is made to proceed with surgery, imaging should include plain radiographs and advanced imaging studies specific to the patient's diagnosis. In the early phase of internal disk disruption, radiographs are essentially normal, with minimal end plate or facet sclerosis, narrowing, or osteophytes.[21,66] In the more advanced phase of degenerative disk disease, radiographs demonstrate loss of disk height, neuroforaminal narrowing, and occasionally segmental instability.[66]

Computed tomography scans are frequently normal in patients with internal disk disruption[1,11,20,66]; however, in cases of advanced disk degeneration, the scan may demonstrate marginal osteophytes, lateral recess or foraminal stenosis, end plate sclerosis, and disk space vacuum signs.[11,66] Magnetic resonance imaging provides additional information but is not always specific for the painful anatomy. Although a "dark disk" (one with loss of signal intensity on T2-weighted images) with annular disruption has the potential to be painful, it is not necessarily so. Disk abnormalities on magnetic resonance imaging have been reported in up to 30% of asymptomatic volunteers.[5] Therefore, imaging results should be

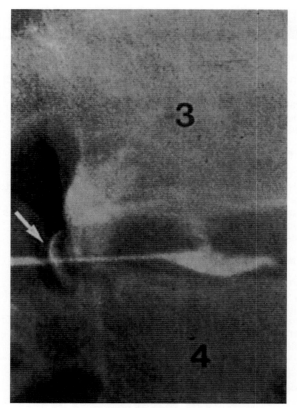

Figure 81–1 Diskogram of the L3-4 level demonstrating contrast material outlining a well-contained herniation *(arrow)*. **No free flow of contrast is noted here.** (From Gleason PL, Maroon JC, Quigley M: Alternative forms of disk excision: Automated percutaneous lumbar discectomy (APLD). In Herkowitz HN, Garfin SR, Balderston RA, et al [eds]: Rothman-Simeone The Spine, 4th ed. Philadelphia, WB Saunders, 1999, p 740.)

correlated with the patient's physical examination and other studies before proceeding with surgery.

Diskography (Fig. 81–1), though controversial, can play a role in confirming the diagnosis of internal disk disruption or degenerative disk disease in patients with diskogenic pain.[1,10,16,36,64,65] A properly performed diskogram should include four criteria (Table 81–2).[3,46] Although all the components must be taken into consideration, the most important is the patient's subjective pain response.[16,44,46,62] In a truly positive diskogram, the injection should exactly reproduce the patient's pain intensity and type (concordant pain). Injections of multiple disks should be done during the same study to obtain nonpainful control levels.[66]

Indications

The indications for laparoscopic procedures are essentially the same as for open anterior lumbar spine surgery. Pathology of the vertebral body and intervertebral disk are particularly amenable to laparoscopic approaches.[18,34,35] This includes biopsy and debridement of infection and tumor,[17,19,52] diskectomy for symptomatic

Table 81–2	Components of an Appropriately Performed Diskogram

Patient's subjective pain response to diskogram
    Concordant pain—suggestive that injected disk is pain
       source
    Discordant pain—unlikely that injected disk is pain source
Disk morphology
    Pooling of dye in centrum of nucleus—normal
    Radial fissures extending from nucleus through annulus—
       abnormal
Injection volume and pressure
    1.5-2.5 mL—normal injection volume
    >3 mL—abnormal, suggestive of complete annular tear
    400-500 kPa—normal peak intradiskal pressure
Lack of concordant pain at adjacent disk levels injected

herniated and degenerative disks, and fusion for pseudarthrosis, instability, and deformity.[2,15,40,68] In some cases, these conditions can be addressed more quickly, more easily, and more safely with laparoscopy than with an open procedure.[2,30,32,66] Other reported benefits include the avoidance of abdominal muscle denervation, decreased risk of hernia formation, quicker recovery and return to work, and overall greater patient satisfaction.[2,13,37,42,49,55-57]

In some cases, a laparoscopic approach may be used to avoid a posterior procedure and the associated morbidity of posterior muscle dissection. Certain posterior spinal pathologies, such as radiculopathy from neuroforaminal impingement, can be addressed indirectly with laparoscopic techniques. By performing an interbody procedure, the disk height can be restored, leading to indirect decompression of the foramen.[6,23,28,45] However, in cases of significant stenosis or a free disk fragment, posterior surgery is required to adequately address the pathology (see Chapter 79).

Surgical Technique

Positioning

The patient is positioned supine on a radiolucent table, with a bolster beneath the lumbar spine to help maintain or enhance lumbar lordosis. The patient is secured to the table so that it can be tilted as necessary during the case. Twenty to 30 degrees of Trendelenburg helps pull the intestinal contents away from the operative site in the lower lumbar region. The abdomen should be prepared and draped widely, and all necessary instrumentation for an open approach should be readily available in case rapid conversion is necessary.

Portal Placement

The primary trocar site can be established with a direct, open technique (Hasson) or by percutaneous access using a blunt-tipped needle (Veres).[4,41,60,61] The Hasson technique involves placement of the blunt trocar under direct visualization after division of the abdominal fascia. The peritoneum is then visualized and incised. Stay sutures are placed through the fascia and peritoneum. Alternatively, the intraperitoneal space can be established percutaneously with the Veres needle. Accurate placement of the needle is confirmed by free passage of fluid through the needle into the intraperitoneal space.[4,57,66]

Diagnostic Laparoscopy

Transperitoneal Approach

The transperitoneal technique uses carbon dioxide to insufflate the intraperitoneal space.[31,49,61] Instruments are introduced through special portals to prevent the insufflating gas from escaping. Because of the excellent visualization of intraperitoneal structures, this technique is ideal for addressing L5-S1 pathology.[15,18,39,47,57,66]

The first portal is generally at the level of the umbilicus. Care is taken to prevent inadvertent penetration of the abdominal viscera. Carbon dioxide is used to insufflate the peritoneum to approximately 15 mm Hg, followed by insertion of the 30-degree laparoscope.

Various configurations are available for the placement of additional portals. Classically, four additional portals are placed under direct laparoscopic visualization. These include two 5-mm portals placed 6 to 8 mm off the midline, midway between the umbilicus and the symphysis pubis, and two working portals placed lateral to the epigastric vessels.[13,40,50,55,66] For instrumentation of the L5-S1 disk space, a suprapubic portal is helpful,[13,55,66] allowing instruments to be introduced parallel to the disk space.

Exposure of the disk space may require mobilization of the sigmoid colon. If necessary, the sigmoid colon can be temporarily tacked to the abdominal wall with intra-abdominal sutures.[13,30,55,66] The bifurcation of the great vessels is an important landmark and generally lies just cephalad to the L5-S1 disk space. In addition, it is important to identify the ureters, the middle sacral vessels, and the presacral autonomic plexus. To expose the L5-S1 disk space, the middle sacral vessels should be ligated and divided. The peritoneum is divided longitudinally, and the prevertebral tissue is bluntly swept to the sides, exposing the disk space.

Retroperitoneal Approach

The laparoscopic retroperitoneal approach attempts to reproduce the same exposure obtained during open retroperitoneal surgery. Therefore, unlike transperitoneal approaches, retroperitoneal surgery can be applied to the entire lumbar spine.[23,37,48,58,63,66] Like the transperitoneal approach, however, meticulous attention to detail is necessary to prevent injury to vital structures.

The viewing portal is established through a small incision in the left flank, just cephalad to the iliac crest. Before introducing any instruments, an index finger should be used to bluntly dissect the retroperitoneal plane.[8,13,22,23,27,63] A dissecting balloon is introduced and insufflated under direct laparoscopic visualization to create a working space and allow access to the lumbar spine. With distention of the balloon, the peritoneal contents are pulled away from the abdominal wall musculature and pushed toward the midline.[22,23,48,55]

Anatomic landmarks should be identified before the placement of additional portals. The iliopsoas muscle should be visualized lying just lateral to the lumbar spine. The pulsations of the aorta can be identified anterior to the lumbar spine. Often, the ureter can be seen lying within the retroperitoneal fat.[29,32] When exposing the lower lumbar spine, the ascending lumbar vein should be identified and may require ligation to prevent heavy bleeding associated with injury to this structure.[32,42] Careful identification of the peritoneal reflection is necessary before placement of the second portal.

The second working portal, located on the anterior aspect of the abdominal wall, is placed to allow instrument access to the lumbar segment of interest. The endoscopic view is used to ensure that this portal lies lateral to the peritoneal reflection. A specialized balloon retractor is used to retract the abdominal contents while a fan lift raises the abdominal wall, creating a gasless retroperitoneal working space to allow access to the lumbar spine over multiple segments.[63]

Working in a fashion analogous to the open retroperitoneal technique, the iliopsoas muscle is retracted laterally and posteriorly along the vertebral bodies. The segmental vessels are identified, ligated, and divided, allowing mobilization of the great vessels from the anterior surface of the spine. This improves exposure to the disks and anterior longitudinal ligament.[8,13,63]

Endoscopically Assisted Mini-Laparotomy

Endoscopically assisted mini-laparotomy combines the benefits of laparoscopy and those of open surgery.[8] It provides access to the entire lumbar spine without the morbidity of a large incision. The primary goal of the endoscopic portion of the procedure is to mobilize the peritoneal sac and develop the retroperitoneal space while minimizing tears to the peritoneum.

Attempts to develop the extraperitoneal space through a small open incision can be challenging and dangerous. Because the peritoneum is adherent to the arcuate line and, in women, to the round ligament as well, maximal mobilization of the peritoneal sac may require a full laparotomy incision.[8,13,32,66] However, with the assistance of an endoscope and balloon dilator, the retroperitoneal space can be developed. The procedure is then converted to a mini-open laparotomy, and the remaining spinal surgery is completed in the standard fashion. One advantage of this procedure is that it is easy to learn because it uses existing techniques already familiar to surgeons performing endoscopic inguinal hernia repair.

The patient is positioned supine on a radiolucent table, with both arms abducted and a small roll under both knees. The viewing portal is established first in the midline, just below the umbilicus. This portal is established in the standard manner, deep to the rectus muscle but above the peritoneum.

The extraperitoneal space is then inflated with carbon dioxide to 12 to 15 mm Hg. Under direct vision, using a combination of blunt dissectors and scissors, a second 5-mm working portal is created approximately 4 to 6 cm inferior to the viewing portal. The arcuate line is identified and carefully dissected off the lateral abdominal wall with the endoscopic scissors. The peritoneal sac, which is adherent to the arcuate line, is mobilized and retracted. At this point, the endoscopic portion of the case is complete, and the endoscopic instruments are removed.

A 4- to 6-cm midline skin incision is made, connecting the two portal incisions. The anterior rectus sheath is opened and, depending on the location of the pathology, the appropriate rectus muscle is retracted laterally. Using blunt finger dissection, the peritoneal sac (which was previously mobilized during the endoscopic dissection) is easily retracted, exposing the retroperitoneal space and the intervertebral disks.

Specific Laparoscopic Pathology

Regardless of the approach to the lumbar spine (transperitoneal, retroperitoneal, or laparoscopically assisted mini-open), the surgical techniques for managing the lumbar pathology are similar. The goal is to address the offending disk or vertebral body and, in some cases, improve spinal stability. In some centers, lumbar fusions are now routinely performed using laparoscopic techniques.[6,8,54,56,59] Laparoscopic anterior or separate posterior instrumentation may also be necessary to address instability and increase fusion rates.

Lumbar Disk Excision

After the surgical approach is established and the disk space is identified, the appropriate level is confirmed radiographically. The annulus is incised, and the end plates are elevated with a Cobb elevator. The disk material is removed with a combination of pituitary rongeurs and curets, similar to open procedures.

The completeness of the diskectomy can be confirmed by direct inspection by inserting the laparoscope into the disk space.[2,12,15] Rotating the angled lens superiorly and inferiorly allows the surgeon to inspect the vertebral end plates. Sometimes a 0-degree scope is inserted to look straight back at the posterior longitudinal ligament and posterior aspect of the annulus or to search for retained or extruded disk material.

Anterior Lumbar Interbody Fusion

When required, an interbody fusion can be performed laparoscopically.[14,23,28,33,37,51] Following the diskectomy, the interbody fusion begins with distraction of the disk space. Various trial wedges are available to assist with disk space distraction. If disk space reaming will be performed for the placement of threaded fusion cages, radiographic control should be used to prevent asymmetrical reaming.

Table 81–3	**Pearls and Pitfalls of Laparoscopic Spine Surgery**

Use of a radiolucent table facilitates intraoperative fluoroscopic and radiographic images

Obtaining a radiograph on the operating table before commencing the operation can help identify surface anatomic landmarks in relation to the lumbar spine

Bolsters beneath the lumbar curve can help maintain and enhance lordosis, which is especially important for interbody fusion

Use of Trendelenburg and reverse Trendelenburg positions can improve intraoperative visibility by pulling intestinal contents away from the operative site

The transperitoneal approach is excellent for L5-S1 pathology but provides limited access to the rest of the lumbar spine; if exposure to multiple or upper lumbar segments is needed, the retroperitoneal or mini-open approach is advised

If necessary, use intraoperative fluoroscopy to place the starting position of the suprapubic portal in line with the L5-S1 disk space

Minimize the use of electrocautery over the L5-S1 disk space to reduce the risk of sympathetic injury and retrograde ejaculation in males

An interbody fusion device is selected and filled with bone graft or an osteoinductive substitute. The implant should be placed to achieve a stable, well-contained position within the disk space.[23,37,51,57,66] With careful attention to detail, the surgeon can generally reestablish lordosis and sagittal plane balance and achieve indirect decompression of the neuroforamen by reestablishing disk height. Depending on the level and type of pathology, posterior segmental instrumentation may be indicated to provide segmental stability and promote a solid fusion.

Pearls and Pitfalls

Table 81–3 lists the pearls and pitfalls of laparoscopic spine surgery.

Postoperative Management

The need for a postoperative drain is dependent on the procedure performed; however, in most instances, a drain is not required. If a drain is used, it should be removed when the output has sufficiently decreased (usually by postoperative day 2). Perioperative antibiotic therapy is routine and should be tailored to the patient and the procedure performed.

Complications

Major laparoscopic complications are rare and occur in less than 1% of all laparoscopic procedures.[32,55] They include intestinal,[32,42] urinary tract,[29] and vascular injuries,[13,42] with overall mortality rates reported at 4 to 8 deaths per 100,000 procedures.[32] Most complications occur as a result of trocar insertion or are secondary to a technical error involving a laparoscopic instrument or the presence of a pneumoperitoneum.[32,40,42]

Both the Hasson and Veres needle techniques have been associated with underlying visceral and vascular injuries.[4,13,31,32,40,42,55] The small bowel is the most frequently injured structure; however, if the injury is discovered and repaired immediately, a good outcome can be expected.[4,13,32,40,66] Injury to retroperitoneal vascular structures can be devastating. These injuries are often overlooked because the bleeding is retroperitoneal rather than overt.

As with other incisions, trocar site complications are possible. Bleeding, infection, and incisional hernia have been described.[13,31,40,55,66] Bleeding from the trocar site into the peritoneal cavity is often secondary to injury to the epigastric vessels and can be controlled intraoperatively with sutures or, if necessary, by enlarging the incision and directly ligating the bleeder.[13,40,42,55,66]

A constant pneumoperitoneum can have both mechanical and chemical physiologic effects on the cardiopulmonary and vascular systems. Newer techniques using gasless retroperitoneal and laparoscopically assisted mini-open procedures eliminate the risks from a constant pneumoperitoneum.[8,23,63]

Summary

Advances in laparoscopic spine surgery are increasing rapidly, and the use of laparoscopy in the management of selected lumbar spine disorders has been shown to be safe and effective. Careful preoperative planning and patient selection are essential components in the management of lumbar pathology. Typically, transperitoneal approaches offer excellent visualization of peritoneal structures and the L5-S1 disk space but provide limited access to the rest of the lumbar spine. The retroperitoneal approach or an endoscopically assisted mini-laparotomy should be considered if wider exposure is necessary.

References

1. Adams MA, Dolan P, Hutton WC: The stages of disc degeneration as revealed by discograms. J Bone Joint Surg Br 68:36-41, 1986.
2. An HS, Andersson G, Lieberman I, et al: Minimally invasive surgery for lumbar degenerative disorders. Part II. Degenerative disc disease and lumbar stenosis. Am J Orthop 29:937-942, 2000.
3. Aprill CN: Diagnostic disc injection. In Frymoyer JW (ed): The Adult Spine: Principles and Practice. New York, Raven Press, 1991, pp 403-442.
4. Bemelman WA, Dunker MS, Busch OR, et al: Efficacy of establishment of pneumoperitoneum with the Veress needle, Hasson trocar, and modified blunt trocar (TrocDoc): A randomized study. J Laparoendosc Adv Surg Tech 10:325-330, 2000.
5. Boden SD, Dais DO, Diana TS, et al: Abnormal magnetic resonance scans of the lumbar spine in asymptomatic subjects. J Bone Joint Surg Am 72:403-408, 1990.
6. Boden SD, Martin GJ Jr, Horton WC, et al: Laparoscopic anterior spinal arthrodesis with rhBMP-2 in a titanium interbody threaded cage. J Spinal Disord 11:95-101, 1998.
7. Bogduk N, Tynan W, Wilson AS: The nerve supply to the human lumbar intervertebral disc. J Anat 132:39-56, 1981.
8. Boos N, Kalberer F, Schoeb O: Retroperitoneal endoscopically assisted minilaparotomy for anterior lumbar interbody fusion: Technical feasibility and complications. Spine 26:1-6, 2001.
9. Bridenbaugh LD, Soderstrom RM: Lumbar epidural block anesthesia for outpatient laparoscopy. J Reprod Med 23:85-86, 1979.
10. Brodsky AE, Binder WF: Lumbar discography: Its value and diagnosis and treatment of lumbar disk lesions. Spine 4:110-120, 1979.
11. Brown MD: The pathophysiology of disc disease: Symposium on disease of the intervertebral disc. Orthop Clin North Am 2:359-370, 1971.
12. Cammisa FP Jr, Girardi FP, Antonacci A, et al: Laparoscopic transperitoneal anterior lumbar interbody fusion with cylindrical threaded cortical allograft bone dowels. Orthopedics 24:235-239, 2001.
13. Chekan EG, Pappas TN: Minimally invasive surgery. In Townsend CM (ed): Sabiston Textbook of Surgery, 16th ed. Philadelphia, WB Saunders, 2001, pp 292-310.
14. Cloward RB: Lesions of the intervertebral discs and their treatment by interbody fusion methods. Clin Orthop 27:51-77, 1963.
15. Cloyd DW, Obenchain TG, Savin M: Transperitoneal laparoscopic approach to lumbar discectomy. Surg Laparosc Endosc Percut Tech 5:85-89, 1995.
16. Collis JS, Gardner WJ: Lumbar discography: An analysis of 1000 cases. J Neurosurg 19:452-461, 1962.
17. Corpataux JM, Halkic N, Wettstein M, Dusmet M: The role of laparoscopic biopsies in lumbar spondylodiscitis. Surg Endosc 14:1086, 2000.
18. Cowles RA, Taheri PA, Sweeney JF, Graziano GP: Efficacy of the laparoscopic approach for anterior lumbar spinal fusion. Surgery 128:589-596, 2000.
19. Craig FS: Vertebral biopsy. J Bone Joint Surg Am 38:93-102, 1956.
20. Crock HV: A reappraisal of intervertebral disc lesions. Med J Aust 1:983-989, 1970.
21. Crock HV: Internal disc disruption: A challenge to disc prolapse fifty years on. Spine 11:650-653, 1986.
22. Debing E, Simoens C, Van den Brande P: Retroperitoneoscopic lumbar sympathectomy with balloon dissection: Clinical experience. J Laparoendosc Adv Surg Tech 10:101-104, 2000.
23. de Peretti F, Hovorka I, Fabiani P, Argenson C: New possibilities in L2-L5 lumbar arthrodesis using a lateral retroperitoneal approach assisted by laparoscopy: Preliminary results. Eur Spine J 5:210-216, 1996.
24. DuBois F, Icard P, Berthelot G, et al: Coelioscopic cholecystectomy: Preliminary report of 36 cases. Ann Surg 211:60-62. 1990.
25. Garry R: Laparoscopic alternatives to laparotomy: A new approach to gynaecological surgery. Br J Obstet Gynaecol 99:629-632, 1992.
26. Gaur DD: Laparoscopic operative retroperitoneoscopy: Use of a new device. J Urol 148:1137-1139, 1992.
27. Gaur DD: Simple nephrectomy: Retroperitoneal approach. J Endourol 14:787-790, 2000.

28. Geerdes BP, Geukers CW, van Erp WF: Laparoscopic spinal fusion of L4-L5 and L5-S1. Surg Endosc 15:1308-1312, 2001.

29. Guingrich JA, McDermott JC: Ureteral injury during laparoscopy-assisted anterior lumbar fusion. Spine 25:1586-1588, 2000.

30. Guiot BH, Khoo LT, Fessler RG: A minimally invasive technique for decompression of the lumbar spine. Spine 27:432-438, 2002.

31. Hannon JK, Faircloth WB, Lane DR, et al: Comparison of insufflation vs retractional technique for laparoscopic-assisted intervertebral fusion of the lumbar spine. Surg Endosc 14:300-304, 2000.

32. Harkki-siren P, Kurki T: A nationwide analysis of laparoscopic complications. Obstet Gynecol 89:108-112, 1997.

33. Hawasli A, Thusay M, Elskens DP, et al: Laparoscopic anterior lumbar fusion. J Laparoendosc Adv Surg Tech 10:21-25, 2000.

34. Heniford BT, Matthews BD, Lieberman IH: Laparoscopic lumbar interbody spinal fusion. Surg Clin North Am 80:1487-1500, 2000.

35. Henry LG, Cattey RP, Stoll JE, Robbins S: Laparoscopically assisted spinal surgery. J Soc Laparoendosc Surg 1:341-344, 1997.

36. Holt EF JR: The question of lumbar discography. J Bone Joint Surg 58:720-726, 1968.

37. Katkhouda N, Campos GM, Mavor E, et al: Is laparoscopic approach to lumbar spine fusion worthwhile? Am J Surg 178:458-461, 1999.

38. Kleeman TJ, Ahn UM, Talbot-Kleeman A: Laparoscopic anterior lumbar interbody fusion with rhBMP-2: A prospective study of clinical and radiographic outcomes. Spine 26:2751-2756, 2001.

39. Lieberman IH, Willsher PC, Litwin DE, et al: Transperitoneal laparoscopic exposure for lumbar interbody fusion. Spine 25:509-514, 2000.

40. Mahvi DM, Zdeblick TA: A prospective study of laparoscopic spinal fusion: Technique and operative complications. Ann Surg 224:85-90, 1996.

41. Marcovich R, Del Terzo MA, Wolf JS Jr: Comparison of transperitoneal laparoscopic access techniques: Optiview visualizing trocar and Veress needle. J Endourol 14:175-179, 2000.

42. McAfee PC, Regan JR, Zdeblick T, et al: The incidence of complications in endoscopic anterior thoracolumbar spinal reconstructive surgery: A prospective multicenter study comprising the first 100 consecutive cases. Spine 20:1624-1632, 1995.

43. McDougall EM, Clayman RV, Fadden DT: Retroperitoneoscopy: The Washington University Medical School experience. Urology 43:446-452, 1994.

44. Moneta GB, Videman T, Kaivanto K, et al: Reported pain during lumbar discography as a function of annular ruptures and disc degeneration: A re-analysis of 833 discograms. Spine 19:1968-1974, 1994.

45. Nibu K, Panjabi MM, Oxland T, Cholewicki J: Intervertebral disc distraction with a laparoscopic anterior spinal fusion system. Eur Spine J 7:142-147, 1998.

46. North American Spine Society: Position statement on discography. Spine 13:1343, 1988.

47. Obenchain TG: Laparoscopic lumbar discectomy: Case report. J Laparoendosc Surg 1:145-149, 1991.

48. Obenchain TG, Cloyd D: Laparoscopic lumbar discectomy: Description of transperitoneal and retroperitoneal techniques. Neurosurg Clin North Am 7:77-85, 1996.

49. O'Dowd JK: Laparoscopic lumbar spine surgery. Eur Spine J 9(Suppl 1):S3-S7, 2000.

50. Onimus M, Papin P, Gangloff S: Extraperitoneal approach to the lumbar spine with video assistance. Spine 21:2491-2494, 1996.

51. Pape D, Adam F, Fritsch E, et al: Primary lumbosacral stability after open posterior and endoscopic anterior fusion with interbody implants: A roentgen stereophotogrammetric analysis. Spine 25:2514-2518, 2000.

52. Parker LM, McAfee PC, Fedder IL, et al: Minimally invasive surgical techniques to treat spine infections. Orthop Clin North Am 27:183-199, 1996.

53. Portis AJ, Elnady M, Clayman RV: Laparoscopic radical/total nephrectomy: A decade of progress. J Endourol 15:345-354, 2000.

54. Regan JJ, Aronoff RJ, Ohnmeiss DD, Sengupta DK: Laparoscopic approach to L4-L5 for interbody fusion using BAK cages: Experience in the first 58 cases. Spine 24:2171-2174, 1999.

55. Regan JJ, Guyer RD: Endoscopic techniques in spinal surgery. Clin Orthop 335:122-139, 1997.

56. Regan JJ, McAfee PC, Guyer RD, et al: Laparoscopic fusion of the lumbar spine in a multicenter series of the first 34 consecutive patients. Surg Laparosc Endosc 6:459-468, 1996.

57. Regan JJ, Yuan H, McAfee PC: Laparoscopic fusion of the lumbar spine: Minimally invasive spine surgery. A prospective multicenter study evaluating open and laparoscopic lumbar fusion. Spine 24:402-411, 1999.

58. Riley LH, Eck JC, Yoshida H, et al: Laparoscopic assisted fusion of the lumbosacral spine: A biomechanical and histologic analysis of the open versus laparoscopic technique in an animal model. Spine 22:1407-1412, 1997.

59. Rodts GE Jr, McLaughlin MR, Zhang J, et al: Laparoscopic anterior lumbar interbody fusion. Clin Neurosurg 47:541-556, 2000.

60. Senagore AJ: Laparoscopic techniques in intestinal surgery. Semin Laparosc Surg 8:183-188, 2001.

61. Staelin ST, Zdeblick TA, Mahvi DM: Laparoscopic lumbar spinal fusion: The role of the general surgeon. J Laparoendosc Adv Surg Tech 10:297-304, 2000.

62. Suseki K, Takahashi Y, Takahashi K, et al: Sensory nerve fibres from lumbar intervertebral discs pass through rami communicantes: A possible pathway for discogenic low back pain. J Bone Joint Surg Br 80:737-742, 1998.

63. Thalgott JS, Chin AK, Ameriks JA, et al: Gasless endoscopic anterior lumbar interbody fusion utilizing the BERG approach. Surg Endosc 14:546-552, 2000.

64. Walsh TR, Weinstein JN, Spratt KF, et al: Lumbar discography in normal subjects: A controlled, prospective study. J Bone Joint Surg Am 72:1081-1088, 1990.

65. Weinstein J, Claverie W, Gibson S: The pain of discography. Spine 13:1344-1348, 1988.

66. Zdeblick TA: Discogenic back pain. In Herkowitz HN, Garfin SR, Balderston RA, et al (eds): Rothman-Simeone The Spine, 4th ed. Philadelphia, WB Saunders, 1999, pp 749-765.

67. Zdeblick TA, David SM: A prospective comparison of surgical approach for anterior L4-L5 fusion: Laparoscopic versus mini anterior lumbar interbody fusion. Spine 25:2682-2687, 2000.

68. Zelko JR, Misko J, Swanstrom L, et al: Laparoscopic lumbar discectomy. Am J Surg 169:496-498, 1995.

Index

Note: Page numbers followed by f indicate illustrations; page numbers followed by t indicate tables.